HAND SURGERY

HAND SURGERY

VOLUME II

Edited by

RICHARD A. BERGER, M.D., PH.D.

Professor and Consultant
Departments of Orthopedic Surgery and Anatomy
Mayo Clinic/Mayo Foundation
Rochester, Minnesota

ARNOLD-PETER C. WEISS, M.D.

Professor of Orthopaedics
Brown Medical School
Rhode Island Hospital
Providence, Rhode Island

LIPPINCOTT WILLIAMS & WILKINS
A **Wolters Kluwer** Company
Philadelphia • Baltimore • New York • London
Buenos Aires • Hong Kong • Sydney • Tokyo

Acquisitions Editor: Robert Hurley
Managing Editor: Tanya Lazar
Developmental Editor: Karen Carter
Supervising Editor: Mary Ann McLaughlin
Production Editors: Holly H. Auten, Kate Sallwasser, and Amanda Yanovitch,
    Silverchair Science + Communications
Manufacturing Manager: Ben Rivera
Cover Designer: Christine Jenny
Compositor: Silverchair Science + Communications
Printer: Walsworth Publishing Company

Library of Congress Cataloging-in-Publication Data
Hand surgery / edited by Richard A. Berger, Arnold-Peter C. Weiss.
    p. ; cm.
    Includes bibliographical references and index.
    ISBN 0-7817-2874-6
    1. Hand--Surgery. 2. Hand--Wounds and injuries. I. Berger, Richard A., 1954- II.
Weiss, Arnold-Peter C.
    [DNLM: 1. Hand--surgery. 2. Orthopedic Procedures--methods. WE 830 H2331 2003]
RD559.H359937 2003
617.5'75059--dc22
                                            2003060625

Care has been taken to confirm the accuracy of the information presented and to describe generally accepted practices. However, the authors, editors, and publisher are not responsible for errors or omissions or for any consequences from application of the information in this book and make no warranty, expressed or implied, with respect to the currency, completeness, or accuracy of the contents of the publication. Application of this information in a particular situation remains the professional responsibility of the practitioner.

The authors, editors, and publisher have exerted every effort to ensure that drug selection and dosage set forth in this text are in accordance with current recommendations and practice at the time of publication. However, in view of ongoing research, changes in government regulations, and the constant flow of information relating to drug therapy and drug reactions, the reader is urged to check the package insert for each drug for any change in indications and dosage and for added warnings and precautions. This is particularly important when the recommended agent is a new or infrequently employed drug.

Some drugs and medical devices presented in this publication have Food and Drug Administration (FDA) clearance for limited use in restricted research settings. It is the responsibility of health care providers to ascertain the FDA status of each drug or device planned for use in their clinical practice.

10 9 8 7 6 5 4 3 2 1

*Richard A. Berger would like to dedicate this text to the memory of his father,
M. Stone, the lifelong support and love of his mother, Donna, the endless source
of pride and joy from his daughter, Andrea, and most of all, the unending
support and love from his lifetime partner, his wife, Evelyn.*

*Arnold-Peter C. Weiss could not possibly have undertaken this project without
the love and unwavering support of his wife, Yvonne, and their five children
(Krista, Schuyler, Petra, Anders, and Barrett). To his parents,
Bernhard and Maria Antoinette Weiss, go the thanks for the countless
lessons of childhood and adolescence and the important direction
and support of what parenting is all about.*

CONTENTS

CONTRIBUTING AUTHORS

Reid A. Abrams, M.D.
Professor of Orthopedics
Department of Orthopedic Surgery
University of California, San Diego,
    School of Medicine
La Jolla, California

Brian D. Adams, M.D.
Professor
Department of Orthopedic Surgery and
    Biomedical Engineering
University of Iowa Roy J. and Lucille A. Carver
    College of Medicine
Iowa City, Iowa

Edward Akelman, M.D.
Professor and Vice Chairman of Department
    of Orthopaedics
Chief of Division of Hand, Upper Extremity,
    and Microvascular Surgery
Department of Orthopaedics
Brown Medical School
Rhode Island Hospital
Providence, Rhode Island

Yousaf Ali, M.D.
Assistant Clinical Professor of Medicine
Department of Medicine
Brown Medical School
Miriam Hospital
Providence, Rhode Island

Edward A. Athanasian, M.D.
Assistant Professor
Cornell University Joan and Sanford I. Weill
    Medical College and Graduate School
    of Medical Sciences
Associate Attending Orthopedic Surgeon
Hospital for Special Surgery
Assistant Attending Surgeon
Memorial Sloan-Kettering Cancer Center
New York, New York

Andrea Atzei, M.D.
Associate Professor of Hand Surgery and Microsurgery
Clinical Coordinator, Master in Hand Surgery
Hand Surgery Unit
Department of Orthopaedic Surgery
University of Verona
Policlinico G. B. Rossi
Verona, Italy

Christopher Bainbridge, M.B., Ch.B., F.R.C.S.
Consultant Hand Surgeon
Pulvertaft Hand Centre
Derbyshire Royal Infirmary
Derby, United Kingdom

Mark E. Baratz, M.D.
Professor and Vice Chairman of Department of Orthopaedics
Director of Division of Upper Extremity
Department of Orthopaedics
Drexel University College of Medicine
Philadelphia, Pennsylvania
Allegheny General Hospital
Pittsburgh, Pennsylvania

Michael S. Bednar, M.D.
Associate Professor of Orthopaedic Surgery
Department of Orthopaedic Surgery and Rehabilitation
Loyola University Chicago Stritch School of Medicine
Foster G. McGaw Hospital
Maywood, Illinois

Richard A. Berger, M.D., Ph.D.
Professor and Consultant
Departments of Orthopedic Surgery and Anatomy
Mayo Clinic/Mayo Foundation
Rochester, Minnesota

Randip R. Bindra, M.D., M.S.Orth., F.R.C.S., M.Ch.Orth.
Associate Professor of Orthopaedics
Director of Hand Surgery
Department of Orthopaedic Surgery
University of Arkansas for Medical Sciences
University of Arkansas for Medical Sciences Medical Center
Little Rock, Arkansas

Allen T. Bishop, M.D.
Professor of Orthopedic Surgery
Chairman of Division of Hand Surgery
Department of Orthopedic Surgery
Division of Hand Surgery
Mayo Medical School
Mayo Clinic
Rochester, Minnesota

Sigrid A. Blome-Eberwein, M.D.
Department of Burns and Reconstructive Surgery
Pennsylvania State University College of Medicine
Hershey, Pennsylvania
Lehigh Valley Hospital, Regional Burn Center
Allentown, Pennsylvania

Leonard S. Bodell, M.D.
Chief of Hand Surgery
Phoenix Orthopaedic Residency Program
Maricopa Medical Center
Phoenix, Arizona

Michael J. Botte, M.D.
Head of Section of Hand Surgery
 and Rehabilitation
Scripps Clinic and Research Foundation
La Jolla, California
Orthopaedic Surgery Service
Department of Surgery
VA San Diego Health Care System
San Diego, California
Clinical Professor
Department of Orthopedic Surgery
University of California, San Diego,
 School of Medicine
La Jolla, California

Dieter Buck-Gramcko, M.D., F.R.C.P.S.(Hon.)
Professor Emeritus
Former Chief of Department of Hand Surgery
Children's Hospital Wilhelmstift
Hamburg, Germany

Peter D. Burge, F.R.C.S.
Consultant Hand Surgeon
Department of Orthopaedic Surgery
University of Oxford
Nuffield Orthopaedic Centre
Oxford, United Kingdom

Frederick W. Burgess, M.D., Ph.D.
Associate Professor of Surgery (Anesthesia)
Department of Anesthesia
Brown Medical School
Rhode Island Hospital
Providence, Rhode Island

Karen L. Carney, O.T.R./L., C.H.T.
Director of Hand Therapy
Department of Hand Therapy
University Orthopedics, Incorporated
Providence, Rhode Island

Paul D. Choi, M.D.
Senior Resident
Department of Orthopaedic Surgery
University of California, San Francisco, School of Medicine
San Francisco, California

Chwei Chin David Chuang, M.D.
Professor of Plastic Surgery
Department of Plastic Surgery
Chang Gung University
Chang Gung Memorial Hospital
Taipei, Taiwan

Mark S. Cohen, M.D.
Associate Professor
Director of Hand and Elbow Section
Director of Orthopaedic Education
Department of Orthopaedic Surgery
Rush-Presbyterian-St. Luke's Medical Center
Chicago, Illinois

William P. Cooney III, M.D., M.S.
Professor of Orthopedic Surgery
Department of Orthopedic Surgery
Mayo Graduate School of Medicine
Mayo Medical School
Mayo Clinic
Rochester, Minnesota

Randall W. Culp, M.D.
Associate Professor of Orthopaedic, Hand, and Microsurgery
Department of Orthopaedics
Jefferson Medical College of Thomas Jefferson University
Thomas Jefferson University Hospital
Philadelphia, Pennsylvania

Tim R. C. Davis, M.B., Ch.B., B.Sc., M.Ch.
Special Professor of Trauma and Orthopaedics
Consultant Hand Surgeon
Department of Trauma and Orthopaedics
University of Nottingham
Queens Medical Centre
Nottingham, United Kingdom

Paul C. Dell, M.D.
Professor of Hand and Microsurgery
Department of Orthopaedics
University of Florida College of Medicine
University of Florida Medical Center
Gainesville, Florida

Dale Dellacqua, M.D.
Assistant Clinical Professor
Department of Orthopaedic Surgery
Indiana University School of Medicine
Indianapolis, Indiana

A. Lee Dellon, M.D., F.A.C.S.
Professor of Plastic Surgery and Neurosurgery
Johns Hopkins University School of Medicine
Baltimore, Maryland
Clinical Professor of Plastic Surgery
    and Neurosurgery
University of Arizona College of Medicine
Tucson, Arizona

Edward Diao, M.D.
Associate Professor
Chief of Division of Hand, Upper Extremity,
    and Microvascular Surgery
Department of Orthopaedic Surgery
University of California, San Francisco,
    School of Medicine
University of California, San Francisco,
    Medical Center
San Francisco, California

Joseph J. Dias, M.D., F.R.C.S., F.R.C.S.(Ed.)
Consultant Orthopaedic and Hand Surgeon
Glenfield General Hospital
Leicester, United Kingdom
Senior Lecturer in Orthopaedic Surgery
Department of Orthopaedics
University of Leicester
Leicester, United Kingdom
Senior Lecturer in Hand Surgery
Pulvertaft Unit
Derby University
Derby, United Kingdom

James H. Dobyns, M.D.
Clinical Professor of Orthopaedics
Department of Orthopaedics
University of Texas Health Science Center
    at San Antonio
Bexar County Medical Center Hospital
San Antonio, Texas
Emeritus Professor of Orthopaedic Surgery
    (A Rating)
United States Air Force Medical Department
Washington, District of Columbia
Emeritus Professor of Orthopedic Surgery
Mayo Medical Center
Mayo Clinic
Rochester, Minnesota

Kazuteru Doi, M.D., Ph.D.
Clinical Professor of Orthopedics
Department of Orthopedic Surgery
Yamaguchi University School of Medicine
President of Ogori Daiichi General Hospital
Ogori, Yamaguchi-ken, Japan

Scott F. M. Duncan, M.D., M.P.H.
Instructor of Orthopedic Surgery
Department of Orthopedic Surgery
Mayo Medical School
Mayo Clinic Hospital Scottsdale
Phoenix, Arizona

Michael J. Dunn, M.D.
Department of Hand Surgery
Allegheny University
Allegheny General Hospital
Pittsburgh, Pennsylvania

Linda T. Dvali, B.A., B.Sc., M.D., M.Sc., F.R.C.S.(C.)
Assistant Professor
Department of Plastic Surgery
University of Toronto Faculty of Medicine
University Health Network, Toronto
    Western Hospital
Toronto, Ontario, Canada

Lee E. Edstrom, M.D.
Professor of Surgery (Plastic)
Department of Surgery
Brown Medical School
Rhode Island Hospital
Providence, Rhode Island

Roslyn B. Evans, O.T.R./L., C.H.T.
Indian River Hand and Upper Extremity
    Rehabilitation, Incorporated
Vero Beach, Florida

Tracy C. Fairplay, B.S.
Licensed Physical Therapist
Consultant
Department of Hand Surgery
Department of Functional Rehabilitation
Policlinico di Modena
Bologna, Italy

Randolph J. Ferlic, M.D.
South Bend Orthopaedics & Sports Medicine
South Bend, Indiana

Guy G. Foucher, M.D.
Professor
Department of Traumatology
University of Las Palmas
Hospital Insular
Las Palmas, Spain

Alan E. Freeland, M.D.
Professor of Orthopaedics
Department of Orthopaedic Surgery
*   and Rehabilitation*
University of Mississippi School of Medicine
University Medical Center
Jackson, Mississippi

Gerard T. Gabel, M.D.
Department of Orthopedic Surgery
Baylor College of Medicine
The Methodist Hospital
Houston, Texas

Marc Garcia-Elias, M.D., Ph.D.
Associate Professor
Department of Physiotherapy
Universitat Internacional Catalunya
Institut Kaplan
Barcelona, Spain

Guenter Germann, M.D., Ph.D.
Professor of Hand and Plastic Surgery
Burn Center
Department of Plastic and Hand Surgery
University of Heidelberg
Heidelberg, Germany
BG-Trauma Center
Ludwigshafen, Germany

Keith A. Glowacki, M.D.
Hand Surgery Specialists/Advanced
*   Orthopaedic Center*
Richmond, Virginia

Felix Göbel, M.D.
Orthopaedic Surgeon
Department of Orthopaedic Surgery
Martin-Luther-University Halle-Wittenberg
Halle/Saale, Germany

Nancy Griffin-Reed, O.T.R./L., C.H.T., M.H.S.
Hand Therapist
University Orthopedics, Incorporated
Providence, Rhode Island

Amit Gupta, M.D., M.S., F.R.C.S., M.Ch.Orth.
Director of Christine M. Kleinert Institute
Kleinert, Kutz and Associates Hand Care Center
Jewish Hospital Hand Care Center
Louisville, Kentucky

Jan-Ragnar Haugstvedt, M.D.
Senior Consultant
Department of Orthopaedics
Division for Hand and Microsurgery
University in Oslo
Rikshospitalet University Hospital
Oslo, Norway

Edward P. Hayes, M.D.
Hand and Upper Extremity Surgery
Department of Orthopedic Surgery
Marshfield Clinic
Eau Claire, Wisconsin

Lior Heller, M.D.
Clinical Instructor
Department of Plastic Surgery
University of Texas Medical School
*   at Houston*
University of Texas M. D. Anderson Cancer Center
Houston, Texas

José Medina Henriquez, M.D.
Professor of Orthopedics
Hand and Upper Surgery Unit
University of Las Palmas
Hospital Insular de Gran Canaria
Las Palmas, Spain

Daniel B. Herren, M.D.
Dipl. NDS ETH
Department of Hand Surgery
Schulthess Clinic
Zurich, Switzerland

Yuichi Hirase, M.D.
Director of Plastic and Reconstructive Surgery
Department of Plastic and Reconstructive Surgery
Saitama Seikeikai Hospital
Higashimatsuyama, Saitama, Japan

Emiko Horii, M.D.
Assistant Professor
Department of Orthopaedics
Nagoya University
Nagoya, Japan

Joseph E. Imbriglia, M.D., F.A.C.S.
Clinical Professor of Orthopaedic Surgery
Department of Orthopaedic Surgery
Director of Hand and Upper Extremity Fellowship Program
University of Pittsburgh School of Medicine
Pittsburgh, Pennsylvania

Michelle A. James, M.D.
Associate Clinical Professor
Department of Orthopaedic Surgery
University of California, Davis, School of Medicine
Davis, California
University of California, San Francisco, School of Medicine
San Francisco, California
Shriners Hospital for Children, Northern California
Sacramento, California

Craig H. Johnson, M.D.
Assistant Professor and Chairman
Department of Plastic Surgery
Mayo Clinic
Rochester, Minnesota

Jesse B. Jupiter, M.D.
Hansjörg Wyss Professor of Orthopaedic Surgery
Department of Hand Surgery
Harvard Medical School
Massachusetts General Hospital
Boston, Massachusetts

Ercan Karacaoglu, M.D.
Fellow in Plastic Surgery
Department of Surgery
Division of Plastic Surgery
Brown Medical School
Rhode Island Hospital
Providence, Rhode Island

Julia A. Katarincic, M.D.
Assistant Professor of Orthopaedic Surgery
Department of Orthopaedic Surgery
Brown Medical School
Rhode Island Hospital
Providence, Rhode Island

Simon P. J. Kay, B.A., B.M., B.Ch., F.R.C.S.,
F.R.C.S.(Plas.), F.R.C.S.E.(Hon.)
Professor
Department of Plastic, Reconstructive, and Hand Surgery
University of Leeds
St. James's University Hospital
Leeds, United Kingdom

Roger K. Khouri, M.D.
Miami Hand Center
Miami, Florida

Thomas W. Kiesler, M.D., M.S.
Department of Orthopaedic Surgery
Hand Care Associates
Warrenville, Illinois

Tadao Kojima, M.D.
Director of Saitama Hand Surgery Institute
Saitama Seikeikai Hospital
Higashimatsuyama, Saitama, Japan

Scott H. Kozin, M.D.
Associate Professor of Orthopaedics
Department of Orthopaedic Surgery
Temple University School of Medicine
Upper Extremity Surgeon
Shriners Hospital for Children
Philadelphia, Pennsylvania

Hermann Krimmer, M.D.
Privatdozent Associated with Department
  of General Surgery
University of Würzburg
Würzburg, Germany
Klinik fuer Handchirurgie
Bad Neustadt, Germany

Ulrich Lanz, M.D., Ph.D.
Professor of Surgery of the Hand
Klinik fuer Handchirurgie
Rhoen-Klinik
Bad Neustadt, Germany

Lisa L. Lattanza, M.D.
Assistant Professor of Orthopaedic Surgery
Department of Orthopaedic Surgery
University of California, San Francisco,
  School of Medicine
University of California, San Francisco,
  School of Medicine Hospital
San Francisco, California
Shriners Hospital for Children,
  Northern California
Sacramento, California

A. Charlotta La Via, M.D.
Santa Monica, California

Donald H. Lee, M.D.
Associate Professor
Division of Orthopedic Surgery
University of Alabama School
  of Medicine
University of Alabama at Birmingham
Birmingham, Alabama

Lisa Leonard, B.A., M.Sc., F.R.C.S.
Orthopaedic Registrar
Department of Orthopaedics
Bath Royal United Hospital
Bath, United Kingdom

Lawrence Scott Levin, M.D., F.A.C.S.
Professor of Plastic and Orthopaedic Surgery
Department of Surgery
Divisions of Plastic and Orthopaedic Surgery
Duke University School of Medicine
Duke University Medical Center
Durham, North Carolina

Ronald L. Linscheid, B.S., N.D., M.S.
Emeritus Professor of Orthopedic Surgery
Department of Orthopedic Surgery
Mayo Medical School
Mayo Clinic
Rochester, Minnesota

Riccardo Luchetti, M.D.
Assistant Professor of Hand Surgery
Department of Plastic and Reconstructive Surgery
and Hand Surgery
School of Medicine of Ancona
Ancona, Italy
Department of Orthopaedics, Traumatology,
and Hand Surgery
State Hospital of San Marino
Republic of San Marino

Susan E. Mackinnon, M.D.
Shoenberg Professor of Surgery
Chief of Division of Plastic and
Reconstructive Surgery
Department of Plastic and Reconstructive Surgery
Washington University School of Medicine
Barnes-Jewish Hospital
St. Louis, Missouri

Anna H. Makowski
Department of Orthopaedics and Rehabilitation
University of Miami School of Medicine
Bascom Palmer Eye Institute
Miami, Florida

Jennifer J. Marler, M.D.
Assistant Professor of Surgery and
Biomedical Engineering
Department of Surgery
University of Cincinnati College of Medicine
Cincinnati Children's Hospital
Medical Center
Cincinnati, Ohio

Victoria R. Masear, M.D.
Clinical Associate Professor of Orthopedics
Department of Surgery
University of Alabama School of Medicine
University of Alabama at Birmingham
Medical Center East
Birmingham, Alabama

Daniel P. Mass, M.D.
Professor of Surgery
Section of Orthopaedics and
Rehabilitation Medicine
Department of Surgery
University of Chicago Pritzker
School of Medicine
University of Chicago Hospitals
Chicago, Illinois

Susan L. Michlovitz, P.T., Ph.D., C.H.T.
Professor of Physical Therapy
Department of Physical Therapy
Temple University School of Medicine
Philadelphia, Pennsylvania

Steven L. Moran, M.D.
Assistant Professor of Surgery
Division of Plastic Surgery
Division of Hand Surgery
Mayo Medical School
Mayo Clinic
Rochester, Minnesota

Peter M. Murray, M.D.
Associate Professor
Department of Orthopedic Surgery
Division of Hand and Microvascular Surgery
Mayo Clinic
Jacksonville, Florida

Daniel J. Nagle, M.D.
Professor of Clinical Orthopaedics
Department of Orthopaedics
Northwestern University Feinberg School of Medicine
Northwestern Memorial Hospital
Chicago, Illinois

David T. Netscher, M.D.
Professor
Division of Plastic Surgery
Baylor College of Medicine
Chief of Hand Surgery
Texas Children's Hospital
Chief of Plastic Surgery
Houston VA Medical Center
Houston, Texas

Robert J. Neviaser, M.D.
Professor and Chairman
Department of Orthopaedic Surgery
George Washington University School of Medicine
George Washington University Hospital
Washington, District of Columbia

Mary Lynn Newport, M.D.
Associate Professor of Orthopaedic Surgery
Department of Orthopaedic Surgery
University of Connecticut Health Center
Farmington, Connecticut

José M. Nolla, M.D.
Department of Orthopedic Surgery
Baylor College of Medicine
Houston, Texas

Fiesky A. Nuñez V., M.D.
Chief of Hand and Upper Extremity Surgery
Department of Orthopaedics and Trauma
Centro Médico Dr. Rafael Guerra Mendez
Valencia, Carabobo, Venezuela

Lewis H. Oster, Jr., M.D.
Hand Surgery Associates, P.C.
Denver, Colorado

A. Lee Osterman, M.D.
Professor of Orthopaedic and Hand Surgery
Department of Orthopaedics
Jefferson Medical College of Thomas Jefferson University
Philadelphia, Pennsylvania
The Philadelphia Hand Center
King of Prussia, Pennsylvania

Elizabeth A. Ouellette, M.D., M.B.A.
Professor of Orthopaedics
Department of Orthopaedics and Rehabilitation
University of Miami School of Medicine
Bascom Palmer Eye Institute
Miami, Florida

Stephen A. Pap, M.D.
Instructor in Surgery
Department of Surgery
Division of Plastic Surgery
Mount Auburn Hospital
Cambridge, Massachusetts

William C. Pederson, M.D.
Clinical Associate Professor of Surgery and
*   Orthopaedic Surgery*
Director of Hand Surgery Fellowship Training
The University of Texas Health Science Center at San Antonio
San Antonio, Texas

Michael Pelzer, M.D.
Department of Hand, Plastic, and Reconstructive Surgery
Burn Center
Department of Plastic and Hand Surgery
University of Heidelberg
Heidelberg, Germany
BG-Trauma Center
Ludwigshafen, Germany

Isabelle Pigeau, M.D.
Fellow in Diagnostic Radiology
Clinical Chief of Radiology and Surgery
Department of Diagnostic Radiology
Hôpital Georges Pompidou
Paris, France

Alastair J. Platt
Specialist Registrar in Plastic Surgery
Department of Plastic, Reconstructive, and Hand Surgery
University of Leeds
St. James's University Hospital
Leeds, United Kingdom

H. Matthew Quitkin, M.D.
Robert E. Carroll Fellow, Hand Surgery
New York Presbyterian Hospital/Columbia Campus
New York, New York
Attending Hand Surgeon
MANUS Center
Vienna, Virginia

Kevin J. Renfree, M.D.
Consultant in Orthopedic Surgery
Department of Orthopedic Surgery
Mayo Clinic Hospital
Phoenix, Arizona

Marco J. P. F. Ritt, M.D., Ph.D.
Professor of Hand Surgery
Department of Plastic, Reconstructive, and Hand Surgery
Vrije Universiteit
Vrije Universiteit Medical Center
Amsterdam, The Netherlands

Melvin P. Rosenwasser, M.D.
Robert E. Carroll Professor of Surgery of the Hand
Columbia University College of Physicians and Surgeons
Chief of Hand and Trauma Services
New York Presbyterian Hospital/Columbia Campus
New York, New York

Kavi Sachar, M.D.
Attending Hand Surgeon
Department of Orthopaedic Surgery
Porter Adventist Hospital
Denver, Colorado

Philippe H. Saffar, M.D.
Institut Français de Chirurgie de la Main
Paris, France

Ioannis Sarris, M.D., Ph.D.
Department of Orthopaedic Surgery, Upper Extremity
Drexel University College of Medicine
Philadelphia, Pennsylvania
Allegheny General Hospital
Pittsburgh, Pennsylvania

Michael Sauerbier, M.D., Ph.D.
Assistant Professor
Department of Hand, Plastic, and Reconstructive Surgery
Burn Center
Department of Plastic and Hand Surgery
University of Heidelberg
Heidelberg, Germany
BG-Trauma Center
Ludwigshafen, Germany

John G. Seiler III, M.D.
Clinical Associate Professor of Orthopaedic Surgery
Department of Orthopaedic Surgery
Emory University School of Medicine
Piedmont Hospital
Atlanta, Georgia

Gontran R. Sennwald, Ph.D.
Consultant Hand Surgeon
Hand Surgery Unit
Medical School of Geneva
Hôpital Cantonal de Genève
Geneva, Switzerland

Adam B. Shafritz, M.D.
Assistant Professor of Orthopedic Surgery
Department of Orthopedic Surgery
University of Vermont College of Medicine
Burlington, Vermont

Randy Sherman, M.D.
Professor of Plastic and Reconstructive Surgery
Department of Surgery
Keck School of Medicine of the University of Southern California
USC University Hospital
Los Angeles, California

Alexander Y. Shin, M.D.
Associate Professor of Orthopedic Surgery
Department of Orthopedic Surgery
Division of Hand Surgery
Mayo Graduate School of Medicine
Mayo Clinic
Rochester, Minnesota

Walter H. Short, M.D.
Clinical Professor of Orthopedics
Department of Orthopedic Surgery
State University of New York Upstate Medical University
Syracuse, New York
Syracuse Orthopedic Specialists
Dewitt, New York

Beat R. Simmen, M.D.
Assistant Professor
Department of Hand Surgery
Schulthess Clinic
Zurich, Switzerland

Divya Singh, M.D.
Orthopedic and Hand Surgeon
Albany General Hospital
Albany, Oregon

Joel S. Solomon, M.D., Ph.D.
Assistant Professor of Plastic Surgery
Department of Surgery
University of Alabama School of Medicine
University of Alabama at Birmingham
University of Alabama Hospitals
Birmingham, Alabama

Panupan Songcharoen, M.D.
Professor of Orthopedic Surgery
Department of Orthopedic Surgery
Mahidol University
Faculty of Medicine
Siriraj Hospital
Bangkok, Thailand

Dean G. Sotereanos, M.D.
Professor of Orthopaedics
Vice Chairman of Department
of Orthopaedic Surgery
Drexel University College of Medicine
Philadelphia, Pennsylvania
Allegheny General Hospital
Pittsburgh, Pennsylvania

David R. Steinberg, M.D.
Associate Professor of Orthopaedic Surgery
Department of Orthopaedic Surgery
University of Pennsylvania
School of Medicine
University of Pennsylvania Health Systems
Chief of Hand Surgery
Department of Surgery
Division of Orthopaedics
Philadelphia VA Medical Center
Philadelphia, Pennsylvania

Scott P. Steinmann, M.D.
Assistant Professor of Orthopedics
Department of Orthopedics
Mayo Clinic
Rochester, Minnesota

James W. Strickland, M.D.
Clinical Professor of Orthopaedic Surgery
Department of Orthopaedic Surgery
Indiana University School of Medicine
St. Vincent Indianapolis Hospital
Indianapolis, Indiana

Stephanie Sweet, M.D.
Clinical Assistant Professor of Orthopaedic Surgery
Attending, Hand Surgery
Department of Orthopaedic Surgery
Jefferson Medical College of
*   Thomas Jefferson University*
Thomas Jefferson University Hospital
Philadelphia, Pennsylvania

Lam-Chuan Teoh, F.A.M.S., F.R.C.S.
Senior Consultant and Advisor
Department of Hand Surgery
Singapore General Hospital
Singapore

Richard M. Terek, M.D.
Associate Professor of Orthopaedic Surgery
Department of Orthopaedic Surgery
Brown Medical School
Rhode Island Hospital
Providence, Rhode Island

Matthew M. Tomaino, M.D., M.B.A.
Professor of Orthopaedics
Chief of Division of Hand and
*   Upper Extremity Surgery*
University of Rochester Medical Center
Rochester, New York

José E. Torres, M.D.
Assistant Professor of Hand Surgery
Department of Orthopaedic Surgery
University of Los Andes
University of Los Andes Hospital
Mérida, Venezuela

Ian A. Trail, M.D., F.R.C.S.
Consultant in Hand and Upper Limb Surgery
Department of Hand and Upper Limb Surgery
Wrightington Hospital
Wigan, England

Joe Upton, M.D.
Associate Professor of Surgery
*   (Plastic/Hand)*
Division of Plastic Surgery
Harvard Medical School
Children's Hospital
Beth Israel Deaconess Medical Center
Boston, Massachusetts

Ann E. Van Heest, M.D.
Associate Professor
Department of Orthopedic Surgery
University of Minnesota Medical School,
*   Twin Cities*
Gillette Children's Specialty Healthcare
Shriners Hospital for Children,
*   Twin Cities Unit*
Minneapolis, Minnesota

Joerg van Schoonhoven, M.D., Ph.D.
Klinik fuer Handchirurgie
Rhoen-Klinik
Bad Neustadt, Germany

David Whitman Vickers, M.B.B.S., F.R.A.C.S.
Clinical Professor
Division of Orthopaedics
Faculty of Medicine
University of Queensland
Brisbane, Australia

John J. Walsh IV, M.D.
Assistant Professor of Orthopaedics
Department of Orthopaedics
University of South Carolina School
*   of Medicine*
Columbia, South Carolina

Robert A. Weber, M.D.
Associate Professor of Surgery
Chief of Section of Hand Surgery
Division of Plastic Surgery
Texas A&M University System Health Science Center
*   College of Medicine*
College Station, Texas
Scott and White Memorial Hospital
*   and Clinic*
Temple, Texas

Denise J. Wedel, M.D.
Professor of Anesthesiology
Department of Anesthesiology
Mayo Foundation
Rochester, Minnesota

Fu-Chan Wei, M.D.
Professor of Plastic Surgery
Department of Plastic Surgery
Dean of College of Medicine
Chang Gung University
Taipei, Taiwan

Andrew J. Weiland, M.D.
Professor of Orthopaedics and Plastic Surgery
Cornell University Joan and Sanford I. Weill
  Medical College and Graduate School
  of Medical Sciences
Hospital for Special Surgery
New York, New York

Jeffrey Weinzweig, M.D.
Assistant Professor of Surgery
  (Plastic Surgery)
Department of Plastic Surgery
Brown Medical School
Rhode Island Hospital
Hasbro Children's Hospital
Providence, Rhode Island

Norman Weinzweig, M.D., F.A.C.S.
Adjunct Attending in Surgery
Department of Plastic Surgery
Rush-Presbyterian-St. Luke's
  Medical Center
Plastic Surgery Attending
John H. Stroger, Jr., Hospital
  of Cook County
Chicago, Illinois

Arnold-Peter C. Weiss, M.D.
Professor of Orthopaedics
Brown Medical School
Rhode Island Hospital
Providence, Rhode Island

Lawrence E. Weiss, M.D.
Adjunct Clinical Assistant Professor of Orthopaedic Surgery
Department of Orthopaedic Surgery
Jefferson Medical College of Thomas Jefferson University
Philadelphia, Pennsylvania
Attending Hand Surgeon
Lehigh Valley Hospital
Allentown, Pennsylvania

J. Hearst Welborn, M.D.
Orthopedic Surgeon
Department of Orthopedics
Kaiser Foundation Hospital
San Rafael, California

Jennifer Moriatis Wolf, M.D.
Assistant Professor of Orthopaedic Surgery
Department of Orthopaedic Surgery
University of Colorado School of Medicine
University of Colorado Health Sciences Center
Denver, Colorado

Scott W. Wolfe, M.D.
Professor of Orthopaedic Surgery
Department of Orthopaedic Surgery
Cornell University Joan and Sanford I. Weill Medical
  College and Graduate School of Medical Sciences
Hospital for Special Surgery
New York, New York

Thomas W. Wright, M.D.
Associate Professor of Orthopaedics
Department of Orthopaedics
University of Florida College of Medicine
Shands Hospital
Gainesville, Florida

Raymond K. Wurapa, M.D.
Attending Hand Surgeon
Department of Orthopedic Surgery
Mount Carmel Medical Center and Children's Hospital
Greater Ohio Orthopedic Surgeons, Incorporated
Columbus, Ohio

PREFACE

It is acknowledged that, historically, a number of useful references have been created on topics related to disorders of the hand, some of which fell out of production, and some of which continued to thrive. All publications that we have reviewed have certainly added significantly to our knowledge and understanding of various aspects of hand surgery. All are written by individuals whom we hold in the highest regard as friends and mentors. As such, one might ask why we should consider adding yet another tome to the shelves of upper extremity textbooks. On careful analysis, we felt that several aspects of previous publications might be improved when considered from a different perspective. These insights were gained from our own perception and from comments made by residents and fellows in training and by colleagues in practice.

The first objective for us was to determine our target readership. We felt that a comprehensive textbook on all aspects of hand surgery was needed to provide a single reference for residents and hand surgery fellows in training, as well as for practicing clinicians, both those formally trained in hand surgery as well as those peripherally trained in hand surgery. To accomplish this, a number of organizational objectives had to be set, one of which was the request to contributing authors that they present as many treatment options as possible, with identification of their preferred method of treatment and development of an algorithm when appropriate. Additionally, chapters dedicated to a review of basic science, conservative care, and postoperative rehabilitation were developed, all with the idea of making this the most comprehensive single-source textbook on hand surgery available.

The book has been organized to facilitate easy location of the topic sought by the reader. It begins with an in-depth review of basic science topics related to hand surgery and progresses through such mainstay topics as trauma, fractures, carpal instability, and tendon injury/reconstruction (among many others) yet includes contemporary issues of arthroscopy, microvascular reconstruction, brachial plexus injuries, and imaging. Every essential topic related to hand surgery is covered. Each chapter is lavishly illustrated with drawings, photographs, and color and full illustrations and contains a comprehensive reference section for further review and reading.

The authors who have contributed chapters to this book represent the very best of modern hand surgery and were chosen carefully from locations around the world. We recognize that the practice of hand surgery is not limited geographically and that regional differences are found in the approach to clinical problems. We want to take advantage of these differences, to actually celebrate them, by presenting different approaches to clinical problems encountered in the practice of hand surgery. We found the authors to be most enthusiastic about the project, and their contributions are nothing short of their very best efforts. We are so proud of their contributions and feel that this special group of authors has come together for a unique opportunity to produce the most comprehensive and contemporary source of information on the topic of hand surgery available to date.

No project of this magnitude would be possible without the dedicated help of certain individuals. The concept was first discussed with and developed through the vision and hard work of Robert Hurley of Lippincott Williams & Wilkins. Working with him have been his assistant, Eileen Wolfberg, and the tireless duo of Developmental Editors, Tanya Lazar and Karen Carter. The artwork was beautifully rendered, and at an unbelievable pace, by Carol Capers. The typesetting and proofs were produced in a timely fashion by Amanda Yanovitch, Kate Sallwasser, and Holly H. Auten at Silverchair Science + Communications and ably managed through production by Mary Ann McLaughlin at Lippincott Williams & Wilkins. Finally, the dedicated work of our secretaries, Natalie Sobotta (R.A.B.) and Jo-Anne Marrapese (A.-P.W.), cannot go unmentioned or forgotten.

This text was produced for active clinicians, whether in training or in practice, treating disorders of the hand. It is to their tireless efforts at providing patients with hand problems the very best care that we have truly dedicated our efforts. It is recognized that these efforts have built on the shoulders of truly wondrous giants.

R.A.B.
A.-P.W.

HAND SURGERY

RECONSTRUCTION FOR ULNAR NERVE PALSY

KAVI SACHAR

Ulnar nerve paralysis most commonly results from traumatic injury. This can be by direct laceration, blunt trauma, severe crush injury, or nerve compression. It can be combined with other peripheral nerve injuries or occur in conjunction with brachial plexus level injuries. Additionally, it can occur in systemic conditions such as Charcot-Marie-Tooth disease and leprosy. The prognosis for recovery is dependent on the nature of the injury, the treatment rendered, and, most important, the age of the patient.

Ulnar nerve paralysis results in a combination of motor and sensory deficits. Because forceful and fine motor manipulation activities may be affected, the limitations may significantly hamper function. Each patient, however, has different needs based on age, sex, and occupation. Anatomic variations, combined lesions, and associated injuries also affect function. A detailed understanding of normal ulnar nerve anatomy allows the physician to localize the level of injury. Knowledge of normal and anomalous innervation patterns allows the physician to document motor and sensory deficiencies. This knowledge, combined with an assessment of the patient's functional limitations, allows the physician and patient to determine the best treatment options. Reconstructive procedures for ulnar nerve paralysis are considered after careful evaluation of the patient's subjective complaints, functional deficit, and potential for recovery from the initial traumatic incident.

ANATOMY

The C8 to T1 nerve roots combine to form the lower trunk, which contributes to both the posterior and medial cords. The medial cord gives rise to the medial pectoral nerve, the medial brachial cutaneous nerve, and the medial antebrachial cutaneous nerve. The medial cord terminates as the ulnar nerve. Although the ulnar nerve derives the majority of its fibers from the C8 and T1 nerve roots, it receives contributions from the seventh cervical nerve and, occasionally, higher nerve roots at least 50% of the time.

This is accomplished through a lateral root derived from the lateral cord or one of its branches (Fig. 1) (1).

At its origin, the ulnar nerve lies medial to the axillary artery, lateral to the axillary vein, and posterior to the medial antebrachial cutaneous nerve. In the upper arm, it lies medial or posterior to the brachial artery. The ulnar nerve pierces the intermuscular septum at approximately the middle of the arm. It then lies on the front of the medial head of the triceps muscle. The medial epicondyle forms the roof of the cubital tunnel, where the nerve is covered by multiple fascial layers. In the cubital tunnel, the nerve lies beneath the fascial arcade formed by the superficial and deep heads of the flexor carpi ulnaris. As it passes between these heads, it comes to lie on the volar surface of the flexor digitorum profundus (FDP) in the middle of the forearm. The nerve lies beneath the flexor carpi ulnaris at the level of the wrist. Both the ulnar nerve and ulnar artery pass lateral to the pisiform and lie volar to the transverse carpal ligament at the wrist. The ulnar nerve ends at the base of the hypothenar eminence by dividing into deep and superficial palmar branches.

The ulnar nerve's first motor branch is usually to the flexor carpi ulnaris muscle, and it originates distal to the medial epicondyle. The nerve then goes on to innervate the ring and small finger components of the FDP tendon. The next branch is the dorsal sensory branch of the ulnar nerve, which originates 7 cm proximal to the radial styloid, providing sensation to the dorsal ulnar aspect of the hand. In the hand, the superficial branch of the ulnar nerve terminates as a common digital nerve to the ring and small web space and a proper digital nerve to the ulnar border of the small finger. As the deep motor branch courses through the hypothenar muscles, it innervates the abductor digiti minimi, flexor digiti minimi brevis, and the opponens digiti minimi. The deep branch then goes on to innervate the two medial lumbricals, all the interossei, the adductor pollicis, and the deep head of the flexor pollicis brevis. The nerve ends by innervating the first dorsal interosseous (FDI). A schematic of normal ulnar nerve motor and sensory innervation is depicted in Figure 2.

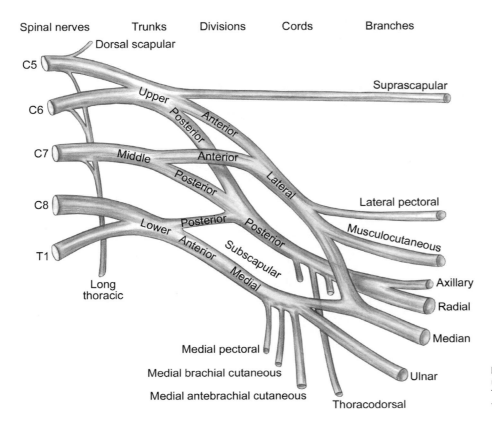

FIGURE 1. The brachial plexus. The ulnar nerve primarily arises from C8 and T1 but occasionally receives branches from higher nerve roots.

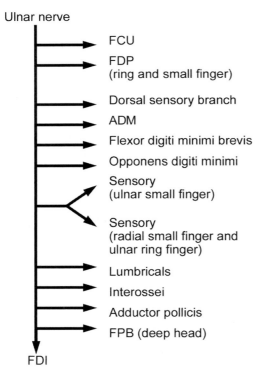

FIGURE 2. Schematic representation of ulnar nerve innervation in sequential fashion. ADM, abductor digiti minimi; FCU, flexor carpi ulnaris; FDI, first dorsal interosseous; FDP, flexor digitorum profundus; FPB, flexor pollicis brevis.

Anomalous innervation patterns occur in the normally innervated ulnar muscles. A forearm ulnar-median communication pattern known as the *Martin-Gruber anastomosis* occurs in 17% of patients (2). Type I connections (60%) send motor branches from the median nerve to the ulnar nerve to innervate "median" muscles. Type II connections (35%) send motor branches from the median to the ulnar nerve to innervate "ulnar" muscles. Type III connections (3%) send motor branches from the ulnar to the median nerve to innervate "ulnar" muscles, and type IV connections (1%) send motor fibers from the ulnar to the median nerve to innervate "ulnar" muscles. Palmar communications also exist and have been described by Riche and Cannieu (3). Additionally, the FDI, third and fourth lumbricals, and adductor pollicis all have been described as having dual innervation. All of these anatomic variants affect the functional deficit that is encountered in ulnar nerve lesions.

CLINICAL EVALUATION

Ulnar nerve palsy results in characteristic clinical signs that reflect the motor loss, sensory loss, and the level of injury. Additionally, specific clinical tests can be performed to demonstrate the functional loss that occurs. The clinical signs can vary based on variant innervation patterns, combined injuries, and generalized ligamentous laxity.

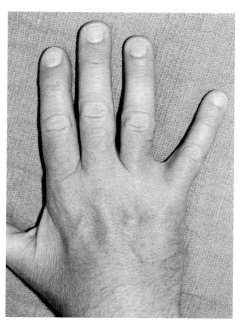

FIGURE 3. Wartenberg's sign. This results from unopposed pull of the small finger extensor tendons.

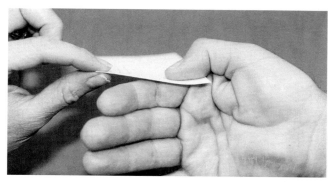

FIGURE 4. Froment's sign. This results from loss of adductor pollicis function with compensatory thumb interphalangeal flexion.

Flattening of the metacarpal arch and hypothenar muscles (Masse's sign) (4,5) results from atrophy of the interossei and opponens digiti quinti. Abductor digiti minimi paralysis allows for unopposed pull of the extensor tendon, which results in small finger abduction (Wartenberg's sign) (Fig. 3) (6,7).

Clawing of the fourth and fifth fingers (Duchenne's sign) occurs due to loss of intrinsic function (8). Without the intrinsics, there is a loss of metacarpophalangeal (MCP) flexion power and proximal interphalangeal (PIP) extension power. This results in an intrinsic minus position of MCP extension and PIP flexion. The median-innervated lumbricals partially protect the index and middle fingers. The clawing is less severe in high ulnar nerve palsy because the loss of the FDP to the ring and small fingers produces less of a flexion force on the distal digits. Patients with more ligamentous laxity may have worse clawing. The MCP volar plate eventually stretches out, accentuating the MCP hyperextension. Early on, the PIP capsule and extensor tendons remain normal. Eventually, however, patients may lose the ability to extend the PIP joint. This is what distinguishes simple from complex clawing and is the basis for Bouvier's test (9). In simple clawing, when MCP hyperextension is corrected, the extensor tendons are able to extend the PIP joints, demonstrating integrity of the extensor apparatus. This is considered to be a positive Bouvier's test. In a negative Bouvier's test, the patient cannot actively extend the PIP joints when MCP hyperextension is corrected, indicating insufficiency of the extensor apparatus. When tendon transfers to correct clawing are planned in a patient with simple clawing (a positive Bouvier's test), the tendon transfer only has to correct the clawing. In complex clawing (a negative Bouvier's test), the tendon transfer must correct the clawing and provide PIP extension.

As clawing becomes more severe, finger extension becomes more difficult. Patients sometimes flex their wrist to extend their digits, taking advantage of extrinsic tenodesis. This is known as the André Thomas sign (10) and is a poor prognostic indicator for successful tendon transfers because the pattern may become ingrained and difficult to change (11).

The clinical tests in ulnar nerve palsy demonstrate both muscle paralysis and loss of functional hand activities. Key pinch relies on adductor pollicis function. In ulnar nerve palsy, key pinch may be diminished as much as 77% to 80% (7,11,12). The flexor pollicis brevis also contributes to key pinch by causing flexion at the MCP joint and preventing MCP hyperextension. In ulnar nerve palsy, adductor pollicis paralysis is compensated for by using the FPL tendon. This results in hyperflexion of the thumb IP joint when attempting key pinch (Froment's sign) (Fig. 4) (13,14). The thumb MCP joint may hyperextend during pinch (Jeanne's sign) (15) if flexor pollicis brevis function is absent (Fig. 5).

Ulnar nerve palsy results in the loss of integration of PIP and MCP flexion (11). This dyssynchronous finger flexion

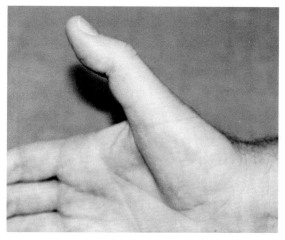

FIGURE 5. Jeanne's sign: hyperextension of the thumb metacarpophalangeal joint.

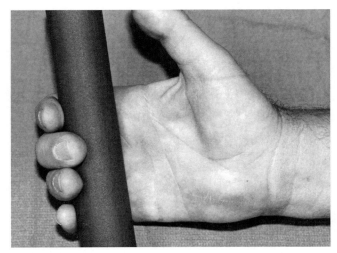

FIGURE 6. Dyssynchronous finger flexion results from loss of intrinsic function and the normal flexion cascade.

results from intrinsic paralysis. In normal gripping, the intrinsics flex the MCP joints before distal interphalangeal flexion, allowing for broad objects to be grasped. In ulnar nerve palsy, ring and small finger MCP joint flexion can occur only after distal joint flexion. Patients therefore tend to push items out of their hands because they cannot secure them in their palms before distal joint flexion (Fig. 6).

Omer described the "cross-your-finger test" to demonstrate paralysis of the first volar interosseous and second dorsal interosseous (16). This test can reveal an inability to cross the flexed long finger dorsally over the index finger or the index finger over the long finger with the hand on a flat surface.

The Pitres-Testut sign is demonstrated by an inability to abduct the middle finger when on a flat surface (7). This tests the second and third dorsal interossei muscles.

In high ulnar nerve palsy, there is an inability to flex the distal interphalangeal joints of the ring and small fingers

TABLE 1. CLINICAL SIGNS AND FINDINGS IN ULNAR NERVE PALSY

Signs	Findings
Masse's sign	Hypothenar atrophy
Wartenberg's sign	Small finger abduction
Duchenne's sign	Ring and small finger clawing
André Thomas sign	Wrist flexion to extend digits
Jeanne's sign	Thumb metacarpophalangeal hyperextension
Froment's sign	Thumb interphalangeal hyperflexion with key pinch
Cross-your-finger test	Inability to cross index and middle finger
Pitres-Testut sign	Inability to abduct middle finger
Pollock's sign	Loss of flexor digitorum profundus to ring and small finger (high ulnar nerve palsy)

due to paralysis of the ulnar innervated FDP tendons (Pollock's sign) (4). These clinical signs and findings are summarized in Table 1. The sensory loss that occurs in ulnar nerve paralysis depends on the level of nerve injury. If the nerve injury is above the mid-forearm, the dorsal sensory branch of the ulnar nerve is affected, resulting in dorsal ulnar hand anesthesia. There is considerable variability in dorsal hand innervation (17). The radial sensory contribution may be large, so a detailed examination is necessary. Palmar sensation is absent over the volar small finger and ulnar one-half of the ring finger (1).

SURGICAL PLANNING

The traumatic or systemic incident that led to the ulnar nerve paralysis should be evaluated in detail. The potential for nerve recovery is variable depending on multiple factors (18–22). The most important prognostic factor for recovery is the age of the patient. For example, a child with a low ulnar nerve laceration that has been repaired acutely has a very good prognosis for recovery and should be followed until sufficient time has passed during which recovery should occur. In contrast, an adult with chronic ulnar nerve compression, established atrophy, and deformity has a poor prognosis for recovery and is a candidate for tendon transfers if appropriate.

The location of the nerve injury and mechanism of injury should be noted. High-energy proximal traction injuries, such as from motorcycles or snowmobiles, have a worse prognosis than low-level, sharp lacerations that have been repaired. It should be noted if the patient had an associated fracture or tendon injuries that may affect available tendons for transfer.

Combined nerve injuries present a special problem because of tendon availability and specific functional needs (23). Careful documentation of available tendons and their motor strength should be made.

In all cases, a chart should be made that documents the functional deficits, tendons available for transfer, their strength, tendon transfer options, and proposed transfers. Patients should be well informed of the proposed procedure and what functional gains should result from the transfers.

All joints to receive transfers should be passively supple. Associated fractures should be healed, and soft tissue wounds should be stable.

SURGICAL MANAGEMENT

Tendon Transfers for Pinch

Key pinch involves forcefully applying the tip of the thumb to the radial border of the index finger. This is primarily accomplished by the adductor pollicis and FDI. The extensor pollicis longus and flexor pollicis longus contribute by providing a small adductor moment. The flexor pollicis brevis provides MCP stability (24,25).

Several tendon transfers have been designed to restore pinch (11,14,16,26–42). Some restore only adductor pollicis function; others restore FDI function as well. The motors that have been described include wrist extensors, the brachioradialis, digital extensors, and digital flexors. Regardless of the motor, most tendon transfers provide only 25% to 50% of normal pinch strength (11).

The decision to restore pinch is based on a patient's functional needs. In a series by Hastings and Davidson, many patients with ulnar nerve palsy were satisfied with their pinch despite significant weakness (11).

Transfers to Restore Adductor Pollicis Function

The tendon motors that are available to restore adductor pollicis function are the extensor carpi radialis brevis (ECRB), flexor digitorum superficialis (FDS), brachioradialis, and extensor digitorum communis.

Extensor Carpi Radialis Brevis

Smith described using the ECRB with a tendon graft to restore adductor pollicis function (24,25). The ECRB is released from its insertion and lengthened with a free palmaris tendon graft. This is then passed through the second metacarpal interspace, dorsal to the adductor pollicis, flexor tendons, and neurovascular structures and volar to the interossei. It is sutured to the adductor pollicis insertion with a tendon weave. Tension is set so that when the wrist is neutral, the thumb lies palmar to the index finger. This transfer has the added benefit of thumb abduction with wrist flexion and thumb adduction with wrist extension through a tenodesis effect (Fig. 7). Omer modified this technique slightly (16). He advocates passing the transfer through the third intermetacarpal space and securing it to the fascia over the abductor tubercle of the first metacarpal. He believes this insertion point improves pronation for pinch (36).

Use of the ECRB offers several advantages to other transfers for pinch. It is an extremely strong motor that is not missed because of the numerous other tendons available for wrist extension. The vector of the transfer recreates the transverse head of the adductor pollicis, which is more functional than restoring the oblique head. It also does not sacrifice a finger flexor in a hand that has already weakened grasp.

Flexor Digitorum Superficialis

The FDS tendons are useful motor donors in low ulnar nerve palsy because they provide a strong motor, have excellent excursion, and are less missed if the FDP tendon

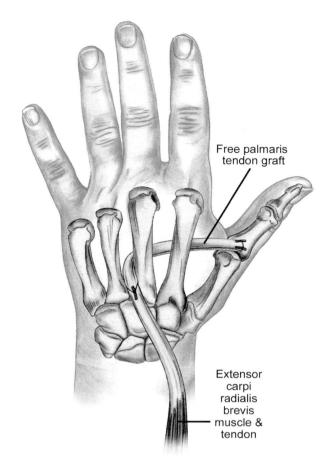

FIGURE 7. Extensor carpi radialis brevis tendon transfer for pinch. The tendon is elongated with a tendon graft and sutured to the adductor pollicis insertion.

is innervated. In low ulnar nerve palsy, the FDS to the ring finger can be sacrificed. In high ulnar nerve palsy, the FDS to the middle finger can be used.

Littler et al. described using the FDS of the ring or middle finger to restore thumb adduction (Fig. 8) (37–39). An oblique incision is made at the base of the finger in the distal palm similar to a trigger finger incision. The finger is flexed, and the FDS tendon is divided distal to the decussation, but the insertion is left to prevent hyperextension deformity of the PIP joint. The tendon is then tunneled to a second incision over the adductor pollicis insertion. The tendon is passed deep to the flexor tendons and neurovascular bundles, paralleling the transverse head of the adductor pollicis. The vertical septae of the palmar fascia serve as a pulley. Littler described passing the transfer into bone with a pullout button. Alternatively, the transfer can be sutured to the adductor pollicis insertion. Tension is set so that with 30 degrees of wrist flexion, the thumb lies in moderate flexion adduction. The hand is immobilized for 3 to 4 weeks and then active motion started. Hamlin and Littler have shown that 70% of pinch power can be restored with this procedure (39).

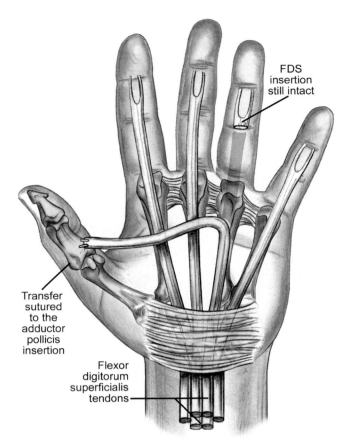

FDS
insertion
still intact

Transfer
sutured
to the
adductor
pollicis
insertion

Flexor
digitorum
superficialis
tendons

FIGURE 8. Flexor digitorum superficialis (FDS) tendon transfer to restore pinch. The palmar fascia serves as a pulley. Alternatively, the FDS to the middle can be used.

Brachioradialis

Boyes described using the brachioradialis tendon as a motor, citing its benefit of functioning in both wrist flexion and extension (40). A lengthy incision from the first dorsal compartment to the mid-forearm allows for mobilization of the tendon and its muscle belly. The muscle is released at the base of the first dorsal compartment. Excursion of up to 30 mm can be obtained by releasing the muscle to the proximal third of the radius. The brachioradialis tendon is elongated with a palmaris longus graft and passed in the same manner as the ECRB transfer as described by Smith.

Extensor Digitorum

When a finger flexor is not available as in combined nerve palsies, the extensor indicis proprius (EIP) can be used as a motor. The tendon is released just proximal to the extensor hood and then passed between the third and fourth metacarpals, dorsal the adductor pollicis. The tendon is brought through the web space and secured to the adductor pollicis insertion (24). Edgerton and Brand have recommended inserting the tendon into the abductor pollicis tendon as a more functional insertion (36).

Bunnel described using the extensor indicis communis tendon because its muscle is stronger than the EIP (40,42). The tendon is elongated with a tendon graft and passed subcutaneous around the ulnar border of the hand and deep to the flexor tendons. It is sutured to the adductor pollicis insertion as previously described.

Restoration of First Dorsal Interosseous

Numerous transfers have been described to restore FDI function (32,40–44), which, when combined with restoration of adductor pollicis function, would truly restore pinch. Most patients, however, can stabilize the index finger against the middle finger, and the true vector of the FDI is difficult to reproduce. These transfers have been reported to improve pinch only 10% to 15%. A strong motor for FDI may produce a "nose-picker finger" with persistent radial deviation of the index finger (11).

Abductor Pollicis Longus Transfer

This transfer is performed by isolating an abductor pollicis longus slip that does not contribute to abduction of the thumb (32). This is usually a more radial slip. The tendon is lengthened with a tendon graft. A dorsal radial incision is made along the FDI, and a dorsal subcutaneous tunnel is created. The tendon graft is woven into the FDI insertion. This transfer does not make the FDI much stronger but does stabilize it during pinch (Fig. 9).

Extensor Digitorum

Bunnel described transfer of the EIP to restore FDI function, and this was later modified by Omer (16,40,42). Omer describes taking the EIP proximal to the extensor hood, withdrawing it at the wrist, and passing it around the radial border of the second metacarpal. The tendon is split so that one slip inserts at the FDI tendon and the other at the adductor pollicis. This transfer does not restore strong power pinch but does stabilize the index finger (16).

The extensor digiti quinti can be used in a manner similar to the EIP (34). The two slips of the extensor digiti quinti are divided and brought distal to the fourth dorsal compartment retinaculum. They are then passed subcutaneously to the insertion of the FDI and adductor pollicis with one slip sewn to each. Although the extensor digiti quinti is a weak motor, recovery of adequate pinch has been reported (34).

Correction of Claw Deformity

The claw deformity in ulnar nerve paralysis is due to loss of intrinsic function. This results in MCP hyperextension and PIP flexion. MCP hyperextension can be corrected with either a static tissue tightening procedure or a dynamic tendon trans-

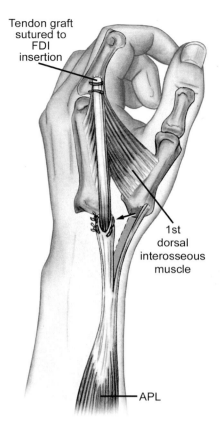

FIGURE 9. Abductor pollicis longus (APL) tendon transfer with graft to restore first dorsal interosseous (FDI) function.

fer. In patients with a positive Bouvier's test, there is no need to restore PIP extension. If the Bouvier's test is negative, a tendon transfer must restore both MCP flexion and PIP extension.

Procedures to improve clawing include bony procedures, soft tissue tightening procedures, and tendon transfers. Tendon transfers use the FDS, extensor carpi radialis longus (ECRL), ECRB, and flexor carpi radialis (FCR) tendons.

Bone and Soft Tissue Procedures for Correction of Clawing

Early attempts at correcting MCP hyperextension involved use of a bone block dorsally over the MCP joint (42,45). These techniques have largely been abandoned as soft tissue techniques have improved.

Bunnel described a procedure that creates bowstringing to increase the flexor moment on the MCP joint (46). He called this a "flexor pulley advancement." The A1 and A2 pulleys are released on both sides but not in the midline to the level of the midproximal phalanx. This allows the flexor tendon to partly bowstring, moving its axis more volar to the MCP joints.

Tightening the volar plate may be useful in patients with mild clawing and good PIP function. Zancolli described proximal advancement of the volar plate (47). Through a longitudinal incision for each digit, the A1 pulley is released, and a distally based rectangular flap is created from the volar plate. The flap is advanced proximally and sutured with the digit in 20 degrees of flexion. Omer modified the procedure by securing the flap to the deep transverse metacarpal ligament (Fig. 10) (16). Leddy et al. recommend securing the proximally advanced volar plate to bone (48).

Brown combined the Bunnel flexor pulley advancement and the Zancolli capsulorrhaphy secured to bone and added the excision of 1.5 cm of skin. He critically evaluated this technique and found a high complication rate. Complications included PIP and distal interphalangeal contractures and a gradual stretching of the capsulorrhaphy. All recurrences occurred within the first year (49).

Flexor Digitorum Superficialis Transfer for Correction of Clawing

There are several variations of the FDS transfer for correction of clawing (50–67). The basic principle is to keep the

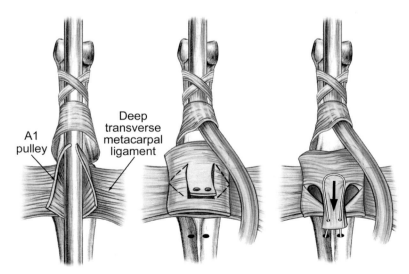

FIGURE 10. Volar plate advancement for correction of clawing. After releasing the A1 pulley **(left)**, a distally based flap of volar plate is developed **(middle)**. The flap is advanced proximally (*arrow*) and secured with a suture anchor to the metacarpal **(right)**.

transferred tendon volar to the deep intermetacarpal ligament, reproducing the vector of the lumbrical. In the Zancolli lasso, the transfer is sewn on itself as a loop (50). In the Stiles-type transfers, the tendon is sewn to the flexor tendon sheath, to the proximal phalanx, or into the lateral band if the Bouvier's test is positive (55).

In general, FDS transfers do not improve power grip because they sacrifice at least one finger flexor. Hastings and McCollam have shown a decrease in grip strength after FDS transfers (62). There is also a high incidence of PIP swan-neck deformities after these transfers (49). The FDS of the ring and small fingers should not be used in high ulnar nerve palsies because these are the only finger motors to the ring and small fingers. Transfers should be performed on all fingers because dynamic clawing may be present in the index and middle fingers as well (16). These transfers do well only in young, ligamentously lax individuals. They are unpredictable in people with stiff hands. Patients with a positive André Thomas sign do not do well with dynamic tendon transfers because of ingrained behavior that makes it difficult to train the transfer (11).

Zancolli Lasso

Zancolli described a tendon transfer that involves using the FDS tendon as a lasso around the A1 pulley (Fig. 11) (50). This provides both static flexion and dynamic flexion strength to the MCP joint. The flexor tendon sheath is exposed through a Bruner incision. The interval between the A1 and A2 pulley is incised, and the FDS tendon is

divided, leaving its insertion to prevent hyperextension. The FDS is then brought volar to the A1 pulley and sutured to itself. The transfer is sutured with the MCP joint in neutral position and the FDS pulled fairly tight. Tension is set so that the MCP joint sits in 40 to 60 degrees of flexion with the wrist in neutral. The small finger tension is set tighter than the ring finger. The MCP joint should be able to be passively extended to 0 degrees with some difficulty with the wrist in neutral but no difficulty with the wrist flexed. A dorsal blocking splint should be used for 6 weeks after surgery. Typically, this procedure is done with the sublimis tendon being used for its own finger. However, if the ring and small finger do not have a strong sublimis tendon or have no active profundus as in high ulnar nerve palsy, the middle finger sublimis can be split and used for both fingers (11). Omer describes looping the FDS around the A2 pulley and performs the procedure on all four fingers (16).

Stiles, Bunnel, Riordan Techniques

Bunnel modified the original Stiles FDS transfer by using all of the FDS tendons and transferring them to both sides of the clawed fingers (46,55). This is considered too strong of a transfer and results in PIP swan-neck deformity (46). The Stiles-Bunnel transfer now involves using one FDS tendon to motor two digits (16).

Midaxial incisions are made on the radial sides of each digit. A midpalmar incision is made to retrieve the FDS donor tendons. The ring finger FDS is harvested through a window between the A1 and A2 pulleys. It is split so that it

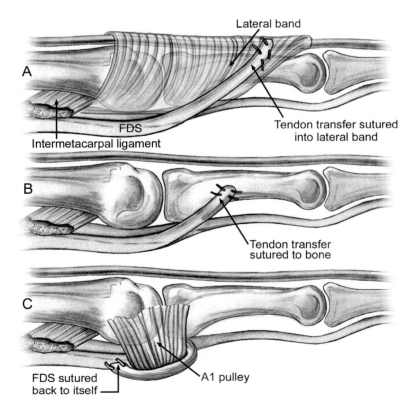

FIGURE 11. Flexor digitorum superficialis (FDS) tendon transfers for correction of clawing. The flexor digitorum superficialis can be sewn to the lateral band **(A)**, to bone **(B)**, or on itself in the Zancolli lasso **(C)**.

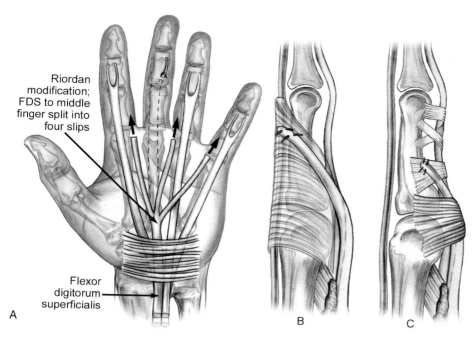

Riordan modification; FDS to middle finger split into four slips

Flexor digitorum superficialis

A   B   C

FIGURE 12. A: Riordan flexor digitorum superficialis (FDS) transfer for correction of clawing. The middle finger flexor digitorum superficialis is split into four slips. The slips are passed volar to the deep transverse metacarpal ligament. If the Bouvier's test is negative, the slips are sewn to a lateral band **(B)**. If the Bouvier's test is positive, the slips are sewn to the flexor tendon sheath **(C)**.

can be used for two fingers. If all four fingers are to be corrected, a second FDS tendon is harvested. Each slip is then passed through the lumbrical canal volar to the deep intermetacarpal ligament. This can be accomplished by passing a Carroll tendon passer from the digital wound proximally into the palmar wound along the path of the lumbrical. With a positive Bouvier's test, the transfer is sutured to the flexor tendon sheath. If the Bouvier's test is negative, the transfer is sewn to the lateral band. Tension is set with the wrist in neutral, the MCP joints in 45 to 50 degrees of flexion, and the IP joints in full extension. One must be careful not to set the tension too tightly and risk PIP hyperextension.

The Riordan modification involves using only the FDS to the middle finger and splitting it into four slips. Omer considers this the standard technique (Fig. 12) (16). The surgical procedure is similar to that described previously.

Wrist Extensor Transfer for Correction of Clawing

When restoration of a strong power grip is as important as correction of clawing, a wrist motor should be used as a tendon transfer. The ECRL, ECRB, FCR, and brachioradialis are all available in an isolated ulnar nerve palsy and can be extremely powerful motors. In addition, the FDS tendons, which serve as weak flexors, do not have to be sacrificed.

All of the wrist motor transfers require a free tendon graft. Donors include the palmaris longus, plantaris, or toe extensors.

Extensor Carpi Radialis Brevis and Extensor Carpi Radialis Longus

Brand describes a dorsal technique using the ECRB tendon (16,58). Through a dorsal incision, the ECRB is released

from its origin. Brand describes using a plantaris tendon, but the palmaris longus may be used. The tendon grafts are secured and passed superficial to the dorsal carpal ligament, through the intermetacarpal spaces, through the lumbrical canal volar to the deep transverse metacarpal ligament, and attached to the radial lateral bands of the middle ring and small fingers and the ulnar lateral band of the index finger. Brand believed that a stronger pinch could be obtained with the index finger stabilized in adduction.

Brand also describes using the ECRL and bringing it volar to the wrist by passing it under the brachioradialis tendon. It is then elongated with tendon grafts, with the grafts being passed through the carpal canal and sutured similarly to the FDS transfers previously described. Omer notes that this may cause a wrist flexion deformity and potentially crowd the carpal canal (16).

Flexor Carpi Radialis

Riordan believed that the FCR could be used as a motor for correction of claw finger and improvement in grip strength (54). He passed the FCR to the dorsal forearm and then proceeded with a technique similar to Brand's dorsal ECRB transfer. The FCR can also be used as a volar motor similar to Brand's volar ECRL transfer (51).

Internal Splint Technique

Omer Superficialis Y Technique

Omer describes an internal splint technique that can improve integration of MCP and IP flexion, key pinch for the thumb, and the flattened metacarpal arch (16). The superficialis Y technique involves using a single superficialis tendon combined with thumb MCP fusion. It combines

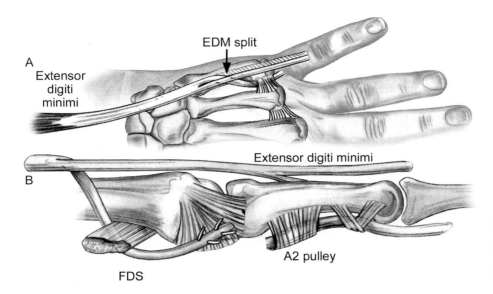

FIGURE 13. Extensor digiti minimi (EDM) transfer for correction of small finger abduction **(A)**. The transfer is sutured to the radial collateral ligaments if no clawing is present **(B)**. FDS, flexor digitorum superficialis.

many of the basic concepts in ulnar nerve reconstruction. The superficialis of the ring finger is used in low ulnar nerve palsy and the superficialis of the middle finger in high ulnar nerve palsy. Thumb MCP fusion is done through a dorsal incision using the surgeon's preferred technique. This fusion improves distal stability for tip pinch. Omer describes harvesting the FDS tendon through a volar Bruner incision. The radial half of the tendon is tenodesed to prevent hyperextension. The ulnar half is released at its insertion. The tendon is split first in half, and then the ulnar half is again divided in half. The radial half is used to restore thumb pinch. It is passed deep to the flexor tendons and neurovascular structures and sutured to the insertion of the abductor pollicis. The pulley for this transfer is the distal edge of the palmar fascia. The ulnar half of the FDS is used as a Zancolli lasso if strength is desired and if Bouvier's test is positive. Omer loops the tendon around the A2 pulley instead of around the A1 pulley. Otherwise, the FDS is used as a Stiles-Bunnell–type transfer inserting in the dorsal extensor apparatus if the Bouvier's test is negative. Tension is set with the wrist in neutral and the hand supinated. The MCP joints of the clawed fingers are placed in 45 degrees of flexion with the PIP joints in 0 degrees' extension. The thumb is adducted so it is parallel to the second metacarpal in an anterior-posterior projection. This position is maintained for 4 weeks until active extension is allowed.

This is not considered a definitive procedure because it divides the strength of a single tendon into multiple insertions. This technique is used as an internal splint after ulnar nerve repair to allow for function during nerve regeneration.

Small Finger Abduction

Wartenberg's sign results from paralysis of the third volar interosseous muscle, resulting in unopposed pull of the extensor digit minimi (EDM). Burge believed that the

deformity also may result from reinnervation of the abductor digiti minimi but not the third volar interosseous (68). Numerous transfers have been described to correct this deformity, most involving transfer of the EDM to the radial side of the finger (68–75). Either the entire EDM or half of the EDM can be used. If the entire EDM is to be used, a functional extensor digitorum communis to the fifth finger must be present (76,77).

Fowler described correction of this deformity and based it on the presence or absence of clawing (77). If clawing is not present, the ulnar slip of the EDM can be released and transferred to the radial collateral ligament of the small finger MCP joint. If clawing is present, it can be transferred more distally to the radial proximal phalanx of the small finger. The tendon is harvested through a dorsal incision and dissected proximally to the dorsal retinaculum. A volar incision is then made, and the tendon is passed through the fourth and fifth metacarpal space into the volar wound. This allows the transfer to pass volar the intermetacarpal ligament. The tendon is tensioned with the wrist in neutral and the MCP joint flexed 20 degrees (Fig. 13).

REFERENCES

1. Hollonshead WH. *Anatomy for surgeons*, 3rd ed. Philadelphia: Harper & Row, 1982.
2. Leibovic SJ, Hastings H 2nd. Martin-Gruber revisited. *J Hand Surg [Am]* 1992;17:47–53.
3. Kaplan EB, Spinner M. Normal and anomalous innervation patterns in the upper extremity. In: Omer GE Jr., Spiner M, ed. *Management of peripheral nerve problems*. Philadelphia: WB Saunders, 1980:75–99.
4. Earle AS, Vlastou C. Crossed fingers and other tests of ulnar nerve motor function. *J Hand Surg [Am]* 1980;5:560–565.
5. Masse L. Contribution à l' étude de l' achon des interosseous. *J Med (Bordeaux)* 1916;46:198.

6. Wartenberg R. A sign of ulnar palsy. *JAMA* 1939;112:1688.

7. Mannerfett L. Studies on the hand in ulnar nerve paralysis. *Acta Orthop Scand (Suppl)* 1966;87:4.

8. Duchenne GB. *Physiology of motion.* Kaplan EB (trans). Philadelphia: JB Lippincott Co, 1949:141–154.

9. Bouvier. Note sur une paralysie partielle des muscles de la main. *Bull Acad Nat Med (Paris)* 1851;18:125.

10. Andre-Thomas T. Le tonus du poignet dans la paralysie du nerf cubital. *Paris Med* 1917;25:473.

11. Hastings H 2nd, Davidson S. Tendon transfers for ulnar nerve palsy. Evaluation of results and practical treatment considerations. *Hand Clin* 1988;4:167–178.

12. Bowden REM, Napier JR. The assessment of hand functions after peripheral nerve injuries. *J Bone Joint Surg Br* 1961;43:481–492.

13. Froment J. La paralysie de l'adducteur du pouce et le signe de la prehension. *Rev Neurol* 1914;28:1236.

14. Brown PW. Reconstruction for pinch in ulnar intrinsic palsy. *Orthop Clin North Am* 1974;2:289.

15. Jeanne M. La deformation du pouce dans la paralysie cubitale. *Bull Med Soc Chir* 1915;41:703.

16. Omer GE. Ulnar nerve palsy. In: Green DP, Hotchkiss WC, Pederson WC, eds. *Green's operative hand surgery*, 4th ed. New York: Churchill Livingstone, 1999:1526–1541.

17. Rowntree T. Anomalous Innervation of the hand muscles. *J Bone Joint Surg Br* 1949;31:505.

18. Omer GE. Evaluation and reconstruction of the forearm and hand after acute traumatic peripheral nerve injuries. *J Bone Joint Surg Am* 1968;50:1454.

19. Brown RE, Zamboni WA, Zook EG, et al. Evaluation and management of upper extremity neuropathies in Charcot-Marie-Tooth disease. *J Hand Surg [Am]* 1992;17:523–530.

20. Omer GE. Timing of tendon transfers in peripheral nerve injury. *Hand Clin* 1988;4:317–322.

21. Trevett MC, Tuson C, de Jager LT, et al. The functional results of ulnar nerve repair. Defining the indications for tendon transfer. *J Hand Surg [Br]* 1995;20:444–446.

22. Smith RJ. Indications for tendon transfers to the hand. *Hand Clin* 1986;2:235–237.

23. Omer GE. Tendon transfers in combined nerve lesions. *Orthop Clin North Am* 1974;5:377–387.

24. Smith RJ. *Tendon transfers of the hand and forearm.* Boston: Little, Brown and Company, 1987:85–133.

25. Smith RJ. Extensor carpi radialis brevis tendon transfer for thumb adduction—a study of power pinch. *J Hand Surg [Am]* 1983;8:4–15.

26. Zancolli EA. *Structural and dynamic basis of hand surgery,* 2nd ed. Philadelphia: JB Lippincott Co, 1978:159–206.

27. Thompson TC. A modified operation for opponens paralysis. *J Bone Joint Surg* 1942;24:632.

28. Bruser P. Motor replacement operations in chronic ulnar nerve paralysis. *Orthopade* 1997;26:690–695.

29. Alnot JY, Masquelet A. Restoration of thumb-index pinch by a double tendon transfer following ulnar nerve paralysis. *Ann Chir Main* 1983;2:202–210.

30. Robinson D, Aghasi MK, Halperin N. Restoration of pinch in ulnar nerve palsy by transfer of split extensor digiti minimi and extensor indicis. *J Hand Surg [Br]* 1992;17:622–624.

31. De Abreu LB. Early restoration of pinch grip after ulnar nerve repair and tendon transfer. *J Hand Surg [Br]* 1989;14:309–314.

32. Neviaser RJ, Wilson JN, Gardner MM. Abductor pollicis longus transfer for replacement of first dorsal interosseous. *J Hand Surg [Am]* 1980;5:53–57.

33. Omer GE Jr. Reconstruction of a balanced thumb through tendon transfers. *Clin Orthop* 1985;195:104–116.

34. Zweig J, Rosenthal S, Burns H. Transfer of the extensor digiti quinti to restore pinch in ulnar palsy of the hand. *J Bone Joint Surg Am* 1972;54:51–59.

35. Reference deleted.

36. Edgerton MT, Brand PW. Restoration of abduction and adduction to the unstable thumb in median and ulnar paralysis. *Plast Reconstr Surg* 1965;36:150–164.

37. Littler JW. Tendon transfers and arthrodesis in combined median and ulnar nerve palsies. *J Bone Joint Surg Am* 1949;31:225–234.

38. North ER, Littler JW. Transferring the flexor superficialis tendon: technical considerations in the prevention of proximal interphalangeal joint instability. *J Hand Surg [Am]* 1980;5:498–501.

39. Hamlin C, Littler JW. Restoration of power pinch. *J Hand Surg [Am]* 1980;5:396–401.

40. Boyes JH. *Bunnell's surgery of the hand,* 5th ed. Philadelphia: JB Lippincott Co, 1970:366.

41. Goldner JL. Replacement of the function of the paralyzed adductor pollicis with the flexor digitorum sublimis—a ten year review. Proceedings of the American Society for Surgery of the Hand. *J Bone Joint Surg Am* 1967;49:583–584.

42. Bunnel S. *Surgery of the hand.* Philadelphia: JB Lippincott Co, 1944.

43. Bruner JM. Tendon transfer to restore abduction of the index finger using the extensor pollicis brevis. *Plast Reconstr Surg* 1948;3:197–201.

44. Hirayama T, Atsuta Y, Takemitsu Y. Palmaris longus transfer for replacement of the first dorsal interosseous. *J Hand Surg [Br]* 1986;11:84–86.

45. Mikhail IK. Bone block operation for clawhand. *Surg Gynecol Obstet* 1964;118:1077–1079.

46. Bunnell S. Surgery of the intrinsic muscles of the hand other than those producing opposition of the thumb. *J Bone Joint Surg* 1942;24:1.

47. Zancolli EA. Claw hand caused by paralysis of the intrinsic muscles. A simple surgical procedure for its correction. *J Bone Joint Surg Am* 1957;39:1076–1080.

48. Leddy JP, Stark HH, Ashworth CR, et al. Capsulodesis and pulley advancement for the correction of claw-finger deformity. *J Bone Joint Surg Am* 1972;54:1465–1471.

49. Brown PW. Zancolli capsulorrhaphy for ulnar claw hand. *J Bone Joint Surg Am* 1970;52:868–877.

50. Zancolli EA. Claw hand caused by paralysis of the intrinsic muscles: a simple surgical procedure for its correction. *J Bone Joint Surg Am* 1957;37:1076.

51. Riordan DC. Intrinsic paralysis of the hand. *Bull Hosp Jt Dis Orthop Inst* 1984;44:435–441.

52. Riordan DC. Rehabilitation and re-education in tendon transfers. *Orthop Clin North Am* 1974;5:445–449.

53. Brandsma JW, Brand PW. Claw-finger correction. Considerations in choice of technique. *J Hand Surg [Br]* 1992;17:615–621.

54. Riordan DC. Tendon transplantation in median nerve and ulnar nerve paralysis. *J Bone Joint Surg Am* 1953;35:312.

55. Stiles HJ, Forreseter-Brown MF. *Treatment of injuries of the spinal peripheral nerves.* London: Fronde & Hodder-Stoughton, 1922:166.

56. Brand PW. Biomechanics of tendon transfers. *Hand Clin* 1988;4:137–154.

57. Brand PW, Beach RB, Thompson DE. Relative tension and potential excursion of muscles in the forearm and hand. *J Hand Surg [Am]* 1981;6:209–219.

58. Brand PW. Paralytic claw hand. *J Bone Joint Surg Br* 1958;40:618.

59. Parkes A. Paralytic claw fingers—a graft tenodesis operation. *Hand* 1973;5:192.

60. Smith RJ. Metacarpal ligament sling tenodesis. *Bull Hosp Jt Dis* 1984;44:466.

61. Brooks AL. A new intrinsic tendon transfer for the paralytic hand. *J Bone Joint Surg Am* 1975;57:730.

62. Hastings H 2nd, McCollam SM. Flexor digitorum superficialis lasso tendon transfer in isolated ulnar nerve palsy: a functional evaluation. *J Hand Surg [Am]* 199419:275–280.

63. Brandsma JW, Ottenhoff-De Jonge MW. Flexor digitorum superficialis tendon transfer for intrinsic replacement. Long-term results and the effect on donor fingers. *J Hand Surg [Br]* 1992;17:625–628.

64. Shah A. Correction of ulnar claw hand by a loop of flexor digitorum superficialis motor for lumbrical replacement. *J Hand Surg [Br]* 1984;9:131–133.

65. Enna CD, Riordan DC. The Fowler procedure for correction of the paralytic claw hand. *Plast Reconstr Surg* 1973;52:352–360.

66. Burkhalter WE, Carneiro RS. Correction of the attritional boutonniere deformity in high ulnar-nerve paralysis. *J Bone Joint Surg Am* 1979;61:131–134.

67. Anita NH. The palmaris longus motor for lumbrical replacement. *Hand* 1969;2:139.

68. Burge P. Abducted little finger in low ulnar nerve palsy. *J Hand Surg [Br]* 1986;11:234–236.

69. Bellan N, Belkhiria F, Touam C, et al. Extensor digiti minimi tendon "rerouting" transfer in permanent abduction of the little finger. *Chir Main* 1998;17:325–333.

70. Voche P, Merle M. Wartenberg's sign. A new method of surgical correction. *J Hand Surg [Br]* 1995;20:49–52.

71. Hoch J. Correction of post-traumatic adduction insufficiency of the small finger by transposition of the tendon of the extensor indicis muscle. *Handchir Mikrochir Plast Chir* 1993;25:179–183.

72. Dellon AL. Extensor digiti minimi tendon transfer to correct abducted small finger in ulnar dysfunction. *J Hand Surg [Am]* 1991;16:819–823.

73. Goloborod'ko SA, Andruson MV, Goridova LD. Method of correcting abduction of the 5th finger after injuries to the ulnar nerve. *Ortop Travmatol Protez* 1985;11:48–50.

74. Blacker GJ, Lister GD, Kleinert HE. The abducted little finger in low ulnar nerve palsy. *J Hand Surg [Am]* 1976;1:190–196.

75. Burge P. Abducted little finger in low ulnar nerve palsy. *J Hand Surg [Br]* 1986;11:234–236.

76. Gonzalez MH, Gray T, Ortinau E, et al. The extensor tendons to the little finger: an anatomic study. *J Hand Surg [Am]* 1995;20:844–847.

77. Fowler SB. Extensor apparatus of digits. *J Bone Joint Surg Br* 1949;31:477.

56

RECONSTRUCTION FOR COMBINED NERVE PALSY

MATTHEW M. TOMAINO

Reconstruction after isolated injury to the radial, median, or ulnar nerve, although challenging, is not only possible but successful. Indeed, Chapters 52 through 54 detail decision-making principles and reconstructive options for treating isolated nerve palsy. Reconstruction for combined nerve palsy, by contrast, is far more challenging because functional impairment is more severe and treatment options are more limited.

By definition, the treatment of palsy suggests that irreversible end-organ muscle atrophy has occurred; hence, only tendon transfers or muscle transplantation exist as options to restore lost function. When expendable donor tendons are not available, unstable intercalary joints may require arthrodesis, or, alternatively, digital motion may be restored by tenodesis. Regrettably, but for the seminal contributions that Dr. George Omer has made to the current literature that addresses the treatment of combined nerve palsy—in large part a reflection of his tremendous personal experience with these problems—there is neither a template for guidance nor abundant options for treatment (1–3).

In that light, patients with combined nerve palsy require our most conscientious attention and creative effort. Indeed, the art and the science of reconstructive hand surgery must be called on. Our surgical game plan must begin with appropriate preoperative assessment and planning and must include not only precise execution, but also appropriate postoperative follow-up.

In this chapter, I do not recapitulate what is known about each individual nerve palsy, as that has been addressed already in Chapters 52 through 54. Rather, my objective in this chapter is to assemble certain fundamental and relevant principles from the literature, which address not only individual peripheral nerve palsies, but also brachial plexus injury and tetraplegia, and to provide a framework that facilitates the potentially difficult navigation through these issues.

PREOPERATIVE EVALUATION AND PLANNING

The goal of reconstruction is function. Having stated the obvious, admittedly, when a patient is left with little func-

tion, even small improvements may be of tremendous value. Accordingly, preoperative assessment must involve conscientious discussion with the patient about expectations. With that as a springboard, physical examination must identify deficit and retained function, and then a list must be developed of potential donors for tendon transfer, which might be used to restore desired function (1). Obviously, fixed contracture, whether it be of individual fingers, the wrist, or the hand, must be prevented and treated, if present at the time of initial presentation. The most successfully executed tendon transfer is not functional if joint mobility is insufficient. If a contracture is not amenable to nonoperative treatment or surgical release, then, sadly, reconstruction of combined nerve palsy may not be advisable.

When first meeting the patient, it is critical to ensure that shoulder and elbow range of motion is adequate to allow the hand to be positioned in space. Before taking inventory—establishing what muscle and tendon function still exists and what has been lost—passive motion of the wrist in the sagittal plane and its effect on the fingers via tenodesis should be assessed. Indeed, at the very least, gravity-assisted wrist flexion, extensor tenodesis, tendon transfer to restore wrist extension, and tendon transfer to extrinsic flexors or flexor tenodesis, for example, may result in a modicum of grasp and simple hand grip (key pinch), as has been described by Moberg (4,5).

If sensation is absent because of median nerve palsy, it must be noted. This sensory deficit, in particular, is perhaps the most devastating to overall hand function, and, yet, visual cues or hearing may substitute if motion can be restored (6). In that light, Omer has emphasized that procedures to restore motor function should be done before procedures to improve sensibility because precise sensibility requires precise motion (1–3), and precise motion requires a favorable soft tissue milieu. Because combined palsy usually results from explosive devices, such as firearms or firecrackers, or mechanical injuries at the workplace, circulation may be impaired and soft tissue fibrosis may result. A favorable soft tissue environment must be restored to ensure that tendon excursion after transfer is satisfactory. In that light, soft tissue augmentation or replacement with free transfer or pedicled tissue rotation may be a wise first stage in the overall reconstruction of combined nerve palsy.

SURGICAL MANAGEMENT

Review of the literature provides few data regarding the results that we might expect after reconstruction of combined palsy. As I have mentioned, quite unlike most other problems in the field of hand and upper extremity surgery, each patient presents a unique challenge. A reconstructive plan ought to be kept simple—one transfer to restore one function—to minimize the need for retraining and the execution of unnecessary surgical procedures with little potential for successful outcome.

When expendable donor muscle–tendon units are available, *tendon transfers* can be performed to eliminate deforming forces that are secondary to imbalance and to replace singular functions, including grasp, pinch, and release. *Tissue transplantation*, free and pedicled, has as its role primarily to restore finger extension or flexion or for the purpose of soft tissue augmentation or replacement. *Nerve transfers* constitute an evolving area within the field of research and clinical care (7). Their role in the reconstruction of combined palsy revolves primarily around sensory reinnervation and reflects the observation that the sensory end-organ is potentially reinnervated long after the peripheral nerve injury. This contrasts markedly with the irreversible atrophy and fatty infiltration that begin to develop after just a few weeks after denervation of a target end-organ that is muscle. *Arthrodesis* may be advisable when a major intercalary joint, such as the wrist, requires stabilization to augment the delivery of power and motion to the fingers. Wrist motion is valuable, however, because tenodesis that accompanies wrist extension and flexion can be used to fuel finger flexion and extension, respectively. Indeed, when precious few donor muscle–tendon units are available for use in tendon transfer, tenodesis may provide a helpful, albeit rudimentary, grasp, release, and pinch. In that light, arthrodesis should be selected as a last resort in most cases.

In the remainder of this chapter, I describe the fundamental functional imperatives to consider while developing a reconstructive plan for different combinations of nerve palsy, including (a) low and (b) high median-ulnar nerve palsy, (c) high median-radial and (d) high ulnar-radial nerve palsy, and, last, (e) high combined radial-median-ulnar nerve palsy. A plethora of alternatives exist for the treatment of each individual palsy; comprehensive discussions for each can be found in Chapters 52 through 54. I also provide a recommended approach to treatment.

Low Median-Ulnar Nerve Palsy

This is the most common combined nerve palsy and reflects how vulnerable our forearms are in a mechanized

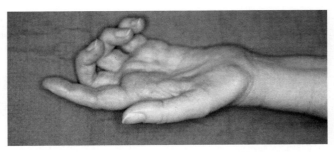

FIGURE 1. Low median-ulnar nerve palsy results in intrinsic paralysis and claw finger deformities. This photograph demonstrates hyperextension deformities of the metacarpophalangeal joints that are secondary to intrinsic paralysis and thenar atrophy, which impairs out-of-plane thumb motion.

work place. Complete loss of palmar sensation and intrinsic motor muscles produces an almost useless claw hand (Fig. 1). Median intrinsic paralysis results in absent thumb opposition—its ability to be drawn out of the plane of the palm, preparatory to grasp. Ulnar intrinsic paralysis results in loss of power pinch (normally afforded by the deep head of the flexor pollicis brevis and the adductor pollicis muscle) and synchronous finger flexion.

Reconstruction of the thumb is extremely important because its contribution to prehension and overall hand function is critical. Hence, special effort must be made to prevent or correct adduction contracture of the thumb–index web (8,9). Although flattening of the transverse palmar metacarpal arch and abduction of the fifth finger accompany low ulnar nerve palsy, their reconstruction, in particular, is not tremendously important to the restoration of overall hand function. The basic requirements include (a) improved key pinch that is provided by stronger adduction of the thumb, (b) restored thumb abduction for opposition, (c) strengthened resistance of the index finger during pinch by restoration of power in the first dorsal interosseous tendon, (d) improved power flexion of the proximal phalanges and metacarpophalangeal joints, and (e) sensory restoration in the distribution that is involved with key or tip pinch.

In the spirit of keeping reconstruction simple, it is not necessarily advisable to restore thumb opposition and adduction, even if donor tendons exist. In the final analysis, neither motion may return as ideally as it would if only one tendon transfer had been performed. In light of the fact that opposition is indeed palmar, abduction and pronation—both of which prepare the thumb for grasp by bringing it out of the plane of the palm—reconstruction should, in my opinion, prioritize power pinch. If the pulley around which the tendon transfer is directed lies within the mid-palm, as it does for the flexor digitorum superficialis (FDS) (10) and the extensor carpi radialis brevis (ECRB) (11) pinch-plasties, then the distal connection can be moved slightly radially, if not all the way to the radial aspect of the

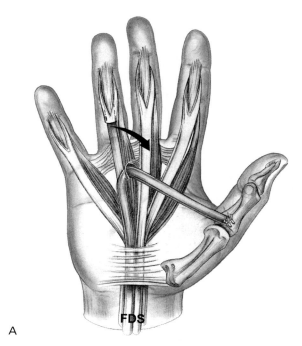

A

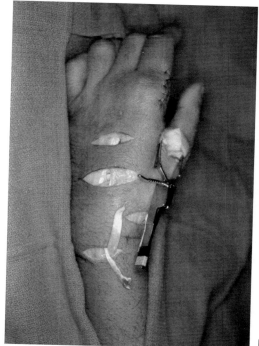

B

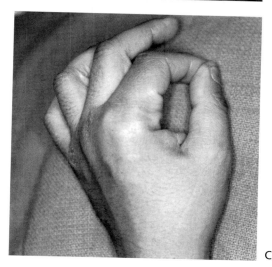

C

FIGURE 2. A: Ring- or long-finger flexor digitorum superficialis (FDS) transfer to the abductor tubercle of the thumb by using the palmar fascia as a pulley restores effective key pinch. **B,C:** Transfer of the extensor carpi radialis brevis, which is extended with a free-tendon graft through the interspace between the third and fourth metacarpals and across the palm volar to the adductor pollicis and dorsal to the finger flexor tendons and neurovascular structures, doubles preoperative key-pinch strength.

thumb, to provide metacarpal pronation, as well as to augment key pinch (Fig. 2). In this situation, I make a volar, rather than ulnar, Brunner incision on the thumb and pass the tendon volar to the flexor sheath. The tendon is woven into the abductor pollicis brevis tendon or attached directly to the radial base of the proximal phalanx itself. Alternatively, the extensor indicis proprius tendon can be used as an opponens transfer, if it appears as though prehension is compromised by inadequate palmar abduction (12).

For low median-ulnar nerve palsy, the radial nerve innervated muscle–tendon units are available for transfer. I prefer Smith's ECRB transfer technique with a free graft between the third and fourth metacarpals to the *abductor*

tubercle of the thumb to restore key pinch and augment opposition (11). Palmaris or plantaris graft can be used. The average key-pinch strength can be doubled by this operation. A tendon graft that is extended from a terminal slip of the abductor pollicis longus tendon—preferably the digastric tendon, as it inserts on the thenar musculature—can be extended subcutaneously to the terminal first dorsal interosseous tendon to augment index finger resistance to pinch from the thumb (13). When claw deformities are mild or include only the ulnar two digits, a Zancolli lasso procedure that using the flexor digitorum sublimis tendons is recommended (14–17) (Fig. 3). If clawing involves all of the fingers, or if improvement in

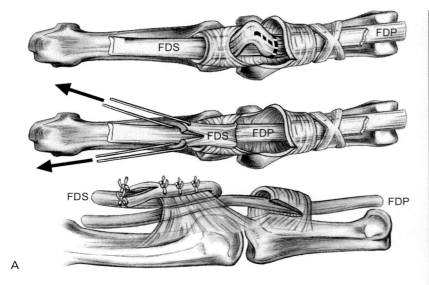

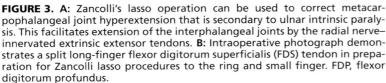

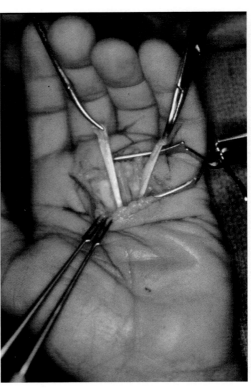

FIGURE 3. A: Zancolli's lasso operation can be used to correct metacarpophalangeal joint hyperextension that is secondary to ulnar intrinsic paralysis. This facilitates extension of the interphalangeal joints by the radial nerve–innervated extrinsic extensor tendons. **B:** Intraoperative photograph demonstrates a split long-finger flexor digitorum superficialis (FDS) tendon in preparation for Zancolli lasso procedures to the ring and small finger. FDP, flexor digitorum profundus.

power grip is needed based on a preoperative assessment that indicates suboptimal grip, a stronger dynamic transfer is more satisfactory. In this case, Brand's extensor carpi radialis longus (ECRL) transfer technique, which uses a four-tailed free graft that is placed between the second and third metacarpals and fourth and fifth metacarpals, is recommended (15,18); however, this necessitates the selection of an alternative pinch-plasty because the ECRB must be retained to provide wrist extension (Fig. 4). In this circumstance, ring- or long-finger FDS pinch-plasty is recommended (10).

Although the sensory deficit that accompanies low median-ulnar nerve palsy results in an anesthetic prehensile surface, visual cueing may nevertheless allow useful function. I have no personal experience with radial-innervated neurovascular-pedicled flap transfer from the proximal index-finger dorsum to the volar thumb tip, but, in unusual circumstances, it may be feasible (19) (Fig. 5). Transfer of the radial sensory nerve to the first common digital, however, might provide sensation to the ulnar aspect of the thumb tip and to the radial aspect of the index finger (20). Indeed, nerve transfer may provide the most reasonable option for sensory reinnervation in this setting, if it is absolutely necessary. Although more proximal donor sources of sensory nerve have been described for median nerve reinnervation in the setting of brachial plexus palsy, including contralateral C7 transfer, these hardly seem advisable in the setting of low palsy and normal eye–hand interaction (21,22).

High Median-Ulnar Nerve Palsy

High median-ulnar nerve palsy is a devastating injury because distance alone from the intrinsic muscles in the hand prohibits reinnervation in most cases, even when acute repair has been performed. Atrophy of the finger pulps discourages power and precise grip, and associated injury to the proximal forearm may weaken or compromise elbow flexion (Fig. 6). In addition to the deficits that accompany low median-ulnar nerve palsy, more proximal injury compromises wrist flexion and finger flexion. These patients bear remarkable similarity to group 3 tetraplegia patients, who have functional brachioradialis (BR) and wrist extensors only (4). In that light, in addition to the reconstructive priorities that were noted previously, finger flexion must be restored if there is any hope for functional grasp. It is unusual to provide a transfer for wrist flexion, however, because the effects of gravity suffice. The ECRL transfer can be used to restore extrinsic finger flexion, and its efficacy has been shown primarily in the setting of Volkmann's ischemic contracture (23) (Fig. 7). Intrinsic balancing, however, augments the extrinsic transfer and is recommended overwhelmingly, in that light (24). BR pinch-plasty is recommended to improve key pinch; mov-

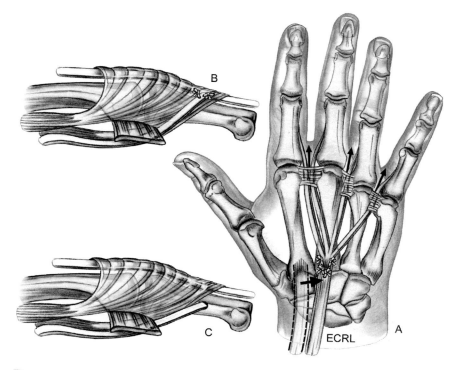

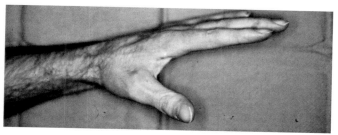

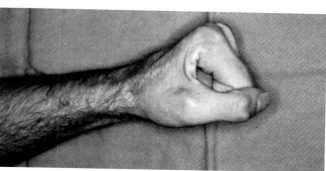

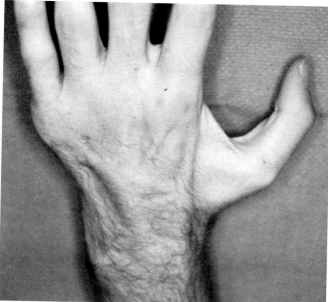

FIGURE 4. Power flexion of the proximal phalanx can be obtained by using an extensor carpi radialis longus (ECRL) transfer that is extended with a free-graft split into four tails **(A)**. The tendon slips are passed volar to the deep transverse metacarpal ligament and transferred into the lateral bands of the dorsal apparatus **(B)** or the bone of the proximal phalanx **(C)**. My preference is the former, and, if I choose not to have the transfer affect proximal interphalangeal joint extension, I divide the wing tendon distal to my transfer. **D:** Postoperative photograph demonstrates the ECRL tendon on the dorsum of the hand. **E:** Correction of clawing has resulted, and **(F)** synchronous metacarpophalangeal flexion is possible, with improved grip strength.

ing its insertion more radially on the thumb promotes thumb opposition, as well (Fig. 8). If longitudinal collapse of the thumb is present, metacarpophalangeal (MCP) capsulodesis and interphalangeal fusion may be required. Zancolli lasso procedures, which use flexor digitorum sublimis for each finger, are probably the simplest way of balancing the intrinsics and correcting the claw deformities (14,16), but extensor indicis proprius or minimi muscle–tendon units, or both, are also potential donors, even though their action is not synergistic with MCP flexion.

When the BR muscle is used to augment key pinch, it is no longer available as a transfer to the flexor pollicis longus (FPL) tendon. In such cases, FPL tenodesis is an option, particularly because wrist extension is retained, unless thumb interphalangeal joint arthrodesis is elected (4,14). If the ECRL transfer is not elected to provide finger flexion—perhaps because key pinch is prioritized in a particular patient—and the ECRB is selected for pinchplasty, pedicled latissimus transfer may provide functional finger flexion (25,26). This transfer is more successful,

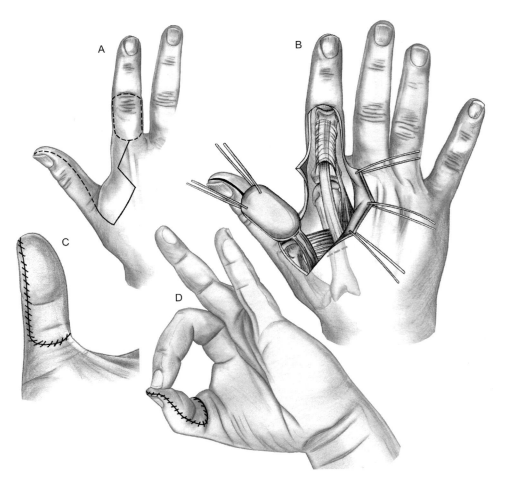

FIGURE 5. **A:** Incisions for a radial-innervated neurovascular-pedicled flap on the first dorsal metacarpal surface of the index finger between the metacarpophalangeal and proximal interphalangeal joints. **B:** Completed dissection of the first dorsal metacarpal artery neurovascular island flap. The flap is elevated with the neurovascular pedicle. **C:** The flap in place on the ulnar–palmar surface of the thumb. **D:** Superficial radial-innervated pinch can be obtained.

however, when it is used to restore finger extension. When the ECRL is selected to restore finger flexion, and the ECRB is selected for key pinch, wrist arthrodesis is necessary. This may reflect the most practical alternative, and, for that reason, it is my recommendation. In this case, BR can be transferred to the FPL, or, if an intercalary collapse deformity is present in the thumb, MCP joint capsulodesis and interphalangeal joint fusion can be performed. Zancolli's two-stage reconstruction for the group 3 tetraplegic patient is worth reviewing, except that digital extension is retained and extensor tenodesis is unnecessary (4,14).

In high median-ulnar nerve palsy, sensibility can be transferred to the distal thumb tip by using a radial-innervated neurovascular flap from the dorsum of the index finger, as was mentioned previously (19). In addition, the distribution of the radial sensory nerve along the index finger dorsum can be used to resurface a broad web between the thumb and long finger, if index ray resection is performed (Fig. 9). Protective sensibility within the new thumb–long finger web may be of benefit in such activities as holding a steering wheel (27,28). Although more heroic attempts at reinnervating the median sensory distribution in the hand have been mentioned (21,22), in reality, there are probably few indications.

High Ulnar-Radial Nerve Palsy

High ulnar-radial nerve palsy is arguably less common than median-ulnar palsy, but more common than median-radial palsy, which is a reflection of ulnar and radial nerve vulnerability to posterior zones of injury. Indeed, the radial

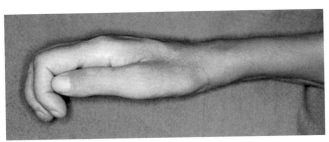

FIGURE 6. Photograph of a hand of a patient with high median-ulnar nerve palsy. Intrinsic and extrinsic paralysis results in impaired pinch and grasp.

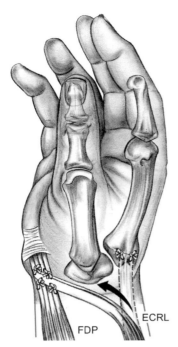

FIGURE 7. Transfer of the extensor carpi radialis longus (ECRL) tendon around the radial aspect of the forearm to the tendons of the flexor digitorum profundus (FDP) results in restoration of finger flexion. Wrist extension augments finger flexion via a tenodesis effect.

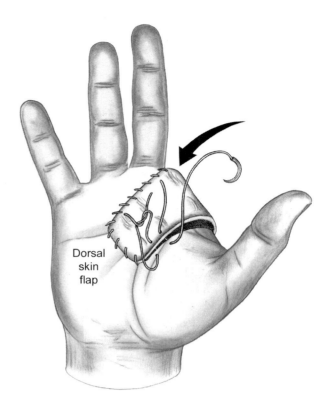

FIGURE 9. A radial-innervated dorsal skin flap can be harvested after index ray amputation to replace insensitive palmar skin with radial-innervated skin in the setting of high median-ulnar nerve palsy.

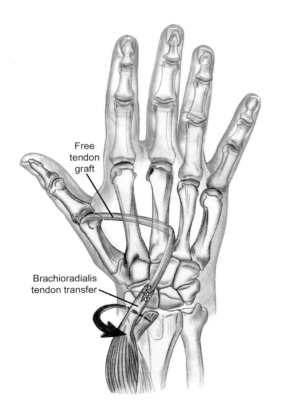

FIGURE 8. Transfer of the brachioradialis, which is extended with a free-tendon graft through the interspace between the third and fourth metacarpals and across the palm volar to the adductor pollicis and dorsal to the finger flexor tendons and neurovascular structures, provides effective key pinch.

and ulnar nerves are relatively posterior at the mid-humeral level. Functional deficits include wrist and finger extension, ring- and small-finger flexion, and ulnar intrinsics. Because median nerve distribution sensibility is retained, intrinsic balancing, correction of claw deformity, and improvement in key-pinch strength can tremendously enhance overall hand function. Median nerve–innervated pronated teres, flexor carpi radialis, FPL, and index- and long-finger flexor digitorum profundus (FDP) ensure, even before reconstruction, at least rudimentary pinch and grasp. Although the absence of active finger extension does not necessarily compromise hand function (29), the inability to extend the wrist leaves the hand in a functionally challenged position and lessens the magnitude of grip strength. This deficit is further compounded by the absence of the synchronous finger flexion that accompanies the intrinsic minus claw deformity.

In that light, restoration of wrist extension and intrinsic replacement constitute the reconstructive priorities for high ulnar-radial nerve palsy. Transfer of the pronator teres to the ECRB is recommended and, for isolated radial nerve palsy, constitutes an extremely successful and reliable transfer (30). Elevation of the periosteal extension of the tendon insertion ensures that length is adequate enough to allow a

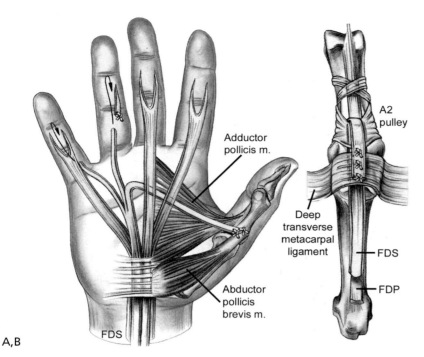

A,B

FIGURE 10. In the setting of high ulnar-radial nerve palsy, augmentation of key pinch and correction of ring- and small-finger clawing are achieved by using the long- or ring-finger flexor digitorum superficialis (FDS) tendon as a split transfer. **A:** One-half of the tendon is transferred to the adductor tubercle, and **(B)** the other half is split into two slips, which are used to perform a Zancolli lasso procedure. The illustration shows the tendons looped around the second annular (A2) pulley, but as is shown in Figure 3, they can be looped over the first annular pulley as well. If all of the fingers are clawed, an alternative median-innervated motor is selected (such as the flexor carpi radialis), and a four-tailed graft can be passed through the carpal canal, or the tendon can be transferred dorsally, and the grafts can be passed through the metacarpal interspaces, as was described in Figure 4. FDP, flexor digitorum profundus; m., muscle.

secure Pulvertaft weave. Augmentation of key pinch and correction of ring- and small-finger clawing are achieved by using the long-finger FDS as a split transfer (Fig. 10). One-half of the tendon is separated into two slips, which are inserted into the flexor sheaths at the level of the first or second annular pulleys (16); the other is passed dorsal to the index flexor sheath, which is on the volar surface of the adductor pollicis muscle, to its insertion at the adductor tubercle of the thumb proximal phalanx (10). Although finger and thumb extension can be restored with the use of ring finger FDS (31), a transfer that was popularized in the rheumatoid patient with multiple extensor ruptures and in isolated radial nerve palsy, this is not advised in the setting of high ulnar-radial palsy, particularly when the long finger FDS is used to restore intrinsic function, as was mentioned previously. Finger and thumb extension lag may not tremendously compromise grasp (29); hence, reconstruction is not always necessary. Two other options exist, nevertheless. First, attachment of the extensor pollicis longus and extensor digitorum communis to the dorsum of the radius can result in functional extension via the tenodesis effect that is afforded by wrist flexion (14). Alternatively, pedicled latissimus dorsi muscle transfer can be used to augment finger extension (25,26). Understandably, it is imperative that full passive extension is present before proceeding with any attempt at restoring finger extension via tendon transfer or tenodesis.

Ring- and small-finger flexion is most easily restored by establishing a side-to-side connection proximal to the wrist with the innervated index- and long-finger flexor digitorum profundus tendons (Fig. 11). Occasionally, the anterior interosseous nerve does not innervate the long-finger FDP muscle. In these cases long-, ring-, and small-finger flexion may not be present, and transfer of these to the intact index finger FDP provides weak and incomplete digital flexion. In this circumstance, I recommend extensor tenodesis (14) and the use of a pedicled latissimus transfer to augment active digital flexion (25,26). I stage this procedure, however, to allow sequential assessment after an initial attempt at restoration of flexion with a side-to-side transfer of the index FDP tendon to the long-, ring-, and small-finger profundus tendons. Although free gracilis or latissimus muscle transplantation is an option for augmenting finger flexion, as has been popularized in the treatment of Volkmann's contracture when tendon transfers are not feasible (32), pedicled transfer obviates the need for microsurgery and nerve regeneration. If a pedicled transfer does not reach, however, neurotization of transplanted muscle is performed by using identifiable branches of the median nerve into the FPL tendon (33). In this case, thumb interphalangeal joint Kirschner wire stabilization or fusion are options.

Nerve transfer provides a valuable option for innervating the ulnar border of the fifth and fourth fingers, if numbness in this region results in functional impairment (34). As has been mentioned, transfers for motor function should precede procedures that are directed at the restoration of sensation because the latter may not be elected by the patient. The third common digital nerve component of the median nerve can be divided distally, leaving the web between the long- and ring-finger anesthetic, and transferred to the common digital nerve that supplies adjacent surfaces of the ring and small finger or to the ulnar

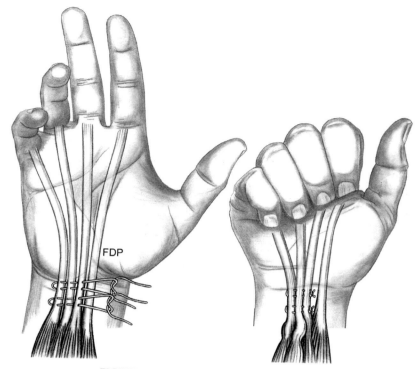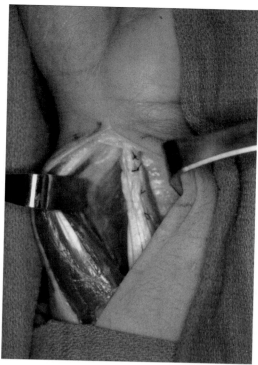

A

B

FIGURE 11. A,B: Ring- and small-finger flexion is most easily restored by establishing side-to-side transfer to the innervated long- and index-finger flexor digitorum profundus (FDP) tendons proximal to the wrist.

digital nerve to the small finger only. In that light, distal double median-to-ulnar nerve transfer has been described in the reconstruction of isolated high ulnar nerve lesions (35). The anterior interosseous nerve may be transferred to the deep motor branch of the ulnar nerve without intercalary nerve graft to restore ulnar-innervated intrinsic function, but this is not recommended if palsy has exceeded 6 months because of irreversible muscle atrophy. The palmar sensory branch of the median nerve has been transferred to the sensory component of the ulnar nerve at the Guyon's canal level with good success. I prefer not to do either of these transfers in the setting of established nerve palsy, but I would entertain the transfer of the third common digital (median) nerve to provide ulnar sensation, if the patient requested it.

High Median-Radial Nerve Palsy

High median-radial nerve palsy is unusual and reflects an injury that, more likely than not, originates laterally and stops just short of the ulnar nerve. As with isolated low median nerve palsy, its most devastating impact lies in the resulting lack of sensibility over the prehensile surfaces of the thumb, index, and long fingers. Nevertheless, reconstruction is advisable, given the preservation of ulnar intrinsic function and at least a modicum of retained key-pinch strength from the deep head of the flexor pollicis brevis and

the adductor pollicis muscles. Wrist flexion is retained because of an innervated flexor carpi ulnaris, but only ring- and small-finger extrinsic flexion is possible. Neither wrist nor finger extension function is retained.

Thumb-index web contracture may need to be corrected before opponensplasty (8,9), but given the retention of key-pinch muscles, a transfer to bring the thumb out of the plane of the palm is advisable, so long as fixed contracture can be managed. Reconstructive priorities also include finger extension and wrist extension or stabilization via arthrodesis.

Because the initial injury may compromise elbow range of motion, it is imperative that the status of the triceps and biceps be assessed; a functional and pain-free elbow range of motion is essential. Indeed, the ultimate salvage for this combined palsy is forearm-level amputation and prosthetic fitting.

Index- and long-finger FDP tendons are sutured side-to-side to the ulnar-innervated ring- and small-finger tendons that are proximal to the wrist, and transfer of the abductor digiti quinti provides time-honored functional opposition for the thumb (36) (Fig. 12). Although Omer has suggested that wrist arthrodesis is indicated in cases of high median-radial nerve palsy (1), this approach negates the potential role of tenodesis for providing finger extension. Indeed, finger extension need only be sufficient enough to allow release, and its strength must overcome only gravity. In that light, pedicled latissimus transfer can be used to restore antigravity wrist extension and to augment grip strength (25,26); retain-

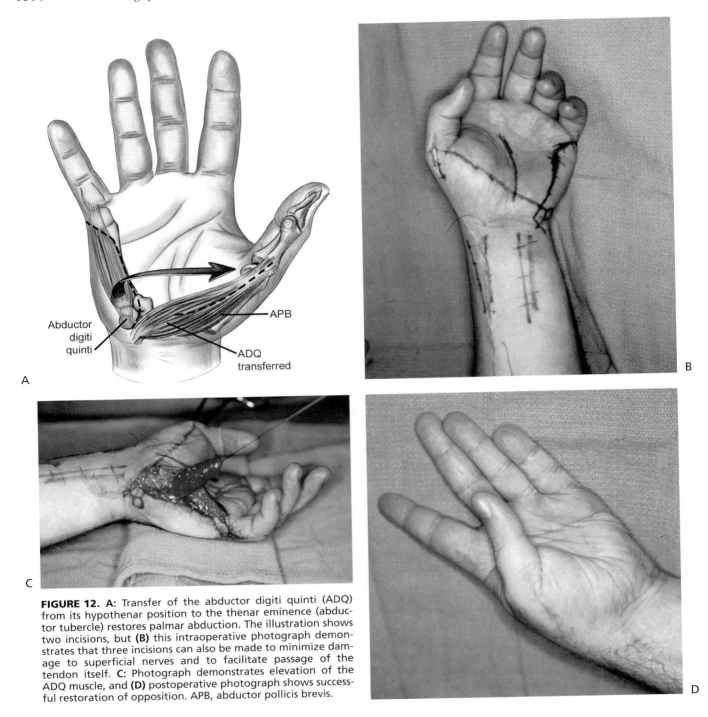

FIGURE 12. A: Transfer of the abductor digiti quinti (ADQ) from its hypothenar position to the thenar eminence (abductor tubercle) restores palmar abduction. The illustration shows two incisions, but **(B)** this intraoperative photograph demonstrates that three incisions can also be made to minimize damage to superficial nerves and to facilitate passage of the tendon itself. **C:** Photograph demonstrates elevation of the ADQ muscle, and **(D)** postoperative photograph shows successful restoration of opposition. APB, abductor pollicis brevis.

ing wrist motion allows wrist flexion to provide finger extension via tenodesis. Alternatively, wrist fusion can be performed, and, if elected by the patient, latissimus transfer can be used to restore finger extension. Generally, the ring- and small-finger profundus provide effective excursion for the index and long fingers after side-to-side transfer, but a stable wrist in slight extension is critical.

My recommendation is to perform wrist arthrodesis in slight extension. In this case, metacarpophalangeal joint extension lags are accepted (29), or latissimus transfer can be used (25,26). Borrowing from the brachial plexus literature, Oberlin's transfer technique (37), which uses the fascicular innervation to the flexor carpi ulnaris (now unnecessary, because the wrist has been fused), can be used to innervate free-muscle transplantation, if pedicled transfer does not reach. This approach results in functional grasp and release and a stable wrist to allow optimal transfer of power distally.

Radial innervated cutaneous transfers are not an option in high median-radial palsy, and median nerve anesthesia may be managed best by visual cueing during prehension. Nevertheless, contralateral C7 transfer is an option, among others that were mentioned previously (21,22), although it is not suggested for this palsy because of the lack of availability of a lengthy, vascularized, ulnar nerve graft. Alternatively, neural anatomy to the fourth-fifth finger web may allow translocation to the common digital nerve, which innervates the ulnar aspect of the thumb and the radial aspect of the index finger and is present 69% of the time (38). However, I do not recommend nerve translocation if it risks leaving the ulnar aspect of the small finger without sensibility.

High Radial-Median-Ulnar Nerve Palsy

Although unusual, combined injury to radial, median, and ulnar nerves at the level of the elbow are possible and devastating. Reconstruction in these cases resembles the complexity and challenge of above-elbow replantation, in which, admittedly, the priority is often to restore a functioning and still-innervated elbow joint. For this combined palsy, prosthetic fitting is clearly an advisable option, and reconstructive priorities should be directed, first and foremost, at restoring functional elbow range of motion. That having been said, there are fundamental reconstructive options that may provide rudimentary hand function and may obviate the need for prosthetic fitting. Indeed, patients may be reluctant to undergo hand amputation.

These options include the provision of a stable wrist via arthrodesis, the use of a pedicled latissimus transfer to provide finger extension (25,26), and the use of a free-muscle transplantation, which is innervated by the median nerve above the elbow, to provide finger flexion (32,33). It is virtually impossible to restore thumb-to-index prehension, however, and complete lack of sensibility in the hand renders these heroic attempts ill-advised, in my opinion, despite their ostensible feasibility. For cases in which some BR function is retained, however, this muscle tendon unit may be used to provide wrist extension, as is often performed in tetraplegia (4). In these cases, gravity-assisted wrist flexion provides finger extension, if extensor tenodesis is performed (14), and a Moberg simple hand-grip (key-pinch) procedure might provide rudimentary pinch (4,14), if pedicled latissimus transfer is performed to provide wrist extension (Fig. 13). If tendon length is a problem, it could be woven into the BR muscle as a so-called conduit, and the BR tendon could then be transferred to the ECRB more distally. Doi et al. (39) have underscored the importance of adequate triceps strength in cases in which a free transfer passes the elbow to prevent unwanted elbow flexion from compromising extension of the more distal joint.

Because these authors applied these techniques to brachial plexus patients with complete avulsion, the objectives of their

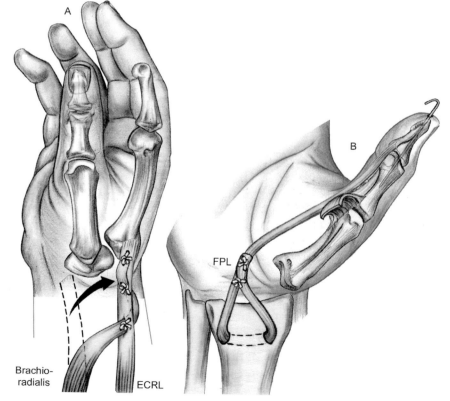

FIGURE 13. A Moberg simple hand-grip (key-pinch) procedure provides rudimentary pinch. **A:** If the brachioradialis is innervated, it can be used to augment wrist extension. If it is not innervated, pedicled latissimus muscle transfer is a potential option. **B:** Interphalangeal stabilization, first annular pulley release, and flexor pollicis longus (FPL) tenodesis result in key pinch when the wrist is extended. ECRL, extensor carpi radialis longus.

first-stage transfer were elbow flexion and digital extension. Therefore, they recommended that the tendon be passed beneath the BR muscle, so that it functioned as a pulley (40). In cases of combined high radial-median-ulnar palsy, this is not necessary, because elbow flexion is present. Although some bowstringing occurs when the elbow is flexed, the risk of tendon adherence is minimized, in my opinion, if the transfer is not passed deep to the BR. As I mentioned, the simplest route might be to weave the latissimus tendon into the BR and transfer its tendon to the ECRB. All this might appear as a so-called long run for a short slide, and if a patient refuses amputation and prosthetic fitting, another alternative might be an externally powered wrist-driven flexor hinge, as is used in the group 0 tetraplegia patient (4).

CONCLUSION

In contrast to the reconstruction of isolated peripheral nerve palsy, in which a number of useful alternative tendon transfers exists, combined palsy challenges even the most innovative of hand surgeons. Although tremendously intimidating at first glance, the development of a reconstructive plan becomes less daunting a task if the surgeon performs an accurate physical examination and develops an inventory of expendable tendon units. The reconstructive plan must be kept simple and practical. Patient motivation, willingness to accept surgery, and appropriate expectations for functional return are integral to overall satisfaction from the patient's perspective and the surgeon's.

Priorities must be established, including grasp and key pinch, and motor transfers should be performed before procedures to improve sensibility. When tendon transfers are not available, the surgeon should familiarize himself or herself with the principles that are involved in reconstruction of the tetraplegic extremity (4,14), in which cases the combinations of arthrodesis and tenodesis may provide at least some ability to perform prehensile functions. The specific details of these operative procedures can be found elsewhere in this text. The impairments with which our patients present and their willingness to endure a reconstructive plan provide for an unparalleled opportunity to be surgeon and artist, and, because of the infrequency of dealing with these devastating injuries, our honest assessment of outcome must be used to guide our future decision making and selection of treatment options.

REFERENCES

1. Omer GE Jr. Combined nerve palsies. In: Green DP, ed. *Operative hand surgery*, 3rd ed. New York: Churchill Livingstone, 1993:1467–1482.
2. Omer GE Jr. Tendon transfers for combined nerve injuries. In: Gelberman RH, ed. *Operative nerve repair and reconstruction*. Philadelphia: JB Lippincott Co, 1991:747–762.
3. Omer GE Jr. Reconstruction of the forearm and hand after peripheral nerve injuries. In: Omer GE, Spinner M, Van Beek AL, eds. *Management of peripheral nerve problems*, 2nd ed. Philadelphia: WB Saunders, 1998:675–705.
4. McDowell CH. Tetraplegia. In: Green DP, ed. *Operative hand surgery*, 3rd ed. New York: Churchill Livingstone, 1993:1517–1532.
5. Moberg E. Surgical treatment for absent single-hand grip and elbow extension in quadriplegia. *J Bone Joint Surg* 1975;57:196–206.
6. Lundborg G, Rosen B, Lindberg S. Hearing as substitution for sensation: a new principle for artificial sensibility. *J Hand Surg* 1999;24:219–224.
7. Mackinnon SE, Novak CB. Nerve transfers: new options for reconstruction following nerve injury. *Hand Clin* 1999;15:643–666.
8. Brown PW. Adduction-flexion contracture of the thumb. Correction with dorsal rotation flap and release of contracture. *Clin Orthop* 1972;88:161–168.
9. Herrick RT, Lister GD. Control of first web space contracture, including a review of the literature and a tabulation of opponensplasty techniques. *Hand* 1977;9:253–264.
10. Hamlin C, Littler JW. Restoration of power pinch. *J Hand Surg* 1980;5:396–401.
11. Smith RJ. Extensor carpi radialis brevis tendon transfer for thumb adduction—a study of power pinch. *J Hand Surg* 1983;8:4–15.
12. Burkhalter W, Christensen RC, Brown P. Extensor indicis proprius opponensplasty. *J Bone Joint Surg* 1973;55:725–732.
13. Neviaser RJ, Wilson JN, Gardner MM. Abductor pollicis longus transfer for replacement of first dorsal interosseous. *J Hand Surg* 1980;5:53–57.
14. Zancolli EA. *Structural and dynamic bases of hand surgery*, 2nd ed. Philadelphia: JB Lippincott Co, 1979:229–262.
15. Brandsma JW, Brand PW. Claw-finger correction: considerations in choice of technique. *J Hand Surg* 1992;17:615–621.
16. Hastings H, McCollam SM. Flexor digitorum superficialis lasso tendon transfer in isolated ulnar nerve palsy: a functional evaluation. *J Hand Surg* 1994;19:275–280.
17. Hastings H, Davidson S. Tendon transfers for ulnar nerve palsy: evaluation of results and practical treatment considerations. *Hand Clin* 1988;4:167–177.
18. Burkhalter WE, Strait JL. Metacarpophalangeal flexor replacement for intrinsic-muscle paralysis. *J Bone Joint Surg* 1973;55:1667–1676.
19. Gaul JS Jr. Radial-innervated cross finger flap from index to provide sensory pulp to injured thumb. *J Bone Joint Surg* 1969;51:1257–1263.
20. Rapp E, Lallemand S, Ehrler S, et. al. Restoration of sensation over the contact surfaces of the thumb-index pinch grip using the terminal branches of the superficial branch of the radial nerve. *Chir Main* 1999;18:179–183.
21. Ihara K, Doi K, Sakai K, et. al. Restoration of sensibility in the hand after complete brachial plexus injury. *J Hand Surg* 1996;21:381–386.
22. Waikakul S, Orapin S, Vanadurongwan V. Clinical results of contralateral C7 root neurotization to the median nerve in brachial plexus injuries with total root avulsions. *J Hand Surg* 1999;24:556–560.

23. Tsuge K. Treatment of established Volkmann's contracture. *J Bone Joint Surg* 1975;57:925–929.

24. McCarthy CK, House JH, Van Heest A, et al. Intrinsic balancing in reconstruction of the tetraplegic hand. *J Hand Surg* 1997;22:596–604.

25. Ihara K, Kido K, Shigetomi M, et al. Experience with the pedicled latissimus dorsi flap for finger reconstruction. *J Hand Surg* 2000;25:668–673.

26. Gousheh J, Arab H, Gilbert A. The extended latissimus dorsi muscle island flap for flexion or extension of the fingers. *J Hand Surg* 2000;25:160–165.

27. Holevich J. A new method of restoring sensibility to the thumb. *J Bone Joint Surg* 1963;45:496–502.

28. Omer GE Jr, Day DJ, Ratcliff H, et al. Neurovascular cutaneous island pedicles for deficient median nerve sensibility. *J Bone Joint Surg* 1970;52:1181–1192.

29. Quaba AA, Elliot D, Sommerlad BC. Long term hand function without long finger extensors: a clinical study. *J Hand Surg* 1988;13:66–71.

30. Reid RL. Radial nerve palsy. *Hand Clin* 1988;4:179–185.

31. Chuinard RG, Boyes JH, Stark HH, et al. Tendon transfers for radial nerve palsy: use of superficialis tendons for digital extension. *J Hand Surg* 1978;3:560–570.

32. Manktelow RT, Zuker RM, McKee NH. Functioning free muscle transplantation. *J Hand Surg* 1984;9:32–39.

33. Manktelow RT. Functioning muscle transplantation. In: Manktelow RT, ed. *Microvascular reconstruction*. Berlin: Springer-Verlag, 1986:151–164.

34. Stocks GW, Cobb T, Lewis RC Jr. Transfer of sensibility in the hand: a new method to restore sensibility in ulnar nerve palsy with use of microsurgical digital nerve translocation. *J Hand Surg* 1991;16:219–226.

35. Battiston B, Lanzetta M. Reconstruction of high ulnar nerve lesions by distal double median to ulnar nerve transfer. *J Hand Surg* 1999;24:1185–1191.

36. Wissinger HA, Singsen EG. Abductor digit quinti opponensplasty. *J Bone Joint Surg* 1977;59:895–898.

37. Oberlin C, Beal D, Leechavengvongs S, et al. Nerve transfer to biceps muscle using a part of ulnar nerve for C5-C6 avulsion of the brachial plexus: anatomical study and report of four cases. *J Hand Surg* 1994;19:232–237.

38. Jolley BJ, Stern PJ, Starling T. Patterns of median nerve sensory innervation to the thumb and index finger: an anatomic study. *J Hand Surg* 1997;22:228–231.

39. Doi K, Muramatsu K, Hattori Y, et al. Restoration of prehension with the double free muscle technique following complete avulsion of the brachial plexus. Indications and long-term results. *J Bone Joint Surg* 2000;82:652–666.

40. Doi K, Kuwata N, Muramatsu K, et al. Double muscle transfer for upper extremity reconstruction following complete avulsion of the brachial plexus. *Hand Clin* 1999;15:757–767.

BRACHIAL PLEXUS INJURY: ACUTE DIAGNOSIS AND TREATMENT

PANUPAN SONGCHAROEN
ALEXANDER Y. SHIN

ANATOMY

The *brachial plexus* is a network of nerves, originating from the spinal cord, that innervates the upper extremity (Fig. 1). The brachial plexus is formed by the ventral rami of the fifth, sixth, seventh, and eighth cervical nerves (C5–C8), along with the first thoracic nerve (T1). In more than half of the cases, the C4 gives off a small branch to the C5 (1). The second thoracic nerve (T2) also contributes directly to the plexus via intrathoracic precostal communication with the T1. Apart from this connection, the T2 always contributes to the innervation of the arm through the intercostobrachial nerve. A *prefixed plexus* refers to a higher position of the plexus relative to the vertebral column. In this condition, there is a significant contribution received from the C4 and an insignificant contribution received from the T1 and T2 (Fig. 2). However, a *postfixed plexus* has a relatively large contribution from the T1, a branch from the T2, a small contribution from the C5, and nothing from the C4 (Fig. 3) (2).

The ventral rami (the roots of the brachial plexus) emerge between the scalenus anterior and the scalenus medius muscles in the posterior triangle of the neck and descend toward the superior portion of the first rib. In the triangle, the plexus is covered by platysma, supraclavicular nerves, and the deep fascia and is crossed by the external jugular vein, the inferior belly of the omohyoid muscle, and the transverse cervical artery. The dorsal rami, which are not part of the brachial plexus, supply the skin and muscles of the posterior part of the neck.

The roots of the brachial plexus travel only a short course in their passage between the scalene muscles. Immediately after entering the posterior triangle, the C5 and C6 join to form the upper trunk, the C7 continues as the middle trunk (Fig. 4), and the C8 and T1 unite to form the lower trunk. The nerve to the subclavius muscle and the suprascapular nerve arise from the upper trunk. The point at which the suprascapular nerve arises from the upper trunk is also known as *Erb's point*.

As the trunks cross the first rib, they lie superior to the first part of the axillary artery before splitting into anterior and posterior divisions just proximal to the clavicular margin. The split is of morphologic significance, as it indicates the separation of the nerve fibers that supply the originally ventral (flexor) parts of the limb from those that supply the dorsal (extensor) parts (2).

Three cords of the plexus are formed by combinations of the anterior and posterior divisions. The lateral cord is formed by the union of the anterior divisions of the upper and middle trunks (C5–C7) and lies on the lateral side of the axillary artery. The medial cord is made up of the anterior division of the lower trunk (C8–T1) and lies on the medial side of the axillary artery. The posterior cord (C5–T1) is formed by the posterior divisions of all three trunks and lies posterior to the axillary artery. The cords form at or just distal to the clavicle. They are invested by the axillary sheath as they descend behind the pectoralis minor tendon. The cords then travel adjacent to the second part of the axillary artery (Fig. 5) into the lower axilla, where they divide into terminal branches.

Lateral Cord

The lateral cord is created by the confluence of the anterior divisions of the upper and middle trunks. It passes superficial and lateral to the second part of the axillary artery and gives off three nerves: the lateral pectoral nerve, the lateral cord contribution to the median nerve, and the musculocutaneous nerve.

The lateral pectoral nerve may arise as a single root from the lateral cord or more often as multiple roots from the anterior division of the upper and middle trunks (1). The nerve contains fibers from the C5, C6, and C7. It leaves the lateral cord lateral to the first part of the axillary artery, crosses the artery anteriorly, and, on occasion, has a loop connection with the medial pectoral nerve. It then pierces the clavipectoral fascia and divides on the deep surface of

The Brachial Plexus

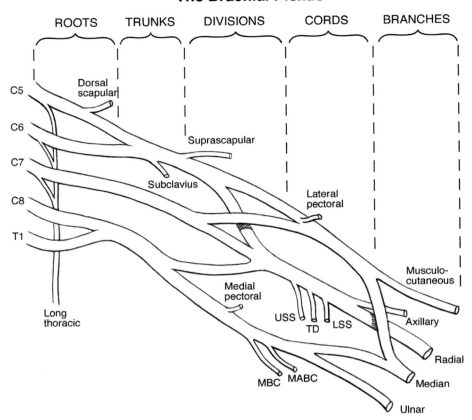

FIGURE 1. The brachial plexus is typically formed from the fifth through eighth cervical nerve (C5–C8) roots, in addition to the first thoracic (T1) root. LSS, lower subscapular nerve; MABC, medial antebrachial cutaneous nerve; MBC, medial brachial cutaneous nerve; TD, thoracodorsal nerve; USS, upper subscapular nerve.

the pectoralis major muscle to innervate the muscle's clavicular head.

The lateral cord contribution to the median nerve (carrying fibers from the C5–C7 roots) descends along the lateral side of the axillary artery to join the medial cord contribution of the median nerve anterior to the third part of the axillary artery or in the proximal part of the upper arm. The lateral cord contribution to the median nerve may be vestigial, in which case the musculocutaneous nerve gives a branch to the median nerve in the proximal part of the arm (3).

The musculocutaneous nerve (the terminal branch of the lateral cord) and the lateral cord contribution to the median nerve divide at the lateral border of the pectoralis minor muscle. The musculocutaneous nerve contains fibers from the C4, C5, and C6 roots. It arises between the axillary artery and the coracobrachialis muscle.

The nerve to the coracobrachialis muscle, arising from the C6 and the C7, is usually incorporated with the musculocutaneous nerve. Alternatively, the coracobrachialis muscle may be innervated by separate branches from the lateral cord or the C7. The musculocutaneous nerve passes through and traverses downward and laterally between the biceps and brachialis muscles, innervating both. It provides an articular branch to the elbow joint, pierces the deep fascia over the front of the elbow between the biceps and bra-

chioradialis, and terminates as the lateral cutaneous nerve of the forearm. In addition, the musculocutaneous nerve also supplies a medullary branch to the humerus, a periosteal branch to the distal end of the humerus, and a branch to the brachial artery.

Medial Cord

The medial cord is formed by the anterior division of the lower trunk. It emerges between the axillary artery and vein and descends medial to the artery, where it gives off the medial pectoral nerve, the medial brachial cutaneous nerve, the medial antebrachial cutaneous nerve, the medial cord contribution to the median nerve, and the ulnar nerve.

The medial pectoral nerve arises from the medial cord of the brachial plexus immediately after its formation. The nerve contains fibers from the C8 and T1 roots. It leaves the medial cord behind the axillary artery and curves anteriorly between the artery and vein, where it occasionally forms a loop of communication with the lateral pectoral nerve. It enters the deep surface of the pectoralis minor muscle, sends branches through, and innervates the pectoralis minor and major (sternal head) muscles.

The medial brachial cutaneous nerve arises from the medial cord of the brachial plexus and the T1 nerve. The nerve contains fibers from the C8 and T1 roots. It leaves

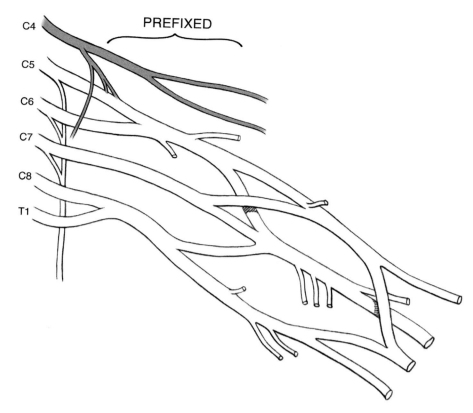

FIGURE 2. When there is a significant contribution from the fourth cervical nerve (C4) root to the brachial plexus, it is called *prefixed*. C5–C8, fifth through eighth cervical nerves; T1, first thoracic nerve.

the medial cord at the lower border of the pectoralis minor muscle, descends into the axilla between the axillary artery and vein, and continues along the medial aspect of the brachial artery and basilic vein in the upper arm. It perforates the deep fascia at mid-arm level to supply the skin and fas-

cia of the proximal half of the upper arm on its medial side. The nerve varies in size. It may be absent, its place being taken by branches of the intercostobrachial nerve or by branches from the posterior cutaneous branch of the radial nerve (4).

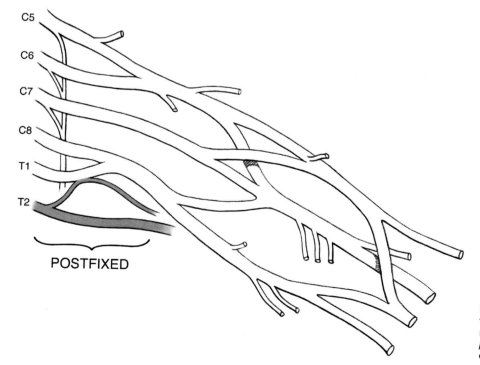

FIGURE 3. When there are contributions from the second thoracic nerve (T2) root to the brachial plexus, it is called *postfixed*. C5–C8, fifth through eighth cervical nerves; T1, first thoracic nerve.

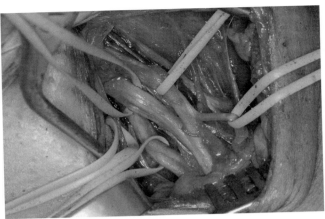

FIGURE 4. A clinical example of the surgical dissection of the fifth through seventh cervical roots and the upper and middle trunks. The vessel loop on the right of the figure holds the suprascapular nerve before the upper trunk splits into its divisions.

The medial antebrachial cutaneous nerve arises from the medial cord of the brachial plexus or the lower trunk. It contains fibers from the C8 and T1 roots. It arises above or below the medial brachial cutaneous nerve, then passes between the axillary artery and vein into the arm. In the proximal half of the arm, it lies superficial to the brachial artery. It becomes cutaneous by piercing the deep fascia at the middle part of the arm on its medial side, accompanying the basilic vein through the distal half. It divides at the front of the elbow into two terminal branches, supplying the skin along the anterior aspect of the arm and the anteromedial aspect of the forearm (5).

The medial cord contribution to the median nerve, containing fibers from the C8 and T1 roots, crosses in front of the terminal part of the axillary artery to join the lateral cord contribution to the median nerve in the proximal part of the upper arm (1). The median nerve therefore receives fibers from all of the cervical and thoracic nerve roots that form the brachial plexus. The median nerve descends through the axilla along the anterolateral aspect of the brachial artery and crosses to the medial aspect in the middle part of the arm. At the elbow, it lies behind the bicipital aponeurosis and the median cubital vein. It passes into the forearm between the two heads of the pronator teres muscle.

The ulnar nerve, the major terminal branch of the medial cord, contains fibers from the C8 and T1 roots. In more than half of the specimens, it received a contribution from either the lateral cord or the lateral cord contribution to the median nerve (the C7 root) (4). It arises deeply between the axillary artery and vein, passes anterior to the teres major and latissimus dorsi muscles, and then descends along the median aspect of the brachial artery anterior to the triceps muscle in the proximal half of the arm. In the distal half of the arm, it pierces the medial intermuscular septum and descends in front of the medial head of the triceps, accompanying the ulnar collateral artery to the cubital tunnel on the medial aspect of the medial condyle of the humerus. It enters the forearm between the humeral and ulnar origins of the flexor carpi ulnaris.

Posterior Cord

The posterior cord is formed by the posterior division of all three trunks. The cord contains fibers from the C5 to T1 roots; however, the contribution from the T1 is often negligible (1). The contributions from each trunk to the posterior cord are not equal. The posterior division of the upper trunk is relatively large, indicating a major contribution from the C5 and C6 roots, especially to the axillary nerve. The posterior division of the middle trunk is larger than the anterior, indicating a significant contribution from the C7 to the posterior cord, particularly to the radial nerve. The posterior division of the lower trunk is usually small, indicating an insignificant contribution from the C8 and T1 roots to the posterior cord. The posterior cord originates superior and lateral to the axillary artery and passes posterior to it. From the posterior cord arise the two subscapular nerves, the thoracodorsal nerve, the axillary nerve, and the radial nerve.

Of the two subscapular nerves, upper and lower, the upper subscapular nerve often has two or three branches. It contains fibers from the C5 and C6 root. It arises from the posterior cord of the plexus behind the axillary artery and passes through the subscapular fascia, where it divides, innervating the upper part of the subscapularis muscle. The lower subscapular nerve contains fibers from the C5 and

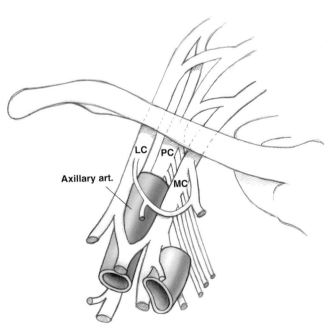

FIGURE 5. Infraclavicularly, the axillary artery is bound by the cords on the lateral, medial, and posterior aspect. A clear understanding of these anatomic relationships is essential when performing surgical explorations of the brachial plexus. art., artery; LC, lateral cord; MC, medial cord; PC, posterior cord.

C6 roots. It arises from the posterior cord behind the axillary artery or, frequently, directly from the axillary nerve. It passes downward behind the axillary vein and the subscapular vessels to the lower border of the subscapularis muscle. It divides into two branches, innervating the lower portion of the subscapularis and teres major muscles.

The thoracodorsal nerve usually arises from the posterior cord between the upper and lower subscapular nerves. Occasionally, it arises from the radial, axillary, or subscapular nerves. It contains fibers from the C6, C7, and C8 roots or from the C7 root only (1). It runs downward and laterally behind the axillary artery between the subscapular nerves. It joins the subscapular artery along the posterior wall of the axilla and innervates the latissimus dorsi muscle on its ventral (deep) surface.

The axillary nerve is a terminal branch of the posterior cord. Occasionally, it arises from the posterior division of the upper or upper and middle trunk. It contains fibers from the C5 and C6 roots. It leaves the posterior cord at the lower border of the subscapularis muscle behind the axillary artery. It leaves the axilla by curving backward, accompanying the posterior circumflex humeral artery adjacent to the inferior border of the shoulder capsule. It passes through the quadrilateral space bounded by the humerus and the subscapularis, triceps (long head), and teres major muscles and divides into anterior and posterior branches. The anterior branch circles the surgical neck of the humerus with the posterior humeral circumflex vessels from the medial to the lateral side. It courses deep to the anterior border of the deltoid, where it divides, sending muscular branches to the muscle and small cutaneous branches to the overlying skin. The posterior branch supplies the teres minor and the posterior part of the deltoid muscle. It curves around the posterior border of the deltoid muscle, then penetrates the deep fascia to the skin over the superolateral aspect of the arm to become the superior lateral brachial cutaneous nerve.

The radial nerve is the largest terminal branch of the brachial plexus and arises from the posterior cord or the posterior division of the upper or upper and middle trunk. It contains fibers from all of the roots that form the posterior cord, the C5 to T1 roots, but the contributions from the C5 and T1 roots are not constant (4). The radial nerve divides from the axillary nerve behind the pectoralis minor muscles. In the axilla, it lies behind the third part of the axillary artery and in front of the subscapularis, teres major, and latissimus dorsi muscles. The posterior cutaneous nerve branch leaves the radial nerve in the axilla, where it innervates the skin on the back of the arm. The radial nerve extends from the axilla and around the back of the humerus. In the arm, it first lies to the medial side of the humerus behind the brachial artery in front of the long head of the triceps. It joins the profunda brachii artery and passes between the long and medial heads of the triceps to the spiral groove. It runs downward and laterally in the groove and around the back of the humerus. It pierces the proximal part of the lateral intermuscular septum and passes in front of the lateral epicondyle of the humerus, where it lies between the brachioradialis and brachialis muscles. Underneath the brachioradialis muscle, it divides into two terminal branches, the posterior interosseous nerve (deep branch) and the superficial radial nerve (superficial), that continue into the forearm.

ETIOLOGY AND CLASSIFICATION

The knowledge about brachial plexus can be traced back to the second century, when Galen accurately described the anatomy of brachial plexus (6). In the early stage, brachial plexus was seen only as a part of the peripheral nervous system and had been treated accordingly for nearly 2 millennia. At the beginning of the nineteenth century, brachial plexus injury became a separate clinical entity from other peripheral nerve lesions (7).

Brachial plexus injury can be caused by a wide variety of circumstances. These etiologic factors can be categorized according to their causative mechanisms as follows:

- Closed injuries
  - Traction
  - Compression
  - Combined lesion
- Open injuries
  - Sharp
  - Gunshot injury
  - Radiation

In closed brachial plexus injuries, the commonly found causative mechanisms are traction and contusion. In some circumstances, the injuries are the result of the combination of traction and contusion. At present, traction is the most frequently found mechanism of brachial plexus injury. In the senior author's (Panupan Songcharoen) series of adult brachial plexus injury, 95% of injuries were caused by traction.

Traction Lesion

Traction lesions result from forceful separation of the neck and shoulder or upper arm and trunk. The nerve pathology occurs between the two anchoring points. The proximal anchoring point is at the spinal cord and nerve root junction, and the distal point is at the neuromuscular junction. The coracoid process is regarded as a temporary lever in forceful hyperabduction of the shoulder. It is not only the direction of the applied force to brachial plexus that determines the severity of the nerve damage, but also the speed of the application of the traction force.

High-velocity traction injury is the overall leading cause of brachial plexus injury in nearly all reports (8,9).

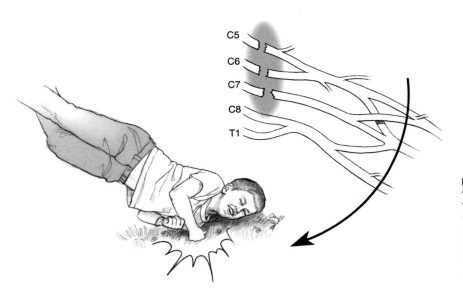

FIGURE 6. Injury to the upper portions of the brachial plexus occurs with widening of the neck–shoulder angle. Such an injury is observed in the patient falling from a motorcycle onto the ground. During this mechanism of injury, the upper portions of the brachial plexus are placed at greatest risk for injury. C5–C8, fifth through eighth cervical nerves; T1, first thoracic nerve.

The majority of traction injuries are a result of motor vehicle crashes. In the senior author's series of 1,173 adult brachial plexus patients, 82% were caused by motorcycle injuries. The individual falls off a speeding motorcycle, landing on the head and shoulder. At the ground impaction, the shoulder is depressed, and the head is forcefully flexed to the opposite side. The sudden widening of the neck–shoulder angle causes a severe traction injury to the clavicle and underlying structures, including the brachial plexus and subclavian vessels. If the clavicle, which is the strongest link between the shoulder and neck, is broken, all of the traction force is transmitted to the neurovascular bundle. This mechanism of injury causes the greatest damage to the upper roots (Fig. 6), whereas hyperabduc-tion of the shoulder or forceful widening of the scapulo-humeral angle mostly affects the C8 and T1 roots (Fig. 7) (10). The high-velocity traction injury can cause nerve root avulsion from the spinal cord, nerve ruptures, or stretch injuries (Fig. 8). The structures protecting the cervical nerve root from traction force are (a) the cone-shaped dural continuation into the epineurium of the cervical spinal nerves and (b) the fibrous attachments between the epineurium of spinal nerves; the C5, C6, and C7 roots; and the cervical transverse process at the neural foramen. The absence of these ligaments at the C8 and T1 roots is the rationale behind the higher incidence of avulsion of these roots compared to the C5 and C6 roots, which sustain a higher incidence of extraforaminal rupture. High-

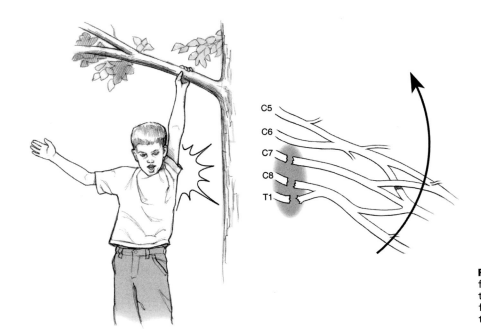

FIGURE 7. Traction injury with the shoulder fully abducted places the lower elements of the brachial plexus at risk for injury. C5–C8, fifth through eighth cervical nerves; T1, first thoracic nerve.

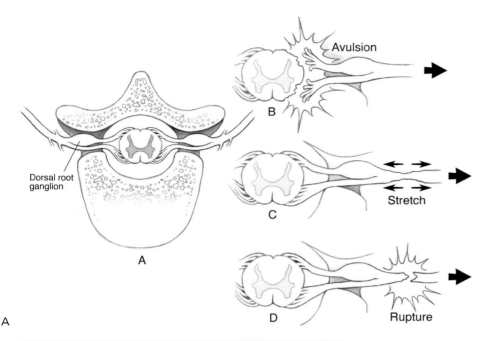

A

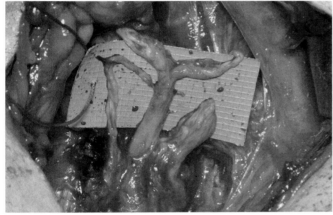

B

FIGURE 8. Anatomy of the brachial plexus roots and types of injury. **A:** The roots are formed by the coalescence of the ventral (motor) and dorsal (sensory) rootlets as they pass through the spinal foramen (*A*). The dorsal root ganglion holds the cell bodies of the sensory nerves, whereas the cell bodies for the ventral nerves lie within the spinal cord. There are three types of injury that can occur: avulsion injuries (*B*) pull the rootlets out of the spinal cord, stretch injuries (*C*) attenuate the nerve, and ruptures (*D*) result in a complete discontinuity of the nerve. When the injury to the nerve is proximal to the dorsal root ganglion, it is called *preganglionic*; when it is distal to the dorsal root ganglion, it is called *postganglionic*. **B:** Clinical example of an avulsion and rupture. The avulsion is the fifth cervical nerve root with the Y split—the dorsal root ganglion is at the left of the Y. The nerve at the right represents a rupture of sixth cervical nerve.

velocity traction injuries are also incurred in speedboat, motor vehicle, and ski crashes.

Low-velocity traction injury has a much lower incidence than higher-velocity injury. In the senior author's series, only 4% of patients had this kind of injury (9). The mechanism of trauma is downward traction or depression of the shoulder. This injury is usually incurred when either the individual falls from a height and lands on his or her shoulder or a heavy object falls on the individual's unprotected shoulder. In industrial situations, a worker's arm may be caught and pulled by a machine, causing a stretch injury to the plexus. In sports, it is not uncommon for a rugby or American football player tackling an opponent with the head and shoulder or a volleyball player practicing overhead smashes to experience transient paresthesia in the upper extremity. These lower-velocity injuries usually produce a lesser degree of brachial plexus pathology.

Improper positioning of the patient in the operating room during general anesthesia can cause traction injuries to the brachial plexus (11,12). The upper trunk can be injured when the patient is in supine or lateral decubitus position, due to prolonged extension and lateral bending of the head to one side. This posture increases the angle between the head and the affected shoulder. Positioning the shoulder on a sandbag or roll can put the brachial plexus under stretch. Suspension of the arm from the operating table screen in the lateral decubitus position may stretch the brachial plexus, especially when the arm is in hyperabduction. Excessive abduction of the arms in either the prone or supine position (e.g., position for spinal procedure) also causes stretching of the brachial plexus.

Compression Lesion

The brachial plexus may be compressed between the clavicle and the first rib. The compression occurs when a traumatic force is exerted on the shoulder in the cephalocaudal direction. The bone fragments from fractures of the cervical transverse processes can compress the cervical nerve roots; the coracoid process fracture can compress the lateral cord and musculocutaneous nerve. Fracture of the neck or scapula, humeral neck fracture, and anteriorly dislocated humeral head can compress the posterior cord and axillary nerve. Fracture of the scapular spine can compress the suprascapular nerve.

In motor vehicle crashes, acute compression by seat belts may also cause brachial plexus injuries. Chronic compression from carrying heavy weights on shoulders may cause a temporary brachial plexus lesion.

Iatrogenic compression injuries to the brachial plexus can occur in the operating room if shoulder pads are improperly placed on an abducted arm while the patient is in a steep Trendelenburg position (11,12). If the shoulder pads are placed medial to the acromioclavicular joint instead of directly over the joint, the pads press the brachial plexus against the first rib. Compression of the brachial plexus can also occur as the arm and shoulder lie between the patient's chest and the operating table in the lateral decubitus position. The bony structures of the shoulder and arm compress the plexus against the rib cage.

Traction and Compression

Complex trauma with multiple fractures of the cervical transverse process, clavicle, scapula, rib, and proximal humerus can cause both compression and traction injury to the brachial plexus. The pathology is usually diffuse, from nerve roots through terminal branches, and disruption of brachial plexus can be found on more than one site. This injury is usually associated with vascular damage.

Open Injury

Open injury of the brachial plexus is much less common in normal practice. In the senior author's series, 4.3% of patients sustained open injury to the brachial plexus (9).

Sharp injury secondary to assault by knife at the neck, chest, and shoulder can directly injure the brachial plexus. The open injury usually involves only part of the plexus. Associated vascular and intrathoracic injuries are commonly found. This kind of injury to the brachial plexus carries a good prognosis. The injured brachial plexus can usually be treated by neurorrhaphy or intraplexal nerve grafting. Iatrogenic sharp injury to the brachial plexus may occur in a brachial plexus anesthetic block or tumor resection at the neck and supraclavicular area. Occasionally, an intact brachial plexus may be damaged during attempts to obtain hemostasis from vascular injury or by insertion of subclavian lines.

Gunshot injuries to the brachial plexus may be encountered in several military and civilian circumstances (13). This kind of injury may be accompanied by life-threatening vascular or thoracic lesions. Gunshot injuries should be considered separately from sharp open injuries because there are significant differences in the extent and character of neural and surrounding tissue damage. In gunshot injuries, the cause of tissue disruption is the high velocity and spin of the bullet. The tissues are first crushed from direct contact with the high-velocity bullet and then stretched via temporary cavitation (14–16). Tissue disruption is dependent on the bullet mass, shape, construction, and striking velocity.

Low-velocity gunshot injury is commonly found in civilian practice and represented 27% of patients in the senior author's series (9). This type of brachial plexus injury, without any associated vascular injury, carries a good prognosis. More than 50% of patients have a significant functional recovery with nonoperative treatment.

High-velocity gunshot injury has a greater tissue penetration and results in a more extensive and diffuse lesion. It is difficult to define the extent of neural tissue damage in the early stages of injury. High-velocity gunshot injury is less common in civilian practice. Spontaneous functional recovery is less likely in this type of injury than it is in cases of low-velocity gunshot injury.

Shotgun injury usually produces extensive tissue damage and contamination. This type of injury also has a lesser chance of spontaneous recovery than does a low-velocity gunshot injury.

Radiation Injury

In general, peripheral nerves are considered to be relatively radioresistant because nerve lies deeper than other tissues and has a low metabolic rate.

Radiation brachial plexus injury is usually found in patients several years after radiation therapy to the ipsilateral breast or axilla for the treatment of breast cancer (17). Patients usually present with progressive motor and sensory deficits that may be caused by radiation, compression of recurrent neoplasm, or both. Investigations and meticulous clinical examination can clarify the diagnosis in some patients, but a number of patients remain undiagnosed until a later stage. Surgical exploration is difficult because of the fibrotic and ischemic nature of the surrounding tissues. Despite the unrewarding results, patients usually insist on surgical exploration because of the intractable pain.

Adult traumatic lesions of the brachial plexus can also be classified according to the anatomic level within the plexus and the relationship to the clavicle. By using the clavicle as a reference, the lesion can be localized at three levels: supraclavicular, retroclavicular, and infraclavicular lesions. To be more specific, the supraclavicular lesions are separated into two types in relation to the dorsal root ganglion: supraganglionic (preganglionic) lesion and infraganglionic (postganglionic) lesion (Fig. 8). Although the clinical significance of this classification is rather limited because of a variety of other factors—such as extent of the lesion, mechanism of injury, multilevel lesion—this anatomic classification helps the brachial plexus surgeon to determine the suitable type of surgical treatment and prognosis of the patient.

CLINICAL EVALUATION

History

Evaluation of the patient with a brachial plexus injury starts with a complete understanding of the nature and mechanism of the injury. The nature (e.g., motor vehicle, penetrating, compression) and mechanism of the injury are helpful in determining its anatomic location and severity. Knowing the exact neck and arm position at the moment of injury greatly assists in predicting the site of the brachial plexus lesion. The downward pull of the shoulder from the cervical column when the arm is in adduction usually results in the injury of the upper roots. The most common mechanism of injury secondary to motorcycle injuries is a fall on the shoulder. Extension of the arm in 90-degree abduction of the shoulder puts maximum tension on the C7 root of the brachial plexus, but with increased force, all nerve roots may be affected. The less frequent mechanism of injury is stretching of the upper extremity in maximal abduction, which usually results in the lesion of the lower roots (8). In penetrating injuries, information about the type of weapon and bullet velocity helps predict the prognosis of the brachial plexus injury.

The patient's medical history is also important. Radiation therapy to the neck, upper chest, and axilla can cause radiation brachial plexitis or fibrosis. Patients usually present with a slowly advancing motor and sensory deficit associated with pain. Iatrogenic compression injuries to the brachial plexus can occur because of improper positioning in the operating room (11,12). An interscalene or axillary brachial plexus block can occasionally injure a portion of plexus. Brachial plexus injury is often underdiagnosed in the presence of cervical spinal cord or head injury. The patient should be asked about alteration of consciousness, motor weakness, and sensory deficit in other extremities.

Physical Examination

The initial physical examination is an important step in determining the anatomic location of the lesion that leads to the treatment plan and prognosis.

General Physical Examination

Contusion and ecchymosis at the suprascapular or deltopectoral area indicate the site of injury in compression lesions of the brachial plexus (Fig. 9). The precise locations of entrance and exit wounds help surgeons make a topographic diagnosis of penetrating brachial plexus injuries. Abrasions on the ipsilateral shoulder and cheek provide strong evidence of traction lesions of the brachial plexus

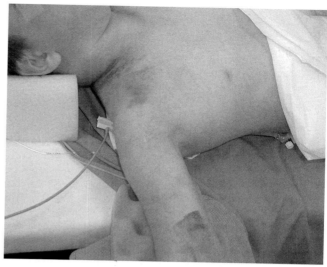

FIGURE 9. Abrasions on the chest wall can give clues to the level of injury of the brachial plexus. In this 12-year-old boy, the abrasions on the cheek and the anterior shoulder give clues to a significant upper brachial plexus injury.

incurred in motorcycle accidents. Posttraumatic cervical scoliosis secondary to massive paracervical muscle paralysis may be observed in a complete root avulsion brachial plexus injury. Winging of the scapula indicates the lesion of the long thoracic nerve.

Neurologic Examination

Motor Examination

According to the Medical Research Council (MRC), every muscle of the affected upper extremity innervated by the brachial plexus must be examined and graded on a scale from 0 to 5 by the manual muscle test. An MRC grade 5 is normal muscle strength, whereas an MRC grade 0 is a flail muscle. The result should be recorded on a special form for follow-up examinations. Testing muscles of the lower extremity and deep tendon reflexes is also required to detect the presence of long tract signs, as brachial plexus root avulsions may be associated with spinal cord injury (18).

Sensory Examination

A complete sensory examination should include both subjective and objective sensory changes. Objective tests of all sensory modalities are performed on each dermatome of the cervical and brachial plexus. Pain, temperature, touch, vibratory sense, and two-point discrimination are tested and recorded.

Disturbances of subjective sensitivity expressed by pain must be carefully evaluated. Neuropathic pain in brachial plexus injury may be present with avulsion lesion of the lower roots. The deafferentation pain from root avulsion usually appears a few weeks after injury. This type of neu-

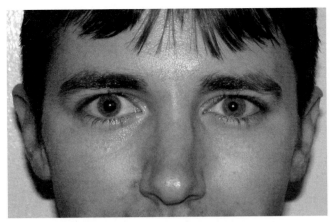

FIGURE 10. Horner's syndrome: With avulsion of the T1 root, the first thoracic sympathetic ganglion is injured. The result is miosis (constricted pupil), ptosis (drooped lid), anhydrosis (dry eyes), and enophthalmos (sinking of the eyeball). This patient demonstrated miosis and ptosis after a lower trunk avulsion injury.

ralgic pain relates to sympathetic nervous system participation. The causalgic pain, which has no precise distribution and appears immediately after injury, is a major therapeutic problem. The pathogenesis of this syndrome is difficult to determine, and a severe long-term deafferentation pain can be expected (7).

The examination of the sympathetic nervous system is also part of the initial clinical evaluation. Avulsion of the lower roots or a high lesion of the corresponding spinal nerves can compromise the ipsilateral sympathetic preganglionic fibers. Vasomotor disturbances, cyanosis, edema of the soft tissues, and trophic lesions should be observed.

Sweating of the affected hand can give useful information about the brachial plexus lesion. Anhydrosis of the anesthetic area suggests a postganglionic lesion. The sweating function can be tested by the ninhydrin test. The presence of Horner's syndrome (anhydrosis, miosis, ptosis, and enophthalmos) is a bad prognostic feature and is associated with T1 root avulsions (Fig. 10) (19).

A complete sensory examination of the lower extremities should be performed to detect signs of spinal cord involvement. Brown-Sequard syndrome can occur in association with massive nerve root avulsion. Clinical examination of patients with this syndrome demonstrates dissociated changes in the lower extremities. The findings in the ipsilateral lower extremity include muscular spasticity in addition to loss of tactile, vibratory, and position senses. The contralateral lower extremity demonstrates loss of pain and temperature senses.

Vascular Examination

Peripheral vascular examination of the affected limb should always be made on initial physical examination. Major vascular injury is found in association with brachial plexus injury in 10% to 16% of cases. Vascular injury can be found with either traction or penetrating brachial plexus lesions (20). Arterial injury usually accompanies an infraclavicular lesion or avulsion of the lower roots of the plexus (Fig. 11). Progressive loss of motor and sensory function of the affected extremity suggests an expanding hematoma or aneurysm compressing the adjacent neural structure. Early detection and prompt surgical treatment rapidly resolve the functional deficit.

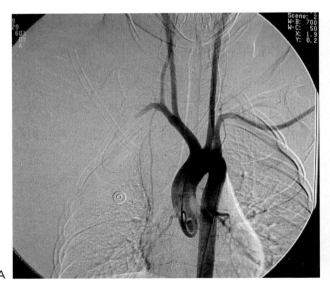

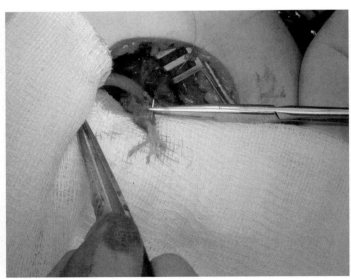

A   B

FIGURE 11. Angiography is indicated in patients with abnormal vascular examination, widened mediastinum, fractures of the first rib, and so forth, to rule out vascular injury. **A:** The angiogram shown here is that of the patient in Figure 9 and demonstrates loss of continuity of the subclavian artery. **B:** At the time of surgical repair of the subclavian artery, nerve root avulsion was identified.

Musculoskeletal Examination

Because the majority of brachial plexus injuries are caused by falls form motorcycles, musculoskeletal injuries are commonly found concomitant with brachial plexus trauma. The associated injuries of the upper extremity can include clavicular fracture, acromioclavicular joint separation, scapula fracture, first rib fracture, cervical transverse process fracture, humeral fracture, glenohumeral dislocation, and scapulothoracic dissociation. Fracture and dislocation around the clavicle indicate a bad prognostic sign (10). Because the clavicle is the only solid structure connecting the shoulder girdle to the neck, its fracture allows all of the traction force to be directed at the underlying soft structures (i.e., brachial plexus and subclavian vessels). Cervical transverse process fractures are commonly found with high ruptures or avulsions of the corresponding nerve roots. Scapulothoracic dissociation is often associated with multiple root avulsions. First rib fracture is often associated with lesion of the lower roots as well as vascular injuries. Fracture of the coracoid process is often found with lateral cord injury, whereas scapular and humeral neck fractures are associated with posterior cord lesion.

INVESTIGATIONS

Radiologic and Imaging Studies

Plain Radiography

Concomitant musculoskeletal injuries are usually found with brachial plexus trauma. Plain radiography of the shoulder girdle, cervical spine, and chest should be made for patients with traumatic brachial plexus lesions. Chest radiography is made to determine whether there is a wid-

ened superior mediastinum, which suggests major vascular injury. Fractures of the first rib are associated with lesion of the lower roots or trunk and arterial injury, whereas fractures of the lower ribs are associated with intercostal nerve injury and pulmonary trauma, which jeopardize the use of intercostal nerves as donors for nerve transfers. Elevation of the hemidiaphragm on inspiration and expiration chest radiography is an indicator of phrenic nerve injury, which prevents the use of phrenic nerves for transfer. Fractures of the transverse process of the cervical spine are strong evidence of intraforaminal lesions of the roots. A scapula fracture around the scapular notch may cause an injury to the suprascapular nerve. Fracture of the coracoid process may be associated with an injury to the lateral cord or the musculocutaneous nerve, which is a common site of second-level lesion in double-lesion brachial plexus injuries.

Myelography and Computed Tomography with Myelography

Traction lesions of the brachial plexus normally result in avulsions of nerve roots and meninges. Myelography is indicated in traction brachial plexus lesions presenting with a persistent complete or partial neurologic deficit. Myelography should be performed no sooner than 3 weeks after injury because the dural tear is still not healed by that time—the visualization of the roots of the brachial plexus is obscured by leakage of contrast media from the injured nerve roots. Myelographic findings that suggest injuries to nerve roots include obliteration of the nerve root sleeve, defect of the root sleeve shadow, and meningeal diverticulum (Fig. 12). The diverticulum is usually referred to as a *traumatic meningocele* or a *pseudomeningocele* (21). Myelog-

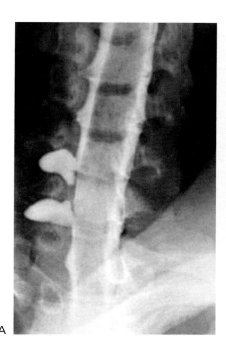

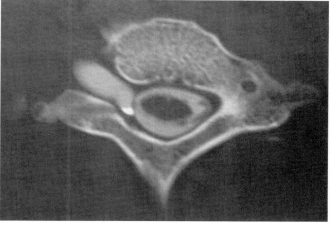

FIGURE 12. Myelography and computed tomography in combination with myelography can be instrumental in determining the level of nerve injury. If a pseudomeningocele is present, there is a greater likelihood of a nerve root avulsion. Demonstrated in the myelogram **(A)** are multiple root avulsions that can be further evaluated by computed tomography **(B)**.

raphy in combination with computed tomography (CT-myelography) improves visualization of the spinal cord and nerve root lesions (Fig. 12). The presence of a pseudomeningocele is a complicating diagnostic factor due to the severity and location of root and rootlet (dorsal and ventral) lesions. According to Sunderland, the ventral (motor) rootlets are thinner and have a lower tensile strength than the dorsal (sensory) rootlets. Therefore, the ventral rootlets are more vulnerable to avulsion injury than the dorsal rootlets.

Nerve root avulsion can be found with a normal myelogram, and a pseudomeningocele can exist with an intact nerve root. When correlated with intraoperative somatosensory evoked potential and extradural inspection, 98% specificity and 95% sensitivity of CT-myelography was found in detection of complete root avulsion. When compared with intradural inspection of roots, the diagnostic accuracy of complete root avulsion was reduced to 75% to 85% of cases (22). However, partial root avulsions are not detected well by CT-myelography because they may not be associated with a pseudomeningocele. The interpretation of CT-myelography has a considerable interobserver variation, which may reduce the reliability of this diagnostic procedure.

Magnetic Resonance Imaging

The application of magnetic resonance imaging (MRI) technology in brachial plexus injuries continues to evolve. Advantages of MRI include the noninvasiveness and lack of radiation. MRI provides a better image of the extraforaminal brachial plexus structures than any other imaging technique, particularly in the nonacute setting. Different kinds of lesions, including injuries, neuroma formation, tumor, and entrapment, can be followed along the length of the plexus. MRI findings associated with intraforaminal plexus lesions include hematomas in the vertebral canal, empty root sleeves, and a shift of the spinal cord away from the midline. However, MRI with axial slices of 3 mm has provided an accurate diagnosis of root avulsion in only 52% of cases when compared with intradural inspection (22). The significant edema that occurs in the acute phase of injury often precludes the effective use of MRI in the early postinjury setting.

Angiography

In adult traumatic brachial plexus lesion, angiography of the upper extremity is recommended in penetrating injuries with or without abnormal neurovascular findings, nonpenetrating injuries with abnormal vascular findings, and nonpenetrating injuries with initial normal neurovascular examination but subsequent progressive neurologic deficit (Fig. 11). Angiography is very helpful in the detection of "silent" vascular lesions that could pose a danger during the surgical exploration and reconstruction of brachial plexus lesions.

Electrodiagnostic Studies

Electromyography

Electromyography gives objective information on motor dysfunction, especially when clinical examination of motor function is difficult. Electromyography is used during the first week after injury to determine whether the lesion is a continuity lesion. The presence of motor unit action potentials across the affected site, in spite of a complete paralysis, indicates a partial lesion. At rest, normal muscle is electromyographically silent, whereas partially or completely denervated muscle generates low electrical potentials. When the axon is injured, degeneration of the distal segment occurs during a 3-week period as wallerian degeneration of the motor axon proceeds, the influence of nerve on muscle is lost, and denervation (fibrillation) potentials appear.

Immediately after leaving the intervertebral foramina, the ventral rami of the C5 to T1 roots unite to become the brachial plexus, and the posterior rami of the corresponding roots course posteriorly to innervate the deep layers of the paracervical muscles and skin. In a preganglionic brachial plexus lesion, denervation potentials can be detected in the deep layers of the paracervical muscles as early as 3 weeks after injury (23). Postganglionic lesion is suggested if a denervation potential is demonstrated in the muscles supplied by the distal part of brachial plexus but the paracervical muscles show no fibrillation potentials at 3 weeks (i.e., normal paracervical muscles). If a denervation potential is demonstrated in the paracervical and peripheral muscles, the injury can be either a preganglionic lesion or a combined preganglionic and postganglionic lesion.

Nerve Conduction Study

In preganglionic lesion, wallerian degeneration occurs in the motor fibers of the injured root. This degeneration is caused by the loss of continuity between the motor fibers and the corresponding motor neurons in the anterior horn of the spinal cord. However, wallerian degeneration does not occur in the sensory fibers because the continuity between the sensory fibers and the sensory neurons in the dorsal root ganglion is still preserved. Thus, after preganglionic injuries, sensory nerve conduction is still normal, whereas motor nerve conduction is absent. Intact sensory nerve conduction with loss of sensation on clinical examination is consistent with preganglionic injuries (i.e., root avulsions). Loss of both sensory and motor conduction can be the result of a postganglionic lesion or a combination of preganglionic and postganglionic lesions.

Somatosensory Evoked Potentials

Somatosensory evoked potentials are a measurement of the somatosensory pathway from a peripheral nerve to the sensory cortex. An electrical stimulus is applied to a peripheral nerve (e.g., the median or ulnar nerve at the wrist) or a digital nerve. If the sensory pathways are intact, scalp electrodes over the cortical representation area of the contralateral sensory cortex record a signal. This pathway can be divided into a smaller segment, and electrodes overlying the pathway for more precise localization perform a recording. When a normal somatosensory evoked potential is measured, a sufficient number of both central and peripheral sensory fibers must be functioning. In the absence of the evoked response, there must be a significant lesion along the pathway. The absence of somatosensory evoked potentials with normal nerve action potential in a clinically nonfunctioning nerve is strong evidence of preganglionic root avulsion (24).

SURGICAL MANAGEMENT

Indications for Surgery

Penetrating Injury

Brachial plexus exploration is indicated for patients with complete or partial neurologic deficit after a penetrating injury. A stab or cut wound secondary to civilian assault by a knife in the neck or shoulder region can directly injure the brachial plexus. An iatrogenic sharp injury to the brachial plexus may occur in lymph node or tumor mass resection at the neck and supraclavicular area, cervical rib or first rib resection for the treatment of thoracic outlet syndrome, and vascular reconstruction of subclavian or axillary vessels. In associated penetrating subclavian vessel and brachial plexus injury, neural repair or reconstruction should be performed at the same time as the vascular procedure to avoid an iatrogenic vascular injury in secondary neural procedures. In general, sharp injuries to the brachial plexus carry a good prognosis. The injured plexus can usually be treated with neurorrhaphy or nerve grafting.

In gunshot injuries, immediate brachial plexus exploration is only indicated when there is an associated major vascular injury. The treatment plan for gunshot injuries should be considered separately from sharp injuries because of the significant differences in the nature and extent of tissue damage. Low-velocity gunshot injury has a good prognosis. Functional recovery occurs in the majority of patients with nonoperative treatment. High-velocity gunshot and shotgun injuries produce extensive tissue damage and have less chance of spontaneous recovery. Surgical exploration should be performed in the first few months if there is no sign of spontaneous functional recovery.

Traction Injury

High-velocity traction injury secondary to a fall from a motorcycle is the leading cause of brachial plexus injury (9). This kind of injury usually causes severe damage to nerve roots. Brachial plexus exploration and surgical repair or reconstruction are indicated in patients who have no spontaneous recovery after 3 months. Time is allowed for the recovery of the low-grade injured neural tissue, subsidence of the swollen surrounding tissue, and completion of the diagnostic investigations. In complete brachial plexus palsy with strong radiologic and electrodiagnostic evidence of complete or multiple root avulsions, early surgery (6 weeks to 3 months after injury) is indicated because the chance of spontaneous recovery is less likely (25).

Low-velocity traction injury should be observed and initially treated by conservative means. Lower-velocity injuries usually have a better prognosis. Surgical exploration is indicated if no spontaneous recovery or progression of Tinel's sign is observed in 3 months.

Radiation Injury

Surgical exploration is occasionally indicated in postradiation brachial plexopathy with progressive neurologic deficit and intractable pain. Surgical exploration is difficult because of the ischemic and fibrotic nature of the surrounding tissue. Results in terms of pain relief and functional improvement cannot be guaranteed. The risk of downgrading the existed limb function should be well considered.

Timing of Surgery

Immediate surgery of the brachial plexus should only be performed in an associated brachial plexus injury (closed or penetrating) with subclavian or axillary vessel injury. A complete exploration to assess the degree of damage to the plexus should be done with emergency vascular reconstruction by a vascular surgeon so that neurorrhaphy or nerve grafting can be performed without the risk of iatrogenic vascular damage. If immediate brachial plexus reconstruction is not possible, the damaged part of the brachial plexus should be identified, and the nerve stumps should be tagged and relocated away from the vascular reconstruction site to minimize the risk of vascular injury in the secondary nerve grafting procedure.

Early surgery (6 weeks to 3 months) should be performed in complete brachial palsy patients with total root avulsion. For incomplete brachial plexus palsy or complete brachial plexus palsy without evidence of root avulsion, exploration should be performed when there is no sign of clinical recovery or the initial recovery stopped after an observation period of 4 to 5 months. The result of operative nerve repair and reconstruction is greatly diminished after a 6-month interval between injury and operation. Six months from the time of injury, free muscle transfers should be considered.

Operative Technique

Patient Preparation and Positioning

The patient should be informed about the operative procedure, postoperative rehabilitation program, success rate, and long recovery time. The routine preoperative evaluation is completed. Autologous blood is donated for intraoperative transfusion in the event of inadvertent injury to blood vessels, although the need is rare.

The operation is performed under general intubation anesthesia without long-acting muscle relaxant. The patient is placed supine on the operating table with the upper part of the body slightly elevated. A flat pillow is placed behind the ipsilateral scapula. The head is turned halfway toward the unaffected side with the neck slightly extended. Prepping and draping should allow extensile exposure of the neck, shoulder, chest, and axilla. The affected arm is draped in such a fashion that allows it to be moved freely. Both lower extremities are also prepared for harvesting of sural nerves, should nerve grafts be required. Well-padded pneumatic tourniquets are placed on both thighs but left uninflated. An indwelling urinary catheter is inserted. The use of an optical aid (i.e., an operating microscope or magnifying loupe) is highly suggested.

Surgical Exposure

The incision begins at a point 3 fingerbreadths below the mastoid process on the posterior border of the sternocleidomastoid muscle and descends along the muscle to the clavicle. It then turns laterally 1 fingerbreadth below and parallel to the clavicle to the coracoid process to enter the deltopectoral groove. The lower limb of the incision can be extended along the anterior axillary fold to the medial aspect of the upper arm if necessary.

The platysma muscle is incised along the skin incision. The skin flap, including the platysma muscle, is carefully raised. The external jugular vein is identified and preserved. The sternocleidomastoid muscle is exposed and retracted medially. The dissection is continued into the prescalene area. The superficial layer of the deep cervical fascia is opened. The cervical fat pad and the omohyoid muscle are retracted downward and medially. The transverse cervical vessels are found crossing over the plexus in the posterior triangle. The vessels are ligated and divided. The anterior and middle scalene muscles are exposed. An intraoperative nerve stimulator on the anterior surface of the anterior scalene muscle can usually identify the phrenic nerve. The nerve runs parallel to the muscle fiber. The phrenic nerve is a helpful landmark in the identification of the C5 root because it can be traced upward to the level of the intervertebral foramen. The phrenic nerve is also used as a medial perimeter of the brachial plexus exploration area. Surgical dissection should not be performed medial to the nerve to prevent iatrogenic injury to vital structures in the neck. Concomitant phrenic nerve and brachial plexus lesions are occasionally found with severe injury to the brachial plexus. The C5 root is usually smaller than the C6 root. The C6 root is inferior, more medial, and less vertical in direction. The C7 root is more medial, more posterior, and horizontal in direction (Fig. 4). The C8 and T1 roots are more inferior

and posterior to the C7 root. They are closely associated with the subclavian artery. Mobilization or osteotomy of the clavicle is needed for better exposure of these two roots.

A tunnel is made from the posterior triangle of the neck under the clavicle to the deltopectoral area by gloved finger. The lateral part of the origin of the pectoralis major muscle is detached from the clavicle. The subclavius muscle is divided and tagged. Special attention should be paid in a patient with a healed clavicle fracture. Blunt dissection underneath the clavicle can be difficult because of the fibrotic nature of the soft tissue. The risk of major vascular and pleural damage must be considered. The middle part of the clavicle is freed from the surrounding soft tissue. The clavicle can be mobilized upward or downward by a retractor. If clavicle ostomy is needed, predrilling of the screws for a plate fixation should be made before division of the clavicle. The infraclavicular exploration is done by further dissection of the deltopectoral interval. The cephalic vein is preserved and retracted laterally. The proximal half of the tendinous insertion of the pectoralis major and clavipectoral fascia is divided. The pectoralis minor muscle is exposed, and its tendinous attachment at the coracoid process is divided and tagged for a later pull-through coracoid process repair. The distal part of the brachial plexus and major vessels are exposed.

Functional Priorities in Brachial Plexus Reconstruction

A complete functional recovery is an ultimate goal in the treatment of brachial plexus injury. However, in most of our patients, this goal cannot be achieved due to the severity of injuries and restriction of donor nerves. The priorities of functional reconstruction in brachial plexus injury have been set as follows (25):

1. Elbow flexion
2. Shoulder abduction
3. Wrist and finger flexion and sensation in the median nerve distribution
4. Wrist and finger extension
5. Intrinsic muscle function

Intraoperative Decision

Lesions in Continuity

Once brachial plexus exploration is performed and lesions in continuity are encountered, neurolysis is indicated. External neurolysis is indicated in Sunderland's first- and second-degree lesions with evidence of external scar compression. Internal neurolysis is indicated in intraneural fibrosis.

Loss of Continuity Lesion

An intraoperative finding of a sharp clean injury of the brachial plexus can be successfully treated with direct neurorrhaphy.

Laceration or rupture at any level of brachial plexus causes a neuroma formation. Nerve grafting is indicated after the neuroma is resected until normal nerve tissue is found on the nerve stump. Root avulsion injury of the brachial plexus cannot be repaired with neurorrhaphy; however, functional reconstruction can be performed by nerve transfer (neurotization) or functional free muscle transfer to muscle function (26).

Surgical Technique

Neurolysis

Although lesions in continuity with evidence of external compression can be successfully treated with neurolysis, the true benefit of this procedure remains controversial because of uncertain and inconsistent results. External neurolysis is performed by microsurgical dissection of the surrounding fibrotic tissue to free the intact neural tissue within the epineurium. A complete disruption of intrafascicular tissue may be undetected under the apparently intact epineurium by performing only external neurolysis. After external neurolysis is completed, internal neurolysis is performed via longitudinal splitting of the fibrotic epifascicular epineurium. If normal fascicles are found, no further dissection is needed. If fascicular and interfascicular fibrosis is present, epifascicular epineurium and interfascicular fibrous tissue are resected. After this procedure, if the fascicular integrity remains doubtful, the segment should be resected and grafted. Intraneural neurolysis carries a risk of devascularization of the fascicle, which may result in recurrent fibrosis.

Neurorrhaphy

Neurorrhaphy is indicated in sharp penetrating brachial plexus injury. The procedure gives a very good result in sharp clean transection. Group fascicular orientation and direct suture can be easily performed if the lesion is treated immediately after injury. In most of the recent studies, few patients sustained this kind of injury.

Nerve Grafting (Intraplexal Grafting)

The most common type of brachial plexus injury has been traction. This kind of injury usually causes root avulsion or rupture of plexal structure. Direct neurorrhaphy is usually impossible because of the nature of neural tissue rupture. The injured nerve stumps must be resected until normal nerve tissue is observed and continuity is restored by intercalated nerve grafting (Fig. 13). The choice of donor nerve for grafting depends on availability and the requirements of the individual patient. The commonly used donors for nonvascularized brachial plexus nerve grafting include the following:

Sural Nerve
The sural nerve of both legs can be used. The skin incision is made from the posterior border of the lateral malleolus to the middle part of the popliteal fossa. Multiple small transverse incisions can be used to avoid unsightly longitudinal scars (Fig. 14). In adults, up to 30 to 36 cm of sural nerve can be harvested from each leg. To maximize revascularization, the sural graft is carefully cleaned of all surrounding tissue, keeping only the epineurium.

Ulnar Nerve of the Ipsilateral Side
In patients with complete avulsion of the lower roots, there is no possibility of spontaneous recovery, and the chance of successful restoration of intrinsic function after nerve reconstruction is very minimal, so the ulnar nerve can be used as a nerve graft. In free nerve grafting, the ulnar nerve

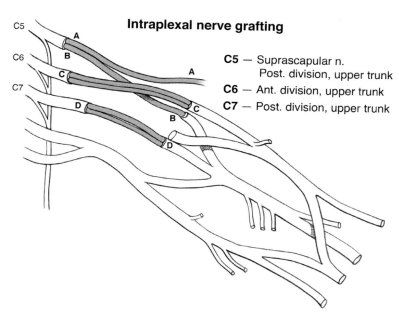

Intraplexal nerve grafting

C5 — Suprascapular n.
      Post. division, upper trunk
C6 — Ant. division, upper trunk
C7 — Post. division, upper trunk

FIGURE 13. In the event that viable and functioning nerve roots are identified (i.e., postganglionic injuries), intraplexal nerve grafting can be performed to target key functions. Illustrated is a postganglionic injury of the fifth, sixth, and seventh cervical nerve (C5–C7) roots. In such a case, the C5 can be used to restore shoulder function [suprascapular nerve (A) and axillary nerve (B) via posterior division of the upper trunk], the C6 can be used for elbow flexion (C), and the C7 can be used for elbow extension and wrist extension (D). Ant., anterior; n., nerve; Post., posterior.

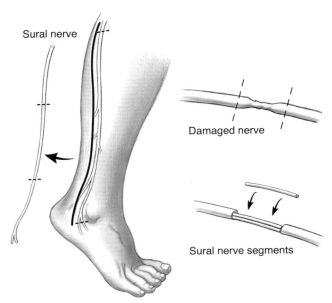

Sural nerve

Damaged nerve

Sural nerve segments

FIGURE 14. Sural nerve graft is harvested from the posterior lateral aspect of the leg. Up to 30 to 35 cm of graft can be easily obtained and used for interposition nerve grafting.

sheath should be divided longitudinally and removed. The nerve is carefully dissected under magnification into fascicle groups, which are used as an individual nerve graft for better revascularization.

Medial Cutaneous Nerve of the Forearm of the Ipsilateral Side

The nerve is harvested through a longitudinal incision on the medial aspect of the arm from its origin at the medial cord adjacent to the ulnar nerve down to the elbow.

Lateral Cutaneous Nerve of the Forearm of the Ipsilateral Side

The cutaneous terminal branch of the musculocutaneous nerve is harvested through a medial longitudinal incision of the affected arm.

Superficial Radial Nerve of the Ipsilateral Side

The superficial radial nerve is the cutaneous continuation of the radial nerve into the forearm. It can be harvested through a longitudinal incision along the anterolateral side of the forearm over the brachioradialis muscle.

Vascularized Nerve Graft

To improve the result of nerve grafting, particularly in situations in which a long nerve graft is required and the tissue bed is heavily scarred with poor vascularity, the technique of free vascularized nerve grafting was introduced. In 1976, Taylor and Ham generated significant interest in the application of this technique to repair lesions of the brachial plexus (27). Since then, experimental and clinical studies

have been performed. However, indications for the use of vascularized nerve grafts in surgical reconstruction of the brachial plexus remain controversial. One of the indications that is widely accepted for the use of vascularized nerve grafts in brachial plexus reconstruction is in the contralateral C7 (hemi- or whole) transfer to the ipsilateral side. In these cases, the gap between nerve endings is often greater than 20 cm.

The donor nerves that have been described for vascularized nerve grafts include the superficial radial nerve, the sural nerve, the superficial peroneal nerve, the anterior tibial nerve, the saphenous nerve, and the ulnar nerve.

The best indication for the use of a vascularized ulnar nerve graft in brachial plexus surgery is a preganglionic injury (avulsion) of the C8 and T1 roots. In such cases, there is no possibility of spontaneous recovery, and the result of nerve transfer for restoration of the ulnar innervated motor and sensory function has generally been very poor. The ulnar nerve can be used as a vascularized pedicle graft based on the superior ulnar collateral artery in the proximal arm or a free vascularized graft using the ulnar vessels as the pedicle (Fig. 15). Before harvesting a free vascularized ulnar nerve graft, it is necessary to establish the patency of the radial artery. The ulnar nerve in the forearm can be taken through a medial longitudinal incision extending from the axilla to the ulnar volar aspect of the wrist.

Nerve Transfer or Neurotization

Nerve transfers can be performed for preganglionic avulsion injuries. Alternatively, they are also increasingly being used to accelerate recovery by decreasing the time for reinnervation to occur by decreasing the distance between the site of nerve repair and the end organ. A functioning but less important nerve is transferred to the distal but more important denervated nerve. Ideally, nerve transfers should be performed before 6 months postinjury but may be better suited than grafting (due to the shortened time frame) in situations after the preferred 6-month time frame.

A variety of donor nerves exist as a source for neurotization. Some of the more common neurotization sources include the spinal accessory nerve (cranial nerve XI), the intercostal nerves (motor and sensory), and the medial pectoral nerve. More recently, the use of a fascicle of a functioning ulnar nerve (Oberlin transfer) or the median nerve in patients with intact C8 and T1 has allowed a rapid and powerful return of elbow flexion. In the 1990s, the use of the phrenic nerve (28) and the contralateral C7 (or hemicontralateral C7) was described (29) in an effort to expand the pool of extraplexal donors and improve outcomes. Some have also reported on the use of other sources, including the deep cervical plexus and hypoglossal nerve (cranial nerve XII).

The average number of myelinated axons in these donor nerves varies. Typically, the spinal accessory nerve has

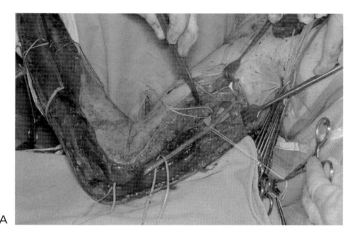

A

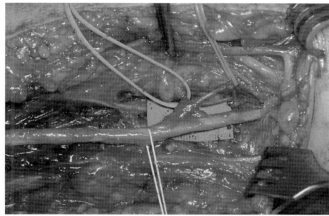

B

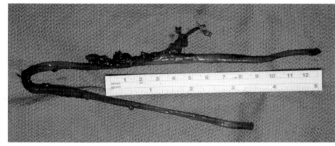

C

FIGURE 15. The ulnar nerve can be used as a vascularized pedicle nerve graft as well as a free vascularized nerve graft. The ulnar nerve is isolated over its entire course **(A)**, and the vascular pedicle based on the superior collateral artery is identified and protected **(B)**. A greater than 20-cm free vascularized ulnar nerve graft can be harvested and used to span significant nerve defects **(C)**.

approximately 1,700 axons, the phrenic has approximately 800 axons, a single intercostal motor nerve has approximately 1,300 axons, and the contralateral C7 has approximately 23,781 axons (30). The goal is to maximize the number of myelinated axons per target function, with as minimal donor site morbidity as possible. Several series have reported an acceptable morbidity of the contralateral C7 and the phrenic nerve, but long-term studies are not available.

Neurotization for shoulder abduction can be easily obtained via nerve transfer of the spinal accessory nerve or the phrenic nerve to the suprascapular nerve. The benefit of these two transfers is that no additional interposition nerve grafts are needed, and a direct coaptation of the nerves is possible (Fig. 16). If additional nerve sources are available, neurotization of the axillary nerve (or nerve grafting from C5) is recommended to give further stability and abduction for the shoulder.

Neurotization for elbow flexion can be performed using intercostal nerves (Fig. 17) directly or the spinal accessory nerve via an interpositional graft. By separating the biceps motor branch from the lateral antebrachial cutaneous nerve in a retrograde manner, the maximum number of motor axons can be transferred directly to the biceps muscle. This technique also helps gain length for the transfer, which eliminates the need for interpositional grafts in the case of intercostal nerves and shortens the length of the graft for the accessory nerve. The phrenic nerve can also be used with an interpositional graft to the musculocutaneous nerve.

In the event of an upper trunk avulsion injury, two popular options exist for reconstruction of elbow flexion. The medial pectoral nerve may be transferred to the musculocutaneous nerve or the biceps branch. Alternatively, a fascicle from the ulnar nerve (Oberlin transfer) can be transferred to the motor branch of the biceps with excellent results (Fig. 18) (31). This technique is an excellent alternative to the previously described neurotizations.

A contralateral or hemicontralateral C7 can be used via a vascularized ulnar nerve graft (in the case of a complete plexus avulsion injury) or via sural nerve grafts to bring a large number of motor axons to the injured side (29,32). When used with the vascularized ulnar nerve graft, a contralateral or hemicontralateral C7 can be used to innervate the median nerve in the hopes of obtaining useful finger flexion and protective sensation in the median nerve distribution (Fig. 19).

Postoperative Care for Nerve Repair and Grafting

The surgically treated limb is immobilized in a Velpeau bandage and shoulder immobilizer for 3 to 4 weeks. The postoperative physiotherapy is started after 4 weeks with passive motion of all the joints of the upper extremity to maintain joint mobility. Maximal passive shoulder movement is avoided for 6 weeks. Electrical stimulation is applied to paralyzed muscles until clinical motor recovery is observed. The patient is evaluated regularly, and if there are early signs of motor recovery, active muscle exercise is begun. The training with biofeedback is useful for patients to have better control of reinnervated muscles in cases of antagonistic cocontraction.

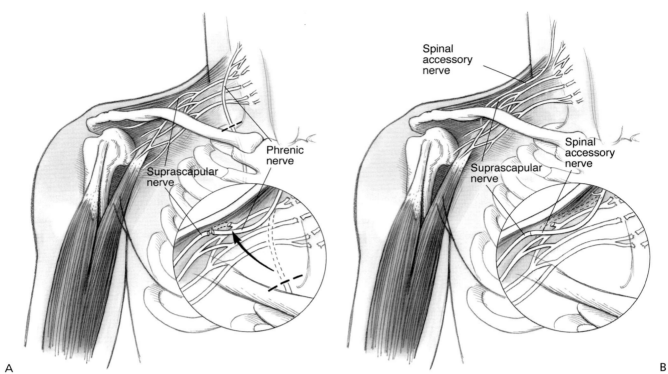

FIGURE 16. Restoration of shoulder abduction can be performed by neurotization of the suprascapular nerve with either the phrenic nerve **(A)** or the spinal accessory nerve **(B)**.

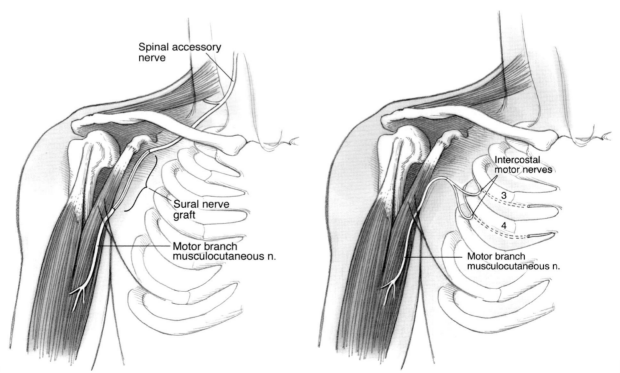

FIGURE 17. Neurotization of the biceps can be performed by use of the spinal accessory nerve with an interposition graft **(A)**, phrenic nerve with graft, or the intercostal motor nerves **(B)**. n., nerve.

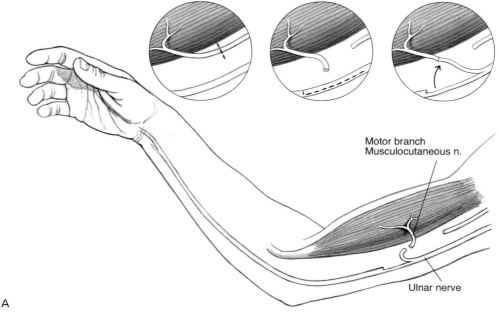

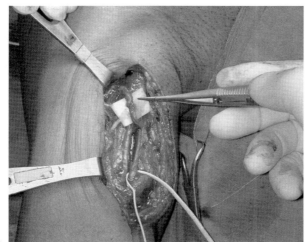

FIGURE 18. A: When the ulnar nerve is normal (i.e., upper trunk injury sparing the eighth cervical and first thoracic nerve), a fascicle can be transferred to the motor branch of the biceps to obtain elbow flexion. **B:** A clinical example demonstrating the fascicles from the ulnar nerve transferred to the motor branch of the biceps. n., nerve.

RESULT

In supraclavicular lesion paralyses affecting the upper roots, nerve repair and nerve grafting give a very good result (75% to 80% MRC grade 3 or better recovery). The involvement of the upper trunk (C5 and C6 roots) in the interscalene region enables nerve repair or nerve grafting with maximum success because the lesions are closer to the motor target, and affected motor functions are generally less complicated than lesions of the lower roots. Results of reinnervation of the proximal muscles of the shoulder and elbow are much better than those obtained by all possible palliative operations. The results of nerve grafting of the middle and lower root lesions are much less favorable.

In retroclavicular and infraclavicular lesions, the results of nerve grafting in lesions relatively close to the innervated muscle, such as suprascapular nerve, axillary nerve, and musculocutaneous nerve lesions, are generally good. A satisfactory (MRC grade 3 or better) motor recovery in 70% to 80% of cases can be expected. The results of nerve grafting in lesions distant from the innervated muscle, such as lateral, medial, and posterior cord and median, radial, and ulnar nerve lesions, are rather uncertain. MRC grade 3 or better motor reinnervation of the wrist and digital flexors and extensors can be expected in 50% to 60% of cases, but no reinnervation of the intrinsic muscles of the hand. MRC grade 3 or better sensory reinnervation in the median nerve area can be expected in 70% to 80% of cases.

Neurotization for elbow flexion and shoulder stability has been demonstrated to be an effective means of restoring muscle function. In a critical metaanalysis of the English literature, Merrell and coauthors evaluated the results of 1,028 nerve transfers in 27 studies to determine the outcome of nerve transfers of the shoulder and elbow (33).

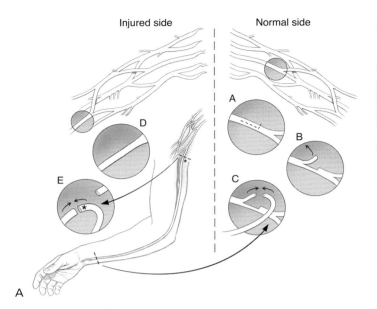

Injured side | Normal side

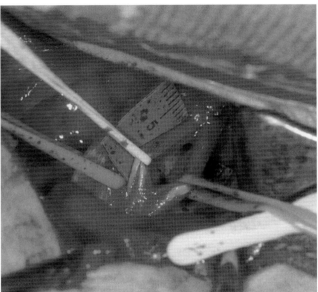

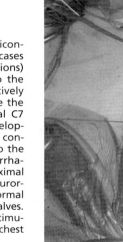

FIGURE 19. Contralateral C7 (or, as the authors prefer, hemicontralateral C7) transfer via a vascularized ulnar nerve graft (in cases of complete fifth cervical through first thoracic nerve avulsions) can be used to bring a large number of motor axons into the injured side. **A:** The hemicontralateral C7 transfer can effectively be used with a vascularized ulnar nerve graft to reinnervate the median nerve for finger flexion and sensation. The normal C7 root is exposed and partially transected (*A*), allowing development of a proximally based fascicular bundle (*B*). The injured contralateral ulnar nerve is transected distally (*D*) and passed to the normal C7 partial transection site, where it undergoes neurorrhaphy to the proximally based C7 fascicular bundle (*C*). The proximal ulnar nerve is transected, and the distal cut end undergoes neurorrhaphy to the median nerve (*E*). **B:** A clinical example of the normal side of the seventh cervical nerve (C7) being split into two halves. The half that results in the least hand motor function when stimulated is used. **C:** A vascularized ulnar nerve reaching across the chest to the contralateral C7 is harvested and mobilized.

For restoration of elbow flexion, 26 studies with 965 nerve transfers were evaluated. Overall, 71% of transfers to the musculocutaneous nerve achieved ≥M3 (antigravity) flexion, and 37% achieved ≥M4 (against gravity, not normal) flexion. The two most common donor nerves were the intercostal (54%) and the spinal accessory (39%). Overall, the intercostal nerves achieved ≥M3 in 72% of patients. If an interposition nerve graft was used, then only 47% achieved ≥M3 results. If a spinal accessory nerve was transferred to the musculocutaneous nerve, 77% of patients had restoration of elbow flexion of ≥M3, and 29% with ≥M4. Oberlin's transfer (two fascicles of the ulnar nerve to musculocutaneous nerve) resulted in 97% ≥M3 flexion, and 94% ≥M4 flexion.

For restoration of shoulder abduction, there were eight studies with 123 transfers. Overall, 73% of patients had

achieved ≥M3 shoulder abduction, and 26% achieved ≥M4 abduction. The spinal accessory nerve was used in 41% and the intercostal nerves in 26%. The spinal accessory nerve (98%) is significantly better than intercostal nerves (56%) in achieving ≥M3 abduction. Good results, however, only provide approximately 45 degrees of shoulder abduction.

REFERENCES

1. Kerr A. Brachial plexus of nerves in man. The variations in its formation and branches. *Am J Anat* 1918;23:285–395.
2. Warwick R, Williams PL, eds. *Gray's anatomy*, 35th ed. Philadelphia: Saunders, 1973:1037–1047.
3. Kaplan E, Spinner M. Normal and anomalous innervation

patterns in the upper extremity. In: Omer G, Spinner M, eds. *Management of peripheral nerve problems.* Philadelphia: Saunders, 1980.

4. Durward A. The peripheral nervous system. In: Romanes GJ, ed. *Cunningham's textbook of anatomy,* 10th ed. London: Oxford University Press, 1964:685–984.
5. Masear VR, Meyer RD, Pichora DR. Surgical anatomy of the medial antebrachial cutaneous nerve. *J Hand Surg [Am]* 1989;14:267–271.
6. McHenry LC. *Garrison's history of neurology.* Spingfield: C.C. Thomas, 1969.
7. Malessy MJA. *Brachial plexus surgery: factors affecting functional recovery.* Den Haag: Pasmans BV, 1999.
8. Alnot JY. Traumatic paralysis of the brachial plexus: preoperative problems and therapeutic indications. In: Terzis JK, ed. Microreconstruction of nerve injuries. Philadelphia: W.B. Saunders, 1987:325–345.
9. Songcharoen P. Brachial plexus injury in Thailand: a report of 520 cases. *Microsurgery* 1995;16:35–39.
10. Sunderland S. Mechanisms of cervical nerve root avulsion in injuries of the neck and shoulder. *J Neurosurg* 1974;41:705–714.
11. Cooper DE. Nerve injury associated with patient positioning in the operating room. In: Gelberman RH, ed. *Operative nerve repair and reconstruction.* Philadelphia: J.B. Lippincott, 1991:1231–1242.
12. Cooper DE, Jenkins RS, Bready L, et al. The prevention of injuries of the brachial plexus secondary to malposition of the patient during surgery. *Clin Orthop* 1988:33–41.
13. Omer G. War wounds of the hand. In: Tubiana R, ed. *The hand,* vol. 3. Philadelphia: W.B. Saunders, 1988:923–924.
14. Fackler ML. Ballistic injury. *Ann Emerg Med* 1986;15:1451–1455.
15. Fackler ML. Civilian gunshot wounds. *Orthopedics* 1986;9:1336–1342.
16. Fackler ML, Bellamy RF, Malinowski JA. Wounding mechanism of projectiles striking at more than 1.5 km/sec. *J Trauma* 1986;26:250–254.
17. Maruyama Y, Mylrea MM, Logothetis J. Neuropathy following irradiation. An unusual late complication of radiotherapy. *Am J Roentgenol Radium Ther Nucl Med* 1967;101:216–219.
18. Chechick A, Amit Y, Shaked I, et al. Brown-Sequard syndrome associated with brachial plexus injury in neck trauma. *J Trauma* 1982;22:430–431.
19. Hentz VR, Narakas A. The results of microneurosurgical reconstruction in complete brachial plexus palsy. Assessing

outcome and predicting results. *Orthop Clin North Am* 1988;19:107–114.
20. Narakas AO. The surgical treatment of traumatic brachial plexus lesions. *Int Surg* 1980;65:521–527.
21. Nagano A, Ochiai N, Sugioka H, et al. Usefulness of myelography in brachial plexus injuries. *J Hand Surg [Br]* 1989;14:59–64.
22. Carvalho GA, Nikkhah G, Matthies C, et al. Diagnosis of root avulsions in traumatic brachial plexus injuries: value of computerized tomography myelography and magnetic resonance imaging. *J Neurosurg* 1997;86:69–76.
23. Bufalini C, Pescatori G. Posterior cervical electromyography in the diagnosis and prognosis of brachial plexus injuries. *J Bone Joint Surg Br* 1969;51:627–631.
24. Sugioka H, Tsuyama N, Hara T, et al. Investigation of brachial plexus injuries by intraoperative cortical somatosensory evoked potentials. *Arch Orthop Trauma Surg* 1982;99:143–151.
25. Narakas A. The surgical management of brachial plexus injuries. In: Daniel RK, Terzis JK, eds. *Reconstructive microsurgery.* Boston: Little, Brown and Co., 1977:443–460.
26. Narakas AO, Hentz VR. Neurotization in brachial plexus injuries. Indication and results [Review]. *Clin Orthop* 1988:43–56.
27. Taylor GI, Ham FJ. The free vascularized nerve graft. A further experimental and clinical application of microvascular techniques. *Plast Reconstruct Surg* 1976;57:413–426.
28. Gu YD, Ma MK. Use of the phrenic nerve for brachial plexus reconstruction. *Clin Orthop* 1996:119–121.
29. Gu YD, Chen DS, Zhang GM, et al. Long-term functional results of contralateral C7 transfer. *J Reconstr Microsurg* 1998;14:57–59.
30. Chuang DC. Neurotization procedures for brachial plexus injuries. *Hand Clin* 1995;11:633–645
31. Oberlin C, Beal D, Leechavengvongs S, et al. Nerve transfer to biceps muscle using a part of ulnar nerve for C5-C6 avulsion of the brachial plexus: anatomical study and report of four cases. *J Hand Surg [Am]* 1994;19:232–237.
32. Songcharoen P, Wongtrakul S, Mahaisavariya B, et al. Hemi-contralateral C7 transfer to median nerve in the treatment of root avulsion brachial plexus injury. *J Hand Surg [Am]* 2001;26:1058–1064.
33. Merrell GA, Barrie KA, Katz DL, et al. Results of nerve transfer techniques for restoration of shoulder and elbow function in the context of a meta-analysis of the English literature. *J Hand Surg [Am]* 2001;26:303–314.

58

BRACHIAL PLEXUS: NEUROTIZATION AND PEDICLE MUSCLE TRANSFER

CHWEI CHIN DAVID CHUANG

Spinal nerve avulsions from the cord surface (true avulsion) (1), or from the intraforaminal roots or rootlet filaments, occur frequently in brachial plexus injuries (2–5), thus leading to a lack of available central connections and becoming irreparable lesions. Nerve transfer (or neurotization), pedicle muscle transfer, or functioning free muscle transplantation possibly produce the only chances for functional restoration. *Neurotization* means transfer of a physiologically active nerve that can be functionally spared to the distal, but more important, irreparable denervated nerve within a time interval after injury in which muscle reactivation is possible. *Pedicle muscle transfer* is a transfer of a regional and functional muscle to replace a denervated and atrophic muscle or muscle group for the major important function, such as shoulder elevation or elbow flexion. *Functioning free muscle transplantation* implies the need for microneurovascular anastomoses to transfer a distant normal muscle to replace the function of a destroyed or chronically denervated muscle or muscle group in the paralyzed limb.

Neurotization (or nerve transfer) has two major categories: intraplexus neurotization and extraplexus neurotization (6,7). *Intraplexus neurotization* is applied in the nonglobal avulsion (one- to four-root avulsion) and implies transfer of a functional spinal nerve or a branch nerve, which may have ruptured, to a more important denervated nerve, such as a proximal C5 spinal nerve–to–median nerve transfer, a long thoracic nerve–to–suprascapular nerve transfer, or part of an ulnar nerve–to–musculocutaneous nerve transfer. *Extraplexus neurotization* means transfer of a non–brachial plexus component nerve to the brachial plexus for neurotization of an avulsed nerve. The reported donor nerves (7,8) in common use are the phrenic (Ph) nerve (9), the spinal accessory nerve (10), the deep motor branches of the cervical plexus (11), the intercostal (IC) nerve (12), the hypoglossal nerve (13), and the contralateral C7 spinal nerve (14). Other donor nerves, which are reported but not popular (7), include the greater occipital nerve, the anterior thoracic nerve, the long thoracic nerve, the thoracodorsal nerve, the inferior ramus of the subscapular nerve, the ramus for leva-tor scapular, and the contralateral pectoral nerves. Other neurotization techniques include neuromuscular neurotization (direct implantation of motor nerve fascicles into denervated muscle), end-to-side neurotization (implanting the distal stump of an irreparably injured nerve into healthy nerve), and sensory neurotization.

From 1986 to 1997 (a 12-year period), 955 adult patients with brachial plexus injury were operated on (based on the operation date) by the same surgeon (D. C. C. Chuang). Seventy-five percent of the cases involved preganglionic root injuries. The author presents in this chapter the author's philosophy of the application of nerve transfer technique in brachial plexus injuries for the restoration of shoulder, elbow, and hand function, comparing its advantages and disadvantages with regional pedicle functional muscle transfer and distant free functioning muscle transplantation.

EXTRAPLEXUS NEUROTIZATION

Anatomy and Surgical Access of the Available Donor Nerves

Intercostal Nerve

IC nerve transfer was introduced by Yeoman and Seddon (12) but was sparked by Japanese doctors (15–17) and the author (18,19). The IC nerve is located beneath the periosteum after dissection through the external and internal IC muscles (Fig. 1). Each IC nerve has two main branches: the deep central and superficial lateral branches. The deep central branch (mostly motor) goes along the rib: in T1 through T3, it is located at the upper margin of the rib; in T4 through T6, it is located at the lower margin and behind the rib; in T7 and lower, it is located in the IC muscles and is inferior to the rib. The superficial lateral branch (mostly sensory) branches out from the deep central branch at the anterior axillary line and courses inferiorly and laterally to the skin. Deep central branches are usually divided

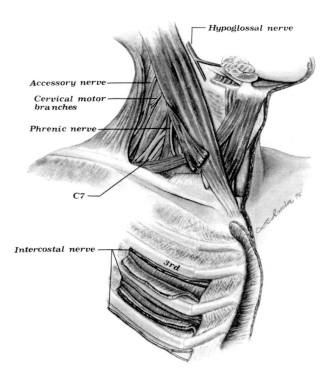

Hypoglossal nerve

Accessory nerve

Cervical motor branches

Phrenic nerve

C7

Intercostal nerve

3rd

FIGURE 1. Anatomic relationship of the available donor nerves and the brachial plexus.

at the costochondral junction and are transferred for neurotization. The IC nerve has often been transferred to neurotize the musculocutaneous nerve or the median nerve or in a functioning free muscle transplantation. The ideal number of IC nerves to use for nerve transfer is unclear. Dolenc (20) used one or two nerves, Seddon (21) used two nerves with nerve grafts, Tsuyama et al. (15) and Nagano et al. (16) used two nerves without nerve grafts, and Narakas et al. (22) used three to four nerves with nerve grafts. The author (18) prefers three nerves without nerve grafts to neurotize the musculocutaneous nerve for elbow flexion. One IC nerve contains 1,200 to 1,300 myelinated fibers, whereas the musculocutaneous nerve contains about 6,000 fibers (23,24). Transfer of three IC nerves without nerve grafts for neurotization of the musculocutaneous nerve and for free muscle transplantation neurotization is recommended (19). Transfer of three to five IC nerves without nerve grafts for median nerve neurotization is recommended. IC nerve transfer to the trunk or cord or IC nerve transfer to the radial or axillary nerve usually ends with poor results (M <3) without definite reasons. There is no difference between using the upper segment IC nerves (T1 through T4) or lower-segment IC nerves (T5 through T7). The T3 IC nerve usually has more terminal branches (two to four), whereas the T4 through T6 nerves have one or two fascicles at the costochondral junction. T3, T4, and T5 IC nerves can be attached with less tension than T2, T6, and T7 nerves and are recommended for transfer.

The author prefers a semicircular incision, extending from the usual incision for brachial plexus exploration, at the anterior border of the axilla onto the infraareolar (in men) or the inframammary fold (in women) to gain access to the IC nerve (18). The mass of adipose tissue is removed from the axillary fossa, which is bounded by the basilar or subclavian vein superiorly, the pectoral minor muscle medially, the anterior thoracic vessel posteriorly, and the subcutaneous layers of the elevated skin flap laterally. This creates a space for subsequent nerve repair. The pectoralis major (PM) muscle is elevated, and the pectoralis minor muscles may be partially detached from their insertions. The rib periosteum is incised along the lower rib margin, and the posterior periosteum is elevated from the rib. The deep central branch of the IC nerve is then easily found by following the linear opening of the periosteum. Direct suture of IC nerves to the target nerve without nerve grafts is the key to good results (M >3). Several techniques have been described to deal with the unequal diameters of the IC nerves and target nerve (15,18,25). The success rate for IC nerve–to–musculocutaneous nerve transfer to gain M4 muscle strength is approximately 70% to 90%, as of 2003. The morbidity that is associated with IC nerve harvest is minimal.

Spinal Accessory (Eleventh Cranial) Nerve

The spinal accessory (eleventh cranial) nerve is the motor nerve of the sternocleidomastoid and trapezius muscles. It is usually, but not always, well protected in trauma that affects the brachial plexus. Proximally, the eleventh cranial nerve can usually be found at the lateral margin of the sternocleidomastoid muscle, at a point within one finger breadth above the emergence point of the greater auricular nerve, which goes in the cephalad direction on the sternocleidomastoid muscle. Multiple divisions of the cervical plexus also emerge from beneath the sternocleidomastoid muscle, travel caudally toward the clavicle, and are all sensory nerves. Nerve stimulation can confirm the identity of the eleventh cranial nerve. This exploration requires upward and posterior extension of the regular **C**-shaped skin incision. Alternatively, the eleventh cranial nerve can also be found subcutaneously on the volar and lateral margin of the trapezius muscle surface, close to the lateral end of the clavicle, by following the regular open wound. Once the eleventh cranial nerve is found, it is dissected as distally as possible. At a level close to the clavicle, two or three terminal muscular rami that enter into the muscle are seen, and the nerve is divided at this point and is moved for transfer. A sensory branch from the cervical plexus, which joins the eleventh cranial nerve before its terminal branching, is usually seen and should be excluded. The branches to the sternocleidomastoid muscle and the first ramus to the upper trapezius are generally spared to preserve the function of the sternocleidomastoid and some part of the trapezius. The eleventh cranial nerve has approximately 2,000 myelinated fibers at the point that is located after the sternocleidomastoid muscle and 1,300 to 1,600 fibers at the point that is located close to the clavicle (7). The eleventh cranial nerve is commonly transferred to the suprascapular nerve or axillary nerve for shoulder function (7,26–28) or to the musculocutaneous nerve to restore elbow flexion (10,17) or to innervate a free muscle transplantation for elbow simultaneous flexion and finger extension (29). Transection of the eleventh cranial nerve distal to the first branch to the trapezius can avoid complete denervation of the trapezius, which is an important stabilizer and rotator of the scapula.

Phrenic Nerve

The Ph nerve is the motor nerve to the diaphragm, originating chiefly from the fourth cervical nerve, and is augmented by fibers from the third and fifth cervical nerves. It lies on the ventral and medial surfaces of the scalene anterior muscle and descends obliquely over the muscle toward the medial clavicle. It is easily encountered during brachial plexus exploration. Nerve stimulation can help identify it. It can be dissected distally down to the medial clavicle by direct visualization by loupe magnification or to the diaphragm by endoscopic assisted technique. It has been frequently used as an effective neurotizer by Chinese surgeons (9,28) but is rarely used in Western countries because of the concern of decrease in pulmonary capacity after its sacrifice (7,10). According to Gu's study (9), pulmonary capacity decreased for 1 year after transection because of limited excursion and constant elevation of the diaphragm. It then recovered to normal values by 2 years postsurgery owing to compensatory mechanisms. The author has also frequently used the Ph nerve for neurotization in adult patients without any significant respiratory problems, even when neurotization was performed concomitantly with IC nerve transfer. In adults, because the diaphragm is fixed to the vertebrae, sacrificing the Ph nerve results in only mild elevation of the diaphragm, without marked respiratory complication except a sense of mild dyspnea that is experienced in the first postoperative night. In infants, however, the diaphragm is not yet fixed to the vertebral bodies, and once the Ph nerve is sacrificed, the diaphragm elevates and occupies one-half of the hemithorax and causes severe respiratory distress. This may necessitate the need for intubation and respiratory machine assistance in the first month postsurgery. Thereafter, a steady improvement is predictable for 1 year postsurgery. After 2 years of age, harvest of the Ph nerve becomes relatively safer.

The Ph nerve is a strong donor nerve and is superior to the eleventh cranial nerve and IC nerve for transfer. The reason for this superiority is not the nerve or fascicle diameter (similar to eleventh cranial) but rather its characteristics of spontaneous rhythmic impulse discharge, which simulates a continuous internal nerve stimulator (or autophysiotherapy) (9,7). The Ph nerve has been used by Gu extensively to neurotize the musculocutaneous, median, radial, or axillary nerves (9). The author has used the Ph nerve more frequently to neurotize the suprascapular nerve or the dorsal division of the upper trunk or the axillary nerve for shoulder elevation or the radial nerve for elbow extension. Endoscopically assisted harvesting of the Ph nerve is possible and may provide an adequate length for transfer to the median nerve or the ulnar nerve at the lower one-third of the forearm or wrist to gain some intrinsic muscle function of the hand.

Motor Branches of Deep Cervical Plexus

While dissecting along the Ph nerve upward to the C4 spinal nerve origin, multiple divisions of the cervical plexus, emerging and coursing downward and superficially to the clavicle, are mostly sensory nerves. Two or three deep branches, which are oriented posterolaterally to innervate the levator scapular, the rhomboid, and part of the trapezius, are motor branches, which can be found by nerve stimulation. Brunelli and Brunelli (11) count the motor fibers to be approximately 2,500 (excluding branches to the sternocleidomastoid muscle) and use the motor branches to neurotize the suprascapular and axillary nerve with nerve grafts. Some used the motor nerve branches for transfer to the long thoracic nerve (7), the pectoral nerve, or the thoracodorsal nerve (26). The author has rarely used the motor branches of the deep cervical plexus (MBCPs) alone as a sole neurotizer in his series; rather, the MBCPs have always been used in company with the eleventh cranial or Ph nerves because of the unpredictable results that are obtained from their use as sole neurotizers (28).

Hypoglossal (Twelfth Cranial) Nerve

The hypoglossal (twelfth cranial) nerve is the motor nerve of the tongue. It is located deep to the tendon of the anterior belly of the digastric muscle. Nerve stimulation can identify it from the nearby lingual nerve (sensory nerve). The twelfth cranial nerve, as a neurotizer, is mentioned briefly by Narakas (13), but no convincing paper has been published yet. The author uses it as a neurotizer only when the Ph nerve is avulsed, but the result is not convincing. It always requires a long nerve graft (greater than 10 cm in length) to the brachial plexus. It is actually a weak nerve for brachial plexus neurotization and therefore is rarely used as a sole neurotizer. The deficits of hypoglossal nerve transection are tongue atrophy and deviation (Fig. 2C), but these conditions do not interfere with eating or drinking at all.

Contralateral C7 Spinal Nerve

The C7 spinal nerve contributes to the posterior and lateral cord and to the pectoral, thoracodorsal, radial, musculocu-

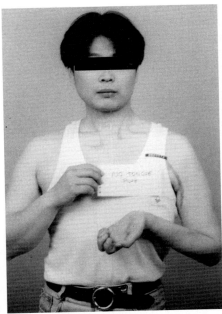
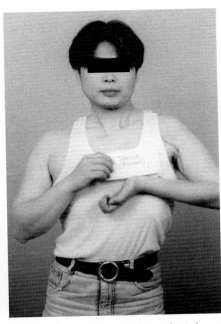
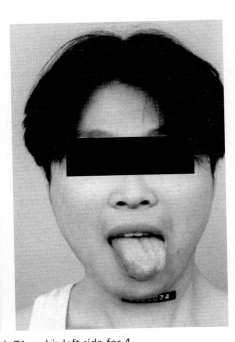

A,B

C

FIGURE 2. A 19-year-old man sustained avulsion injuries of C4 through T1 on his left side for 4 months. His eleventh cranial nerve was injured, too. He received a hypoglossal nerve–to–suprascapular nerve transfer and three intercostal nerve–to–musculocutaneous nerve transfers. **A,B:** Results of shoulder abduction and elbow flexion 2 years after surgery. **C:** Permanent deficit of tongue deviation and atrophy, which did not interfere with eating or drinking.

taneous, and median nerves (14,30). C7-innervated muscles have cross-innervation with other spinal nerves (mainly with C6 and C8 and less with C5 and T1). Because of this fact, isolated C7 severance does not result in significant loss of any specific muscle function. This has been proven by Gu (14) and Chuang (31). The contralateral neck is explored through a small **C**-shaped, curved incision along the posterior margin of the sternocleidomastoid muscle to the clavicle. The whole spinal nerves from C5 to T1 should be identified to avoid any anatomic variation and error. The predominant response from C7 stimulation causes forearm pronation, elbow extension, and shoulder adduction without any wrist and finger flexion or extension. After identifying the C7 spinal nerve, it is dissected as long as possible down to the division and is cut after the division. The proximal stump is turned upward and is fixed to the margin of the sternocleidomastoid muscle with 6-0 Prolene suture. A vascularized ulnar nerve graft can be a pedicle type or a free type and is routinely used for contralateral C7 elongation (32). A free vascularized ulnar nerve graft is preferred over a pedicled type, because the graft length that is required is shorter. A segmental ulnar nerve, including its associated ulnar vessels, is harvested from the forearm of the paralyzed limb and is approximately 20 cm in length in free graft but 30 cm in length in pedicled graft if it goes to the median nerve. It can be placed in antegrade or retrograde fashion, but a retrograde (or reverse) vascularized ulnar nerve graft is basically performed to avoid axons from sprouting out through the branches and wasting. This phenomenon

sometimes depends on the recipient vessel availability. The ulnar nerve graft can be placed through a subcutaneous tunnel or through the prevertebral space. The latter option, being more direct, can spare a length of 5 cm or more, thus reducing the regeneration period. A pedicled reverse vascularized ulnar nerve graft, which is based on the superior ulnar collateral vessel, is usually applied in cases in which the brachial plexus had been explored previously to avoid passing through the scar or is indicated in a child in whom the vessels are still rather small. The ulnar nerve is dissected from the proximal wrist, including the deep motor branch, the superficial volar digital branches, and the dorsal digital branches, upward to the proximal arm level. The ulnar artery and vein are dissected together with the ulnar nerve, are ligated, and are cut at the palmar level distally and at the upper one-third of the forearm proximally. The inferior ulnar collateral artery is also divided. The pedicled vascularized ulnar nerve is then reversed and passed through the subcutaneous tunnel from the axillary fossa to the exposed contralateral neck wound. A supercharging anastomosis of the distal ulnar artery to the contralateral transverse cervical artery is performed before coaptation of the reverse distal ulnar nerve stump to the proximal C7 stump. If the pedicled vascularized ulnar nerve graft is going to neurotize the median nerve, epineurotomy of the ulnar nerve and division of the fascicles are performed under a microscope at a suitable point in the paralytic upper arm level. The epineural tissue is kept in continuity. The median nerve is then completely transected and transferred to the epineurotomy site of the ulnar nerve and is coapted to the distal stumps of the fascicles. Gu et al. (14) used the contralateral C7 nerve to the selected nerves of the affected limb in a two-stage procedure with an interval of 8 to 12 months. We prefer to transfer the C7 to the median nerve in a one-stage procedure to restore function below the elbow in the paralytic limb for finger sensation and flexion (8,32).

INTRAPLEXUS NEUROTIZATION

Intraplexus neurotization implies application in nonglobal root avulsion, in which at least one of the spinal nerves is still available for transfer. In the global neuropathy (not total root avulsion), the proximal stumps of the ruptured spinal nerve can be transferred to the distal irreparable, but important, nerves. For example, in the case of a ruptured upper trunk that is associated with root avulsion of C7 through T1, a looped vascularized ulnar nerve graft is frequently applied to connect the proximal upper trunk to the distal musculocutaneous and median nerves (4,5). In the case of a rupture of the C5 and avulsion of the C6, the proximal C5 is frequently transferred to the anterior division of the upper trunk, instead of to the posterior division of the upper trunk, to achieve elbow flexion. Branches from the intact spinal nerves are also available for intraplexus transfer, for instance, branches from the pectoral nerves (6), branches from the long thoracic nerve (7), and fascicles from the ulnar or median nerves (33). Such intraplexus neurotization is individualized depending on the patient's condition and requirements and the surgeon's facility and philosophy.

RECONSTRUCTIVE STRATEGIES FOR NEUROTIZATION AND RESULTS

The author's result evaluation is based on the Medical Research Council scale grading system: motor (M) results range from M0 to M5, and sensory (S) results range from S0 to S4 (34). Some modifications on M3 and M4 are applied: in M1, muscle contraction is palpable or visible, but there is no movement; in M2, movement with gravity is eliminated; in M3, there is muscle contraction against gravity; in M3+, there is movement against one-finger resistance, but it occurs for less than 30 seconds; in M4, there is movement against one-finger resistance for more than 30 seconds (M4 is really a useful function; the patient uses the achieved function for daily activity); and in M5, there is movement against four-finger resistance. A successful or good result is defined as M4.

The author's experience in this article is based on 247 IC nerves, 228 spinal accessory nerves, 143 Ph nerves, 60 contralateral C7s, 26 MBCPs, 11 hypoglossal nerve extraplexus, and 29 intraplexus transfers.

Reconstructive strategies for neurotization procedures have maintained pace with time. The surgeon's philosophy

and facilities; the patient's severity of injury, age, motivation, cooperation, and rehabilitation; and the therapist's facilities and aggressiveness are all determining factors for this strategy change and evolution.

GENERAL PRINCIPLES FOR NEUROTIZATION

1. In brachial plexus injury, nerve reconstruction is always superior to palliative tendon or muscle transfer (4,35). This is why the brachial plexus injury should be explored and nerve transfer should be done in the early stages, within 5 months after the injury (8,18,28).
2. In neurotization, transfer with direct repair is always superior to nerve graft.
3. In extraplexus neurotization for shoulder abduction, the priority of choice of donor nerve is the Ph nerve, the eleventh cranial nerve, the MBCPs, and then the twelfth cranial nerve. The priority of choice of the recipient nerve is the distal C5 (Fig. 3A,B), the suprascapular nerve (Fig. 4), the dorsal division of the upper trunk (Fig. 5A), and then the axillary nerve. In extraplexus neurotization for elbow flexion, the IC nerve is always the first choice (Figs. 2B, 3D, 4B, 5B), followed by the Ph nerve, the eleventh cranial nerve, and the contralateral C7 spinal nerve, respectively. For hand function, the contralateral C7 is the first choice, followed by the Ph nerve and the IC nerve, respectively. The recipient nerve for hand function is the median nerve, followed by the radial nerve. The result from hypoglossal nerve transfer is not effective (Fig. 2A,B).
4. Ipsilateral neurotization is superior to contralateral nerve transfer. For example, ipsilateral C5– or C6–to–median nerve transfer ends with better results than contralateral C7–to–median nerve transfer (Figs. 6A,B and 7A,B).
5. In intraplexus neurotization, whether the donor nerve is healthy is the determining factor. For example, using the long thoracic nerve (from the C5, C6, and C7) to neurotize the suprascapular nerve (due to C5 and C6 palsy) is probably not a wise transfer and ends with questionable results.
6. The patient's motivation and cooperation are important. All neurotization patients need induction exercise, once the muscle has achieved M1 grade. For example, after IC or Ph nerve transfer, patients are directed and encouraged to run, walk, or climb hills to encourage deep breathing to induce more exercise of the reinnervated muscles. Exercise is always superior to electric stimulation. Similarly, shoulder-up or bend-back exercises in spinal accessory nerve transfer, tongue-to-palate push-up exercises in hypoglossal nerve transfer, and shoulder grasp exercises of the

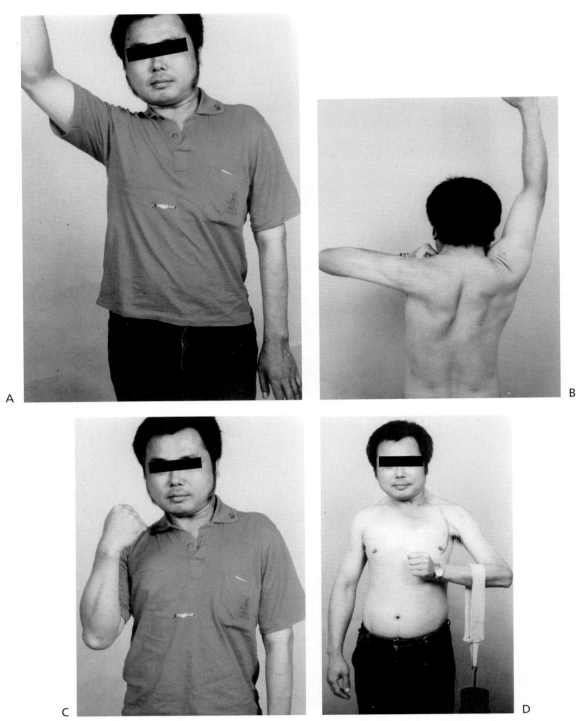

FIGURE 3. **A:** A 36-year-old man had an avulsion injury of the left C5, C6, and C7 for 4 months. **B:** 90 degrees of shoulder abduction were achieved 4 years after the combined transfer of the phrenic nerve, the motor branches of the deep cervical plexus, and the eleventh cranial nerve to the distal C5. **C:** Initially, there was no elbow flexion. **D:** The patient could elevate a 5.5-kg weight 4 years after a transfer of the T3 through T5 three intercostal nerves (T3–T5) to the musculocutaneous nerve.

healthy limb (donor limb) in contralateral C7 transfer are all exercises to induce the reinnervated muscle to exercise more. The realization of the importance of these exercises is crucial, as good results are commonly achieved by psychologically strong and ambitious patients who cooperate well in their rehabilitation programs, whereas poor results are often obtained by lazy or uncooperative patients.

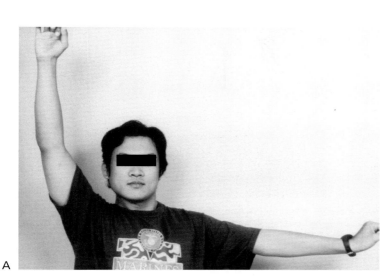
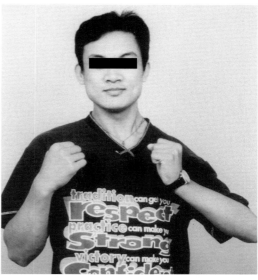

A

B

FIGURE 4. A: A 24-year-old man had left C5 and C6 root avulsion for 2 months. He received multiple nerve transfers: the eleventh cranial nerve to the suprascapular nerve, the phrenic nerve to the dorsal division of the upper trunk, and T3 through T5 intercostal nerves to the musculocutaneous nerve. The patient achieved 90 degrees of shoulder abduction and M4 elbow flexion **(B)** (lifting 5 kg of weight) 3 years after nerve reconstruction.

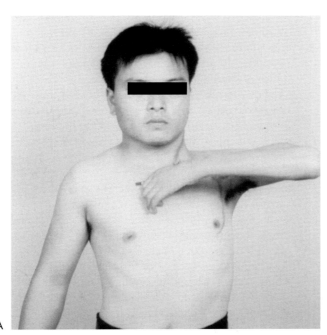
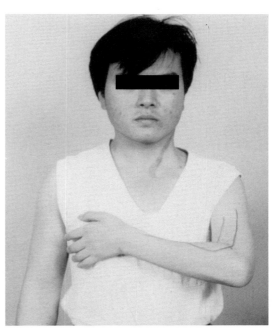

A

B

FIGURE 5. A: A 22-year-old man had a left brachial plexus injury with total root avulsion for 3 months. He received surgery with multiple nerve transfers: the eleventh cranial nerve to the suprascapular nerve, the phrenic nerve and motor branches of the deep cervical plexus to the dorsal division of the upper trunk, and T3 through T5 intercostal nerves to the musculocutaneous nerve. The patient achieved 90 degrees of shoulder abduction and M4 elbow flexion **(B)** 7 years after nerve transfers.

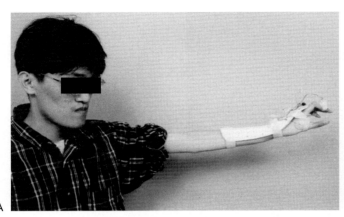
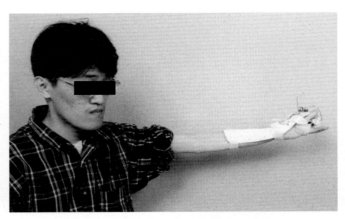

A   B

FIGURE 6. A,B: Example of results 3 years after C6 free vascularized ulnar nerve graft of the median nerve for hand function, which was impaired owing to rupture of C5 and C6, and was accompanied by C7 through T1 root avulsion. The patient needs help with interphalangeal joint extension and has a dynamic splint for hand prehension. His shoulder abduction and elbow extension were achieved by C5 intraplexus neurotization.

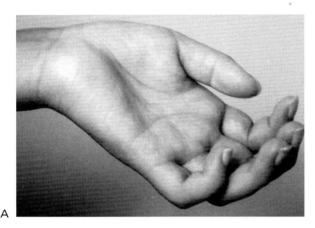

A

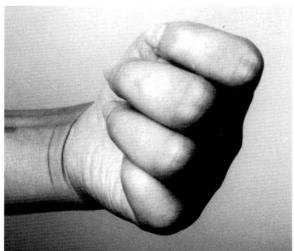

B

FIGURE 7. A,B: Example of results after C5 and C6 graft (free vascularized ulnar nerve graft) to the median nerve. The patient achieved wrist and finger flexion 2 years after intraplexus neurotization.

RATIONALE

Whether shoulder abduction or shoulder adduction is an important priority for reconstruction varies based on the surgeon's philosophy. Shoulder adduction can increase shoulder grasp power, but strong shoulder abduction can provide greater range of motion for the arm and forearm. Shoulder fusion is technically difficult, and the limited range of shoulder excursion that is achieved is not appreciated by patients. Therefore, shoulder abduction is preferred for reconstruction. However, shoulder abduction is a complex mechanism that requires synchronous coupled movements of the scapula and humerus. At least eight muscles are involved in the achievement of full abduction of the shoulder. Neurotization in upper plexus avulsion (C5, C6, or C7, or a combination of these) usually has better results than it does in global total root avulsion.

In the author's experience, if suprascapular and axillary nerves are innervated simultaneously, an average of 60 degrees of shoulder abduction in patients with total root avulsion and an average of 90 degrees or more of shoulder abduction in patients with upper root avulsion are often achieved. Because direct axillary nerve reinnervation is always required, a long nerve graft (greater than 10 cm), from the eleventh cranial or the Ph nerve, is used. The author shifts the target nerve to the dorsal division of the upper trunk, which can spare the necessity of nerve graft, and the axillary nerve reinnervation can be achieved (the axillary nerve comes from the dorsal division of the upper trunk). The Ph nerve is a strong donor nerve. When it neurotizes the dorsal division of the upper trunk, not only the deltoid muscle but also the triceps and extensor carpi radialis can be reinnervated (usually at the third year after transfer of the Ph nerve to the dorsal division of the upper trunk).

Another strategy is eleventh cranial nerve application. Doi et al. (36) developed the use of a free muscle transplantation for replacement of the extensor digitorum communis (EDC), which is innervated by the eleventh cranial nerve, and got impressive results in 1993. The author also had the same good results. Since then, in cases of total root avulsion, the eleventh cranial nerve is now spared while performing brachial plexus exploration and nerve reconstruction for free muscle transplantation of the EDC replacement in the late stage.

IC nerve transfer has been proven effective in providing musculocutaneous nerve reinnervation by the author since 1992, after his first report (18). The success rate (M >3) now ranges from 70% to 90%, with an average of 80%. Three IC nerves are still recommended as the donor nerves. The target nerve—the musculocutaneous nerve—is cut at the point at which it leaves the lateral cord, excluding the branch to the coracobrachialis muscle. The distal stump of the musculocutaneous nerve is then moved to the axillary fossa for suture to the IC nerves. Five clinical signs of functional recovery appear at different times during the postoperative course. The first earliest sign is biceps squeezing, which induces chest pain, and usually appears in the first 3 months postoperatively. The second recovery sign is biceps contraction without elbow joint movement (M1), especially during deep inspiration. This sign usually appears 3 to 6 months postoperatively. Induction exercise is then encouraged, and 2 km of walking or running per day is a minimal requirement. The third recovery sign is elbow movement with elbow support (gravity eliminated, M2) and usually appears in the second 6 months postoperatively. The fourth recovery sign is elbow flexion against gravity (M3) and appears in the third 6 months postoperatively. Once the muscle strength has reached M3, power can be increased by resistance exercises, and muscle strength steadily increases 0.5 kg every 6 months to a maximum strength of 3 to 6 kg of weight lifting (Fig. 3D).

IC nerves to innervate a free muscle transplant for elbow flexion are still a good option in the chronic cases (19). The success rate is similar to the IC nerve–to–musculocutaneous nerve transfer—close to 80%. IC nerve–to–median nerve transfer is effective in children with obstetric brachial plexus but poor in adult patients.

The IC nerve is also not suitable to radial nerve, axillary nerve, or more proximal spinal nerve reinnervation, and its use usually ends in poor results with unclear reasons.

The author has used the Ph nerve for neurotization in more than 150 patients since 1986. In most instances, it was used for shoulder abduction, with transfer to the C5 (Fig. 3), the suprascapular nerve, the dorsal division of the upper trunk (Figs. 4 and 5), or the axillary nerve. Some were transferred to the radial nerve for elbow and wrist extension (Fig. 8), and some were used as adjuvant nerves that were accompanied with C5 or C6 spinal nerves to the median nerve. The results from those transfers were effective and significantly improved the author's clinical results.

Some results were unexpected. For example, direct transfer of the Ph nerve to the dorsal division of the upper trunk achieved improved shoulder abduction (M3 deltoid muscle) and, unexpectedly, elbow extension (M3 triceps) and wrist extension (M2 to M3 of extensor carpi radialis longus). With the endoscopic assisted technique, harvest of the Ph nerve is possible to gain more length for neurotization. The author's animal rat study proves that the Ph nerve can reach the lower one-third of the forearm or the wrist level, which can be transferred for more function of the hand. The disadvantages of Ph nerve transfer include (a) hemidiaphragm paralysis and elevation, which might cause respiratory distress, especially in children who are younger than 2 years of age; and (b) easy fatigue of the reinnervated muscle. This is why Ph nerve transfer is good for shoulder abduction but not good for elbow flexion without long duration for weight lifting. Respiratory distress in adult patients after Ph nerve transection is usually subclinical and temporary. Ph nerve transection is strongly contraindicated in the child who is younger than 2 years of age.

MBCPs were used as neurotizers in a small number of patients (only 26). MBCPs might be transferred to the C5, the suprascapular nerve, or the dorsal division of the upper trunk, but all of them accompany the Ph nerve or the eleventh cranial nerve, or both, for multiple neurotization. Shoulder abduction of more than 60 degrees was achieved in 20 patients (20 of 26, 77%). This adjuvant neurotizer seems to be supportive and has improved the author's results. Recently, the author has tried to use it as a sole neurotizer, mainly to the suprascapular nerve, to replace the eleventh cranial nerve. The eleventh cranial nerve is then spared for late reconstruction with free muscle transplantation for elbow flexion and finger extension.

Hypoglossal (twelfth cranial) nerve transfer was only applied in 11 patients. In most cases, it was used as a substitute to the avulsed Ph nerve. It always required a nerve graft of more than 10 cm to reach the target nerve of the brachial plexus, such as the dorsal division of the upper trunk, alone or in company with the eleventh cranial nerve, for neurotization. The result was not impressive: In 8 of 11 patients (73%), the shoulder abduction was less than 60 degrees.

Between 1989 and 1997, the author performed contralateral C7 transfer on 60 patients with brachial plexus injuries. Forty-seven patients have been followed for at least 2 years after complete reconstruction. Management strategies were different with three groups of patients: (a) immediate contralateral C7 transfer in the early stage (27 patients), (b) immediate contralateral C7 transfer in the early stage followed by functioning free muscle transplantation (two-stage procedure, 9 patients), and (c) delayed contralateral C7 transfer followed by functioning free muscle transplantation (two-stage procedure, 11 patients). The main nerve for reinnervation was the median nerve. The main part for reconstruction was finger flexion. The average success rate was 55% (with a range of 54% to 57%) to gain finger sen-

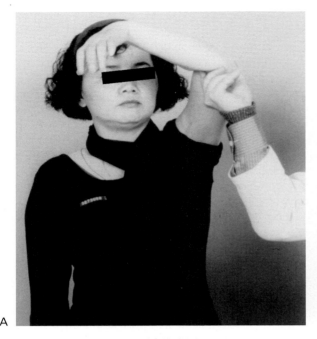

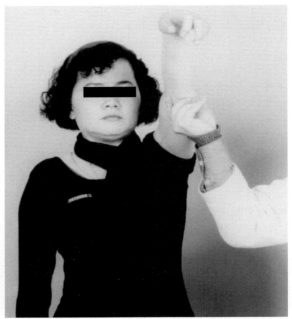

A

B

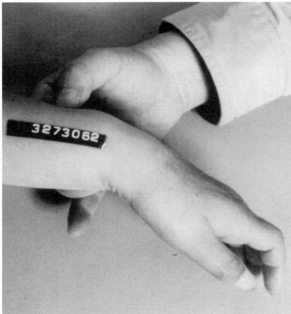

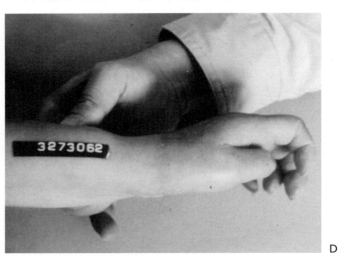

C

D

FIGURE 8. Example of results of 2 years after transfer of phrenic nerve grafts to the radial nerve. The patient could extend the elbow **(A,B)** and the wrist **(C,D)**.

sation and flexion. Single-stage neurotization appears to promote quicker motor and sensory recovery than the two-stage procedure. Many factors influence its success, including the timing of surgery; the patient's age, motivation, and cooperation; the surgeon's skill; and rehabilitation. Contralateral C7 transfer can only resolve some hand problems in complete preganglionic brachial plexus injuries. All of the author's patients required a dynamic splint for interphalangeal joint extension or another free muscle transplantation (using the eleventh cranial nerve as a neurotizer) for finger extension. A significant potential still exists for further investigation to define more precisely the role of con-

tralateral C7 transfer in brachial plexus reconstruction. Contralateral entire-C7 transection is a safe procedure, although subclinical, and some not significantly clinical, findings are observed. The symptoms and signs usually disappear within 3 to 6 months after C7 transection.

Intraplexus transfer is only indicated in non-total root–avulsed patients. Twenty-nine patients had this reconstruction: C5 transfer was performed in ten patients; C6 transfer was performed in six patients; and C5 and C6 or upper trunk transfer was performed in 13 patients. One patient, who had upper trunk rupture that was associated with C7 and T1 root avulsion, received C5 transfer to the anterior division of the upper trunk for elbow flexion and C6 transfer to the median nerve for hand function. A vascularized ulnar nerve was frequently used as a trunk graft for interposition by pedicle or by free type (4,5). From the author's experience, intraplexus spinal nerve transfer for hand function is always superior to the contralateral C7 transfer: Not only is the surgical technique easier and recovery quicker, but also rehabilitation is faster owing to brain adaptation in control of movement (Figs. 6 and 7). The average success rate was higher, approximately 71%.

STRATEGY OF SURGICAL MANAGEMENT FOR DIFFERENT ROOT INJURIES

Combined Intra- and Extraplexus Neurotization (Author's Recommended Technique)

Root avulsion was present in 75% of cases in the author's series. Five situations were found intraoperatively, and management strategies were recommended as described in the following sections.

Single Root Avulsion

- C5 single root avulsion: multiple nerve transfer of the Ph, eleventh cranial, and MBCP nerves directly to the C5 spinal nerve without nerve grafts (Fig. 3A–C).
- C6 single root avulsion, usually associated with C5 rupture: C5 is transferred to the anterior division of the upper trunk for elbow flexion, the Ph nerve and MBCPs are transferred to the posterior division, and the eleventh cranial nerve is transferred to the suprascapular nerve for shoulder abduction.
- C7 single root avulsion, usually associated with C5, C6, or upper trunk rupture: only repair of the upper trunk without C7 reinnervation.

Two Root Avulsion

- C5 and C6 root avulsion: the Ph nerve and MBCPs are transferred to the dorsal division of the upper trunk, the eleventh cranial nerve is transferred to the suprascapular nerve for shoulder abduction, and three IC nerves are transferred to the musculocutaneous nerve for elbow flexion (Figs. 4 and 5).
- C6 and C7 root avulsion, usually associated with C5 rupture: C5 is transferred to the anterior division of the upper trunk for elbow flexion, and the Ph nerve, eleventh cranial nerve, and MBCPs are transferred for shoulder abduction.
- C8 and T1 root avulsion, usually associated with C5 through C7 rupture: C5 is transferred for shoulder abduction, C6 is transferred to the median nerve for hand function, IC nerves are transferred to the musculo-

cutaneous nerve for elbow flexion, and the eleventh cranial nerve is transferred to functioning free muscle transplantation for EDC.
- C7 nerve graft; indirect nerve repair with nerve grafts owing to its higher incidence of root injury, too.

Three Root Avulsion

- C5, C6, and C7 root avulsion: Ph nerve, MBCPs, and eleventh cranial nerve transfer for shoulder abduction; IC nerve transfer for elbow flexion.
- C7, C8, and T1 root avulsion, usually associated with C5 and C6 rupture: C5 transfer for shoulder abduction; C6 transfer to the C8 or to the median nerve for hand function; IC nerve transfer to the musculocutaneous nerve for elbow flexion (Fig. 6).

Four Root Avulsion

- C6 through T1 four-root avulsion, usually associated with C5 rupture. Two situations may be encountered: (a) If the C5 stump is healthy: C5–to–median nerve transfer for hand function; Ph nerve and MBCP transfer for shoulder abduction; IC nerve transfer for elbow flexion. The eleventh cranial nerve is spared for late-stage functioning free muscle transplantation for EDC. (b) If the C5 stump has questionable health: C5–to–dorsal division transfer, Ph nerve–to–suprascapular nerve transfer for shoulder abduction; IC nerve transfer for elbow flexion; contralateral C7 vascularized ulnar nerve graft for hand function.
- The eleventh cranial nerve is spared for late-stage free muscle transplantation for EDC.

Five Root Avulsion

- Ph nerve and MBCP transfer for shoulder abduction; IC nerve transfer for elbow flexion; contralateral C7 transfer for hand function; eleventh cranial nerve transfer for late-stage free muscle transplantation for EDC replacement.

Pedicle Muscle Transfer

When sequelae deformities persist after the maximal recovery, spontaneously or after nerve reconstruction, palliative reconstruction can be considered. *Maximal recovery* means that the patient has already been without evidence of recovery for more than 2 years postinjury. These patients have entered the chronic state in which no further recovery is anticipated. The sequelae lesions are permanent. Palliative reconstruction includes pedicle muscle transfer, functioning free muscle transplantation, tendon transfer, tenodesis, arthrodesis, and osteotomy (37–52).

With muscle or tendon transfer in brachial plexus injuries, the prerequisites of joint mobility, adequate soft tissue and skin coverage, and absence of edema must be satisfied. In

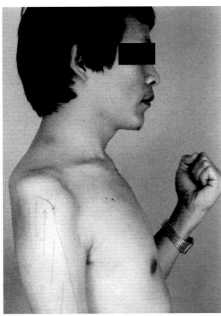 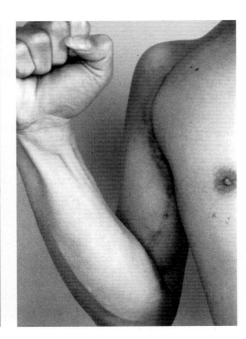

A,B

FIGURE 9. Before **(A)** and after **(B)** latissimus dorsi bipolar myocutaneous flap transfer for right elbow flexion after 3 years of palsy. The patient's elbow flexion strength is M3 (he could not flex his elbow against the examiner's one-finger resistance).

addition, the donor muscle must be of adequate strength and amplitude of excursion, which are especially crucial in brachial plexus–injured patients. This might be only indicated in patients with pure upper plexus or pure lower plexus injuries but is not indicated in a global plexopathy. In other words, muscles that are innervated by upper and lower plexus components (C6, C7, and C8) are always suspicious and should be treated carefully. For example, pedicled latissimus dorsi (LD) muscle or myocutaneous flap transfer, which is used more frequently for elbow flexion and less frequently for elbow extension or finger flexion, is quite a tricky procedure in the brachial plexus injury because results are often disappointing (Fig. 9A,B) (usually M3 or less, but not M4 results), despite careful preoperative evaluation. The reason is that the LD is innervated by C6, C7, and C8. During transfer of the muscle to provide elbow flexion, the elbow flexors have been persistently paralyzed owing to upper plexus injury (C5 and C6, plus or minus C7). The maximal recovery of the muscle is actually no longer equivalent to a healthy muscle. Most tendon transfers result in a loss of one grade of strength. Transfer of initially denervated and maximal recovery muscles always ends in an M4 result. Once transferred, these muscles result in an M3 rating and cannot actually support daily activity.

In pedicle muscle transfer, with one or two pedicles based on the reposition of the origin or insertion of the muscle, or both, it seems that the extraplexus-innervated muscle transfer is more reliable than intraplexus-innervated muscle transfer. However, extraplexus-innervated muscle transfers, such as trapezius (innervated by the spinal accessory nerve) transfer for shoulder abduction (38) and sternocleidomastoid (innervated by the spinal accessory nerve) transfer for elbow flexion (39), have not achieved popularity owing to their excursion and appearance limits. Most reconstructive surgeons today regard the procedures as mainly of historic interest.

In intraplexus-innervated muscle transfer, pure upper plexus palsy or pure lower plexus palsy is more suitable for pedicle muscle or tendon transfer, including L'Episcopo procedure (40) for shoulder external rotation, PM transfer (41,42), LD transfer (42), triceps transfer (43), or Steindler flexoplasty (44) for elbow flexion. In obstetric palsy, many patients recover by aberrant reinnervation (45). The principle of muscle transfer is quite different from the adult brachial plexus injury. Release of antagonistic muscle and transfer to the paretic (not complete palsy) muscle for augmentation in obstetric palsy usually create good results (46).

L'Episcopo Procedure

L'Episcopo procedure is a posterolateral rerouting of the insertion of the LD and teres major to enhance active lateral rotation of the shoulder. It is particularly useful in cases of recovery by aberrant reinnervation, such as a penetrating injury of the upper plexus, or obstetric palsy. It is characterized by contracture of the internal rotators and weakness (paresis) of the external rotators. L'Episcopo procedure may be performed simultaneously with release of the anterior capsule, subscapularis, and PM tendons or even external rotational osteotomy of the humerus (47–49). The procedure is effective and usually significantly improves shoulder external rotation but not shoulder abduction.

Pectoralis Major Transfer

The PM muscle has two portions: the clavicular part of the PM, which is innervated by lateral pectoral nerves (branches from anterior divisions of the upper and middle trunk) and the sternal part of the PM, which is innervated by medial pectoral nerves (branches form the posterior divisions of the middle and lower trunk). In pure upper plexus palsy, the sternal part of the PM may be useful to restore elbow flexion. The PM muscle may be used as a monopolar (41) or bipolar transfer (41,42). It may help by elevating a segment of rectus abdominis sheath: The origin may be located at the coracoid process or at the acromion in bipedicle fashion. The insertion is at the distal biceps tendon. The disadvantages of this muscle transfer include a big chest scar and prominent bulk in the upper arm.

Latissimus Dorsi Transfer

The LD muscle is innervated by the thoracodorsal nerve, a branch from the posterior cord that comes from C6, C7, and C8. The LD muscle transfer may be performed as a unipolar (50) or bipolar (42) transfer, but bipolar is preferred. Determining the subtle weakness of the LD preoperatively is somewhat difficult on motor testing alone. This is why some patients need a secondary procedure, such as Steindler flexoplasty, for augmentation (35).

Triceps Transfer

Triceps transfer for elbow flexion (43) is effective for elbow flexion but sacrifices elbow extension and results in elbow flexion contracture that is due to muscle imbalance if the patient does not perform daily stretching exercises. This muscle transfer has been abandoned by the author.

Steindler Flexoplasty (Flexor-Pronator Muscle Group Advancement)

Central or lateral advancement of the flexor-pronator muscle group (44) to the humerus bone actually produces weak elbow flexion strength. At least 5 cm of advancement proximal to the medial epicondyle and fixation into the bone, not the periosteum, are advocated. This procedure is useless as a main procedure in complete paralysis of elbow flexion (M0 to M1) but is most helpful in supplementing power in patients with some preexisting elbow flexion (M2 to M3), such as incomplete recovery of the elbow flexion after nerve reconstruction or after other pedicle muscle transfer (34). A flexion contracture of the elbow (range from 15 to 40 degrees) was an adverse consequence of this procedure.

Functioning Free Muscle Transplantation

Using functioning free muscle transplantation in brachial plexus peripheral reconstruction is effective and has become more and more popular (51–53). It is actually a type of extraplexus-innervated muscle transfer and is more reliable and effective. The muscle comes from a distant site but is a fresh muscle. The donor nerve is the eleventh cranial nerve, the IC nerve, or the contralateral nerve. The only disadvantage is that this procedure is technically demanding. The results seem to be more satisfactory than

they are in pedicle muscle transfer, especially for elbow and hand function restoration in the global plexopathy.

REFERENCES

1. Bonney G. In: Birch R, Bonney G, Wynn Parry CB, eds. *Surgical disorders of the peripheral nerve.* Edinburgh: Churchill Livingstone, 1998:157–158.
2. Alnot JY. Traumatic brachial plexus lesions in the adult. *Hand Clin* 1995;11:623–631.
3. Narakas AO. Lesions found when operating traction injuries to the brachial plexus. *Clin Neurol Neurosurg* 1993;95:S56–S64.
4. Terzis JK, Vekris MD, Soucacos PN. Outcomes of brachial plexus reconstruction in 204 patients with devastating paralysis. *Plast Reconstr Surg* 1999;104:1221–1240.
5. Chuang DCC. Management of traumatic brachial plexus injuries in adults. *Hand Clin* 1999;15:737–755.
6. Gilbert A. Long-term evaluation of brachial plexus surgery in obstetrical palsy. *Hand Clin* 1995;11:583–595.
7. Narakas AO. Neurotization in the treatment of brachial plexus injuries. In: Gelberman R, ed. *Operative nerve repair and reconstruction.* Philadelphia: JB Lippincott, 1991:1329–1358.
8. Chuang DCC. Neurotization procedures for brachial plexus injuries. *Hand Clin* 1995;11:633–645.
9. Gu YD. Phrenic nerve transfer for brachial plexus motor neurotization. *Microsurgery* 1989;10:287–289.
10. Allieu Y, Privat JM, Bonnel F. Paralysis in root avulsion of the brachial plexus. Neurotization by the spinal accessory nerve. *Clin Plast Surg* 1984;11:133–137.
11. Brunelli G, Brunelli F. Use of anterior nerves of cervical plexus to partially neurotize the avulsed brachial plexus. In: Brunelli G, ed. *Textbook of microsurgery.* Milan, Italy: Masson, 1988:803–807.
12. Yeoman PM, Seddon HJ. Brachial plexus injuries: treatment of the flail arm. *J Bone Joint Surg* 1961;43:493–500.
13. Narakas AO. Neurotization or nerve transfer in traumatic brachial plexus lesions. In: Tubiana R, ed. *The hand.* Philadelphia: WB Saunders, 1987:656–683.
14. Gu YD, Zhang GM, Chen DS, et al. Seventh cervical nerve root transfer from the contralateral healthy side for treatment of brachial plexus root avulsion. *J Hand Surg* 1992;17:518–521.
15. Tsuyama N, Hara T, Nagano A. *Intercostal nerve crossing as a treatment of irreparably damaged whole brachial plexus. Recent developments in orthopedic surgery.* Manchester, England: Manchester University Press, 1987:169–174.
16. Nagano A, Tsuyama N, Ochiai N, et al. Direct nerve crossing with the intercostal nerve to treat avulsion injuries of the brachial plexus. *J Hand Surg* 1989;14:980–985.
17. Kawai H, Kawabata H, Masada K, et al. Nerve repairs for traumatic brachial plexus palsy with root avulsion. *Clin Orthop* 1988;237:75–86.
18. Chuang DCC, Yeh MC, Wei FC. Intercostal nerve transfer of the musculocutaneous nerve in avulsed brachial plexus injuries: evaluation of 66 patients. *J Hand Surg* 1992;17:822–828.
19. Chuang DCC, Carver N, Wei FC. Results of functioning free muscle transplantation for elbow flexion. *J Hand Surg* 1996;21:1071–1077.

20. Dolenc VV. Intercostal neurotization on the peripheral nerves in avulsion plexus injuries. In: Terzis JK, eds. *Microreconstruction of nerve injuries.* Philadelphia: WB Saunders, 1987:425–445.

21. Seddon HJ. Nerve grafting. *J Bone Joint Surg* 1963;45:447–461.

22. Narakas AO. Surgical treatment of avulsion type injuries of the brachial plexus. In: Brunelli G, ed. *Textbook of microsurgery.* Milan, Italy: Masson, 1988:781–787.

23. Narakas AO. Brachial plexus surgery. *Orthop Clin North Am* 1981;12:303–323.

24. Narakas A, Hentz V. Neurotization in brachial plexus injuries, indications and results. *Clin Orthop* 1988;237:43–56.

25. Minami M, Ischiis S. Satisfactory elbow flexion in complete (preganglionic) brachial plexus injury: produced by suture of third and fourth intercostal nerves to musculocutaneous nerve. *J Hand Surg* 1987;12:1114–1118.

26. Millesi H. Brachial plexus injury in adults: operative repair. In: Gelberman R, ed. *Operative nerve repair and reconstruction.* Philadelphia: JB Lippincott, 1991:1285–1301.

27. Terzis JK, Maragh H. Strategies in the microsurgical management of brachial plexus injuries. *Clin Plast Surg* 1989;16:605.

28. Chuang DCC, Lee GW, Hashem F, et al. Restoration of shoulder abduction by nerve transfer in avulsed brachial plexus injury: evaluation of 99 patients with various nerve transfers. *Plast Reconstr Surg* 1995;96:122–128.

29. Doi K, Sakai K, Kuwata N, et al. Reconstruction of finger and elbow function after complete avulsion of the brachial plexus. *J Hand Surg* 1991;16:796–803.

30. Chuang DCC, Wei FC, Norrdhoff MS. Cross-chest C7 nerve grafting followed by free muscle transplantations for the treatment of total avulsed brachial plexus injuries: a preliminary report. *Plast Reconstr Surg* 1993;92:717–725.

31. Chuang DCC, Cheng SL, Wei FC, et al. Clinical evaluation of C7 spinal nerve transection: 21 patients with at least 2 years' follow-up. *Br J Plast Surg* 1998;51:285–290.

32. Chuang DCC. Contralateral C7 transfer (CC-7T) for avulsion injury of the brachial plexus. *Tech Hand Upper Extrem Surg* 1999;3:185–192.

33. Oberlin C. Nerve transfer to biceps muscle using a part of ulnar nerve for C5–6 avulsion of the brachial plexus—anatomical studies and report of four cases. *J Hand Surg* 1994;19:232–237.

34. Tubiana R. Clinical examination and functional assessment of the upper limb after peripheral nerve lesions. In: Tubiana R, ed. *The hand.* Philadelphia: WB Saunders, 1988:453–488.

35. Chuang DCC, Epstein MD, Jeh MC, et al. Functional restoration of elbow flexion in brachial plexus injuries: results in 167 patients (excluding obstetric brachial plexus injury). *J Hand Surg* 1993;18:285–291.

36. Doi K, Sakai K, Ihara K, et al. Reinnervated free muscle transplantation for extremity reconstruction. *Plast Reconstr Surg* 1993;91:872–883.

37. Leffert RD. Brachial plexus. In: Green DP, ed. *Operative hand surgery.* New York: Churchill Livingstone, 1993:1483–1516.

38. Aziz W, Singer RM, Wolff TW. Transfer of the trapezius for flail shoulder after brachial plexus injury. *J Bone Joint Surg* 1990;72:701–704.

39. Bunnell S. Restoring flexion to the paralytic elbow. *J Bone Joint Surg* 1951;33:566–571.

40. L'Episcopo JB. Restoration of muscle balance in the treatment of obstetrical paralysis. *N Y State J Med* 1939;39:357–363.

41. Clark JM. Reconstruction of biceps brachii by pectoral muscle transplantation. *Br J Surg* 1946;34:180.

42. Schottstaedt ER, Larsen LJ, Bost FC. Complete muscle transposition. *J Bone Joint Surg* 1955;37:897–919.

43. Carroll RE, Hill NA. Triceps transfer to restore elbow flexion: a study of 15 patients with paralytic lesions and arthrogryposis. *J Bone Joint Surg* 1970;52:239–244.

44. Steindler A. Operative reconstruction work on hand and forearm. *N Y Med J* 1918;108:1117–1119.

45. Chuang DCC, Ma HS, Wei FC. A new evaluation system to predict the sequelae of late obstetric brachial plexus palsy. *Plast Reconstr Surg* 1998;101:673–685.

46. Chuang DCC, Ma HS, Wei FC. A new strategy of muscle transposition for treatment of shoulder deformity caused by obstetric brachial plexus palsy. *Plast Reconstr Surg* 1998;101:686–694.

47. Henry AM. The treatment of residual paralysis after brachial plexus injury. *J Bone Joint Surg* 1949;31:42–49.

48. Price AE, Grossman JA. A management approach for secondary shoulder and forearm deformities following obstetrical brachial plexus injury. *Hand Clin* 1995;11:607–617.

49. Richards RR. Operative treatment for irreparable lesions of the brachial plexus. In: Gelberman RH, ed. *Operative nerve repair and reconstruction.* Philadelphia: JB Lippincott Co, 1991:1303–1327.

50. Hovnanian AP. Latissimus dorsi transplantation for loss of flexion or extension at the elbow. A preliminary report of technique. *Ann Surg* 1956;143:493–499.

51. Doi K, Sakai K, Kuwata N, et al. Double-muscle technique for reconstruction of prehension after complete avulsion of brachial plexus. *J Hand Surg* 1995;20:408.

52. Chuang DCC. Functioning free muscle transplantation for brachial plexus injury. *Clin Orthop* 1995;314:104–111.

53. Chuang DCC. Results of functioning free muscle transplantation for elbow flexion. *J Hand Surg* 1996;21:1071–1077.

59

BRACHIAL PLEXUS: FREE COMPOSITE TISSUE TRANSFERS

KAZUTERU DOI

Brachial plexus injuries (BPIs) affect active young individuals. They cause devastating neurologic dysfunction and result in considerable disability. Although restoration of normality in the affected limb cannot be expected, refinement of microsurgical techniques over the past three decades have improved functional outcome. Most pioneers in this field focused on using nerve grafting and nerve-transfer techniques for reconstruction of proximal limb functions, such as elbow flexion or shoulder rotation. These aggressive procedures provided some functions such as lifting with the forearm or arm–trunk prehension for patients with complete avulsion of the brachial plexus (1–4). The reconstructed upper limb was still relatively useless because it did not have prehensile function, the basic function of the human hand.

The results of nerve-crossing procedures (2,4) for reinnervation of forearm muscles to restore prehension are far from satisfactory. The strength of the reinnervated forearm muscles is insufficient to perform daily activities. Reliability of reinnervation is also poor because of several factors. It takes a long time for the regenerating axons to reach the muscle, as the distance between the site of the nerve crossing and the neuromotor units of the forearm muscles is too far. By the time regenerating axons reach the muscle, increased denervation time results in atrophy of the targeted muscle. Misdirection of the regenerating axons occurs frequently because of the numerous motor branches of the repaired distal nerve. At present, simple nerve-crossing procedures are indicated only for reconstruction of shoulder and elbow function and not for reconstruction of finger function after BPIs.

In contrast, functioning free muscle transfer can provide reliable and powerful motor recovery for finger function as the denervation time is reduced because the neuromotor units of the free muscle are in the upper arm and misdirection of regenerating axons is reduced as the nerve to the muscle has only a motor component (5–12). Free muscle transfer had been used to reconstruct elbow flexion in delayed cases of complete paralysis secondary to BPI. To improve prehensile function after BPIs, the focus has shifted from the previous simple nerve-crossing procedures to recent functioning free muscle transfer with multiple nerve crossings.

The purpose of this chapter is to describe the operative technique of the muscle transfer for upper extremity reconstruction and secondary reconstructions after BPI, based on the personal experience of the author.

Functioning free muscle transfer in BPI has been used for reconstruction of elbow flexion in delayed cases of complete paralysis or upper-type paralysis of brachial plexus and prehensile reconstruction after complete paralysis. These two options of free muscle transfers are described under separate headings.

Terms such as *free muscle transfer* and *free transfer* are used in this chapter for convenience. These words actually mean functioning free muscle transfer.

PROCEDURE 1: FREE MUSCLE TRANSFER FOR ELBOW FLEXION IN DELAYED CASES (SUPPLEMENTAL PROCEDURE: SIMULTANEOUS RECONSTRUCTION OF ELBOW FLEXION AND SHOULDER FLEXION OR WRIST EXTENSION)

Indication

In a complete or upper type of BPI, free muscle transfer for only elbow flexion is indicated for patients with absence of available regional muscles of adequate strength for tendon transfer and a time interval of more than 9 months from injury. This procedure is technically demanding. However, the younger the patient, the better the recovery. Children older than age 2 years are candidates for the free muscle transfer. Satisfactory results are not obtained in patients older than 50 years because of the poor reinnervation of the transferred muscles and other problems such as joint contracture and causalgia.

Donor Muscle Selection

The latissimus dorsi muscle, gracilis, and rectus femoris muscle are used as the donor muscles when the reconstruction is planned only for elbow flexion and not for finger function. The ipsilateral latissimus dorsi can be used as a pedicled flap based on vascular pedicle for this purpose. Nerve crossing of the thoracodorsal nerve to the donor motor nerve, spinal accessory nerve, or intercostal nerves will be needed if the latissimus dorsi is affected in the BPI. If the duration of injury is longer than 1 year, the ipsilateral latissimus dorsi may have become atrophic; the contralateral latissimus dorsi muscle is used as a donor muscle for functioning free muscle transfer, which needs neurovascular anastomoses.

The rectus femoris muscle is also a powerful muscle and can be used to supplement elbow flexion. Transient reduction of knee extension occurs following harvest of the rectus femoris muscle. The gracilis is the best choice as a donor muscle. There is no postoperative functional deficit after its harvest. It provides sufficient strength to act as an elbow flexor.

Donor Nerve Selection

The most frequently used donor motor nerves are the third to sixth intercostal nerves. When the intercostal nerves have been already used previously as donor motor nerves for nerve crossing to the musculocutaneous nerve, the lower intercostal nerves than those previously used can be used. Fracture of the corresponding ribs might have injured the intercostal nerve. This should be taken into consideration when deciding to use the intercostal nerves.

The spinal accessory nerve is the donor motor nerve of our choice if it has not been used for nerve crossing to the suprascapular nerve. We prefer to transfer the terminal branch of the spinal accessory nerve, which innervates the middle and lower portion of the trapezius muscle.

Operative Procedure

Exploration of the Recipient Site

For elbow flexion by free muscle transfer, the nutrient vessels of the transferred muscle are anastomosed with the thoracoacromial artery and the cephalic veins or with the thoracodorsal artery and vein when thrombosis of the subclavicular artery is present.

Donor Nerve Dissection

Intercostal Nerves

A curved incision is taken from the parasternal area to the axilla along the infraareolar margin or inframammary fold. Two of the third to sixth intercostal nerves are used. After raising the skin flaps, the costal origin of the lower part of the pectoralis major muscle is divided to facilitate the dissection. The periosteum is separated from the ribs. The intercostal nerve, artery, and vein are located at the inferior edge of the rib. The lateral cutaneous sensory branch of the intercostal nerve is found at a point between the anterior and posterior axillary line and dissected proximally where the main trunk runs and the medial motor branch bifurcates. Use of a nerve stimulator makes the identification of motor and the sensory lateral cutaneous branch of the intercostal nerve easier. The medial motor branch is harvested up to the mid-clavicular line and transferred to the axillary region with the lateral cutaneous sensory branch, where neurorrhaphy will be performed to the motor branch of the transferred muscle and respective nerve for sensory reinnervation. Two intercostal nerves are usually sufficient for coaptation with the motor nerve of the transferred muscle. Before coaptation, the periosteum is reapposed over the ribs.

Spinal Accessory Nerve

An incision is made from the anterior axillary fold to the posterior to the acromion. The clavicular attachment of the trapezius muscle is divided and retracted posteriorly. In the areolar tissue anterior to the trapezius muscle, the transverse cervical artery and vein are easily found. Along these vessels, the cervical nerves and the spinal accessory nerve, which join together, are found, running inferiorly anterior to the trapezius muscle (Fig. 1). Use of a nerve stimulator helps to distinguish the motor nerve and the supraclavicular sensory nerve. At the anterior border of the trapezius, the spinal accessory nerve pierces the deep fascia covering the deep surface of the muscle and continues for the remainder of its course between the muscle and fascia. The spinal accessory nerve is traced inferiorly to its bifurcation. The terminal branch of the spinal accessory nerve distal to the branch innervating the upper fibers of the trapezius is dissected, divided, and transferred to the supraclavicular region, where neurorrhaphy will be performed with the motor branch of the transferred muscle. Care is taken not to injure the comitant vessels and to prevent excessive tension on the nerve. The lower terminal branch supplies the middle and lower fibers of the trapezius; thus, morbidity after its division is less noticeable.

Donor Muscle Harvest

Latissimus Dorsi Muscle

The entire latissimus dorsi muscle with a paddle of skin is dissected through an incision along its anterior margin and surrounding skin paddle over the muscle. The fascial origin of the muscle attached to the posterior crest of the ilium should be included with the musculocutaneous flap. The insertion of the muscle is detached from the humerus. The neurovascular pedicle is preserved when the ipsilateral latis-

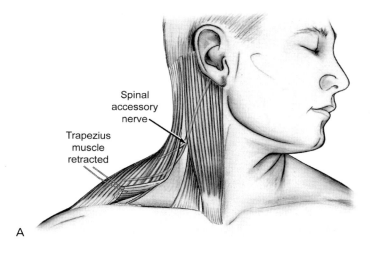

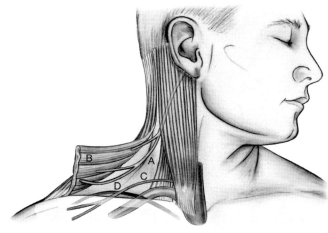

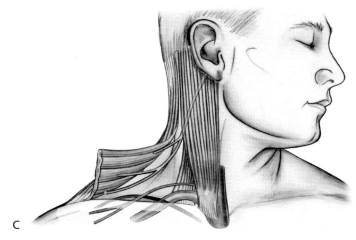

FIGURE 1. Spinal accessory nerve transfer. **A:** The clavicular attachment of the trapezius muscle is divided and retracted posteriorly. **B:** In the areolar tissue anterior to the trapezius muscle (*B*), the transverse cervical artery (*C*) and vein (*D*) are easily found, and along these vessels, the cervical nerves and the spinal accessory nerve (*A*), which join together, are found running inferiorly anterior to the trapezius muscle. **C:** The spinal accessory nerve is traced deeply to the bifurcation of the proximal branch innervating the upper part of the trapezius and the distal branch innervating the middle and lower part. The distal branch is dissected distal to the bifurcation and divided and transferred to the supraclavicular area for coaptation to the motor nerve of the gracilis.

simus dorsi muscle is being transferred. After elevation of the flap, the skin defect is closed primarily.

Rectus Femoris Muscle

The entire rectus femoris muscle with a small paddle of skin over the proximal third of the muscle is harvested through an incision along the central axis of the muscle extending from the anterior superior iliac spine to the patella encircling the skin paddle. The orientation of the vascular pedicle allows dissection of the muscle from the ipsilateral thigh. The neurovascular pedicle enters from the undersurface of the muscle proximally and should be protected.

Gracilis Muscle

The donor gracilis muscle from the contralateral side has been selected because the ultimate location of its neurovascular bundle matches the site of the recipient vessels. The length of the donor muscle, from its pubic bone origin to its tibial insertion, is measured to verify that it will span the distance from the acromion to the mid-forearm without excessive tension. The donor muscle is then harvested from its proximal origin to the distal attachment. To avoid a long

and cosmetically unacceptable scar, endoscopic harvesting of the gracilis muscle may be considered (13).

Muscle Transfer

After division of its neurovascular pedicle, the muscle is then transferred to the recipient site. The tendon of origin is secured to either the coracoid process or the clavicle with polyamide interrupted sutures or with soft tissue anchoring sutures. Muscle is revascularized by anastomosis of its vascular pedicle to the thoracoacromial artery and cephalic vein when the nerve is being coapted to the spinal accessory nerve or to the thoracodorsal artery and comitant vein when coaptation is being done to the intercostal nerves. The motor branch of the muscle is passed deep to the clavicle to the supraclavicular space and is coapted to the spinal accessory nerve before revascularization. When coaptation is done to the intercostal nerves, the corresponding two intercostal nerves are transferred to the axillary region and coapted to the motor nerve of the muscle. The muscle is then placed in the subcutaneous tunnel created earlier and the distal tendinous portion is passed toward the elbow and

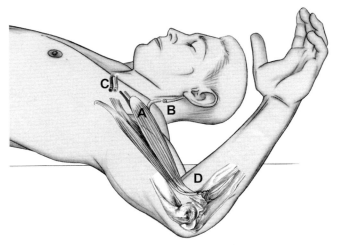

FIGURE 2. Free muscle transfer for reconstruction of elbow flexion. The motor branch of the gracilis (*A*) is connected to the branches of the spinal accessory nerve (*B*), and the nutrient vessels are anastomosed to the thoracoacromial artery (*C*) and veins. The gracilis is sutured to the acromion and lateral portion of the clavicle proximally and to the tendinous portion of the biceps distally (*D*).

is secured to the biceps tendon under tension, using an end-weave technique and interrupted sutures of No. 2-0 polyamide sutures (Fig. 2). The elbow is immobilized postoperatively for 6 weeks in a position of 60 to 75 degrees of abduction and

15 degrees of anterior flexion of the shoulder and 100 degrees of elbow flexion and supination of the forearm. After 6 weeks, passive elbow flexion is permitted, but extension beyond 30 degrees of flexion is avoided for at least 3 months. Reeducation and strengthening exercise using the electromyographic biofeedback technique are initiated when evidence of muscle contraction is observed (Fig. 3).

Supplemental Procedure

The free muscle transfer can move multiple joints simultaneously such as elbow flexion and shoulder flexion or elbow flexion and wrist extension by changing the proximal attachment of the muscle and the distal tendon suture. The rationale and concept of reconstruction are almost the same as those of the double free muscle transfer and are described below.

PROCEDURE 2: FREE MUSCLE TRANSFER FOR PREHENSILE RECONSTRUCTION AFTER COMPLETE AVULSION OF BRACHIAL PLEXUS

Rationale for the Surgical Approach

Several surgical approaches have been developed to restore prehension after complete brachial plexus avulsion (7,14).

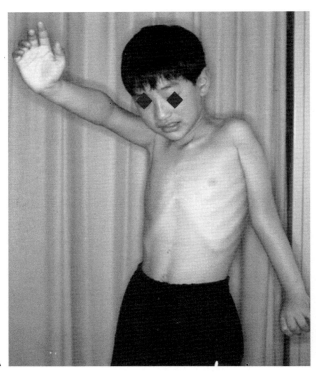
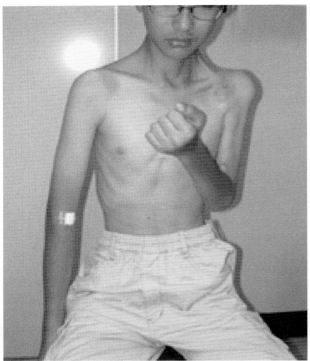

FIGURE 3. A 9-year-old boy suffered complete paralysis of C5 and C6 nerve roots secondary to an obstetric injury. **A:** The patient could not elevate the right upper extremity or flex his elbow, although he could extend the elbow joint and had normal function of the wrist and fingers. Electromyography showed no innervation of the deltoid, biceps brachii, supraspinatus, infraspinatus, and serratus anterior. The patient underwent a free muscle transfer described in the section Muscle Transfer for reconstruction of elbow flexion April 19, 1996. **B:** The patient could flex his elbow fully 12 months after the operation.

In these patients, to restore key pinch in a Moberg type of simple hand grip reconstruction, functioning free transfer was needed, as simple nerve crossing failed to achieve reliable activation of forearm muscles (5,6). However, finger flexion was weak, as it was achieved by synergistic action. These patients have a contralateral normal upper limb and can perform most of the activities of daily living. Few important activities will need a powerful grip independent of the contralateral limb and use of both hands, such as lifting a heavy box with both hands or holding a bottle while opening its cap. Direct activation of finger flexion is imperative for a powerful grip. The author's previous procedure successfully achieved this goal (9,11).

Grasp release is also necessary for useful prehension. Release reconstructed by secondary tenodesis of the finger extensor tendons as in Moberg-type reconstruction will need gravity-aided wrist flexion (14–16) and can be accomplished only with the elbow flexed. This synergistic action cannot be accomplished when the elbow is extended. To achieve voluntary finger extension independent of elbow position, a second free muscle transfer is essential.

Stability of the shoulder and elbow joints is necessary for proper transmission of power of the transferred muscle to achieve effective hand function. Shoulder stabilization can be achieved by the glenohumeral arthrodesis when shoulder instability persists after double free muscle transfer that supplementally stabilizes the glenohumeral joint. Stability of the elbow is extremely important for optimal use of the hand in day-to-day activities. Many authors (5,6) dismissed the significance of elbow stabilization because of technical difficulty and reconstructed finger flexion or extension function without providing some form of elbow stabilization. Their patients, in spite of achieving powerful wrist extension or finger flexion, could not use their fingers optimally in daily activities, as their elbow was unstable. In addition to finger extension or finger flexion, all the transferred muscles in this double muscle technique simultaneously cause elbow flexion, similar to the transferred brachioradialis muscle in cases of spinal cord injury. In this situation without elbow extensor function, the patient stabilizes the unstable elbow with the contralateral normal hand, a useless maneuver in daily activities. Reconstruction of elbow extension is imperative whenever prehension is being reconstructed by the transfer of one muscle that moves multiple joints simultaneously (17). The available intercostal nerves are used to neurotize the triceps brachii muscle via the radial nerve for elbow extension. This enables the patient to stabilize the elbow independently without the need of the contralateral hand and to use powerful finger flexion effectively.

Claw finger deformity frequently develops after reconstruction of finger flexion and extension. It should be prevented to achieve useful prehension. The lasso operation described by Zancolli (18,19) prevents this deformity by synergistic action of gravity-aided wrist flexion and is effective only in the flexion position of the elbow. Reconstructive procedures that require synergistic action are not useful in patients with BPI who have a normal contralateral upper extremity. Claw finger deformity is due to an imbalance between the strength of extrinsic finger flexor and extensor motors. In my experience with 120 free muscle transfers in the brachial plexus, the free muscle reinnervated by the spinal accessory nerve is more powerful than that reinnervated by the intercostal nerves. I use the spinal accessory nerve as the motor nerve for finger extension and the intercostal nerves for finger flexion to prevent claw finger deformity. I also use a plastic static volar splint, with the wrist in neutral position and the proximal and distal interphalangeal joints in full extension postoperatively, to facilitate interphalangeal joint contracture and to create a stable wrist and to prevent claw finger deformity.

Basic sensory functions such as protective sensation and position sense should be restored when the motor function is being reconstructed in a severely paralyzed limb. The supraclavicular or intercostal nerve-crossing procedures provide limited sensibility of the hand after double muscle transfer.

Indications and Contraindications

The most important prerequisites for this procedure are the patient's motivation and financial support to continue the postoperative rehabilitation for at least 1 year (20). Other factors such as the interval between injury and operation and the patient's age also play an important role in recovery. The triceps brachii undergoes severe atrophy when the duration between injury and operation is more than 1 year. Incomplete recovery of triceps brachii strength produces loss of elbow stability. No patients who had this procedure more than 1 year after the injury restored useful prehension. This procedure should be performed within 6 months after the injury. Patients older than age 40 years cannot obtain satisfactory results because of the poor reinnervation of the transferred muscles and other problems such as joint contracture and causalgia.

Subclavicular artery injury is a contraindication for this procedure because the recipient vessels for anastomoses to the nutrient vessels of the transferred muscle may have been injured, resulting in an increased risk of thrombosis in the anastomosed vessels.

Finger and elbow joint mobility, undamaged tendons in the hand and forearm, and good skin coverage over the upper extremity are other important prerequisites for this transfer.

Donor Muscle Selection

The gracilis muscle is the best choice for the donor muscle. The latissimus dorsi muscle, gracilis, and rectus femoris muscle have all been used as the donor muscle in the initial period of reconstruction by this technique. Long-term results have shown that the latissimus dorsi does not provide satisfactory finger function because of adhesion of the muscle to the fabricated pulley system and rupture of its tendon due to ischemic necrosis of the portion distal to the pulley. The rectus femoris is a bipennate muscle and has reduced excursion, resulting in poor finger function.

Donor Nerve Selection

Simultaneous reconstruction of two functions by the transfer of a single long muscle resolves the discrepancy between the number of available motor nerves and the number of basic functions that require restoration. Elbow flexion and finger extension are restored by a single free muscle transfer innervated by the spinal accessory nerve. Finger flexion is restored by a second free muscle neurotized by the fifth and sixth intercostal nerves. The third and fourth intercostal nerves are coapted to the motor branch of the triceps brachii muscle to restore elbow extension. This stabilizes the elbow and helps in positioning the hand in space and prevents the tendency of elbow flexion that may occur when the fingers are extended.

Sensory recovery is better when the intercostal nerves are used for reconstruction compared with the supraclavicular nerves.

Technique

The double free gracilis muscle transfer technique consists of five established but modified reconstructive procedures: (a) exploration of the brachial plexus and repair of the disrupted motor nerves, if possible; (b) the first free muscle transfer, neurotized by the spinal accessory nerve, for elbow flexion and finger extension; (c) the second free muscle transfer, neurotized by the fifth and sixth intercostal nerves for finger flexion; (d) a nerve-crossing procedure using the third and fourth intercostal nerves to neurotize the motor branch of the triceps brachii muscle for elbow extension, done simultaneously with the second muscle transfer; and (e) the intercostal sensory rami coapted to the medial cord of the brachial plexus to restore sensibility of the hand. In addition, (f) a sixth set of procedures for secondary reconstruction, such as arthrodesis of the glenohumeral joint, carpometacarpal joint of the thumb, and the wrist joint, to increase stability, and if the power strength of the triceps brachii muscle is too weak to stabilize the elbow joint, tendon transfer of the reinnervated infraspinatus muscle may be indicated. Tenolysis of the transferred muscle and tendons may also be necessary.

Timing of the various reconstructive procedures is important and is guided by several criteria. Procedures (a) and (b) are performed at the first stage of the operation, and procedures (c) to (e) are performed at the second stage,

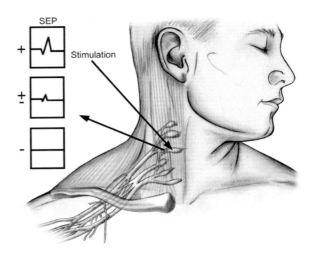

FIGURE 4. Exploration of the brachial plexus, measurement of spinal-evoked potential (SEP), and nerve repair. SEP was elicited by nerve root stimulation and the response was recorded from an electrode placed in the epidural space of the cervical spine. When the amplitude of SEP is more than 5 μV, the nerve root will be used as a source of motor nerve for repair of respective nerve using nerve graft.

usually 2 or 3 months after the first operation. Procedure (f) is done, depending on the condition of recovery, approximately 1.5 years after the first stage of the operation.

Brachial Plexus Exploration

All patients undergo initial surgical exploration of the brachial plexus. Spinal-evoked potentials and sensory nerve action potentials are recorded intraoperatively to confirm the diagnosis and to define the pattern and level of injury (Fig. 4). Reconstruction is undertaken only after confirming the diagnosis of complete brachial plexus palsy secondary to avulsion of the C5 to T1 nerve roots. In case of rupture of the C5 nerve root, nerve grafting should be done between the proximal remnant of the C5 root and the suprascapular nerve to restore shoulder function (Fig. 5). When the C5 nerve root is not available for nerve repair, I prefer the contralateral C7 nerve root for repair of suprascapular nerve using vascularized ulnar nerve graft. This is important, as shoulder stability and minimal movement of shoulder flexion and external rotation are essential for optimal function for prehension.

First Muscle Transfer

In the first stage, simultaneous elbow flexion and finger extension are reconstructed with a free muscle transfer using the spinal accessory as the motor nerve (Fig. 6) (21).

The donor gracilis muscle from the contralateral thigh is selected because the orientation and location of its neurovascular bundle matched the site of the donor vessels. The length of the gracilis muscle should be sufficient to

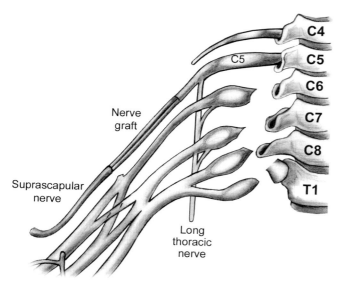

FIGURE 5. Nerve reconstruction using C5 nerve root. C5 nerve root is coapted to the suprascapular nerve using nerve graft.

span the distance between the acromion and mid-forearm without tension. It is verified by measuring the length of the gracilis muscle from its pubic origin to tibial insertion. The donor muscle is then harvested from its proximal origin to the distal attachment.

Correct muscle tension is critical for good postoperative function. Before detaching the muscle, the resting length of

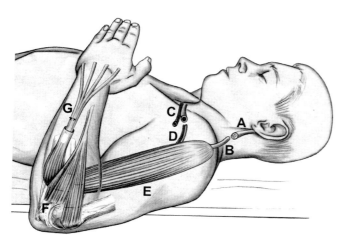

FIGURE 6. The initial operative procedure for reconstruction of prehension after complete brachial plexus avulsion is a free muscle transfer to restore elbow flexion and finger extension simultaneously. The gracilis is transferred and innervated by the spinal accessory nerve. A, accessory nerve; B, motor branch of the muscle transplant; C, thoracoacromial artery and branches of the cephalic vein; D, nutrient artery and veins of the muscle transplant; E, muscle transplant; F, the brachioradialis and wrist extensors serving as a pulley; G, extensor digitorum communis tendon. (Redrawn from Doi K, Muramtsu K, Hattori Y, et al. Reconstruction of upper extremity function brachial plexopathy using double free gracilis flaps. *Tech Hand Upper Extremity Surg* 2000;4:34–43.)

the muscle is recorded by placing black silk ligatures on the surface of the muscle at 5-cm intervals, as described by Manktelow and colleagues (22,23).

The distal portion of the spinal accessory nerve is dissected, divided, and transferred. The motor nerve of the transferred muscle is passed behind the clavicle and coapted to the distal branch of the spinal accessory nerve in the supraclavicular area. The nutrient vessels of the free gracilis muscle are then anastomosed to the thoracoacromial artery and vein or to the cephalic vein. The transferred muscle is placed superficially over the anterior part of the deltoid and is sutured to the acromion with nonabsorbable sutures or by a soft tissue anchoring system. A simple and straight route for the free muscle is created from its new origin to final insertion to maximize the force of contraction. It is placed on the anterolateral aspect of the arm and dorsal surface of the forearm. To prevent bowstringing, the free muscle is passed deep to the brachioradialis and radial wrist extensor muscles, just distal to the elbow. This position of the muscle is optimal for elbow flexion and finger extension. However, the grip strength may weaken when the elbow is flexed. Correct muscle tension is reproduced in the upper limb before final suturing of the muscle to the finger extensors. The original muscle length is restored by stretching the muscle until the distance between the markers is once again 5 cm. Tension is adjusted with the shoulder in 60 degrees of abduction and 15 degrees of anterior flexion, the elbow in 150 degrees of flexion, the wrist in neutral, and the fingers in full extension. After adjusting the tension, the position of coaptation is marked over the tendon of the extensor digitorum communis and the donor muscle tendon. The elbow is flexed to 90 degrees, and with the wrist in neutral and the fingers fully flexed, the tenorrhaphies between the donor muscle tendon and the extensor digitorum communis tendon are completed at the previously marked sites. The appropriateness of tension in the transfer is evaluated using the tenodesis principle.

Second Free Muscle Transfer

Finger flexion reconstruction is done by using a second free muscle transfer (Fig. 7). It is performed 2 to 3 months after the first operation after improvement of postoperative contracture of the elbow and finger joints. The third to sixth intercostal nerves are dissected as far as the midclavicular line and transferred to the axillary region. The fifth and sixth intercostal nerves are used as the donor motor nerve for the second gracilis muscle transplant. The gracilis is harvested from the ipsilateral thigh, after ensuring that it will reach the mid-forearm from the second rib. The proximal end is sutured to the second and third ribs. To activate finger flexion, it is placed on the medial aspect of the upper arm and forearm so as not to be a secondary elbow flexor.

The muscle is passed deep to the pronator teres and long wrist flexor muscles, just distal to the elbow. The distal portion of the gracilis muscle is tendinous and thin and can easily be passed through the small hiatus deep to the fore-

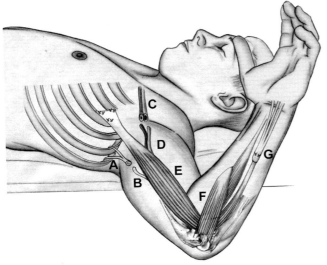

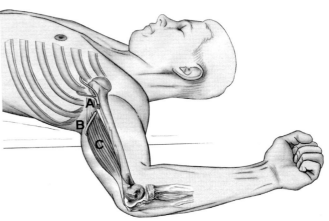

FIGURE 7. The second operative procedure for reconstruction of prehension after complete brachial plexus avulsion is a second free muscle transfer to restore finger flexion. The transferred gracilis is reinnervated by the fifth and sixth intercostal nerves. A, fifth and sixth intercostal nerves; B, motor branch of the muscle transplant; C, thoracodorsal artery and vein; D, nutrient artery and veins of the muscle transplant; E, muscle transplant; F, pronator teres and wrist flexors serving as a pulley; G, long finger flexor tendons. (Redrawn from Doi K, Muramtsu K, Hattori Y, et al. Reconstruction of upper extremity function brachial plexopathy using double free gracilis flaps. *Tech Hand Upper Extremity Surg* 2000;4:34–43.)

FIGURE 8. Nerve crossing of the third and fourth intercostal nerves to the motor branch of the triceps brachii muscle to restore elbow extension and stabilization after complete brachial plexus avulsion. A, third and fourth intercostal nerves; B, motor branch of the triceps brachii muscle; C, triceps brachii muscle. (Redrawn from Doi K, Muramtsu K, Hattori Y, et al. Reconstruction of upper extremity function brachial plexopathy using double free gracilis flaps. *Tech Hand Upper Extremity Surg* 2000;4:34–43.)

arm flexor muscles. The distal tendinous portion of the gracilis is coapted to the flexor digitorum profundus tendons. Muscle tension is determined with the principles described previously. While adjusting the tension, the shoulder, elbow, and wrist are in the same position as described above. Fingers are kept in full flexion. The nutrient vessels are anastomosed to the thoracodorsal artery and vein. The fifth and sixth intercostal nerves are coapted without tension to the motor nerve of the second muscle transplant.

Nerve Crossing to the Motor Branch of the Triceps Brachii Muscle

The third and fourth intercostal nerves are coapted to the motor branch of the triceps brachii muscle to activate the elbow extensors. Coaptation is performed before the second muscle is detached from the thigh (Fig. 8).

Sensory Reconstruction

To restore hand sensibility, the sensory rami of intercostal nerves are sutured to the medial cord of the brachial plexus at the second operation (Fig. 9). The sensory-dominant fascicles of the medial cord can be easily distinguished from the motor-dominant fascicles by measuring the sensory nerve action potentials. Sensory nerve fibers do not undergo wallerian degeneration, as most dorsal ganglion cells survive after preganglionic injury to the nerve roots.

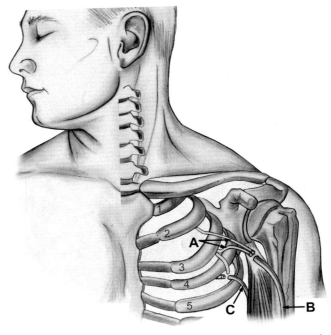

FIGURE 9. Nerve crossing of the supraclavicular nerve at the first free muscle transfer or the sensory rami of the second, third, and fourth intercostal nerves to the median or ulnar nerve component of the medial cord at the second free muscle transfer to restore sensibility to the hand. A, sensory rami of the second, third, and fourth intercostal nerves; B, ulnar nerve or median nerve; C, motor branch of the triceps brachii muscle. (Redrawn from Doi K, Muramtsu K, Hattori Y, et al. Reconstruction of upper extremity function brachial plexopathy using double free gracilis flaps. *Tech Hand Upper Extremity Surg* 2000;4:34–43.)

Postoperative Management

The upper limb is immobilized without tension on the transferred muscles, motor nerves, and nutrient vessels for 4 weeks postoperatively. The rehabilitation programs are described below.

Secondary Reconstruction

Elbow Extension (Dynamic Stability)

Elbow instability after intercostal nerve neurotization ruins prehension function even if the strength of the reinnervated transferred muscles is enough to move the fingers. Supplemental reinforcement of elbow extension by transferring the reinnervated infraspinatus to the triceps or tenodesis of the triceps brachii when the infraspinatus has not recovered enough for transfer is an optional procedure to provide stability of the elbow (Fig. 10) (17).

Tenolysis

Some cases of double free muscle transfer result in gliding insufficiency of the transferred muscle in spite of satisfactory contraction of the muscle due to adhesion to surrounding structures and needed tenolysis. Under local anesthesia, tenolysis of the transferred gracilis and distal tendons is performed to allow full evaluation from the proximal musculotendinous junction of the gracilis to the distal insertion of the tendon. Adhesions within the pulley system are also carefully released.

Carpometacarpal Arthrodesis of the Thumb

After recovery of the active finger motion, arthrodesis of the thumb carpometacarpal joint may be helpful. In addition, intentional flexion of the metacarpophalangeal joint and interphalangeal joint of the thumb and proximal and distal interphalangeal joints of the fingers may augment stable pinch function.

Glenohumeral Arthrodesis

The muscle transfer procedures may provide stability to shoulder joint. If instability persists, at a later stage after reinnervation of the transferred muscle is maximal, arthrodesis of the glenohumeral joint may be performed to allow the scapulothoracic joint to be moved by the remnant of the trapezius muscle. This allows proper control of the upper limb and prevents dispersion of power of the transferred muscles. Glenohumeral arthrodesis should be performed last in the reconstructive program because it makes subsequent reconstructive procedures difficult to perform in the position of the shoulder adduction.

COMPLICATIONS

Vascular Compromise

The muscle flap may develop vascular insufficiency from ischemia or congestion due to arterial or venous thrombosis, respectively. The accompanying skin paddle with the muscle flap helps in monitoring the circulatory status of the underlying muscle flap. If vascular problems are suspected, prompt (emergent) exploration of the anastomosed vessels is carried out to enhance survival of the transferred muscle. After revision of the anastomosed vessel, not only fresh bleeding from the muscle but also muscle contraction to electrical stimulation should be confirmed. Otherwise, the muscle will develop ischemic necrosis, leading to a poor result, and another free muscle transfer will be required.

Delayed or Nonreinnervation of the Transferred Muscles and Triceps Brachii Muscle

Depending on the donor motor nerve used, electromyographic reinnervation of the transferred muscle is detected 3 to 10 months after surgery. Muscles reinnervated by the spinal accessory nerve recover significantly earlier (mean of 3.9 months) than the muscles reinnervated by the intercostal nerves (mean of 4.8 months; $p < .05$). Voluntary contraction

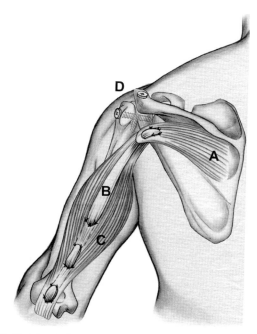

FIGURE 10. The infraspinatus-to-triceps transfer. After arthrodesis of the glenohumeral joint, the fascia latae tendon graft is sutured to the distal end of the infraspinatus muscle, which had been reinnervated by the repaired postganglionic C5 nerve root and the triceps aponeurosis. A, infraspinatus muscle; B, fascia latae tendon graft; C, triceps brachii muscle; D, glenohumeral arthrodesis. (Redrawn from Doi K, Muramtsu K, Hattori Y, et al. Reconstruction of upper extremity function brachial plexopathy using double free gracilis flaps. *Tech Hand Upper Extremity Surg* 2000;4:34–43.)

usually ensues 2 months later. Reinnervation of the triceps muscle occurs even much later than the reinnervation of the transferred muscle by the intercostal nerve (mean of 8.2 months; p <.001). Nonreinnervation or delayed reinnervation later than the time described previously indicates poor functional prognosis. Even if reinnervation occurs, after a long delay, muscle atrophy of the target muscle adversely affects the activation of joint motion. In such situations, further reconstructive plans should be abandoned.

Adhesion of the Transferred Muscle

Adhesion of the transferred muscle to the surrounding tissue occurs to some degree in all cases. Approximately one-third of the cases will require a subsequent tenolysis procedure. Tenolysis is indicated when active finger function is not achieved despite strong contraction of the transferred muscle. The latissimus dorsi transfers develop recurrent adhesions. In my experience, all the gracilis transfers have improved range of finger motion postoperatively because of reduced adhesion formation.

Instability of the Proximal Joints

The double free muscle transfer imparts motion to multiple joints simultaneously. The first free muscle transfer is designed to generate both finger extension and elbow flexion. The second free muscle transfer also flexes the elbow simultaneously with finger flexion, even though it is not placed in the flexion–extension plane of the elbow and is not intended for elbow flexion. Hence, without recovery of elbow flexion antagonists, simultaneous elbow flexion occurred with finger movement (either flexion or extension). The third and fourth intercostal nerves are coapted to the motor branch of the triceps brachii muscle to restore elbow extension and to stabilize the elbow by negating the tendency of elbow flexion with finger movement. Even if the power of the triceps brachii is weak, it contributes to stability of the elbow with the aid of gravity. If reinnervation of the triceps brachii fails, secondary reconstruction—e.g., reinnervated infraspinatus transfer to the triceps brachii or tenodesis of the triceps brachii—is recommended to restore elbow stability.

The reinnervated free muscle and the triceps brachii and shoulder girdle muscles without arthrodesis can achieve stability of the glenohumeral joint. During exploration of the brachial plexus, the C5 nerve root, if available, should be crossed to the suprascapular nerve with the nerve graft. This not only improves shoulder function, but also contributes to reinnervation of paralyzed muscles for use as possible donor muscles for transfer if the triceps brachii does not recover. If the glenohumeral joint remains unstable even after recovery of these muscles, glenohumeral arthrodesis is to be performed, although it may limit several activities— e.g., turning over during sleep. Care must be taken to prevent fractures of the proximal humerus.

No Sensibility of the Hand

Restoration of basic modalities (e.g., protective sensation and position sense) is imperative when prehensile function is reconstructed for irreparable BPI. Half of the patients recover sensibility of the palm and adequate position sense. However, protective sensation in the ulnar side of the hand and finger does not recover in half of the patients. Minor injury and burn can easily occur in these parts of the hand.

Pain Syndrome

None of our patients had severe causalgia that could not be controlled by the usual analgesics.

REHABILITATION

Initial Stage (before Electromyographic Evidence of Reinnervation to the Transferred Muscles)

The use of electrical stimulation for the transferred muscles and nerve-repaired muscles remains controversial. However, we prefer to use electrical stimulation for the paralyzed target muscles such as two transferred gracilis muscles, the triceps brachii, and the supraspinatus and infraspinatus, if the suprascapular nerve has been repaired. Low-intensity electrical stimulation started during the third postoperative week and is continued until electromyographic reinnervation is detected in the muscles.

Functional orthoses are used to immobilize the reconstructed upper limb. We prefer the airbag type of orthosis (Nakamura Brace, Shimane, Japan) to immobilize the shoulder and elbow joints. A plaster of paris long arm cast is used for immobilization of the wrist and finger joints. The long arm cast is removed 4 weeks postoperatively, and only passive flexion of the elbow joint is commenced. During the early postoperative period, a plastic static splint is used to maintain the wrist in a neutral position and the proximal and distal interphalangeal joints in extension to allow these joints to contract in this position. At the sixth postoperative week, while protecting overtension at the muscle–tendon suture site of the transferred muscle by wrist extension after the first free muscle transfer or flexion after the second free muscle transfer, passive extension of the elbow is started. Only the metacarpophalangeal joints are moved passively because the transferred muscles are intended to move the single joint to decrease the effect of claw finger deformity. At the ninth postoperative week, the airbag orthosis is removed, and an elbow sling orthosis is applied to prevent subluxation of the shoulder.

Late Stage (after Reinnervation)

After electromyographic documentation of reinnervation of the transferred muscle, usually 3 to 8 months post-

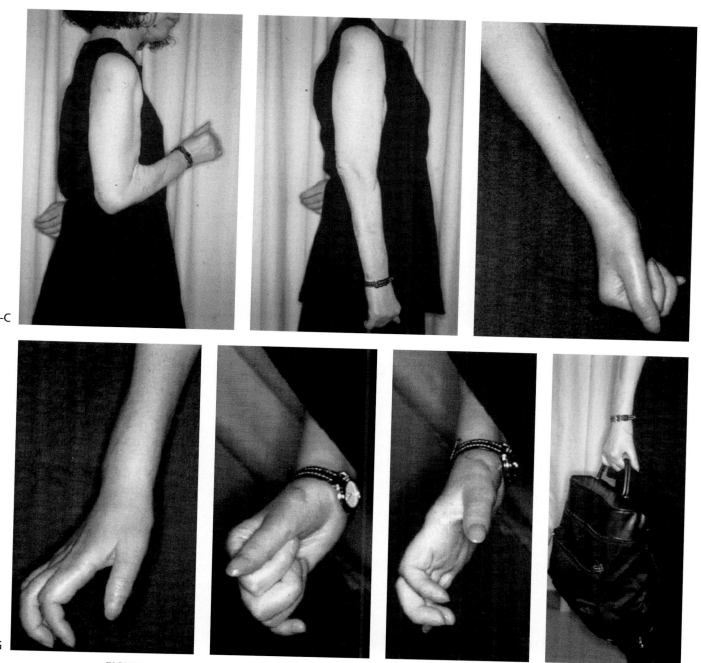

A–C

D–G

FIGURE 11. A 30-year-old female sustained complete avulsion of C5 to T1 of right brachial plexus and underwent double free muscle transfer procedure, although she had no nerve repair of C5 root. Postoperative motor function 36 months after the initial procedure. Elbow flexion **(A)** and extension **(B)**; finger flexion **(C)** and extension **(D)** with the elbow in extension. Finger flexion **(E)** and extension **(F)** with the elbow in flexion; and carrying a bag **(G)**. (From Doi K, Sakai K, Fuchigami Y, et al. Reconstruction of irreparable brachial plexus injuries with reinnervated free-muscle transfer. Case report. *J Neurosurg* 1996;85:174–177, with permission.)

operatively, electromyographic biofeedback techniques are started to train the transferred muscles to move the elbow and fingers.

Muscle reeducation is indicated when patients display minimal active contraction with an identified muscle or muscle group. The initial goal of reeducation is for patients to reactivate voluntary control of the muscle. When the patient is working with a weak muscle, the intensity of motor unit activity and the frequency of the muscle contraction are emphasized. Treatment sessions should be short and end when fatigue is noted by a decreasing ability of the patient to achieve the set goal level.

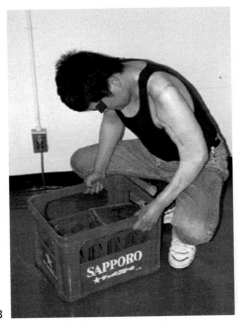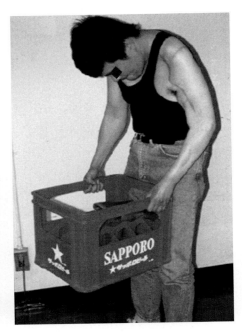

A,B

FIGURE 12. Result of reconstruction by double free muscle transfer. A 24-year-old man sustained complete avulsion of C5 to T1 of the left brachial plexus. **A,B:** Reconstruction of prehension permits lifting of a 13-kg weight using both hands.

GENERAL FUNCTIONAL OUTCOME

Twenty-six of 32 patients reconstructed by the double free muscle procedure and followed up for more than 24 months after the second free muscle transfer (mean follow-up, 40 months) were assessed for long-term outcome of universal prehension, including motion and stability of the shoulder and elbow, voluntary and independent motion of fingers, sensibility, and activities-of-daily-living functions (20). Functional outcome of prehension according to the

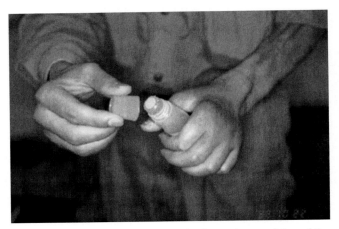

FIGURE 13. Another patient, who had complete avulsion of the left brachial plexus and underwent the double free muscle transfer procedure, is shown lifting a 5-kg container with both hands at 36 months postoperatively. (From Doi K, Muramatsu K, Hattori Y, et al. Restoration of prehension with the double free muscle technique following complete avulsion of the brachial plexus: indications and long-term results. *J Bone Joint Surg Am* 2000;82:652–666, with permission.)

author's classification was excellent in four (restoration of more than 90 degrees of elbow flexion, dynamic stability of the elbow while moving fingers, and more than 60 degrees of total active motion of fingers), good in 10 (same as excellent, except total active motion of fingers is 30 to 60 degrees), fair in two (total active motion of fingers is less than 30 degrees), and poor in 10. Satisfactory results (excellent and good) were obtained in 14 of the 26 patients (54%) and they obtained more than 90 degrees of elbow flexion, dynamic stability of the elbow, voluntary finger motion at any position of the elbow, and more than 30 degrees of total active motion of fingers. They also used their reconstructed hand for hand activities such as holding a bottle while opening a cap and lifting a heavy object. All the patients who had satisfactory results were younger than 32 years of age with a shorter interval between injury and surgery (less than 8 months); a longer follow-up (more than 55 months); no serious accompanied injuries of the subclavicular artery, spinal accessory nerve, or spinal cord; reconstruction with both the gracilis muscles; and successful restoration of elbow stability with nerve-crossing or secondary tendon transfer. Satisfying these prerequisites, the double free muscle procedure should provide reliable and useful prehensile function for the patient with complete avulsion of the brachial plexus to be able to use his or her otherwise useless limb (Figs. 11–13).

REFERENCES

1. Krakauer JD, Wood MB. Adult injuries and salvages. In: Peimer C, ed. *Surgery of the hand and upper extremity.* New York: McGraw-Hill, 1996:1411–1442.

2. Millesi H. Brachial plexus injuries: management and results. In: Terzis JK, ed. *Microreconstruction of nerve injuries.* Philadelphia: WB Saunders, 1987:247–260.

3. Nagano A, Tsuyama N, Ochiai N, et al. Direct nerve crossing with the intercostal nerve to treat avulsion injuries of the brachial plexus. *J Hand Surg [Am]* 1989;14:980–985.

4. Narakas AO, Hentz VR. Neurotization in brachial plexus injuries: indication and results. *Clin Orthop* 1988;237:43–56.

5. Akasaka Y, Hara T, Takahashi M. Free muscle transplantation combined with intercostal nerve crossing for reconstruction of elbow flexion and wrist extension in brachial plexus injuries. *Microsurgery* 1991;12:346–351.

6. Berger A, Flory PJ, Schaller E. Muscle transfers in brachial plexus lesions. *J Reconstr Microsurg* 1990;6:113–116.

7. Doi K. Obstetric and traumatic pediatric palsy. In: Peimer C, ed. *Surgery of the hand and upper extremity.* New York: McGraw-Hill, 1996:1443–1463.

8. Doi K. New reconstructive procedure for brachial plexus injury. *Clin Plast Surg* 1997;24:75–85.

9. Doi K, Ihara K, Sakamoto T, et al. Functional latissimus dorsi island pedicle musculocutaneous flap to restore finger function. *J Hand Surg [Am]* 1985;10:678–684.

10. Doi K, Sakai K, Fuchigami Y, et al. Reconstruction of irreparable brachial plexus injuries with reinnervated free-muscle transfer. Case report. *J Neurosurg* 1996;85:174–177.

11. Doi K, Sakai K, Kuwata N, et al. Reconstruction of finger and elbow function after complete avulsion of the brachial plexus. *J Hand Surg [Am]* 1992;16:796–803.

12. Doi K, Sakai K, Kuwata N, et al. Double-muscle technique for reconstruction of prehension after complete avulsion of brachial plexus. *J Hand Surg [Am]* 1995;20:408–414.

13. Doi K, Hattori Y, Tan S-H. Endoscopic harvesting of the gracilis muscle for reinnervated free-muscle transfer. *Plast Reconstr Surg* 1997;100:1817–1823.

14. Moberg E. Surgical treatment for absent single-hand grip and elbow extension in quadriplegia. *J Bone Joint Surg Am* 1975;57:196–206.

15. Moberg E. Reconstructive hand surgery in tetraplegia, stroke and cerebral palsy: some basic concepts in physiology and neurology. *J Hand Surg [Am]* 1976;1:29–34.

16. Moberg E. *The upper limb in tetraplegia.* Stuttgart: George Thieme, 1978.

17. Doi K, Shigetomi M, Kaneko K, et al. Significance of elbow extension in reconstruction of prehension with reinnervated free-muscle transfer following complete brachial plexus avulsion. *Plast Reconstr Surg* 1997;100:364–372.

18. Zancolli EA. *Structural and dynamic bases of hand surgery,* 2nd ed. Philadelphia: JB Lippincott Co, 1979.

19. Zancolli EA. Surgery for the quadriplegic hand with active strong wrist extension preserved. A study of 97 cases. *Clin Orthop* 1975;112:101–113.

20. Doi K, Muramatsu K, Hattori Y, et al. Restoration of prehension with the double free muscle technique following complete avulsion of the brachial plexus, indications and long-term results. *J Bone Joint Surg Am* 2000;82:652–666.

21. Doi K, Muramtsu K, Hattori Y, et al. Reconstruction of upper extremity function brachial plexopathy using double free gracilis flaps. *Tech Hand Upper Extremity Surg* 2000;4:34–43.

22. Manktelow RT, McKee NH. Free muscle transplantation to provide active finger flexion. *J Hand Surg [Am]* 1978;3:416–426.

23. Manktelow RT, Zuker RM, McKee NH. Functioning free muscle transplantation. *J Hand Surg [Am]* 1984;9:32–39.

60

RECONSTRUCTION OF THE SPASTIC HAND

ANN E. VAN HEEST

HAND SPASTICITY

Definition and Classification

Spasticity in the hand is a secondary peripheral manifestation of primary central nervous system (CNS) dysfunction. Classification of the spasticity depends on the type of primary CNS lesion, most commonly cerebral palsy, stroke, and traumatic brain injury. The peripheral effects of cerebral palsy, stroke, and traumatic brain injury are classified based on the topographic involvement and the type of tone that is present (1). *Topographic involvement* means the number of limbs that are involved: monoplegia (one limb), hemiplegia (one arm, one leg), diplegia (both legs), quadriplegia (both arms and both legs), and total body involvement (quadriplegia with mental retardation). The type of muscle tone disorder that is clinically manifested further classifies the disorder. Manifestations of CNS dysfunction can include spasticity, dystonia (athetosis), flaccidity, or mixed dysfunction. The amount of CNS control of the peripheral muscles is variable and is important prognostically; isolated or combined spasticity, dystonia, and flaccidity can be present.

Incidence and Natural History

Cerebral palsy is a nonprogressive CNS dysfunction that occurs in the perinatal period. Cerebral palsy is associated most commonly with prematurity and low birth weight (2) but can be due to neonatal asphyxia, intrauterine stroke, CNS malformation, infections, such as neonatal meningitis, kernicterus (Rh incompatibility), or postnatal brain injury that is due to closed head trauma or anoxic events.

Stroke is most common in individuals owing to a cerebral vascular accident that affects the middle cerebral artery, injures the motor and sensory strip in the brain, and leads to a hemiplegic pattern of deformity. Strokes affect 1 in 1,000 individuals per year, causing 200,000 deaths per year, and are a major cause of hemiplegia in adults in the United States. If the patient survives the initial 6 months after stroke, the average subsequent survival is more than 6 years. Within 6 months after stroke, recovery is usually stable for surgical assessment (3–6).

Traumatic brain injury affects 1 to 2 per 1,000 individuals per year in the United States, with most affected individuals younger than 40 years of age, and occurring secondary to motor vehicle accidents. Eleven percent of individuals with traumatic brain injury die. Traumatic brain injury is assessed by Glasgow Coma Scale, with younger patients with higher Glasgow Coma Scale scores having the best chances for survival. Patients who emerge from coma within 2 weeks have the best chance for neurologic recovery. Improvement in motor function improves at as long as 18 months after injury, with cognitive function continuing beyond 18 months (6).

In cerebral palsy, cerebral vascular accidents, and traumatic brain injury, a pattern of spastic hemiplegia is the most common manifestation of the CNS deficiency. This chapter focuses on the most common form of spasticity in the hand: spastic hemiplegia due to cerebral palsy. In general, the principles that are used to treat this disorder can be applied to other disorders that cause similar spasticity deformities.

Pathogenesis

Spasticity is characterized by a velocity-dependent increase in muscle tone. In upper motor neuron lesions, such as cerebral palsy, traumatic brain injury, and stroke, the normal inhibitory function is lost. Many neural pathways control stretch reflex excitability, and a malfunction in any of them could produce spasticity. At the present time, the underlying mechanism is understood to be a loss or decrease in the presynaptic Ia inhibition, which leads to an increase in exaggeration of the reflex with resultant spasticity (7). Increased muscle spasticity then leads to musculoskeletal impairment through muscle imbalance across the joints, which leads to impaired function acutely, and chronic joint contractures with skeletal deformation.

Clinical Significance

Because of the CNS injury, patients with CNS dysfunction can have significant functional impairment of their upper limbs. In the past, most evaluation and treatment of cerebral palsy centered on the lower extremities and the patient's ability to walk. In the twenty-first century, with improved motorized wheelchair controls, public handicapped accessibility, and increased opportunities for individuals to access computers and assistive communication devices, treatment emphasis has now swung more toward maximizing functional use of the upper extremities.

PATIENT EVALUATION

History, Physical Examination, and Testing

Evaluation of children with cerebral palsy has evolved to an integration of our assessment for each aspect of manifestation of cerebral palsy: mentation, motivation, functional use patterns, sensation, static and dynamic deformities, and motor control. Evaluation of a patient's baseline involvement in each of these areas allows formulation of realistic treatment goals and can allow measurement of treatment outcomes.

Assessment of the patient's mentation includes evaluating the extent of musculoskeletal involvement and the degree of generalized central involvement, along with the presence or absence of seizures. *Mentation* can be measured by intelligence quotient testing or, for the higher functioning child, by school performance.

Motivation assessment is important for the higher functioning child, particularly with tendon transfer reconstructive surgery, which may require a highly motivated child to participate with postoperative therapy.

The child's *functional use* of the hand can be quantified by using House's classification of upper extremity functional use (Table 1). In this nine-level classification, functional use is classified into the following categories: does not use, passive assist (poor, fair, good), active assist (poor, fair, good), and spontaneous use (partial, complete). Functional use patterns can be determined through questioning the parent and child regarding use in daily activities, as well as through observation of child play (for the younger child) or the carrying out of daily activities of dressing or tying shoes (for the older child). This provides a baseline that can be used to help the physician communicate the functional goals of the surgery with the parents. The functional use can then be reassessed postoperatively by using this scale to assess for functional improvement.

Sensation can be evaluated by stereognosis, two-point discrimination, and proprioception. In our review of 40 children with spastic hemiplegia (8), we have found that stereognosis is the most sensitive discriminator of the degree of sensibility impairment, as is shown in Table 2. We found that 97% had a stereognosis impairment when using the 12 objects that are shown in Table 3. The five objects that are listed on the left

TABLE 1. CLASSIFICATION OF UPPER EXTREMITY FUNCTIONAL USE

Level	Category	Description
0	Does not use	Does not use
1	Poor passive assist	Uses as stabilizing weight only
2	Fair passive assist	Can hold object placed in hand
3	Good passive assist	Can hold object and stabilize it for use by other hand
4	Poor active assist	Can actively grasp object and hold it weakly
5	Fair active assist	Can actively grasp object and stabilize it well
6	Good active assist	Can actively grasp object and manipulate it
7	Spontaneous use, partial	Can perform bimanual activities and occasionally uses the hand spontaneously
8	Spontaneous use, complete	Uses hand completely, independently, without reference to the other hand

From Van Heest AE, House JH, Cariello, C. Upper extremity surgical treatment of cerebral palsy. *J Hand Surg [Am]* 1999;24:324, with permission.

column of the table discriminate gross motor function, and the seven objects that are listed on the right column of the table discriminate fine motor function. These children demonstrated recognition of 12 out of 12 objects on the unaffected side, verifying that they understood the test. Furthermore, we found that those children with severe sensibility impairment had a significant size discrepancy when the affected side was compared to the unaffected side. The shortened limb can be a useful clue to underlying sensibility deficiency, particularly in the child who is too young or too retarded to reliably perform a sensibility assessment. Children with sensibility deficiencies need to be coached to use the eyes, rather than touch, for afferent feedback. Several studies have indicated that poor sensation is *not* a contraindication for surgery (9). In fact, one study has reported an improvement in sensibility function after surgical intervention (10), presumably associated with increased postoperative functional use.

Physical examination begins with evaluation for *static deformity* by examining the limb for passive range of motion of the shoulder, elbow, forearm, wrist, and hand, evaluating for joint contractures. Passive range of motion needs to be done slowly to overcome muscle tone. Contractures can exist

TABLE 2. SENSIBILITY IMPAIRMENT IN SPASTIC HEMIPLEGIA

Stereognosis impairment	No. of objects correctly identified	% of children
Intact	12	3
Mild	9–11	22
Moderate	5–8	40
Severe	0–4	35

TABLE 3. OBJECTS FOR ASSESSMENT OF STEREOGNOSIS FUNCTION

Gross	Fine
Cube	Safety pin
Key	Paper clip
Pencil	Penny
Marble	Pin
Spoon	Button
	Rubber band
	String

in the joints or the muscles, or both. Note that the finger and thumb flexor muscles are *biarticular muscles*, which means that they cross the wrist and finger joints. Wrist joint contractures can be checked first with the fingers flexed to assess if contractures exist in the joint itself and then with fingers extended to assess if the finger and thumb flexor muscles are contracted. If there is full passive mobility of each joint and muscle, no static deformity exists, and assessment proceeds to dynamic deformities by looking at motor function.

In addition to sensibility testing, the occupational therapist can be helpful in the evaluation of *motor function*. In the higher functioning child, the pediatric Jebsen-Taylor standardized test can be used as a baseline from which to measure the effect of subsequent treatment and also as a screen of which subtest functions have the greatest impairment (e.g., pinching small objects versus grasping large cans). Videotaping allows assessment of the spasticity that is encountered during routine activities of daily living and eliminates the stress of performance on demand in the physician's office. Observation of the child carrying out functional tasks on videotape, as well as in the office, allows assessment of the *dynamic deformities* that are present. Identification of the specific spastic muscle can be determined by the joint position; for example, excessive dynamic wrist flexion with ulnar deviation identifies the flexor carpi ulnaris (FCU) as the spastic deforming force. Palpation of specific spastic muscles also localizes the source of the dynamic imbalance. Voluntary control of the muscle also needs assessment. Additionally, spasticity (increased muscle tone) versus dystonia (lack of CNS control with position of dynamic deformity, varying with time) should be noted.

Dynamic electromyography (EMG) testing is another diagnostic tool that has been used to help assess motor tone and phasic control of specific muscles (11,12). In major centers that have motion labs for gait analysis, the same technology can be used for upper extremity assessment. For example, Kozin et al. (13) have shown that biceps or brachialis spasticity, or both, can lead to elbow flexion deformity; preoperative dynamic EMG can assess spastic tone and phase control of each muscle to direct treatment to the specific offending muscles. Differences in phasic control of muscles versus continuous spastic activation can be assessed, as well as determination of central control of muscles, as children are viewed carrying out functional tasks.

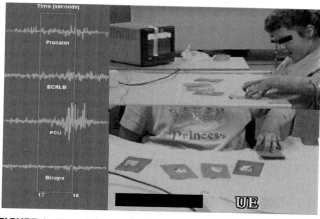

FIGURE 1. Use of the motion laboratory in assessment of upper extremity activities. The two video frames on the right show a front and side view of the child performing the pediatric Jebsen-Taylor hand test. Looking at the two angles simultaneously allows assessment of the deformity in both the sagittal and coronal planes. For example, this child can be seen to demonstrate a wrist flexion and ulnar deviation deformity. The electromyography (EMG) data on the left show 3 seconds of electrical-myographic activity of four muscles: the biceps, the pronator teres, the flexor carpi ulnaris, and the extensor carpi radialis longus/brevis. Needle electrodes are used for the pronator teres and the flexor carpi radialis. Surface electrodes are used for the biceps and the radial wrist extensor muscles. The box encompassing the central one-third of the EMG data highlights the 1 second of activity that is simultaneously shown on the video frames on the right. This motion analysis study allows for assessment of the spasticity patterns of the muscles and whether the child is able to actively control the muscles for functional use.

In our motion lab, experience shows that children need to be at least 7 years of age to appropriately cooperate with the motion lab analysis. The children have tolerated the placement of the fine needle electrodes through the use of topical anesthetic cream for 1 hour before electrode placement. The protocol that is used in our motion laboratory is demonstrated in Figure 1.

In summation of the evaluative process, the physician needs to integrate the results of the assessment of mentation, motivation, sensibility testing, static and dynamic deformities, and clinical and dynamic EMG motor testing to synthesize an overall treatment plan, taking into account the child's capabilities, disabilities, and potential in the context of the child's age. Discussion with the parents and the child is imperative in formulating the individualized treatment plan and its expected outcome.

NONOPERATIVE TREATMENT

Options and Indications

Options for treatment in cerebral palsy include occupational therapy, medications, injections, and neurosurgical procedures.

Occupational therapy includes the use of splints, stretching and strengthening programs, and active functional use activities, and many therapists may now administer electrical stimulation programs. Two types of *splints* can be used: nighttime serial static splinting is used for treatment of muscle or joint contractures, and daytime splints are used for prepositioning the hand to improve active function. The indication for *nighttime splinting* is contracture; if no contractures of the muscles or joints exist, nighttime splinting is not necessary and is a waste of time and money for the child and family. If contractures *do* exist at the elbow, serial static splints can be used. If contractures exist at the wrist or fingers and thumb, a nighttime forearm-based wrist–hand orthosis may be helpful. Pronation contractures are difficult to splint and are usually treated with passive stretching. *Daytime splints* are usually used to preposition the wrist in a neutral to slight "cock-up" position to help improve grasp and to preposition the thumb out of the palm to help improve pinch. If the splint is bulky or cumbersome, it interferes with rather than enhances function, thus defeating its purpose. Care should be given to ensure proper fit of the splint, so that its purpose can be achieved. *Stretching and strengthening programs*, along with *active functional use activities*, are carried out by the therapist and are taught to the parents and child as a home program. The efficacy of these treatments has been documented in limited studies (14–16), but no controlled studies have been done. *Electrical stimulation* is a modality that is administered by therapists as neuromuscular electrical stimulation, threshold electrical stimulation, or functional electrical stimulation. Neuromuscular electrical stimulation and functional electrical stimulation involve stimulation that produces a muscles contraction with the goal of strengthening and training a muscle. Threshold electrical stimulation involves low-intensity stimulation below the level that causes a muscle contraction and is used, while the patient sleeps, on muscles that are antagonists to the affected spastic muscles. Strengthening any muscle has been shown to improve the individual's ability to control the muscle, but does not reduce spasticity (17). Lasting outcomes have not been reported (16).

For patients with more global tone problems, appropriate consultation or multispecialty evaluation, or both, with the rehabilitation physicians, a neurologist, or a neurosurgeon, or a combination of these, is indicated. The treatment pros and cons need to be explored for the options of tone-reducing medications (Valium, baclofen), tone-reducing injections (botulinum toxin, phenol), or tone-reducing neurosurgical interventions (baclofen pumps, selective dorsal rhizotomy), or a combination of these options. For the quadriplegic patient with overall tone control problems, medications or neurosurgical interventions should be used and stabilized before hand surgery intervention. Selective dorsal rhizotomy has been shown, in studies in the 1990s, to have an indirect tone-reducing effect on the upper extremities, in addition to its primary direct effect in the lower extremities (18,19).

For patients with more focal muscle-tone imbalance, botulinum toxin type A injections (Botox, Allergan Pharmaceuticals, Irvine, CA) have been shown to be effective in reducing spasticity in the muscles that are injected and in improving hand function (20–24). Botulinum toxin type A locally blocks the release of acetylcholine at the neuromuscular junction with a reversible action that lasts for an average of 3 to 4 months. During this period, assessment of the antagonist muscles can be made, possible surgical benefits can be assessed, antagonist muscles can be strengthened, and spastic muscles can be stretched, with the benefits lasting beyond the direct effects of the medication. For the mildly involved child, treatment with botulinum toxin type A injections may obviate the need for surgical intervention.

Author's Preferred Treatment: Techniques, Personal Series, and Results

For patients with spastic hemiplegia that is secondary to cerebral palsy, the typical deformity includes shoulder internal rotation, elbow flexion, forearm pronation, wrist flexion with ulnar deviation, and thumb-in-palm, swanneck, or clenched fist deformities. Optimal surgical candidates are patients who are at least 7 years of age (or mature enough to comply with postoperative regimens) with a joint-positioning deformity that interferes with active functional use of the arm. After children are diagnosed with cerebral palsy, there exists a period of, usually, 7 years before children can even be considered surgical candidates; in the meantime, children are, by definition, treated nonoperatively. Most of the nonoperative regimen revolves around parent and child education in active functional use of the affected arm to the extent that the child is able to perform.

Annual or biannual monitoring by the physician is important to assess for the development of contractures and overall developmental progress regarding age-appropriate use of the arm. For example, babies are assessed for their ability to weight bear on the arm for sitting and crawling; young children are assessed for bimanual gross motor skills, such as dressing and ball catching; school-age children are assessed for fine motor skills, such as buttoning and shoe tying; and all children are assessed for the development of contractures with growth. If failure to meet developmental milestones is encountered, a specific therapy protocol is instituted to help keep the child as close to normal developmental progress as their physical disabilities allow. Therapists are in a unique position to develop a relationship with the family and child through patient education regarding use patterns and adaptive patterns, and their services can be an integral part of the delivery of medical attention to these children.

For children with fixed deformities, nighttime static splints are prescribed, as described previously in the section Options and Indications. For children with dynamic deformities, daytime functional splints *may* be helpful but need to be carefully assessed as to whether they are in fact improving function rather than immobilizing and promoting patterns of the child ignoring the limb. If the daytime splints are counterproductive, they should be discontinued.

A treatment option for dynamic deformities due to spastic imbalance across a joint is botulinum toxin injection.

TABLE 4. SURGICAL TREATMENT OPTIONS IN THE SPASTIC UPPER EXTREMITY[a]

Procedures	Deformity				
	Elbow flexion	Forearm pronation	Wrist flexion/ulnar deviation	Finger deformity	Thumb-in-palm
Soft tissue releases	Biceps lengthenings (42) Brachialis lengthenings (42)	PT releases (26) Biceps aponeurosis releases PQ release	FCR lengthenings (43) Flexor pronator slides (29,30) FCU lengthenings (43)	FDS lengthenings (43)	Adductor and/or first dorsal interosseous releases (35) First web Z-plasty
Tendon transfers		PT rerouting (27)	BR to ECRB/L (44,45) ECU to ECRB/L FCU to ECRB/L FCR to ECRB/L (46,47) PT to ECRL	FCU to EDC BR to EDC FDS tenodesis (33) Lateral band reroutings (31) Spiral oblique retinacular ligament reconstruction (32)	FPL lengthenings FCR to APL PL to APL (34) PL to EPB BR to APL BR to EPB
Bone/joint stabilization		Rotational osteotomies	Wrist fusion with PRC PRC (48)	Palmar plate capsulodesis PIP fusions Distal interphalangeal joint fusions	PL to EPL EPL reroutings (38) BR to EPL FCR to EPB Accessory muscle of APL to EPB MCP fusions (37) MCP capsulodesis (36) Interphalangeal joint fusions

APL, abductor pollicis longus; BR, brachioradialis; ECRB/L, extensor carpi radialis brevis and/or longus; ECU, extensor carpi ulnaris; EDC, extensor digitorum communis; EPB, extensor pollicis brevis; EPL, extensor pollicis longus; FCR, flexor carpi radialis; FCU, flexor carpi ulnaris; FDS, flexor digitorum superficialis; FPL, flexor pollicis longus; MCP, metacarpophalangeal joint; PIP, proximal interphalangeal joint; PL, palmaris longus; PQ, pronator quadratus; PRC, proximal row carpectomy; PT, pronator teres.
[a]The numbers refer to the reference for the surgical technique.
From Van Heest AE, House JH, Cariello, C. Upper extremity surgical treatment of cerebral palsy. *J Hand Surg [Am]* 1999;24:325, with permission.

My series (24) of 51 children who were treated with 107 botulinum injections at an average of 10.5 years of age (with a range from 2 to 34 years of age) showed 7 of 12 quadriplegic patients exhibiting successful diminution of contractures and 32 of 39 hemiplegic and triplegic patients exhibiting improved function, as measured by range of motion, pediatric Jebsen-Taylor hand testing, and functional questionnaire evaluations. For the hemiplegic child with no fixed joint contractures, botulinum toxin injections into the FCU (for wrist flexion deformities due to a spastic FCU with active, but weak, wrist extensors) and into the pronator teres (for forearm pronation due to a spastic pronator teres with an active, but weak, supinator) are effective in improving function.

SURGICAL MANAGEMENT

Options and Indications

Surgical Principles

The surgical principles for treatment of spastic deformities in cerebral palsy are the following:

1. Release or lengthen the spastic or contracted muscles.
2. Augment (tendon transfers into) the weak or flaccid antagonist muscles.
3. Stabilize the joint for severe joint instability or severe fixed contractures.

The major goal in surgical reconstruction is *balance* across the affected joints. Surgical treatment targets joint imbalance to prevent fixed deformity and to improve functional use. Ideally, joint balance can be achieved through appropriate releases or lengthenings of the spastic muscles, with tendon transfers to augment the weak antagonist muscles, as necessary. If severe fixed deformity is already present, joint stabilization procedures may be necessary.

The surgeon is required to carefully assess the type of deformity and its treatment at each joint separately and then to synthesize them together to organize a comprehensive surgical reconstructive plan. Adequate shoulder, elbow, and forearm function are necessary for the patient to be able to appropriately position the limb in space; adequate wrist, finger, and thumb function are necessary for the patient to appropriately grasp, pinch, and release. Surgical treatment options for each of the deformities are listed in Table 4.

Shoulder

The most *common* deformity at the shoulder is internal rotation and adduction, which usually is not symptomatic, as this positions the arm effectively by the side. The most *symptomatic* deformity at the shoulder is external rotation and abduction. The arm interferes with normal balance or may strike objects, such as when the patient comes through a doorway. If the patient is wheelchair bound, wheelchair adaptations to restrain the arm in adduction can be tried. If conservative measures fail, a slide of the deltoid insertion for abduction deformity or an internal humeral derotational osteotomy for external rotation deformity can be performed. If the movement is primarily athetotic, surgical management is not recommended.

Elbow

The most common deformity at the elbow is flexion. The primary muscles that contribute to this deformity are the biceps and the brachialis. The secondary offenders are the brachioradialis (BR) and flexor pronator wad muscles, as these muscles cross the elbow joint but are not primary elbow flexors. The primary procedure that is used to treat elbow flexion deformity is Z-lengthening of the biceps tendon with fractional lengthening of the brachialis muscle. If severe contracture exists, the BR may need to be released off its origin as well. A flexor pronator slide, as treatment for a wrist and finger flexion deformity, has a secondary effect of lessening the elbow flexion deformity.

Elbow flexion deformities of less than 45 degrees rarely functionally impair use of the limb and are usually treated nonoperatively. Elbow flexion deformities of greater than 90 degrees should be approached with caution, as the neurovascular bundle may be shortened and may limit the amount of surgical correction that is possible. Improvement of 40 degrees has been reported as an average result after biceps and brachialis lengthening (25).

Forearm

The most common deformity of the forearm is pronation, which can severely limit the child's ability to position the arm in space for grasping objects or for bringing the palms of the hands together for two-handed activities. The offending muscles are primarily the pronator teres and, secondarily, the pronator quadratus.

There are several surgical procedures to lessen forearm pronation (26,27). Two procedures that directly address the problem are pronator teres release and pronator teres rerouting. The pronator teres release works primarily through release of a deforming spastic muscle and relies on the biceps or the supinator, or both, to provide active supination after the deforming force of pronation is released. This operation is indicated if the child exhibits a severely spastic pronator teres

with little control of its activity. The pronator teres is released off its insertion on the middle one-third of the radius.

The pronator rerouting procedure not only releases the pronator teres as a deforming pronation force, but also transfers the pronator back to the radius as a supinator force. This operation provides greater correction, as it releases the agonist and augments the antagonist, but care needs to be taken not to overcorrect.

Several procedures provide forearm supination as a secondary effect. The flexor pronator slide diminishes the strength of the pronator teres by releasing it off its origin. Transfer of the FCU to the extensor carpi radialis longus (ECRL) or extensor carpi radialis brevis (ECRB) provides a supination moment arm, which is greatest if the FCU is released two-thirds of the length of the forearm, as it wraps around the ulna onto the dorsum of the wrist (28). Take note that, conversely, transfer of the flexor carpi radialis (FCR) around the radius to the ECRL or brevis provides a pronation moment arm; this transfer exacerbates the forearm pronation deformity and should be avoided as a wrist tendon transfer in this population.

Wrist

The most common deformity of the wrist is flexion, often with ulnar deviation, as well. This is probably the most functionally disabling deformity, as it significantly interferes with grasp and release function. Several different surgical options exist, with the choice dependent on the degree of deformity and the extent of volitional control of each muscle involved. Application of the surgical principles that were listed previously is necessary and is part of the art of designing a successful reconstructive plan: Release or lengthen the deforming spastic muscles (FCU, FCR), transfer tendons to augment the weak antagonist muscles (ECRL, ECRB), and stabilize the joint only for the severe, fixed, nonfunctioning wrist (wrist fusion).

If the wrist flexion deformity is mild, and wrist extensor control exists, weakening the wrist flexors through fractional lengthening may be sufficient. If the mild wrist flexion deformity exhibits concomitant wrist ulnar deviation, the FCU would be lengthened. If the mild wrist flexion deformity exhibits concomitant finger flexion and pronator spasticity, the entire flexor pronator mass can be lengthened by using a flexor pronator slide (29,30).

If the wrist flexor deformity is more severe, and wrist extensors are not functional, then tendon transfer surgery to augment wrist extension may be necessary. Muscles that can be transferred into wrist extensors include the BR, the extensor carpi ulnaris (ECU), or the FCU. Using the BR or the ECU as the donor tendon has the advantage of leaving both flexor tendons intact, thus avoiding overcorrection; yet, the disadvantage is not achieving balance, unless the wrist flexors are lengthened, if their spasticity is significant. Using the ECU tendon has the advantage of correction of the ulnar deviation deformity, although this may require FCU lengthening concomitantly; yet, the disadvantage is not providing significantly more wrist extension force than is already present. Using the FCU tendon has the advantage of removing its force as a spastic wrist flexor and ulnar deviator while transferring its forces into wrist extension; yet, the disadvantage is overcorrection if the deformity is not severe or if the transfer is tensioned too tightly, particularly in the younger child.

In all cases of transfer into the wrist extensors, finger function must be assessed preoperatively with the wrist in neutral, the desired postoperative position. If the finger flexors are too tight when the wrist is brought into neutral, then a finger flexor lengthening is necessary as part of the procedure. If the patient does not have finger extensor control to allow for release of grasped objects, then a transfer into the finger extensors (extensor digitorum communis) may be indicated.

If the patient has severe wrist joint contracture that limits functional use of the hand (even as a paperweight!), consideration should be given to a proximal row carpectomy to shorten the skeletal column across the wrist joint or to a wrist fusion to hold the wrist in a fixed, more functional position. The proximal row carpectomy is used in combination with tendon transfers and releases in those cases in which passive mobility of the wrist cannot be achieved into extension. Passive mobility of the wrist is a necessary prerequisite to tendon transfer surgery, which aspires to improve active mobility, as well.

Wrist fusion predictably maintains the wrist in fixed position and is usually indicated only for improved cosmesis and use of the hand as a paperweight in the skeletally mature individual. The proximal carpal row can be removed as part of the wrist fusion to facilitate positioning of the wrist into slight extension. Wrist fusion is contraindicated in the individual who uses wrist flexion tenodesis for release function, as this function would be lost if the wrist were to be fixed in a single position.

Fingers

The most common finger deformities are spastic flexion deformity and swan-neck deformity. Spastic flexion deformities are addressed in the previous section on wrist deformities, as these muscles are biarticular muscles, crossing the wrist and finger joints. Thus, they need to be lengthened in concert with the wrist flexion deformity correction, as part of the flexor pronator slide or with selective fascial lengthenings.

Swan-neck deformity of the fingers is due to dynamic imbalance of the muscles that act on the proximal interphalangeal (PIP) joint. Swan-neck finger deformity is characterized by PIP joint hyperextension with distal interphalangeal joint flexion. Swan-neck deformities can be due to a variety of causes; in cerebral palsy, swan-neck deformities are due to intrinsic muscle spasticity and often are augmented by overactivity of the extrinsic finger extensors. Many patients with cerebral palsy have better volitional control of their extrinsic finger extensors than they have of their wrist extensors. Thus, patients attempt to extend their wrists through activation of their extrinsic finger extensors. Overactivity of the extrinsic finger extensors causes metacarpophalangeal (MCP) joint hyperextension and can contribute to PIP joint hyperextension (swan-necking).

The overactivity of the extrinsic finger extensors combines with spasticity in the intrinsics to cause swan-necking. Due to cerebral palsy, the intrinsic muscles in the hand are often spastic. Spasticity of the intrinsic muscles causes overpull of the lateral bands, thus accentuating PIP joint extension. With chronic intrinsic spasticity, overpull of the lateral band causes incompetence of the transverse retinacular ligament, stretching of the PIP joint volar plate, and resultant dorsal subluxation of the lateral bands. The finger has a swan-neck deformity, as is shown in Figure 2. Excessive lengthening or surgical release of the flexor digitorum superficialis (FDS), such as is used in the superficialis-to-profundus transfer, often unmasks intrinsic spasticity that results in significant swan-neck deformities.

The indication for surgical correction of swan-neck deformities is a locking swan-neck deformity (usually greater than 40 degrees) that is not responsive to splinting and that interferes with function as part of the generalized assessment of upper limb function. For the patient with significant wrist flexion deformities and only mild swan-necking, surgical correction of wrist position alone may be adequate for treatment. For

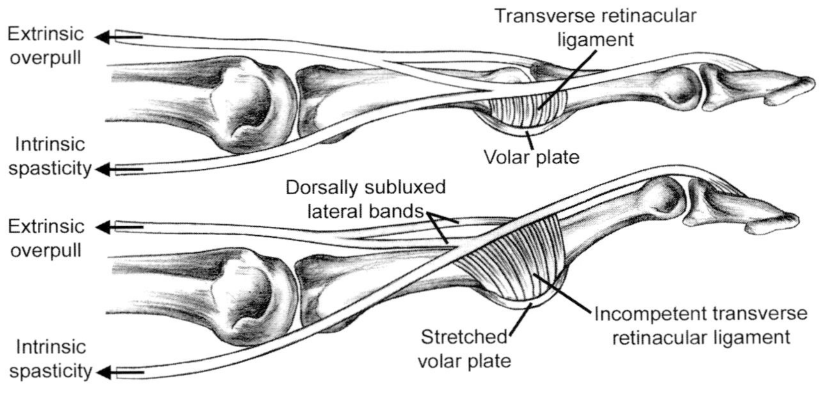

FIGURE 2. Pathophysiology of proximal interphalangeal (PIP) joint hyperextension in cerebral palsy. In cerebral palsy, the extrinsic finger extensors may be overactive in their attempt to augment wrist extension if a wrist flexion deformity exists. The intrinsic muscles are often spastic. Overactivity of the extrinsic finger extensors and spasticity of the finger intrinsics can both contribute to PIP hyperextension with resultant incompetency of the transverse retinacular ligament and volar plate. PIP hyperextension concentrates the extension forces at the PIP joint with slackening of the terminal tendon, allowing distal interphalangeal joint flexion posturing. A swan-neck deformity is characterized by PIP joint hyperflexion with distal interphalangeal joint flexion. (From Van Heest A. Lateral band re-routing in the treatment of swan-neck deformities due to cerebral palsy. *Tech Hand Upper Extrem Surg* 1997;1, with permission.)

Labels on figure:
Extrinsic overpull
Intrinsic spasticity
Transverse retinacular ligament
Volar plate
Dorsally subluxed lateral bands
Stretched volar plate
Incompetent transverse retinacular ligament

the patient with severe swan-necking (greater than 40 degrees), rebalancing of the muscle forces at the PIP joint is necessary. Surgical options include lateral band rerouting (31), lateral band tenodesis, spiral oblique ligament reconstruction (32), intrinsic muscle slide, a resection of the ulnar nerve motor branch in Guyon's canal (6), or superficialis tenodesis (33). The author's preferred method is the lateral band rerouting procedure, because it requires less extensive dissection and rebalances the intrinsic and extrinsic tendons as deforming forces.

Thumb

The most common deformity for the thumb is in the palm. Thumb-in-palm deformity is the most complex of the deformities in the upper extremity. Treatment requires a thorough understanding of the actions of the nine muscles that act on the thumb and how these can be surgically rebalanced to provide pinch function.

Many different surgical combinations exist, with the choice dependent on the degree of deformity and the extent of volitional control of each muscle involved. Application of the surgical principles that were listed previously is necessary and part of the art of designing a successful reconstructive plan: Release or lengthen the deforming spastic muscles (flexor pollicis longus, adductor pollicis, flexor pollicis brevis), transfer tendons to augment the weak antago-

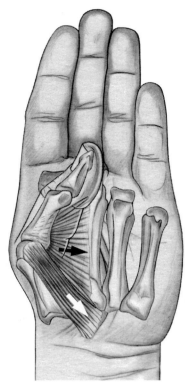

FIGURE 4. The type 2 thumb-in-palm deformity. In addition to the thumb metacarpal adduction deformity from the adductor pollicis muscle spasticity, the type 2 thumb-in-palm deformity additionally has a thumb metacarpophalangeal joint flexion deformity due to flexor pollicis brevis spasticity.

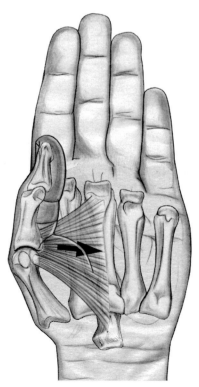

FIGURE 3. The type 1 thumb-in-palm deformity. Spasticity in the adductor pollicis causes significant adduction of the first metacarpal, narrowing the first web and limiting grasp. The adductor pollicis is the primary deforming force.

nist muscles (extensor pollicis brevis, abductor pollicis longus), and stabilize the joint for instability (MCP capsulodesis or fusion).

Common patterns of thumb deformity have been described (34) and help determine which muscles are the deforming forces that need to be lengthened or released and which muscles are the deficient antagonists that need to be augmented.

Four types of thumb-in-palm deformity have been described. In all types, the thumb adductor is a spastic deforming force. In the *type 1 thumb-in-palm deformity* (Fig. 3), spasticity in the adductor pollicis causes significant adduction of the first metacarpal, narrowing the first web and limiting grasp. The adductor pollicis is the primary deforming force. In the *type 2 thumb-in-palm deformity* (Fig. 4), not only does adductor pollicis spasticity cause significant adduction of the first metacarpal, but also flexor pollicis brevis spasticity causes significant thumb MCP joint flexion deformity. In the *type 3 thumb-in-palm deformity* (Fig. 5), prolonged adductor pollicis spasticity with metacarpal adduction leads to secondary deformity, with the thumb extension and abduction *through* the MCP joint; this leads to secondary MCP joint instability, subluxation, and dislocation. The MCP becomes dorsally unstable with an incompetent volar plate. In the *type 4 thumb-in-*

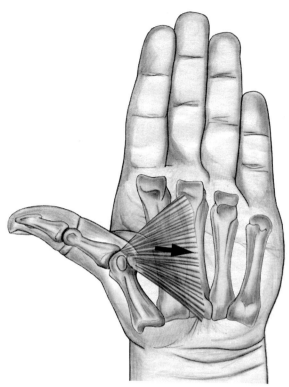

FIGURE 5. The type 3 thumb-in-palm deformity. With prolonged adductor pollicis spasticity, the thumb will extend and abduct through the metacarpophalangeal (MCP) joint (i.e., secondary MCP joint instability, subluxation, and dislocation). The MCP joint becomes dorsally unstable with an incompetent volar plate.

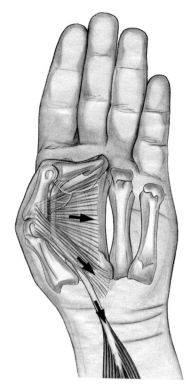

FIGURE 6. The type 4 thumb-in-palm deformity. In addition to the thumb metacarpal adduction deformity due to adductor pollicis spasticity and the metacarpophalangeal joint flexion due to flexor pollicis brevis spasticity, the type 4 thumb-in-palm deformity has interphalangeal joint flexion deformity due to flexor pollicis longus spasticity.

palm deformity (Fig. 6), in addition to the thumb metacarpal adduction deformity that is due to adductor pollicis spasticity and the MCP flexion that is due to flexor pollicis brevis spasticity, the interphalangeal joint has a flexion deformity that is due to flexor pollicis longus spasticity.

In each of these types of deformities, the offending spastic muscle needs to be released or lengthened. In the type 1 deformity, two options exist for decreasing the spastic forces of the adductor pollicis muscle, as are shown in Figures 7 and 8: the Matev (35) adductor slide or the partial adductor myotomy. In the Matev release, a palmar incision is used, and the origin of the transverse head of the adductor pollicis is elevated off the third metacarpal. The thumb is immobilized postoperatively, with the first metacarpal held in abduction, so that the adductor pollicis origin heals radially in a lengthened position. In the partial adductor myotomy, a first web Z-plasty (standard or four part) is used to increase the width of the first web skin for grasp function. Through this incision, the transverse head of the adductor pollicis is released near its insertion. The oblique head of the adductor pollicis is left intact to preserve pinch function.

In the type 2 deformity, the adductor is released in the same manner as in the type 1 deformity, and the flexor brevis is released, as well. Using the Matev incision, it is extended proximally, and the flexor pollicis brevis (FPB) origin of the thenar eminences is elevated off its origin. Using the first web incision, the FPB is released off its insertion.

In the type 3 deformity, the adductor is released in the same manner as in the type 1 deformity. Additionally, the thumb MCP joint is stabilized through a radial mid-lateral incision by using a capsulodesis technique (36) or fusion (37).

In the type 4 deformity, the adductor and FPB are released in the same manner as was described for the type 2 deformity, but the flexor pollicis longus is also lengthened in the forearm.

For the milder deformities, when antagonist control is present, a release or lengthening of the spastic muscles is indicated without additional procedures. For more severe deformities without sufficient antagonist control, tendon transfers into the abductor pollicis longus or extensor pollicis brevis are indicated. The exception is that transfers into the extensor pollicis brevis are not indicated for the type 3 thumb-in-palm deformity, unless the joint is fused, as a strong MCP extensor exacerbates the MCP extension instability.

Tendon transfers to augment extension and abduction of the thumb include transfers into the abductor pollicis longus and extensor pollicis brevis or rerouting of the extensor pollicis longus (EPL) into the first dorsal compartment. Donor tendons for transfer include the FCR (if the FCU is not transferred as part of the wrist correction), the

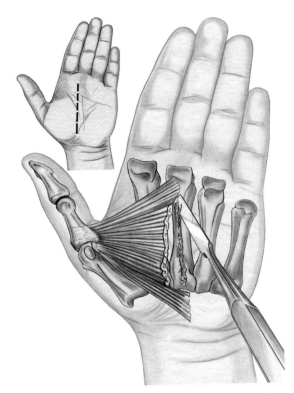

FIGURE 7. Type 1 thumb-in-palm deformity Matev release (35). Through a palmar incision, the origin of the transverse head of the adductor pollicis is elevated off the third metacarpal. The thumb is immobilized postoperatively with the first metacarpal held in abduction so that the adductor pollicis origin heals radially in a lengthened position.

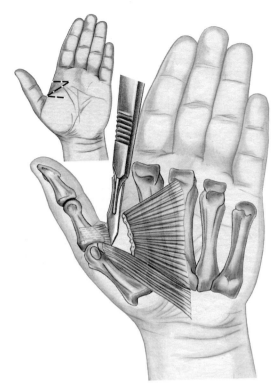

FIGURE 8. Thumb-in-palm partial adductor myotomy. Through a first web Z-plasty incision, used to increase the width of the first web skin for grasp function, the transverse head of the adductor pollicis is released near its insertion. The oblique head of the adductor pollicis is left to preserve pinch function.

BR, and the palmaris longus. If satisfactory tendon donors are not available, tenodeses can be carried out in the lower-functioning hand. Rerouting of the EPL from the third dorsal compartment, where it acts as a secondary thumb adductor, into the first dorsal compartment, converts it into a thumb extensor abductor (38).

Results and Outcome, Review of the Literature, and Factors That Affect Outcome

A review of the literature documents overall functional improvement of children with spastic hemiplegia after operative treatment (9,39,40). Nylanders (39) documented that functional improvement was achieved by 6 months postsurgery and was maintained at a 4.5-year follow-up in 24 children. Eliassion (40) reported on 32 children who were treated with tendon transfers and muscle releases and showed functional improvement in all children regardless of the degree of preoperative impairment. He noted that the extent of improvement was based on preoperative functional level. I reported on 134 patients who were treated with soft tissue release, tendon transfer, and joint stabilization procedures (9). Most commonly, all deformities were

corrected during one operation, with an average of four procedures performed per surgery. Surgical results showed an average improvement of 2.6 level according to House's classification of upper extremity functional use (Table 1). This functional improvement was not affected by level of mentation, two-point discrimination, stereognosis function, or type of cerebral palsy. (Note that only three athetoid patients were treated surgically over 25 years.) Patients with poor motor control did have less improvement in functional use. Most patients who were treated surgically were highly motivated.

Author's Preferred Treatment: Techniques, Personal Series, and Results

The challenge of upper extremity reconstructive surgery for spastic conditions is that there is no single surgical solution that is applicable to all patients. Each patient has varying degrees of fixed contractures and varying degrees of spasticity that causes dynamic deformity. Spasticity causing muscle imbalance across joints limits function to the greatest extent in the wrist and in the thumb. Thus, surgical planning usually targets the wrist and thumb, as surgical reconstruction of these joints provides the greatest functional improvement.

For the child younger than 7 years old or uncooperative for tendon transfer surgery, I prefer nonoperative management as discussed above. For the child older than 7 years old and cooperative, this is an optimum time for surgical intervention, before the development of fixed contractures.

In my practice, I would recommend a motion laboratory analysis before surgical intervention for tendon transfer surgery. At the present time, I use fine needle electrodes in the pronator teres and FCU muscles (Fig. 1). If either muscle shows significant spasticity with continuous electrical activity and no evidence of selective control, then I would recommend a release or lengthening of the muscle. If either muscle shows appropriate phasic control of its electrical activity, then I would recommend tendon transfer using that muscle. For example, if the pronator teres is continuously spastic, then I would perform a pronator teres release; if the pronator teres is under phasic control, then I would perform a pronator teres rerouting. Another example, if the FCU is continuously spastic, then I would perform an FCU lengthening and transfer the BR or ECU for wrist extension; if the FCU is under phasic control, then I would perform an FCU tendon transfer for wrist extension.

Surgical Technique

For tendon transfer surgery, including the elbow, the patient is positioned supine with a sterile tourniquet to allow for tourniquet removal before tensioning of the biceps lengthening. For all other forearm, wrist, and hand surgeries, a standard tourniquet is used.

For biceps and brachialis lengthening, an anterior "lazy S" incision is used across the antecubital fossa with the proximal limb extending medially and the distal limb extending laterally toward the biceps insertion. After identification and protection of the lateral antebrachial nerve, the biceps tendon is isolated, and the lacertus fibrosis is released. The biceps tendon is lengthened using a step-cut Z-lengthening technique. The brachialis is lengthened using a series of transverse incisions through the fascial layers. The biceps is repaired in a lengthened position at the conclusion of surgery when the sterile tourniquet is deflated.

For the pronator teres release or rerouting, a longitudinal radial incision is used along the middle one-third of the radius. Dissection is carried down onto the radial insertion of the pronator teres, with careful protection of the radial artery and superficial radial nerve. For the pronator teres release, the tendon is released along its radial insertion and its fascial attachments to the extent that retraction of the muscle can be verified. For pronator teres rerouting, the muscle is freed off its volar insertion with a long periosteal extension and tagged with 0-0 nonabsorbable suture. A window is then made in the interosseous membrane of sufficient size and position to pass the pronator teres. The pronator teres is passed through the window, dorsally around the radius, back onto its insertion, and, if tendon length allows, back onto the volar aspect of the radius to provide maximum supination (41). The tendon is sewn firmly onto periosteum or attached with bone anchors or bone drill holes. The arm is immobilized postoperatively for both procedures in maximum supination.

For the wrist tendon transfers, the FCU is transferred to the ECRB (Fig. 9A) through a long ulnar-sided incision. Dissection is carried down along the FCU insertion on the pisiform with careful identification and protection of the ulnar nerve and artery. The FCU is transected at its pisiform insertion and tagged with a 2-0 nonabsorbable grasping suture. The muscle is mobilized off its ulnar origin and fascial investments over the distal two-thirds of the ulna to maximize its excursion (Fig. 9B). The most distal ulnar motor nerve branch to the FCU can be sacrificed if necessary to facilitate excursion. A dorsal incision is then made over the ECRB just proximal to the extensor retinaculum. A fascial window is cut over the ECRB just distal to the thumb outcropper muscles. A subcutaneous tunnel is then made from the proximal end of the ulnar incision to the dorsal radial incision, and the FCU tendon is passed around the ulnar border of the forearm (Fig. 9C). Three Pulvertaft weaves of the FCU end-to-side into the ECRB tendon are then made and sewn in place with tensioning so that at rest, in a gravity-dependent position, the wrist sits at neutral (Fig. 9D). Passive elongation of the muscle should allow for wrist flexion, and active firing of the muscle should allow for wrist extension. After the wounds are closed, the wrist is immobilized in slight wrist extension.

For the fingers and thumb, there is no "cookbook" formula that can be used for the spastic hand. Use of the surgical principles outlined above is imperative with customization to the reconstruction plan and the degree of spasticity and/or deformity. In the fingers, the superficialis to profundus transfer for finger flexion deformity is used for the nonfunctional hand to help with hygiene problems. A volar forearm incision is used with identification of the FDS superficially, protection of the median nerve in the intermediate layer, and identification of the flexor digitorum profundus (FDP) in the deep layer. A 2-0 nonabsorbable suture is used to sew the four FDS tendons together in their resting cascade, and the tendons are then transected at their distal-most end, just proximal to the carpal tunnel, with the fingers in full flexion to deliver the most amount of tendon into the wound. A 2-0 nonabsorbable suture is used to sew the FDP tendons together in their resting cascade, and the tendons are then transected at the proximal end, just at the musculotendinous junction. The distal end of the FDS tendons are then woven into the proximal ends of the FDP tendons using 2-3 Pulvertaft weaves on each of the four fingers' tendons. Care is taken to maintain the normal cascade and tension so that the hand at rest lays flat.

For the thumb, I prefer to lengthen the adductor pollicis muscle through a first web Z-plasty incision (Fig. 8), using

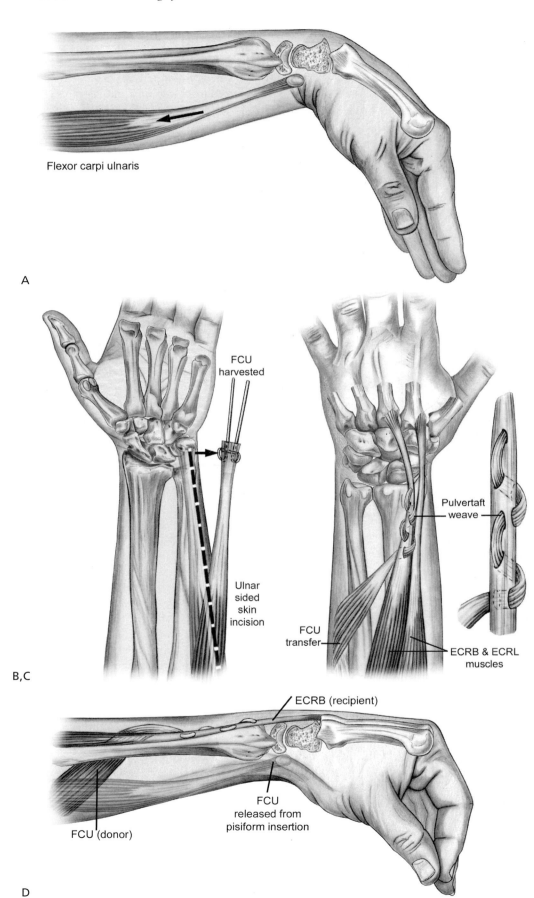

A

Flexor carpi ulnaris

B,C

FCU harvested

Ulnar sided skin incision

FCU transfer

Pulvertaft weave

ECRB & ECRL muscles

D

ECRB (recipient)

FCU released from pisiform insertion

FCU (donor)

FIGURE 9. The flexor carpi ulnaris (FCU) to extensor carpi radialis brevis (ECRB) tendon transfer. **A:** For the severe wrist flexion deformity, the FCU can be released as a deforming force and transferred to the ECRB to augment weak or absent wrist extension. **B:** Through a long ulnar-sided incision, the FCU is harvested from its pisiform insertion and tagged with a 2-0 nonabsorbable grasping suture. The muscle is mobilized off its origin and fascial investments over the distal two-thirds of the ulna to maximize its excursion. **C:** The FCU tendon is passed through a subcutaneous tunnel from the ulnar incision into a dorsal incision over the ECRB, just proximal to the extensor retinaculum. Three Pulvertaft weaves are sewn in place with 2-0 nonabsorbable sutures. **D:** The transfer is tensioned so that at rest, in a gravity-dependent position, the wrist sits at neutral. Passive elongation of the muscle should allow for wrist flexion, and active firing of the muscle should allow for wrist extension. ECRL, extensor carpi radialis longus.

a four-part **Z**-plasty for the more severely contracted skin. A complete release of the fascia and a partial release of the transverse head allow first metacarpal abduction without precluding pinch. If the metacarpal joint is dorsally unstable, I prefer an MCP capsulodesis. A radial midlateral incision is made with dissection carried directly to an MCP capsulotomy. The volar plate insertion is usually attenuated. Both the metacarpal neck and the sesamoids are abraded. Either a bone suture anchor or a periosteal stitch is used to bring the sesamoids into direct contact with the metacarpal neck. The MCP joint should sit in 20 to 30 degrees of flexion, and should come to neutral with passive stretch. The joint is then pinned in 20 to 30 degrees of flexion. If the extensors or abductors are weak, augmentation is performed through tendon transfer. If the EPL is well controlled, a transfer of the EPL from the third compartment into the first compartment with shortening of the tendon, using the dorsal wrist incision from concomitant wrist tendon transfer, is my preferred technique.

I advocate multiple simultaneous upper extremity procedures for multilevel correction of the spastic limb in cerebral palsy. Postoperatively, a well-padded cast that allows for swelling but maintains intraoperative positioning is applied. The cast is removed 4 weeks later, and the patient is fitted with a custom Orthoplast splint. The splint is worn full-time for 4 weeks, with the patient removing it for active range of motion, light at-table activities, and hygiene. After 4 weeks of full-time wear, if the patient is maintaining the position of joint correction and learning active range of motion, then the patient is progressed to part-time use protection during sleep and activities (e.g., school and sports) and is started on strengthening exercises with gentle passive range of motion if needed for mobility.

After this 3-month postoperative program, a long-term upper extremity functional use protocol, encouraging long-term bimanual skills, is recommended.

Algorithm for Evaluation and Management (Based on the Author's Preferred Treatment)

Based on the author's preferred treatment, the algorithm outlined in Figure 10 has been developed.

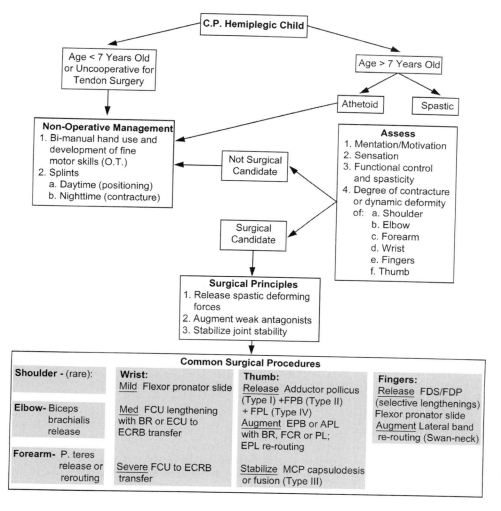

FIGURE 10. Algorithm of author's preferred treatment. APL, abductor pollicis longus; BR, brachioradialis; C.P., cerebral palsy; ECRB, extensor carpi radialis brevis; ECU, extensor carpi ulnaris; EPB, extensor pollicis brevis; EPL, extensor pollicis longus; FCR, flexor carpi radialis; FCU, flexor carpi ulnaris; FDP, flexor digitorum profundus; FDS, flexor digitorum superficialis; FPB, flexor pollicis brevis; FPL, flexor pollicis longus; MCP, metacarpophalangeal; O.T., occupational therapy; P., pronator; PL, palmaris longus.

COMPLICATIONS

All surgical procedures carry risk, which must be weighed against the potential benefits that most commonly are achieved. Multiple simultaneous upper extremity procedures can be safely performed with meticulous attention to pre-, intra-, and postoperative details.

Preoperatively, patients must be screened for anesthetic complications, including a bleeding screen for patients on long-term Depakote antiseizure medications; screening for bladder and lung infections, particularly for patients with poor urinary or pulmonary control; and assessment of nutritional status (height and weight percentiles for age).

Intraoperative attention to wound care is imperative to avoid wound healing problems, particularly in Z-plasty approaches. Large wounds should be treated with a postoperative drain to prevent hematoma formation. Nerve and artery injury due to overzealous correction of joint position is to be avoided.

Postoperatively, the splint or cast should be adequate to allow for postoperative swelling and should be split if excessive swelling is encountered. Many children with spasticity do not have a normal preoperative sensory or motor examination and may not have normal mentation, so normal parameters cannot be used to monitor for compartment syndrome. Premature removal of the cast or splint, as well as overzealous patient activities, can lead to tendon rupture or attenuation. Excessive immobilization can lead to excessive adhesion formation, diminishing the eventual functional use.

Long-term problems most commonly center around loss of the balance achieved at the time of the surgery. Many children have tendon transfers as young as 7 years old and, with continued skeletal growth, may have recurrent deformity. Overcorrection can also occur with the "opposite" deformity occurring. Additionally, further "fine tuning" surgery may be necessary to address complications that develop after correction of the original deformity. For example, after corrective lengthening of the finger and wrist extensors, intrinsic spasticity in the hand may be unmasked. This may be assessed through an ulnar nerve motor block in Guyon's canal; if successful, an ulnar motor neurectomy can be performed. Recurrent over- or undercorrection can be treated with stretching, splinting, and nonoperative measures as outlined in Nonoperative Treatment.

Principles that help prevent these complications include

1. Do not overcorrect deformity, particularly in the younger child.
2. Leave options to reverse the surgical correction if necessary.
3. Keep functional grasp and release as your highest priority in your surgical planning.
4. Avoid wrist arthrodesis as this precludes the tenodesis effect of the wrist for finger use.

Surgical expectations should be realistically discussed with your patients and their parents to avoid unrealistic expectations. In general, using the functional use scale in Table 1, an average of two and one-half functional levels of improvement can be achieved with surgical intervention. Most commonly, this would mean that a child who presents with a severely flexed wrist with a thumb-in-palm deformity that limits use of the limb to a good passive assist could be improved to a fair to good active assist with better wrist and thumb positioning.

As surgeons, we must remember that we are treating only the secondary peripheral manifestations of a primary CNS dysfunction that persists.

REFERENCES

1. Minear WL. A classification of cerebral palsy. *Pediatrics* 1956;18:841.
2. Dunin-Wasowicz D, Rowecka-Trzebicka K, Milewska-Bobula B, et al. Risk factors for cerebral palsy in very low birth weight infants in the 1980s and 1990s. *J Child Neurol* 2000;15:417–420.
3. Fuchs Z, Blumstein T, Novikov I. Morbidity, comorbidity, and their association with disability among community-dwelling oldest-old in Israel. *J Gerontol A Biol Sci Med Sci* 1998;53:447–455.
4. Lackland DT, Bachman DL, Carten TD. The geographic variation in stroke incidence in two areas of the southeastern stroke belt: the Anderson and Pee Dee Stroke Study. *Stroke* 1998;29:2061–2068.
5. Sacco RL, Boden Albala B, Gan R. Stroke incidence among white, black and Hispanic residents of an urban community: the Northern Manhattan Stroke Study. *Am J Epidemiol* 1998;147:259–268.
6. Trumble TE, Van Heest A. Stroke, traumatic brain injury, and cerebral palsy. In: Trumble TE, ed. *Principles of hand surgery and therapy*. Philadelphia: WB Saunders, 2000:361–375.
7. Katz R. Presynaptic inhibition in humans: a comparison between normal and spastic patients. *J Physiol* 1999;93:379–385.
8. Van Heest AE, House J, Putnam M. Sensibility deficiencies in the hands of children with spastic hemiplegia. *J Hand Surg* 1993;18:278–281.
9. Van Heest AE, House JH, Cariello C. Upper extremity surgical treatment of cerebral palsy. *J Hand Surg* 1999;24:323–330.
10. Dahlin LB, Komoto-Tufvesson Y, Salgeback S. Surgery of the spastic hand in cerebral palsy. Improvement in stereognosis and hand function after surgery. *J Hand Surg* 1998;23:334–339.
11. Hoffer MM. The use of the pathokinesiology laboratory to select muscles for tendon transfers in the cerebral palsy hand. *Clin Orthop* 1993;288:135–138.
12. Hoffer MM, Perry J, Melkonian G. Postoperative electromyographic function of tendon transfers in patients with cerebral palsy. *Dev Med Child Neurol* 1990;32:789–791.

13. Kozin SH, Keenan MH. Using dynamic electromyography to guide surgical treatment of the spastic upper extremity in the brain-injured patient. *Clin Orthop* 1993;288:109–117.

14. Nogen AG. Medical treatment for spasticity in children with cerebral palsy. *Child Brain* 1976;2:304–308.

15. Hines AE, Crago PE, Villian C. Functional electrical stimulation for reduction of spasticity in the hemiplegic hand. *Biomed Sci Instrum* 1993;29:259–266.

16. Carmick J. Clinical use of neuromuscular electrical stimulation for children with cerebral palsy. Part II: upper extremity. *Phys Ther* 1993;73:514–527.

17. Steinbok P, Reiner A, Kestle JR. Therapeutic electrical stimulation following selective posterior rhizotomy in children with spastic diplegic cerebral palsy: a randomized clinical trial. *Dev Med Child Neurol* 1997;39:515–520.

18. Beck AJ, Gaskill SJ, Marlin AE. Improvement in upper extremity function and trunk control after selective posterior rhizotomy. *Am J Occup Ther* 1993;47:704–707.

19. Loewen P, Steinbok P, Holsti L, et al. Upper extremity performance and self-care skill changes in children with spastic cerebral palsy following selective posterior rhizotomy. *Pediatr Neurosurg* 1998;29:191–198.

20. Fehlings D, Rang M, Glazier J, et al. An evaluation of botulinum-A toxin injections to improve upper extremity function in children with hemiplegic cerebral palsy. *J Pediatr* 2000;137:300-303,331–337.

21. Autti-Ramo I, Larsen A, Peltonen J, et al. Botulinum toxin injection as an adjunct when planning hand surgery in children with spastic hemiplegia. *Neuropediatrics* 2000;31:4–8.

22. Wall SA, Chait LA, Temlett JA, et al. Botulinum A chemodenervation: a new modality in cerebral palsied hands. *Br J Plast Surg* 1993;46:703–706.

23. Van Heest AE. Applications of botulinum toxin in orthopaedics and upper extremity surgery. *Tech Hand Upper Extrem Surg* 1997;1:27–34.

24. Van Heest AE. A prospective evaluation of treatment of the upper extremity in spastic hemiplegia using botulinum toxin. In: Ogino T, ed. *Congenital differences of the upper limb.* Kyoto: Yamagata University School of Medicine; 2000:307–320.

25. Mital MA, Sakellarides HT. Surgery of the upper extremity in the retarded individual with spastic cerebral palsy. *Orthop Clin North Am* 1981;12:127–141.

26. Strecker WB, Emanuel JP, Dailey L, et al. Comparison of pronator tenotomy and pronator rerouting in children with spastic cerebral palsy. *J Hand Surg* 1988;13:540–543.

27. Sakellarides HT, Mital MA, Lenzi WD. Treatment of pronation contractures of the forearm in cerebral palsy by changing the insertion of the pronator radii teres. *J Bone Joint Surg* 1981;63:645–652.

28. Van Heest AE, Murthy NS, Sathy MR, et al. The supination effect of tendon transfer of the flexor carpi ulnaris to the extensor carpi radialis brevis or longus: a cadaveric study. *J Hand Surg* 1999;24:1091–1096.

29. Inglis AE, Cooper W. Release of the flexor-pronator origin for flexion deformities of the hand and wrist in spastic paralysis. *J Bone Joint Surg* 1966;48:847–857.

30. White WF. Flexor muscle slide in the spastic hand: the Max Page operation. *J Bone Joint Surg* 1972;54:453–459.

31. Tonkin MA, Hughes J, Smith KL. Lateral band translocation for swan-neck deformity. *J Hand Surg* 1992;17:260–267.

32. Littler JW. The finger extensor mechanism. *Surg Clin North Am* 1967;47:415–432.

33. Swanson AB. Surgery of the hand in cerebral palsy and the swan neck deformity. *J Bone Joint Surg* 1960;42:951–964.

34. House J, Gwathmey F, Fidler M. A dynamic approach to the thumb-in-palm deformity in cerebral palsy. *J Bone Joint Surg* 1981;63:216–225.

35. Matev I. Surgery of the spastic thumb-in-palm deformity. *J Hand Surg* 1991;16:346–348.

36. Filler BC, Stark HH, Boyes JH. Capsulodesis of the metacarpophalangeal joint of the thumb in children with cerebral palsy. *J Bone Joint Surg* 1976;58:667–670.

37. Goldner JL, Koman LA, Gelberman R, et al. Arthrodesis of the metacarpophalangeal joint of the thumb in children and adults: adjunctive treatment of thumb-in-palm deformity in cerebral palsy. *Clin Orthop* 1990;253:75–89.

38. Manske PR. Redirection of extensor pollicis longus in the treatment of spastic thumb-in-palm deformity. *J Hand Surg* 1985;10:553–560.

39. Nylanders G, Carlstrom C, Adolfsson L. 4.5 year follow-up after surgical correction of upper extremity deformities in spastic cerebral palsy. *J Hand Surg* 1999;24:719–723.

40. Eliassion AC, Ekholm C, Carlstedt T. Hand function in children with cerebral palsy after upper-limb tendon transfer and muscle release. *Dev Med Child Neurol* 1998;41:284–285.

41. Van Heest AE, Sathy M, Schutte L. Cadaveric modeling of the pronator teres rerouting tendon transfer. *J Hand Surg* 1999;24:614–618.

42. Mital MA. Lengthening of the elbow flexors in cerebral palsy. *J Bone Joint Surg* 1979;61:515–522.

43. Zancolli EA. *Structural and dynamic bases of hand surgery,* 2nd ed. Philadelphia: Lippincott Williams & Wilkins, 1968.

44. House JH, Gwathmey FW. Flexor carpi ulnaris and the brachioradialis as a wrist extension transfer in cerebral palsy. *Minn Med* 1978;61:481–484.

45. McCue FC, Honner R, Chapman WC. Transfer of the brachioradialis for hands deformed by cerebral palsy. *J Bone Joint Surg* 1970;52:1171–1180.

46. Green WT. Tendon transplantation of the flexor carpi ulnaris for pronation-flexion deformity of the wrist. *Surg Gynecol Obstet* 1942;75:337–342.

47. Green WT, Banks HH. Flexor carpi ulnaris transplant and its use in cerebral palsy. *J Bone Joint Surg* 1962;44:1343–1352.

48. Omer GE, Capen DA. Proximal row carpectomy with muscle transfers for spastic paralysis. *J Hand Surg* 1976;1:197–204.

61

BURNS OF THE HAND AND UPPER EXTREMITY

JEFFREY WEINZWEIG
NORMAN WEINZWEIG

The burned hand represents a complex problem. Optimal management requires careful consideration of a number of crucial variables, such as the need for escharotomy or fasciotomy in the acute setting, the method of wound débridement, internal and external splinting, the choice of dressings, the timing of burn wound excision and grafting, additional soft tissue reconstruction, and subsequent rehabilitation. Each of these factors plays a critical role in contributing to the ultimate function of the hand that is achieved after burn injury.

Because the hand is involved in a myriad of occupational, recreational, and daily activities, it is not surprising that the upper extremity is the most frequently injured anatomic structure (1). In a study that was conducted by the U.S. Consumer Product Safety Commission, it was estimated that 39% of burn wounds that were associated with product-related injuries involved some portion of the hand or upper extremity (2). Therefore, a thorough understanding of the appropriate management of these relatively common injuries is a mandatory component of the hand surgeon's armamentarium. Proper initial management of burns of the hand with subsequent diligent therapy and rehabilitation can result in normal hand function in 97% of patients with superficial injuries and 81% of patients with deep dermal injuries (3).

SURGICAL ANATOMY AND BIOMECHANICS

An ever-present menace in hand surgery is the decided tendency for the hand to stiffen and to stiffen in the position of nonfunction (4).

Contracture is the enemy of function. Nowhere is it demonstrated better than in the patient with severe hand burns. Prevention of joint contracture and deformity is perhaps the most important component in the restoration of hand function. Adequate wound closure, including skin grafting and soft tissue reconstruction, is also an integral part of the

equation. In 1956, Sterling Bunnell astutely emphasized the propensity of the hand to stiffen with resultant functional loss (4).

Injury, infection, excessive immobilization, and inadequate splinting of the hand all predispose a patient to the development of joint stiffness and the ensuing adverse sequelae. The initial response to any insult to the hand is localized edema. Fluid resuscitation in the management of severe burns produces systemic edema that is due to increased capillary permeability. This edema is prominent in the pulmonary system and extremities.

The accumulation of fluid or hematoma within the capsular structures of the joint or within the synovial space acutely impairs joint function and subsequently promotes joint stiffness and contracture (5). An increase in the fluid content of the articular capsule and collateral ligaments effectively shortens these structures, whereas excess fluid within the synovial space distends the capsule. The *intrinsic minus* hand, which consists of interphalangeal (IP) joint flexion, metacarpophalangeal (MCP) joint extension, thumb adduction, and wrist flexion, is the resultant deformity.

The MCP joint is key to the development of the intrinsic minus hand. When nearly fully extended, the MCP joint has maximal capsule and collateral ligament laxity, as well as intracapsular fluid capacity. Potential abduction, adduction, and rotation are maximal, the joint contact surface area is minimized, and the joint is relatively unstable. When fully flexed, the intracapsular fluid capacity of the MCP joint is minimal and the joint is stable, thus allowing minimal abduction, adduction, or rotation. In this position, the collateral ligaments are taut with a broad, full-width joint contact surface area (Fig. 1). After injury, edema fluid hydraulically drives the MCP joints into extension. This position increases flexor tension and decreases extensor tension. As a result, the fingers flex at the proximal interphalangeal (PIP) and distal IP joints. There is only minimal change in the anatomy and fluid capacity of the flexed versus extended IP joints, and there is no hydraulic

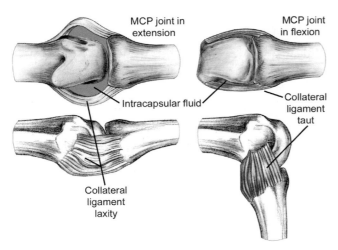

FIGURE 1. Collateral ligament anatomy. The anatomy of the extended metacarpophalangeal (MCP) joint differs significantly from that of the fully flexed MCP joint. In extension, the bone contact surface area is minimal. The collateral ligaments are loose, the intracapsular fluid space is at a maximum, and the joint is relatively unstable. The proximal phalanx rotates, abducts, and adducts on the metacarpal. In full flexion, the metacarpal condylar surface is broad, and the contact area is maximal between the metacarpal and proximal phalanx. The collateral ligaments are tight, secondary to a cam effect and the necessity of the collaterals to pass around the metacarpal head prominences. The intracapsular fluid space is minimal, and the joint is highly stable secondary to bone and ligament configurations in the flexed position. (From Watson HK, Weinzweig J. Stiff joints. In: Green DP, Hotchkiss RN, Pederson WC, eds. *Operative hand surgery,* 4th ed. New York: Churchill Livingstone, 1998, with permission.)

drive, as compared to the MCP joints. The positional changes in the IP joints are therefore secondary to changes in the MCP joints. The total power capacity of the flexor tendons significantly exceeds that of the extensor tendons; thus, slight wrist flexion is usually present in a neglected, edematous hand (6).

PATHOPHYSIOLOGY

Burn wounds that involve greater than 20% total body surface area (TBSA) typically produce a systemic inflammatory response with resultant capillary leak (7). An outpouring of protein-rich fluid occurs that initiates an inflammatory response that leads to increased fibrous protein synthesis (8). Extracapillary efflux of this protein-rich fluid is accompanied by the extracellular fluid shifts that necessitate replacement to maintain fluid balance and homeostasis.

Appropriate fluid resuscitation can be estimated by the Parkland formula:

$$\text{Fluids for first 24 hours} = 4\,\text{mL} \times \frac{\text{patient weight}}{\text{in kilograms}} \times \frac{\%\ \text{TBSA}}{\text{that is burned}}$$

One-half of the fluid, usually lactated Ringer's solution, is administered over the first 8 hours from the time of injury.

The second half is given over the remaining 16 hours. Adjustment of the quantity of fluid that is administered is based on continuous patient monitoring, including urine output, heart rate, blood pressure, and acid–base status. After the initial 24-hour period, fluids are provided as indicated by these systemic parameters. It is important to note that, although burn resuscitation protocols vary among burn units, especially with respect to provision of albumin during the early postburn period, there is agreement that albumin must not be provided in the first 24 hours when capillary leak is maximal and exacerbated one-third spacing of protein-rich fluid increases the likelihood of resultant pulmonary edema.

The pathophysiology of burn injuries predisposes the burned hand to the development of severe contracture and functional limitation unless appropriate prophylactic measures are taken in the acute setting to avert disability and deformity. Fluid shifts within the capsular and ligamentous structures of the hand result in positional changes that predispose to contracture and functional loss. Such fluid shifts within a nondistensible structure, as occur after severe burns of the hand and upper extremity, predispose to compartment syndrome, vascular compromise, Volkmann's contracture, and intrinsic muscle necrosis. Additional factors, apart from the initial injury, contribute to postburn deformity and functional loss, including persistent edema, wound infection, improper or prolonged immobilization, and delayed or inadequate skin coverage (9). Each of these factors can result in a prolonged period of inflammation with resultant increases in fibrosis of normal, initially uninjured structures.

The most comfortable position for the burned hand in the acute setting is typically the position of deformity with adduction of the thumb, flexion of the PIP joints, hyperflexion of the MCP joints, and flexion of the wrist. This position permits laxity of the collateral ligaments of the MCP joints with resultant shortening and fibrosis. Shortening of the transverse metacarpal ligaments results in loss of the transverse metacarpal arch. MCP joint hyperextension impairs flexor tendon function at the MCP joint level, whereas adhesion and scarring of the sagittal bands further limit the excursion of the central slip of the extensor tendon. Unopposed flexor tendon activity at the PIP joint level soon results in these joints becoming fixed in flexion. Persistent flexion of the PIP joint, or direct burn injury to the extensor mechanism at this level, can result in volar migration of the lateral bands below the axis of the joint with resultant hyperextension of the distal IP joint and the development of a boutonnière deformity. Every attempt must be made in the acute postburn setting to prevent the evolution of such devastating deformities.

EVALUATION

The burn patient is a trauma patient and must be treated as such. A myriad of injury mechanisms can produce burns of the hand and upper extremity. The particular mechanism that is involved must be quickly identified as that information often directs treatment. Ng et al. (10) reported a large series of occupational causes of hand burns that included electrical (29.5%), flame (24.4%), flash (9.8%), tar and asphalt (9.3%), scale (7.8%), chemical (5.1%), steam (4.7%), and grease (1%). Nonoccupational causes include house fires, cooking mishaps, and motor vehicle accidents. Almost 90% of patients with major burns have burns that involve the hands (11).

With this in mind, evaluation of the patient with burns of the hand begins with a comprehensive assessment for associated and, in particular, more serious injuries that must be addressed first. As with all trauma patients, burn patients require a thorough airway, breathing, and circulation assessment. Potential life-threatening injuries, such as those involving the cervical spine or those with an inhalation component, must be ruled out before commencing with a focused evaluation of the hand and upper extremity.

Evaluation of the burned hand commences with an assessment of the depth and extent of the injury. In general, partial-thickness burns are red and hypersensitive and are associated with blistering, which occurs at the dermal-epidermal junction. In contrast, full-thickness burns are often white, waxy, and leatherlike in appearance and usually are insensitive. A number of variables affect the ultimate depth of a particular burn, such as location, etiology, and age. A burn on the dorsum of the hand, where the skin is much thinner, is likely to be deeper than one on the volar surface of the hand, certainly in a child. Similarly, a short-exposure scald burn is more likely to produce a partial-thickness injury than a flame burn, which is more often a full-thickness injury (9). However, there is no uniform means of assessing burn depth, and it is often difficult to determine whether a burn is partial or full thickness at the time of injury. Serial observation and proper management permit determination of the depth of most burns. Desiccation, infection, and improper early treatment may cause conversion of a partial-thickness burn, which may have been managed nonoperatively, to a full-thickness burn that requires excision and grafting.

The skin of the hand is exceptionally important because of its physical qualities, sensory properties, and microcirculation. The relationship of surface area to volume of the hand is comparable only to that of the brain, whose surface is proportionately much greater than its total volume. A volume of 1 cm^3 in the digit corresponds to a skin surface area of 2.5 cm^2, whereas in the forearm, the value drops to 0.5 cm^2 (12).

The skin of the hand can be divided into two types—the thin, mobile, dorsal skin that permits free articular motion in flexion and the specialized, thick, palmar (glabrous) skin that is resistant to pressure, stabilizes the grip, and has important sensory functions. The palmar skin does not possess a pilosebaceous system and is thus referred to as *glabrous skin*, but it does have an abundance of exocrine sweat glands (400 per cm^2). This glabrous skin possesses papillary ridges that are responsible for the cutaneous striations that form fingerprints. The papillary ridges, which are designed for prehensile grip and are moistened by eccrine sweat glands, overlie the fat pads of the fingertips, the thenar and hypothenar eminences, and the metacarpal heads.

These pads and ridges are endowed with the highest density of sensory end-organs in the body and supply texture and grip surface to the hand. Free nerve endings and Merkel cell complexes are found in the epidermis and function as mechanoreceptors with slow adaption. Meissner's, Krause's, Ruffini's, and pacinian corpuscles are found in the dermis. Meissner's, pacinian and Krause's corpuscles function as mechanoreceptors with rapid adaptation, whereas Ruffini's corpuscles function as mechanoreceptors with slow adaptation.

With such a complex network of sensory end-organs in the hand, it is easy to understand why disruption of this system by burn injuries can produce severe impairment in sensibility. However, pain is an unreliable indicator that a burn is not full thickness, as the injury may exhibit components of superficial and deep partial-thickness (second-degree) burns and full-thickness (third-degree) burns. Therefore, the presence of pain does not rule out full-thickness injury.

In the immediate setting, it is crucial to detect vascular compromise in the patient with circumferential burns. Pain due to vascular ischemia must be differentiated from that due to the cutaneous burn itself. In addition, the absence of a pulse does not necessarily indicate vascular compromise due to the burn. Inadequate fluid resuscitation and relative hypovolemia can result in markedly diminished peripheral pulses in an attempt to perfuse vital organs while maintaining cardiac output and venous return to the heart. Therefore, systemic perfusion should be assessed by means of central venous pressure catheters and urine output. Swan-Ganz catheter assessment of pulmonary artery wedge pressures may be indicated in the elderly or in the severely burned patient in whom significant fluid shifts are anticipated and must be closely monitored. The absence of pulses in a patient with circumferential burns who is adequately resuscitated may be due to vascular compromise that is secondary to edema in a nondistensible extremity and presents an indication for escharotomy.

NONOPERATIVE TREATMENT

The first 24 hours after a severe burn injury are crucial. In this relatively brief period, accurate serial assessment of the adequacy of fluid resuscitation and the perfusion of an involved limb must be made. Appropriate fluid resuscitation ensures adequate circulating volume and limb perfusion. However, significant edema results secondary to increased capillary permeability and the massive fluid loads that are required to maintain intravascular volume. The effect of edema on vasculature compression is substantially compounded by the tourniquet effect of an unyielding circumferential burn eschar (11). The result is tissue ischemia, which must be expediently addressed by escharotomy (see the section Escharotomy).

Local Wound Care

In the stable patient without vascular compromise, attention should be directed toward wound closure and prevention of deformity and loss of function. To accomplish this, proper assessment of the wound is mandatory. By definition, the presence of blistering represents separation of the skin at the dermal-epidermal junction and therefore indicates a partial-thickness injury. However, the exact depth of the partial-thickness, or second-degree, burn, and the propensity for the injury to progress to a full-thickness, or third-degree, burn, is often not readily determined at the time of initial evaluation. Factors that serve to minimize the likelihood of conversion of a burn from partial thickness to full thickness include bacteriologic control of the wound and prevention of desiccation. This is accomplished by the application of a number of topical antibacterial agents.

After débridement of blisters and other nonviable tissue, mechanically or enzymatically (13,14), 1% silver sulfadiazine cream (Silvadene) is commonly used and is applied twice daily. A custom fit can be achieved by using gauze strips and elastic netting while permitting maximal movement of the extremity (11). The application of topical antibacterial agents can be facilitated by using a glove that is created from products such as Biobrane, Gore-Tex, or OpSite (15–17). These gloves permit easy movement of the hand and optimize healing conditions by providing a moist environment and maximizing contact with antibacterial topical agents. The Biobrane glove fits and adheres well and can be left in place during the healing process for partial-thickness burns of the hand that do not require débridement (11). However, prolonged application of Biobrane and other synthetic dressings must be administered with careful monitoring, as infection beneath these products can culminate in toxic shock syndrome (18).

Splinting

Preservation of function is the most important aspect of burn management of the hand. A functionless hand is a worthless hand. In fact, it is a hindrance. The burn claw deformity consists of MCP joint extension, PIP joint flexion, thumb adduction, and wrist flexion. This deformity can be prevented if attention is paid to properly splinting the hand on the day of injury and securing the involvement of a hand therapist to immediately institute active and passive range-of-motion exercises (19). Armed with the knowledge of how the collateral ligaments shorten when they are improperly managed, doctors should place all patients in splints that maintain the MCP joints at 70 to 80 degrees of flexion with the IP joints fully extended. Owing to the sig-

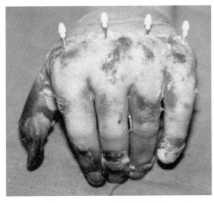

FIGURE 2. Kirschner wire fixation of the metacarpophalangeal joints in flexion and the interphalangeal joints in extension minimizes the incidence of collateral ligament shortening and joint contracture.

nificant swelling that occurs shortly after a major burn, it is often necessary to initially flex the MCP joints as much as is possible or tolerable by the patient and, subsequently, to modify the splint daily as additional flexion is feasible. Continual elevation of the hand helps to reduce edema. Customized splints that are fashioned from thermoplastic materials are generally the most effective and easiest to modify on a daily basis.

With severe burns of the hand, it is often necessary to place Kirschner wires across the PIP and MCP joints to ensure proper joint positioning to minimize the incidence of joint contracture (Fig. 2). This is usually done within the first several days of the injury, with the ultimate goal of maintaining the Kirschner wires for no more than 2 to 3 weeks, during which time the edema resolves, and the skin coverage is usually completed.

SURGICAL MANAGEMENT

Escharotomy

The combination of edema and circumferential injury with resultant unyielding circumferential eschar should lead one to consider performing an escharotomy. Circulatory compromise to the upper extremity at any level is an absolute indication for escharotomy. Although this may not be necessary within the first 24 hours after injury, edema continues to progress over the next 12 to 24 hours, and close observation is mandatory during this period, should the need for release become evident. Delay can lead to severe muscular necrosis with resultant Volkmann's contracture and functional loss.

Assessment of the burned extremity to determine the need for escharotomy must focus on quantitative monitoring of subcutaneous pressures, as circulatory compromise can occur even in the presence of palpable pulses. This is best done using a Stryker pressure gauge or, more simply, a manometer that is connected to an arterial line setup. Filling pressures of 30 mm Hg or greater on two separate readings indicate the need for escharotomy. If the hand, wrist, or forearm is tight on clinical examination, one should always err on the side of performing an escharotomy (11).

In the presence of vascular compromise, escharotomy of the upper extremity should include release of the burned arm, wrist, intrinsic compartments, and each involved finger. Escharotomy can be performed at the bedside by using an electrocautery, which also facilitates hemostasis and minimizes blood loss. The escharotomy incision is typically made in the midlateral plane, extending from the most proximal portion of the circumferential injury, across the entirety of the constricting burn, distally down to the wrist, and then across the midlateral plane of the hand and onto the thenar and hypothenar eminences (9) (Fig. 3). A radially or ulnarly based flap should be incorporated into the incision design at the level of the wrist to ensure adequate coverage of the median nerve. Similarly, incision design at the level of the medial epicondyle should be made anterior to the epicondyle to avoid injury to the ulnar nerve.

Dorsal incisions between the metacarpals permit exposure of the dorsal interossei (Fig. 4). A hemostat can be used to spread the edematous tissue, thus permitting division of the investing fascia with a scalpel. Complete release of the intrinsic compartments is crucial, as intrinsic muscle ischemia and necrosis can result in significant postburn disability of the hand (1). Longitudinal division of the investing fascia allows for decompression of the intrinsic musculature. Digital release is usually accomplished with a single incision along the midaxial plane of each finger. It usually is not necessary to make an incision along both sides of each finger, unless the burns are severe, and a single-sided incision does not provide adequate release. When possible, it is preferable to make incisions along the nondominant side of each finger. Thus, midlateral incisions should be performed along the ulnar aspect of the index, middle, and ring fingers to minimize the possibility of a painful scar at the point at which the thumb opposes the fingers (11). Although the incisions should not be deep enough to expose the neurovascular bundles, which might subject the digital nerves to desiccation, it is still the authors' preference not to use electrocautery for these incisions, thereby minimizing the likelihood of iatrogenic nerve injury. After escharotomy, the hand and arm are elevated. The wounds can be treated openly with a topical chemotherapeutic agent in a similar fashion to other burn wounds. When appropriately performed and subsequently managed, excellent hand function can be preserved long-term after escharotomy (Fig. 5).

Excision and Skin Grafting

The decision to excise and graft a burn is based on the determination that it will not heal satisfactorily within 2 to 3 weeks. Early excision and grafting minimize the incidence of hypertrophic scarring and contracture formation while facilitating early mobilization and rehabilitation. Early excision of a full-thickness burn wound may be performed at any time after injury, as it does not heal by conservative means and surely results in hypertrophic scarring and deformity. In addition, excision of a full-thickness eschar within 4 to 5 days after injury minimizes the incidence of significant bacterial invasion and infection (19).

Full-thickness eschar excision is usually performed to the level of the peritendinous fatty tissue or to the fascia. This is followed by autografting, when possible, or the application of allograft or other biologic dressings in severe burns in which sufficient donor sites are unavailable. Tangential excision of a burn wound, using a Weck or Goulian knife or dermatome, removes necrotic tissue in layers until healthy bleeding tissue is reached. In cases in which tangential excision is performed down to the level of the dermis, adequate epithelial elements should be present to permit spontaneous healing without grafting. Such wounds may be covered with a biologic or synthetic dressing that can be replaced every 4 to 5 days until healing is completed. However, reepithelialization occurs more rapidly beneath a bio-

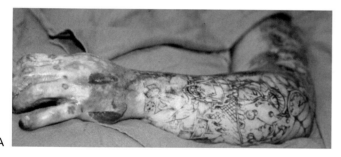

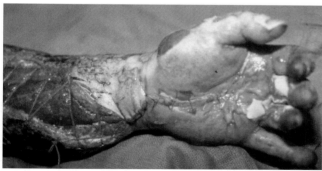

FIGURE 3. A: Escharotomy of the hand usually includes release of the thenar and hypothenar compartments, the intrinsic compartments (via a dorsal approach), and the individual digits. **B:** Release of the volar surface of the hand or forearm should include radially or ulnarly based flaps to ensure coverage of the median and ulnar nerves. Decompression of the carpal tunnel and Guyon's canal is also recommended to prevent damage to the median and ulnar nerves at the level of the wrist. Use of a Jacob's ladder, in which a vessel loop is secured in zigzag fashion by using staples at the edges of the wound, facilitates wound closure after release as the edema subsides.

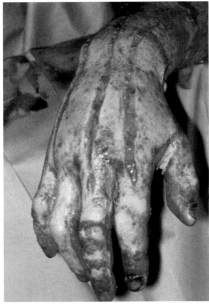
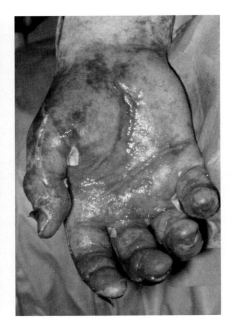

FIGURE 4. A: Release of the intrinsic compartments is performed by using dorsal longitudinal incisions over the metacarpals. Proximal extension of these incisions can be performed to release a circumferential burn of the wrist, as is shown in this case. **B:** Digital escharotomy should initially use incisions along the nondominant side of each finger. If these prove inadequate, incisions are then made along both sides of each finger. Whenever possible, the surgeon should avoid longitudinal incisions along the radial aspect of the index finger, the ulnar aspect of the thumb, and the ulnar aspect of the little finger. However, one should never compromise the vascularity to the digit if additional incisions are necessary.

A,B

logic dressing (e.g., allograft) than it does beneath a synthetic dressing (e.g., Biobrane) with less risk of bacterial invasion (19). When a burn wound is tangentially excised down to the level of subcutaneous tissue, the equivalent of a full-thickness excision autografting must be done.

Skin graft donor sites should be selected based on color and texture match, availability, and ease of concealment. Typical donor sites include the upper thighs and buttocks. With severe burns that involve a significant percent of TBSA, in which multiple regions require grafting, donor sites from which thin grafts have been obtained (0.010 to 0.012 in.) can generally be reharvested in 2 to 3 weeks. Of course, thicker grafts contract less than thinner grafts, a feature that supports their use for the hand. In such cases, it is occasionally necessary to harvest skin from the scalp, which is a source of thick skin that can be reharvested without difficulty.

Skin grafts to the hand are usually not meshed, as an unattractive permanent fishnet pattern often results after healing of the interstices of the graft. In addition, meshed grafts contract to a greater extent than unmeshed grafts. For grafting relatively small defects of the volar surface of the hand and fingers, as well as for release of burn contractures and syndactyly, Park et al. (20) recommend the use of full-thickness skin grafts that are harvested from the ulnar aspect of the wrist with direct closure of the donor site. In a series of 20 patients, they reported restoration of normal function in each case and a resultant scar that was inconspicuous.

The goal of skin grafting of the dorsum of the hand is to adequately resurface the area and restore normal hand function without development of secondary deformities. The common "safe" position of the hand, with the MCP joints flexed to 80 to 90 degrees, the IP joints extended, and the wrist extended to 20 to 30 degrees, has been commonly used for immobilization of the hand after grafting. However, this position specifically protects hand function; it does not ensure adequate skin grafting of the dorsum of the

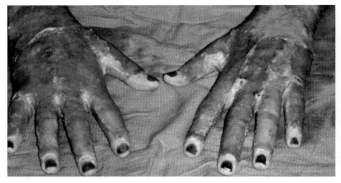
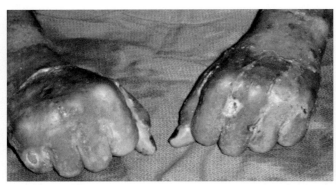

A

B

FIGURE 5. A,B: Three months after escharotomies, there is excellent functional recovery of both hands. Aggressive hand therapy is paramount in achievement of these results.

hand. Split-thickness skin grafts contract by as much as 30% to 50% of the original size owing to secondary contraction. Insufficient skin graft increases the propensity for contracture deformity of the dorsal hand (21).

Burm and Oh (22) advocate the "fist" position in which all MCP and IP joints of the fingers and the wrist are flexed, thereby maximally stretching the dorsal surface of the hand before skin grafting. Compared to the safe position, the fist position produces increases in lengths of the dorsal surface of the hand of 11% to 20% and of the dorsal surface of the finger of 12% to 17%. This position was maintained for 7 to 9 days after skin grafting with excellent function and cosmetic results obtained in the authors' report.

ELECTRICAL INJURIES

High-voltage electrical injuries produce an arc of current that passes from an entrance wound through a pathway of least resistance to an exit wound. As a result, these injuries are more prone to producing devastating soft tissue injury and loss (23,24). The hand and upper extremity are the most frequent sites of entry in electrical injuries, which are usually job related and the result of inadvertent contact with a high-voltage source. These injuries are often associated with other serious injuries that may be due to falling from heights while working on power poles or roofs. Therefore, all victims of high-voltage electrical trauma must be treated aggressively until more severe injuries, such as cervical fractures, have been ruled out. All victims of high-voltage electrical trauma should be admitted to a trauma or burn intensive care unit. Muscular destruction that is secondary to electrical injury often produces myoglobinuria, which is an indicator of rhabdomyolysis and myonecrosis. If left untreated, myoglobinuria is associated with intratubular deposition of pigments, which leads to acute renal failure. Urine flow in the range of 75 to 100 mL hour must be maintained by administering a sufficient volume of lactated Ringer's solution or by inducing diuresis with mannitol or furosemide and alkalinizing the urine by sodium bicarbonate infusion to maintain pigment solubility. Electrical injury can also produce refractory cardiac arrhythmias and serum electrolyte derangements, which can prove fatal if they are not adequately assessed and managed.

A small skin defect may be associated with massive damage to underlying muscles, nerves, or vessels (11). Indeed, variable skeletal, muscle, neural, and vascular tissue injury is typically distributed along the path of the current (25). Several decades ago, limb amputation rates were reported as high as 71% (26). Today, the ability to reconstruct anatomic defects and to restore function has dramatically increased the rate of limb salvage after such devastating injuries.

Limb swelling usually accompanies significant deep soft tissue injury. Suspicion of compartment syndrome based on clinical manifestations of muscle or nerve ischemia or tenseness on palpation should be confirmed with serial measurement of compartment pressures every 6 to 8 hours for the first 24 hours postinjury. When compartment pressures exceed 30 mm Hg, fasciotomy should be performed by using similarly placed incisions as those that were described for escharotomy. A low threshold for fasciotomy should be maintained in these patients, as the consequences that result after inadequately treated compartment syndrome are devastating. Serial débridements are usually necessary to determine the extent of devitalized tissue, which is often not apparent during the initial débridement procedure. The need for subsequent débridements can often be guided by performing quantitative wound cultures. After each débridement, the application of allografts or topical antimicrobial agents to the wounds is generally performed.

Reconstructive requirements after electrical injury are often more extensive and more complex than those after thermal burns. Once a limb has been satisfactorily débrided without evidence of residual necrotic tissue or infection, skin grafts, local skin flaps, fasciocutaneous flaps, or microvascular free flaps can be used to cover the wound and salvage the injured extremity.

CHEMICAL INJURIES

Chemical injuries can be categorized into four groups: acid burns, alkali burns, phosphorus burns, and chemical injection injuries. Although alkalis, as a group, are the most common chemicals that are involved in cutaneous burns, the most frequent single chemical agent that is involved is sulfuric acid (27). Chemical injection injuries can result from industrial accidents, including subcutaneous injection of oil, paint, and other substances, or from intravenous extravasation injuries, including passage of chemotherapeutic and other medicinal agents into the soft tissue compartments of the hand. In fact, more than 60% of chemical injuries are the result of work-related mishaps (28). Acid burns cause coagulation necrosis; alkaline burns cause saponification followed by liquefaction necrosis and, in general, penetrate more deeply and carry a greater risk of severe systemic toxicity. Mechanisms of injury and methods of treatment differ among the four groups, although some similarities exist. Because most injuries occur during the handling of chemical substances, the hand and upper extremity are affected most often. Moreover, these injuries, which typically result in a much smaller percentage of TBSA that is involved compared to thermal injuries, often result in greater morbidity, as a greater percent of these injuries produce full-thickness burns.

Chemical injuries produce tissue destruction not as the result of a burning process but rather as a result of tissue protein coagulation with resultant necrosis. The major difference between thermal and chemical injuries is the length of time of tissue destruction. Thermal burn injuries are the result of momentary exposure, whereas chemical injuries

TABLE 1. MANAGEMENT OF COMMON CHEMICAL INJURIES

Commercial types	Chemical compound	Treatment
Batteries	Sulfuric acid, Li^{2+}	Water irrigation
Toilet bowl cleaners	Sulfuric acid, hydrochloric acid (muriatic acid)	Water irrigation
Pool cleaners	Hydrochloric acid	Magnesium oxide, soaps
Rust removers	Hydrofluoric acid (H^+Fl^-), chromic acid	Water irrigation, calcium-magnesium ($Ca^{2+}Mg^{2+}$) slurry
Petroleum solvents	Organics	Dilute soaps, water irrigation
Bleach	Sodium hypochlorite	Water irrigation
Drain clog removers, oven cleaners	Lye (sodium hypochlorite), sodium hydroxide	Water irrigation
Tile cleaners	Ammonium chloride (alkali)	Water irrigation
Cement	Lye	Water irrigation

Adapted from Reilly DA, Garner WL. Management of chemical injuries to the upper extremity. *Hand Clin* 2000;16:215–224.

continue to cause damage until the offending agent is entirely removed or neutralized. Therefore, the most important steps in the initial management of a chemically injured patient are (a) removal of any clothing articles that are contaminated with the offending agent and (b) immediate, copious, and continuous irrigation with water. This serves to dilute the chemical agent, minimize contact and tissue penetration, decrease the rate of chemical reaction, decrease tissue metabolism, and restore normal skin pH (28). Only injuries due to elemental sodium, potassium, and lithium should not be irrigated with water, which causes ignition and additional thermal injury.

The agents that are most commonly responsible for chemical-related injuries are listed in Table 1. Injuries resulting from exposure to hydrofluoric acid are among the most painful of the chemical injuries. This may be attributable to its bimodal mechanism of action. The H^+ ion that is released, as with all acid burns, must be rapidly neutralized to minimize tissue necrosis. Subsequently, the powerful Fl^- ion is released and binds with tissue cations, calcium and magnesium, in particular (28). Tissue damage and bony decalcification progress until the ion is neutralized. Treatment is therefore directed at absorption of the negative ions. This is initially done with irrigation of the wound with water followed by application of a 2.5% calcium gluconate gel. Cessation of pain is indicative of adequate treatment. Persistent symptoms indicate the need for injection of the wound with 10% calcium gluconate or magnesium sulfate solutions, which are administered at 0.5 mL per cm². Intraarterial infusion of calcium gluconate is advocated if the exposure area is greater than 2% TBSA or if symptoms remain after other forms of treatment of smaller wounds. Using a radial arterial line, a solution of 2 g of calcium gluconate in a solution of 250 mL dextrose 5% in water is infused over 4 hours and usually repeated in 6 to 8 hours. Cardiac monitoring for signs of hypocalcemia and serum calcium level monitoring are crucial (11).

Débridement of blisters, bullae, and all necrotic tissue is performed after adequate irrigation and management of the involved extremity. At this point, wound care consists of the application of topical antimicrobial agents, such as 1% silver sulfadiazine dressings twice a day, until healing has occurred for partial-thickness injuries or excision and skin grafting or flap reconstruction for full-thickness injuries.

RECONSTRUCTION OF THE BURNED HAND

Proper initial management of the burned hand is crucial to ensure a favorable long-term outcome. However, the complex nature of burn injuries and the resultant tissue destruction invite a host of potential complications or sequelae of the initial injury. In the best of cases, in which adequate soft tissue coverage is achieved shortly after the burn injury and healing progresses without infection or other acute adverse consequences, most patients, after significant burns, must contend with skin and soft tissue contractures, including web space contractures and adduction contractures of the thumb web space. In addition, syndactylism, claw deformities, and hypertrophic scarring can also occur after burn injuries and must be addressed if adequate function is to be preserved or restored. The reconstructive burn surgeon must possess an armamentarium of procedures with which to address these complex problems.

Skin and Soft Tissue Contractures

The most common problem after burn injuries of the hand is the development of skin and soft tissue contractures, which may be the result of skin grafts of inadequate size or thickness, hypertrophic scar or keloid formation, inadequate postinjury splinting, or an inadequate physical therapy rehabilitation program (1).

Contractures of the palm after burns to the volar surface of the hand occur commonly when the hand has not been properly splinted after injury. The propensity for flexion contractures of the wrist and fingers and adduction contractures of the thumb necessitates splinting the hand with the wrist in hyperextension, the thumb fully abducted, and all fingers flexed at the MCP joints and

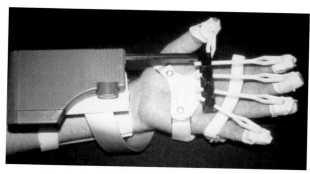

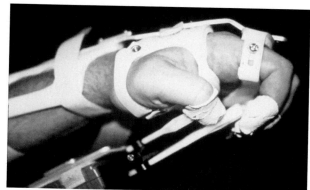

FIGURE 6. A,B: A variety of continuous passive motion devices are currently used to prevent contractures and to maximize hand function after burns.

extended at the IP joints for at least a portion of the day. The immediate use of a fitted Jobst garment can significantly decrease the extent of hypertrophic scarring and contracture formation. Prevention of contracture is essential. Once contracture has developed, surgical release and split-thickness or full-thickness skin grafting of the palm are necessary (29). Incisions parallel to the distal palmar and thenar creases often provide sufficient release. The groin crease or lower abdominal wall usually provides adequate full-thickness skin graft donor sites. In addition, a contracted PIP joint volar plate may require incision and release to permit finger extension.

Adequate splinting and an aggressive therapy program after contracture release play a crucial role in the prevention of contracture recurrence. A regimen that includes night splinting for 1 year with the wrist and fingers fully extended and the early use of pressure garments is necessary to maintain mobility and function. The use of continuous passive motion devices has also been advocated for this purpose (30) (Fig. 6).

Contractures of the dorsum of the hand can be just as debilitating as those of the volar surface. Tightness, MCP joint hyperextension or even dislocation, and limitation of flexion of the fingers can result and necessitate excision and grafting of the dorsum of the hand. In cases with severe contracture, the extensor tendons may be markedly shortened, severely scarred, and unamenable to tenolysis or step-cut lengthening (1). Such cases may require ten-

don transection or excision to allow MCP joint flexion. Once good passive range of motion of the MCP joints has been reestablished, adequate soft tissue coverage that enables subsequent tendon gliding and prevents recurrence of contracture must be provided (Fig. 7). A variety of approaches, including the use of groin flaps (Fig. 8), abdominal wall flaps, radial forearm fasciocutaneous flaps, and free flaps, can be used in these cases with excellent results (31–34).

Hypertrophic Scars and Keloids

The development of hypertrophic scars and the formation of keloids remains poorly understood from a physiologic perspective. Indeed, although these two entities behave quite different clinically, they are virtually identical histologically. The best means of addressing these complex problems is prevention, as, once they have developed, they are almost impossible to correct without extensive surgery. The Jobst glove pressure garment remains the best method of prevention and should be used in any patient who has undergone skin grafting of the hand or in patients in whom burn wounds have taken longer than 14 days to heal spontaneously. Scar massage and application of various oil preparations, such as Lubriderm (Pfizer, New York, NY), minimize the occurrence of ulceration and new scar formation. Injection of thickened scars along graft suture lines with triamcinolone acetonide (Kenalog) often yields some degree of improvement.

Web Space Contracture

Contracture of the web space is the most common deformity of the web space after burns (11). Thickened scar or graft contracture along the dorsal edge of the web can produce dorsal hooding or "distal creep." Without the use of splints, which are infrequently used, to maintain the fingers in an abducted position, the fingers usually assume an adducted position at rest. As a result, the burned web often heals in a state of contracture (1). Z-plasty release is often adequate to release the simpler web space contracture. However, more extensive contractures, in which the "creeping" web space has extended from one-half to three-fourths the distance from the MCP joint to the PIP joint, benefit from a V-M–plasty, in which five flaps are created in the web space to reconstitute the proximal position of the web (35). Advanced web space contractures that require significant release and flap advancement may also require a skin graft on the lateral aspects of the involved fingers.(11).

Burn Syndactyly

Syndactyly that occurs after a severe burn and that resembles congenital syndactyly, with skin loss along the entire length of the lateral digits, is uncommon. When it does occur, it is

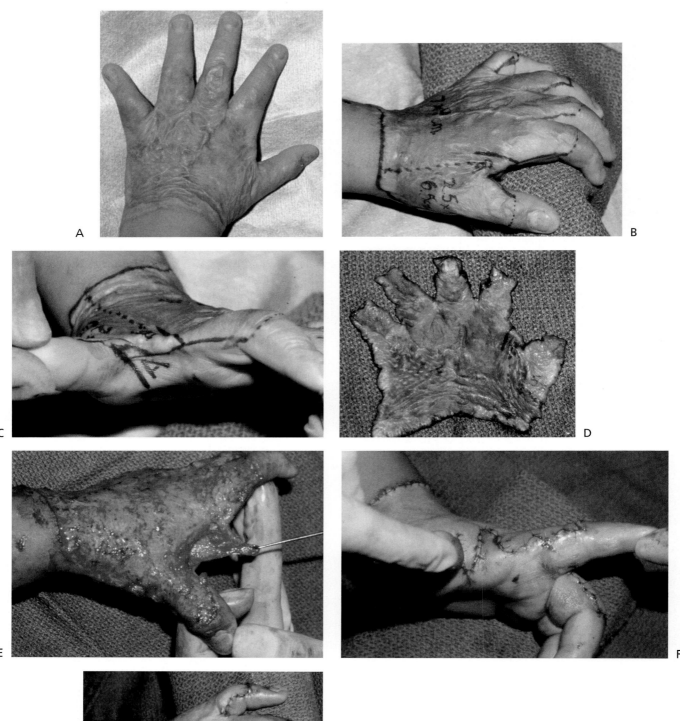

FIGURE 7. **A–C:** Release of dorsal hand and web space contractures requires complete excision of all restrictive scar tissue and resurfacing with soft, pliable tissue. Thick split-thickness or full-thickness sheet skin grafts are often used; flap coverage is performed when skin grafting cannot provide adequate coverage of vital structures. **D,E:** The dorsal burn scar is excised. **F:** A volar flap is transposed into the first web space. **G:** The dorsum is grafted with a thick split-thickness sheet graft with darting along the mid-lateral aspects of the digits.

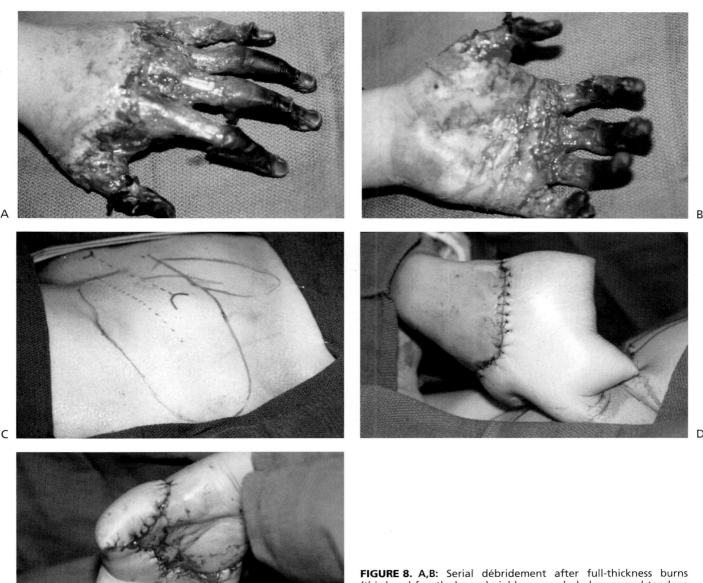

FIGURE 8. A,B: Serial débridement after full-thickness burns (third and fourth degree) yields exposed phalanges and tendons that require soft tissue coverage. Distal digital amputations are often necessary. **C:** A groin or epigastric flap is designed based on the superficial inferior epigastric artery or superficial circumflex iliac artery. **D,E:** The fasciocutaneous flap is elevated and inset to cover all exposed structures of the hand. The groin flap is usually divided 2 to 3 weeks later.

treated by release and skin grafting. Flap design may be a bit more complicated than that performed to release a congenital syndactyly case, as this condition is the result of extensive scarring rather than failure of digital separation.

Adduction Contracture of the Thumb

An adduction contracture of the thumb involves the first web space. It is a complex deformity, as it involves not only scarring of the skin of the first web but also fibrosis of the adductor muscle and the first dorsal interosseous muscle (36). Therefore, it is unlikely, except in rare circumstances,

that a Z-plasty alone can provide adequate release of an adductor contracture. MCP joint hyperextension is often associated with adductor contracture that is secondary to dorsal scarring. Therefore, the releasing incision should extend dorsally from over the MCP joint through the web space and volarly along the thenar crease to adequately release the MCP joint as well (1). Care must be taken during release of the adductor contracture to avoid the sensory branch of the radial nerve, as well as the neurovascular bundles to the thumb and radial side of the index finger. Fascia and muscle are released until an adequate web space has been created. Four-flap Z-plasties (Fig. 9) and five-flap

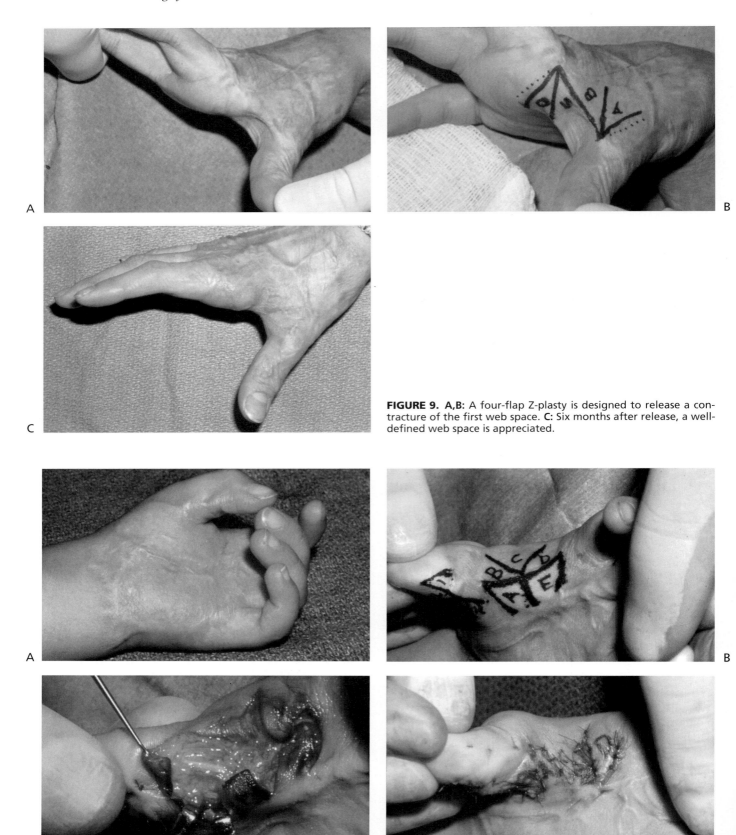

FIGURE 9. A,B: A four-flap Z-plasty is designed to release a contracture of the first web space. **C:** Six months after release, a well-defined web space is appreciated.

FIGURE 10. A,B: A five-flap Z-plasty is designed to release an adductor contracture that involves not only skin but also underlying muscle. **C:** Flap elevation reveals the underlying neurovascular bundles that require coverage. **D:** The flaps are then transposed and sutured in place.

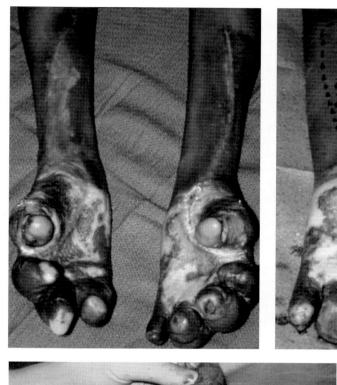
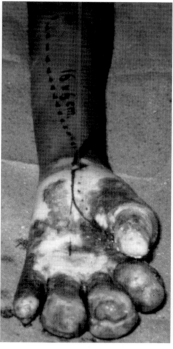
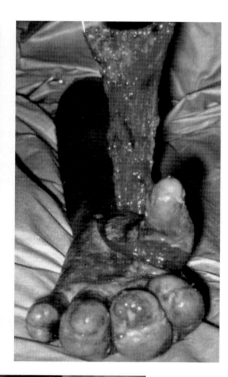

A,B

C

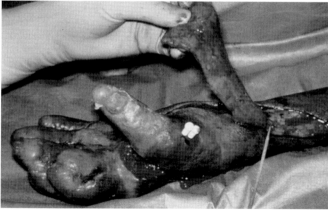

D

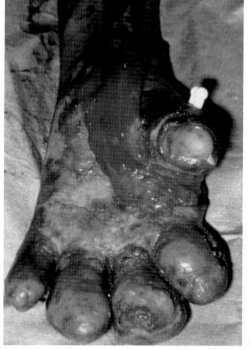

E

FIGURE 11. A: One year after severe bilateral burns, reconstruction is undertaken to release a severe adductor contracture of the left hand. Before this, the patient underwent groin flap coverage of the dorsum of the hand and digits, followed by digitalization. **B:** A distally based radial forearm fascial flap is designed. **C,D:** The contracture is released. **E:** The flap is then elevated based on the distal perforators of the radial artery. It is transposed into the first web space after Kirschner wire fixation of the first and second metacarpals in abduction.

Z-plasties (Fig. 10) are often designed to release contractures of the first web space. When deeper structures have not been exposed, resurfacing of the web space with a skin graft is often sufficient; coverage of deeper structures is often accomplished with a groin flap or a distally based radial forearm flap, when it is available (Fig. 11). Before grafting or flap coverage is performed, the first and second metacarpals are abducted and pinned apart to maintain the breadth of the web space, and the MCP joint is pinned in maximum flexion to optimize subsequent joint mobility.

CONCLUSION

Proper management of burns of the hand and upper extremity requires an aggressive approach that incorporates the efforts of the hand surgeon, the physical and occupational therapists, and the patient to preserve complex anatomic structures and to maximize long-term functional recovery. The importance of appropriate splinting, determination of the need for escharotomy, and timing of burn wound excision and skin grafting cannot be overemphasized. Reconstruction of web space and adduction contractures and other sequelae after burn injuries often necessitates various types of Z-plasty procedures, as well as the use of local, regional, and free flaps. Familiarity with these techniques is essential in the reconstruction of such secondary problems.

REFERENCES

1. Salisbury RE, Dingeldein GP. The burned hand and upper extremity. In: Green DP, ed. *Operative hand surgery,* 3rd ed. New York: Churchill Livingstone, 1993:2007–2031.
2. Consumer Product Safety Commission. Consumer Product-related injuries treated in hospital emergency rooms. Jan. 1–Dec. 31, 1976. U.S. Consumer Product Safety Commission; April 1978; Washington, DC.
3. Sheridan RL, Hurley J, Smith MA. The acutely burned hand: management and outcome based on a ten-year experience with 1047 acute hand burns. *J Trauma* 1995;38:406–411.
4. Bunnell S. Splinting the hand. In: Bunnell S, ed. *Surgery of the hand,* 3rd ed. Philadelphia: JB Lippincott Co, 1956.
5. Watson HK, Weinzweig J. Stiff joints. In: Green DP, Hotchkiss RN, Pederson WC, eds. *Operative hand surgery,* 4th ed. New York: Churchill Livingstone, 1998:552–562.
6. Brand PW. *Clinical mechanics of the hand.* St. Louis: CV Mosby, 1985:61–87.
7. Flowers KR, Pheasant SD. The use of torque angle curves in the assessment of digital joint stiffness. *J Hand Ther* 1988;1:69–74.
8. Pruitt BA, Goodwin CW, Pruitt SK. Burns. In: Sabiston, DC, Lyerly HK, eds. *Textbook of surgery: the biological basis of modern surgical practice,* 15th ed. Philadelphia: WB Saunders, 1997.
9. Salisbury RE. Acute care of the burned hand. In: McCarthy JG, ed. *Plastic surgery.* Philadelphia: WB Saunders, 1990:5399–5417.
10. Ng D, Anastakis D, Douglas LG, et al. Work-related burns: a 6-year retrospective study. *Burns* 1991;17:151–154.
11. Achauer BM. The burned hand. In: Green DP, Hotchkiss RN, Pederson WC, eds. *Operative hand surgery,* 4th ed. New York: Churchill Livingstone, 1998:2045–2060.
12. Morel Fatio D. Surgery of the skin. In: Tubiana R, ed. *The hand.* Philadelphia: WB Saunders, 1961:224–225.
13. Hansbrough JF, Achauer BM, Dawson J, et al. Wound healing in partial-thickness burn wounds treated with collagenase ointment versus silver sulfadiazine cream. *J Burn Care Rehabil* 1995;16:241–247.
14. Gant TD. The early enzymatic debridement and grafting of deep dermal burns to the hand. *Plast Reconstr Surg* 1980;66:185–190.
15. Bache J. Clinical evaluation of the use of Op-Site gloves for the treatment of partial thickness burns of the hand. *Burns* 1988;14:413–416.
16. Smith DJ, McHugh TP, Phillips LG, et al. Biosynthetic compound dressings—management of hand burns. *Burns* 1988;14:405–408.
17. Terrill PJ, Edwards SM, Lawrence JC. The use of Gore-Tex bags for hand burns. *Burns* 1991;17:161–165.
18. Weinzweig J, Gottlieb LJ, Krizek TJ, Toxic shock syndrome associated with use of Biobrane in a scald burn victim. *Burns* 1994;20:180–181.
19. Boswick JA Jr. Early management of burns of the hand. In: Boswick JA Jr, ed. *The art and science of burn care.* Rockville, MD: Aspen Publishers, 1987:347–352.
20. Park S, Hata Y, Ito O, et al. Full-thickness skin graft from the ulnar aspect of the wrist to cover defects on the hand and digits. *Ann Plast Surg* 1999;42:129–131.
21. Burm JS, Chung CH, Oh SJ. Fist position for skin grafting on the dorsal hand. I. Analysis of length of the dorsal hand surface in hand positions. *Plast Reconstr Surg* 1999;104:1350–1355.
22. Burm JS, Oh SJ. Fist position for skin grafting on the dorsal hand. II. Clinical use in deep burns and scar contractures. *Plast Reconstr Surg* 2000;105:581–588.
23. Lee RC. Injury by electrical forces: pathophysiology, manifestations, and therapy. *Curr Probl Surg* 1997;34:677–765.
24. Lee RC, Astumian RD. The physiochemical basis for thermal and nonthermal "burn" injuries. *Burns* 1996;22:509–519.
25. Danielson JR, Capelli-Schellpfeffer M, Lee RC. Upper extremity electrical injury. *Hand Clin* 2000;16:225–234.
26. Rouse RG, Dimick AR. The treatment of electrical injury compared to burn injury: a review of pathophysiology and comparison of patient management protocols. *J Trauma* 1978;18:43–47.
27. Sykes RA, Mani MM, Hiebert JM. Chemical burns: retrospective review. *J Burn Care Rehabil* 1986;7:343–347.
28. Reilly DA, Garner WL. Management of chemical injuries to the upper extremity. *Hand Clin* 2000;16:215–224.
29. Pensler JM, Steward R, Lewis SR, et al. Reconstruction of the burned palm: full-thickness versus split-thickness skin grafts—long-term follow-up. *Plast Reconstr Surg* 1988;81:46–49.
30. Bentham JS, Brereton WD, Cochrane IW, et al. Continuous passive motion device for hand rehabilitation. *Arch Phys Med Rehabil* 1987;68:248–250.
31. Gao JH, Hyakusoku H, Inoue S, et al. Usefulness of narrow pedicled intercostal cutaneous perforator flaps for coverage of the burned hand. *Burns* 1994;20:65–70.
32. Park C, Shin KS. Total palmar resurfacing with scapular free flap in a 26-year contracted hand. *Ann Plast Surg* 1991;26:183–187.
33. Quaba AA, Davision PM. The distally-based dorsal hand flap. *Br J Plast Surg* 1990;43:28–39.
34. Shen TY, Sun YH, Cao DX, et al. The use of free flaps in burn patients: experiences with 70 flaps in 65 patients. *Plast Reconstr Surg* 1988;81:352–357.
35. Alexander JW, MacMillan BG, Martel L. Correction of postburn syndactyly: an analysis of children with introduction of the V-M-plasty and postoperative pressure inserts. *Plast Reconstr Surg* 1982;70:345–352.
36. Kurtzman LC, Stern PJ, Yakuboff KP. Reconstruction of the burned thumb. *Hand Clin* 1992;8:107–119.

62

FROSTBITE

LEWIS H. OSTER, JR.

Frostbite injury occurs when the body is exposed to cold and localized tissue freezes (1). Tissue freezes at 28°F or −2°C (2). Frostbite injury can result from any environmental factor that facilitates the transfer of heat away from the tissues. The more rapidly heat is transferred, the less time is needed to cause cellular damage and death. Factors that enhance the development of frostbite include wind chill (3), water immersion (4), high altitude (5), consumption of alcohol or drugs (6,7), vascular dehydration (8,9), fatigue (10), inactivity (11), previous cold injury (12), and chemical agent exposure (13).

Military campaigns have provided a rich historic perspective of cold and frostbite injury that has been sustained by human beings. Xenophon described the severe cold injuries that were incurred by Spartan soldiers who retreated across the Carduchian mountains after they left Alexander's armies (4). Aurelius Cornelius Celsus, in his *Compendium de Medicina*, provided one of the first pathologic descriptions of frostbite (4): "Cold is hurtful to an older or slender man; to his ears, hips, private parts, teeth, bones, nerves, and brain; it renders the surface of the skin pale, dry, hard, and black." Ten percent of George Washington's army perished during the winter campaigns of 1778 due to exposure to extreme cold (14). Similar effects were seen in Napoleon's army during its retreat from Moscow (15). Trench foot was seen in epidemic proportions throughout World War I as a result of soldiers who stood in rain-filled trenches (4,16). American soldiers who served in World War II and the Korean War experienced a new etiology of cold injury from high-altitude flying (17).

Currently, frostbite continues to be a common problem not only in military personnel, but also in the increasing population that is involved in winter outdoor recreational sports. The incidence of frostbite is unknown due to a lack of documentation in a central registry.

PATHOPHYSIOLOGY

Definition

There is a spectrum of cold injury that begins with tissue cooling or frostnip and concludes with tissue freezing or frostbite. The mildest form of cold injury is frostnip. Frostnip is the only reversible cold injury to tissue (2). Frostnip is characterized by blanching and numbness of the affected skin. There is no damage to the dermal or subcutaneous tissue if rewarming is initiated immediately. If rewarming is not begun promptly, frostnip can progress to frostbite. Chilblain, or *pernio*, is more severe than frostnip and can occur in nonfreezing temperatures (18). This condition is a recurrent chronic vasculitis that occurs on exposed extremities after repeated cold exposure. Trench foot, or immersion foot, results from prolonged exposure to wet and cold conditions between 30° and 50°F for periods of 4 hours or longer (4,19). This also can occur in upper extremities. Tissue freezing or frostbite is the most severe type of cold injury (2). The severity of frostbite injury is dependent on the rate of heat loss from the tissue, the tissue temperature, the intensity of the initial exposure, and the length of time before adequate circulation can be restored to the affected area (20,21).

Classification

Several types of classification systems for frostbite can be found in the literature. The traditional classification system describes frostbite in terms of four different degrees (22). The zone of injury is described as being edematous and erythematous in first-degree injury. Patients who incur second-degree injury develop blistering of the affected skin and partial-thickness skin loss. Third-degree injury patients experience full-thickness skin loss and skin necrosis. Fourth-degree cold injury results in necrosis of not only the skin but also the deep tissues, including bone and muscle.

The two-degree classification is a more clinically useful system that describes the frostbite as superficial or deep (23). Superficial frostbite is injury to the skin and subcutaneous tissue (23). There is minimal tissue loss. The affected tissue is supple when it is depressed and painful after rewarming. Minimal to moderate edema often develops after rewarming. Clear blisters and reactive hyperemia cover the affected tissues. Patients with superficial frostbite often experience a permanent hypersensitivity to cold. Deep frostbite is cold injury that extends to the deep structures of the extremities (23). Injury occurs not only to the skin but also to tendon, bone, and muscle. The affected tissue or extremity is firm when it is depressed and anesthetic after rewarming. Large amounts of edema often develop after rewarming the extremity with deep frostbite. Hemorrhagic blisters cover the affected tissues, and the skin is blue-gray. Patients experience extensive tissue loss that often requires amputation of the affected extremity after an episode of deep frostbite. Patients are also at risk for the development of gangrene. It is often difficult to ascertain the extent of frostbite injury on initial examination of the patient. Subsequent physical examinations are required to determine the extent of injury.

Pathogenesis

The human's initial physiologic response to cold is peripheral vasoconstriction (24). This is a protective neurologic response to maintain and to preserve the core temperature of the body. The vasoconstrictive response is dynamic, rather than static, in nature. The vasculature of the extremities vasodilates through arteriovenous shunting in an effort to rewarm the tissue. This is known as the *Hunting response*, and it repeats itself every 7 to 10 minutes until the body's core temperature begins to fall (24). When the core temperature falls, the extremity vasoconstriction becomes static. This results in tissue cooling, until freezing occurs at –2°C. When all tissue is frozen, the temperature of the extremity falls to the environmental temperature.

Tissue injury and death are believed to occur not only while the affected extremity is cooling and freezing, but also during rewarming (25). Clinically, it is best advised that an extremity be left frozen rather than rewarmed and frozen again. The freeze-thaw-freeze scenario causes repeated cell injury and is more detrimental to the patient.

Cell death during the cooling phase is believed to be a consequence of prolonged vasoconstriction (25). The sludging of blood that occurs during vasoconstriction in the extremity can lead to cell ischemia and death. The ischemic process triggers chemically and cellularly mediated pathways that induce an inflammatory response. Examples of chemical mediators involved in the process are prostaglandins (26), bradykinins (27), thromboxane (26), and histamine (28). Examples of cell mediators are leukocytes (29) and platelets (30).

Cell death during the freezing phase is believed to result from cellular dehydration (31). Prolonged exposure to cold causes the extracellular or interstitial fluid to freeze first. As the water in the interstitial space crystallizes, a hypertonic solution is created in the interstitium. The ionic gradient that is created draws the water out of the cell, thus causing an intercellular dehydration to occur. This dehydration results in cellular dysfunction. If exposure to the cold continues, the remaining water within the cell crystallizes and further inhibits cell function. Finally, ice crystals form within the cell membrane itself. The result is loss of membrane integrity and cell death.

Tissue death after rewarming is believed to be a consequence of a localized toxic environment. Rapid rewarming of the extremity causes the extremity temperature to rise above –2°C. The resultant endothermic reaction causes the ice crystals to melt. The chemical mediators that are frozen within the ice crystals are free to continue the inflammatory response that was triggered during the freezing phase. The integrity of the cell membrane is lost during freezing and is dysfunctional after rewarming. The resultant localized toxic environment is thought to contribute to necrosis of adjacent viable tissue.

EVALUATION

History

History taking is important in assessment of the depth and degree of frostbite injury. All patients with frostbite injury present for medical treatment with a history of exposure to cold. The severity of the frostbite injury is proportionate to the temperature and duration of exposure to cold. The amount of heat that is lost from the tissues is a critical concept in understanding why parts of the body are at different levels of risk for frostbite. Extremities tend to be more at risk for the development of frostbite.

History taking should include assessment of host and environmental factors to determine the patient's degree of risk of development of frostbite. Host medical risk factors are poor general health, peripheral vascular disease, diabetes, tobacco use, consumption of alcohol or drugs, alteration of mental status, and sensitivity to cold from previous exposure. Environmental factors include the temperature during exposure to cold, the time of exposure, the force of the wind or wind chill factor, and the relative humidity in the air. It is important to ascertain whether the affected area was in contact with better heat conductors than air, such as water or metal. It is important to ask the patient if his or her clothing was wet during exposure to cold. Wet clothing, shoes, and other body coverings are 20 times less warm than the same dry items of clothing.

Physical Examination

Physical examination of the patient with frostbite injury includes inspection and palpation of the affected extremity. Superficial frostbite occurs most often on the face and results in minimal skin and subcutaneous tissue loss. The skin may appear waxy-looking, with a blanching or whitening in color (32). The injury site is supple and painful after rewarming, with minimal to moderate edema. Large clear blisters appear early. The blisters often extend to the tips of the digits. In addition, the injured tissue exhibits a reactive hyperemia after thawing. Deep frostbite occurs most commonly in the lower extremities and causes significant tissue loss to the deep structures of bone, muscle, and tendon. It is slightly less common in the upper extremities and is rare in the head and neck. The injury site is firm when it is depressed and anesthetic after rewarming, with pronounced edema. The affected skin has a bluish-gray appearance. Hemorrhagic blisters develop with deep frostbite injury. These blisters reflect the damage to the subdermal structures that has occurred. It is important to distinguish between superficial and deep frostbite injury, because the proper classification has prognostic and therapeutic implications for treatment.

Imaging Studies

Various imaging techniques have been tried to more accurately determine the extent and severity of frostbite injury. The goal of imaging studies is to determine the level of demarcation as early as possible. Early identification of demarcation facilitates prompt intervention and recovery and avoids the pitfall of further tissue loss that is secondary to complications, such as infection and metabolic imbalances.

Plain radiographic films are of little value in the determination of the severity of frostbite injury. However, the value of plain films in the frostbitten upper extremity lies in the ability to assess concomitant trauma that may have occurred because of an anesthetic extremity. Roentgenograms are also useful to determine the degree of injury in growth plates of children after frostbite injury. Children with open growth plates at the time of frostbite injury experience long-term growth disturbances (33,34).

Xenon 133 has been used to predict the amount of tissue loss after frostbite injury (35). The scan measures the local soft tissue blood flow but not bone blood flow. It also has been criticized for increasing injured-tissue pressure.

Angiography has been used to assess vascular changes after frostbite injury, to choose proper therapy, and to determine the extent of amputation that is required (36). However, arteriograms that are obtained soon after injury do not sufficiently clarify levels of viability (21). The addition of vasodilator pharmacologic agents during early arteriography has been useful in predicting demarcation (36,37). Angiography is invasive and expensive and does not allow for imaging of vessels at the arteriolar or capillary levels. Doppler ultrasound and digital plethysmography may be used to assess local blood flow after frostbite (38). Neither of these techniques is able to assess microcirculation or capillary function.

The standard imaging study that is used within a few days of injury is the technetium 99m pyrophosphate scintigraphy, which allows for the evaluation of the microcirculation of the soft tissue and the bone (39). Many clinicians have used this imaging technique to determine the level of amputation (1). Bone scans at 48 hours after admission have been advocated (40). Nonoperative treatment is recommended in patients with normal scans. Early ablation is advocated in patients with absent, delayed images (40).

The techniques of magnetic resonance imaging and magnetic resonance angiography (MRA) compare well to bone scan in their ability to directly image vascularity of cold-injured tissue (41). Both imaging methodologies define the extent of tissue ischemia well before clinical signs of necrosis occur. T2-weighted images in MRA show increased signal intensity in cold-injured muscle tissue (41). This is believed to represent disruption of cellular membranes and increased extracellular water. It is considered to be an indication of cellular death. MRA scanning may be of little use in evaluation of digital injuries because of the lack of striated muscle.

As of 2003, there is no prognostic imaging technique that predicts death at the cellular level in the immediate postinjury period. "A delay of two or three weeks is still necessary to exceed the period of transitory vascular instability before any radiologic technique can reliably distinguish the line of demarcation and the required level of débridement or amputation" (21).

MANAGEMENT OF FROSTBITE

Field Management

Initial treatment in the field focuses on the protection of the affected extremity from mechanical trauma and avoidance of rewarming, until definitive rewarming can be performed (21). Cyclic thawing and cooling or inadequate rewarming can worsen a frostbite injury (25). The extremity is placed in a well-padded splint in a functional position for protection. The patient's overall condition should be assessed, and a complete history and physical should be performed.

Hospital Care

Nonoperative Intervention

The measurement of core body temperature on patient arrival to the hospital is imperative (42). Treatment of rewarming of the affected extremity should not commence until the core body temperature rises above 35°C. At this temperature, peripheral vascular vessel beds reopen. The result is an influx of cold blood to the core body that can cause a paradoxic decrease in body temperature. Rapid rewarming of the extremity is superior to slow thawing of the extremity, because it decreases tissue necrosis and the overall period of freezing (43).

The ideal temperature at which the cold-injured part should be rewarmed is between 40° and 42°C (44). Rewarming of the affected extremity is best accomplished in a hydrotherapy tub (i.e., a Hubbard tank), which is commonly found in physical therapy or burn units. It is important to stay within this narrow temperature range for two reasons. First, rewarming at a lower temperature leads to greater thawing time and is less beneficial to tissue survival. Second, rewarming at higher temperatures could compound the tissue injury by resulting in a burn injury to the affected area.

Rewarming should be continued for 15 to 30 minutes or until thawing is complete. Warming should be completed when a red or purple appearance and pliable texture of the affected extremity occur. This means the end of vasoconstriction in the injured extremity. Active motion during rewarming is helpful, but massage is not recommended.

The patient's initial treatment should include antitetanus prophylaxis, 600 mg of penicillin by intravenous administration every 6 hours for 2 to 3 days, and 400 mg of ibuprofen by mouth every 6 hours (45). Pain management should be accomplished by using opiates that are appropriate to the case. Frostbite injury itself usually does not demand intravenous fluid resuscitation. Intravenous fluid may be required to treat associated conditions, such as dehydration and, occasionally, rhabdomyolysis, which results in possible renal failure. All organ systems should be monitored and treated in accordance with the individual's general medical condition.

Operative Intervention

It is difficult to determine viable from nonviable tissue in the early stages of superficial and deep frostbite injury. The only absolute indication for early débridement is uncontrollable infection (2). White or clear blisters suggest superficial frostbite injury and require débriding to prevent further contact with the high levels of prostaglandins and thromboxane in the blister exudates (26). The blisters are "unroofed," and topical aloe vera is applied to the affected area (45). Aloe vera has been shown to be an effective thromboxane inhibitor and results in less tissue loss when it is added to the protocol that is outlined here (46). Hemorrhagic blisters are representative of structural injury to the dermal plexus (21). There is controversy over whether to drain or débride these blisters (46). Wound care includes wrapping the affected extremity in sterile dressings and splinting the extremity in a functional position. Fingers should be splinted in the intrinsic plus position to prevent late deformities that are secondary to intrinsic muscle contracture.

Mummification and black eschar occur at approximately 3 to 6 weeks postinjury (17). Amputation is generally deferred for 6 to 8 weeks. At this time, the affected extremity often appears to be *autoamputating*, and a clear line of demarcation occurs. The adage "freeze in January, amputate in July" is often used because of the time that it takes for clear demarcation (47). Amputation that is performed at the time of mummification is usually done in the operating room, initially without the use of a tourniquet. The lack of tourniquet enables the surgeon to determine the level of viable tissue during surgery. Tissue is removed to the extent that the tissue edges exhibit capillary bleeding or when viable muscle contraction is observed, or both. The key to success is to remember that amputation levels should be conservative, because any remaining hyperemic tissues tend to heal quickly (42). Skin grafts, local flaps, and free tissue transfers have been used for wound coverage and in an effort to preserve extremity function.

Adjunctive Therapies

A number of adjunctive therapies have been studied in an attempt to reduce the amount of cellular ischemia that is seen in frostbite. One focus to limit ischemia is by preventing thrombosis. Weatherly-White et al. (48) reported that tissue loss was reduced compared to control rabbits after the administration of dextran.

Anticoagulation with heparin and dextran has been suggested as a method to improve tissue perfusion and survival (48–50). Investigative studies that have used anticoagulants have thus far been inconclusive in their influence on the degree of tissue loss (51).

Injection of vasodilators has been used as a method to improve tissue vascular supply (52,53). The use of many different vasodilators in combination with anticoagulants has failed to exhibit improved tissue survival compared to rapid rewarming alone.

Studies continue to demonstrate that thrombolysis is a key element in the recognition of the progression of frostbite injury. The use of thrombolytic agents, such as streptokinase, tissue plasminogen factor, and urokinase, has been investigated and suggests a beneficial role in frostbite treatment (54–56).

Surgical sympathectomy has been used as a method to treat frostbite. There is evidence that edema pain resolution, return of sensation, demarcation, and healing of ulcers occurs more rapidly after surgical sympathectomy (57–59). However, it has not been shown that sympathectomy decreases the amount of tissue loss after frostbite injury.

Hyperbaric oxygen therapy's role in the treatment of frostbite remains unclear. It is a theoretically attractive modality because of its ability to deliver increased dissolved oxygen to the plasma and tissues (60,61). Hyperbaric oxygen therapy has been associated with acceleration of capillary formation (62) and improved white cell function (63). However, its clinical efficacy remains in conflict, but no deleterious effect has been reported in the treatment of frostbite (21).

ALGORITHM FOR TREATMENT

The author's preferred treatment protocol is presented in Table 1.

COMPLICATIONS OF FROSTBITE

Early common complications of frostbite injury are infection and gangrene. Frequent late sequelae after frostbite are

TABLE 1. AUTHOR'S PREFERRED TREATMENT PROTOCOL FOR FROSTBITE

Rapidly rewarm extremity in whirlpool bath.
  Temperature: 40–42°C, 104–108°F.
  Duration: 15–30 min or until thawed.
  Repeat whirlpool daily.
Initiate pain management therapy.
Blisters.
  Clear: Débride.
  Dark: Leave intact.
  Culture wounds, then apply aloe vera, sterile dressing, and a
    splint in a functional position, and elevate.
Tetanus prophylaxis.
Ibuprofen, 400 mg by mouth every 12 h.
Penicillin G, 500,000 U by i.v. administration q6h for 3 d.
No tobacco products.
If at altitude, daily hyperbaric oxygen therapy.
  1 h q6h for 3 d.
Débride or amputate, if the necrotic area becomes infected.
  Otherwise, observe for a definitive margin of demarcation.

Adapted from McCauley RL, Hing DN, Robson MC, et al. Frostbite injuries: a rational approach based on the pathophysiology. *J Trauma* 1983;23:143–147.

residual pain and cold intolerance of the affected site (17). Less common complications include hyperhidrosis, pigment changes, and skin atrophy (64). Localized osteoporosis and pronounced subchondral bone loss have been reported as early as 4 weeks postinjury and as late as several months later (65). Physeal injury with subsequent growth disturbance has been observed in children (33,34,66,67). Long-term complications that involve joints and soft tissue injury result in a deforming joint contracture and, occasionally, spontaneous fusion. These may occur as late as 16 months after the initial insults.

REFERENCES

1. Su CW, Lohman R, Gottlieb LJ. Frostbite of the upper extremity. *Hand Clin* 2000;16:235–247.
2. Vogel JE, Dellon AL. Frostbite injuries of the hand. *Clin Plast Surg* 1989;16;565–576.
3. Danielsson U. Wind chill and the risk of tissue freezing. *J Appl Physiol* 1996;81:2666–2673.
4. Schechter DC, Sarot RA. Historical accounts of injuries due to cold. *Surgery* 1968;63:527–535.
5. Ward M. Frostbite. *BMJ* 1974;1:67–70.
6. Dembert ML, Dean LM, Nodden EM. Cold weather morbidity among US Navy and Marine Corps personnel. *Milit Med* 1981;146:771–775.
7. Valnicek SM, Chasmar LR, Clapson JB. Frostbite in the prairies: a 12-year review. *Plast Reconstr Surg* 1993;92:633–641.
8. Candler WH, Ivey H. Cold-weather injuries among U.S. soldiers in Alaska: a 5-year review. *Milit Med* 1997;162:788–791.
9. Cattermole TJ. The epidemiology of cold injury in Antarctica. *Aviat Space Environ Med* 1999;70:135–140.
10. Boswick JA, Thompson JD, Jonas RA. The epidemiology of cold injury. *Surg Gynecol Obstet* 1979;149:326–332.
11. Lapp NL, Juergens JL. Frostbite. *Mayo Clin Proc* 1965;40:932–948.
12. Flatt AE. Frostbite of the extremities: a review of current therapy. *J Iowa Med Soc* 1962;52:53–55.
13. Wegener EE, Barraza KR, Das SK. Severe frostbite caused by Freon gas. *South Med J* 1991;84:1143–1146.
14. Thatcher J. *Military journal during the American revolutionary war from 1776 to 1783.* Boston: Richardson and Lord, 1923.
15. Larrey DJ. *Memoirs of military surgery,* vol 2. Baltimore: Joseph Cushing, 1814.
16. Welch GS, Gormley PJ. Frostbite of the hands. *Hand* 1974;6:33–39.
17. Orr KD, Fainer DC. Cold injuries in Korea during winter of 1950–1951. *Medicine* 1952;31:177–220.
18. Jacob JR, Weisman JH, Rosenblatt SI. Chronic pernio. A historical perspective of cold-induced vascular disease. *Arch Intern Med* 1986;146;1589–1592.
19. Purdue GF, Hunt JL. Cold injury: a collective review. *J Burn Care Rehabil* 1986;7:331–342.
20. Granberg DO. Freezing cold injury. *Arctic Med Res* 1991;50[Suppl 6]:76–79.
21. Murphy JV, Banwell PE, Roberts AH, et al. Frostbite: pathogenesis and treatment. *J Trauma Inj Infect Crit Care* 2000;48:171–178.
22. Ervasti E. Frostbites of the extremities and their sequelae. *Acta Chir Scand* 1962;299:7.
23. Mills WJ, Whaley R, Fish W. Frostbite: experience with rapid rewarming and ultrasonic therapy. *Ala Med* 1960;2:1–3, 114–122.
24. Lewis T. Observations upon the reaction of vessels of human skin to cold. *Heart* 1930;15:177–208.
25. Washburn B. Frostbite. *N Engl J Med* 1962;266:974–989.
26. Robson MC, Heggers JP. Evaluation of frostbite blister fluid as a clue to pathogenesis. *J Hand Surg* 1981;6:43–47.
27. Back N, Jainchill M, Wilkens HJ, et al. Effect of inhibitors of plasmin, kallikrein and kinin on mortality from scalding in mice. *Med Pharmacol Exp Int J Exp Med* 1966;15:597–602.
28. Ozyazgan I, Tercan M, Melli M, et al. Eicosanoids and tissue inflammatory cells in frostbitten tissue: prostacyclin, thromboxane, polymorphonuclear leukocytes, and mast cells. *Plast Reconstr Surg* 1998;101:1881–1886.
29. Marzella L, Jesudass RR, Marson PN, et al. Morphologic characterization of acute injury to vascular endothelium of skin after frostbite. *Plast Reconstr Surg* 1989;83:67–75.
30. Zook N, Hussmann J, Brown R, et al. Microcirculatory studies of frostbite injury. *Ann Plast Surg* 1989;40:246–253.
31. Meryman HT. Mechanics of freezing in living cells and tissues. *Science* 1956;124:515–521.
32. McKinley Health Center. Frostbite. Available at: http://www.mckinley.uiuc.edu. Accessed February 17, 2002.
33. Bigelow DR, Ritchie GW. The effects of frostbite in childhood. *J Bone Joint Surg* 1963;45:122–131.
34. Dreyfuss JR, Glimcher MJ. Epiphyseal injury following frostbite. *N Engl J Med* 1955;253:1065–1068.
35. Sumner DS, Boswick JA, Criblez T, et al. Prediction of tissue loss in human frostbite with xenon-133. *Surgery* 1971;69:899–903.

36. Gralino BJ, Porter JM, Rosch J. Angiography in the diagnosis of therapy and frostbite. *Radiology* 1976;119:301–305.

37. Erikson U, Ponten B. The possible value of arteriography supplemented by a vasodilator agent in the early assessment of tissue viability in frostbite. *Injury* 1974;6:150–153.

38. Rakower SR, Shahgoli S, Wong SL. Doppler ultrasound and digital plethysmography to determine the need for sympathetic blockade after frostbite. *J Trauma Inj Infect Crit Care* 1978;18:713–718.

39. Greenwald D, Cooper B, Gottlieb L. An algorithm for early aggressive treatment of frostbite with limb salvage directed by triple-phase scanning. *Plast Reconstr Surg* 1997;102:1069–1074.

40. Mehta RC, Wilson MA. Frostbite injury: prediction of tissue viability with triple-phase bone scanning. *Radiology* 1989;170:511–514.

41. Barker JR, Haws MJ, Brown RE, et al. Magnetic resonance imaging of severe frostbite injuries. *Ann Plast Surg* 1997;38:275–279.

42. McAdams TR, Swenson DR, Miller RA. Frostbite: an orthopedic perspective. *Am J Orthop* 1999;28:21–26.

43. Mills WJ. Comments on this issue of Alaska medicine—from then (1960) until now (1993). *Ala Med* 1993;35:70–87.

44. Entin MA, Baxter H. The influence of rapid re-warming on frostbite in experimental animals. *Plast Reconstr Surg* 1952;9:511–515.

45. McCauley RL, Hing DN, Robson MC, et al. Frostbite injuries: a rational approach based on the pathophysiology. *J Trauma* 1983;23:143–147.

46. Heggers JP, Robson MC, Manavalen K, et al. Experimental and clinical observations on frostbite. *Ann Emerg Med* 1987;16:1056–1062.

47. Britt LD, Dascombe WH, Rodriguez A. New horizons in management of hypothermia and frostbite injury. *Surg Clin North Am* 1991;71:345–370.

48. Weatherly-White RC, Paton BC, Sjostrom B. Experimental study in cold injury: III. Observations on the treatment of frostbite. *Plast Reconstr Surg* 1965;36:10–18.

49. Mundth ED, Long DM, Brown RB. Treatment of experimental frostbite with low-molecular-weight dextran. *J Trauma* 1964;4:246–257.

50. Lange K, Weiner D, Boyd LJ. Frostbite: physiology, pathology and therapy. *N Engl J Med* 1947;237:383–389.

51. Lazarus HM, Hutto W. Electronic burns and frostbite: patterns of vascular injury. *J Trauma* 1982;22:581–585.

52. Porter JM. Intra-arterial sympathetic blockade in the treatment of clinical frostbite. *Am J Surg* 1976;132:625–630.

53. Snider RL, Porter JM. Treatment of experimental frostbite with intra-arterial sympathetic blocking drugs. *Surgery* 1975;77:557–651.

54. Salimi Z, Wolverson MK, Herbold DR, et al. Treatment of frostbite with streptokinase: an experimental study in rabbits. *AJR Am J Roentgenol* 1987;149:773–776.

55. Skolnick AA. Early data suggest clot-dissolving drugs may help save frostbitten limbs from amputation. *JAMA* 1992;267:2008–2010.

56. Zdeblick TA, Field GA, Shaffer JW. Treatment of experimental frostbite with urokinase. *J Hand Surg* 1988;13:948–953.

57. Golding MR, DeJong MR, Sawyer PN, et al. Protection from early and late sequelae of frostbite by regional sympathectomy: mechanism of "cold sensitivity" following frostbite. *Surgery* 1963;53:303–308.

58. Kyosola K. Clinical experiences in the management of cold injuries: a study of 110 cases. *J Trauma* 1974;14:32–36.

59. Schumacker HB. Sympathectomy in the treatment of frostbite. *Surg Gynecol Obstet* 1951;93:727–734.

60. Bassett BE, Bennett PB. Introduction to the physical and physiological basis of hyperbaric therapy. In: Hunt TK, Davis JC, ed. *Hyperbaric oxygen therapy.* Bethesda, MD: Undersea Medical Society Inc, 1977:11–24.

61. Wells CH, Hart GB. Tissue gas measurements during hyperbaric oxygen exposure. In: Smith G, ed. Proceedings of the sixth international congress on hyperbaric medicine. Aberdeen, Scotland: Aberdeen University Press, 1977:118–124.

62. Hunt TK, Zederfeldt B, Goldstick TK. Oxygen and healing. *Am J Surg* 1969;118:521–525.

63. Mader JT. Phagocytic killing and hyperbaric oxygen: antibacterial mechanisms. *HBO Review* 1981;2:37–49.

64. Suri ML, Vijayan GP, Puri HC, et al. Neurological manifestations of frostbite. *Indian J Med Res* 1978;67:292–299.

65. Tishler JM. The soft-tissue and bone changes in frostbite injuries. *Radiology* 1972;102:511–513.

66. Hakstian RW. Cold-induced digital epiphyseal necrosis in children. *Can J Surg* 1972;53:303–308.

67. Selke AC. Destruction of phalangeal epiphyses by frostbite. *Radiology* 1969;93:859–860.

63

DUPUYTREN'S CONTRACTURE

JENNIFER MORIATIS WOLF

PATHOPHYSIOLOGY

Dupuytren's contracture is characterized by the development of contracture due to the formation of nodules and cords in the hand and fingers. The nodules represent sites of active contraction of tissues. The cords are made up of normal fascia that connect the nodules to the skin and other tissues.

The origin of the abnormal tissue of Dupuytren's contracture remains unknown. Normal palmar fascia is composed of primarily type I collagen, with a small amount of type III collagen. Bazin et al. (2) studied the abnormally thickened palmar fascia in Dupuytren's contracture patients and found that the ratio of type III collagen to type I collagen is increased in patients with Dupuytren's contracture. The basic cell type in Dupuytren's contracture is the myofibroblast (3). This cell, which shares the characteristics of fibroblasts as well as smooth muscle cells, is the active cell type in the production of abnormally thickened tissues.

On the molecular level, components of the extracellular matrix are postulated to have an effect on myofibroblasts. Prostaglandin $F_2\alpha$ and lysophosphatidic acid have been shown to increase myofibroblast contraction, whereas prostaglandin E_1 and $E_2\alpha$, as well as calcium channel blockers, cause relaxation of myofibroblasts (4). There is some theoretical evidence that Dupuytren's contracture fibroblasts are more sensitive to growth factors, such as basic fibroblast growth factor and platelet-derived growth factor (5).

History

Dupuytren's contracture is a disease of the palmar fascia that causes thickening of the soft tissues and joint contracture of the hand. Felix Platter of Basel, Switzerland, first described this entity in 1614. Platter postulated that contracture of the ring and small fingers was due to flexor tendon shortening. In 1777, Henry Cline of London dissected two cadaveric hands with this disease. He noted that the palmar fascia was the cause of the contractures and proposed fasciotomy as the treatment (1).

Baron Guillaume Dupuytren was a well-known physician and lecturer in France in the early 1800s. It is thought that his name was given to this disease of palmar fascia because of his extensive lectures on the subject. Dupuytren demonstrated a fasciotomy, by using a transverse palmar incision, to treat a patient with contractures (1).

Clinical Presentation and Natural History

Dupuytren's contracture is diagnosed by nodular thickening of the palm with associated progressive contracture of the metacarpophalangeal (MCP) and proximal interphalangeal (PIP) joints (Fig. 1). The ulnar side of the hand is most commonly involved, with contractures of the small finger being most common (6). This is a disease of middle age, most commonly presenting in adult men who are between 40 and 60 years of age.

Genetics

The overall incidence of Dupuytren's contracture has shown geographic variation. Studies in Norway and Britain have shown a prevalence of Dupuytren's contracture that is between 16% and 28% in men who are older than 65 years of age (7,8). A study by Egawa et al. (9) in Japan of a sample size of more than 6,000 subjects showed a similar prevalence but less severity of the disease, which may indicate a different phenotype of disease. A recent study compared the prevalence of Dupuytren's contracture in Norwegians to that in the Sami (Lapp) aboriginal population, an ethnically distinct group that lives in the far north of Norway. There was a lower prevalence of Dupuytren's contracture in all age groups in the Sami population, although the difference was not statistically significant (10). A study performed with U.S. Veterans Affairs patients showed that of 9,938 patients with Dupuytren's contracture, 9,071 were white, 412 were African American, 234 were Hispanic, 11 were Native American, and 8 were Asian, with 202 of unknown background (11). These studies support the commonly held view that the prevalence of Dupuytren's contracture is highest in persons of northern European descent.

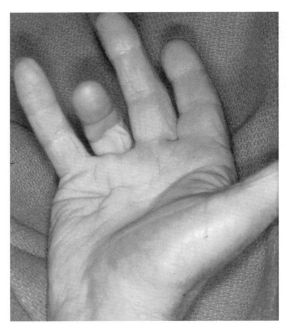

FIGURE 1. Clinical appearance of palmar Dupuytren's contracture.

Gender Distribution

Dupuytren's contracture is seen predominantly in men, with a reported male to female ratio of almost 6:1 (12). Zemel (13) reported a higher recurrence rate and greater risk of a flare reaction to surgery in women. However, a study by Wilbrand et al. (12) disputed the issue of recurrence, showing that 18% of women, compared to 24% of men, went on to a second surgery for Dupuytren's contracture. Sennwald (14) reported that 40% of women developed reflex sympathetic dystrophy as a complication of surgery for Dupuytren's contracture, compared to 15% of men. The authors recommended the use of sympathetic blockade intraoperatively in women to prevent this complication.

Genetic Inheritance

A genetic influence in Dupuytren's contracture is evident from the multiple reports of its occurrence in family clusters. However, investigation of the details of genetic transmittal of Dupuytren's contracture has shown mixed results. Twin studies have shown conflicting data. Lyall's report (15) in 1993 noted that previous literature reported Dupuytren's contracture in both persons of multiple twin pairs. Lyall described two sets of identical twins with one of each twin pair affected and the other examined with no evidence of contracture.

Ling's study (16) from 1963 provides compelling evidence of the inheritance of Dupuytren's contracture. The author examined the relatives of Dupuytren's contracture patients and noted that 34 of 50 patients in Scotland had affected relatives. Eight hundred thirty-two relatives were then examined; 101 persons, or 12%, were determined to

have Dupuytren's contracture. Pedigree studies reported by Matthews (17) showed evidence of autosomal-dominant inheritance with incomplete penetrance, in a cluster with a high rate of female involvement.

Dupuytren's Diathesis

Dupuytren's diathesis, a term that was coined by Hueston, describes a more severe form of Dupuytren's contracture, which is characterized by a younger age at onset, bilateral involvement, a strong family history of Dupuytren's contracture, and rapidly progressing disease. Patients with a strong Dupuytren's diathesis are noted to have ectopic lesions, including plantar fibromatosis (Lederhosen disease), penile fascial thickening (Peyronie's disease), and thickened knuckle pads (Garrod's disease). Hueston (18) noted a higher rate of recurrence and extension in his series of patients.

SURGICAL ANATOMY

Normal and Pathologic Anatomy

The palmar and digital fascia are the tissues that are involved by Dupuytren's contracture. The fibers that make up the palmar aponeurosis run in longitudinal, transverse, and vertical axes to the plane of the palm (19). The longitudinal fibers, which originate from the tendon of the palmaris longus, are most predominantly involved in Dupuytren's contracture. These fibers split into the pretendinous bands that go to each digit (20).

In the distal palm, the longitudinal palmar aponeurosis divides into three layers: superficial, intermediate, and deep. The superficial layer inserts into the dermis distal to the level of the MCP joint and can be involved by nodules that cause pitting of the skin. The intermediate layer passes deep to the natatory ligament and neurovascular bundles to insert into the longitudinal fibers of the finger, which are known as the *lateral digital sheet* (21). Involvement of these bands leads to the formation of a spiral cord (Fig. 2). The deep layer passes on the side of the flexor tendon sheath and inserts near the extensor tendon (22).

The transverse fibers of the palmar fascia include the natatory ligament, which runs across the base of the digits and has attachments to the overlying skin as well as deeper structures, and the transverse ligament of the palmar aponeurosis. The vertical fibers connect the palmar fascia to the dermis and insert into the volar plates of the MCP joints. The septa of Legueu and Juvara form fibroosseous compartments as part of the vertical fibers (23).

In Dupuytren's contracture, nodules and cords make up the pathologic anatomy that involve changes in normal structures (19). In the palm, the pretendinous cords develop from the pretendinous bands and cause MCP

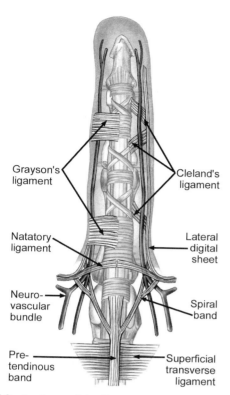

FIGURE 2. Anatomy of the ligaments and bands in the digit.

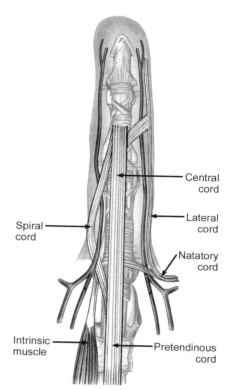

FIGURE 3. Anatomy of the pathologic cords of Dupuytren's contracture.

joint flexion posture (22). In the transition between palm and digit (called the *palmodigital fascia*), the spiral cord develops as an abnormal thickening of the pretendinous band distally as it blends into the spiral band, running deep and then lateral to the neurovascular bundle. This complex then inserts into the lateral digital sheet and then into Grayson's ligament. As the cord tightens, it tends to displace the nerve and artery more superficially and toward the midline (Fig. 3). The natatory cord arises from the natatory ligament (22).

In the digit, central, lateral, digital, and retrovascular cords can be identified. Central cords lie in the midline and generally do not affect the course of the neurovascular bundles. Central cords involve the superficial fascia and often attach to the dermis. The lateral cord represents the diseased lateral digital sheet, originating at the natatory ligament, and generally does not cause PIP joint contracture, except when the cord attaches to the abductor digiti minimi (ADM) cord in the small finger (24). This ADM cord is known as the digital cord, which generally originates at the ADM tendon and lies superficial to the neurovascular bundle. The digital cord has a variable insertion in the middle phalanx or on the distal phalanx, causing PIP or DIP joint contracture, respectively (25). Finally, the retrovascular cord was described by McFarlane (26) as a structure arising from the retrovascular band and running deep to the neurovascular bundle.

ETIOLOGY

An association between Dupuytren's contracture and various diseases or other factors has been postulated. Diabetes, alcohol abuse, smoking, seizure disorders, and heavy manual labor have all been reported as risk factors for the development of Dupuytren's contracture (Table 1). Arkkila et al. (27) studied a group of young type 1 diabetics and noted that the incidence of newly diagnosed Dupuytren's contracture was 2% a year, which correlated significantly with increasing age and duration of diabetes. Another study of a diabetic population revealed a significantly higher prevalence of Dupuytren's contracture, limited joint motion, carpal tunnel syndrome, and tenosynovitis when compared to a nondiabetic control group, which possibly indicates that abnormalities in the soft tissues of diabetic patients predispose them to these entities (28).

An association between Dupuytren's contracture and the amount of alcohol intake has been described in many studies.

TABLE 1. PROPOSED ETIOLOGIES OF DUPUYTREN'S CONTRACTURE

Tobacco use	Epilepsy and antiepileptic drugs
Alcohol use and abuse	Manual labor
Diabetes mellitus	

The investigation by Burge et al. (29) of patients who underwent surgery for contracture showed that the relative risk of developing Dupuytren's contracture in heavy drinkers (at least 21 units of alcohol a week) was approximately twice that of a control group. However, the Reykjavik study investigators analyzed a group of 193 self-reporting Icelandic men and demonstrated no difference between those with Dupuytren's contracture and those without the disease, in terms of alcoholism or alcohol intake (30). Due to the difficulty in quantifying alcohol consumption over time, the classic correlation between alcohol use and Dupuytren's contracture has been based on anecdotal evidence and has not been proven definitively.

Tobacco use has also been implicated as a risk factor. The Reykjavik study found a significant correlation between smoking and Dupuytren's contracture in a large population sample in Iceland (31). Similarly, the study by Burge et al. (29) showed an almost three times greater relative risk for the development of Dupuytren's contracture in smokers, as compared to nontobacco users.

The association between epilepsy and Dupuytren's contracture was described by Lund (32), who noted a high incidence of Dupuytren's contracture in patients with seizure disorders. Later literature suggested that the effect was mediated by antiepileptic drugs that were taken over a period of time (33). Arafa et al. (34) compared two groups of epileptics with a control group of nonepileptics and found a 38% incidence of Dupuytren's contracture in one group of epileptics, compared to 12% in the control group. There was a trend toward significance in the amount of antiepileptic drugs that were taken by those with Dupuytren's contracture compared to those without Dupuytren's contracture.

Finally, the association between heavy labor and trauma to the hand and Dupuytren's contracture has been fairly controversial. The pathophysiologic explanation is that microtrauma to the palmar fascia stimulates the differentiation of fibroblasts to myofibroblasts and begins the nodular formation of Dupuytren's contracture (35). Early's study (7) showed no difference in the prevalence of Dupuytren's contracture between manual laborers and office workers. In contrast, the Icelandic population studies have shown a highly significant correlation between manual work and Dupuytren's contracture (31). Other studies have shown an equal incidence of Dupuytren's contracture in manual and nonmanual workers (36) and have noted an absence of the disease in people who apply continued heavy stress to their hands (37).

EVALUATION

History and Physical Examination

The typical patient with Dupuytren's contracture presents with painless thickening or nodularity of the tissues of the palm or finger, with a varying degree of contracture noted.

The differential diagnosis with a presentation of hand nodules includes palmar ganglion cysts, inclusion cysts, rheumatoid nodules, and soft tissue tumors of the hand (38). Joint contractures can be due to stenosing tenosynovitis and tendon injury.

A patient who presents with Dupuytren's contracture should be queried for the presence of risk factors for the disease, including heavy alcohol use, smoking, epilepsy, diabetes, and heavy occupational work. The presence of a family history of disease should also be ascertained. It is important to learn about previous surgery on the extremity and the presence of deposits of thickened skin elsewhere, including the feet and penis.

In examining the extremity, the location and extent of Dupuytren's contracture cords and nodules, as well as precise measurement of the flexion contractures of the MCP and PIP joints, are integral parts of the exam. For longitudinal follow-up, the location of disease should be drawn as a picture in the chart. Most patients are able to flex fully into the palm, but extension contractures should be noted if they are present.

Workup and Imaging Studies

The use of magnetic resonance imaging (MRI) as an imaging modality in Dupuytren's contracture has been described (39). In a recent study, preoperative MRI findings were correlated with intraoperative pathology. The authors showed that cords and nodules had different imaging characteristics based on level of cellularity; cords tended to be hypocellular, whereas nodules were more variable but had higher cellularity characteristics. They postulated that MRI imaging might have prognostic significance in terms of recurrence occurring in more cellular lesion areas.

NONOPERATIVE THERAPY

Options

Dupuytren's contracture is generally observed when patients have nodules without contracture or mild contracture that does not impair hand function significantly. Treatment is generally recommended when patients can no longer place their palm flat on a table surface (the "table-top test") (40), to avoid the complications of treating severe contractures.

Although many nonoperative modalities have been proposed for Dupuytren's contracture, only a few have shown long-term success. Radiotherapy (41,42), dimethylsulfoxasole (42), ultrasound (43), and steroid injection (44) have all been described for treatment, mostly with limited results. Gamma-interferon has shown some preliminary success in decreasing the size of Dupuytren's contracture nodules when injected intralesionally in one study (45).

The use of injected collagenase has shown great promise as a nonoperative therapy for Dupuytren's contracture. Hurst and Badalamente (46) have described the treatment of Dupuytren's cords with associated contractures of the

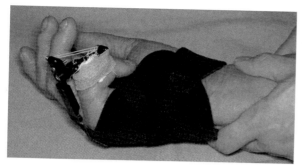

FIGURE 4. Skeletal extension device in place, with traction applied through rubber band tensioning.

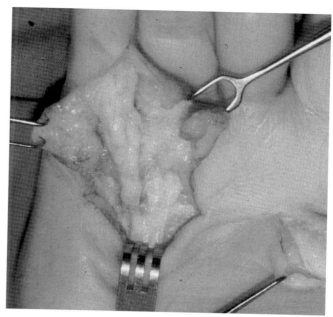

FIGURE 5. Subtotal fasciectomy with exposure of Dupuytren's contracture cord.

MCP and PIP joints with 10,000 units of purified collagenase as an office procedure, which is known as *enzymatic fasciotomy*. The cord is injected and then manually ruptured approximately 18 hours later. A recent study demonstrated maintenance of correction of MCP joint contractures at 0 to 5 degrees at 4 years, with a recurrence rate of 22% (47). PIP contractures showed similar correction at 3.8 years in five of seven patients who were treated, with four patients going on to recurrence (57%). Multicenter clinical trials are currently ongoing.

Finally, a minimally invasive treatment for Dupuytren's contracture uses the technique of skeletal traction for gradual correction of flexion contracture. Messina's TEC (technicadi extensa continua) device (48) used a frame that applied traction through pins in the phalanges to gradually extend the digits. Later devices (49–51) have applied similar principles of gradual elongation of the tissues followed by surgery (46). These devices show promise as an adjunct to other treatments (Fig. 4).

SURGICAL TREATMENT

Surgery is the mainstay of treatment for Dupuytren's contracture. Many surgeons use the table-top test as a guide for patients when advising surgery; when the patient's hand cannot be placed flat on a table, the functional limitations of joint contracture become more significant and warrant surgery. There is no definitive amount of contracture that warrants surgery, although common indices are an MCP contracture of 30 degrees or greater or a PIP contracture of 20 degrees or greater (52).

Options: Incisions

A variety of incisions have been described for the treatment of Dupuytren's contracture. Longitudinal incisions broken up by Z-plasties, Bruner Z-incisions, local rotation flaps, and V-Y plasties have all been demonstrated for extensile exposure of Dupuytren's nodules and cords (6,53). Many surgeons use a combination of these incisions to gain work-able exposure in surgery. The open palm technique, described further in the next section, uses transverse incisions, which are not closed, across the palm (54).

Options: Surgical Approach

The general approach to the surgical treatment of Dupuytren's contracture is fasciectomy or the removal of the diseased fascia. *Radical fasciectomy*, which is defined as the removal of *all* palmar fascia in the effort to prevent future disease recurrence, had early popularity (55) but lost favor owing to patient symptoms of pain with grip and loss of palmar protection (56). Thus, subtotal fasciectomy with removal of as much diseased tissue as possible is common practice (Fig. 5). Moermans (57) described the technique of segmental aponeurectomy or removal of discontinuous portions of diseased tissues through multiple small incisions.

The open palm technique, originally described by McCash (54), uses transverse incisions in the palm that are left open after surgery for healing by secondary intention (Fig. 6). The open incision decreases the flexion force of skin closure, thus allowing full digital extension without tension. The wound is allowed to granulate and generally is closed within 3 to 5 weeks (58).

Dermofasciectomy, or the addition of skin grafting to disease resection, was recommended by several surgeons. Hueston (59) described full-thickness skin grafting to cover skin defects to allow tension-free closure. Donor sites that are used include the groin, forearm, or foot (58,60). The disadvantage of this technique is that immobilization is required until skin graft viability can be evaluated (58).

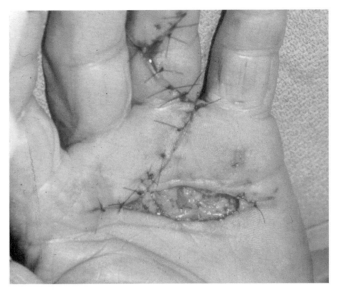

FIGURE 6. Wound closure with the McCash technique of leaving the transverse limbs open.

Surgical Results

In considering the outcomes of surgery, Hunter and Ogdon (61) noted that correction of MCP joint contracture was generally more successful than correction of PIP joint contracture. This observation has been confirmed in the literature. A series by McFarlane and Botz (62) had a recurrence and extension rate of 50% to 60% in a group of 1,074 patients. This large group was comprised of surgical treatment populations that received local fasciotomy, regional fasciectomy, extensive fasciectomy, and dermofasciectomy. Although this mixed-treatment group makes interpretation of these results difficult, McFarlane and Botz identified variables that contributed significantly to recurrence and extension. These included early onset of disease, other areas of involvement, and involvement of three or more rays.

Rodrigo et al. (63) compared the results of fasciotomy to fasciectomy and showed that fasciectomy had a lower rate of recurrence. In 65 hands that were treated with fasciectomy, 63% had recurrence, but only 15% required further surgery, and the gains in extension were durable. In comparison, in 47 hands that had fasciotomy, all had recurrence, and 43% underwent further surgery. Moermans' series (64) of 173 hands that were treated with segmental aponeurectomy showed that 45% had no flexion contracture at the 3-year follow-up. This study noted extension of disease to unoperated areas in 16% and a recurrence of disease in 38%. Most recurrences occurred at the PIP joint. A much lower recurrence rate was found by Jabaley (65), who reported a series of nearly 200 fasciectomies with a recurrence rate of 2% to 3% at 5- to 10-year follow-up.

Lubahn et al. (66) compared the use of the open palm technique to standard closure and noted better total active movement and complication rates in the open palm group. The total active movement improved 17% in the patients who were treated with open palm surgery, in contrast to 10% improvement in those who were closed primarily. There was a 19% complication rate in the standard closure group. Schneider et al. (67) performed a similar review of the open palm method in 49 hands with an average follow-up of 5 years. All open wounds healed at an average of 4 weeks. The recurrence rate was 34%, with a rate of extension of 48%.

Dermofasciectomy was reported to have excellent results by Ketchum et al. (68), who noted that, in 36 hands of 24 patients, there was no recurrence at the 3.9-year average follow-up. Full-thickness grafts were used to cover most of the palm in an effort to decrease extension. The extension rate outside the graft areas was 8% in this study. Brotherston et al. (69) used dermofasciectomy to treat recurrent disease in 46 patients, who similarly showed no recurrence under the graft at an average 8-year follow-up. Residual flexion contracture at the PIP joint was 0 to 15 degrees.

Proximal Interphalangeal Joint

The contracture of the PIP joint presents a particularly difficult problem in Dupuytren's contracture, because the chronicity of flexion deformity often leads to secondary changes in the joint structures. Crowley and Tonkin (70) noted that multiple structures, including skin nodules, tightening of the flexor sheath and shortening of the flexor musculature, volar plate adhesions, and contractures of the collateral ligaments, are contributory in secondary joint contracture. To address contracture at the PIP joint, capsulectomy and release of the volar plate, including pathologic checkrein ligaments, as well as opening the flexor sheath, have been recommended by some authors (70,71). However, Weinzweig et al. (72) found no statistically significant difference in the outcomes of PIP flexion contractures that were treated with standard fasciectomy compared to those treated with capsuloligamentous release combined with fasciectomy.

Breed and Smith (73) reported on 188 PIP joints that were evaluated after standard fasciectomy. In this study, 40% of patients required treatment for residual flexion contracture postoperatively. Patients were treated with gentle passive manipulation followed by splinting and reoperation for joint release or with splinting alone. The best outcome was seen in the group that was treated with gentle passive motion, with improvement of flexion contracture from an average of 88 to 14 degrees.

The use of skeletal traction as a surgical adjunct has been reported to have had good results in the correction of PIP joint contracture. Rajesh et al. (74) focused on 34 patients with PIP flexion contractures that were greater than 70 degrees that were treated with limited palmar fasciotomy and placement of a joint extension device for 6 weeks. Standard fasciectomy was then performed 2 weeks after device removal. At 30-month follow-up, the authors noted a residual PIP flexion contracture that averaged 22 degrees and an average joint correction of 67 degrees. A series by Citron and Messina (50) showed similar improvement after joint extension and fasciectomy, with a 29-degree average contracture at 18 months.

When the PIP contracture does not respond to additional surgical measures, salvage procedures include fusion, PIP joint arthroplasty, and amputation. Moberg (75) recommended that arthrodesis be performed with 25 degrees of flexion to provide optimal function at the PIP joint. PIP joint replacement has been described as a salvage procedure to avoid amputation, which should be considered as end-stage salvage only (76).

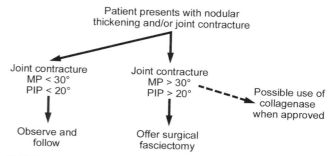

FIGURE 7. Algorithm for evaluation and treatment of Dupuytren's contracture. MP, metacarpophalangeal; PIP, proximal interphalangeal.

Author's Preferred Treatment

The author's preferred surgical treatment of Dupuytren's contracture is a standard open fasciectomy, using a combination of the open palm technique and longitudinal incisions for the digits. General or axillary block anesthetic is used, and an Esmarch bandage is used to exsanguinate the arm. The patient is treated with preoperative antibiotic prophylaxis.

The incisions combine transverse incisions on the palm that are placed at a location at which release of contracted skin and fascia results in the skin being difficult to close. Longitudinal extensions from the palmar incision are placed to resect the diseased fascia from the digit and palm.

The most important surgical principle, to which the author rigidly adheres, is to identify the neurovascular structures in normal tissue and then to follow the nerve and artery into the abnormal fascial tissue. The Dupuytren's contracture–related tissue may extend from the dorsal portion of the flexor sheath, and one must take care to palpate the tissues and skin to resect as much diseased fascia as possible.

The tourniquet is released before closure to inspect the vascularity of the digits. Hemostasis is obtained with cautery, and a Penrose drain is used if the transverse incisions are closed. This is removed in the office the following day, if the procedure was performed on an outpatient basis. The patient is splinted in extension postoperatively and remains in this position until suture removal at 10 days after surgery. At this time, the patient is referred to hand therapy for fabrication of a resting hand-based splint that extends to the fingertips to maintain full extension and that is worn primarily at night. The patient is started on active range-of-motion exercise as the wound tolerates. If the transverse incisions are left open, the patient begins hand therapy earlier for dressing changes, wound monitoring, and range of motion.

A proposed algorithm for the management of Dupuytren's contracture is shown in Figure 7.

Complications

The complications that can occur with surgical treatment of Dupuytren's contracture include nerve injury, vascular injury, postoperative hematoma, Dupuytren's contracture flare or reflex sympathetic dystrophy, and infection. Iatrogenic injury to the neurovascular bundle is one of the most significant complications in Dupuytren's contracture surgery, owing to the proximity of these structures during surgical dissection. The formation of a spiral cord around the nerve and artery can cause displacement of these structures in a more midline, superficial position. The study by Umlas et al. (77) of 66 digits showed that more than one-half of the digits had spiral nerves (a neurovascular structure that is affected by a spiral cord), in contrast to the earlier work of Short and Watson (78), which showed a spiral nerve incidence of only 16% in 276 patients. Both of these studies showed that a PIP flexion contracture was a strong predictor for the presence of a spiral nerve, particularly in association with a soft tissue mass between the distal palmar confluence and proximal digital crease.

Lack of perfusion to a digit after fasciectomy is most commonly due to vasospasm, particularly after correction of severe flexion deformity (79). The other cause is direct vessel laceration. It is imperative to assess the vascularity of the digits by tourniquet release before closure. Vasospasm may be treated with local smooth muscle relaxants (lidocaine or papaverine), which allow the digit to flex, and systemic anticoagulation (79). It is rare that both digital arteries experience injuries, but, if this occurs, repair or interpositional vein grafting is necessary to restore flow to the digit.

Hematoma can cause skin necrosis or loss if it is not recognized and addressed. Meticulous cautery after tourniquet release and the use of suction drains can decrease the risk of blood accumulation in a closed wound. The open palm technique has the advantage of allowing drainage directly into the dressing and has been shown to decrease the incidence of hematoma formation (58).

The Dupuytren's contracture flare reaction and reflex sympathetic dystrophy are part of a spectrum of postoperative pain syndromes that are described as complications of surgical fasciectomy. Flare reaction is an inflammatory state that presents 2 to 3 weeks postoperatively with erythema, pain, stiffness, and hyperesthesia (52). It is postulated that acute carpal tunnel syndrome and flexor tenosynovitis may be contributing factors (79). Early identification of a pain syndrome's evolution is a key part of the treatment. If a specific cause can be localized, prompt treatment, such as carpal tunnel release or first annular pulley release, should be performed. Otherwise, symptomatic therapy to decrease pain and increase motion should be instituted. This includes sympathetic blockade, hand therapy that is focused on stress loading, and oral medications, including corticosteroids and neuroregulatory agents (79).

Finally, infection is a risk in any surgical procedure. In cases that involve Dupuytren's contracture fascial resection, the risk of infection is higher in patients with diabetes mellitus or peripheral vascular disease. Early recognition, prompt treatment with antibiotics, and surgical débridement are the mainstays of therapy for this complication.

Recurrence

Although recurrence of Dupuytren's contracture often complicates the postoperative management of this entity, recurrence is not considered strictly a complication of surgery. Because the goals of surgery are the control of disease and the restoration of hand function, not the complete eradication of abnormal tissue, it is often inevitable that some disease is left behind. Additionally, the genetic influences of Dupuytren's contracture may contribute to reformation of myofibroblastic tissue. The rate of recurrence is reported to range from 0% to 71% in the literature (80,81).

The surgical treatment of recurrent Dupuytren's contracture carries a much higher risk of neurovascular injury and a much lower rate of improvement than primary surgery. A study by Roush and Stern (82) presented the results of surgery on 19 patients with 28 fingers that were operated on for a recurrent contracture. Only 32% of digits had normal sensation, as tested by Semmes-Weinstein monofilaments. Three digits were anesthetic. Only the subgroup that was treated with fasciectomy and local flap had a significant increase in total motion. No vascular injuries, infections, or flap or graft necrosis occurred, and there was a high rate of patient satisfaction.

REFERENCES

1. Elliot D. The early history of Dupuytren's disease. *Hand Clin* 1999;15:1–11.
2. Bazin S, LeLouis M, Duance V, et al. Biochemistry and histology of the connective tissue of Dupuytren's disease lesions. *Eur J Clin Invest* 1980;10:9–16.
3. Tomasek JJ, Vaughan MB, Haaksma CJ. Cellular structure and biology of Dupuytren's disease. *Hand Clin* 1999;15:21–34.
4. Badalamente MA, Hurst LC. The biochemistry of Dupuytren's disease. *Hand Clin* 1999;15:35–45.
5. Alioto RJ, Rosier RN, Burton RI, et al. Comparative effects of growth factors on fibroblasts of Dupuytren's tissue and normal palmar fascia. *J Hand Surg* 1994;19:442–452.
6. McGrouther DA. Dupuytren's contracture. In: Green DP, Hotchkiss RN, Pederson WC, eds. *Green's operative hand surgery*, 4th ed. New York: Churchill Livingstone, 1999:563–591.
7. Early PF. Population studies in Dupuytren's contracture. *J Bone Joint Surg* 1962;44:602–613.
8. Mikkelson OA. Epidemiology in a Norwegian population. In: McFarlane RM, McGrouther DA, Flint MH, eds. *Dupuytren's disease*, 5th ed. Edinburgh: Churchill Livingstone, 1990:191–200.
9. Egawa T, Senrui H, Horiki A, et al. Epidemiology of the Oriental patient. In: McFarlane RM, McGrouther DA, Flint MH, eds. *Dupuytren's disease*, 5th ed. Edinburgh: Churchill Livingstone, 1990:239–245.
10. Finsen V, Dalen H, Nesheim J. The prevalence of Dupuytren's disease among two different ethnic groups in Northern Norway. *J Hand Surg* 2002;27:115–117.
11. Sabobeiro AP, Pokorny JJ, Shehadi SI, et al. Racial distribution of Dupuytren's disease in department of Veterans Affairs patients. *Plast Reconstr Surg* 2000;106:71–75.
12. Wilbrand S, Ekbom A, Gerdin B. The sex ratio and rate of reoperation for Dupuytren's contracture in men and women. *J Hand Surg* 1999;24:456–459.
13. Zemel NP. Dupuytren's contracture in women. *Hand Clin* 1991;7:707–711.
14. Sennwald GR. Fasciectomy for treatment of Dupuytren's disease and early complications. *J Hand Surg* 1990;15:755–761.
15. Lyall HA. Dupuytren's disease in identical twins. *J Hand Surg* 1993;18:368–370.
16. Ling RS. The genetic factor in Dupuytren's disease. *J Bone Joint Surg* 1963;45:709–718.
17. Matthews P. Familial Dupuytren's contracture with predominantly female expression. *Br J Plast Surg* 1979;32:120–123.
18. Hueston JT. Dupuytren diathesis. In: McFarlane RM, McGrouther DA, Flint MH, eds. *Dupuytren's disease*, 5th ed. Edinburgh: Churchill Livingstone, 1990:246–249.
19. McGrouther DA. The microanatomy of Dupuytren's contracture. *Hand* 1982;14:215–236.
20. Holland AJ, McGrouther DA. Dupuytren's disease and the relationship between the transverse and longitudinal fibers of the palmar fascia: a dissection study. *Clin Anat* 1997;10:97–103.
21. Gosset J. Dupuytren's disease and the anatomy of the palmodigital aponeuroses. In: Hueston JT, Tubiana R, eds. *Dupuytren's disease,* 2nd ed. Edinburgh: Churchill Livingstone, 1985:13–26.
22. Rayan GM. Palmar fascial complex anatomy and pathology in Dupuytren's disease. *Hand Clin* 1999;15:73–86.
23. Legueu F, Juvara E. Des aponeurosis de la paume de la main. *Bull Soc Anat Paris Serie* 1892;6:383–400.
24. McGrouther DA. Dupuytren's contracture. In: Green DP, Hotchkiss RN, Pederson WC, eds. *Green's operative hand surgery*, 4th ed. New York: Churchill Livingstone, 1999:563–591.
25. Barton NJ. Dupuytren's disease arising from the abductor digiti minimi. *J Hand Surg* 1984;9:265–270.
26. McFarlane R. The anatomy of Dupuytren's disease. In: Hueston J, Tubiana R, eds. *Dupuytren's disease,* 2nd ed. Edinburgh: Churchill Livingstone, 1985:54–71.

27. Arkkila PE, Kantola IM, Viikari JS, et al. Dupuytren's disease in type I diabetic patients: a five-year prospective study. *Clin Exp Rheum* 1996;14:59–65.

28. Chammas M, Bousquet P, Renard E, et al. Dupuytren's disease, CTS, trigger finger, and diabetes mellitus. *J Hand Surg* 1995;20:109–114.

29. Burge P, Hoy G, Regan P, et al. Smoking, alcohol, and the risk of Dupuytren's contracture. *J Bone Joint Surg* 1997;79:206–210.

30. Gudmundsson KG, Arngrimsson R, Jonsson T. Dupuytren's disease, alcohol consumption, and alcoholism. *Scand J Prim Health Care* 2001;19:186–190.

31. Gudmundsson KG, Armgrimsson R, Sigfusson N, et al. Epidemiology of Dupuytren's disease: clinical, serological, and social assessment. The Reykjavik study. *J Clin Epidemiol* 2001;53:291–296.

32. Lund M. Dupuytren's contracture and epilepsy. *Acta Psych Neurol Scand* 1941;16:465–468.

33. Crutchley EM, Vakil SD, Hayward HW, et al. Dupuytren's disease in epilepsy: result of prolonged administration of anticonvulsants. *J Neurol Neurosurg Psych* 1976;39:498–503.

34. Arafa M, Noble J, Royle SG, et al. Dupuytren's disease and epilepsy revisited. *J Hand Surg* 1991;17:221–224.

35. Skoog T. Dupuytren's contraction. *Acta Chirurgica Scand* 1948;96:109–134.

36. Hueston J. Dupuytren's contracture and occupation. *J Hand Surg* 1987;12:657–658.

37. McFarlane R. Dupuytren's disease: relation to work and injury. *J Hand Surg* 1991;16:775–779.

38. Erdmann MW, Quaba AA, Sommerlad BC. Epithelioid sarcoma masquerading as Dupuytren's disease. *Br J Plast Surg* 1995;48:39–42.

39. Yacoe ME, Bergman AG, Ladd AL, et al. Dupuytren's contracture: MR imaging findings and correlation between MR signal intensity and cellularity of lesions. *AJR Am J Roentgenol* 1993;160:813–817.

40. Leclercq C. Clinical aspects. In: Tubiana R, Leclercq C, Hurst LC, et al., eds. *Dupuytren's disease,* 1st ed. London: Martin Dumitz Ltd., 2000.

41. Keilholz L, Seegerschmiedt M, Sauer R. Radiotherapy for prevention of disease progression in early-stage Dupuytren's contracture: initial and long-term results. *Int J Radiat Oncol Biol Phys* 1996;36:891–897.

42. Weinzierl L, Flugle M, Geldmacher J. Lack of effectiveness of alternative nonsurgical treatment procedures of Dupuytren's contracture. *Chirurg* 1993;64:492–494.

43. Stiles R. Ultrasonic therapy in Dupuytren's contracture. *J Bone Joint Surg* 1966;48:452–454.

44. Ketchum L. Dupuytren's contracture: triamcinolone injection. *Am Soc Surg Hand Newslett* 1983;2.

45. Pittet B, Rubbia-Brandt L, Desmouliere A, et al. Effect of γ-interferon on the clinical and biologic evolution of hypertrophic scars and Dupuytren's disease: an open pilot study. *Plast Reconstr Surg* 1994;93:1224–1235.

46. Hurst LC, Badalamente MA. Non-operative treatment of Dupuytren's disease. *Hand Clin* 1999;15:97–107.

47. Badalamente MA, Hurst LC, Hentz VR. Collagen as a clinical target: nonoperative treatment of Dupuytren's disease. *J Hand Surg* 2002;27:788–798.

48. Messina A, Messina J. The TEC treatment (continuous extension technique) for severe Dupuytren's contracture of the fingers. *Ann Hand Surg* 1991;10:247–250.

49. Hodgkinson P. The use of skeletal traction to correct the flexed PIP joint in Dupuytren's disease. *J Hand Surg* 1994;19:534–537.

50. Citron N, Messina JC. The use of skeletal traction in the treatment of severe primary Dupuytren's disease. *J Bone Joint Surg* 1998;80:126–129.

51. Agee JM. Unstable fracture dislocations of the proximal interphalangeal joint: treatment with the force couple splint. *Clin Orthop* 1987;214:101–112.

52. Saar JD, Grouthaus PC. Dupuytren's disease: an overview. *Plast Reconstr Surg* 2000;106:125–134.

53. King EW, Exeter MH, Bass EM, et al. Treatment of Dupuytren's contracture by extensive fasciectomy through multiple V-Y plast incisions: short-term evaluation of 170 consecutive operations. *J Hand Surg* 1979;4:234–241.

54. McCash CR. The open palm technique in Dupuytren's contracture. *Br J Plast Surg* 1964;17:271–280.

55. McIndoe A, Beare RL. The surgical management of Dupuytren's contracture. *Am J Surg* 1958;95:197–203.

56. Skoog T. The transverse element of the palmar aponeurosis in Dupuytren's contracture. *Scand J Reconstr Surg* 1967;1:51–63.

57. Moermans JP. Segmental aponeurectomy in Dupuytren's disease. *J Hand Surg* 1991;16:243–254.

58. Lubahn JD. Open-palm technique and soft tissue coverage in Dupuytren's disease. *Hand Clin* 1999;15:127–136.

59. Hueston JT. The control of recurrent Dupuytren's contracture by skin replacement. *Br J Plast Surg* 1975;22:152–156.

60. Gonzalez RI. Open fasciotomy and full thickness skin graft in a correction of digital flexion deformity. In: Hueston JT, Tubiana R, eds. *Dupuytren's disease,* 2nd ed. Edinburgh: Churchill Livingstone, 1985:158–163.

61. Hunter JA, Ogdon C. Dupuytren's contracture, II, scanning electron microscope observation. *Br J Plast Surg* 1975;28:19–25.

62. McFarlane RM, Botz JS. The results of treatment. In: McFarlane RM, McGrouther DA, Flint MH, eds. *Dupuytren's disease,* 5th ed. Edinburgh: Churchill Livingstone, 1990:387–412.

63. Rodrigo JJ, Niebauer JJ, Brown RL, et al. Treatment of Dupuytren's contracture. *J Bone Joint Surg* 1976;58:380–387.

64. Moermans JP. Long-term results after segmental aponeurectomy for Dupuytren's disease. *J Hand Surg* 1996;21:797–800.

65. Jabaley ME. Surgical treatment of Dupuytren's disease. *Hand Clin* 1999;15:137–147.

66. Lubahn JD, Lister GD, Wolfe T. Fasciectomy and Dupuytren's disease: a comparison between the open-palm technique and wound closure. *J Hand Surg* 1984;9:53–58.

67. Schneider LH, Hanklin FM, Eisenberg T. Surgery of Dupuytren's disease: a review of the open method. *J Hand Surg* 1986;11:23–27.

68. Ketchum LD, Hixson FP. Dermofasciectomy and full-thickness grafts in the treatment of Dupuytren's contracture. *J Hand Surg* 1987;12:659–664.

69. Brotherston TM, Balakrishnan C, Milner RH, et al. Long term follow-up of dermofasciectomy for Dupuytren's contracture. *Br J Plast Surg* 1994;47:440–443.

70. Crowley B, Tonkin MA. The proximal interphalangeal joint in Dupuytren's disease. *Hand Clin* 1999;15:137–147.

71. Michon J. Operative difficulties and postoperative complications in the surgery of Dupuytren's disease. In: Hueston JT, Tubiana R, eds. *Dupuytren's disease,* 2nd ed. Edinburgh: Churchill Livingstone, 1985:177–183.

72. Weinzweig N, Culver JE, Fleegler EJ. Severe contractures of the proximal interphalangeal joint in Dupuytren's disease: combined fasciectomy with capsuloligamentous release versus fasciectomy alone. *Plast Reconstr Surg* 1996;97:560–566.

73. Breed CM, Smith PJ. A comparison of methods of treatment of PIP joint contractures in Dupuytren's disease. *J Hand Surg* 1996;21:246–251.

74. Rajesh KR, Rex C, Mehdi H, et al. Severe Dupuytren's contracture of the proximal interphalangeal joint: treatment by two stage technique. *J Hand Surg* 2000;25:442–444.

75. Moberg E. Three useful ways to avoid amputation in advanced Dupuytren's contracture. *Orthop Clin North Am* 1973;4:1001–1005.

76. Tonkin MA, Lennon WP. Dermofasciectomy and proximal interphalangeal joint replacement in Dupuytren's disease. *J Hand Surg* 1985;10:351–352.

77. Umlas ME, Bischoff RJ, Gelberman RH. Predictors of neurovascular displacement in hands with Dupuytren's contracture. *J Hand Surg* 1994;19:664–666.

78. Short WH, Watson HK. Prediction of the spiral nerve in Dupuytren's contracture. *J Hand Surg* 1982;7:84–86.

79. Boyer MI, Gelberman RH. Complications of the operative treatment of Dupuytren's disease. *Hand Clin,* 1999;15:161–166.

80. Gordon S. Dupuytren's contracture: recurrence and extension following surgical treatment. *Br J Plast Surg* 1957;51:286–288.

81. Norotte G, Apoil A, Travers V. A ten-year follow-up of the results of surgery for Dupuytren's disease. *Ann Chir Main* 1988;7:277–281.

82. Roush TF, Stern PJ. Results following surgery for recurrent Dupuytren's disease. *J Hand Surg* 2000;25:291–296.

64

FINGERTIP AND NAILBED INJURIES

ADAM B. SHAFRITZ
EDWARD P. HAYES

The fingertip is the most common site of trauma to the hand. The goal of treatment for fingertip injuries is to restore a durable fingertip that is free from pain yet has normal or near-normal sensation and appearance.

SURGICAL ANATOMY AND PHYSIOLOGY OF THE FINGERTIP

Normal

The fingertip is comprised of soft tissue: osseous and specialized nail-supporting and -producing tissues distal to the level of the flexor and extensor tendon insertions (1). The epidermal skin overlying the fingertip pulp is thick with deep papillary ridges and terminates distally as the hyponychium beneath the distal edge of the nail plate. The fingertip pulp is composed of highly vascular fibrofatty tissue stabilized by fibrous septa extending from the dermis to the distal phalanx periosteum (2). In humans, the fingernail protects the fingertip and enhances both dexterity and sensation. The rate of nail growth is more accelerated in the longer fingers and during the warmer months. Nail growth declines with age. The perionychium is composed of the nailbed and the surrounding soft tissue, called the *paronychium* (Fig. 1).

The nailbed histologically has an intimate, convoluted attachment to the periosteum of the distal phalanx, a relationship that resists traumatic nailbed avulsion. The nailbed consists of the germinal and sterile matrices. The germinal matrix lies on the palmar floor of the nail fold and terminates at the distal extent of the lunula. Compared to the remainder of the nailbed, the germinal matrix has enhanced vascularity. By the process of gradient perikaratosis, the germinal matrix produces nearly all (90%) of the nail volume. Germinal matrix cells originate as basilar cells near the periosteum, duplicate, and are driven dorsally in columns toward the nail. Once the cell columns meet the resistance of the nail, the cells flatten and stream distally, effecting longitudinal nail growth. The nailbed and the nail plate are a continuum in all stages of nail production.

The sterile matrix is that portion of the nailbed distal to the lunula and has a variable contribution to nail production. Cells originating from the germinal matrix enlarge, flatten, and elongate. The large cells eventually break down and become incorporated in the nail. At the sterile matrix, the nail is securely anchored to the underlying linear ridges in the squamous epithelium. The nail is less adherent to the germinal matrix.

The paronychium is the lateral border of the nail and the fold of skin that extends over the nail (3). The hyponychium is the junction of the sterile matrix of the nailbed with the fingertip skin. It consists of a keratinous plug with abundant neutrophils and lymphocytes and is an effective barrier of defense in preventing microbial invasion of the subungual area (2). The nail fold is an anatomic transition between the nailbed and the paronychium. The germinal matrix comprises the palmar floor. The portion of the nailbed that imparts nail shine is located on the dorsal roof, opposing the nail plate. This portion of the dorsal nail roof can produce symptomatic spicules of nail if left behind during nail ablation procedures. The most distal and dorsal portion of the nail fold is the eponychium where the nail fold attaches to the surface of the nail. At this junction, a thin veil of tissue, called the *nail vest*, is formed.

In one cadaveric study, the average distance from the terminal extensor tendon origin to the germinal matrix was 1.2 mm (4). The authors concluded that when the extensor tendon insertion is seen during exposure of the distal dorsal finger, care should be taken to avoid injury to the germinal matrix. As a corollary, visualization of the extensor tendon ensures complete excision when ablation of the nailbed is to be performed.

Two dorsal branches from the digital artery nourish the nailbed (5). One branch enters the proximal portion of the nail fold, and another larger branch enters the mid-nailbed and then continues on to the pulp of the finger. There is an abundant network of draining veins proximal to the nail fold. The digital nerve trifurcates just distal to the distal interphalangeal (DIP) joint, with one branch to the nail fold, one to the fingertip, and one to the pulp. The vascular supply to the pulp has been demonstrated by Rose et al. (6). Proximal and distal arches were defined, as was a pulp

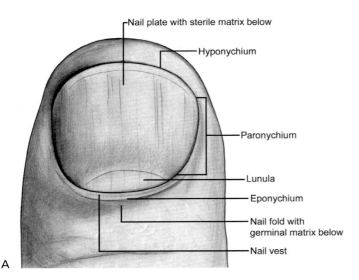

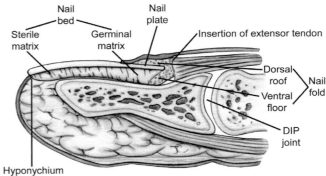

FIGURE 1. A: Topographical view of the fingertip and nailbed. **B:** Cross-sectional view of the fingertip and nailbed. DIP, distal interphalangeal. (Redrawn from Guy RJ. The etiologies and mechanisms of nailbed injuries. *Hand Clin* 1990;6:9–19, with permission.)

artery. Numerous fine capillary communications and venous networks were defined.

Pathologic

A subungual hematoma is the result of some degree of trauma to the nailbed (7). In the event of nailbed injury, primary healing after accurate approximation of the nail matrix is essential for regrowth of a normal-appearing nail (2). Gaps heal by granulation tissue formation, leading to scar and nail deformity or nonadherence. The nail fold, composed of the dorsal roof and the ventral floor, must be maintained by some sort of stent to prevent adherence of the two surfaces by scar tissue. The replaced nail functions best for this purpose. The consequence of nail fold adherence is a split nail or a painful and inflamed nail as the nail cuts through the adhesions.

Distal phalanx fractures usually disrupt the nailbed but may leave the nail plate unaffected (7). A distal phalangeal fracture with palmar angulation combined with a transverse nailbed laceration can deliver the proximal nail plate out of the dorsal nail fold. The Seymour fracture involves a similar nailbed injury occurring with an apex dorsal-angulated Salter-Harris I injury of the distal phalanx (8).

PATHOPHYSIOLOGY OF NAILBED AND FINGERTIP INJURY

Definition and Classification

The various mechanisms of nailbed injuries have led to their classification as simple lacerations, stellate lacerations, severe crush injuries, and avulsions (9). All of these options may or may not also include distal phalangeal fractures and additional soft tissue fingertip injury. A classification of nailbed injuries that assists in treatment decisions and prognosis has been developed (7). Type I injuries involve small (25%) subungual hematomas. Type II injuries have larger (50%) subungual hematomas. Type III injuries are nailbed lacerations with associated distal phalangeal fractures. Nailbed fragmentation is the hallmark of type IV injuries. Type V injuries have nailbed avulsion. For each of these types, there can be further subclassification into whether the injury predominantly involves the sterile or germinal matrix. All of these options may or may not include injury to the paronychium and other fingertip soft tissues.

Incidence of Nailbed and Fingertip Injury

The hand is the most frequently injured body part, and the fingertip is the most commonly involved region of the hand. Nailbed injuries usually require significant force (9). The nailbed is sandwiched between the distal phalanx and the nail plate. A force substantial enough to disrupt one of these structures is usually necessary for a nailbed injury. Blunt impact over a broad area tends to shatter the nailbed into multiple pieces, whereas sharper objects may focus forces enough to cause lacerations. Power equipment, such as saws, lawnmowers, and drills have both crush and laceration components of injury. Abrading tools, such as belts and sanders, produce avulsion injuries. Snowblower injuries occur during an attempt to unclog wet snow manually and frequently affect the dominant hand (10). Multiple digit involvement, amputations, and combined injuries involving bone, fingertip pulp, perionychium, nerves, and tendons are common. Fractures are the most frequent injury, followed by nailbed injuries and amputations.

In a retrospective study of 268 nailbed injuries, most patients were children or young adults (11). Males predominated. Most injuries involved both the nailbed and the fingertip, and half were associated with distal phalangeal fractures. The most common etiologies were door slams or a crush between two objects. Children younger than the age of 4 years are common victims of fingertip and nailbed trauma caused by doors (12). In one large series, 25% of the injuries involved avulsion of the nail from the nailbed or amputation of part of the fingertip, which caused considerable distress to both children and parents.

Evaluation and Management

The evaluation and management of fingertip injuries follow basic surgical principles. A thorough history of the mechanism of injury gives expectations of the degree of soft tissue injury and contamination. The examination often requires some degree of analgesia and removal of the nail plate. Inspection of the neurovascular status of the fingertip and the flexor and extensor tendon function should be performed before administration of local anesthetics. The injury should be thoroughly described and documented with diagrams or photographs. The common incidence of distal phalangeal fractures mandates plain radiographs.

NAILBED INJURIES: NONOPERATIVE TREATMENT

Options and Indications

Nailbed injuries present with, at the very least, a subungual hematoma. In the event of an intact nail plate and nail margin, the pressure of the hematoma can cause marked throbbing pain (7). According to Zook and Brown, a subungual hematoma involving at least 25% to 50% of the nail surface area may represent a significant nailbed injury and warrants removal of the nail plate for nailbed inspection and repair (13). A lesser procedure, trephination of a fingernail and evacuation of the subungual hematoma, can be performed safely with cautery, a heated paper clip, an 18-gauge needle, or an 11-scapel blade (1).

The traditional teaching mandating nailbed exploration and repair has been challenged in a recent prospective study of childhood fingernail crush injuries randomized into operative and nonoperative treatment groups (14). All patients had a subungual hematoma with an intact nail plate and paronychium and no previous nail abnormality. There was no notable difference in outcome between children treated with nailbed repair and those treated conservatively regardless of hematoma size, presence of fracture, injury mechanism, or age. Monetary charges were substantially higher for the operative group. The authors concluded that nail removal and nailbed exploration is not indicated or justified for children with subungual hematoma, an intact nail, and nail margin.

Authors' Preferred Treatment and Techniques

In the case of a small subungual hematoma (less than 50% of the nail surface area), the authors generally reserve treph-

ination for those patients with moderate to severe pain despite analgesics. For a painful subungual hematoma with an intact nail plate and paronychial tissues and no fracture, trephination using an 11-scapel blade or a 16- to 20-gauge hypodermic needle in a twirling fashion is performed to perforate the nail plate over the hematoma. If more than 50% of the nail is undermined by the hematoma and if a high-energy injury mechanism is involved, consider nail plate removal and nailbed exploration and repair. Often, a stellate and displaced nailbed injury is found under these circumstances.

NAILBED INJURIES: SURGICAL MANAGEMENT

Options and Indications

Clear indications for surgical intervention are a nailbed injury with associated displaced distal phalangeal fracture, disruption of the dorsal nail fold or other paronychial tissues, or a disrupted or avulsed nail plate (7).

Results, Review of the Literature, and Factors Affecting Outcome

The standard principles of establishing a sterile surgical field as well as antibiotic and tetanus prophylaxis apply in surgical management of nailbed injuries. For adults, metacarpal block anesthesia is usually adequate. General anesthesia may be required for children. A blood-free field maintained by a digital tourniquet and the use of loupe magnification are essential for good results (1). Lacerations are repaired after removal of the nail plate. The nail plate is usually quite adherent to the sterile matrix. A careful, atraumatic technique helps avoid iatrogenic injury to the nailbed (7). The use of tenotomy scissors has been described for this process, but a Freer elevator or a small hemostat is a gentler and less risky instrument to introduce under the nail plate for exposure of the sterile matrix.

Aggressive irrigation and débridement are to be avoided; all nailbed tissue should be preserved (1). Reduction and internal fixation of a displaced or unstable distal phalanx fracture should proceed first. If fracture fragments are large enough, Kirschner wire fixation can be used (Fig. 2). Usually, a .028- or .035-in. wire will suffice. If possible, avoid transfixing the DIP joint. Care must be taken to avoid iatrogenic nailbed injury by too dorsal placement of the wire. A nondisplaced or highly comminuted fracture may be adequately stabilized with a combination of soft tissue repair and replacement of the nail plate. Using the replaced nail plate as a native splint after nailbed repair is also effective in restoring stability to open epiphyseal fractures of the distal phalanx in children.

Supplemental fixation can also be achieved with a dorsal tension band suture placed after nailbed repair and replace-

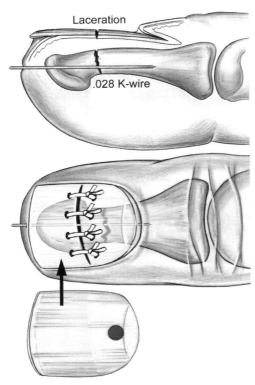

FIGURE 2. Repair of the fingertip and nailbed. The nail plate is gently removed. Unstable fractures of the distal phalanx are reduced and held with a Kirschner wire (K-wire). The nailbed is repaired using fine resorbable suture. Any associated injury to the paronychium and eponychium is also repaired. Pulp injuries are addressed. A drainage hole is placed into the nail plate before reinsertion and fixation with a suture. (Redrawn from Van Beek AL, Kassan MA, Adson MH, et al. Management of acute fingernail injuries. *Hand Clin* 1990;6:23–38, with permission.)

ment of the nail plate (15). The nonabsorbable monofilament suture is placed proximally in a transverse manner superficial to the germinal matrix through the dorsal nail fold and distally in the opposite transverse direction through the fingertip pulp just distal to the nail. The suture forms a figure-of-eight loop crossing dorsally over the replaced nail. The suture is removed at approximately 3 weeks postoperatively.

The best way to achieve a smooth nailbed healed by primary intention is to accurately approximate the edges of lacerations using fine suture (6-0 or 7-0 chromic gut) under magnification (1,2). If the laceration involves the germinal matrix, exposure is obtained by incisions through the dorsal nail fold at perpendicular angles from the eponychial border. These nail fold incisions are also helpful when the proximal nail plate is displaced out of the dorsal nail fold, usually seen with a distal phalangeal fracture or epiphyseal injury and a transverse nailbed laceration. Paronychial lacerations, usually involving the lateral nail folds, should be repaired using 5-0 nylon. Associated injuries of the paronychium and the dorsal nail fold must be meticulously repaired, as they serve as "runners" guiding new nail growth along the appropriate

path. If available, the cleaned nail should be placed over the bed and into the nail fold. This additionally splints fractures, protects soft tissue repairs, provides a template for new nail growth, and prevents adhesion formation between the nailbed and the dorsal nail fold.

Adherent dressings on the raw nailbed are difficult and painful to remove (16). If the nail plate is not available, a silicone sheet or a carefully contoured piece of foil from suture packaging serves the purpose. Replacement of a fractured nail plate repaired with tissue adhesives has also been described (9).

As expected, crush and avulsion injuries, especially those associated with phalangeal fractures, have a worse prognosis than isolated simple and stellate lacerations. Associated injuries to the paronychium and the fingertip pulp also portend a poorer outcome (1). A proximally detached and avulsed germinal matrix is replaced deep to the dorsal nail fold and secured with horizontal mattress sutures tied over the dorsal skin of the nail fold (17). Completely avulsed pieces of sterile or germinal matrix can be sutured into place in the defect directly on the cortex of the distal phalanx. All retrievable pieces of nailbed should be used as grafts, and this includes grafts from unsalvageable digits in severe trauma. In cases of loss of matrix tissue, the nail plate should be inspected for pieces of adherent nailbed. The avulsed tissue can be carefully removed with a scalpel to serve as a graft for repair. When a small fragment of nail plate is adhered to a similar-sized avulsed piece of nailbed, the nail plate along the margins can be trimmed, leaving exposed nailbed, and the composite graft can be sutured to the defect. Shepard reported 85% good results with these techniques of repair of nailbed avulsions (17). The repairs of germinal matrix avulsions were associated with more nail deformity than those of the sterile matrix.

When tissue is not available for repair of defects of the sterile matrix, split thickness nail grafts can be raised from a donor bed (18). The donor site may be from an uninjured portion of the sterile matrix on the affected digit (rarely possible), from an unsalvageable amputated digit, or from the great toe. To avoid a donor site deformity, the graft must be very thin, on the order of seven to ten thousandths of an inch. Expecting some degree of contracture, the graft should be 1 to 2 mm larger than the defect. The longitudinal axis of the graft should be parallel to the defect. The replaced nail plate and an overlying firm dressing are applied. Split-thickness sterile matrix grafts represent a substantial improvement over previous treatments for nailbed tissue loss, including allowing healing with granulation tissue, skin grafts, dermal grafts, reversed dermal grafts, and xenografts.

Loss of the nail plate, nailbed, and periosteum over the exposed distal phalanx can be reconstructed by a split-thickness nailbed graft placed directly on granulating decorticated bone (19). Loss of germinal matrix, provided the defect is not too extensive, can be treated by local rotational or bipedicle flaps (13,17). Local rotation of the full-thickness germinal and sterile matrices on proximally based flaps have been used with success to cover devitalized bone graft to the distal phalanx, a tribute to the robust vascularity of the proximal nailbed. Although the vascular germinal matrix tissues can withstand undermining, they do not advance very far. Larger defects involving greater than one-third of the germinal matrix can be treated with split-thickness germinal matrix grafts from an adjacent area or from the great toe. Split- or full-thickness germinal matrix grafts are not as successful as sterile matrix grafts; both the donor and recipient sites often have some degree of residual deformity. Finally, whole, free, vascularized toenail transfers for reconstruction of congenital and traumatic nailbed defects have been described and, in small series, achieve excellent cosmetic results while maintaining normal hand function (20).

When confronted with loss of dorsal nail fold tissue, the surgeon must remember that the dorsal nail fold has specialized epithelium in direct contact with the nail (1,21). This specialized matrix tissue has some contribution to nail formation and also imparts the shine seen on the nail surface. The contribution of the dorsal nail fold to nail production can sometimes be seen after fingertip amputations when the retained dorsal fold tissues produce painful nail spicules. Reconstruction of tissue loss to the dorsal nail fold is best accomplished with a dorsal rotational skin flap or a reversed cross-finger flap (22). Reconstruction of the specialized matrix of the dorsal nail fold has been successfully achieved using a layer of split-thickness sterile matrix graft sutured to the undersurface of a local rotational skin graft (17).

Authors' Preferred Treatment, Techniques, Surgical Pearls, and Pitfalls

The described principles of nailbed injury care are commonly used in the authors' practices. Careful attention to detail in the treatment of these common injuries is suggested. The majority of these procedures can be performed under digital block anesthesia in a well-equipped procedure room. To decrease the risk of subungual contamination and subsequent infections, including osteomyelitis, the affected digit should have a standard surgical scrub before nail removal or trephination. Twenty-four hours of oral antibiotics is generally recommended, but the benefit of prophylactic antibiotics is not proven under these circumstances.

A frequently seen pitfall is iatrogenic injury to the remaining nailbed by too aggressive and impatient removal of the nail plate. After the nailbed repair, we place a small drainage hole in the replaced nail plate to facilitate drainage of any hematoma. The nail plate is sutured proximally deep to the dorsal nail fold and distally to the fingertip pulp with horizontal mattress nylon sutures. The dorsal tension band suture technique is an effective and minimally invasive means of fixation of associated distal phalangeal fractures. Kirschner wire fixation for very unstable fractures is used. Unless there is special concern about tissue viability or

infection, the operative dressing is generally left in place for 7 to 10 days. Earlier dressing removal is unnecessarily painful and risks avulsion of the replaced nail plate. Long-term follow-up, on the order of 1 year, is needed to adequately assess and learn from the results of treatment of these injuries. The surgical repair is best reflected in the appearance of the resulting nail plate.

Postoperative Rehabilitation

Scar reduction techniques and fingertip desensitization begin roughly 2 weeks from injury, once the wounds have stabilized (7). The replaced nail plate or other stent under the dorsal nail fold will be pushed out by the new nail at 2 to 3 weeks. In the event of no fracture or only a minimal tuft fracture, early range of motion is preferable. Generally, 3 to 4 weeks of protected immobilization of the DIP joint is allowed if there is an unstable distal phalanx fracture. Kirschner wire removal occurs at 4 weeks. A custom fingertip protector can be fashioned to allow early return to work and activities of daily living.

Complications: Etiology, Prevention, Incidence, and Classification

Iatrogenic nailbed deformities have resulted from too vigorous nail plate trephination and removal (9,23). Anatomic repair of a nailbed injury usually results in minimal scar and no significant disruption between the continuum of cells from the nailbed into the nail plate. A wide scar inhibits the cellular continuity over the scarred area and frequently along the entire nailbed distal to the scar. Gaps heal by granulation formation, leading to scar and nail deformity or nonadherence. Distal nonadherence results in loss of the protective hyponychium, leading to the accumulation of foreign material under the nail and predisposing to infection. Proximal nonadherence is even more troublesome, leading to an unstable nail prone to being torn loose. The use of slowly absorbing and large sutures for nailbed repair may cause nail ridging and nonadherence.

Associated distal phalangeal fractures require accurate reduction, as poor alignment of the dorsal cortex leads to nailbed irregularities. Care must also be taken with Kirschner wire placement; superficial wire placement and nailbed injury can lead to longitudinal nail ridging. In the event of distal phalangeal bone loss, care must be taken to ensure adequate distal bone support for the nailbed; otherwise, a hooked or beaked nail can result.

Clinical History, Physical Examination, Office Tests, and Imaging Studies

The distal phalanx must be imaged when faced with nail deformities (24). Nailbed deformities are most often the sequelae of trauma. Malalignment of a distal phalanx fracture or a bone spur commonly leads to nonadherence and other nail deformities. Occasionally, axial cuts of a CT scan through the distal phalanx are beneficial.

Operative Management

Excessive nail matrix scar is the cause of nonadherence. The treatment is excision of the scar (23,24). Closing the defect should not be done under tension and usually necessitates a split-thickness sterile or germinal matrix graft. Malreduced distal phalanx fractures and exostoses commonly lead to nonadherence or ridging of the nail plate. The underlying bone abnormality must be assessed and corrected (Fig. 3).

A longitudinal scar in the germinal or sterile matrices, or both, can cause a split nail plate. The treatment is similar to above with complete excision of the intervening scar (often requiring a microscope) and split-thickness grafting of sterile matrix. More than minimal loss of the germinal matrix requires a local rotational flap, or, more commonly, a germinal matrix graft from the toe. A sterile matrix graft, even if full thickness, will not suffice for a germinal matrix defect.

Adhesions between the dorsal nail fold and the germinal matrix can produce split nails. Reconstructions for loss of tissue or adhesions of the dorsal nail fold must take into account the unique epithelium lining the undersurface of the dorsal nail fold. This tissue assists in nail formation and imparts shine to the nail. Successful reconstructions of split nails have been reported using split-thickness sterile matrix grafts to the undersurface of the dorsal nail fold, coupled with careful postoperative stenting of this space to prevent adhesions.

A crooked nail plate curves to one side during longitudinal growth (24). This is caused by sterile matrix scar contracture on one side. After scar excision, the defect requires a full-thickness nail matrix graft. The use of partial-thickness grafts or allowing healing by secondary intention results in excessive contracture and recurrence of the crooked nail deformity.

The hooked nail can result from congenital deficiency of the fingertip, but it most often is a posttraumatic deformity. The usual cause is insufficient bone support of the sterile matrix. A common error in the treatment of fingertip amputations with an associated nailbed injury is to pull the nailbed tissue distally over the exposed distal phalanx. Prevention is the key. Because the shape of the nail plate follows the contour of the nailbed, the nail plate curves palmarly over the fingertip pulp. Healing by secondary intention can allow for significant contracture of the dorsal soft tissues and draw the nailbed distally. The hooked nail deformity can be avoided by ensuring adequate distal bone support of the nailbed and by avoiding tension in reapproximating the dorsal and palmar soft tissues.

The distal edge of the sterile matrix should be at least 2 mm proximal to the distal extent of the distal phalanx bone stock. Two steps may be necessary to address this problem. First is correction of the mismatch between the distal phalanx and the nailbed. Options include shortening the nailbed, releasing the nailbed and allowing it to retract dorsally, and lengthening or osteotomy of the distal phalanx. After correction of the nailbed-bone relationship, soft tissue coverage for the fingertip is needed. Options include advancement of local tissues, full-thickness skin grafts, and regional or distant flaps (25).

FINGERTIP INJURIES: OVERVIEW

Fingertip injuries can include a wide variety of injuries and can be successfully managed by a spectrum of options from simple nonoperative treatments to rather complicated reconstruction techniques. As summarized by Ma et al. (26), regardless of the treatment option chosen and the experience and/or level of training of the treating surgeon, the results of many treatments yield similar good results. This portion of the chapter focuses primarily on both nonoperative treatments of fingertip injuries with or without associated nailbed injuries and simple operative procedures (flaps) on the fingertip.

For fingertip amputations and injuries, a wide variety of classification schemes exist (27–33). These classification

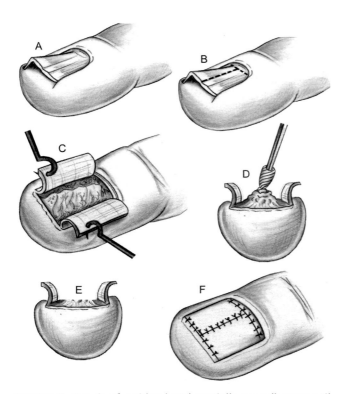

FIGURE 3. Repair of a ridged and partially nonadherent nail. **A:** The sterile matrix is exposed. **B,C:** Scar tissue is excised. **D:** The distal phalanx is recontoured. **E,F:** The sterile matrix is repaired primarily and grafted if necessary. (Redrawn from Shepard GH. Nail grafts for reconstruction. *Hand Clin* 1990;6:79–103, with permission.)

systems are based on amputation level, obliquity, nailbed involvement, and/or bone exposure. A practical simplification divides these injuries into two main categories of amputations and fingertip injuries: those that include skin and/or pulp loss but do not involve exposed bone, and those that involve exposed bone. This simple classification system helps to guide the surgeon's treatment options and decisions, especially if replantation is not considered to be a viable option.

Nonoperative Treatment: Results and Outcome, Review of the Literature, and Factors Affecting Outcome

Options and Indications

Numerous methods have been devised and reported over the years for nonoperative treatment of pulp and skin loss on the tip of the digit. Usually, nonoperative treatment is recommended for injuries that do not involve exposed bone. The simplest method of nonoperative therapy involves simple mechanical débridement followed by the application of an antibiotic ointment to the fingertip, a nonadherent sterile dressing, tube gauze, and fingertip protector cap. Examples of these nonadherent dressings include OpSite (Smith and Nephew), Xeroform (Sherwood Medical), Adaptic (Johnson and Johnson Medical), Vaseline gauze (Sherwood Medical), and Owens (Davis and Geck).

The results of simple open treatment have been reported with the use of an OpSite dressing (34,35). Mennen and Wiese reported on 200 fingertip injuries treated simply with an OpSite over the injured fingertip after local irrigation and débridement (34). The theory behind the treatment protocol is that a semi-occlusive dressing provides a temporary "skin" that would allow for healing of the underlying soft tissues in an optimal environment, thereby promoting earlier granulation tissue formation and epithelialization of the wound. In their study, the authors found that the use of a simple weekly dressing change of an OpSite resulted in near normal pulp shape and useful epithelium of an injured fingertip within a period of 20 to 30 days. They thought that the dressing should not be changed any more frequently than once per week, as this would slow healing. This method was used regardless of whether bone of the distal phalanx was exposed. They had no complications requiring surgery, and no patients developed a significant hook nail deformity. Patients recovered and regenerated a nearly normal pulp with excellent tactile sensation. In a similar study, Williamson et al. reported favorable results using similar materials on 40 patients (36).

Using a different technique, Fox et al. reported on 18 adults treated nonoperatively with a simple wound cleansing followed by coverage with an occlusive dressing made from sterile aluminum foil and gauze (37). Dressing changes were performed on the third, fifth, and seventh day, and then weekly until the wound healed. They reported that although at 2 weeks into the treatment the wound did not appear aesthetically pleasing, healing of the amputated fingertip occurred within 4 weeks, and the resultant fingertip had excellent sensory perception. Normal digital range of motion was noted, and acceptable cosmetic appearance was the rule. They thought that this outcome was satisfactory to all and resulted in less than 10 days lost from work.

A study by Buckley et al. reviewed the results of patients treated conservatively with silver sulfadiazine dressing changes performed on 21 digits, six of which had exposed bone (38). An occlusive dressing of Vaseline gauze with silver sulfadiazine covered by a finger portion of a disposable rubber glove was fashioned. The dressing was changed every other day during the first week and then on an as-needed basis until healed (range, 19 to 90 days). The cases were reviewed at an interval of 2 to 8 years after injury. All of the patients were satisfied with the treatment and the cosmetic appearance. Complications included minor nail abnormalities in 29% of patients, scar tenderness in 19%, and variable degrees of cold intolerance in 38%. Two-point discrimination was normal in all. All preferred the results obtained versus a revision amputation, digital shortening, and primary closure.

Ipsen et al. reported a prospective investigation of 81 consecutive fingertip injuries in which conservative treatment was used (39). The fingertip injuries were defined as greater than or equal to 1 cm × 2 cm in the distal phalanx without any joint or tendon injuries. All of the wounds were cleansed and covered with simple Vaseline gauze. If bone was exposed, 2 to 3 mm of bone was removed with a rongeur, and the wound was dressed in the same manner. Dressings were changed to fresh Vaseline gauze via soaks on day 5 and then weekly until healed. The average healing time was 25 days, with complications of scar tenderness in 26% of patients, cold intolerance in 36%, and nail deformities in 58%. In a similar study, Lamon et al. studied 25 fingertip amputations treated by débridement and application of bacitracin ointment and simple gauze dressings (40). The dressings were changed after 48 hours and then a three-times daily program of warm soaks in mild soapy water for 10 minutes followed by application of bacitracin and gauze dressing was instituted. This regimen was continued until the wound healed. Exposed bone was present in six cases. The average time to healing was 29 days. Those patients who were able to return to work (those who could keep their fingers clean and dry) were able to do so after 24 hours. Three patients had minimal sensory changes, there were no infections, and there were no significant complications reported with the use of this technique.

The use of Mepitel silicone net dressing (SCA Molnlycke Ltd, Bedfordshire, UK) was recently reported by O'Donovan et al. (41). They compared the silicone dressing to traditional dressings used on fingertip injuries in children ages 6 months to 11 years. During the first 3 weeks of dressing changes, the Mepitel net prevented adherence of the wound to the outer dressing and therefore significantly reduced the pain and anxiety suffered by the children associated with wound care. There was no difference in time of wound healing associated with this method when compared to other methods.

The use of chitin as a biologic dressing for fingertip injury has been reported (42,43). Hyphecan artificial skin membrane (Hainan Kangda Marine Biomedical Corp., China) is an occlusive fingertip dressing made of a chitin derivative (1-4,2-acetamide-deoxy-beta-D-glucan) that is extracted from shellfish exoskeleton. It is nonantigenic and thus does not cause systemic allergic reactions. It is semipermeable and maintains a sterile environment without wound dehydration. The protocol for its use requires a simple local irrigation and débridement and application of the Hyphecan cap and sterile gauze over the cap. The cap is not changed. It is slowly cut away as it dries and separates from the wound as it heals. Excellent results have been reported in 276 fingertip injuries treated in such a manner (42,43). No significant complications were reported, and all patients were satisfied with form and function of the injured finger. No revision surgery was needed in any case.

Finally, Ma et al. (26) reported on the treatment of fingertip injuries using a simple dressing, split-thickness skin grafting, full-thickness skin grafting, V-Y advancement flaps (both Kutler and Atasoy), revision amputation and primary closure, and cross-finger flap. In their series of 200 randomized patients, they found little difference in the ultimate results among any of the methods used.

Authors' Preferred Method of Treatment

If nonoperative treatment is going to be accepted by the physician and patient, these injuries are easily treated and serially followed until healing is assured. It is probably not appropriate to elect nonoperative treatment if a skin defect larger than 1 cm × 2 cm is present, and/or if there is exposed bone present. The patient is evaluated in the emergency department or office, and a digital block is used to allow for adequate débridement of the fingertip injury in a painless fashion. After adequate débridement is performed, Bactroban ointment (2% Mupirocin ointment, SmithKline Beecham Pharmaceuticals, Philadelphia, PA) is applied to the wound and covered by Xeroform nonadherent dressing. The finger is then covered with gauze, and a simple fingertip tube–type dressing is applied. A metal cap fingertip protector is placed over the dressing to prevent the patient from inadvertently injuring the finger. This dressing is kept clean and dry until the patient is reevaluated. Mild narcotics and oral antibiotics (cephalexin or clindamycin if patient is allergic to penicillin) are usually prescribed for a short course but have not been shown to affect outcome.

A wound check is performed at 2 or 3 days. The old occlusive dressing can be soaked off in a sterile saline solution. The fingertip is then reevaluated for further demarcation of injury and necrosis. Further débridement may be performed in the office. A repeat application of a similar dressing is then placed, and the patient is examined at weekly intervals with weekly dressing changes. As the wound gradually begins to granulate, the patient can perform dressing changes as necessary at home, unsupervised.

If an adequate débridement cannot be obtained from a single time in the emergency department or office (e.g., if there is grease or other organic matter embedded in the pulp), the patient is referred to the hand therapy unit for sterile whirlpool débridement of the fingertip. This treatment is begun after the patient has been seen for the first follow-up examination and is performed on a daily basis. After each treatment session, the fingertip is dressed with antibiotic ointment, nonadherent dressing, and clean gauze. The patient is reassessed twice weekly until there is evidence of granulation without any evidence of infection. Once this is accomplished, the patient can then be monitored on a weekly basis, and the patient can be instructed on home dressing changes. Depending on size of the involved skin loss and pulp loss, the patient may need to be followed conservatively over 4 to 6 weeks. Many patients need reassurance that the wound will heal and that good results are the rule (Fig. 4).

Surgical Management: Results and Outcome, Review of the Literature, and Factors Affecting Outcome

Options and Indications

If nonoperative therapy is not acceptable to the patient and/or if there is exposed bone with soft tissue and skin loss as well as nailbed injury, then surgical management is considered. Six commonly used methods of acute fingertip reconstruction are reviewed. Four of these procedures can be performed in the emergency department or a well-equipped procedure room. These include the "cap" procedure or composite grafting, the Kutler repair, the Atasoy V-Y advancement flap, and revision amputation and primary closure. The cross-finger flap and thenar flap and its variations are also discussed; however, it is recommended that this operative procedure be performed formally in the operating room. Finally, some special situations and alternative local flaps are reviewed.

"Cap" Technique (Composite Grafting)

The "cap" technique is nonmicrosurgical reattachment of fingertip amputations (6). This method of treatment is effectively used in children and adults who have amputated

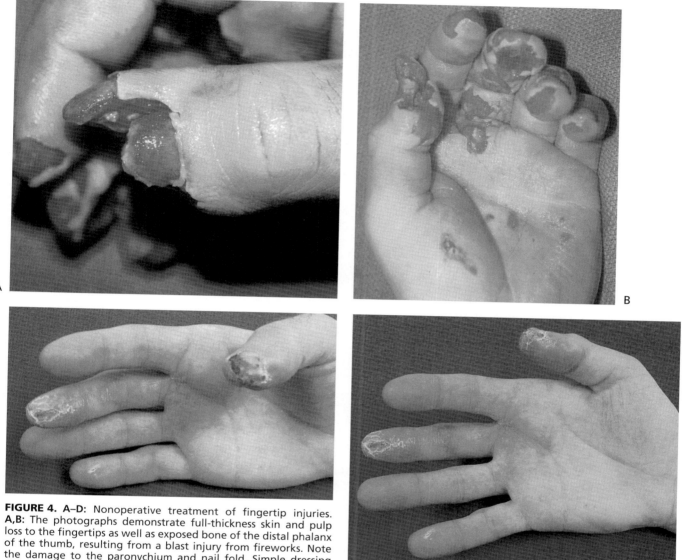

FIGURE 4. A–D: Nonoperative treatment of fingertip injuries. **A,B:** The photographs demonstrate full-thickness skin and pulp loss to the fingertips as well as exposed bone of the distal phalanx of the thumb, resulting from a blast injury from fireworks. Note the damage to the paronychium and nail fold. Simple dressing changes were performed for 2 months. The results at 2 months are shown in panels **C** and **D**.

their fingertip through the mid-level or distal to the nail-bed, either by a guillotine-type amputation or by avulsion. The technique can be performed in the setting of a dirty wound that would not be suitable for formal replantation. The procedure requires the presence of the amputated part for reattachment. For young children, it is recommended to proceed to the operating room so that adequate anesthesia and sedation can be achieved. It is important to explain to family members and the patient (if appropriate age) that this procedure is not a true replantation, rather that it is a way of reattaching the amputated part to form a "biologic dressing" or scab. This procedure allows for granulation tissue to form underneath the amputated part as the body naturally heals the fingertip over time. The patient and/or family members must be informed that the replanted part

will undergo necrosis and desiccation. Eventually, over the course of 4 to 6 weeks, it will form a scab and fall off, leaving behind a well-healed fingertip. This procedure is quite effective at restoring, overall, a normal looking fingertip. However, this fingertip will not be identical to its uninjured counterparts.

Operative Procedure. Composite grafting may be performed in the emergency department or in the operating room with digital anesthesia and the use of a finger tourniquet. After adequate débridement of both the injured finger and the recovered fingertip, the nail plate is removed from the amputated part as well as from the digit. If bone is present in the amputated part, it is cleared using a rongeur or a knife. Excess fat and subcutaneous tissue are removed from the

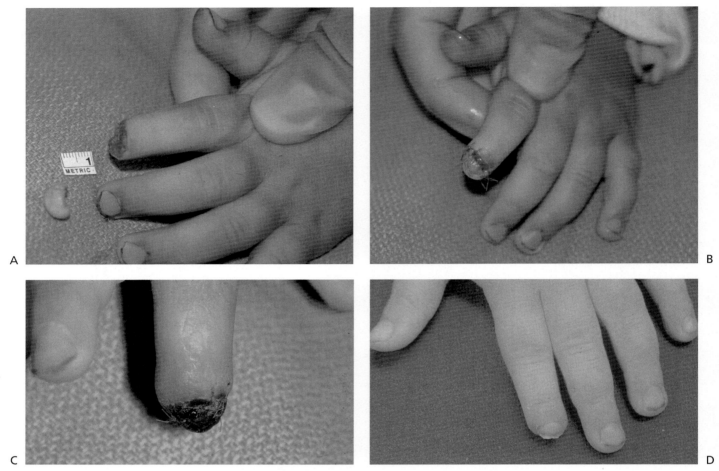

FIGURE 5. **A–D:** Composite grafting ("cap" technique). A 2-year-old boy sustained an amputation through the mid-nailbed **(A)**. The wound was grossly contaminated with grease on presentation. After débridement, the fingertip was reattached **(B)**. It underwent necrosis and desiccation as expected **(C)** and fell off 2 months later. His results at 5 months are shown **(D)**.

amputated part. The skin edges, subcutaneous tissue, and bony end of the finger are débrided. The fingertip and amputated portion are simply sutured using a resorbable stitch such as 6-0 chromic gut (Fig. 5). The nailbed is repaired to itself as well, if possible. Once the portion of the digit has been reattached, sterile dressings are applied after release of the finger tourniquet. Reevaluation occurs at 5 to 7 days.

The results of this technique were evaluated by Rose et al., and they reported on seven adults treated in this manner (6). They found that this procedure was effective at returning the fingertip to a near-normal appearance, that the mean two-point discrimination was 6.5 mm, and though the finger was shortened an average of 6 mm, it did give the illusion of a normal fingertip. There were no infections, and, overall, satisfactory results were the rule.

Atasoy Volar V-Y Advancement Flap

The Atasoy volar V-Y advancement flap has been attributed to Tranquilli-Leali (44) as described in 1935, but gained its commonly used eponym when Atasoy et al. published their

results in 1970 (45). The flap may be used with transverse or dorsal oblique injuries to the fingertip involving both the nailbed and the pulp with exposed bone. It is less useful when a palmar oblique fingertip amputation is encountered. The technique is based on a V-Y full-thickness advancement of the digital pulp over the tip of the finger. It is important when considering this technique to remove any excess or redundant nailbed to avoid the hooked nail deformity. Atasoy et al. reported on their results in 1970 and found that 56 of 61 of patients had near-normal motion and sensibility in their fingertip (45). However, these findings were contradicted by Tupper and Miller when they reported decreased sensibility in 15 of 16 patients and that 50% of patients developed cold intolerance after the Atasoy V-Y flap was performed (46). Three patients had a mild hook nail deformity, and 2 of the 16 patients (12.5%) were dissatisfied with their final results.

Operative Procedure. The Atasoy volar V-Y advancement flap can be performed in the emergency department with a simple digital block and digital tourniquet. After surgical prep and drape, excess sterile matrix is removed 1 to 2 mm proximal to the bone of the distal phalanx. The bone may need to be shortened using a rongeur (Fig. 6). Next, a full-thickness skin flap of digital pulp is brought up, with care not to injure the flexor digitorum profundus attachment and the vascular supply to the flap. The procedure should be carried out with loupe magnification to ensure preservation of the small-caliber vessels supplying the flap during division of the fibrous connections securing the flap. Care must also be taken to avoid crossing the DIP flexion crease; otherwise, a contracture may ensue. The palmar flap is mobilized distally and dorsally, and a nailbed repair directly to the distal edge of the flap is performed using a 6-0 chromic gut suture. The medial and lateral portions of this flap are then sutured to the remaining digital pulp using either

an absorbable or nonabsorbable suture (a 4-0 nylon or Prolene stitch is sufficient). Finally, the more proximal portion of the V is closed on itself using this same suture.

Kutler Lateral V-Y Flaps

William Kutler described his procedure of creating two lateral V-Y flaps to close fingertip amputations in 1947 (47). It remains useful in treating transverse amputations of the distal phalanx through the level of the nail and nailbed. Like the Atasoy flap, it can be performed under digital anesthesia in the emergency department. Two simple lateral V-Y advancement flaps are created to meet in the midline of the digit. The procedure is thus suitable for dorsal oblique and transverse amputations, but is less applicable to palmar oblique amputations. This procedure is described below and shown in Figure 7.

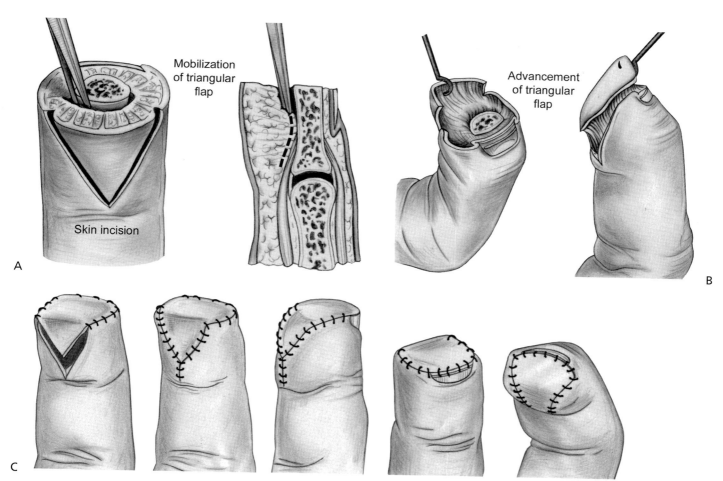

FIGURE 6. The Atasoy volar V-Y advancement flap. **A:** The fingertip is débrided, and bone is shortened if necessary. **B:** A full-thickness triangular palmar flap is developed and advanced to the sterile matrix. The skin is then closed as illustrated **(C)**. [Redrawn from Atasoy E, Ioakimidis E, Kasdan M, et al. Reconstruction of the amputated finger tip with a triangular volar flap. *J Bone Joint Surg* 1970;52(A):921–926, with permission.]

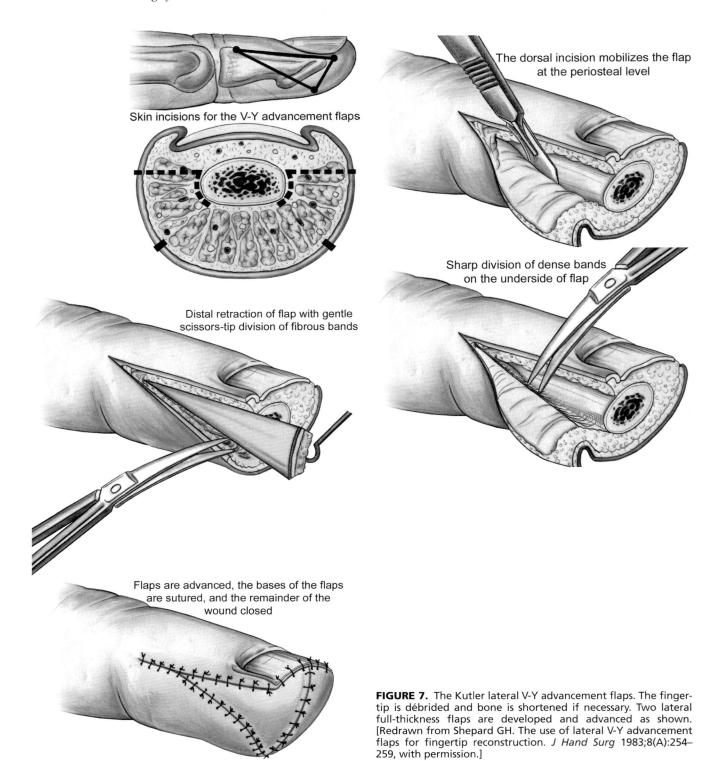

Skin incisions for the V-Y advancement flaps

The dorsal incision mobilizes the flap at the periosteal level

Distal retraction of flap with gentle scissors-tip division of fibrous bands

Sharp division of dense bands on the underside of flap

Flaps are advanced, the bases of the flaps are sutured, and the remainder of the wound closed

FIGURE 7. The Kutler lateral V-Y advancement flaps. The fingertip is débrided and bone is shortened if necessary. Two lateral full-thickness flaps are developed and advanced as shown. [Redrawn from Shepard GH. The use of lateral V-Y advancement flaps for fingertip reconstruction. *J Hand Surg* 1983;8(A):254–259, with permission.]

Operative Procedure. Two triangular lateral radial and ulnar flaps are made down to the level of the DIP flexion crease in Kutler lateral V-Y advancement flaps. Care is taken not to cross this crease or disrupt the blood supply to the overlying skin. As with the Atasoy flap, the procedure should be carried out under loupe magnification. The two lateral flaps are then advanced to meet in the midline of the digit. Bony shortening of the distal phalanx may be necessary to align the sterile matrix properly to prevent a hook nail deformity. The nailbed is repaired distally to the flaps using a resorbable suture such as a 6-0 chromic gut. The palmar skin is also sutured to the radial and ulnar flaps. Finally, the more proximal portions of the flaps are primarily repaired to themselves.

The results of this technique were reported by Shepard (48) and by Freiberg and Manktelow (49). They have reported studies of 37 and 30 patients, respectively, and 50% of those patients complained of cold intolerance and tenderness to percussion when the Kutler V-Y technique was used , thus yielding results similar to those obtained for the Atasoy V-Y flap. Others have reported similar results in their series (50–52).

Cross-Finger Flap

The cross-finger flap was first described by Gurdin and Pangman in 1950 (53). The technique is useful when maintaining digital length is critical. The procedure is considered when an amputation has occurred in palmar oblique fashion to the tip of the index finger or ring finger. The middle finger is then used as a donor site for the cross-finger flap. The basis of the cross-finger flap is that the skin and soft tissue from the adjacent finger are used to cover the bony and soft tissue defect on the injured finger without necessitating primary bone shortening to obtain wound closure.

Ideally, this procedure should be performed in the operating room under local anesthesia. The patient should be counseled preoperatively that skin will be removed from the "bikini-line" area around the hip and thigh to use as a skin graft for the finger. It is also important to explain to the patient that two fingers will be sewn together for 2 to 3 weeks. If the patient is willing to undergo these inconveniences, then digital length can be maintained.

Operative Procedure. The injured finger is prepped and draped in the usual sterile fashion and so is the ipsilateral inguinal region, similarly to draping during an iliac crest bone graft procedure. Local anesthesia is infiltrated in the superior region of the iliac crest before skin graft harvest. After débridement of the injured finger, a full-thickness skin flap is developed off the dorsal aspect of the middle phalanx of the long finger with a base adjacent to the injured digit (Fig. 8). This flap should be large enough to

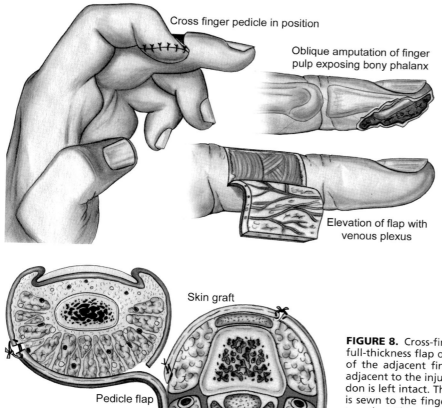

FIGURE 8. Cross-finger flap. The injured finger is débrided. A full-thickness flap of skin and subcutaneus tissue is developed off of the adjacent finger over the middle phalanx. The pedicle is adjacent to the injured finger. The paratenon of the extensor tendon is left intact. The injured finger is flexed slightly, and the flap is sewn to the fingertip; thus, both fingers are temporarily sewn together. Skin graft taken from a hairless portion of the "bikini-line" is sewn over the soft tissue defect created in the adjacent donor finger. A bolster gently holds the skin graft down, allowing for proper adherence. The fingers are separated at 2 to 3 weeks. (Redrawn from Kleinert HE, McAlister CG, MacDonald CJ, Kutz JE. A critical evaluation of cross finger flaps. *J Trauma* 1974;14:756–761, with permission.)

cover the injured digit without any tension being placed on the graft. Care is taken to cauterize the dorsal veins of the digit and not to enter the extensor tendon sheath, but rather to leave the paratenon of the extensor tendon sheath intact. Preservation of the paratenon allows for skin grafting over this skin and soft tissue defect. After the cross-finger flap is mobilized and sewn into place over the injured amputated digit, the full-thickness skin graft is obtained from the hip and thigh region. If at all possible, a hairless region should be obtained for this graft, as hair follicles will continue to grow in the new location on the finger.

Once the graft has matured at 3 weeks, the bridging piece or pedicle (the fourth side of the square) is surgically released. This procedure can be performed under local anesthesia in the office using a digital block. After the two fingers are separated, the wound is sutured closed. It is important to reassure the patient that an almost normal contour of the dorsal aspect of the long finger will be obtained over time as the grafted area fills.

Results of the cross-finger flap were reported by Nishikawa and Smith in 1985 (54). They reviewed 54 patients who had undergone a cross-finger flap. Although 92% of the patients were satisfied with their results, 53% reported cold intolerance of the digit. All of the flaps had diminished sweating and a raised threshold for electrical stimulation. None of the patients had recovery of tactile sensation over the tip even though patients had protective sensation. Other authors have reported similar good results over the years (55–62). Recently, Paterson et al. (63) reported on donor finger morbidity associated with the procedure. Ten of 16 patients (63%) complained of cold intolerance in the donor finger, 8 of 16 (50%) had joint stiffness, and 50% had poor cosmetic results associated with the skin graft over the extensor surface. Although overall digital length is maintained, it is done so at a cost to the donor finger.

Thenar Flap

Similar to the cross-finger flap, if faced with a palmar oblique amputation of the index or long finger, a surgeon may elect to perform a thenar flap (64). Originally described in the hand surgery literature by Flatt, the concept is quite similar to the cross-finger flap (65). The donor skin and soft tissue come from the thenar region of the palm, rather than the dorsal aspect of the long or radially adjacent finger.

Operative Procedure. The thenar flap procedure should be performed ideally in the operating room. The entire arm is prepped and draped. Local anesthesia is used for a digital block and for procuring a forearm skin graft. The "bikini-line" skin graft site may also be used. The finger is débrided. The finger is bent to meet the palm, and a template of the site for the flap is left behind in blood. According to Flatt, the length should not be more than twice the width, and two-thirds of the subcutaneous fat should be carried on the

flap, with the remaining third serving as a bed for the skin graft (65). A split-thickness skin graft is obtained from a hairless portion of the forearm or "bikini-line." This graft is sewn into the thenar bed using a chromic gut suture. The fingertip is flexed down, and the flap is sewn to the tip of the finger. Radial and ulnar sutures are placed, but care must be taken to avoid damaging the vascular supply of the flap. A bolster is placed over the skin graft site to ensure success. Finally, the digit is held in a flexed position using an aluminum and foam malleable splint. The dressing is changed every fourth day. At 2 weeks, the thenar flap is divided under local anesthesia and sutured to the fingertip. Digital range of motion exercises are begun.

In a review of 150 cases using the thenar flap, Melone et al. reported excellent results in 98% of patients (66). Average two-point discrimination was 7 mm in adults and 3.5 mm (normal) in children younger than 10 years of age. Donor site morbidity was extremely low (3%) and consisted of scar tenderness. Joint contractures occurred in 4%. Ninety-four percent of patients resumed their former work after an average time off of 14 weeks.

Revision of Amputation and Primary Closure

When the surgeon is faced with significant soft tissue injury from a severe crush or degloving-type injury associated with severe bony injury, especially to the base of the distal phalanx into the DIP joint, consideration of revision amputation with disarticulation at the DIP joint and primary closure may be warranted (67). There are some practical points to remember if this treatment is chosen (Fig. 9). If the nail is to be ablated, make sure all of the germinal matrix is removed from the fingertip; otherwise, painful and problematic nail cysts will develop, requiring further ablative surgery. If a finger disarticulation is performed at the level of the DIP joint, the flexor digitorum profundus tendon should be divided and allowed to retract into the finger and hand. One should not suture the flexor digitorum longus over the tip of the finger to the extensor tendon, as doing this will lead to the quadriga effect and reduce motion, power, and excursion of adjacent digits, especially in the ulnar three digits. A late lumbrical plus finger deformity may arise and may require a release of the lumbrical to the affected digit. The head of the middle phalanx should be rounded and debulked slightly to prevent a bulbous amputation stump. Finally, the terminal branches of the digital nerves should be identified and sharply divided, and transposed away from the suture line to prevent a painful neuroma from forming in the scar. Soderberg et al. (68) evaluated shortening and primary closure compared with nonoperative treatment. The surgical group had an overall shorter healing time but had a higher morbidity associated with this type of treatment. They found that one-third of those patients treated surgically developed minor infections, whereas none of those treated nonoperatively developed infections.

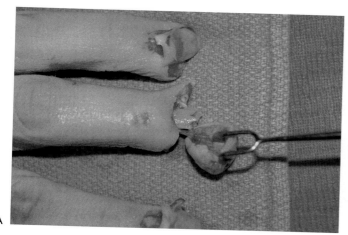

A

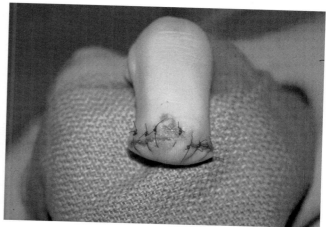

B

FIGURE 9. Revision of amputation and primary wound closure just distal to the distal interphalangeal joint in a patient who sustained an avulsion and crush injury of the fingertip from a dumpster lid **(A)**. Complete ablation of the nail fold and sterile matrix avoids potential nail cyst formation **(B)**. Visualization of the extensor tendon insertion helps to ensure a complete ablation of nail-producing tissues.

Other Methods

Numerous case reports and small series have been reported using variations on the themes presented in this chapter. They are presented and referenced here for further investigation. The authors have limited specific experience with any of these techniques.

Russell et al. reviews the use of the side finger flap to cover thumb and proximal finger amputation (69). The principles of this procedure are similar to the cross-finger flap and the thenar flap. Beasley reviewed local and distant flaps to the hand, including the groin flap (70).

Biddulph has described a modification of the Kutler V-Y flaps whereby unilateral or bilateral triangular flaps are elevated on the neurovascular pedicle and advanced over an amputation stump for closure (71). The technique was successful in restoring normal two-point discrimination in eight patients, and was an overall success in all 18 patients reported on in this series. There were two complications of hook nail deformity in two patients. Others have reported on and developed similar local neurovascular island flaps (72–78).

Furlow reported on an extended volar V-Y advancement flap with cupping of the distal end to re-create the digital pulp on three patients (79). There were no complications and no finger contractures even though the skin crease of the DIP was crossed and skin advanced.

Robbins reported on the use of the "jam roll flap" for fingertip reconstruction (80). He presented a case of an oblique fingertip amputation treated by a modification of the reverse cross-finger flap, the "jam roll," to restore a near-normal contour to a fingertip that would otherwise have required acute shortening and closure.

Many other methods to transfer pulp and/or nailbed to oblique fingertip amputations have also been reported (18,81–88). Finally, we believe that more proximally based homo-digital or cross-digital neurovascular island flaps and their variations are more appropriate for thumbtip reconstruction than for fingertip reconstruction (89–95.)

Authors' Preferred Method of Treatment

Because numerous methods are available to treat fingertip amputations, and they all have similar results, one method is not necessarily better than any other. The clinical situation that is presented usually dictates the treatment. For example, the self-employed laborer may not wish to be off work for 4 to 6 weeks while wound healing by secondary intention occurs, or even to be off work for a month while a cross-finger flap matures and heals. Such a person may elect to have a primary bony shortening and closure using volar or lateral flaps, whichever is easier to perform given the nature of the wound, so that he or she might return to work in 2 weeks when the sutures are removed. On the other hand, a palmar oblique amputation through the fingertip is best treated by a cross-finger flap in most situations. Given a pure transverse amputation through one of the ulnar three digits, the Atasoy volar V-Y advancement is simpler to perform and more reliable than Kutler V-Y advancement technique, as one large flap needs to survive rather than two smaller flaps. A cross-finger flap is usually not needed for such injuries, and a thenar flap is not feasible for the ulnar digits. Finally, for highly contaminated, complex, intraarticular injuries involving the DIP joint with significant soft tissue loss, a primary disarticulation through the DIP joint and skin closure may be warranted.

Regardless of the procedure performed, patients are usually given a single dose of cefazolin (vancomycin if allergic to penicillin) intravenously and a tetanus booster in the emergency room. Cephalexin (clindamycin if penicillin allergic) is given orally for 3 days for relatively clean wounds. A longer period of oral antibiotics may be necessary for more severe wounds that might be prone to infection. Patients are also dismissed with a low-potency narcotic for pain control. Follow-up in the office is partially dictated by the severity of the injury and the integrity of the repair, with a usual date being 5 to 7 days post injury. Patients are usually followed weekly until healed and are seen at 2 to 3 months to assure full recovery. It might be necessary to refer a patient to hand therapy for scar desensitization or range of motion exercise. Overall, the results are acceptable for both patient and surgeon no matter what treatment is used.

COMPLICATIONS

In discussions of management principles, complications associated with nailbed and fingertip trauma are outlined in this chapter. As can be appreciated, the treatment of these common injuries is controversial, as no perfect technique has been developed to ensure a normal-appearing, sensate, painless, and fully functional fingertip after trauma has occurred. A broad spectrum of treatment ideas and options for these injuries is presented, and the drawbacks of any given treatment plan are outlined.

Complications of such injuries and their management have been reviewed by Browne (96). The complications associated with fingertip injury overlap with those associated with nailbed injury to a large extent. Neuromas, cold intolerance, fingertip pain and hypersensitivity, loss of fine sensation, poor cosmetic appearance, nail deformity, finger shortening, stiffness of neighboring joints, and donor site morbidity are all possible complications that are potentially unavoidable regardless of the method of treatment used. In this chapter, common pitfalls that might lead to the development of a complication are outlined in the hope that the surgeon will be cognizant of such situations. The complications of reduced fine tactile sensation and finger shortening have no solution. Cold intolerance is treated by avoidance and protective garments (gloves or mittens). Hypersensitivity, joint stiffness, and fingertip pain are managed with varying degrees of success by hand therapists. Painful neuromas can be resected. The management of nail deformities has been discussed. As of this writing, aside from revision surgery directed at a particular anatomic site, there is no panacea for any or all of the potential complications that may be encountered with fingertip and nailbed injuries no matter how they are initially managed.

REFERENCES

1. Fassler PR. Fingertip injuries: evaluation and treatment. *J Am Acad Orthop Surg* 1996;4:84–92.
2. Zook EG. Anatomy and physiology of the perionychium. *Hand Clin* 1990;6:1–7.
3. Zaias N. *The nail of health and disease.* Lancaster, England: SP Medical and Scientific Books, 1980:31–34.
4. Shum C, Bruno RJ, Ristic S, et al. Examination of the anatomic relationship of the proximal germinal nail matrix to the extensor tendon insertion. *J Hand Surg* 2000;25A:1114–1117.
5. Strauch B and de Moura W. Arterial system of the fingers. *J Hand Surg* 1990;15A:148–153.
6. Rose EH, Norris MS, Kowalski TA, et al. The "cap" technique: nonmicrosurgical reattachment of fingertip amputations. *J Hand Surg* 1989;14(A):513–518.
7. Van Beek AL, Kassan MA, Adson MH, et al. Management of acute fingernail injuries. *Hand Clin* 1990;6:23–38.
8. Seymour N. Juxta-epiphyseal fractures of the terminal phalanx of the finger. *J Bone Joint Surg* 1966;48B:347–349.
9. Guy RJ. The etiologies and mechanisms of nail bed injuries. *Hand Clin* 1990;6:9–19.
10. Chin G, Weinzweig N, Weinzweig J, et al. Snowblower injuries to the hand. *Ann Plast Surg* 1998;41(4):390–396.
11. Zook EG, Guy RJ, Russell RC. A study of nail bed injuries: causes, treatment, and prognosis. *J Hand Surg* 1984;9A:247–252.
12. Macgregor DM, Hiscox JA. Fingertip trauma in children from doors. *Scott Med J* 1999;44(4):114–115.
13. Zook EG, Brown RE. The perionychium. In: Green DP, Hotchkiss RN, Pederson WC, eds. *Green's operative hand surgery*, 4th ed. New York: Churchill Livingstone, 1999:1353–1380.
14. Roser SE, Gellman H. Comparison of nail bed repair versus nail trephination for subungual hematomas in children. *J Hand Surg* 1999;24A(6):1166–1170.
15. Bindra RR. Management of nail-bed fracture-lacerations using a tension-band suture. *J Hand Surg* 1996;21A(6):1111–1113.
16. Dove AF, Sloan JP, Moulder TJ, et al. Dressings of the nailbed following nail avulsion. *J Hand Surg* 1988;13(B):408–410.
17. Shepard GH. Management of acute nail bed avulsions. *Hand Clin* 1990;6:39–58.
18. Saito H, Suzuki Y, Fujino K, et al. Free nail bed graft for treatment of nail bed injuries of the hand. *J Hand Surg* 1983;8(A):171–178.
19. Matsuba HM, Spear SL. Delayed primary reconstruction of subtotal nail bed loss using a split-thickness nail bed graft on decorticated bone. *Plast Reconst Surg* 1988;81:440–443.
20. Shibata M, Seki T, Yoshizu T, et al. Microsurgical toenail transfer to the hand. *Plast Reconstr Surg* 1991;88:102–109.
21. Kleinert HE, Putcha SM, Ashbell TS, et al. The deformed fingernail, a frequent result of failure to repair nail bed injuries. *J Trauma* 1967;7:177–190.
22. Atasoy E. Reversed cross-finger subcutaneous flap. *J Hand Surg* 1982;7(A):481–483.
23. Zook EG, Russell RC. Reconstruction of a functional and esthetic nail. *Hand Clin* 1990;6:59–68.
24. Shepard GH. Nail grafts for reconstruction. *Hand Clin* 1990;6:79–103.
25. Kumar VP, Satku K. Treatment and prevention of "hook nail" deformity with anatomic correlation. *J Hand Surg* 1993;18(A):617–620.
26. Ma GF, Cheng JC, Chan KT, et al. Finger tip injuries: a prospective study on seven methods of treatment on 200 cases. *Ann Acad Med Singapore* 1982;11:207–213.

27. Allen MJ. Conservative management of finger tip injuries in adults. *Hand* 1980;12:257–265.

28. Tamai S. Twenty years experience of limb replantation: review of 293 upper extremity replants. *J Hand Surg* 1982;7(A):549–556.

29. Yamano Y. Replantation of the amputated distal part of the fingers. *J Hand Surg* 1985;10(A):211–218.

30. Ishikawa K, Ogawa Y, Soeda H, et al. A new classification of the amputation level of the distal part of the finger. *J Jpn Soc Microsurg* 1990;3:54–62.

31. Foucher G, Norris RW. Distal and very distal digital replantations. *Br J Plast Surg* 1992;45:199–203.

32. Merle M, Dautel G. Advances in digital replantation. *Clin Plast Surg* 1997;24:87–105.

33. Hirase Y. Salvage of fingertip amputated at nail level: new surgical principles and treatments. *Ann Plast Surg* 1997;38:151–157.

34. Mennen U, Wiese A. Fingertip injuries management with semi-occlusive dressing. *J Hand Surg* 1993;18(B):416–422.

35. Shabat S, Sagiv P, Stern A, Nyska M. Polyurethane film (OpSite) for superficial fingertip avulsion injuries (letter). *Plast Reconstr Surg* 2000;106:512.

36. Williamson DM, Sherman KP, Shakespeare DT. The use of semipermeable dressings in fingertip injuries. *J Hand Surg* 1987;12(B):125–126.

37. Fox JW, Golden GT, Rodeheaver G, et al. Nonoperative management of fingertip pulp amputation by occlusive dressings. *Am J Surg* 1977;133:255–256.

38. Buckley SC, Scott S, Das K. Late review of the use of silver sulphadiazine dressings for the treatment of fingertip injuries. *Injury* 2000;31:301–304.

39. Ipsen T, Frandsen PA, Barfred T. Conservative treatment of fingertip injuries. *Injury* 1987;18:203–205.

40. Lamon RP, Cicero JJ, Frascone RJ, Hass WF. Open treatment of fingertip amputations. *Ann Emerg Med* 1983;12:358–360.

41. O'Donovan DA, Mehdi SY, Eadie PA. The role of Mepitel silicone net dressings in the management of fingertip injuries in children. *J Hand Surg* 1999;24(B):727–730.

42. Halim AS, Stone CA, Devaraj VS. The Hyphecan cap: a biological fingertip dressing. *Injury* 1998;29:261–263.

43. Lee LP, Lau PY, Chan CW. A simple and efficient treatment for fingertip injuries. *J Hand Surg* 1995;20(B):63–71.

44. Tranquilli-Leali E. Ricostruzione dell'apice delle falangi ungruali mediante autoplastica volare peduncolata per scorrimento. *Infort Traum Lavaro* 1935;1:186–193.

45. Atasoy E, Ioakimidis E, Kasdan M, et al. Reconstruction of the amputated finger tip with a triangular volar flap. *J Bone Joint Surg* 1970;52(A):921–926.

46. Tupper J, Miller G. Sensitivity following volar V-Y plasty for fingertip amputations. *J Hand Surg* 1985;10(B):183–184.

47. Kutler W. A new method for finger tip amputation. *JAMA* 1947;133:29–30.

48. Shepard GH. The use of lateral V-Y advancement flaps for fingertip reconstruction. *J Hand Surg* 1983;8(A):254–259.

49. Freiberg A, Manktelow R. The Kutler repair for fingertip amputations. *Plast Reconstr Surg* 1972;50:371–375.

50. Gaber M. Kutler repair for the amputated fingertip. *Ann R Coll Surg Engl* 1979;61:298–300.

51. Haddad RJ. The Kutler repair of fingertip amputation. *South Med J* 1968;61:1264–1267.

52. Rothwell AG. Finger tip amputations: the Kutler technique of repair. *N Z Med J* 1970;71:212–214.

53. Gurdin M, Pangman WJ. The repair of surface defects of fingers by trans-digital flaps. *J Plast Reconstr Surg* 1950;5:368–371.

54. Nishikawa H, Smith PJ. The recovery of sensation and function after cross-finger flaps for fingertip injury. *J Hand Surg* 1992;17(B):102–107.

55. Atasoy E. The cross thumb to index finger pedicle. *J Hand Surg* 1980;5:572–574.

56. Johnson RK, Iverson RE. Cross-finger pedicle flaps in the hand. *J Bone Joint Surg* 1971;53(A):913–919.

57. Kappel DA, Burech JG. The cross-finger flap: an established reconstructive procedure. *Hand Clin* 1985;1:677–683.

58. Kleinert HE, McAlister CG, MacDonald CJ, Kutz JE. A critical evaluation of cross finger flaps. *J Trauma* 1974;14:756–761.

59. Nicolai JPA, Hentenaar G. Sensation in cross-finger flaps. *Hand* 1981;13:12–16.

60. Souquet R, Souquet JR. The actual indications of cross finger flaps in finger injuries. *Ann Chir de la Main* 1986;5:43–53.

61. Spokevicius S, Gupta A. The modified cross finger flap for finger pulp and nail bed reconstruction. *J Hand Surg* 1997;22(B):745–749.

62. Sucur D, Radivojevic M. Cross finger flap: a new technique. *J Hand Surg* 1985;10(B):425–429.

63. Paterson P, Titley OG, Nancarrow JD. Donor finger morbidity in cross-finger flaps. *Injury* 2000;31:215–218.

64. Gatewood. A plastic repair of finger defects without hospitalization. *JAMA* 1926;87:1479.

65. Flatt AE. The thenar flap. *J Bone Joint Surg* 1957;39(B):80–85.

66. Melone CP, Beasley RW, Carstens JH. The thenar flap—an analysis of its use in 150 cases. *J Hand Surg* 1982;7:291–297.

67. Weston PA, Wallace WA. The use of locally based triangular skin flap for the repair of finger tip injuries. *Hand* 1976;8:54–58.

68. Soderberg T, Nystrom A, Hallmans G, Hulten J. Treatment of fingertip amputations with bone exposure. *Scand J Plast Reconstr Surg* 1983;17:147–152.

69. Russel RC, Van Beek AL, Zook EG. Alternative hand flaps for amputations and digital defects. *J Hand Surg* 1981;6:399–405.

70. Beasley RW. Principles of soft tissue replacement for the hand. *J Hand Surg* 1983;8:781–784.

71. Biddulph SL. The neurovascular flap in finger tip injuries. *Hand* 1979;11:59–63.

72. Elliot D, Moiemen NS, Jigjinni VS. The neurovascular Tranquilli-Leali flap. *J Hand Surg* 1995;20(B):815–823.

73. Foucher G, Dallaserra M, Tilquin B, et al. The Hueston flap in reconstruction of fingertip skin loss: results in a series of 41 patients. *J Hand Surg* 1994;19(A):508–515.

74. Inoue G. Fingertip reconstruction with a dorsal transposition flap. *Br J Plast Surg* 1991;44:530–532.

75. Lanzetta M, Mastropasqua B, Chollet A, Brisebois N. Versatility of the homodigital triangular neurovascular island flap in fingertip reconstruction. *J Hand Surg* 1995;20(B):824–829.

76. Shibu MM, Tarabe MA, Graham K, et al. Fingertip reconstruction with a dorsal island homodigital flap. *Br J Plast Surg* 1997;50:121–124.

77. Tsai TM, Yuen JC. A neurovascular island flap for volar-oblique fingertip amputations. *J Hand Surg* 1996;21(B):94–98.

78. Venkataswami R, Subramanian N. Oblique triangular flap: a new method of repair for oblique amputations of the fingertip and thumb. *Plast Reconstr Surg* 1980;66:296–300.

79. Furlow LT. V-Y "cup" flap for volar oblique amputation of fingers. *J Hand Surg* 1984;9(B):253–256.

80. Robbins TH. The "jam roll" flap for fingertip reconstruction. *Plast Reconstr Surg* 1988;81:109–111.

81. Brown RE, Zook EG, Russell RC. Fingertip reconstruction with flaps and nail bed grafts. *J Hand Surg* 1999;24(A):345–351.

82. Dautel G, Corcella D, Merle M. Reconstruction of fingertip amputations by partial composite toe transfer with short vascular pedicle. *J Hand Surg* 1998;23(B):457–464.

83. Deglise B, Botta Y. Microsurgical free toe pulp transfer for digital reconstruction. *Ann Plast Surg* 1991;26:341–346.

84. Elliot D, Jigjinni VS. The lateral pulp flap. *J Hand Surg* 1993;18(B):423–426.

85. Hirase Y, Kojima T, Matsui M. Aesthetic fingertip reconstruction with a free vascularized nail graft: a review of 60 flaps involving partial toe transfers. *Plast Reconstr Surg* 1997;99:774–784.

86. Koshima I, Inagawa K, Urushibara K, et al. Fingertip reconstructions using partial-toe transfers. *Plast Reconstr Surg* 2000;105:1666–1674.

87. Lee HB, Tark KC, Rah DK, Shin KS. Pulp reconstruction of fingers with very small sensate medial plantar free flap. *Plast Reconstr Surg* 1998;101:999–1005.

88. Netscher DT, Meade RA. Reconstruction of fingertip amputations with full-thickness perionychial grafts from the retained part and local flaps. *Plast Reconstr Surg* 1999;104:1705–1712.

89. Adani R, Busa R, Castagnetti C, et al. Homodigital neurovascular island flaps with "direct flow" vascularization. *Ann Plast Surg* 1997;38:36–40.

90. Chao JD, Huang JM, Wiedrich TA. Local hand flaps. *J Am Soc Surg Hand* 2001;1:25–44.

91. Del Bene M, Petrolati M, Raimondi P, et al. Reverse dorsal digital island flap. *Plast Reconstr Surg* 1994;93:552–557.

92. Han SK, Lee BI, Kim WK. The reverse digital artery island flap: clinical experience in 120 fingers. *Plast Reconstr Surg* 1998;101:1006–1111.

93. Lai CS, Lin SD, Tsai CC, Tsai CW. Reverse digital artery neurovascular cross-finger flap. *J Hand Surg* 1995;20(A):397–402.

94. Sapp JW, Allen RJ, Dupin C. A reversed digital artery island flap for the treatment of fingertip injuries. *J Hand Surg* 1993;18(A):528–534.

95. Tonkin MA, Ahmad TS. The reconstruction of a dorsal digital defect using a reverse homodigital island flap incorporating vascularized tendon. *J Hand Surg* 1997;22(B):750–751.

96. Browne EZ. Complications of fingertip injuries. *Hand Clin* 1994;10:125–137.

65

SKIN GRAFTS AND TISSUE EXPANDERS

GUENTER GERMANN
SIGRID A. BLOME-EBERWEIN

Skin grafting has been the most commonly used technique for reconstruction of cutaneous defects over the last decades. Numerous variations, such as mesh graft, cultured epithelial autografts, and combined alloautograft techniques (sandwich technique), have significantly enhanced the therapeutic spectrum of the traditional skin graft technique, especially in the treatment of severely burned upper extremities. The introduction of tissue expansion has added a new dimension for secondary scar corrections or the treatment of neoplastic skin lesions that are not suitable for excision and primary closure. As in all surgical procedures, correct indications, a well-designed treatment plan, good selection of the proper technique, and excellent technical execution are the keys to success in reconstruction of major and minor defects of the skin of the arm and hand.

SURGICAL ANATOMY

Skin of the Hand

Distinct qualities of the dorsal and palmar hand skin make them especially suited for their different tasks. Although both have in common an irregular border between the basal layer of the epidermis and the dermis, the epidermis (keratin layer) in the palmar skin with its thick *stratum corneum* is approximately three times as thick as it is in dorsal skin. This structure is responsible for the enormous capacity of spontaneous healing in abrasion injuries, burns, or contusion injuries. There are no hair follicles or sebaceous glands on the palmar side of the hand. Instead, specialized encapsulated nerve endings are found. Meissner's corpuscles are present in dermal papillae, and Vater-Pacini corpuscles are present in the deep dermis. The submacroscopic structure resembles the honeycomb architecture of the plantar skin. The aponeurotic system with its structural arrangement of fibrous and elastic fibers provides stability and resistance to shear forces.

All other features, such as epidermal rete ridges, intraepidermal nerve endings that terminate in Merkel cell neurite complexes, a dense network of blood vessels, sensory and autonomic nerve fibers, and sweat glands, which are located in the base of the dermis, as well as subcutaneous fat, are found in dorsal and palmar skin (Figs. 1 and 2) (1–5).

Skin of the Arm

The skin of the arm resembles the skin in any other part of the body. In general, the inner-flexor side skin contains fewer hair follicles, and the dermis is thinner than the outer-extensor side skin.

Superficial Nerves

Seven nerves provide sensibility for the skin of the arm and hand. In the shoulder region that overlies the deltoid muscle, the axillary nerve is supplying the skin. The upper arm is supplied by the medial cutaneous brachii nerve (upper inner arm and axilla) and the medial cutaneous antebrachii nerve (upper and lower inner arm). The radial nerve and its branches (cutaneous brachii posterior nerve, cutaneous antebrachii posterior nerve, ramus superficialis, digitales dorsales nerves) supply the upper and lower lateral aspect of the arm, as well as the dorsum of the hand up to the metacarpophalangeal joints of the index, middle, and ring fingers and the dorsum of the thumb.

The musculocutaneous nerve and its branch (cutaneous antebrachii lateralis nerve) reach the radial flexor side of the lower arm, including the thumb, and up to the proximal interphalangeal joints of the index and middle fingers. The cutaneous branches of the median and ulnar nerves provide sensibility and tactile gnosis for both aspects of the digits (3–5).

PATHOPHYSIOLOGY

Skin Defects of the Fingers, Hand, Wrist, and Arm

Cutaneous defects of the hand and wrist most commonly result from trauma (including burns) or its sequelae. Tumor

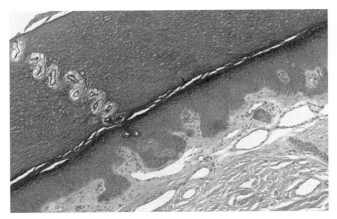

FIGURE 1. Light microscopic histologic section of palmar skin. Note the thickness of the keratin layer and the transiting sweat pore.

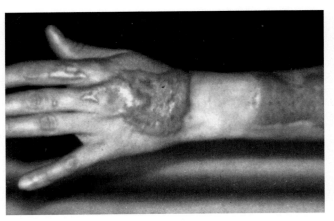

FIGURE 3. Typical hypertrophic scars resulting from burns. Not only do the scars cross the joint lines, but also the reduced compliance of scar tissue limits motion by reducing excursion of the skin.

resection or the sequelae of extravasation of intravenous drug applications are less frequent causes for skin defects. Secondary skin losses can result from operative procedures in traumatized hands, Dupuytren's contracture release, or the treatment of congenital deformities (e.g., syndactyly, club hand). Skin grafts are the easiest method of coverage for skin defects. The type of skin graft that is used depends on the type of defect, the characteristics of the wound, the personal profile of the patient, and the aesthetic requirements of the individual patient (see Skin Grafts). In the case of exposed or destroyed important functional structures, such as tendons, bones, or joints, different reconstructive techniques have to be considered (see Fig. 9) (6).

Scars

The process of scar formation is complicated and is not yet completely understood. Wound healing proceeds in three stages, beginning with the inflammatory phase, followed by

the proliferative phase, and then followed by contraction and maturation with rearrangement of the collagen fibrils in a more organized way. In hypertrophic scarring, the appropriate end point for continuous collagen production is neglected by the tissues, and the orientation of fibrils is unorganized (7). Hypertrophic scars are common over joints, in burns, and in scars that are perpendicular to the resting skin tension lines (Fig. 3).

Keloids display different properties. They grow beyond the limits of the scar into healthy tissue and exhibit tumor-like growth properties. They have a higher incidence in very fair and dark skin.

The disruption of the ideal wound healing process is caused by multiple factors, such as ischemia (8), hypovolemia (9), infection, and mechanical forces. Some nutritional deficiencies, such as deficits in protein, vitamins C and E, zinc, and copper, can also cause disturbances in the wound healing process. There are a few hereditary diseases (e.g., factor XIII deficiency, protein C and A deficiencies) that interfere with wound healing, and drug-related disturbances of the normal healing process may occur (e.g., glucocorticoid therapy) (10).

CLINICAL SIGNIFICANCE (INCIDENCE)

Skin defects of the tips of fingers are common owing to the exposed location. In most cases, superficial, as well as deeper, lesions without exposure of bone or tendons heal spontaneously under moist or occlusive dressings. Complex defects can usually be reconstructed with some type of local or regional flap (11).

In the authors' patient population, the authors treat approximately 300 burn patients per year, of which 80% demonstrate involvement of the hand. Approximately 50% of these patients require some form of skin grafting to the hand. In Dupuytren's contracture release, only 0.5% of all procedures leave a skin defect that requires

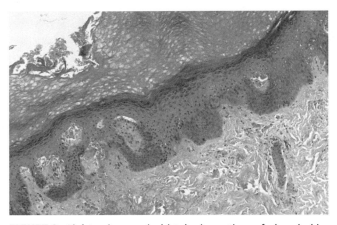

FIGURE 2. Light microscopic histologic section of dorsal skin. Note the thinness of the keratin layer compared to the palmar skin in Figure 1 but the otherwise similar histologic organization.

skin grafting. Approximately 50 cases per year are treated with skin grafting for skin defects that are caused by infection or some other complication from trauma or with surgical intervention. In syndactyly release, skin grafting is indicated in 80% of the cases. Compound defects are usually treated by pedicled or microvascular flap transfer (approximately 250 cases per year).

NATURAL HISTORY

Only superficial skin defects, such as in first-degree burns (also known as *superficial partial-thickness burns*), heal spontaneously without scar formation. However, changes in skin pigmentation may occur, especially in very fair- or dark-skinned patients. Usually, reepithelialized areas remain reddish or pink in color for several months, until the underlying hyperemia resolves, and the skin color returns to the preinjury tan. Deeper (partial-thickness burns) skin defects of the upper extremity, if left untreated, heal by secondary intention through the formation of granulation tissue and consecutive wound edge contracture. Deeper defects of the fingertips are the exception. They usually heal under occlusion dressings without scarring, and even the fingerprint may be regenerated. Because normal function of the joints largely depends on a supple soft tissue envelope, secondary healing leads to the development of severe contractures that result in marked functional losses. The same holds true for hypertrophic scars and keloids. Keloids in general tend to become worse over time and with the number of attempts of keloid excision, if no further adjunctive treatment is applied [i.e., radiation, corticoid injection, pressure garment application, percutaneous silicone sheet application(12,13)]. Unstable scars are another sequel of spontaneously healing larger defects. Recurrent ulceration, diminished resistance for shear forces, and impaired healing of ulcerated areas are typical characteristics. Ultimately, Marjolin's ulcer may evolve (14).

EVALUATION

Physical Examination

The physical examination of skin defects in the upper extremity includes the determination of the exact location and size of the defect, the assessment of viability of underlying and surrounding tissues, the presence of chronically unstable areas, the extent of functional limitation, the skin quality in the vicinity of the defect, the overall appearance of the patient, and the patient's personal profile.

Scars are described by size and as being pale, hyperemic or blue, hyper- or hypopigmented, soft and pliable or hard and rigid, and at or above the level of the surrounding tis-

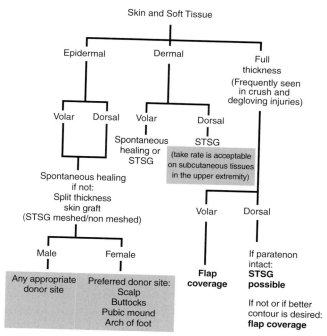

FIGURE 4. Flowchart of patient factors that must be considered when contemplating treatment options for scar tissue. STSG, split-thickness skin graft.

sue and by whether they constitute a limitation to movement. The skin quality of the individual needs to be taken into consideration (e.g., age, gender, and drug therapy, such as corticoids or blood thinners) (Fig. 4).

Imaging Studies

In case of scar contractures, especially after major burns or in polytrauma patients, conventional x-ray studies should be taken to exclude heterotopic ossification or secondary bony deformities. Computed tomography scan or magnetic resonance imaging is usually indicated only in cases of malignant soft tissue tumors; angiography or magnetic resonance angiography is required only in vascular malformations or after severe trauma.

NONOPERATIVE TREATMENT

There is no nonoperative treatment option for deeper skin defects in the upper extremity, except in defects of the fingertips. Fingertip defects epithelialize over a period of time under moist or occlusive dressings and yield better sensitivity and appearance than grafted fingertips (15).

Hypertrophic scars respond well to nonoperative measurements, which represent the foundation of scar treatment. The stepwise concept includes a primary application of pressure garments or bandages. This can be combined with a cutaneous application of silicone gel sheets, silicone cream,

TABLE 1. CONSERVATIVE (NONOPERATIVE) TREATMENT OPTIONS FOR SCAR AND DYSPIGMENTED TISSUE

Hypertrophic scar	Scar contracture	Surface and pigmentation irregularities
Pressure garments	Physical therapy:	Peelings
Silicone gel sheets	Stretching	Coblation
Face mask	Massage	Dermabrasion
Intralesional injection of cortisone	Pressure garments	Permanent makeup (tattoo)
Anticytokine injection	Silicone gel sheets	Camouflage makeup
Massage		

or adhesive silicone foils. It is important to monitor the perfect fit, and the patient has to wear his or her pressure garment 23 hours per day for at least 6 months after trauma. This treatment has to be initiated early after complete epithelialization, because matured hypertrophic scars usually do not respond to this treatment. The effects of pressure or percutaneous silicone application have not yet been completely understood. When the relative hypoperfusion under pressure garments is made responsible for the prevention of hypertrophic scarring, no comprehensive explanation has been found for the efficacy of silicone application.

Intralesional injection of cortisone is another conservative measure that can be combined with pressure therapy. Injections with anticytokines are still under clinical investigation and, their efficacy has not yet been proven.

Physical therapy, including scar massage and electrostimulation, can resolve or prevent joint contractures in many cases by softening the areas that are involved. Scar massage always has to be directed perpendicular to the course of the scar to prevent or break the collagen fibril organization. This is of special importance in deeper burns, in which the deeper subcutaneous layers may also be contracted. The therapist has to be familiar with the special needs of a patient whose limitation results from skin and subdermal contractures rather than from isolated joint stiffness.

Laser treatment, peelings, coblation, and dermabrasion are other adjunctive procedures that may resolve dyspigmentation or smooth rippled skin surfaces, and some patients can be helped with permanent makeup (tattooing) to ameliorate the effects of dyspigmentation (Table 1).

SURGICAL MANAGEMENT

Tissue Expansion

History

The first expandable air-filled tissue expander was reported in 1957 by Neumann (16). Radovan reported about the use of an expansion device to stretch the periau-

ricular skin for the purpose of ear reconstruction (17). Despite all technical improvements, increasing knowledge about the tissue reactions, and the geometric responses to expanders of different shape, the principles of skin stretching have remained the same. With improved technology, the principle gained a widespread popularity for scar correction or defect closure after skin tumor resection in the 1980s. The initial enthusiasm surrounding their use in reconstructive surgery was soon dampened by a considerable complication rate, including infection, extrusion of the expander, or skin breakdown (18–24). The analysis of these inherent complications led to a better definition of the indications. The main applications today include correction of alopecia, head and neck reconstruction, scar correction in the trunk after burns or trauma, or breast reconstruction combined with alloplastic implants. Provided suitable indications, tissue expansion may be a reasonable alternative to serial excision, local flaps, or regional pedicled flaps, and it avoids an additional donor site. The newly gained tissue matches the color and texture of the surrounding tissue and remains sensate. The use of tissue expansion in the upper extremity has only been occasionally reported (18,25–28). The method has been proposed in this location for scar corrections, contracture release, coverage of tumor resection defects, and congenital anomaly corrections (i.e., syndactyly), but actual numbers in the literature are small (29–31). An interesting method of tissue expansion for the treatment of syndactyly has been proposed by Ogawa et al. (32). They applied outside pressure to the to-be-created interdigital space with a pincer device and created enough laxity of the skin to perform the syndactyly operation with local flaps only. This way they spared the patient a second operation and skin graft coverage.

Principle

Tissue expansion uses the ability of the skin that is adjacent to a scar or a future defect (for instance, in tumor resection) to stretch to mechanical forces. The effect is achieved by placing a silicone-shelled balloon into a subcutaneous pocket that is adjacent to the area to be reconstructed. The incision for this pocket should be perpendicular from the edge of the soft tissue–deficient area to minimize the risk of extrusion. Endoscopically assisted expander placement can eliminate this problem (33). The balloon is sequentially filled with saline through an integrated portal system, or a remote port is used that is placed into another pocket at some distance from the expander. The remote port is the safer solution, because the risk of incidental injection into the expander with subsequent deflation is considerably higher in integrated ports (34). Expansion is delayed in this concept for 2 to 3 weeks to allow proper soft tissue healing and to prevent skin breakdown or extrusion of the balloon. The expansion is then progressively continued, usually over a period of 6 to 12 weeks, always according to the individual patient's tolerance.

The expanded skin is thinned; despite an epidermal hypertrophy, the vascularity of the expanded tissue is also enhanced owing to a delaylike phenomenon. A membrane with pseudoendothelium is formed around the silicone balloon. This membrane is well vascularized and may serve as a gliding surface in upper extremity reconstructions that use preexpanded free flaps. After removal of the expander, shrinkage of 25% of the expanded surface has to be expected due to the elastic properties of the expanded skin. Therefore, many surgeons tend to leave the maximally inflated expanders in place for another 4 weeks to reduce this phenomenon, whenever the patients tolerate this.

There are many different shapes and sizes of expanders with various geometric responses of the expanded tissue. The bottom plate determines the size in two planes; the actual tissue gain is created by the projected height of the expander, which has to be considered during the planning. Ideally, the bottom plate is placed on a hard resistant surface, such as the skull, in which the expansion is only directed toward the skin. In concave areas or in areas with a soft bed, the expansion may also be directed into the underlying tissues and does not sufficiently stretch the skin. In children, it has to be considered that bony impressions, for instance, in the ribs or the skull, are possible (35).

The advantages of tissue expansion include the close match in tissue texture and color and the fact that sensible innervation is maintained. The disadvantages of tissue expansion include the risk of extrusion, infection, and skin breakdown, as well as the fact that it always includes a minimum of two operative procedures with insertion of the expander, and subsequent expander removal and scar correction. In selected cases, in which the primary tissue gain is not sufficient, the expander can be reinserted, and repeated expansion can be initiated. Multiple clinic visits for wound control and expander filling are time and cost consuming for the patient and physician.

Operative Technique

Careful planning of the procedure is the most important key to success. The scar has to be measured in all dimensions, and a corresponding expander has to be chosen. The incision for placement of the expander should be made perpendicular to the long edge of the scar. It has to be included into the actual scar excision and the spreading of the expanded skin. This requires some experience with tissue handling and knowledge of the skin resting-tension lines. In the upper extremity, it also must be considered not to create straight lines across joints and to design the expanded skin flaps in a way to conceal the resulting scar on the medial side of the arm. Contrary to the most common recommendation, the authors prefer placement of the expander in the arm epifascially, more precisely in the *fascial cleft* (36). The pocket is usually created by sharp and blunt dissection with an instrument like the Korn tongs. The pocket has to be large enough to fit the expander without wrinkles at the bottom plate. A separate pocket is created for the port, well away from the expander, to avoid accidental puncture of the expander or even coverage of the port by the inflated device. After meticulous hemostasis, the cavity is rinsed with diluted iodine solution, and the device is tested for leakage by inflating it with air and holding it under diluted iodine solution (1:10). After this test, all air is aspirated, and the expander is inserted after glove change. Folds and wrinkles in the pouch have to be removed before wound closure. The device is slightly filled to smooth any residual wrinkles, to avoid dead spaces, and to provide additional hemostasis. Wrinkles promote uneven distribution of pressure during the expansion process, which predisposes for skin irritation with subsequent infection or perforation. The skin is closed in two layers.

Inflation may be started after wound healing (from 8 to 10 days to 2 to 3 weeks after insertion). Once or twice weekly, the port is punctured under sterile conditions with a 22-gauge needle, and sterile saline or Ringer's lactate solution is injected until the patient feels pain or until the skin above the expander blanches. At this point, 2 mL are removed, and the needle is withdrawn. Intraluminal pressures can exceed capillary closing pressures without affecting skin capillary refill (28).

Endoscopically assisted expander placement has significantly improved the tissue expansion procedure. After a small incision that is remote from the projected expander pocket, the fascial cleft is identified and a "spacemaker" balloon is inserted through a small canal of approximately 3 to 5 cm in length. This is an inflatable device that is inserted with a guiding rod. The balloon is then filled with air and creates its own optical cavity to incorporate the expander. The cavity can then be endoscopically inspected for bleeders, and hemostasis can also be achieved with endoscopic instruments. The combination of a small incision and an insertion canal creates a "bottleneck effect." This prevents extrusion of the expander through the incision line and allows for a significantly greater initial filling volume than with the conventional technique. Often, as much as 30% of the nominal expander volume can be filled during expander placement without waiting for wound healing. This is a major advantage, especially in children, because it causes less pain, requires fewer filling sessions, and abbreviates the total reconstruction period.

The initial patient consultation deserves special attention. The necessity for weekly fillings, the temporary deformity caused by the expansion, the duration of the process, the necessity for two surgical procedures, as well as possible complications have to be discussed in detail with the patient to obtain the necessary compliance for the process (Fig. 5).

Skin Grafts

History

The concept of autologous skin grafting was not reported until 1838 (37) and 1845 (38). Reverdin (39) and Thiersch

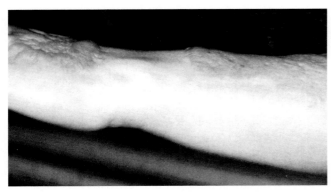

FIGURE 5. Lateral view of a hand with hypertrophic scar before surgical intervention.

reported successful transplantation of split-thickness skin in 1869 and 1874 (40). In 1875, Krause (41) and Wolfe (42) established full-thickness grafts. Since then, these techniques have become the backbone of reconstructive procedures. However, there are indications in medical history that skin grafting was used by Hindu surgeons as well as Greek surgeons long before a medical literature existed.

Type of Graft

The best choice for a skin graft depends on the location of the defect or scar, the properties that are expected of the grafted skin, the expected aesthetic appearance, the size of the defect or scar, the donor availability, and the donor site morbidity. In general, two histologic types of skin grafts can be distinguished, *split-thickness* and *full-thickness* grafts. Split-thickness grafts include dermal components, depending on the thickness of the harvested graft, but they do not include the full dermal layer. Full-thickness skin grafts include all layers of the skin, so that the donor site has to be primarily closed or, in rare cases, grafted with a thinner graft itself. This distinction is, although principally correct, nevertheless insufficient. First, the donor site for the graft determines how many skin appendages are included into the graft. This means that various skin grafts can be differently composed, although they have been harvested with the same dermatome adjustments. Second, there is not much scientific evidence that a groin full-thickness graft has better properties, with respect to contraction, pliability, and aesthetic appearance, than a thick split-thickness graft from the back. It can certainly be said that a standard 0.001- to 0.002-in. setting on the dermatome, which is recommended in most of the literature, does not guarantee a histologically standardized graft. Inter- and intraindividual variations in skin thickness, which is dependent on age, gender, and constitution, as well as possibly medication (e.g., glucocorticoids), require some routine in skin grafting to choose the ideal graft for a defect or scar correction. In most of the literature, full-thickness grafts are preferred for palmar hand defects, and split-thickness grafts are preferred for defects on the arm and the dorsum of the hand. It can be generally stated that the thinner the graft, the better the take of the graft, but the higher the incidence of resulting graft contracture.

Graft healing proceeds through a series of stages that are unique to skin grafting. The first 24 hours are called *plasmatic imbibition* (43). During these hours, the graft is attached by fibrin to the wound bed and takes up wound exudate, gaining up to 40% of its weight. This prevents drying out and keeps the vessels inside the graft open. Eventually, the fibrin is replaced by granulation tissue, and revascularization proceeds. The first "neovessels" are formed within 72 hours [inosculation (44)]. Subsequently, vascular proliferation occurs in the graft and its bed. Full circulation is restored to the graft within 4 to 7 days (45). Restoration of lymphatic vessels parallels restoration of the vascular supply during the first week; reinnervation may start as early as 2 to 4 weeks after grafting, although full sensation is usually not achieved. Epidermal proliferation and hyperplasia are seen on and after the fourth postoperative day and persist for weeks (45).

Even after the blood supply has been reestablished, many factors can still interfere with graft take. The graft is vulnerable to infection, shear forces, and ischemic periods (e.g., through cigarette smoking), so that meticulous care and control are needed, and the graft has to be protected from mechanical forces for another 1 to 3 weeks, until secure graft take and healing are secured. Especially in full-thickness grafts in the hand, shear forces may disrupt the vulnerable neovascularization, may lead to hematoma, and may cause secondary graft loss. A careful balance has to be maintained between graft protection and urgently indicated physical therapy during this time, and only experienced physical therapists should be trusted with this task.

Operative Technique

Preparation of the Wound Bed

To guarantee secure graft take, the wound bed has to be clean, free of residual necroses, and well vascularized. This applies for burn wounds, as well as for traumatic defects. In burn wounds, skin defects predominantly result from tangential or epifascial burn eschar excision. If the excision is performed down to layers of healthy, well-perfused tissues, skin grafting can be performed immediately after meticulous hemostasis.

In trauma defects, wound conditioning is sometimes required when tissue of questionable viability remains in the wound or when perfusion disturbances occur after severe contusion or avulsion injuries or in débrided, infected areas. Contamination should be avoided, and, in case of infection, the wound has to be topically treated before grafting is considered. It has been shown that bacterial counts of more than 10^6 per gram of wet weight lead almost inevitably to graft loss. Topical treatment may consist in soaking the wound with antiseptic solutions, topical antibacterial creams, or repeated surgical débridement.

Conditioning the wound to promote growth of granulation tissue can be achieved with moist dressings, frequent rinsing, mechanical débridement of the wound, temporary wound closure with xenograft or allograft, and the application of intermittent or constant vacuum over polyurethane foam dressing in a hermetically sealed wound. It has been shown that application of *vacuum-assisted closure* generates granulation tissue, reduces bacterial contamination, and enhances the vascularity of the wound bed. However, this technique should be used solely for wound preparation over a short period of time, before definitive closure is achieved. Prolonged application over tendons, joints, or bony surfaces leads to significant stiffness of the joints and severely limited tendon excursion.

Donor Site Choice

The selection of the donor site is essential to achieve the best possible results. The closer the donor site is to the defect, the better the color and texture match. However, there are only limited sites for full-thickness grafts in the upper extremity. The upper inner arm usually has excess skin that can be used for full-thickness grafts; the elbow crease is another possible site, but it has the potential risk of scar contracture. The area between *rascetta* and *restricta* at the wrist can be used as a donor site for finger defects. However, incisions at the volar aspect of the wrist should only be considered in rare cases, because patients have reported that they have been suspected of attempted suicide when their environment registered the scars. The ulnar side of the hypothenar has recently been described as a donor site for palmar defects of the hand (46). Patients in general prefer donor sites at which scars can be hidden, such as under a watchband or a T-shirt. This needs to be discussed before surgery.

For split-thickness grafts, in general, convex areas of the body are easier to harvest than concave areas. Depending on the size of the defect, the thighs or upper arms may be used (Fig. 6). Bony prominences have to be avoided, as do areas that overlie bone or tendon (e.g., anterior tibial crest, Achilles tendon, radial head). The lower arms and legs should be avoided as donor sites because of unsightly pigment disturbances and delayed healing. The back and the scalp are excellent donor sites for split-thickness grafts. The back skin is thick, and the donor site can usually be concealed with clothing. The scalp is a perfect donor site, because there remains no visible scar, the hair growth is usually not affected, and the dermis contains a large number of hair follicles, so that healing is accelerated. Disadvantages are the limited accessibility when the patient is in the supine position (back skin) and the necessity for general anesthesia. When performing a reconstructive procedure on one hand, it may be much more practical to use the

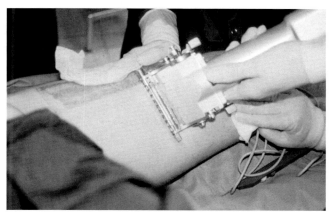

FIGURE 6. Harvesting a split-thickness skin graft from the anterolateral thigh with a dermatome.

same arm as a donor site for skin grafts, regardless of possible advantages of other areas. However, cosmetic appearance is of increasing importance, so that, especially in young women or children, the donor sites should be as inconspicuous as possible.

Difficult donor sites can be prepared by injection of large volumes of sterile saline solution. Blood loss can be limited by injecting epinephrine in saline $1:10^6$, and the authors have had excellent experience with adding a long-lasting local anesthetic for postoperative pain control.

After the donor site has been chosen and prepped, the skin is lubricated (with mineral oil, Vaseline, or saline), and the graft of the desired thickness is harvested. For small grafts, a Weck knife can be used; larger grafts are more evenly cut with a dermatome. When using a dermatome, it is important to pay special attention, before every use, to the adjusted thickness, the fixation of the blade, and the correct width of the graft, so that the graft does not inadvertently turn into a full-thickness graft or a narrow or disrupted graft. Particularly in children and people with atrophic skin, this is of utmost importance. The thickness of the graft can also be altered by the pressure that is applied to the instrument while cutting.

Once the graft has been taken, local epinephrine is applied for hemostasis, and a dressing is chosen. Because there are hundreds of dressings available for fresh donor sites, and every user swears by his or her preferred dressing, the authors only mention the basic principles of dressing use here. There are nonadhesive dressings, which are based on Vaseline gauze and silicone films; tanning and air drying have been used, as well as hydrogels. In general, it is essential for rapid healing to maintain a moist and clean environment. Healing does not occur if the wound becomes infected or if the newly epithelialized surface is disrupted by a dressing change every other day. According to these principles, the authors use a Vaseline gauze that is soaked with scarlet red, which has bactericidal properties. The dressing is left in place until it can be peeled off easily after healing has occurred (10 to 14 days). The gauze allows secretions from the wound to drain into the overlying dressing material. Our experience with silicone film has not been as satisfactory, because fluid collects frequently underneath the film, which may prompt superinfection.

When preparing the graft for transplantation, it is important to keep it moist, but soaking in saline should be avoided. The saline may be absorbed, and the keratinocytes swell and burst. Split-thickness grafts can be prepared as sheet grafts, for example, in digital defects, or as mesh grafts, when larger surface areas have to be covered. It is recommended to punch little draining holes into a sheet graft by using a no. 11 blade to facilitate drainage of wound fluid. The graft can be secured with sutures or staples. A tie-over bolster dressing is applied over multilayered gauze to generate a moist environment with some pressure. Control for graft take is usually performed on the fifth day posttransplantation. In case of suspected infection or hematoma, a dressing change has to be scheduled earlier.

Full-thickness graft donor sites are usually closed primarily. Secondary split-thickness transplantation for donor site coverage should be avoided whenever possible. The graft is then defatted until the dermis with the skin appendices is clearly visible (Fig. 7). This can be done by extending the graft over one finger of the surgeon to create a convex surface or wrapping it around one of the cylindrical containers for needles on the operating room table. The graft is harvested a little smaller than the defect. This allows suturing of the graft under slight tension, so that it nicely adheres to the underlying wound bed. This creates slight pressure for better hemostasis and better contact with the wound bed. Full-thickness grafts have higher metabolic demands than split-thickness grafts. Therefore, meticulous hemostasis is mandatory in full-thickness grafts. Accumulation of fluid prevents adhesion of the graft and leads to impaired neovascularization and subsequent graft loss.

The graft should also be perforated with a no. 11 blade for fluid drainage. Fixation is usually performed with sutures to guarantee a perfect fit. Skin staples, fibrin glue, and OpSite spray (Smith & Nephew, London) have been

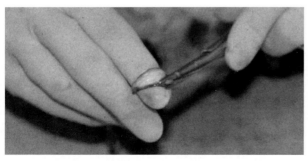

FIGURE 7. An elliptical full-thickness skin graft is defatted with scissors before placement on the recipient site.

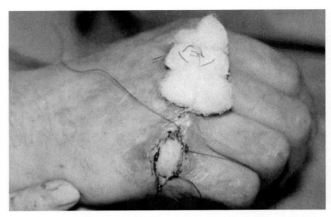

FIGURE 8. Full-thickness skin grafts are secured with peripheral sutures to the recipient site. Compression is achieved with the application of cotton bolsters.

suggested as alternatives or adjunctives to suture. A tie-over bolster dressing over multiple gauze layers is then applied (Fig. 8). Immobilization is indicated to secure graft take for 5 days until the first dressing change. Depending on the clinical appearance, immobilization may be prolonged if a secure graft take has not yet occurred.

Postoperative Care

Although early mobilization is the key principle in most reconstructive procedures in the upper extremity, skin grafts require immobilization of the involved segments until the graft has securely healed. To minimize additional functional loss, the best possible positions have to be selected. For the hand, this means the so-called intrinsic plus position, that is, the wrist extended to 30 degrees, metacarpophalangeal joints flexed to 90 degrees, and the proximal interphalangeal and distal interphalangeal joints fully extended. This position leads to minimal ligamentous shrinking and joint stiffness. However, to gain maximum skin length after grafting, a fist position has been recommended for 7 to 9 days (47).

The wrist is best immobilized in 30 degrees of extension; the elbow is best immobilized in 70 degrees of extension. Rarely, adjacent joints have to be immobilized, so that physical therapy is immediately initiated in all joints that do not require immobilization. Physical therapy of the grafted areas is usually started after 5 days, when the take of the graft is secure. This applies for traumatic defects, as well as for burn defects. Applications of stress and shear forces have to be avoided during this period until 2 to 3 weeks posttransplantation, when they cannot lead to graft disruption. After complete graft healing, it is recommended to keep the grafted area supple by application of moisturizing creams. Pressure garments are frequently indicated to prevent scar hypertrophy. Alternatives and adjunctive methods are external application of silicone films, silicone cream, or silicone gel sheets (13).

Complications

Complications of Skin Expansion

In discussing a certain operative plan with the authors' patients, the authors have to be aware and to talk about the most common complications in detail. The complication rate with tissue expansion is reported in the literature to be between 10% and 50%, depending on the location and indication (18,22,24,48–50). All studies report a steep learning curve, with the complication rate significantly dropping with the experience of the surgeon. Strict antisepsis and minimal handling of the devices, as well as the tissues, seem to be important factors in the prevention of infection. There are certain conditions and age groups in which tissue expansion appears to be especially difficult. For the correction of burn sequelae, a higher than usual complication rate has been reported; likewise, a higher complication rate has been reported for preschool- to adolescent-age children.

Hematoma is reported to be an infrequent event with expander placement. It can be prevented by placing it in the interfascial plane, with meticulous hemostasis and placement of drains for 1 to 3 days. Further complications include infection, extrusion, damage to the expander, insufficient skin gain, and aesthetically disadvantageous scar placement (with the scar producing another functional deficit).

Complications of Skin Grafting

Complications include complications of the graft and of the donor sites. Loss, or partial loss, of the graft can be caused by infection, mechanical shear forces, or collection of fluids (51,52). There are no studies in the literature that describe the incidence of graft loss. If the wound bed is prepared according to the criteria mentioned previously, the graft is protected from shear forces, the incidence of massive infections is low, the patient doesn't smoke, and no other factors that could interfere with normal wound healing are present, graft take may be expected to reach 100%. Because of the multiple factors that influence the healing of skin grafts, it is difficult to assess a definitive complication rate.

Donor site problems are usually caused by superinfection or by excessively deep graft harvesting due to too much pressure or wrong settings on the dermatome. Pain can become a problem if grafts have been harvested from areas such as the back or buttocks.

Late complications of skin grafting include graft contractures, keloid formation, hypertrophic scarring, and unstable scars with the potential for the development of Marjolin's ulcer.

Treatment of Complications

Control of the complications is an essential part of successful surgery. Many complications, such as inflammatory reactions in tissue expansion or beginning graft infections, can be controlled by proper conservative management. Immobilization of the affected area for a few days, oral antibiotics, and anti-inflammatory drugs may be indicated. If complications in graft take are suspected, early dressing change is recommended. Thereafter, fluid accumulation can be evacuated, superinfection can be treated topically with a diluted iodine preparation, mafenide acetate, or silver nitrate, and nonadhering parts can be excised. These measures can salvage many grafts from complete loss. Donor site complications are also treated by local wound care, and, in the case of nonhealing donor sites, they may have to be overgrafted with thin partial-thickness skin grafts themselves.

Severe complications, such as expander extrusion or complete graft loss, need retreat strategies. In the case of extrusion of the expander, removal of the expander and usage of the already-gained expanded skin for limited correction is appropriate. The expander pocket can be left in place, including its capsule. After an interval of 3 to 6 months, a new expander can be reinserted, and expansion is started over again.

A defect expander is removed, the pocket is rinsed with saline and antiseptic solutions, and a new expander is inserted. In some instances, a leakage has occurred at the connection between the port and the tubing to the expander. The authors routinely place a suture around the connecting part for extra safety. Leakage has also been reported from the port itself. Repeated puncture with large bore needles may cause a permanent opening in the puncture membrane. This can be avoided only by using sharp small bore needles (22 gauge) (28). In the case of pocket infection, removal of the expander and rinsing of the pocket often suffice to primarily solve the problem. After an interval of 3 to 6 months, the insertion of another expander can be attempted with acceptable risk. Careful and compassionate guiding of the patient during this period is of utmost importance to maintain the patient's compliance.

In the case of graft loss, the treatment options are usually straightforward. Conservative or surgical débridement of the wound bed, cleansing and reduction of bacterial contamination, generation of a well-vascularized wound bed, prevention of hypergranulation, and regrafting are the essential steps. In rare cases, alternative treatment options like Integra artificial skin (Integra LifeSciences, Plainsboro, NJ) or foam suction dressing may be used to treat complications of skin grafting and tissue expansion. They can be used to help create a granulating wound bed or to cover untransplantable tissues, such as tendons and bone, in case there are no alternatives (e.g., in burn patients, cases of necrotizing fasciitis, or severe peripheral vascular disease, which precludes free flap coverage) (Fig. 9). As already mentioned previously, patient guidance is important in these situations.

Hypertrophic scar management can become a challenge during follow-up of patients who received skin grafts, as

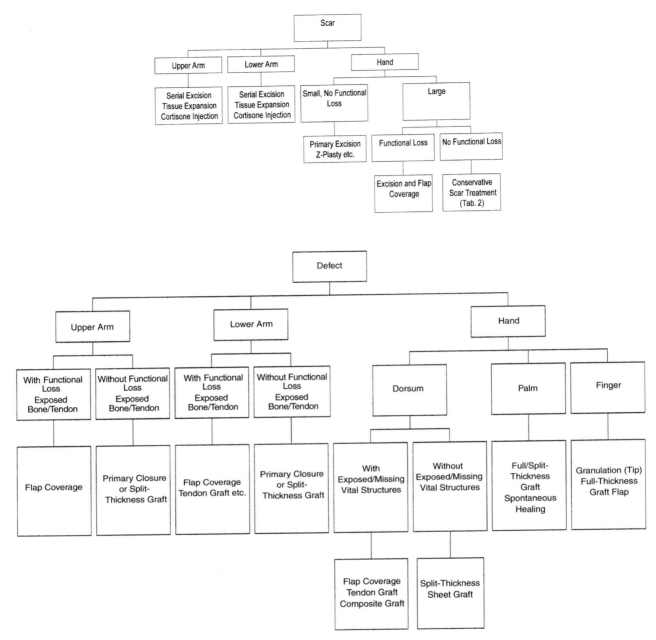

FIGURE 9. Algorithm for the treatment of scar tissue.

well as scar contracture, which may require secondary reconstruction. The whole repertoire of plastic and reconstructive procedure options may be required, from Z-plasty and glucocorticoid injections, to local and distant flap coverage, to free tissue transfer.

Prevention of Complications

Most of the complications of skin grafting can be avoided by proper selection of the donor site, such as the back as opposed to the lower leg in elderly patients and the scalp as opposed to the extremities in children to avoid hypertrophy of the donor site; selection of the right thickness of graft; and proper preparation of the wound bed. A bacterial count of 10^5 or greater always causes major graft infection and has to be reduced before grafting (51). Obviously, sterile technique is of utmost importance, and the graft should be touched as little as possible (41).

After grafting, the area has to be immobilized for at least 5 to 7 days, depending on the age of the patient and the area grafted (47). Joints and pressure points need longer protection from shear forces. In children, it has proven advantageous to immobilize the whole extremity rather than just one joint or to use tie-over dressings. In elderly patients, it may speed healing time to apply continuous suction dressing over the graft for 5 to 10 days. If there is any suspicion of contamination of the grafted area, early dressing change and wet soaks with antiseptic solution (e.g., Lavasept, mafenide acetate) may prevent graft loss. Unstable scarring may be prevented by using a slightly thicker graft, provided that there is sufficient donor site.

To prevent complications of tissue expansion in the upper extremity, the aseptic technique should be used when placing the expander and when filling it. Care should be taken not to overexpand the balloon. This is recognized by prolonged blanching of the skin that overlies the expander, and it may cause necrosis and subsequent extrusion of the device. If at all possible, a healthy area of skin should be selected for expansion. For successful tissue expansion, proper and careful planning of incisions and expected tissue gain is essential. Even if premature removal becomes necessary, a good final result can still be achieved in 90% of cases via a repeated expansion. In general, complication rates are higher in burn patients and children of certain ages (48). Careful monitoring and extensive preoperative counseling of patients and their parents are paramount for success.

REFERENCES

1. Gray H, Williams PL, et al., eds. *Gray's anatomy,* 37th ed. Edinburgh: Churchill Livingstone, 1989.
2. Green DP, Hotchkiss RN, Pederson WC. *Green's operative hand surgery,* 4 ed. Edinburgh: Churchill Livingstone, 1999.
3. Kahle W. *Atlas der Anatomie,* band 3. 1978.
4. Pansky B. *Review of gross anatomy.* New York: Collier Macmillan, 1984.
5. Schmidt HM, Lanz U. *Chirurgische Anatomie der Hand.* 1992.
6. Germann G, Sherman R, Levin LS. *Decision-making in reconstructive surgery: upper extremity.* Springer-Verlag, 2000.
7. Ratner D. Skin grafting. *Dermatol Clin* 1998;16:75–90.
8. Hunt TK, Pai MP. The effect of varying ambient oxygen tensions on wound metabolism and collagen synthesis. *Surg Gynecol Obstet* 1972;153:561–567.
9. Forrester JC. Wound healing. *J R Soc Med* 1982;75:820–823.
10. Hunt TK. Basic principles of wound healing. *J Trauma* 1990;30:122.
11. Levin LS, Germann G. Local flap coverage about the hand. *Atlas Hand Clin* 1998;3:2.
12. Agbenorku P. Triple keloid therapy: a combination of steroids, surgery and silicone gel strip/sheet for keloid treatment. *Eur J Plast Surg* 2000;23:150–151.
13. Robson MC, Barnett RA, Leitch IO, et al. Prevention and treatment of postburn scars and contracture. *World J Surg* 1992;16:87–96.
14. Hahn SB, Kim DJ, Jeon CH. Clinical study of Marjolin's ulcer. *Yonsei Med J* 1990;31:234–241.
15. Martin C, Gonzales del Pino J. Controversies in the treatment of fingertip amputations. *Clin Orthop* 1998:63–73.
16. Neumann CG. The expansion of an area of skin by progressive distension of a subcutaneous balloon. *Plast Reconstr Surg* 1957;19:124.
17. American Society of Plastic and Reconstructive Surgeons. *Adjacent flap development using an expandable Silastic implant.* 1976.
18. Aubert JP, Paulhe P, Magalon G. Forum: l'expansion tissulaire. L'expansion cutanee au membre superieur. *Ann Chir Plast Esthet* 1993;38:34–40.
19. Favarger N, Deglise B, Krupp S. Tissue expansion in children. *Z Kinderchir* 1988;43:220–221.
20. Gibstein LA, Abramson DL, Bartlett RA, et al. Tissue expansion in children: a retrospective study of complications. *Ann Plast Surg* 1997;38:358–364.
21. Hagerty RC, Zubowitz VN. Tissue expansion in the treatment of hypertrophic scars and scar contractures. *South Med J* 1986;79:432–436.
22. Iconomou TG, Michelow BJ, Zuker RM. Tissue expansion in the pediatric patient. *Ann Plast Surg* 1993;31:134–140.
23. Sharpe DT, Burd RM. Tissue expansion in perspective. *Ann R Coll Surg Engl* 1989;71:175–181.
24. Youm T, Margiotta M, Kasabian A, et al. Complications of tissue expansion in a public hospital. *Ann Plast Surg* 1999;42:396–401.
25. Casanova D, Bardot J, Magalon G. Quoi de neuf dans l'expansion cutanee au membre superieur? *Ann Chir Plast Esthet* 1998;43:618–620.
26. Meland NB, Smith AA, Johnson CH. Tissue expansion in the upper extremities. *Hand Clin* 1997;13:303–314.
27. Morgan RF, Edgerton MT. Tissue expansion in reconstructive hand surgery: case report. *J Hand Surg* 1985;10:754–757.
28. Van BA, Adson MH. Tissue expansion in the upper extremity. *Clin Plast Surg* 1987;14:535–542.
29. Ashmead D, Smith PJ. Tissue expansion for Apert's syndactyly. *J Hand Surg* 1995;20:327–330.
30. d'Arcangelo M, Maffulli N. Tissue expanders in syndactyly: a brief review. *Acta Chir Plast* 1996;38:11–13.
31. Fernandez-Villoria JM, Abad MJ. Tissue expansion for thumb and first web space reconstruction. *J Hand Surg* 1994;19:663–664.
32. Ogawa Y, Kasai K, Doi H, et al. The preoperative use of extra-tissue expander for syndactyly. *Ann Plast Surg* 1989;23:552–559.
33. Levin LS, Rehnke R, Eubanks S. Endoscopic surgery of the upper extremity. *Hand Clin* 1995;11:59–70.
34. Meland NB, Loessin SJ, Thimsen D, et al. Tissue expansion in the extremities using external reservoirs. *Ann Plast Surg* 1992;29:36–39.
35. Schmelzeisen R, Schimming R, Schwipper V, et al. Influence of tissue expanders on the growing craniofacial skeleton. *J Craniomaxillofac Surg* 1999;27:153–159.
36. Levin LS, Rehnke R, Eubanks S. Endoscopy of the upper extremity. *Hand Clin* 2001;11:59–70.
37. Ammon FA, Baumgarten M. *Die plastische Chirurgienach ihren bisherigen Leistungen.* Berlin: G. Reimer, 1842.
38. Dieffenbach JF. *Die operative Chirurgie.* 1845.
39. Reverdin JL. Greffe epidermique. *Bull Soc Imp Chir* 1869;10:493–511.
40. Rogers BO. Historical development of free skin grafting. *Surg Clin North Am* 1959;39:289–311.
41. Krause F. Über die Transplantation grosser ungestielter Hautlappen. *Verh Dtsch Ges Chir* 1893;22:46–51.

42. Wolfe JR. A new method of performing plastic operations. *Br Med J* 1875;2:360–361.

43. Converse JM, Uhlschmid CK, Ballantyne DL. "Plasmatic circulation" in skin grafts. *Plast Reconstr Surg* 1969; 43:495.

44. Converse JM, Smahel J, Ballantyne DL, et al. Inosculation of vessels of skin graft and host bed: a fortuitous encounter. *Br J Plast Surg* 1975;28:274.

45. Smahel J. The healing of skin grafts. *Clin Plast Surg* 1977;4:409–424.

46. Park S, Hata Y, Ito O, et al. Full thickness skin graft from the ulnar aspect of the wrist to cover defects on the hand. *Ann Plast Surg* 1999;42:129–131.

47. Burm JS, Chung CH, Oh SJ. Fist position for skin grafting on the dorsal hand: I. Analysis of length of the dorsal hand surgery in hand positions. *Plast Reconstr Surg* 1999;104:1350–1355.

48. Elias DL, Baird WL, Zubowicz VN. Applications and complications of tissue expansion in pediatric patients. *J Pediatr Surg* 1991;26:15–21.

49. Governa M, Bonolani A, Beghini D, et al. Skin expansion in burn sequelae: results and complications. *Acta Chir Plast* 1996;38:147–153.

50. Neale HW, High RM, Billmire DA, et al. Complications of controlled tissue expansion in the pediatric burn patient. *Plast Reconstr Surg* 1988;82:840–848.

51. Bacchetta CA, Magee W, Rodeheaver G, et al. Biology of infections of split thickness skin grafts. *Am J Surg* 1975;130:63–67.

52. Browne EZ. Complications of skin grafts and pedicle flaps. *Hand Clin* 1986;2:353–359.

66

SKIN AND SOFT TISSUE: PEDICLED FLAPS

STEVEN L. MORAN
CRAIG H. JOHNSON

Without adequate soft tissue coverage, even the most elegant hand reconstruction is destined for failure. Stable soft tissue coverage is a cornerstone for successful hand reconstruction, allowing for hand mobilization and rehabilitation. Pedicled flaps play a critical role in providing this soft tissue coverage. Since the 1970s, there have been several advancements in the understanding of the vascular anatomy of the upper extremity, and the hand surgeon is now able to choose from an array of pedicled flaps for wound reconstruction. Many of these flaps can provide vascularized tendon and bone, thus allowing the surgeon to reconstruct complex tissue deficits.

WHAT IS A PEDICLED FLAP?

A flap is a unit of skin and other tissue that maintains its own circulation while being transferred from its donor site to the injured area. A pedicled flap is dependent on its arterial and venous leash for survival. A skin graft, in comparison, does not bring its own blood supply, and its survival is dependent on the vascularity of the recipient site. Each artery within the upper extremity terminates in a zone of osseous, muscular, or cutaneous perforators. These perforators supply a block of tissue, which is termed an *angiosome* (1,2). Between two vascular territories, or angiosomes, there is a watershed region, which contains a system of reduced-caliber choke arteries and arterioles. The venous territories in each angiosome match the arterial territories. Where angiosomes are linked with choke arteries, the venous territories are linked by veins that are devoid of valves, which allow bidirectional flow. These have been termed the *oscillating veins*. If one angiosome is divided and elevated on its source artery, it can carry some of the adjacent angiosome with it; this occurs through the dilatation of choke vessels and venous return through the oscillating veins (3,4).

One may choose to harvest all or part of the source artery's angiosome when elevating a flap. Thus, pedicled flaps may consist of skin, fascia, muscle, or bone. Arterial inflow may pass directly to the skin, in which case the flap is termed a *cutaneous flap*, such as the groin flap. It may pass through the investing fascia, in which case the flap is termed a *fasciocutaneous flap*, such as the lateral arm flap. The artery may supply muscle first, which may be taken alone or with the overlying skin; in this case, the flap is referred to as a *myocutaneous flap*, such as a latissimus muscle flap with a skin island.

WHY USE A PEDICLED FLAP?

Pedicled flaps lie in the middle to upper portion of the classical reconstructive ladder (Fig. 1). Progressing up this ladder tends to increase the complexity of the surgical operation. The classic teaching was to use the simplest procedure to provide soft tissue coverage; however, current thinking favors proceeding directly to the procedure that provides the best reconstructive outcome. Although pedicled flaps may be a more aggressive surgical procedure than delayed closure or skin grafting, there are times when the patient's situation calls for well-vascularized, immediate coverage.

Pedicled flaps offer several advantages over skin grafts and random pattern flaps. Their axial blood supply allows for more predictable flap survival. Axial blood flow provides more resistance against bacterial inoculum (5,6). The isolation of the flap on its pedicle allows for easier positioning and insetting. Because of their proximity to the injured site, many pedicled flap procedures may be performed by using regional blocks, thus avoiding general anesthesia. In comparison to free tissue transfer, pedicled flaps avoid the need for microsurgical anastomoses and are usually less time consuming. The major disadvantages of local flaps, however, can be their limited availability, their inability to fill large or deep defects, and the detrimental effects of flap harvest on an already injured extremity.

MANAGEMENT STRATEGIES

In elective cases, a general history and examination are critical to determine the best flap options. Systemic diseases,

free tissue transfer

pedicle flaps

local random flaps

skin grafting

secondary intention

delayed primary closure

primary closure

FIGURE 1. The reconstructive ladder starts with primary closure and progresses to free tissue transfer. Progression up the ladder usually increases the complexity of the reconstruction.

such as diabetes, renal failure, and peripheral vascular disease, which may hinder wound healing and the success of free tissue transfer, should be evaluated. Medications, such as corticosteroids, which inhibit wound healing, should be noted. A careful inspection of the wound site is made to get a rough idea of tissue type and size requirements. In oncologic cases, patient examination is best done with the extirpative surgeon, so that incisions may be planned jointly. This avoids the inadvertent division of vascular pedicles.

A careful vascular examination should be performed, with direct palpation of the brachial, radial, and ulnar arteries. A hand-held Doppler can be used to assess the quality of the perfusion; triphasic signals indicate normal flow, whereas monophasic or biphasic signals herald arterial disease. If there is any question about perfusion and the availability of specific vessels, noninvasive vascular studies should be pursued. Abnormal results warrant arteriography. Contrast dye before flap procedures has not been shown to adversely effect outcome (7). Magnetic resonance imaging at many centers can also provide valuable information on vascular status if angiogram is prohibited due to renal status or dye allergies.

In the case of trauma, thorough inspection and evaluation of the wound are best done in the operating room under anesthesia. Attention is directed to the size of the defect, its location, and associated damaged structures. Tendon injury, nerve injury, and the need for vascular repair must be noted. Certain pedicled flap options may be prohibited owing to the extent of the vascular injury. The presence of exposed vital structures, such as joints, tendons, and neurovascular structures, may necessitate early or even immediate coverage.

The timing of definitive coverage, in the case of contaminated wounds, is often difficult to assess. Falling bacteria counts and an intact wound healing mechanism are heralded by the presence of granulation tissue and the absence of purulence within the wound bed. One gains a great deal of information from inspection of the dressing materials. Decreasing exudate tends to imply an improving wound milieu. There are no definite rules to determine the number of hours or days before coverage. Early soft tissue coverage, however, allows one to initiate physical therapy sooner,

which helps maintain range of motion, while decreasing edema, pain, and scarring. Many wounds, if they are not grossly contaminated or the result of high-energy trauma, can often be covered within 24 hours (8). Lister and Scheker (9) and others have recommended immediate wound closure, if possible (10,11). The success of immediate wound coverage is dependent on the ability of the surgeon to remove all nonviable and marginally viable tissue.

Although the benefits of early coverage have been clearly documented, one should not blindly rush wound closure. The unhealthy wound that is covered too soon leads to wound breakdown and possible flap loss. Caution should be exercised in cases of crush, press, or farming injuries in which the extent of devitalized tissue may not be apparent for several days (12–14). Serial débridements back to healthy tissue should be performed in the operating room at 24- to 48-hour intervals, until the wound is clean. The authors have also found whirlpool and vacuum-assisted closure dressing changes helpful in decreasing edema and increasing granulation tissue formation in preparation for definitive closure (15,16).

Only after adequate débridement can one determine the options for wound coverage. Skin grafting is an option for well-vascularized wound beds. Exposure of poorly vascularized structures, such as bone, hardware, or tendon without paratenon, certainly requires flap coverage, as skin grafts do not provide stable coverage in these situations. In addition, skin grafts become adherent to their bed. Thus, they are not appropriate in areas that require large amounts of excursion. Finally, local wound factors, such as radiation and infection, may make attempts at primary closure and skin grafting less reliable.

Postoperative requirements, such as staged reconstructive procedures, including tendon transfers or bone grafting, are facilitated with a pedicled flap, which may be reelevated easily. Pedicled flaps can provide for smooth gliding surfaces in cases of tendon reconstruction and avoid late contracture, which is often seen in primary closure or skin-grafted closures. In general, pedicled flaps are required when (a) a wound bed is unsuitable for the placement of a skin graft; (b) vital structures need protection, such as nerve, bone, or hardware; or (c) there is a requirement for subcutaneous tissue in addition to skin (17).

A back-up plan also needs to be formulated, should the primary reconstruction not sufficiently work or fail completely. The time to formulate this back-up plan is preoperatively. This avoids erroneous placement of incisions and ligation of branches that may preclude the future use of other flaps.

ANATOMY

The proper use and selection of upper extremity pedicled flaps is predicated on a thorough understanding of the vascular anat-

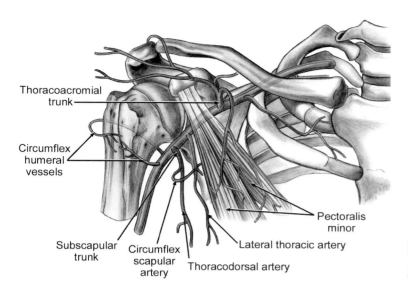

Thoracoacromial trunk

Circumflex humeral vessels

Subscapular trunk

Circumflex scapular artery

Thoracodorsal artery

Lateral thoracic artery

Pectoralis minor

FIGURE 2. The axillary artery is divided into three portions, based on the course of the pectoralis minor. The proximal portion contains the thoracoacromial trunk; the distal segment contains the subscapular trunk.

omy of the upper extremity. Most axial and pedicled flaps use a major arterial branch with its surrounding soft tissue. There can be significant variation in the arm's arterial anatomy. Familiarity with major arterial variants is crucial for flap design and modification, should variations appear intraoperatively (18).

Starting in the axilla, the axillary artery begins at the outer border of the first rib. The axillary artery is divided into three major portions in relation to the course of the pectoralis minor. It has proximal, posterior, and distal segments. The proximal portion contains the thoracoacromial trunk and the superior thoracic artery (Fig. 2). The thoracoacromial trunk provides arterial flow to the pectoralis major, the pectoralis minor, and the deltoid. Beyond the pectoralis minor, the axillary artery gives off the subscapular trunk, in addition to the lateral thoracic artery. The subscapular trunk terminates in the circumflex scapular vessels and the thoracodorsal vessels. The circumflex scapular vessels provide flow to the parascapular flap and the subscapular flaps, which can provide pedicle coverage for the axilla and shoulder. The thoracodorsal vessel provides the vascular inflow to the latissimus dorsi and the serratus anterior muscle. The latissimus may be pedicled on the thoracodorsal vessels to provide arm and shoulder coverage.

The axillary artery turns into the brachial artery at the lower border of the teres major. The deep brachial artery leaves the brachial artery to course with the radial nerve in the upper one-third of the humerus. The deep brachial artery branches into the medial collateral and radial collateral arteries. The medial collateral artery runs with the triceps and is a major pedicle for the anconeus muscle flap. Distally, this artery connects with the recurrent posterior interosseous artery (PIA) (19). The radial collateral artery terminates in an anterior and posterior branch. The anterior branch accompanies the radial nerve between the brachialis and the brachioradialis, whereas the posterior radial collateral branch enters the intermuscular septum between

the brachioradialis and the triceps. This artery provides perforators to the lower lateral skin of the arm and is the arterial inflow for the lateral arm flap (Fig. 3). The superior ulnar collateral artery arises from the brachial artery, below

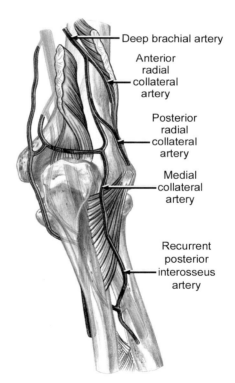

Deep brachial artery

Anterior radial collateral artery

Posterior radial collateral artery

Medial collateral artery

Recurrent posterior interosseus artery

FIGURE 3. Diagram of the course of the radial collateral artery and the medial collateral artery in the arm. The anterior radial collateral artery follows the radial nerve between the brachialis and brachioradialis, whereas the posterior radial collateral branch enters the intermuscular septum between the brachioradialis and triceps. The medial collateral artery travels with the triceps to the forearm, where it anastomoses with the recurrent posterior interosseous artery.

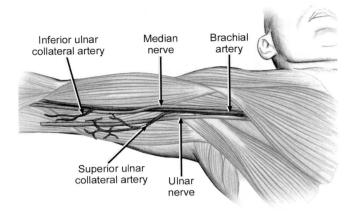

FIGURE 4. The superior ulnar collateral artery follows the course of the ulnar nerve in the upper arm.

the middle of the humerus. It then follows the ulnar nerve to the level of the lower humerus, supplying perforators to the medial arm, and is the source vessel for the medial arm flap (20,21) (Fig. 4).

At the level of the elbow, the brachial artery divides into the radial and ulnar arteries. The radial artery, after leaving the brachial artery, runs between the brachioradialis and the flexor carpi radialis. Cutaneous perforators to the overlying skin continue within the intermuscular septum and run between the two muscles (Fig. 5). Through these perforators, the artery supplies most of the palmar skin of the forearm. In addition, the radial artery provides multiple nutrient branches to the metaphyseal and diaphyseal portion of the distal radius. Variations in radial arterial anatomy are abundant. A common anomaly is a supracondylar takeoff of the radial artery (22). In a series of 750 adult cadaver arms, the origin of the radial artery was found to be in the upper arm in 14% of specimens (23). Reports have also described no radial artery in the presence of a dominant median artery, in addition to pure ulnar dominant cutaneous perforators to the forearm (24–27). Variations in arterial formation may be associated with significantly different angiosomal distributions to the muscles and overlying skin; one should exercise caution in raising radial forearm flaps, if such anomalies are encountered (22).

The ulnar artery at its origin gives off the common interosseous artery. Following this, the ulnar artery continues into the forearm between the flexor carpi ulnaris (FCU) and flexor digitorum superficialis. Cutaneous perforators are found within the septum between the flexor digitorum superficialis and FCU (28). Two to 6 cm proximal to the pisiform, a dorsal ulnar artery leaves the main trunk and runs beneath the FCU tendon. This artery gives off several branches: one supplies the dorsal ulnar skin of the forearm, one joins the dorsal carpal arch, one goes to the pisiform, and one is the muscular pedicle for the FCU. The ulnar dorsal cutaneous branch allows one

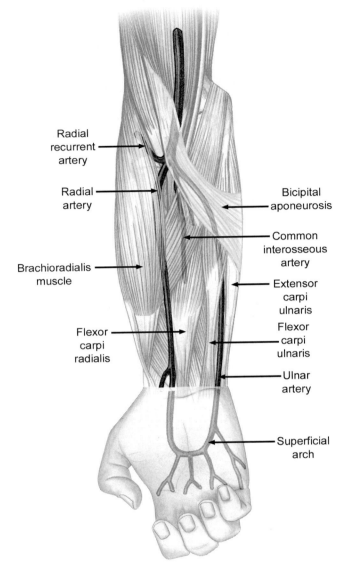

FIGURE 5. Diagram of the arterial anatomy of the forearm. Note the large arterial circuit that is formed between the ulnar and radial arteries and the posterior and anterior interosseous arteries. The radial artery travels between the brachioradialis and the flexor carpi radialis, whereas the ulnar artery travels between the flexor carpi ulnaris and extensor carpi ulnaris.

to harvest an ulnar-sided fasciocutaneous flap without sacrifice of the ulnar artery (29–31).

After leaving the ulnar artery, the common interosseous artery divides into the anterior and posterior interosseous arteries. These arteries then run on either side of the interosseous membrane with their corresponding nerves. These arteries, in most patients, form a loop through their common origin and distal anastomosis (32). There are some cases in which this anastomosis is not present, which possibly contributes to the unfavorable results that are seen with the retrograde posterior interosseous (PIO) flap (33,34). The anterior interosseous artery supplies the skin on the extensor surface of the distal one-third of the forearm (28,35). The anterior interosseous artery divides into two terminal branches; one joins the dorsal carpal network and the other completes the arterial loop with the PIA (36). The PIA perforates the interosseous membrane approximately 6 cm distal to the lateral epicondyle. It then runs from the distal edge of the supinator in the intermuscular septum between the extensor carpi ulnaris (ECU) and extensor digiti minimi muscle bellies. Its cutaneous perforators supply the dorsal proximal two-thirds of the forearm (37,38). Although this artery is consistent in its location, there is variability in its diameter, which can result in inability to carry the overlying skin island as a pedicled flap (39).

At the level of the wrist, the arterial blood supply turns from an axial pattern to a pattern of transverse arches. There are three dorsal and three volar arterial arches, with the ulnar, radial, and anterior interosseous arteries contributing to the majority of the blood flow (Figs. 6 and 7). The PIA is a minor contributor to the arterial supply of the wrist (36). These carpal arterial arches are the basis for many described pedicled vascularized bone flaps (40–43). In addition, the volar arterial arches allow for the use of the pronator quadratus as a pedicled muscle flap. The pronator quadratus may be pedicled on its ulnar or radial contributions or on the anterior interosseus artery.

Distal to the wrist, the major arterial supply to the dorsal and volar surfaces of the hand is through the ulnar and radial arteries. A deep and superficial arterial arch is created in the palm, with the radial artery providing the major inflow to the deep arch and the ulnar artery contributing to the superficial

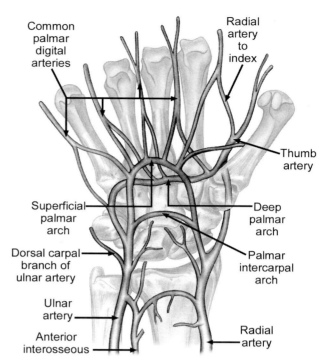

FIGURE 7. Diagram of the arterial anatomy of the palmar surface of the hand.

arch. There has been some disagreement regarding each artery's contribution to the blood supply of specific digits (44–46). Within the palm, the superficial arch gives rise to the common digital arteries. These, in turn, divide into the proper digital arteries at the level of the web space. Just proximal to the web space, the common digital artery is joined by a branch from the dorsal and palmar metacarpal arteries. The dorsal metacarpal arteries' connections with the volar blood supply allow the dorsal metacarpal arteries to be used in a retrograde fashion for the design of pedicled flaps for coverage about the fingers (36). The palmar and dorsal metacarpal arteries communicate through anastomosis at the level of the metacarpal base neck and head (36,47). The four dorsal metacarpal arteries may run deep or superficial to the interosseous fascia. These arteries supply the dorsal skin over the proximal phalanx and at the level of the web space, in addition to providing perforators to the extensor tendons and metacarpals (48–51). The dorsal metacarpal arteries divide into two dorsal digital arteries at the level of the metacarpal heads. These arteries run down the ulnar and radial aspects of the finger to the level of the middle phalanx, where they contribute to the subdermal plexus and anastomose with dorsal branches of the proper palmar digital artery (52). Strauch believes that the proximal interphalangeal (PIP) joint is the level at which the major anastomoses exist between the dorsal and volar digital blood supplies (53). The dorsal arterial anatomy provides an abundant and reliable source of pedicled tissue. The perfusion to the dorsum of the thumb is supplied by the dorsal artery, which perfuses to the level of the inter-

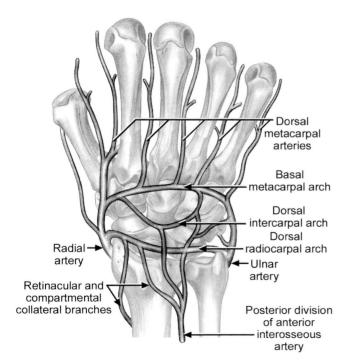

FIGURE 6. Diagram of the arterial anatomy of the dorsum of the hand.

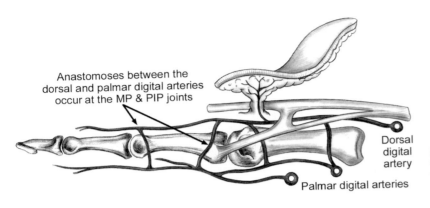

Anastomoses between the
dorsal and palmar digital arteries
occur at the MP & PIP joints

Dorsal
digital
artery

Palmar digital arteries

FIGURE 8. Anastomoses between the palmar digital arterial system and the dorsal digital arterial system occur at the level of the metacarpophalangeal (MP) and proximal interphalangeal (PIP) joints.

phalangeal (IP) joint (54) (Fig. 8). Anastomoses between the radial and ulnar digital arteries are seen as transverse aches at the volar base and neck of each phalanx. The vincular vessels stem from these transverse arches (36,53).

The hand's venous system is arranged in a series of sagittal and transverse aches that allow for the drainage of blood, generally from palm to the dorsum of the hand and from superficial to deep. There are three venous systems within the hand. The first is the superficial epifascial system, which consists of the cephalic and basilic veins with their interconnections. The second is the deep system, which encompasses the paired venous comitantes that runs with the major arteries within the hand and forearm (55–57). Often, there is no venous comitantes with the digital artery distal to the PIP joint. Finally, there are a series of perforating veins that connect the deep and superficial venous system (58). Valves have been identified in veins with a caliber of at least 0.2 mm (36). The valves within the communicating system are unicuspid in nature and may be less consistent in position, allowing for some retrograde flow (59–61).

The capability of the venous system to allow for retrograde flow allows the hand surgeon to use many pedicled flaps in a retrograde fashion, such as the radial arm flap and the PIO flap. Several authors have studied the mechanism that permits retrograde venous flow. Initially, it was believed that small bridging veins that were found between the venous comitantes allowed blood to bypass the valves within the deep venous system (59). Timmons (62) later found that a component of retrograde flow was due to the denervation of the veins during flap dissection. Torii et al. (63) have also shown than there is reflux through the valves due to valvular incompetence, which results from increased venous back-pressure. Thus, it appears that retrograde venous flow is due to several factors, but the important points to emphasize are that increased venous back-pressure overcomes valvular competence in the deep and communicating venous systems and that the denervation of veins during dissection decreases sympathetic tone, which contributes to venous incompetence (64).

With this arterial roadmap, the authors now examine those pedicled muscle and fasciocutaneous flaps that have stood the

test of time for hand and wrist coverage. Because pedicled flaps are tethered to a fixed point on the extremity, coverage options are largely considered on the basis of location on the arm, forearm, and hand. We subdivide coverage options into four categories: the axilla and the upper arm, the elbow, the forearm and the wrist, and the hand and the fingers.

GENERAL FLAP TYPES

Muscle Flaps

Muscle pedicled flaps were originally described for closure of complicated wounds in the lower extremity by Ger (65). Muscle provides bulk for obliteration of dead space, as well as a robust blood supply that can help with the eradication of infection and the possible revascularization of ischemic bone (5,6,66,67). The benefits of muscle flaps have been shown in many types of infected wounds, including osteomyelitis and infected prosthetic grafts (68–71). In addition, muscles, such as the latissimus, can be reinserted to produce function and thus reconstruct forearm flexors, triceps, or the external rotator of the shoulder.

Mathes and Nahai described the different types of perfusion to the human muscle system (71a). Five different types of perfusion were identified in the human body and are described in reference to their vascular pedicles:

1. One major vascular pedicle
2. One dominant pedicle and one minor pedicle
3. Two dominant pedicles
4. Several segmental pedicles
5. One dominant pedicle and peripheral pedicles.

Types 1, 2, 3, and 5 lend themselves to effective creation of island flaps (72) (Fig. 9). The dominant pedicle can support the entire muscle if the other pedicles are ligated. Type 4 muscles have segmental perfusion; each arterial branch supplies a distinct and discreet part of the muscle. Type 4 muscle perfusion is quite prevalent in the upper extremity, thus limiting the number of pedicle muscle flaps that are available for use (28).

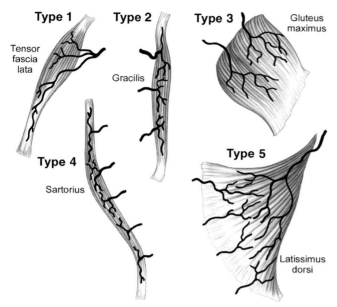

FIGURE 9. The Mathes classification of musculocutaneous flaps.

Fasciocutaneous Flaps

The major pedicled fasciocutaneous flaps of the hand and forearm are the radial forearm flap, the PIO flap, and the ulnar artery flap. These flaps all provide thin pliable coverage when muscle bulk is not required. Although the lateral arm flap has broad applicability as a free flap, its use as a pedicled flap is limited due to its short pedicle length and inconsistent survival when it is used in a retrograde fashion. Pedicled fascial flaps have been shown to increase their blood flow after transfer and can help decrease bacterial counts in wound beds, but not to the same extent as muscle flaps (67). For severely contaminated wounds, muscle flaps remain the standard coverage option.

The fasciocutaneous flaps have been classified according to their vascular patterns (73,74):

Type A: Multiple unnamed fasciocutaneous perforators enter the base of the flap. These random-pattern fasciocutaneous flaps may be based on the vascular plexus of the deep forearm fascia. The usefulness of these random fascial flaps has been shown in lower extremity reconstruction and, more recently, in upper extremity reconstruction (60,75). Lai et al. (76) described the adipofascial turnover flap for the resurfacing of dorsal wrist defects, as well as dorsal finger defects. These flaps are random in nature and follow length to width ratios of 1:1 to 1.0:1.5 but can provide coverage for exposed tendons and distal interphalangeal injuries.

Type B: These flaps are based on single fasciocutaneous perforators of large diameter. The perforators tend to have a consistent location and may be mobilized as pedicled flaps or free flaps. The antecubital forearm flap is an example. This flap is based on the inferior cubital artery (77).

Type C: These flaps have several perforators along the length of the source artery. These perforators reach the skin through a septum that runs between the muscles. Examples include the radial forearm flap.

COVERAGE BY ANATOMIC LOCATION

Axilla and Shoulder

The shoulder girdle, like the elbow, helps position the hand in space. Soft tissue coverage may be needed for exposed vital structures, soft tissue loss after tumor extirpation, or release of contractures. The two major muscle flaps that are used for coverage in this area are the latissimus dorsi and the pectoralis major. The ipsilateral latissimus dorsi muscle offers broad coverage capabilities owing to its large surface area. Its usefulness in and around the shoulder girdle, axilla, triceps region, and elbow is well documented (78–80). The length of the thoracodorsal vascular leash is typically 10 to 11 cm (81). The muscle is typically harvested via an oblique incision on the posterolateral back but can be raised endoscopically to minimize donor site morbidity (82,83). The vascular pedicle runs underneath the latissimus muscle. Flap dissection is greatly facilitated by identifying the anterior margin of the muscle at the interdigitation of the serratus muscle (Fig. 10). The lateral anterior border is then traced cephalad above the level of the nipple. Here it is easier to identify the thoracodorsal vessels. Care must be taken not to injure the teres major or posterior serratus slips during dissection, as intramuscular tethers are found in both areas. The branch that supplies the serratus anterior needs to be ligated, unless the serratus is being taken for additional bulk and coverage. The thoracodorsal artery divides into two distinct branches before entering the muscle in 94% of specimens. One branch runs 3.5 cm from the superior margin of the muscle and supplies the medial portion of the muscle. The second branch runs 2.5 cm from the lateral margin of the muscle and supplies the lateral portion. This arterial design allows the surgeon to split the muscle, should only a narrow component be required for reconstruction. Splitting the muscle also allows for preservation of neural input into either segment of muscle (84,85).

Donor site morbidity may include seroma formation and hypertrophic scarring. Some upper extremity weakness may also develop. In a series of 24 patients who underwent latissimus transfer, Russell et al. (86) found mild to moderate shoulder weakness and some loss of motion. Most patients improved over the course of several months. The authors stated that upper extremity disability in strength and shoulder motion should be anticipated after latissimus dorsi transfer. Clough et al. (87) found 13% of patients had difficulty pushing downward with a fist, 13% found it impossible to push up from a chair, and 46% had some limitation in upward mobility of the hand after pedicled myocutaneous latissimus transfer. Other studies have failed to show a clear loss of function with its use (88). The authors have found that the majority of patients have minimal postoperative weakness owing to the recruitment of synergistic muscle units; however, vigorous range-of-motion exercises after sur-

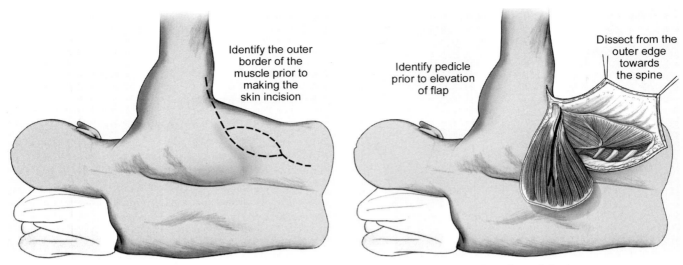

FIGURE 10. Standard incision for the latissimus dorsi flap. The muscle may be split, and the lateral aspect of the muscle may be taken for smaller defects.

gery should be encouraged to minimize adhesions and joint capsule stiffness. Caution should be exercised in using this muscle in patients who are confined to a wheelchair or who require prolonged rehabilitation on crutches.

The pectoralis major muscle flap has comparable anterior upper extremity coverage capabilities. The muscle that is pedicled on its thoracoacromial trunk can cover the shoulder girdle, axilla, and anterior arm (79,89). The latissimus and the pectoralis may be used to restore shoulder or elbow function, in addition to providing soft tissue coverage; however, the anterior hemithorax distortion and malposition of the breast and nipple after pectoralis transfer can be aesthetically unpleasant (90–93). More acceptable scars can be produced after latissimus transfer, especially if this is done with the aid of the endoscope.

The pectoralis and latissimus may be taken with skin islands; however, pure fasciocutaneous flaps may be taken from the scapular or parascapular regions (94,95). The parascapular and scapular flaps are fasciocutaneous flaps, which are supplied by the circumflex scapular artery, a branch of the subscapular system. These flaps are particularly good for resurfacing the axilla after scar contracture release (96,97). The donor site can be closed primarily, if flap orientation is planned carefully (Fig. 11).

Elbow

The elbow is covered by thin, pliable skin with minimal subcutaneous tissue. This soft tissue envelope can be compromised by fracture, septic olecranon bursitis, tumor, burns,

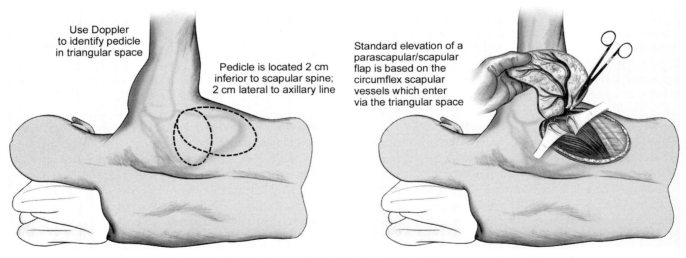

FIGURE 11. Diagram of the standard elevation technique for the parascapular and scapular flaps. These flaps are based on the circumflex scapular vessels, which enter through the back through the triangular space.

and failed extensor origin release (98). Flaps may be pedicled proximal or distal to the elbow and include muscle and fascial flaps.

Muscle options begin with the latissimus, which can be pedicled to reach the elbow. The latissimus provides the additional benefit of reconstructing lost biceps or triceps function. The latissimus has been used for biceps, triceps, and forearm flexor reconstruction with good success (90,99–103). Recently, Ihara has described the use of the latissimus to restore active finger flexion and extension in cases of brachial plexus injuries and replanted arms (104). The pectoralis has also been classically described for restoration of elbow flexion in cases of plexus injury (93).

Alternatives for muscle flap coverage of the elbow include the anconeus flap. The anconeus flap has been described for cases of recurrent olecranon bursitis and lat-

eral epicondylitis (19,105). The flap has three arterial branches: the medial collateral artery, the recurrent PIO, and a terminal branch of the radial collateral artery, which more proximally supplies the lateral arm flap (19,106). The nerve to the anconeus travels with the medial collateral artery. The muscle may be spared after open reduction and internal fixation of the elbow, if fracture exposure involves elevation of the anconeus off the ulna. This spares the proximal neurovascular pedicle and leaves the anconeus attached to the triceps. Anatomic dissection by Schmidt's group suggests that this flap can provide coverage of the radiocapitellar joint, olecranon and the distal triceps tendon when the flap is based on the medial collateral artery (19) (Fig. 12).

The brachioradialis forearm flap has also been described for use around the elbow, forearm, antecubital fossa, and lat-

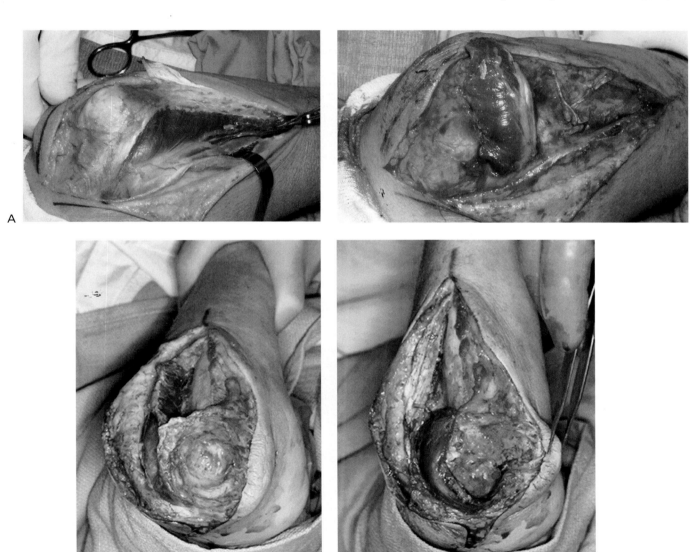

FIGURE 12. Anconeus flap that was used to treat a case of recurrent olecranon bursitis. **A:** Flap exposure. **B:** Flap elevation. **C:** Course of the medial collateral artery. **D:** Insetting with obliteration of dead space.

eral epicondyle. McGeorge et al. (107) have described it as a myocutaneous flap, whereas Lai et al. (108) and Lalikos et al. (109) have described its use as a distally based flap. In the majority of reports, it is pedicled on the radial recurrent artery (RRA) (107–111). Cadaveric studies that were performed by Sanger et al. (112) note that the major pedicle to the proximal portion of the flap may come from the brachial, the RRA, or the radial artery. Rohrich et al. (113) noted that the major vascular pedicles were located 4.2 cm proximal and 4.7 cm distal to the elbow flexion crease, with the major pedicle arising from the RRA in 58% of specimens. Sanger et al. (112) found that the dominant perforator arose from the RRA in only 33% of specimens. In this study, the dominant perforator was found to arise from the radial artery in 39% and from the brachial artery in 27% of specimens. Leversedge et al. (22) found that the RRA perfused only 41% of the length of the muscle; however, inclusion of the radial arterial perforators 3 cm immediately distal to RRA origin improved flap survival, with perfusion to more than 90% of the muscle.

Fasciocutaneous options for elbow coverage include the radial forearm flap. This is one of the most versatile flaps for upper extremity coverage. This flap has been successfully applied to many types of elbow defects (114). The ability to design orthograde and retrograde flow allows the flap to cover areas from above the elbow to the dorsum of the hand.

The radial forearm flap was described initially for hand coverage by the Chinese in 1978 and was later reported by Yang et al. in 1981 (115,116) and Song et al. in 1982 (117,129). The cutaneous territory of the radial artery extends over the radial two-thirds of the forearm (77,118). The flap may be harvested as a compound flap, including the flexor carpi radialis, the palmaris longus, and the lateral or medial antebrachial cutaneous nerves (119–123). It may also be taken with a portion of the radius, as an osteocutaneous flap (124–127). Its arc of rotation, when based proximally, is limited by the radial artery origin approximately 1 to 4 cm distal to the intracondylar line of the elbow (62,128). The maximal amount of tissue can be as much as 15 cm × 35 cm, but most defects are significantly smaller (129,130). Defects larger than 8 cm × 4 cm usually require a skin graft to cover the donor site (118,131).

The flap is elevated after an Allen's test confirms adequate distal circulation with the radial artery occluded. The course of the radial artery can be marked with the aid of a hand-held Doppler. A template of the defect can aid in flap design. The flap is made slightly larger than the defect site to prevent a tight closure. Templates that are placed more distally result in a greater area of exposed tendon at the donor site. This may result in skin graft loss if the paratenon is at all violated during flap elevation. The flap is then raised with the tourniquet inflated to the level of the flexor carpi radialis and then to the level of the brachioradialis. Alternatively, the portion of the flap margin that overlies the radial artery, closest to the wrist crease, is opened first, and the radial artery is identified. A vascular clamp

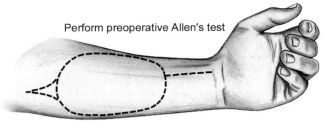

Identify and mark vessel course preoperatively

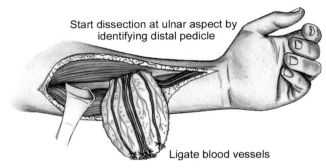

FIGURE 13. Elevation of a radial forearm flap. Epifascial dissection is carried to level of the flexor carpi radialis and the brachioradialis. Dissection is started by identification of the pedicle distally. The cephalic vein, in addition to the medial and lateral antebrachial nerves, can be included in the dissection.

may be placed on the artery, and the tourniquet can be deflated to evaluate the collateral flow to the hand. Once adequate perfusion has been confirmed, dissection may resume. Dissection preserves the radial nerve but includes the cephalic vein to aid in flap drainage. The lateral antebrachial cutaneous branch is also included within the flap. The artery may then be ligated, and flap elevation proceeds to the pivot point (Figs. 13 and 14).

There are two main disadvantages to the radial forearm flap. One is the sacrifice of the radial artery. The second is the frequent donor site complications (132,133). If the radial artery is sacrificed, and the patient has an incomplete arch, ischemia may develop in the radial fingers, particularly the thumb (134,135). Gellman et al. (45) found a 15% incidence of incomplete superficial arches in which no anastomosis was seen between the radial or ulnar arteries. However, studies from the cardiovascular literature have found that, although the superficial arch was continuous between the ulnar and radial arteries, in only 34% of patients, a major tributary that was capable of collateral flow did exist in all patients (136). Several authors have attempted to evaluate the vascular morbidity that is associated with elevation of the radial forearm flap. Kleinman and O'Connel (137) found an 18% delay in reconstitution of normothermia after cold stress testing in patients who had undergone radial forearm flap transfer in comparison to controls. Braun et al. (138) found cold intolerance in 75% of patients who had undergone radial forearm flaps; however, these symptoms disappeared after two winters.

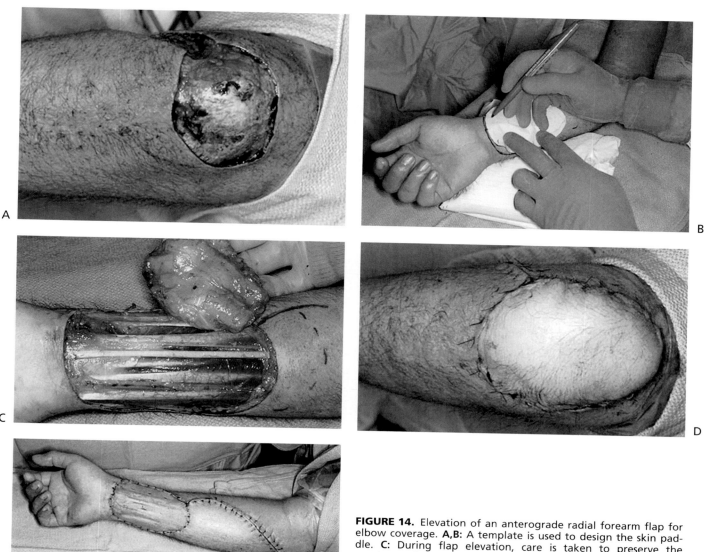

FIGURE 14. Elevation of an anterograde radial forearm flap for elbow coverage. **A,B:** A template is used to design the skin paddle. **C:** During flap elevation, care is taken to preserve the paratenon that overlies the tendons. Insetting **(D)** and donor site coverage **(E)** with unmeshed skin graft from the thigh.

Temperature measurements in a study by Meland et al. (139) showed a delay in early rewarming of the radial side of the hand at 1 minute, but this resolved by 5 minutes. There was no significant difference in thumb and index finger temperature and thumb and little finger temperature in the donor hand compared to the contralateral side. Transcutaneous oxygen values and cutaneous blood flow measured by Doppler laser flowmeter did not show any significant differences between hands. In addition to this work, other studies have found a compensatory increase in collateral flow after radial artery sacrifice. Suominen et al. (140) found an increase in ulnar flow velocity after radial forearm flap elevation. Ciria-Llorens et al. (141) also found compensatory flow through the ulnar and interosseous arteries after flap elevation. The anterior interosseous artery showed the greatest increase in blood (from 8.2 to 67.7 mL per minute), reaching a relative flow percentage (33%)

close to that of the radial artery before its excision (39%). Results of this study and others indicate that another major vascular axis, which is based on the anterior interosseous artery, develops after sacrificing the radial artery and that global arterial inflow to the hand is not impaired (141–143). Based on these data, it appears that vein grafting for arterial reconstruction need not be done on a routine basis.

Other complications after radial forearm flap elevation can include a decrease in radial nerve sensation, delayed healing at the skin graft site, decreased range of motion, and fractures of the radius after osteocutaneous flap elevation. Richardson et al. (144) found, in a series of 100 patients, that 13% experienced exposed tendons, 19% had delayed healing over the donor site, and 32% had decreased sensation in the radial nerve distribution. Raising the flap with a portion of the radius has been associated with a high incidence of postoperative fractures (145,146).

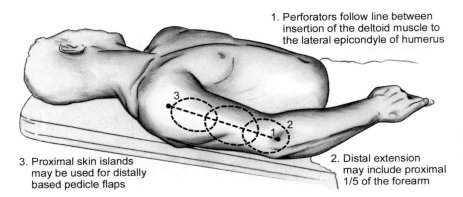

1. Perforators follow line between insertion of the deltoid muscle to the lateral epicondyle of humerus

3. Proximal skin islands may be used for distally based pedicle flaps

2. Distal extension may include proximal 1/5 of the forearm

FIGURE 15. Location of the skin island for a lateral arm flap may vary depending on whether the flap is to be based in an antero-grade or retrograde fashion. The flap is most often used as a free flap.

Attempts at limiting donor site morbidity have included modifications in flap elevation. The flap may be elevated as a pure fascial flap, allowing for primary closure of the donor site (147–149). The flap may also be elevated suprafascially; this allows for fewer donor site complications with enhancement of skin graft take and elimination of tendon exposure (150–152). Further improvement to the donor site may be made by placing tissue expanders before or after flap transfer to help with primary closure of the donor site (153–155). Also, ulnar-based skin islands have been used to close the donor site (156,157).

Other fasciocutaneous options for elbow coverage include the lateral arm flap and the reverse lateral arm flap. The lateral arm flap is based on the posterior radial collateral vessel. The septal perforators from this vessel supply the skin of the distal one-half of the lateral forearm and the proximal dorsal portion of the forearm. Although the lateral arm flap is usually used as a free flap, the flap may be raised with the incorporation of a distal forearm fasciocutaneous extension for transposition and coverage of anterior and posterior elbow defects (158,159) (Fig. 15).

The reverse lateral arm flap is nourished in a retrograde fashion through the septal perforators of the posterior radial collateral artery, which obtains its blood supply from the interosseous recurrent artery (160–162). The distal vascular pedicle should contain a sufficient amount of subcutaneous fat and underlying fascia to enhance the arterial input and the venous drainage to the flap. If the flap is less than 4 cm, or if it is taken as a pure adipofascial flap, the donor site can be closed primarily without tension (163,164). The major advantage of this flap is that it does not sacrifice any of the major arteries to the hand and allows for immediate mobilization of the elbow. In trauma-related defects of the posterior elbow, a preoperative angiogram is important before raising this flap (165).

A remaining fasciocutaneous option for elbow coverage is the antecubital forearm flap. Originally described by Lamberty and Cormack (166), this is an axial fasciocutaneous flap that is based on the inferior cubital artery. The inferior cubital cutaneous artery is the terminal division of the anterior radial collateral artery. This artery provides a large fasciocutaneous perforator 4 cm distal to the midpoint of the anterior interepicondylar line. This perforator

lies in the interval between the pronator teres and the brachioradialis and parallels the course of the cephalic vein. The flap may be used as a rotational flap or may be pedicled on the inferior cubital artery. Flap elevation proceeds from distal to proximal deep to the fascia (98,166,167) (Fig. 16).

Forearm and Wrist

For closure of defects within the forearm and wrist, the reverse radial forearm flap is an excellent choice (Fig. 17). In 1984, Lin et al. (59) proposed a reverse radial forearm flap that was based on retrograde flow through the palmar arch and ulnar artery. Venous drainage was provided by

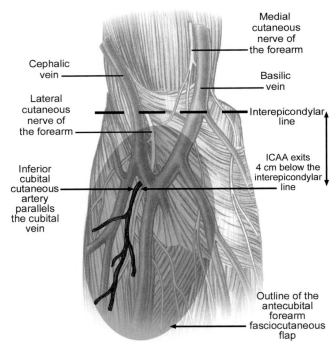

Cephalic vein

Lateral cutaneous nerve of the forearm

Inferior cubital cutaneous artery parallels the cubital vein

Medial cutaneous nerve of the forearm

Basilic vein

Interepicondylar line

ICAA exits 4 cm below the interepicondylar line

Outline of the antecubital forearm fasciocutaneous flap

FIGURE 16. The antecubital forearm fasciocutaneous flap, as described by Lamberty and Cormack, is based on the inferior cubital cutaneous artery (ICAA), a branch of the radial recurrent artery. The vessels parallel the cephalic vein and exit 4 cm below the interepicondylar line.

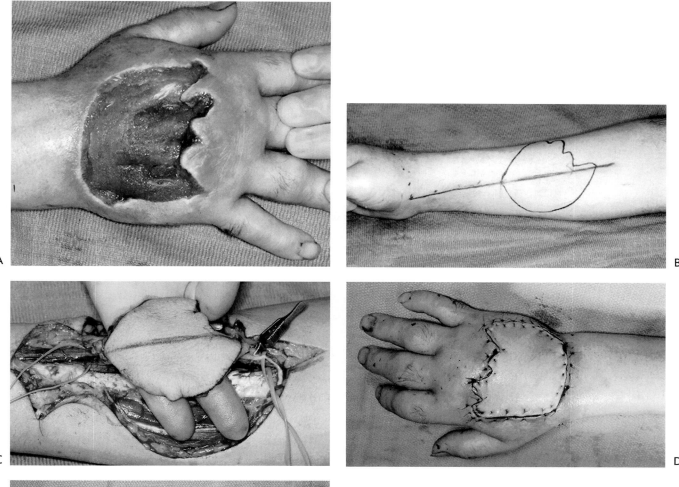

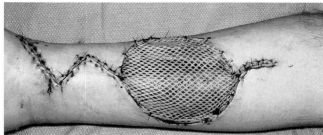

FIGURE 17. A dorsal hand defect that was covered with a reverse pedicled radial forearm flap. **A:** Defect location. **B:** Flap design. **C:** Flap elevation. **D:** Insetting. **E:** Donor site after placement of a meshed split-thickness skin graft.

communicating branches in the venae comitantes that cross over and bypass the valves. Timmons (62) later found that a component of retrograde flow was due to the denervation of the veins during flap dissection. Torii et al. (63) have also shown than there is reflux through the valves due to valvular incompetence. The reverse radial forearm flap has been used successfully in cases of palmar trauma in which the palmar arches have been injured. This is most likely due to the volar and dorsal carpal arterial arches that communicate with the radial artery (168,169). In addition, a radial forearm fascial flap may be elevated for distal forearm and wrist coverage. Six to ten septocutaneous perforators in the area of the anatomical snuffbox supply this flap. These vessels provide the vascular supply to the forearm fascia and can be

mobilized without the sacrifice of the radial artery proper; in addition, this facial flap does not result in a significant cosmetic deformity of the skin. The skin flaps over the forearm maintain perfusion through the subdermal plexus and may be closed primarily (170) (Fig. 18).

Other options for forearm and wrist reconstruction include the PIO flap. This flap came into existence in 1986, after the development of the radial forearm flap. The PIO flap attempted to recreate a distally based flap that would not sacrifice the radial artery (37,38). The flap is based on the PIA, which originates beneath the supinator muscle. It runs with the radial nerve between the two heads of the supinator. It then divides into two branches, a branch that ascends to the elbow and constitutes the distal pedicle of the lateral arm

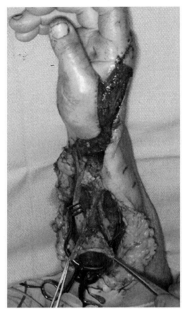

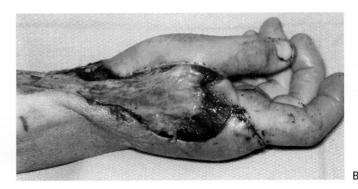

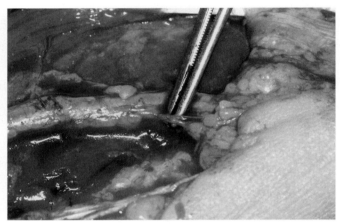

FIGURE 18. Use of a retrograde radial forearm fascial flap for coverage of the first web space. **A:** Flap harvest. **B:** Insetting. **C:** The perforators are located approximately 1.5 to 3.0 cm proximal to the radial styloid (the perforator is seen running above the forceps).

flap and a descending branch that follows the septum between the extensor digiti quinti and the ECU muscle. The deep branch of the radial nerve accompanies the artery. This descending branch gives off perforators to the skin, the most important of which is the first branch (171). In this area, the radial nerve gives off several branches to the extensor digitorum communis and ECU and a deeper branch to the extensor pollicis longus, abductor pollicis longus, extensor pollicis brevis, and extensor indicis proprius (171,172). The branches to the extensor digitorum communis and ECU are the most prone to injury, when elevating the flap.

Flap design is centered over a line that is drawn from the lateral epicondyle to the ulnar styloid with the elbow held at 90 degrees of flexion. This line corresponds with the axis of the septocutaneous perforator. The PIA arises at the junction of the proximal and middle two-thirds of this line. There are usually 7 to 14 perforators that run along this line. These may be identified with a hand-held Doppler preoperatively. The most proximal perforator arises at the proximal and middle two-thirds junction. The central portion of the flap should be designed distal to this site. The PIA anastomoses with the dorsal wrist arcade 2 cm proximal to the radiocarpal joint. Dissection is usually started distally to ensure integrity of the PIA, if the flap is to be used in a retrograde fashion. Flaps as wide as 6 to 7 cm have been reported (Fig. 19).

Despite reports that cite the PIO flap's propensity to undergo venous congestion, many large series have empha-

sized the usefulness of this flap (32,39). Costa et al. (173) presented a series of 81 clinical cases, finding the flap particularly useful in cases in which there was injury to the radial and ulnar arteries. Costa et al. used the flap for soft tissue deficits of the dorsal hand up to the metacarpal joints, the first web space up to the IP joint of the thumb, and the ulnar border of the hand. Brunelli et al. (174) reported the use of this flap in 113 cases. Flaps survived completely in 98 patients. Twelve patients had superficial necrosis of the distal part of the flap, which did not require additional surgical procedures. Six patients demonstrated paralysis of the motor branch to the extensor muscles of the wrist or fingers (generally to the ECU, the extensor digiti quinti, or the extensor pollicis longus). All recovered completely within 6 months. There were major anatomic variations that precluded the use of the flap twice in this series. Venous congestion can be due to inconsistent venous comitantes (175). This could account for the flap's propensity for vascular congestion and persistent edema (176).

Similar to the radial forearm flap, the ulnar artery flap can be based proximally or distally to cover defects of the elbow, forearm, or hand (177–181). This flap offers advantages over the radial forearm flap. The transferred flap has less hair, the donor site overlies muscle rather than tendon, and the donor site may often be closed primarily. The major disadvantage to this flap is the sacrifice of the major arterial inflow to the hand in addition to ulnar nerve dysesthesia that can develop after flap elevation (182).

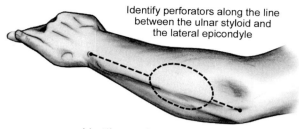

Identify perforators along the line
between the ulnar styloid and
the lateral epicondyle

Identify vessel course with Doppler

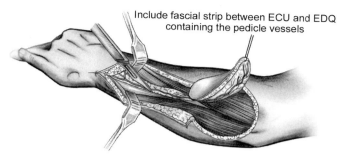

Include fascial strip between ECU and EDQ
containing the pedicle vessels

FIGURE 19. The skin paddle for the posterior interosseous flap is centered over the proximal one-third, with a line drawn between the lateral epicondyle and the ulnar styloid. The perforators should be identified with a Doppler before flap design. Preservation of subcutaneous veins allows for venovenous anastomosis, should venous congestion occur after flap elevation and insetting. ECU, extensor carpi ulnaris; EDQ, extensor digiti quinti.

A modification of the ulnar artery flap may be made that does not sacrifice the ulnar artery. In 1992, Becker and Gilbert (35) described a flap that was based on the dorsal ulnar artery for defects of the dorsal and palmar hand. The dorsal skin flap can be as large as 20 cm in length by 9 cm in width (183). The origin of the dorsal branch of the ulnar artery arises 2 to 5 cm proximal to the pisiform. This is initially identified through an incision that is 2 cm proximal to the pisiform. The FCU is the retracted to reveal the artery. The flap is centered along the axis of the ulna, with the palmaris longus representing the volar limit of the flap, whereas the fourth dorsal compartment marks the limit of dorsal dissection (Fig. 20). A modification of this technique by Karacalar and Ozcan (29,30) dissects the flap back to the anastomosis of the dorsal ulnar artery with the dorsal carpal arch. This allows division of the dorsal branch of the ulnar artery. The flap receives arterial flow through the dorsal carpal arch. This increases pedicle length, thus allowing for easier insetting.

Other options for recurrent or recalcitrant irritation of the median nerve or small palmar wrist wounds within zone 4 is the hypothenar fat pad flap. This adipofascial flap may be pedicled on perforators from the ulnar artery after release of Guyon's canal (184–186) (Fig. 21). As an alternative, the adductor digiti minimi may be pedicled on its proximal blood supply and moved into the carpal canal (187–189). Finally, the pronator quadratus may also be pedicled on its ulnar or radial attachments or on the anterior interosseous artery to provide coverage of small defects at the level of the wrist. The pronator quadratus flap has also been described for recalcitrant carpal tunnel and for defects at the level of the wrist (190–192). These flaps are reliable but small and do not have broad application throughout the forearm.

Hand and Wrist

Defects about the dorsum of the hand and fingers may often be covered with the use of the radial forearm flap or other flaps that are used for forearm coverage. For smaller defects, however, flaps that are based on the dorsal metacarpal arterial system can provide excellent coverage with minimal donor site defects. In addition, these flaps do not compromise the arterial supply to the remaining hand.

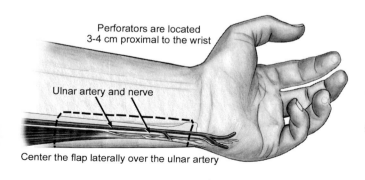

Perforators are located
3-4 cm proximal to the wrist

Ulnar artery and nerve

Center the flap laterally over the ulnar artery

FIGURE 20. Reverse ulnar perforator flap is based on the dorsal branch of the ulnar artery, exiting 2 to 5 cm proximal to the pisiform.

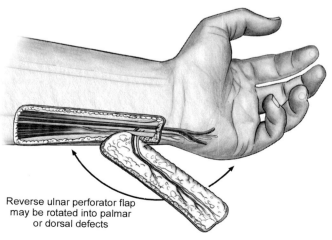

Reverse ulnar perforator flap
may be rotated into palmar
or dorsal defects

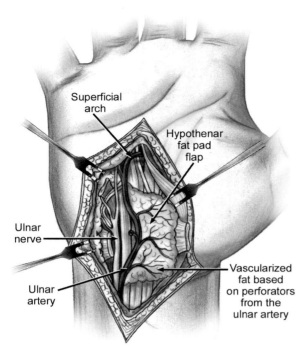

FIGURE 21. The hypothenar fat pad flap is a vascularized adipofascial flap that is based on the perforators from the ulnar artery. Full release of Guyon's canal is required for adequate flap mobilization.

Holevich (193) originally described the first dorsal metacarpal artery (FDMA) island flap in 1963 for resurfacing of the thumb. The flap has since been applied to a broad array of dorsal hand defects (194–198). The flap is based on perforators that arise at the level of the metacarpal head. The FDMA arises from the radial artery at the apex of the angle between the first and second metacarpals (Fig. 22). The course of the artery parallels the second metacarpal. It may run on top of or beneath the fascia of the first interosseous muscle; the artery may run within the muscle in as many as 15% of patients (199–201). Planning of the flap is aided by Doppler identification of the vessel's course (202). The pedicle can be prone to spasm, and paleness in the flap is not always correlated with tension (203–206). Inclusion of the fascia of the interosseous muscle is crucial for flap success.

The flap presents problems with cortical interpretation when it is used for palmar thumb coverage. In addition, the flap does not carry glabrous skin to replace the thumb tip. Foucher et al. (199,207) have reported disappointing results with attempts at neurotization of the radial nerve branch with the ulnar collateral nerve of the thumb. Variations in the flap have included the dissection of the distal veins over the proximal phalanx of the index finger and the use of these veins to drain blood from an amputated thumb with large dorsal skin loss. In addition, the flap may be extended by elevating the skin from the dorsum of the index and middle fingers for large defects. The flap may also be used as a free flap (208–211) (Fig. 23).

The second dorsal metacarpal artery, as detailed by Early (204,212), can also be used in resurfacing of the hand. This artery is present in 92% to 97% of patients (204,213,214). The origin of the artery is variable, and it has been reported to originate from the deep palmar arch, the radial artery, the FDMA, and the PIA. It runs on or under the fascia of the second dorsal interosseous muscle and terminates near the metacarpophalangeal (MCP) joint. The artery supplies perforators to the skin of the dorsum of the second web space and first phalanges of the index and long finger. It may be larger than the FDMA in more than 33% of specimens (199). It has been used for sensory resurfacing of the thumb (215). The flap's vascular pedicle may also be extended to the dorsal branch of the radial artery by including the dorsal carpal arch in flap elevation (214). Use of the third and fourth dorsal metacarpal flaps has been reported, but the third and fourth dorsal metacarpal arteries may be absent in 17% to 30% of patients (44,50,216).

Retrograde flaps may be designed on any of the dorsal metacarpal arteries. These flaps are perfused through the interconnections between the terminal branch of the dorsal metacarpal arteries, the deep palmar metacarpal arteries, and the palmar digital arteries (52,217). The skin paddle is outlined at the apex of the interosseous angle and is pivoted at the radial side of the neck of the associated metacarpal (50,199,206,216). These flaps can provide coverage for distal digital defects (Fig. 24).

Additional coverage options for distal defects can be provided with the use of the reverse dorsal digital island flaps. These flaps are based on the arterial branches that anastomose the palmar and dorsal arterial network (218,219). These *boomerang flaps*, as termed by Legaillard et al. (220), are based on retrograde blood flow through the vascular arcade between the dorsal and palmar digital arteries. The flap is useful in covering injuries to the dorsum of the distal phalanx. In comparison to the homodigital island flap, it does not sacrifice volar blood supply in an already injured digit (221).

HETERODIGITAL ISLAND FLAPS

Alternatives for palmar finger reconstruction include the use of heterodigital island flaps. These flaps provide sensate glabrous skin but do sacrifice one digital nerve and vessel to the donor finger. The neurovascular island flaps were originally described for coverage of the insensate thumb. In the original description by Littler (222), the donor defect was created at the ulnar aspect of the ring or long fingers. Since its initial description, multiple studies have described its use in treating thumb pulp defects (223–230).

Markley and Littler (230) suggest that dissection start at the level of the web space to ensure that there are no anomalies in the corresponding digits' vascular supply. A perivascular cuff must be taken with the digital vessels to preserve venous outflow. The bundle is dissected to the level of the

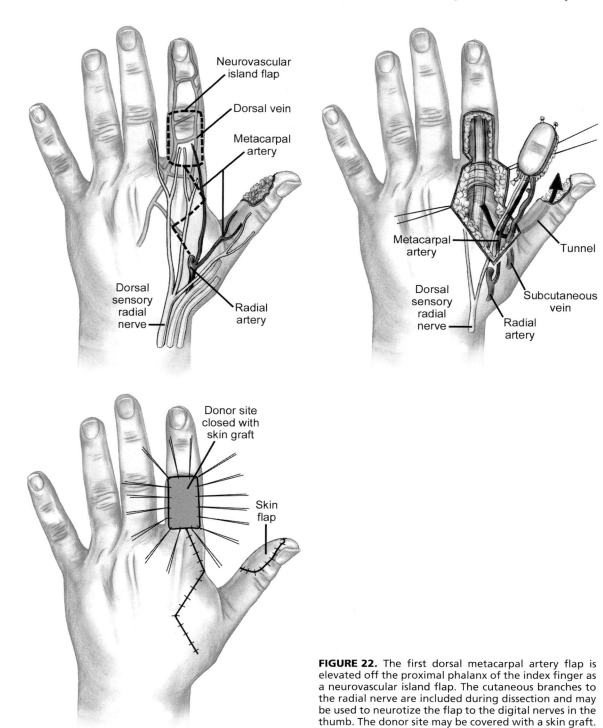

FIGURE 22. The first dorsal metacarpal artery flap is elevated off the proximal phalanx of the index finger as a neurovascular island flap. The cutaneous branches to the radial nerve are included during dissection and may be used to neurotize the flap to the digital nerves in the thumb. The donor site may be covered with a skin graft.

superficial arch. For the flap to reach the tip of the thumb, intrafascicular neural dissection needs to be performed, sometimes to the level of the median nerve (Fig. 25).

Straight transfer of the digital nerve may make sensory reeducation difficult, especially if the patient is older than 50 years of age (231). Failure to achieve cortical reorientation has been reported in some series to be as high as 25% (232,233). Dividing the donor digital nerve and anasto-

mosing it to the recipient site nerve have been suggested as means of avoiding reorientation and the double sensation phenomenon (234). *Double sensibility* refers to the perception of stimuli at the donor or recipient area or to the donor area alone. In a comparative study, Adani et al. (229) found that double sensibility was improved in their reanastomosed patients; however, two-point discrimination was not as good as that obtained in their patients who under-

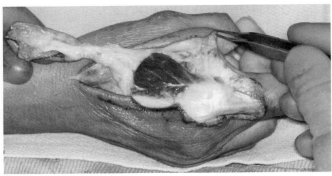

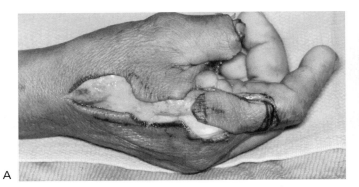

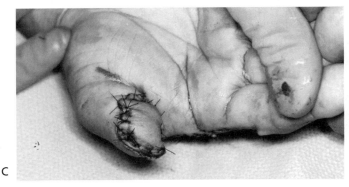

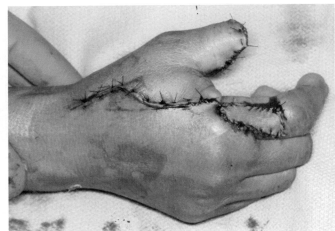

FIGURE 23. A,B: Use of the first dorsal metacarpal artery island flap for coverage of a thumb avulsion injury at the level of the interphalangeal joint. Dissection is carried deep to the fascia to include the vessel. **C,D:** Result after insetting.

went the classic Littler technique. Most complaints in this study, however, were not related to sensation discrepancies but rather to donor site problems, including cold intolerance and hypertrophic scarring. Oka (228), in a similar comparative study, found that all patients recognized the thumb in the modified Littler procedure; however, only 60% of patients recognized sensation as coming from the thumb with the original Littler procedure. All of the patients with the classic Littler procedure experienced a

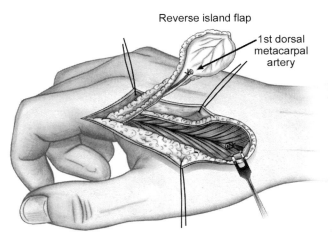

FIGURE 24. Design and elevation of a reverse first dorsal radial forearm flap.

component of the double sensation phenomenon. Some long-term outcome studies have shown poor preservation of long-term sensation (234). To improve postoperative sensibility, Markley and Littler (230) stress the importance of including the entire sensory zone of the proper digital nerve. Flaps that are designed too proximally or too small may overtension the pedicle, which may, in turn, limit the sensation that is obtained in the reconstructed digit.

We have found this flap to be useful in the coverage of the radial borders of the index and long fingers. The flap provides an increase in finger vascularity, good sensation, and a well-padded flap for fingertip reconstruction. The flap is easy to raise and is reliable, as long as a perivascular cuff remains around the neurovascular bundle.

Another heterodigital flap is the C-ring cross finger flap or Turkish flap. This flap is based on the digital vascular bundle of a corresponding finger and can be based distally or proximally. The flap is based on the dorsal skin and may include the volar skin of the middle phalanx, as well. The flap does not include the digital nerve. The flap is dissected above the paratenon of the extensor and flexor mechanism. The flap can be mobilized to cover an adjacent finger or the same digit (235) (Fig. 26).

Hirase et al. (236) and Joshi (237) described the dorsal middle phalangeal finger flap. The flap is taken from the dorsum of the long finger. This flap has the potential to provide sensate coverage of the fingers but not the thumb. The flap requires a normal contralateral digital vessel, as verified by

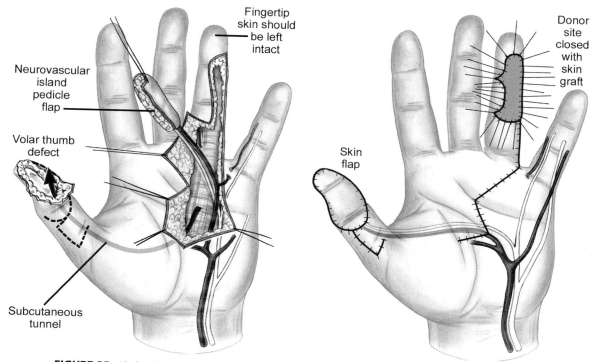

FIGURE 25. Littler flap. The flap is elevated from the ulnar aspect of the ring or long finger and used classically for reconstruction of thumb defects, although the flap can be used for sensate glabrous skin coverage over any digit. The donor site is skin grafted.

digital Allen's test. The flap is designed like a cross finger flap, but the base includes the vascular bundle. The dorsal sensory branch is taken as an interposition graft for reconstruction of digital nerve defects in the affected finger. Pedicle length is obtained by dissecting proximally to the common digital artery or the palmar arch. Again, one should avoid skeletonization of the pedicle during elevation, as the small venous comitantes surround the arterial pedicle.

HOMODIGITAL ISLAND FLAPS

Finger

The most immediate source of tissue for finger reconstruction is the same finger. This provides the benefit of limiting injury to a single site and prevents the immobilization of other joints. Because the ulnar and radial digital arteries are connected at the level of the volar plate by transverse venous and arterial arcades, flaps from the middle and proximal phalanx may be mobilized to cover distal defects or exposed tendons on the dorsal or volar surface. These flaps necessitate sacrifice of one digital artery and rely on retrograde flow through the intact anastomosis at the contralateral normal artery (238–241). These flaps should only be used in isolated sharp injuries, without crush or significant soft tissue injury to the surrounding finger.

The reverse vascular pedicle digital island flap was described in 1989 by Lai et al. (238) and later by Kojima et al. (242). The flap sacrifices one of the digital vessels with preservation of the digital nerve. The flap is usually elevated off the middle phalanx and pedicled distally to cover pulp defects. The flap is elevated from a proximal to distal direction, attempting to keep the pedicle within the soft tissue of the flap. The digital vessels

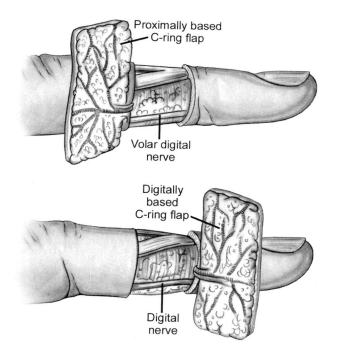

FIGURE 26. Steps in the elevation of the C-ring digital flap.

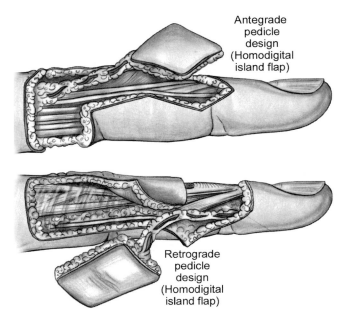

FIGURE 27. Homodigital island flaps require the sacrifice of one digital artery. The flap may be used to cover defects at the level of the distal phalanx.

must be elevated with their perivascular fat to preserve venous outflow. Flaps may be combined with portions of the lateral band if terminal extensor tendon reconstruction is required (243). These reverse flaps require neurorrhaphy of a dorsal nerve branch for optimal return of sensibility (244,245). Lai et al. (239) found that the average two-point discrimination of the reconstructed fingertip was 6.8 mm in noninnervated flaps compared to 3.9 mm in innervated flaps (Fig. 27).

Thumb

The thumb has the benefit of having a significant dorsal blood supply that allows for bipedicle advancement of the volar skin without concern for compromising the dorsal skin of the thumb. The advancement of the volar skin allows for the preservation of glabrous skin and immediate sensation, as opposed to reinnervation through grafts, as with the first metacarpal artery island flap, or through sensory reeducation, as is seen with the Littler flap.

Moberg (246) first described his advancement flap for thumb reconstruction in 1964. Dissection carries down to the flexor sheath, and the flap is then elevated off the flexor sheath. The MCP crease is the limit of dissection. Resultant IP joint contracture is the most common complication after this procedure and can impede function. Designing the proximal portion of the flap in a V-Y fashion can facilitate closure and limit IP contractures. Defects as large as 10 mm may be covered with this flap (247–249). O'Brien (250) has modified this procedure by using an islandized bipedicled advancement flap (251). This may decrease the IP contracture that is produced through pure Moberg advancement. The resulting proximal defect must be skin grafted, but con-

tracture rates are improved. Advancement of 10 to 15 mm can usually be achieved. A rectangular incision is made from mid-lateral to mid-lateral line. Proximal extension of the incisions allows for identification and mobilization of vessels first. Once this is accomplished, dissection of the flap can be carried out at the level of Cleland's ligament, just dorsal to the neurovascular bundle. The authors believe that if more than 45 degrees of IP flexion are required for closure with a standard Moberg flap, then relaxing incisions should be made by using the O'Brien modification or a V-Y incision. The flap may then be advanced on its two vascular pedicles with a V-Y closure of the proximal base. Hynes (252) has described bringing the base of the V to the thenar eminence. He mobilizes the finger at 14 days (Fig. 28).

When applied to general fingertip reconstruction, the Moberg flap may produce dorsal tip necrosis in addition to an unstable pulp scar (253). The dorsal blood supply to the finger is supplied through perforating branches from the palmar arteries at the MCP and PIP joints; these vessels are divided when using the classic Moberg technique. Macht and Watson (254), however, preserved the dorsal perforating branch in a modification of the digital volar advancement flap through a "spreading-dissecting" technique. They reported no skin loss or joint stiffness in 69 transfers with two-point discrimination within 2 mm of the contralateral finger.

DISTANT PEDICLED FLAPS

Groin Flap

The workhorse flap before the advent of microsurgery was the groin flap. This flap is based on the superficial femoral circumflex artery. This vessel arises from the femoral artery along with the superficial inferior epigastric artery in the femoral triangle. The superficial femoral circumflex artery is present in more than 95% of patients on angiogram (255,256). The superficial femoral circumflex vessel initially runs below the deep fascia of the thigh; it then pierces the fascia at the medial border of the sartorius muscle. At this level, the artery gives off a deep branch to the sartorius muscle and a cutaneous vessel to the skin. The vessel then runs approximately 2 cm below and parallel to the inguinal ligament. The vascular territory extends laterally beyond the anterior iliac spine (257).

The flap has shown great versatility. The flap may include the lateral cutaneous branch of the femoral nerve or the subcostal nerve to the twelfth thoracic nerve if a neurotized flap is required (258). The flap may be combined with the abdominohypogastric flap for large defects, or the flap may be expanded before transfer (259,260). If bone is required, a portion of the iliac crest may be harvested (261–263). The flap may also be split longitudinally to cover defects on both aspects of the hand (260).

The midline of the flap is designed 2 cm inferior and parallel to the inguinal ligament. The width of the pedicle

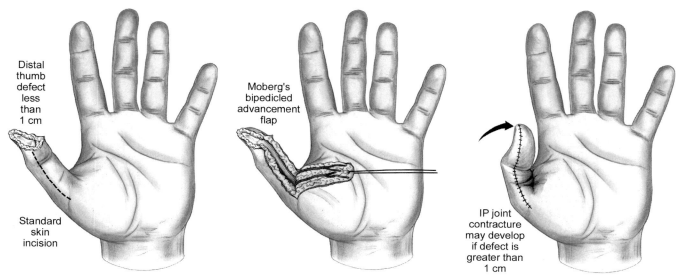

FIGURE 28. Standard elevation technique for the Moberg flap. Defects greater than 1 cm can produce significant interphalangeal (IP) joint contractures.

to be tubed is designed out to the level of the anterior superior iliac spine. The flap is often more difficult to tube in larger patients with more abdominal fat. If the proximal portion of the pedicle is too large to tube safely, moist dressings may be applied to the deep surface of the flap to prevent desiccation. The wound bed needs to be clean before transfer, as any contamination leads to an increased risk of flap necrosis (264,265) (Fig. 29).

The flap is normally incised at its edges down to the deep fascia, and dissection then proceeds from lateral to medial. Care is taken at the edge of the sartorius fascia to include the superficial femoral circumflex vessels as it runs beneath the fascia (182,266). External fixation between the iliac crest and the radius has been recommended by some to prevent shearing forces on the flap (267). This, however, greatly enhances postoperative stiffness (182).

The flap can often be divided safely at 3 weeks, especially if the wound is well healed at the flap's distal margin. Any compromise to the arm's vascularity, such as preoperative radiation or electrical injury, may prolong the period of revascularization. Division as early as 8.5 days has been reported with the use of ischemic preconditioning and

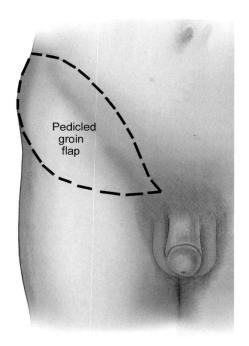

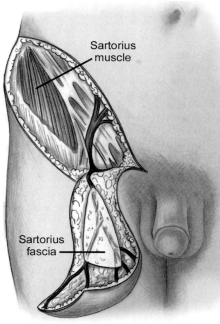

FIGURE 29. The pedicled groin flap is designed on a line that is drawn 2 cm inferior and parallel to the inguinal ligament. The vascular pedicle arises deep to the deep fascia below the inguinal ligament. Do not include the deep fascia until the sartorius muscle is encountered. From this point, the deep fascia should be included to preserve the superficial circumflex iliac artery.

Doppler laser flowmeter measurements of pedicle flow (268). If there is doubt about the vascularity of the flap before division, the pedicle may be occluded with a tourniquet. Other options include fluorescein injections into the flap to verify viability (269,270). Division can be staged by dividing the pedicle alone, dividing one-half of the tube, or dividing the flap and waiting to perform the final insetting (182). Secondary defatting procedures are required in as many as 85% of patients (271).

Use of the groin flap does require the hand to be immobilized for as long as 3 to 4 weeks. This can result in stiffness, edema, and possible infection. Complication rates as high as 25% have been reported by several authors (271,272). Death and pulmonary embolism have also been associated with this flap in patients who are older than 50 years of age; this is most likely due to the prolonged period of patient immobilization (271). The institution of early physical therapy has been shown to avoid the postoperative stiffness that is seen frequently in the elderly population (273).

In addition to the groin flap, other distant axial-pattern flaps include the thoracoepigastric, lateral thoracic, external oblique, pectoralis major, and rectus abdominus muscle pedicled flap (274–278). The use of these flaps has largely been superseded by the development of the free flap. The groin flap, however, still remains a reliable means of providing soft tissue coverage for large hand wounds without the need for microvascular experience (279).

COMPLICATIONS

With any pedicled flap, there is the potential for total or partial flap loss. Infection, hematoma, anatomic abnormalities, and technical errors in flap elevation design or insetting may all lead to flap loss. Arterial and venous insufficiency are early signs of impending flap failure. Immediate arterial insufficiency may be manifested as pallor within the skin paddle, poor capillary refill, lack of punctate bleeding after needle stick, or poikilothermia. Intraoperatively, if arterial insufficiency is present after flap transfer, one may attempt to rewarm the patient or to use papaverine on the arterial pedicle to help resolve any vascular spasm. If arterial ischemia is not resolved, the pedicle may need to be examined for any signs of kinking. If repositioning the flap does not improve arterial inflow, and there is no other external compression on the pedicle, such as a tight skin tunnel, one should place the pedicle back into its native bed. If arterial inflow returns, it is probably best to delay the flap transfer. Delay allows the choke vessels within the flap to dilate, thus helping one to carry additional tissue with the flap (280–282). If none of these methods resolves arterial insufficiency, one must consider the possibility of irreparable arterial injury due to trauma or intimal flap formation. In these cases, the flap may need to be converted to a free tissue transfer for salvage.

Venous congestion is manifested by brisk bleeding from the muscle edges, firmness and fullness within the draining veins, and swelling and blue discoloration within the skin paddle. Early venous congestion presents as hyperemia within the skin paddle, which then progresses to blue discoloration. Venous congestion may be due to overlying compression of the superficial veins or kinking at the pedicle pivot site (283). In drastic situations, free tissue transfer or supercharging of a pedicled flap may be necessary to salvage congested portions.

Multiple adjuncts have been described to monitor pedicled flaps and free tissue transfers. These include pH monitoring, fluorescein, Doppler ultrasonography, Doppler laser flowmeter, color spectrophotometry, and photoplethysmograph (284–295). Postoperatively, edema, bulky dressings, and surrounding ecchymosis can obscure signs of arterial insufficiency. It is best if one minimizes the amount of postoperative dressings to allow for easier flap monitoring. The authors have found that clinical judgment and a trained nursing unit that is familiar with flap management are the most effective means of flap monitoring.

Postoperative compromise of undetermined etiology needs exploration. Often, kinks or obstruction to outflow through hematoma, tight dressings, or tight stitches may be easily eliminated, thus allowing for flap salvage (296). For flaps that have experienced an ischemic insult, there are several methods that can maximize flap survival. These include keeping the flap moist, keeping the ambient temperature elevated, and the institution of supplemental oxygen (297–302). It is also critical to ensure that the patient has adequate volume resuscitation and an adequate blood pressure; this prevents peripheral vasoconstriction and an increased blood viscosity. Adequate volume resuscitation also helps maximize oxygen delivery to the flap (303). Pharmacologic methods, such as free radical scavengers, have not been clearly shown to increase flap survival in randomized human studies. In the future, pharmacologic methods may help further improve flap survival.

CONCLUSION

Pedicled flaps can provide reliable coverage for the majority of traumatic and acquired hand defects. These flaps require little microsurgical experience and can be elevated in relatively little time. Familiarity with these flaps is crucial for the hand surgeon in providing successful hand reconstruction.

REFERENCES

1. Taylor GI, Palmer JH. The vascular territories (angiosomes) of the body: experimental study and clinical applications. *Br J Plast Surg* 1987;40:113–141.
2. Morris SF, Taylor GI. Predicting the survival of experimental skin flaps with a knowledge of the vascular architecture. *Plast Reconstr Surg* 1993;92:1352–1361.

3. Watterson PA, Crock JG. The venous territories of muscles: anatomical study and clinical implications. *Br J Plast Surg* 1988;41:569–585.

4. Taylor GI, Watterson PA, Crock JG, et al. The venous territories (venosomes) of the human body: experimental study and clinical implications. *Plast Reconstr Surg* 1990;86:185–213.

5. Calderon W, Mathes SJ, et al. Comparison of the effect of bacterial inoculation in musculocutaneous and fasciocutaneous flaps. *Plast Reconstr Surg* 1986;77:785–794.

6. Chang N, Mathes SJ. Comparison of the effect of bacterial inoculation in musculocutaneous and random-pattern flaps. *Plast Reconstr Surg* 1982;70:1–10.

7. Yaremchuk MJ, Sedacca T, May JW Jr, et al. The effect of preoperative angiography on experimental free-flap survival. *Plast Reconstr Surg* 1981;68:201–207.

8. Godina M. Early microsurgical reconstruction of complex trauma to the extremities. *Plast Reconstr Surg* 1986;78:285–292.

9. Lister G, Scheker L. Emergency free flaps to the upper extremity. *J Hand Surg* 1988;13:22–28.

10. Mackinnon SE, Godina M, et al. Immediate forearm reconstruction with a functional latissimus dorsi island pedicle myocutaneous flap. *Plast Reconstr Surg* 1983;71:700–710.

11. Breidenbach WC. Emergency free tissue transfer for reconstruction of acute upper extremity wounds. *Clin Plast Surg* 1989;16:505.

12. Brown H. Closed crush injuries of the hand and forearm. *Orthop Clin North Am* 1970;1:253–259.

13. Simpson SG. Farm machinery injuries. *J Trauma* 1984;24:150–152.

14. Buchler U. Traumatic soft-tissue defects of the extremities. Implications and treatment guidelines. *Arch Orthop Trauma Surg* 1990;109:321–329.

15. DeFranzo AJ, Marks MW, Molnar JA, et al. The use of vacuum-assisted closure therapy for the treatment of lower-extremity wounds with exposed bone. *Plast Reconstr Surg* 2001;108:1184–1191.

16. DeFranzo AJ, Argenta LC, Genecov DG, et al. Vacuum-assisted closure for the treatment of degloving injuries. *Plast Reconstr Surg* 1999;104:2145–2148.

17. Beasley RW. Principles of soft tissue replacement for the hand. *J Hand Surg* 1983;8:781–784.

18. Rodriguez-Niedenfuhr M, Nearn L, Ferreira B, et al. Variations of the arterial pattern in the upper limb revisited: a morphological and statistical study, with a review of the literature. *J Anat* 2001;199:547–566.

19. Schmidt CC, Greenberg JA, Kann SE, et al. The anconeus muscle flap: its anatomy and clinical application. *J Hand Surg* 1999;24:359–369.

20. Gao XS, Yang ZN, Wang BB, et al. Medial upper arm skin flap: vascular anatomy and clinical applications. *Ann Plast Surg* 1985;15:348.

21. Kaplan EN, Pearl RM. An arterial medial arm flap-vascular anatomy and clinical applications. *Ann Plast Surg* 1980;4:205.

22. Leversedge FJ, Payne SH, Seiler JG III, et al. Vascular anatomy of the brachioradialis rotational musculocutaneous flap. *J Hand Surg* 2001;26:711–721.

23. McCormack LJ, Anson BJ, et al. Brachial and antebrachial arterial patterns: a study of 750 extremities. *Surg Gynecol Obstet* 1953;96:43.

24. Madaree A, McGibbon IC. Anatomic variation in the blood supply of the radial forearm flap. *J Reconstr Microsurg* 1993;9:277–279.

25. Small JO, Millar R. The radial artery forearm flap: an anomaly of the radial artery. *Br J Plast Surg* 1985;38:501–503.

26. Funk GF, McCulloch TM, Graham SM, et al. Anomalies of forearm vascular anatomy encountered during elevation of the radial forearm flap. *Head Neck* 1995;17:284–292.

27. Porter CJ, Mellow CG. Anatomically aberrant forearm arteries: an absent radial artery with co-dominant median and ulnar arteries. *Br J Plast Surg* 2001;54:727–728.

28. Inoue Y, Taylor GI. The angiosomes of the forearm: anatomic study and clinical implications. *Plast Reconstr Surg* 1996;98:195–210.

29. Karacalar A, Ozcan M. Preliminary report: the distally pedicled dorsoulnar forearm flap for hand reconstruction. *Br J Plast Surg* 1999;52:453–457.

30. Karacalar A, Ozcan M. The distally based ulnar artery forearm flap supplied by the dorsal carpal arch. *Ann Plast Surg* 1998;41:304–306.

31. Bertelli JA, Pagliei A. The neurocutaneous flap based on the dorsal branches of the ulnar artery and nerve: a new flap for extensive reconstruction of the hand. *Plast Reconstr Surg* 1998;101:1537–1543.

32. Dadalt Filho LG, Penteado CV, et al. Absence of the anastomosis between the anterior and posterior interosseous arteries in a posterior interosseous flap: a case report. *J Hand Surg* 1994;19:22–25.

33. Hu W, Foucher G, Baudet J, et al. Le lambeau interosseux anterieur. *Ann Chir Plast Esthet* 1994;39:290–300.

34. Giunta R, Lukas B. Impossible harvest of the posterior interosseous artery flap: a report of an individualized salvage procedure. *Br J Plast Surg* 1998;51:642–645.

35. Becker C, Gilbert A. Le lambeau cubital. *Ann Chir Main Memb Sufer* 1988;7:136–142.

36. Nystrom A, Zoldos J, et al. Intrinsic vascular anatomy of the hand. *Atlas Hand Clin* 1998;3:1–32.

37. Penteado CV, Cheverel JP, et al. The anatomical basis of the fascia cutaneous flap of the posterior interosseous artery. *Surg Radiol Anat* 1986;8:209–215.

38. Zancolli EA, Angrigiani C. Posterior interosseous island forearm flap. *J Hand Surg* 1988;13:130–135.

39. Costa H, Martins A, Rodrigues J, et al. Further experience with the posterior interosseous flap. *Br J Plast Surg* 1991;44:449–455.

40. Sheetz KK, Berger RA, et al. The arterial blood supply of the distal radius and ulna and its potential use in vascularized pedicled bone grafts. *J Hand Surg* 1995;20:902–914.

41. Fontaine C, Blancke D, Mestdagh H, et al. Anatomic basis of pronator quadratus flap. *Surg Radiol Anat* 1992;14:295–299.

42. Hurlburt PT, Lee KH, et al. A cadaveric anatomic study of radial artery pedicle grafts to the scaphoid and lunate. *J Hand Surg* 1997;22:408–412.

43. Shin AY, Bishop AT. Pedicled vascularized bone grafts for disorders of the carpus: scaphoid nonunion and Kienböck's disease. *J Am Acad Orthop Surg* 2002;10:210–216.

44. Coleman SS, et al. Arterial patterns in the hand based upon a study of 650 specimens. *Surg Gynecol Obstet* 1961;113:409.

45. Gellman H, Shankwiler J, Gelberman RH, et al. Arterial patterns of the deep and superficial palmar arches. *Clin Orthop* 2001;383:41–46.

46. Kleinert JM, Abel CS, Firrell J. Radial and ulnar artery dominance in normal digits. *J Hand Surg* 1989;14:504–508.

47. Gelberman RH, Taleisnik J, Baumgaertner M, et al. The arterial anatomy of the human carpus. Part I: the extraosseous vascularity. *J Hand Surg* 1983;8:367–375.

48. Yousif NJ, Sanger JR, Arria P, et al. The versatile metacarpal and reverse metacarpal artery flaps in hand surgery. *Ann Plast Surg* 1992;29:523–531.

49. Yuceturk A, Tuncay C, Tandogan R, et al. Treatment of scaphoid nonunions with a vascularized bone graft based on the first dorsal metacarpal artery. *J Hand Surg* 1997;22:425–427.

50. Quaba AA, Davison PM. The distally-based dorsal hand flap. *Br J Plast Surg* 1990;43:28–39.

51. Mathoulin C, Brunelli F. Further experience with the index metacarpal vascularized bone graft. *J Hand Surg* 1998;23:311–317.

52. Valenti P, Begue T, et al. Anatomic basis of a dorsal commisural flap from the 2nd, 3rd, and 4th intermetacarpal spaces. *Surg Radiol Anat* 1990;12:235–239.

53. Strauch B, de Moura W. Arterial system of the fingers. *J Hand Surg* 1990;15:148–154.

54. Brunelli F. Le lambeau dorso-cubital du pouce. *Ann Chir Main* 1993;12:105–114.

55. Nystrom A, Friden J, Lister GD, et al. The palmar digital venous anatomy. *Scand J Plast Reconstr Surg* 1990;24:113–119.

56. Nystrom A, Lister GD, et al. Deep venous anatomy of the human palm. *Scand J Plast Reconstr Surg* 1991;25:233–239.

57. Nystrom A, Lister GD, et al. Venous anatomy of the thumb and thenar area. *Scand J Plast Reconstr Surg Hand Surg* 1992;26:155–160.

58. Birkbeck DP, Moy OJ. Anatomy of upper extremity skin flaps. *Hand Clin* 1997;13:175–187.

59. Lin SD, Chiu CC, et al. Venous drainage in the reverse forearm flap. *Plast Reconstr Surg* 1984;74:508–512.

60. Tolhurst DE, Zeeman RJ, et al. The development of the fasciocutaneous flap and its clinical applications. *Plast Reconstr Surg* 1983;71:597–606.

61. Wee JT. Reversed venous flow in the distally pedicled radial forearm flap: surgical implications. *Handchirurgie* 1988;20:119–123.

62. Timmons MJ. The vascular basis of the radial forearm flap. *Plast Reconstr Surg* 1986;77:80–92.

63. Torii S, Mori R, et al. Reverse-flow island flap: clinical report and venous drainage. *Plast Reconstr Surg* 1987;79:600–609.

64. Wee JT. Venous flow in the distally pedicled radial forearm flap. In: Gilbert A, Heintz V, et al., eds. *Pedicled flaps of the upper limb.* Boston: Little, Brown and Company, 1992:101.

65. Ger R. The operative treatment of the advanced stasis ulcer: a preliminary communication. *Am J Surg* 1966;111:659.

66. Stein H, Horer D, et al. Vascularized muscle pedicle flap for osteonecrosis of the femoral head. *Orthopedics* 2002;25:485–488.

67. Gosain A, Mathes S, Hunt TK, et al. A study of the relationship between blood flow and bacterial inoculation in musculocutaneous and fasciocutaneous flaps. *Plast Reconstr Surg* 1990;86:1152–1162.

68. Ger R. Muscle transposition for treatment and prevention of chronic post-traumatic osteomyelitis of the tibia. *J Bone Joint Surg* 1977;59:784–791.

69. Stark WJ. The use of pedicled muscle flaps in the surgical treatment of chronic osteomyelitis resulting form compound fractures. *J Bone Joint Surg* 1946;28:343.

70. Perler BA, Dufresne CR, Williams GM, et al. Can infected prosthetic grafts be salvaged with rotational muscle flaps? *Surgery* 1991;110:30–34.

71. Mixter RC, Smith DJ Jr, Acher CW, et al. Rotational muscle flaps: a new technique for covering infected vascular grafts. *J Vasc Surg* 1989;9:472–478.

71a. Mathes SJ, Nahai F. Classification of the vascular anatomy of muscles: experimental and clinical correlation. *Plast Reconstr Surg* 1981;67:177–187.

72. McCraw JB, Carraway JH, et al. Clinical definition of independent myocutaneous vascular territories. *Plast Reconstr Surg* 1977;60:341–352.

73. Cormack GC, Lamberty BG. A classification of fasciocutaneous flaps according to their patterns of vascularisation. *Br J Plast Surg* 1984;37:80.

74. Cormack GC, Lamberty BG. *The arterial anatomy of skin flaps,* 2 ed. Edinburgh: Churchill Livingstone,1994.

75. Fix RJ, Vasconez LO. Fasciocutaneous flaps in reconstruction of the lower extremity. *Clin Plast Surg* 1991;18:571–582.

76. Lai CS, Yang CC, Chou CK, et al. The adipofascial turnover flap for complicated dorsal skin defects of the hand and finger. *Br J Plast Surg* 1991;44:165–169.

77. Cormack GC, Lamberty BG. Fasciocutaneous vessels in the upper arm: application to the design of new fasciocutaneous flaps. *Plast Reconstr Surg* 1984;74:244–250.

78. Cohen BE. Shoulder defect correction with island latissimus dorsi flap. *Plast Reconstr Surg* 1984;74:650–656.

79. Dowden RV, McCraw JB. Muscle flap reconstruction of shoulder defects. *J Hand Surg* 1980;5:382–390.

80. Mendelson BC, Masson JK. Treatment of chronic radiation injury over the shoulder with a latissimus dorsi myocutaneous flap. *Plast Reconstr Surg* 1977;60:681–691.

81. Bartlett SP, Yaremchuk MJ, et al. The latissimus dorsi muscle: a fresh cadaver study of the primary neurovascular pedicle. *Plast Reconstr Surg* 1981;67:631–636.

82. Lin CH, Levin LS, Chen MC, et al. Donor-site morbidity comparison between endoscopically assisted and traditional harvest of free latissimus dorsi muscle flap. *Plast Reconstr Surg* 1999;104:1070–1077.

83. Cho BC, Ramasastry SS, Baik BS, et al. Free latissimus dorsi muscle transfer using an endoscopic technique. *Ann Plast Surg* 1997;38:586–593.

84. Tobin GR, Perterson GH, Nichols G, et al. The intramuscular neurovascular anatomy of the latissimus dorsi muscle: the basis of splitting the flap. *Plast Reconstr Surg* 1981;67:637–641.

85. Tobin GR, Dubou RH, Weiner LJ, et al. The split latissimus dorsi myocutaneous flap. *Ann Plast Surg* 1981;7:272–280.

86. Russell RC, Zook EG, Leighton WD, et al. Functional evaluation of latissimus dorsi donor site. *Plast Reconstr Surg* 1986;78:336–344.

87. Clough KB, Fitoussi A, Couturaud B, et al. Donor site sequelae after autologous breast reconstruction with an extended latissimus dorsi flap. *Plast Reconstr Surg* 2002;109:1904–1911.

88. Laitung JK, Peck F. Shoulder function following the loss of the latissimus dorsi muscle. *Br J Plast Surg* 1985;38:375–379.

89. Freedlander E, Vandervord JC, et al. Reconstruction of the axilla with a pectoralis major myocutaneous island flap. *Br J Plast Surg* 1982;35:144–146.

90. Doyle JR, Larsen LJ, Ashley RK, et al. Restoration of elbow flexion in arthrogryposis multiplex congenita. *J Hand Surg* 1980;5:149–152.

91. Atkins RM, Sharrard WJ, et al. Pectoralis major transfer for paralysis of elbow flexion in children. *J Bone Joint Surg* 1985;67:640–644.

92. Brooks DM, et al. Pectoral transplant for paralysis of the flexors of the elbow. *J Bone Joint Surg* 1959;41:36–43.

93. Tsai T, Burns J, Kleinert HE, et al. Restoration of elbow flexion by pectoralis major and pectoralis minor transfer. *J Hand Surg* 1983;8:186–190.

94. Dimond M, Barwick W. Treatment of axillary burn scar contracture using a arterialized scapular island flap. *Plast Reconstr Surg* 1983;72:388–390.

95. Dos Santos LF. The vascular anatomy and dissection of the free scapular flap. *Plast Reconstr Surg* 1984;73:599–603.

96. Teot L, Bosse JP. The use of scapular skin island flaps in the treatment of axillary postburn scar contractures. *Br J Plast Surg* 1994;47:108–111.

97. Maruyama Y. Ascending scapular flap and its use for the treatment of axillary burn scar contracture. *Br J Plast Surg* 1991;44:97–101.

98. Bishop AT. Soft tissue loss about the elbow: selecting optimal coverage. *Hand Clin* 1994;10:531–542.

99. Brones MF, Lesavoy MA, et al. Restoration of elbow function and arm contour with the latissimus dorsi myocutaneous flap. *Plast Reconstr Surg* 1982;69:329–332.

100. Schottstaedt ER, Bost FC, et al. Complete muscle transposition. *J Bone Joint Surg* 1955;37:897–919.

101. Stern PJ, Gregory RO, Kreilien JG, et al. Latissimus dorsi myocutaneous flap for elbow flexion. *J Hand Surg* 1982;7:25–30.

102. Takami H, Ando M, et al. Latissimus dorsi transplantation to restore elbow flexion in the paralyzed limb. *J Hand Surg* 1984;9:61–63.

103. Zancolli E, Mitre H. Latissimus dorsi transfer to restore elbow flexion. *J Bone Joint Surg* 1973;55:1265–1275.

104. Ihara K, Shigetomi M, Kawai S, et al. Experience with the pedicled latissimus dorsi flap for finger reconstruction. *J Hand Surg* 2000;25:668–673.

105. Almquist EE, Bach AW, et al. Epicondylar resection with anconeus muscle transfer for chronic lateral epicondylitis. *J Hand Surg* 1998;23:723–731.

106. Parry SW, Mathes SJ, et al. Vascular anatomy of the upper extremity muscles. *Plast Reconstr Surg* 1988;81:358–365.

107. McGeorge DD, Stilwell JH, et al. The distally-based brachioradialis muscle flap. *Br J Plast Surg* 1991;44:30–32.

108. Lai MF, Pelly AD, et al. The brachioradialis myocutaneous flap. *Br J Plast Surg* 1981;34:431–434.

109. Lalikos JF, et al. Brachioradialis musculocutaneous flap closure of the elbow utilizing a distal skin island: a case report. *Ann Plast Surg* 1997;39:201–204.

110. Binns M, Pho RW, et al. Brachioradialis forearm flap in a case of traumatic bone and skin loss at the elbow. *J Hand Surg* 1990;15:317–319.

111. Balakrishnan C, Nyitray J, et al. The use of the brachioradialis muscle flap for the coverage of burns of the acute elbow joint. *J Burn Care Rehabil* 1999;20:265–266.

112. Sanger JR, Yousif NJ, Matloub HS, et al. The brachioradialis forearm flap: anatomy and clinical application. *Plast Reconstr Surg* 1994;94:667–674.

113. Rohrich RJ, et al. Brachioradialis muscle flap: clinical anatomy and use in soft-tissue reconstruction of the elbow. *Ann Plast Surg* 1995;35:70–76.

114. Meland NB, Wood MB, et al. Pedicled radial forearm flaps for recalcitrant defects about the elbow. *Microsurgery* 1991;12:155–159.

115. Yang GF, Gao YZ, Liu XY, et al. Forearm free skin flap transplantation. *Natl Med J China* 1981;61:139.

116. Yang GF, Gao YZ, Liu XY, et al. Forearm free skin flap transplantation: a report of 56 cases. 1981. *Br J Plast Surg* 1997;50:162–165.

117. Song R, Song Y, et al. The forearm flap. *Clin Plast Surg* 1982;9:21–26.

118. Lamberty BG, et al. The forearm angiosomes. *Br J Plast Surg* 1982;35:420–429.

119. Hallock GG. Soft tissue coverage of the upper extremity using the ipsilateral radial forearm flap. *Contemp Orthop* 1987;15:15–23.

120. Foucher G, Merle N, et al. A compound radial artery forearm flap in hand surgery: an original modification of the Chinese forearm flap. *Br J Plast Surg* 1984;37:139–148.

121. Muhlbsuer W, Stock W, et al. The forearm flap. *Plast Reconstr Surg* 1982;70:343–344.

122. Yajima H, Shono M, Tamai S, et al. Radical forearm flap with vascularized tendons for hand reconstruction. *Plast Reconstr Surg* 1996;98:328–333.

123. Podlewski J, Jankiewicz L, et al. Dorsal hand injury repair with vascularized tendon graft using a radial forearm flap—case report. *Acta Chir Plast* 1988;30:58–62.

124. Foucher G, Merle M, Michon J. Single stage thumb reconstruction by a composite forearm island flap. *J Hand Surg* 1984;9:245–248.

125. Matev I. The osteocutaneous pedicle forearm flap. *J Hand Surg* 1985;10:179–182.

126. Brotherston TM, Lamberty BG, et al. Digital reconstruction using the distally based osteofasciocutaneous radial forearm flap. *J Hand Surg* 1987;12:93–95.

127. Reid CD, et al. One-stage flap repair with vascularized tendon grafts in a dorsal hand injury using the "Chinese" forearm flap. *Br J Plast Surg* 1983;36:473–479.

128. Hoang P, Maldague P, Burke FD, et al. Radial forearm flaps in surgery of the hand. *Atlas Hand Clin* 1998;3:119–146.

129. Chang TS, et al. Forearm flap in one-stage reconstruction of the penis. *Plast Reconstr Surg* 1984;74:251–258.

130. Waterhouse N, Townsend PL, et al. Lower limb salvage using an extended free radial forearm flap. *Br J Plast Surg* 1984;37:394–397.

131. Fatah MF, et al. The radial forearm island flap in upper extremity limb reconstruction. *J Hand Surg* 1984;9:234–238.

132. McGregor AD. The free radial forearm flap: the management of the secondary defect. *Br J Plast Surg* 1987;40:341–352.

133. Timmons MJ, Pode MD, et al. Complications of radial forearm flap donor sites. *Br J Plast Surg* 1986;39:176–178.

134. Jones BM, et al. Acute ischaemia of the hand resulting from elevation of a radial forearm flap. *Br J Plast Surg* 1985;38:396–397.

135. Higgins JP, Chang P, Serletti JM, et al. Hypothenar hammer

syndrome after radial forearm flap harvest: a case report. *J Hand Surg* 2001;26:772–775.

136. Ruengsakulrach P, Fahrer C, Fahrer M, et al. Surgical implications of variations in hand collateral circulation: anatomy revisited. *J Thorac Cardiovasc Surg* 2001;122:682–686.

137. Kleinman WB, O'Connel S. Effects of the fasciocutaneous radial forearm flap on vascularity of the hand. *J Hand Surg* 1993;18:953–958.

138. Braun FM, Merle M, Van Genechten F, et al. Technique and indications of the forearm flap in hand surgery. A report of thirty-three cases. *Ann Chir Main* 1985;4:85–97.

139. Meland NB, Hoverman VR, et al. The radial forearm flap donor site: should we vein graft the artery? A comparative study. *Plast Reconstr Surg* 1993;91:865–870, 1993.

140. Suominen S, Asko-Seljavaara S, et al. Donor site morbidity of radial forearm flaps. A clinical and ultrasonographic evaluation. *Scand J Plast Reconstr Surg Hand Surg* 1996;30:57–61.

141. Ciria-Llorens G, et al. Hand blood supply in radial forearm flap donor extremities: a qualitative analysis using Doppler examination. *J Hand Surg* 2001;26:125–128.

142. Ciria-Llorens G, Talegon-Melendez A, et al. Analysis of flow changes in forearm arteries after raising the radial forearm flap: a prospective study using color duplex imaging. *Br J Plast Surg* 1999;52:440–444.

143. Talegon-Melendez A, Gomez-Cia T, Mayo-Iscar A, et al. Flow changes in forearm arteries after elevating the radial forearm flap: prospective study using color duplex imaging. *J Ultrasound Med* 1999;18:553–558.

144. Richardson D, Vaughan ED, Brown JS, et al. Radial forearm flap donor-site complications and morbidity: a prospective study. *Plast Reconstr Surg* 1997;99:109–115.

145. Boorman JG, Sykes PJ, et al. Morbidity in the forearm flap donor arm. *Br J Plast Surg* 1987;40:207–212.

146. Swanson E, Mulholland RS, et al. The radial forearm flap: a biomechanical study of the osteotomized radius. *Plast Reconstr Surg* 1990;85:267–272.

147. Jin YT, Shi TM, Quian YL, et al. Reversed island forearm fascial flap in hand surgery. *Ann Plast Surg* 1985;15:340–347.

148. Reyes FA, et al. The fascial radial flap. *J Hand Surg* 1988;13:432–437.

149. Smith PJ, et al. Tubed radial fascial flap and reconstruction of the flexor apparatus in the forearm. *J Hand Surg* 1993;18:959–962.

150. Chang SC, Halbert CF, Yang KH, et al. Limiting donor site morbidity by suprafascial dissection of the radial forearm flap. *Microsurgery* 1996;17:136.

151. Lutz BS, Chang SC, Yang KH, et al. Donor site morbidity after suprafascial elevation of the radial forearm flap: a prospective study in 95 consecutive cases. *Plast Reconstr Surg* 1999;103:132–137.

152. Avery CM, Brown AE, et al. Suprafascial dissection of the radial forearm flap and donor site morbidity. *Int J Oral Maxillofac Surg* 2001;30:37–41.

153. Hallock GG. Refinement of the radial forearm flap donor site using skin expansion. *Plast Reconstr Surg* 1988;81:21–25.

154. Hallock GG. Free flap donor site refinement using tissue expansion. *Ann Plast Surg* 1988;20:566–572.

155. Masser MR. The preexpanded radial free flap. *Plast Reconstr Surg* 1990;86:295–301.

156. Juretic M, Zambelli M. The radial forearm free flap: our experience in solving donor site problems. *J Craniomaxillofac Surg* 1992;20:184–186.

157. Bardsley AF, Elliot D, Batchelor AG, et al. Reducing morbidity in the radial forearm flap donor site. *Plast Reconstr Surg* 1990;86:287–292.

158. Kincaid CB, et al. The lateral arm flap: free tissue transfer of pedicled flap? In: Gilbert A, Heintz V, et al., eds. *Pedicled flaps of the upper limb.* London: Martin Dunitz Ltd., 1992:53.

159. Sherman R. Soft-tissue coverage for the elbow. *Hand Clin* 1997;13:291–302.

160. Lai CS, Chou CK, Tsai CC. The reverse lateral arm flap, based on the interosseous recurrent artery, for cubital fossa burns. *Br J Plast Surg* 1994;47:341–345.

161. Lai CS, Liao KB, Lin SD, et al. The reverse lateral arm adipofascial flap for elbow coverage. *Ann Plast Surg* 1997;39:196–200.

162. Kostakoglu N, et al. Upper limb reconstruction with reverse flaps: a review of 52 patients with emphasis on flap selection. *Ann Plast Surg* 1997;39:381–389.

163. Coessens B, De Mey A, et al. Clinical experience with the reverse lateral arm flap in soft-tissue coverage of the elbow. *Plast Reconstr Surg* 1993;92:1133–1136.

164. Maruyama Y, et al. The radial recurrent fasciocutaneous flap: reverse upper arm flap. *Br J Plast Surg* 1986;39:458–461.

165. Tung TC, Fang CM, Lee CM, et al. Reverse pedicled lateral arm flap for reconstruction of posterior soft-tissue defects of the elbow. *Ann Plast Surg* 1997;38:635–641.

166. Lamberty BG, Cormack G. The antecubital fasciocutaneous flap. *Br J Plast Surg* 1983;36:428–433.

167. Van Landuyt K, Monstrey SJ, Blondeel PN, et al. The antecubital fasciocutaneous island flap for elbow coverage. *Ann Plast Surg* 1998;41:252–257.

168. Naasan A, et al. Successful transfer of two reverse forearm flaps despite disruption of both palmar arches. *Br J Plast Surg* 1990;43:476–479.

169. Cavanagh S, et al. The reverse radial forearm flap in the severely injured hand: an anatomical and clinical study. *J Hand Surg* 1992;17:501–503.

170. Weinzweig N, Chen ZW, et al. The distally based radial forearm fasciosubcutaneous flap with preservation of the radial artery: an anatomic and clinical approach. *Plast Reconstr Surg* 1994;94:675–684.

171. Masquelet AC. The posterior interosseous forearm flap in surgery of the hand. *Atlas Hand Clin* 1998;3:109–118.

172. Germann G, Levin LS, et al. *Decision-making in reconstructive surgery (upper-extremity).* Berlin: Springer-Verlag, 2000:181–221.

173. Costa H, Vranchx J, Cunha C, et al. The posterior interosseous flap: a review of 81 clinical cases and 100 anatomical dissections—assessment of its indications in reconstruction of hand defects. *Br J Plast Surg* 2001;54:28–33.

174. Brunelli F, Dumontier C, Panciera P, et al. The posterior interosseous reverse flap: experience with 113 flaps. *Ann Plast Surg* 2001;47:25–30.

175. Chen HC, Chuang D, Wei FC, et al. Microvascular free posterior interosseous flap and a comparison with the pedicled posterior interosseous flap. *Ann Plast Surg* 1996;36:542–550.

176. Mazzer N, Cortez M, et al. The posterior interosseous forearm island flap for skin defects in the hand and elbow. A prospective study of 51 cases. *J Hand Surg* 1996;21:237–243.

177. Glasson DW, et al. The ulnar island flap in hand and forearm reconstruction. *Br J Plast Surg* 1988;41:349–353.

178. Jawad AS, et al. The island sensate ulnar artery flap for reconstruction around the elbow. *Br J Plast Surg* 1990;43:695–698.

179. Guimberteau JC, Panconi B, Schuhmacher B. The reverse ulnar artery forearm island flap in hand surgery: 54 cases. *Plast Reconstr Surg* 1988;81:925–932.

180. Sakai S, Endo T, Shojima M, et al. Distally based ulnar artery island forearm flap for the large defect of the ulnar side of the hand. *Ann Plast Surg* 1989;23:266–268.

181. Li ZT, Cao YD, et al. The reverse flow ulnar artery island flap: 42 clinical cases. *Br J Plast Surg* 1989;42:256–259.

182. Lister GD, et al. Skin flaps. In: Green DP, Pederson WC, eds. *Green's operative hand surgery.* New York: Churchill Livingstone, 1999:1783–1850.

183. Holevich-Madjarova B, Topkarov V, et al. Island flap supplied by the dorsal branch of the ulnar artery. *Plast Reconstr Surg* 1991;87:562–566.

184. Giunta R, Lanz U, et al. The hypothenar fat-pad flap for reconstructive repair after scarring of the median nerve at the wrist joint. *Chir Main* 1998;17:107–112.

185. Strickland JW, Lourie GM, Plancher KD, et al. The hypothenar fat pad flap for management of recalcitrant carpal tunnel syndrome. *J Hand Surg* 1996;21:840–848.

186. Plancher KD, Lourie GM, Strickland JW, et al. Recalcitrant carpal tunnel. The hypothenar fat pad flap. *Hand Clin* 1996;12:337–349.

187. Spokevicius S, et al. The abductor digiti minimi flap: its use in revision carpal tunnel surgery. *Hand Clin* 1996;12:351–355.

188. Reisman NR, et al. The abductor digiti minimi muscle flap: a salvage technique for palmar wrist pain. *Plast Reconstr Surg* 1983;72:859–865.

189. Milward TM, Kleinert HE, et al. The abductor digiti minimi muscle flap. *Hand* 1977;9:82–85.

190. Pizzillo MF, Tomaino MM, et al. Recurrent carpal tunnel syndrome: treatment options. *J South Orthop Assoc* 1999;8:28–36.

191. Adani R, Battiston B, Marcoccio I, et al. Management of neuromas in continuity of the median nerve with the pronator quadratus muscle flap. *Ann Plast Surg* 2002;48:35–40.

192. Dellon AL, et al. The pronator quadratus muscle flap. *J Hand Surg* 1984;9:423–427.

193. Holevich J. A new method of restoring sensibility to the thumb. *J Bone Joint Surg* 1963;45:496.

194. Small JO, et al. The first dorsal metacarpal artery island neurovascular island flap. *J Hand Surg* 1988;13:136–145.

195. Yang JY. The first dorsal metacarpal flap in first web space and thumb reconstruction. *Ann Plast Surg* 1991;27:258–264.

196. Paneva-Holevich E, et al. Further experience with the bipedicled neurovascular island flap in thumb reconstruction. *J Hand Surg* 1991;16:594.

197. Shi SM, et al. Island skin flap with neurovascular pedicle from the dorsum of the index finger for reconstruction of the thumb. *Microsurgery* 1994;15:145–148.

198. Ratcliffe RJ, Scerri GV, et al. First dorsal metacarpal artery flap cover for extensive pulp defects in the normal length thumb. *Br J Plast Surg* 1992;45:544–546.

199. Foucher G, et al. Island flaps based on the first and second dorsal metacarpal arteries. *Atlas Hand Clin* 1998;3:93–108.

200. Foucher G, et al. A new island flap transfer from the dorsum of the index to the thumb. *Plast Reconstr Surg* 1979;63:344–349.

201. Kuhlmann N. Contributuin a l'etude de la vascularization du dos de la main. Son interet pratique. *Ann Chir* 1978;32:587–591.

202. Healy C, Earley MJ, Woodcock J, et al. Focusable Doppler ultrasound in mapping dorsal hand flaps. *Br J Plast Surg* 1990;43:296–299.

203. Chang LY, Wie FC, et al. Reverse dorsal metacarpal flap in digits and web space reconstruction. *Ann Plast Surg* 1994;33:281–289.

204. Early MJ, et al. Dorsal metacarpal flaps. *Br J Plast Surg* 1987;40:333–341.

205. Foucher G, et al. A new island flap transfer from the dorsum of the index to the thumb. *Plast Reconstr Surg* 1979;63:344–349.

206. Schoofs M, Leps P, et al. The reverse metacarpal flap from the first web. *Eur J Plast Surg* 1993;16:26–29.

207. Foucher G, Merle M, et al. La technique du "debranchement-rebranchement" du lambeau en ilot pedicule. *Ann Chir* 1981;35:301–303.

208. Foucher G, et al. Digital reconstruction with island flaps. *Clin Plast Surg* 1997;24:1–32.

209. Gebhard B, et al. An extended first dorsal metacarpal artery neurovascular island flap. *J Hand Surg* 1995;20:529–531.

210. German G, et al. Intrinsic flaps in the hand. *Tech Hand Upper Extrem Surg* 1997;1:48–61.

211. German G, Raff T, et al. Two new applications for the first dorsal metacarpal artery pedicle in the treatment of severe hand injuries. *J Hand Surg* 1995;20:525–528.

212. Early MJ. The arterial supply of the thumb, first web space and index finger and its surgical application. *J Hand Surg* 1986;11:163–174.

213. Ikeda A, Kazihara Y, Hamada N, et al. Arterial patterns in the hand based on a three-dimensional analysis of 220 cadaver hands. *J Hand Surg* 1988;13:501–509.

214. Hao J, Bao-Feng G, et al. The second dorsal metacarpal flap with vascular pedicle composes of the second dorsal metacarpal artery. *Plast Reconstr Surg* 1993;92:501–506.

215. Small JO, et al. The second dorsal metacarpal artery neurovascular island flap. *Br J Plast Surg* 1990;43:17–23.

216. Maruyama Y, et al. The reverse dorsal metacarpal flap. *Br J Plast Surg* 1990;43:24–27.

217. Dautel G, et al. Dorsal metacarpal reverse flaps. Anatomical basis and clinical application. *J Hand Surg* 1991;16:400–405.

218. Bene MD, Raimondi R, Tremolada C, et al. Reverse dorsal digital island flap. *Plast Reconstr Surg* 1994;93:552.

219. Pelissier P, Bakhach J, Martin D, et al. Reverse dorsal digital and metacarpal flaps: a review of 27 cases. *Plast Reconstr Surg* 1999;103:159–165.

220. Legaillard P, Casoli V, Martin D, et al. Le Lambeau bommerang: vertiable lambeau cross finger pedicule en un temps. *Ann Chir Plast Esthet* 1996;41:251–258.

221. Chen SL, Chen SG, Cheng TY, et al. The boomerang flap in managing injuries of the dorsum of the distal phalanx. *Plast Reconstr Surg* 2000;106:834–839.

222. Littler JW. Neurovascular pedicle transfer of tissue in reconstructive surgery of the hand. *J Bone Joint Surg* 1956;38:917.

223. Reid DA. The neurovascular island flap in thumb reconstruction. *Br J Plast Surg* 1966;19:234–244.

224. Tubiana R, et al. Restoration of sensibility in the hand by neurovascular skin island transfer. *J Bone Joint Surg* 1961;43:474.

225. Luppino T, Balli A, Ligabue A, et al. Neurovascular island flaps in the emergency reconstruction of the terminal phalanx of the thumb. *Ital J Orthop Traumatol* 1980;6:67–76.

226. Cook FW, Pollock MA, et al. Local neurovascular island flap. *J Hand Surg* 1990;15:798–802.

227. Thompson JS. Reconstruction of the insensate thumb by neurovascular island transfer. *Hand Clin* 1992;8:99–105.

228. Oka Y. Sensory function of the neurovascular island flap in thumb reconstruction: comparison of original and modified procedures. *J Hand Surg* 2000;25:637–643.

229. Adani R, Castagnetti C, Lagana A, et al. A comparative study of the heterodigital neurovascular island flap in thumb reconstruction, with and without nerve reconnection. *J Hand Surg* 1994;19:552–559.

230. Markley J, Littler JW. The composite neurovascular skin island graft in surgery of the hand. *Atlas Hand Clin* 1998;3:59–76.

231. Krag C, et al. The neurovascular island flap for defective sensibility of the thumb. *J Bone Joint Surg* 1975;57:495–499.

232. Murray JF, Gavelin GE, et al. The neurovascular island pedicle flap: an assessment of late results in sixteen cases. *J Bone Joint Surg* 1967;49:1285–1297.

233. Henderson HP, et al. Long term follow-up of neurovascular island flaps. *Hand* 1980;12:113–122.

234. Stice RC, et al. Neurovascular island skin flaps in the hand: functional and sensibility evaluation. *Microsurgery* 1987;8:162–167.

235. Chao JD, Wiedrich TA, et al. Local hand flaps. *J Am Soc Surg Hand* 2001;1:25–44.

236. Hirase Y, Matsuura S, et al. A versatile one-stage neurovascular flap for fingertip reconstruction: the dorsal middle phalangeal finger flap. *Plast Reconstr Surg* 1992;90:1009–1015.

237. Joshi BB. A local dorsolateral island flap for restoration of sensation after avulsion injury of fingertip pulp. *Plast Reconstr Surg* 1974;54:175–182.

238. Lai CS, Yand CC, et al. The reverse digital artery flap for fingertip reconstruction. *Ann Plast Surg* 1989;22:495–500.

239. Lai CS, Chou CK, Tsai CW, et al. A versatile method for reconstruction of finger defects: reverse digital artery flap. *Br J Plast Surg* 1992;45:443–453.

240. Sapp JW, Dupin C, et al. A reversed digital artery island flap for the treatment of fingertip injuries. *J Hand Surg* 1993;18:528–534.

241. Niranjan NS, et al. A homodigital reverse pedicle island flap in soft tissue reconstruction of the finger and the thumb. *J Hand Surg* 1994;19:135–141.

242. Kojima T, Hirase Y, et al. Reverse vascular pedicle digital island flap. *Br J Plast Surg* 1990;43:290–295.

243. Tonkin MA, et al. The reconstruction of a dorsal digital defect using a reverse homodigital island flap incorporating vascularized tendon. *J Hand Surg* 1997;22:750–751.

244. Endo T, Hirase Y, et al. Vascular anatomy of the finger dorsum and a new idea for coverage of the finger pulp defect that restores sensation. *J Hand Surg* 1992;17:927–932.

245. Lai CS, Chou CK, Tsai CW, et al. Innervated reverse digital artery flap through bilateral neurorrhaphy for pulp defects. *Br J Plast Surg* 1993;46:483–488.

246. Moberg E. Aspects of sensation in reconstruction surgery of the upper extremity. *J Bone Joint Surg* 1964;46:817–825.

247. Elliot D, et al. V-Y advancement of the entire volar soft tissue of the thumb in distal reconstruction. *J Hand Surg* 1993;3:399–402.

248. Bang H, Hayashi H, et al. Palmar advancement flap with V-Y closure for thumb tip injuries. *J Hand Surg* 1992;17:933–934.

249. Dellon AL. The extended palmar advancement flap. *J Hand Surg* 1983;8:190–194.

250. O'Brien B. Neurovascular island pedicle flaps for terminal amputations and digital scars. *Br J Plast Surg* 1968;21:258–261.

251. Snow JW. The use of a volar flap for repair of fingertip amputations: a preliminary report. *Plast Reconstr Surg* 1967;40:163–168.

252. Hynes DE. Neurovascular pedicle and advancement flaps for palmar thumb defects. *Hand Clin* 1997;13:207–216.

253. Snow JW. Volar advancement skin flap to the fingertip. *Hand Clin* 1985;1:685–688.

254. Macht SD, Watson H. The Moberg volar advancement flap for digital reconstruction. *J Hand Surg* 1980;5:372–376.

255. Smith PJ, McGregor IA, Jackson IT, et al. The anatomical basis of the groin flap. *Plast Reconstr Surg* 1972;49:41–47.

256. Katai K, Numaguchi Y, et al. Angiography of the iliofemoral arteriovenous system supplying free groin flaps and free hypogastric flaps. *Plast Reconstr Surg* 1979;63:671–679.

257. Chuang DC, Chen HC, Wei FC, et al. Groin flap design and versatility. *Plast Reconstr Surg* 1989;84:100–107.

258. Joshi BB. Neural repair for sensory restoration in a groin flap. *Hand* 1977;9:221–225.

259. DeHaan MR, Mann RJ, et al. Controlled tissue expansion of a groin flap for upper extremity reconstruction. *Plast Reconstr Surg* 1990;86:979–982.

260. Smith PJ. The Y-shaped hypogastric-groin flap. *Hand* 1982;14:263–270.

261. Reinisch JF, Puckett CL, et al. The use of the osteocutaneous groin flap in gunshot wounds of the hand. *J Hand Surg* 1984;9:12–17.

262. Finseth F, Smith RJ, et al. Composite groin flap with iliac bone for primary thumb reconstruction. Case report. *J Bone Joint Surg* 1976;58:130–132.

263. Button M, et al. Segmental bony reconstruction of the thumb by composite groin flap: a case report. *J Hand Surg* 1980;5:488–491.

264. Chow JA, Hui P, Hall RF, et al. The groin flap in reparative surgery of the hand. *Plast Reconstr Surg* 1986;77:421–426.

265. Boyd JB, et al. An evaluation of the pedicled thoracoumbilical flap in upper extremity reconstruction. *Ann Plast Surg* 1989;22:236–242.

266. Lister GD, Jackson IT, et al. The groin flap in hand injuries. *Injury* 1973;4:229–239.

267. Nappi JF, et al. External fixation for pedicled flap immobilization: a new method providing limited motion. *Plast Reconstr Surg* 1983;72:243–245.

268. Cheng MH, Wei FC, See LC, et al. Combined ischemic preconditioning and laser Doppler measurement for early division of pedicled groin flap. *J Trauma* 1999;47:89–95.

269. McGrath MH, Finseth F, et al. The intravenous fluorescein test: use in timing of groin flap division. *J Hand Surg* 1979;4:19–22.

270. Wray RC, Young VL, Weeks PM, et al. The groin flap in severe hand injuries. *Ann Plast Surg* 1982;9:459–462.

271. Arner M, et al. Morbidity of the pedicled groin flap. A retrospective study of 44 cases. *Scand J Plast Reconstr Surg Hand Surg* 1994;28:143–146.

272. Graf P, et al. Morbidity of the groin flap transfer: are we getting something for nothing? *Br J Plast Surg* 1992;45:86–88.

273. Buchman SJ, Robertson BC, et al. Pedicled groin flaps for upper-extremity reconstruction in the elderly: a report of 4 cases. *Arch Phys Med Rehabil* 2002;83:850–854.

274. Fisher J. External oblique fasciocutaneous flap for elbow coverage. *Plast Reconstr Surg* 1985;75:51–61.

275. Davis WM, Carraway JH, et al. Use of a direct transverse thoracoabdominal flap to close difficult wounds of the thorax and upper extremities. *Plast Reconstr Surg* 1977;60:526–533.

276. Webster JP. Thoraco-epigastric tubed pedicles. *Surg Clin North Am* 1937;17:145.

277. Sbitany U, et al. Use of the rectus abdominus muscle flap to reconstruct an elbow defect. *Plast Reconstr Surg* 1985;77:988–989.

278. Burstein FD, Stahl RS, et al. Elbow joint salvage with the transverse rectus island flap: a new application. *Plast Reconstr Surg* 1989;84:492–497.

279. Freedlander E, McGrouther DA, et al. The present role of the groin flap in hand trauma in the light of a long-term review. *J Hand Surg* 1986;11:187–190.

280. Taylor GI, Caddy CM, Zelt RG, et al. An anatomic review of the delay phenomenon: II. Clinical applications. *Plast Reconstr Surg* 1992;89:408–416.

281. Callegari PR, Caddy CM, Minabe T, et al. An anatomic review of the delay phenomenon: I. Experimental studies. *Plast Reconstr Surg* 1992;89:397–407.

282. Morris SF, et al. The time sequence of the delay phenomenon: when is a surgical delay effective? An experimental study. *Plast Reconstr Surg* 1995;95:526–533.

283. Smith PJ. The importance of venous drainage in axial pattern flaps. *Br J Plast Surg* 1978;31:233–237.

284. Raskin DJ, Erik Y, Spira M, et al. Critical comparison of transcutaneous PO_2 and tissue pH as indices of perfusion. *Microsurgery* 1983;4:29–33.

285. Kerrigan CL, et al. Monitoring acute skin flap failure. *Plast Reconstr Surg* 1983;71:519–524.

286. McCraw JB, Shanklin KD, et al. The value of fluorescein in predicting the viability of arterialized flaps. *Plast Reconstr Surg* 1977;60:710–719.

287. Dibbell DC, Mcgraw JB, Rankin JH, et al. A quantitative examination of the use of fluorescein in predicting viability of skin flaps. *Ann Plast Surg* 1979;3:101–105.

288. Hickerson WL, Proctor KG, et al. Regional variations of laser Doppler blood flow in ischemic skin flaps. *Plast Reconstr Surg* 1990;86:319–326.

289. Jones JW, Hillman WC, et al. Remote monitoring of free flaps with telephonic transmissions of photoplethysmograph waveforms. *J Reconstr Microsurg* 1989;5:141–144.

290. Jones BM, Greenhalgh RM, et al. Differential thermometry as a monitor of blood flow in skin flaps. *Br J Plast Surg* 1983;36:83–87.

291. Jones BM, Greenhalgh RM, et al. Monitoring skin flaps by color measurements. *Br J Plast Surg* 1983;36:88–94.

292. Dooley TW, Puckett CL, et al. Noninvasive assessment of microvessels with the duplex scanner. *J Hand Surg* 1989;14:670–673.

293. Fischer JC, Shaw WW, et al. Comparison of two laser Doppler flowmeters for the monitoring of dermal blood flow. *Microsurgery* 1983;4:164–170.

294. Scheker LR, Firrell JC, Lister GD, et al. The value of the photoplethysmograph in monitoring skin closure in microsurgery. *J Reconstr Microsurg* 1985;2:1–4.

295. Svenson H, Holmberg J, Jacobsson S, et al. Detecting arterial and venous obstruction in flaps. *Ann Plast Surg* 1985;14:20–23.

296. Mulliken W, et al. Pathogenesis of skin flap necrosis from an underlying hematoma. *Plast Reconstr Surg* 1979;63:540–546.

297. Sasaki S, Soeda S, et al. Attempts to increase the surviving length in skin flaps by a moist environment. *Plast Reconstr Surg* 1979;64:526–531.

298. McGrath MH. How topical dressings salvage "questionable" flaps: experimental study. *Plast Reconstr Surg* 1981;67:653–659.

299. Tan CM, Myers RA, Hoopes JE, et al. Effects of hyperbaric oxygen and hyperbaric air on the survival of island slaps. *Plast Reconstr Surg* 1984;73:27–28.

300. Zamboni WA, Russel RC, Nemiroff PM, et al. The effects of acute hyperbaric oxygen therapy on axial pattern skin flap survival when administered during and after total ischemia. *J Reconstr Microsurg* 1989;5:343–347.

301. Kauffman T, et al. Systemic and local oxygen effects on rat axial pattern flap survival. *Chir Plast* 1983;7:201–209.

302. Awwad AM, Webster MH, Vance JP, et al. The effects of temperature on blood flow in island and free skin flaps: an experimental study. *Br J Plast Surg* 1983;36:373–382.

303. Awwad AM, Lowe GD, Forbes CD, et al. The effects of blood viscosity on blood flow in experimental saphenous flap model. *Br J Plast Surg* 1983;36:383–386.

67

FREE TISSUE TRANSFERS FOR COVERAGE

LIOR HELLER
LAWRENCE SCOTT LEVIN

The introduction of the operating microscope for anastomosis of blood vessels, which was described by Jacobson and Suarez (1) in 1960, marked the beginning of the microsurgery era for extremity reconstruction. After the beginning of microsurgical repair of digital arteries and digital replantation in the 1960s (2,3), microsurgical composite tissue transplantation began in the 1970s and still continues to evolve. Today, free tissue transfers are routine procedures and are used frequently as the reconstructive option of choice, alone or as a part from a more complex treatment. Combined procedures, including simultaneous management of fractures and associated soft tissue injury—the so-called orthoplastic approach—are now accepted treatment for upper extremity trauma. Expeditious repair of the soft tissue, which is enabled by free tissue transfer, allows for optimal repair processes for bone and soft tissue to take place, and it facilitates further reconstruction, such as tendon transfers or bone grafting. In many cases, free tissue transfer for coverage of upper extremity soft tissue defects is only a part of a team effort, which includes coordination among orthopedic surgeons, oncologists, vascular surgeons, traumatologists, and plastic surgeons, to salvage a limb. Communication and careful preoperative planning are important to ensure successful reconstruction. Sir Harold Gillies, who is considered to be one of the fathers of modern reconstructive plastic surgery, used the motto "replace like with like." The interpretation of this principle with regard to free tissue transfer is that the reconstructive surgeon transplants autogenously vascularized tissue into defects that are the result of trauma, tumor, infection, or congenital defects. The ability of the reconstructive surgeon to deliver the correct tissue at the correct time with the correct composite nature represents the art and the challenge of microsurgery in hand reconstruction.

INDICATIONS

Indications for free flaps for hand coverage are situations in which the other options that are included in the reconstructive ladder cannot be used or in which the result of their use may give an undesirable result, such as the following situations:

- To avoid the complications of edema and stiffness that are incurred by dependency, such as in the use of a groin flap.
- For a variety of large defects that involve the hand and forearm or unavailable local tissue for wound coverage.
- To avoid sacrificing a major artery, such as occurs with the reverse radial forearm flap, which requires cutting the radial artery proximally. In an already traumatized hand, this would cause further deprivation of blood supply. A free flap with end-to-side arterial anastomosis can cover a large defect without sacrificing a major artery.
- To avoid the increase of scar of the hand or the forearm that is caused by using a flap that is adjacent to the wound. The donor site of a free flap can be selected, thus resulting in a scar in a concealed area.
- To avoid the bulkiness that is caused by some conventional flaps that result in a limited range of movement. In contrast, a carefully selected free flap is able to facilitate a good functional as well as aesthetic result.

PREOPERATIVE PLANNING

In few other areas of hand surgery is careful preoperative planning so important. Like planning for tendon transfers, all possible permutations and combinations should be considered for their advantages and disadvantages. One must start with a clear idea of what has been lost, what is needed ideally for a given defect, the options available for restoration of each part and the one that should be selected, and the best time for performance of the transplant. It is important to realize that this a is a multistep procedure that includes preparation of the recipient site, harvest of the flap, transfer and revascularization of the flap, as well as inset of the tissue, and, in some cases, reconstruction of tendons, or stabilization of vascularized bone, such as in osteocutaneous or tendocutaneous flaps.

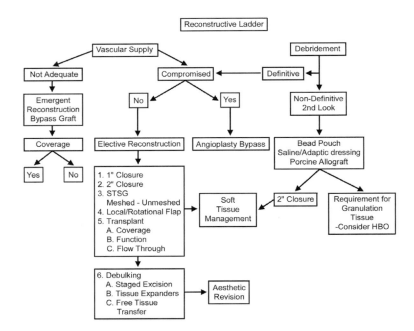

FIGURE 1. The reconstructive ladder for soft tissue. HBO, hyperbaric oxygen; STSG, split-thickness skin graft.

PERSONALITY OF SOFT TISSUE INJURY IN UPPER EXTREMITY TRAUMA

Evaluation of the soft tissue injury of the upper extremity and preparation of the wound are mandatory to enhance the success of the free tissue transfer. The time of injury, mechanism, energy absorption, fracture configuration, systemic injuries, damage to the soft tissue envelope, vascularity of the extremity, and sensibility should be noted in cases of trauma reconstruction. The mechanism of injury is important in determining how soft tissue should be treated and what part of the reconstructive ladder should be applied (Fig. 1). For example, electrical injuries that are associated with fracture may appear innocuous but may involve significant damage to soft tissue, as well as bone. In any high-energy wound, recognition of the zone of injury is of critical importance in determining the extent of débridement and the need for tissue (preferably imported) from a site that is outside the zone of injury for reconstruction of the soft tissue envelope (4). In acute cases, repetitive examinations of an open wounds should be done in an sterile environment to decrease the rates of wound infections and osteomyelitis. Prophylactic antibiotics should be administered on a regular basis, until definitive wound débridement and fracture stabilization can be performed. The presence of systemic shock, hemorrhage, and systemic injuries influence the soft tissue response of the injured hand and may jeopardize the reconstruction process. Underlying systemic diseases, such as cardiac disease or diabetes, may influence the approach to the reconstructive option that is offered to the patient. Once these considerations are dealt with, a reconstructive treatment plan can be formulated for the individual patient.

To understand the role of free tissue transfer in upper extremity reconstruction, one must understand the concept of the *reconstructive ladder* (Fig. 1). It represents an increasingly complex solution for soft tissue problems, with the ultimate goal being reconstitution of soft tissue. This algorithm should be used in the setting of acute or chronic soft tissue envelope damage. The reconstructive algorithm or ladder is used to select treatment for an injury, with or without fractures. In addition, it can be applied to chronic conditions, such as osteomyelitis, nonunion, or tumors (5).

Coverage can be in the form of a skin graft, local tissue transfer, adjacent tissue transfer, regional tissue transfer, or free tissue transfer, which represents the most complex rung on the reconstructive ladder and is the subject of this chapter. Free flaps represent solutions to complex soft tissue problems, with the ultimate goal being reconstitution of the soft tissue envelope (6). They can be used possibly in combination with lower rungs of the ladder, such as skin closure, skin grafting, or rotational flaps. The first rung in the reconstructive ladder is débridement and preparation of the wound for reconstruction.

DÉBRIDEMENT

The French term *débridement* implies the removal of soft tissues and bone that are nonviable. The purpose of débridement is to prevent infection. In the past, surgeons were reluctant to make the traumatic defects larger by radical débridement. Today, free tissue transfer of large, well-perfused flaps is readily available and allows radical débridement and removal of necrotic tissue. Débridement is required in acute trauma situations and for chronic wounds that have resulted from the improper handling of soft tissue or infection.

In an acute wound, the débridement can be done with the tourniquet up or down. Our preference is to begin the débridement with the tourniquet up, because hemorrhage and oozing can stain tissue, which makes it difficult to appreciate true bleeding and viability of tissue. The border of the débrided wound should include healthy tissue. Avulsed skin muscle and fascia should be removed from the base of avulsed flaps. Damaged tissue is recognized by the presence of foreign bodies, irregular tissue consistency, and irregular distribution of dark red stains, which represent hematomas. All nonviable tissue is removed preferably with a knife. It is not possible to do exact débridement with scissors. Scissors should be used only when dissecting important structures, such as nerves, vessels, or tendons. Releasing the tourniquet allows the surgeon to determine viability of tissue by observing the bleeding, color, and consistency of a tissue, such as muscle. Exposed bone should be washed with antibiotic solution. Severed vessels are ligated and, if they are not vital, are excised to normal appearing margins. If they are vital, continuity should be restored with interposition vein grafts. Nerves are the only structures in which the débridement is more conservative. Epineurium can be removed, with fascicles remaining intact. Occasionally, the bed of the wound remains irregular after débridement. With additional incisions, it can be made regular in shape, provided that the irregularity is not caused by tissue of functional importance. This maneuver serves to eliminate dead space by permitting free flaps close contact with the wound bed, thus preventing hematoma and subsequent formation of scar.

Chronic Wounds

Débridement of a chronic wound is also done with the limb exsanguinated. The goal of treatment for the chronic wound is to treat the wound as a tumor and to excise it in its entirety to the level of normal tissue planes. All scar tissue should be excised. Bone débridement can be difficult, because it can be difficult to distinguish the viable bone and callus from necrotic and inflamed areas of the medullary canal. Studies, such as computed tomography, bone scans, and magnetic resonance imaging, may be helpful in preoperative planning for bone débridement. At the conclusion of wound débridement, normal tissue planes should be visualized. If this is not possible, then a second-look procedure in which the débridement process is repeated is strongly advised. This should be done no later than 48 hours after the initial débridement, preferably at 24 hours after the initial débridement (7).

In compromised wounds, hyperbaric oxygen can be used to promote granulation tissue and to stimulate angiogenesis (8). In addition to exposure to hyperbaric oxygen, wound dressings are changed under sterile conditions by chamber personnel and further improve wound conditions, so that closure can be performed directly or with grafting, depending on the coverage needs.

Vacuum-assisted closure is a recently developed tool that uses subatmospheric pressure and promotes formation of granulation tissue. It has proven to be extremely effective in the treatment of a wide spectrum of wounds (9). The negative pressure that is applied to the wound helps to remove the excess fluid from the interstitium at the wound periphery, thus decreasing the local interstitial pressure and restoring blood flow to vessels that are compressed or collapsed by the excess pressure. The removed fluid contains factors that inhibit healing.

INDICATIONS FOR FREE TISSUE TRANSFER IN THE UPPER EXTREMITY: TRAUMA, SEPSIS, AND TUMOR

Trauma patients are the main group that benefits from free tissue transfer for soft tissue defects. The recognized importance of proper soft tissue coverage to maintain the vascularity of bone fragments leads to the simultaneous management of soft tissue injury and fractures, the so-called orthoplastic approach. This coordinated repair process for bone and soft tissue protects against the adverse sequelae of exposed fixation, bone sepsis, and possible amputation. The initial treatment should include débridement of the devitalized and contaminated tissue and stabilization of fractures. The need for an arteriogram should be based on the clinical assessment and the mechanism of injury. The anastomosis should be located outside of the zone of injury to decrease the incidence of thrombosis.

The concept of *zone of injury* refers to the inflammatory response, which extends beyond the gross wound and results in perivascular changes in the blood vessels, of the soft tissue of the limb. These changes include increased friability of the vessels and increased perivascular scar tissue, which can contribute to a higher failure rate, especially in lower limb free tissue transplantation, presumably due to a higher rate of microvascular thrombosis (10). Most surgeons avoid the zone of injury by extensive proximal dissection of the recipient vascular pedicle or use of vascular grafts. Isenberg and Sherman (4) demonstrated that clinical acceptability of the recipient pedicle (vessel wall pliability and the quality of blood from the transected end of the vessel) were more important than the distance from the wound. The choice of flap to be used for wound coverage is determined by the size of the wound, the type of tissue deficit, the state of the wound (e.g., colonization, amount of cavitation), the location of the injury, and the length of the pedicle that is needed.

Advanced age should not be a contraindication to microvascular limb salvage procedures. Careful preoperative patient evaluation and perioperative monitoring can effectively decrease morbidity and mortality rates to those equal to rates of younger patients. Microvascular reconstruction can be performed safely and successfully in the elderly patient (11).

TIMING OF FREE TISSUE TRANSFER

The timing of the wound closure by using microsurgical techniques is important. In severe injuries of the extremity with associated soft tissue defects, early aggressive wound débridement and soft tissue coverage with a free flap within 5 days were found to reduce postoperative infection and decrease the incidence of flap failure, nonunion, and chronic osteomyelitis (12,13). It also allows early mobilization of the extremity after injury, thus decreasing limb edema and postoperative stiffness. Godina (14) emphasized the pathophysiology of the high-energy trauma and the emergency (during the first operation) or the importance of radical débridement and early tissue coverage within the first 72 hours. Lister and Scheker (15) reported the first case of an emergency free flap transfer to the upper extremity in 1988, and they defined the emergency free flap as a "flap transfer performed either at the end of primary débridement or within 24 hours after the injury." Yaremchuk et al. (16) recommended that flaps should be transferred between 7 and 14 days after injury and several débridements. The argument in favor of this approach is that the zone of injury, which often may not be apparent at presentation, can be determined by serial débridements that are performed in the operating room over several days.

The keys factors that should be considered when deciding to do an early closure with a free flap of a hand soft tissue defect are the presence of an exposed vital structure, the risk of infection, and the possibility for early mobilization of the extremity; in these cases, early closure decreases limb edema and postoperative stiffness. An *exposed vital structure* is defined as "one that will rapidly undergo necrosis if not covered by adequate soft tissue" (17). The decision of what constitutes a vital structure depends on circumstances. Tissues, such as vessels, nerves, joint surfaces, tendons, and bone that is denuded of periosteum, may lose function and may create an environment that results in infection when they are left exposed for long periods of time. In the decision-making process, the surgeon must consider the risk of leaving the vital structure exposed, its functional importance, and the probability of differential recovery of function, depending on primary or delayed primary coverage.

The risk of infection should be also considered because it may jeopardize the limb, the quality of the functional recovery, or the free flap. As the risk of infection increases, the wisdom of primary closure with a free flap is reduced. Débridement of the wound is the most powerful tool of the surgeon to reduce the risk of infection of the wound. If radical débridement is not possible, it is not considered safe to consider a primary free flap transfer. Another perspective is that the capability to perform free tissue transfer allows the surgeon increased freedom to perform radical débridement and may actually reduce the risk of infection (18). Factors such as the mechanism of injury, the elapsed time, and the degree of contamination of the wound should be considered to better evaluate the degree of wound infection. In an acute, sharp, noncontaminated injury, for which closure would be routinely performed if there were no skin loss, there seems to be little reason not to consider an emergency free flap.

AMPUTATION VERSUS SALVAGE PROCEDURE

In complex extremity injuries, the treating physician must always determine first whether limb salvage is feasible. This can be done based on mangled score scales such as MESS (Mangled Extremity Severity Score) (19). Before complex and prolonged reconstructions are started on a limb that ultimately may function poorly or not at all, a well-fitted prosthesis should be seen as an excellent option, and early amputation should be considered. Lange (20) and Hansen (21) have delineated a sound algorithm for these difficult wounds. The questions that should be asked before beginning a long reconstructive process are if neurovascular structures are injured, are they repairable? Is normal sensibility obtainable? Does a compartment syndrome exist? Without its recognition, muscle ischemia and death occur, converting potentially viable soft tissue to infarcted muscle and scar. This ultimately increases the need for large block resections and tissue replacement, thus demanding a higher rung on the reconstructive ladder. Although the evolution of sophisticated microsurgical reconstructive techniques has created the possibility of successful limb salvage in even the most extreme cases, it has become painfully obvious that the technical possibilities are double-edged swords. Hansen (21), in analyzing his vast personal experience with managing open fractures, noted that protracted limb salvage attempts might destroy a person physically, psychologically, socially, and financially, with adverse consequences for the entire family, as well. In spite of the best attempts, the functional results are often worse than an amputation. Thus, enthusiasm for limb salvage techniques must be tempered by a realistic assessment of the results, not just for the injured part but for the patient as a whole (20). Donor site morbidity should also be considered with free tissue transfer, when approaching a limb reconstruction. Indicators for a poor prognosis for limb salvage, in order of significance, are (a) massive crush injuries, (b) other high-energy soft tissue injuries, (c) a warm ischemia time that is longer than 6 hours, (d) severely comminuted or segmental fracture patterns, (e) major arterial injury, (f) prolonged severe hypovolemia shock, and (g) age older than 50 years.

When an amputation is performed, coverage should be planned meticulously. In these cases in which a local flap is not available, free flaps should be considered. These flaps can provide coverage of the stump, and, if microneural anastomosis is performed, sensation of the stump can be achieved, which may assist proprioception within the prosthesis. A free *fillet flap* may represent an ideal solution in these cases. *Classic fillet flaps* are defined as axial pattern flaps that are harvested from amputated, discarded, or otherwise nonfunctioning or nonsalvageable parts. These flaps can cover finger stumps, as well as more proximal parts of the upper extremity, depending on the amputated part and the size of the stump that needs to be covered (22).

ORTHOPEDIC SEPSIS: OSTEOMYELITIS AND INFECTED JOINT PROSTHESIS

Hand infections with loss of soft tissue and osteomyelitis are now treatable diseases. The management of dead space after sequestrectomy relies heavily on the technique of free tissue transfer (23). Free muscle flaps provide coverage for the débrided bone and soft tissue, obliterate dead space, improve vascularity, and enhance leukocyte function (24–26).

Other advantages of free muscle flaps, such as latissimus dorsi (27), serratus anterior (28), and rectus abdominis (29), compared to the local muscle flaps are that they provide greater bulk (filling larger wounds), have longer pedicles (increasing flexibility in muscle positioning), and carry larger-diameter vessels (facilitating the microanastomoses).

Exposure of plates and screws may occur after open reduction and internal fixation of fractures. This occurs commonly when there is a significant tissue edema, thus creating difficulty in skin closure. When exposed, orthopedic prosthetic materials become colonized with bacteria, and, in the majority of these cases, rapid intervention is required to salvage the extremity and to prevent osteomyelitis. Removal of the prosthesis, débridement, closure with a muscle flap, and delayed insertion of a new prosthesis constitute the preferred treatment. Free muscle transfers not only provide coverage of the defect but also provide a well-vascularized tissue in close proximity to the new prosthesis. Fasciocutaneous flaps, such as the anterolateral thigh, can provide good coverage for exposed plates.

TUMORS

Upper extremity tumors that involve compartment resections that leave large soft tissue defects are best treated with free tissue transfer, specifically free muscle or free skin flaps. In soft tissue sarcoma, in which entire compartments are resected, microsurgical transplantation replaces

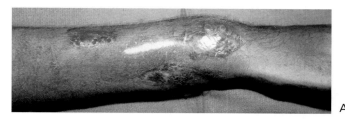

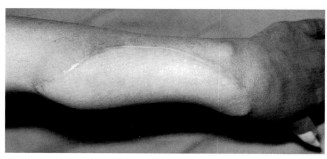

FIGURE 2. A: Sarcoma of the forearm. **B:** Scapula fasciocutaneous flap after resection of the tumor.

components of muscle and skin to maintain limb contour and to aid in healing. In radiated wounds, import of well-vascularized tissue that is provided by the free flaps results in more rapid wound healing and may improve local circulation in radiated areas. For this reason, many centers have adopted the policy that immediate microsurgical reconstruction be performed after tumor extirpation. The results of immediate microsurgical transfers in these cases have been well substantiated and have led to decreased hospital time, decreased costs, decreased morbidity, increased rate of limb salvage, and high patient satisfaction (30) (Fig. 2).

SOFT TISSUE CHARACTERISTICS

Dorsal Surface

The tissue on the dorsum of the hand is nonglabrous, hirsute, thin, and mobile to allow individual movements of the joints of the hand. A thin layer of the areolar tissue that covers extensor tendons permits easy tendon gliding. The ideal replacement tissue should also be thin and supple and should permit motion and tendon gliding.

Palmar Surface

The glabrous skin of the palmar surface of the hand represents specialized epithelium that is extremely difficult to replace after full-thickness loss. The normal surface is thick, hairless, cornified, and elastic to provide protection and support. The concentration of sensory mechanoreceptors in the palm is higher than it is on any other surface of the body. There is an abundance of exocrine sweat glands that lubricate the skin and indirectly aid in sensation. Anchored to the underlying system of fascia by fibrous septae, the palmar hand is immobile yet malleable.

The ideal replacement for full-thickness palmar defects is tissue that is thin, durable, relatively immobile, hairless, and sensate. In contrast to dorsal defects, the requirement for sensation is more important in the palm.

FLAP SELECTION

There are numerous flaps that have a place in hand reconstruction. Each flap has advantages and disadvantages. We discuss these flaps that, based on our experiences, come closest to fulfilling the tissue requirements of the dorsal or palmar surface of the hand or any other surface of the upper extremity. The commonly used fasciocutaneous free flaps are the lateral arm flap, radial forearm flap, scapular flaps, dorsalis pedis, and groin flaps.

Lateral Arm Flap

This flap can serve as innervated fasciocutaneous flap or as deepithelized subcutaneous fascial flap. The lateral arm flap is based on the posterior radial collateral artery, which is a direct continuation of the deep brachial artery and venae comitantes. The dimensions of the skin flap can be as large as 8×15 cm^2 with a pedicle length of as large as 7 cm. The anatomy of this vascular pedicle is constant, in contrast with the medial arm flap, which has a more variable vascular supply (Fig. 3). The lateral arm flap is innervated by the posterior brachial cutaneous nerve, a proximal branch of the radial nerve (C5 and C6), which gives the flap potential as a sensate flap. Additional sensory supply comes from the posterior antebrachial cutaneous nerve, which divides at the distal upper arm, with the upper branch supplying the posterior inferior upper arm and the lower branch supplying the lateral side of the arm and elbow (31). The deep fascia is included in the flap, and this kind of flap can be advantageous in cases in which thin well-vascularized coverage is required and for coverage of areas in which tendon gliding is required (32), as well as for the dorsum of the hand (33). The periosteal blood supply from the posterior radial collateral artery allows a vascularized bony segment that is 10 cm long and 1 cm wide to be included with the skin flap. Concerning its dimension for primary closure, the width should be less than 6 cm for primary closure. In cases in which a thinner flap is needed, such as finger coverage, the lateral arm fascia flap can provide the desired tissue. The fascia can be covered with a skin graft (34) (Fig. 4).

Radial Forearm Flap

This is a thin well-vascularized fasciocutaneous flap on the ventral aspect of the arm that was used widely in China,

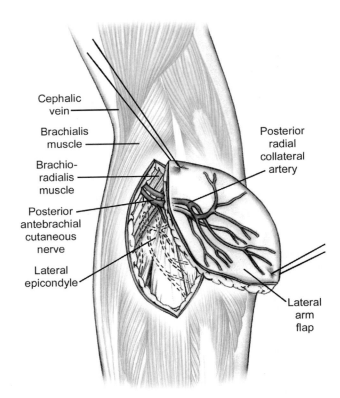

FIGURE 3. Surgical anatomy of the lateral arm flap.

before it was popularized in the Western literature (35,36). The flap is based on the radial artery, which can achieve a 20-cm-long pedicle. This length of the pedicle facilitates the microsurgical anastomosis out of zone of injury. The venous drainage is through the venae comitantes of the radial artery, but the flap can include the cephalic vein or the basilic vein, or both. The flap can contain the lateral antebrachial cutaneous nerve or the medial antebrachial cutaneous nerve and serves as a neurosensory flap. The size of the flap can be 10×40 cm^2. A portion of the radius can be included as a vascularized bone with this flap (37). Preliminary tissue expansion increases the flap dimensions, and, more importantly, it allows direct closure of the donor defect (38). In most of the cases, the donor site requires a skin graft for closure, thus leaving a scar in a visible place. The radial forearm is used less today for closure of defects in the hand, because its elevation causes a decrease of blood flow to the hand (Fig. 5).

Scapular Flap

The scapular flap is a thin, usually hairless, skin flap from the posterior chest and can be used when large defects should be covered. The primary indication for the scapular flap is a defect that requires a relatively thin, large, cutaneous flap (39). The flap is perfused by the cutaneous branches of the circumflex scapular artery and is drained by its venae comitantes. The circumflex scapular artery is the

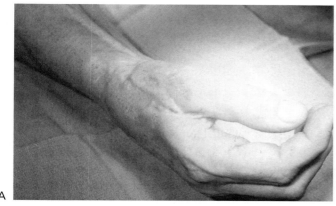

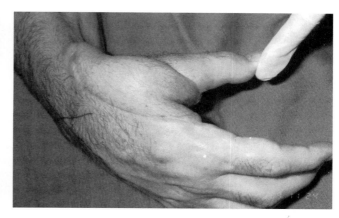

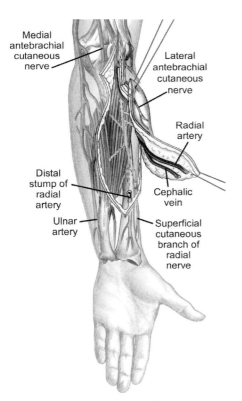

FIGURE 4. A: Constriction of the first web space. **B:** Lateral arm flap after release of the constriction. **C:** Lateral arm donor site.

main branch of the subscapular artery, and it is the main blood supply to the scapula, the muscles that attach to the scapula, and the overlying skin. The length of the pedicle is 5 cm. The vascular pattern of this territory makes it possible to raise multiple skin flaps on a single vascular pedicle

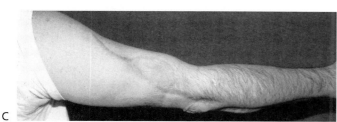

FIGURE 5. Surgical anatomy of the radial forearm flap.

Medial antebrachial cutaneous nerve

Lateral antebrachial cutaneous nerve

Radial artery

Distal stump of radial artery

Cephalic vein

Ulnar artery

Superficial cutaneous branch of radial nerve

or to harvest the lateral border of the scapula as an osteo-cutaneous flap for a complex reconstruction. The cutaneous territory can be 20×7 cm^2 and can be divided in two components: a horizontal territory (horizontal scapular flap) and a vertical territory (parascapular flap), based on the branches of the circumflex scapular artery, after the vessel courses through the triangular space. Innervated by the lateral posterior cutaneous branches of the intercostal nerves, this flap has no potential for use as a sensate flap. Preliminary expansion of the territory of the scapular flap increases the flap dimensions and permits direct donor site closure. This flap can be combined with other flaps, based on subscapular blood supply, and may greatly facilitate certain complex reconstructions. These include the latissimus dorsi and serratus anterior flaps, which can supply additional skin, muscle, and bone (rib), if necessary (40–42) (Fig. 6).

Anterolateral Thigh Flap

The anterolateral thigh flap was reported first as a septo-cutaneous perforator-based flap in 1984 (43). The dominant pedicle is based on branches from the descending branch of lateral circumflex femoral artery and venae comitantes and can achieve a length of 12 cm. The branches can enter the fascia through a septocutaneous or intramuscular pathway. Additional blood supply originates in branches from the transverse branch of lateral circumflex femoral artery and venae comitantes. The size this flap can reach is 12×20 cm^2.

The advantages of this flap are its moderate thickness and the large cutaneous area that allows aesthetic and

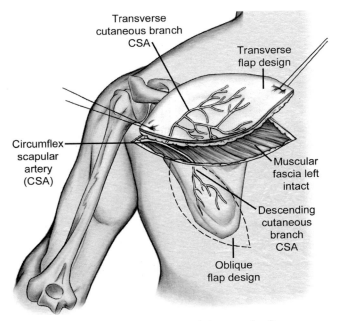

FIGURE 6. Surgical anatomy of the scapular flap.

functional refinements. The anterolateral thigh flap can also be combined with neighboring tissue and other free flaps. A flow-through type of anterolateral thigh flap has also been developed to reconstruct defects of soft tissue and major vessels (44). This flap can provide coverage of large soft tissue defects, and, when the fascia of vastus lateralis is included in the flap, it can be used for tendon reconstruction. The lateral cutaneous femoral nerve, when it is included in the flap, can provide sensation (Fig. 7).

Dorsalis Pedis Flap

The dorsalis pedis flap is a thin sensate fasciocutaneous flap from the dorsum of the foot that is based on the dorsalis pedis artery and its venae comitantes (45). The length of the pedicle is 6 to 10 cm. The nerve supply comes from the branches of deep and superficial peroneal nerves. The size of the flap is 6×10 cm², and it can be raised as a skin flap alone or in combination with the second metatarsal bone as an osteocutaneous flap or in com-

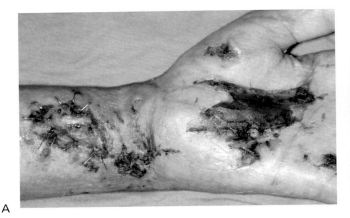

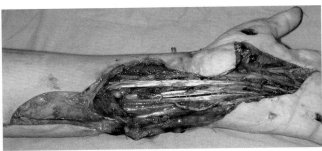

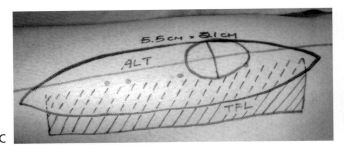

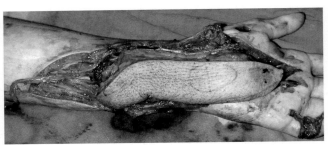

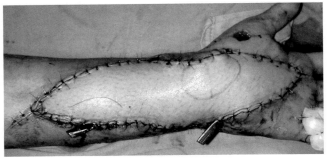

FIGURE 7. A: Left hand and forearm injury after an industrial accident. **B:** The hand and forearm after débridement. **C:** The donor site and plan of anterolateral thigh flap. **D:** Inset of the flap on the injury site. **E:** The flap after it was inset.

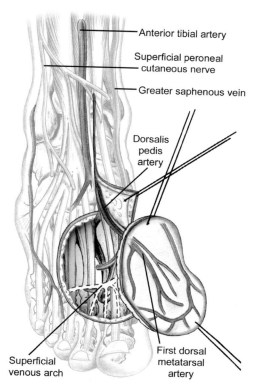

FIGURE 8. Surgical anatomy of the dorsalis pedis flap.

Labels on figure:
Anterior tibial artery
Superficial peroneal cutaneous nerve
Greater saphenous vein
Dorsalis pedis artery
First dorsal metatarsal artery
Superficial venous arch

bination with first and second toe transfer (46). With vascularized tendons of the toe extensor, it can provide simultaneous coverage and tendon reconstruction (47). The flap can be used in the upper extremity to cover joins and tendons and in microvascular transplants of metacarpophalangeal joints in children (48). The donor site morbidity is of concern in this flap, and it can include difficulties in primary healing, with a need for skin grafts, lymphedema, and hypertrophic scars (49). For this reason, this flap is used less now (Figs. 8 and 9).

Groin Flap

The groin flap provides a large skin and subcutaneous tissue territory that is based on superficial circumflex iliac artery and vein. The length of the pedicle is 2 cm, and the diameter is 1.5 mm. The dimension of the flap can be as large as 10×25 cm^2. Preliminary expansion of the lateral groin skin beneath the deep groin fascia expands flap dimensions and allows direct donor site closure. This flap is used mainly in acute settings to provide temporary coverage of a hand wound before a definite reconstruction procedure is done. Some of the disadvantages of this flap are its complexity of the vascular anatomy and the small diameter of the superficial circumflex iliac artery, which make this a less popular flap compared to other free skin flaps (50) (Fig. 10).

Temporoparietal Fascial Flap

The temporoparietal fascial flap can be used as a fascial or fasciocutaneous flap. The fascia covers the temporal muscle, which extends over the temporal fossa, and lies superficial to the deep temporal fascia, which covers the temporalis muscle. It continues as the galea beyond the limits of the temporal fossa. The blood supply is based on the superficial temporal artery, and the length of the pedicle is 4 cm. The course of the vessels is on the fascia from the preauricular into the temporal fossa. The sensory nerve supply comes from the auriculotemporal nerve. The size of the flap is 12×9 cm^2 (51). This flap is ideally suited for covering small defects of the hand. The minimal thickness of this well-vascularized flap prompts some authors to describe the technique as a "microvascular transplantation of a recipient bed" (52). This flap was found to be useful in cases of burns, particularly when joint spaces or tendons were exposed after débridement (53) (Fig. 11).

Thenar Fasciocutaneous Flap

The thenar fasciocutaneous flap is located at the radial aspect of the thenar area. The flap can be 3×5 cm^2 in size. Its vascular pedicle is the superficial palmar branch of the radial artery. The venous drainage is the superficial vein at the dorsal border of the thenar area. The nerve supply originates from the radial nerve branch and a branch from the lateral antebrachial cutaneous nerve (Fig. 12).

Muscle Flaps

The classification of muscle type is based on five patterns of muscle blood circulation (54). A muscle for free tissue transfer must be able to survive on one vascular pedicle that is dominant and that supports the entire muscle mass. Classification is as follows:

- Type 1: one vascular pedicle (extensor digitorum brevis, tensor fascia latae)
- Type 2: dominant pedicle and minor pedicles (abductor hallucis longus, gracilis)
- Type 3: two dominant pedicles (rectus abdominis, serratus anterior)
- Type 4: segmental vascular pedicles (sartorius)
- Type 5: one dominant and secondary vascular pedicles (latissimus dorsi, pectoralis major, pectoralis minor)

Unclassified potential transfers include fillet flaps and combination flaps, such as the latissimus dorsi serratus anterior muscle flap that is based on one dominant pedicle (thoracodorsal artery).

Latissimus Dorsi

The latissimus dorsi is a type 5 muscle (major pedicle and multiple segmental vessels). The dominant pedicle contains

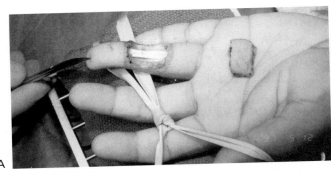

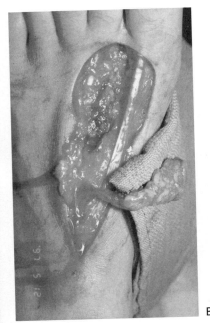

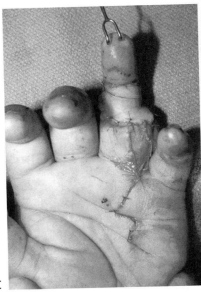

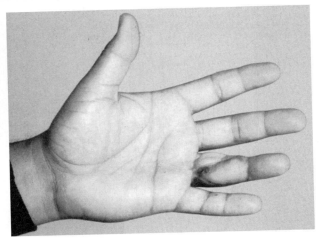

FIGURE 9. A: Defect caused by tumor excision. **B:** Dorsalis pedis flap. **C:** Inset of the flap. **D:** The flap after 4 months.

the thoracodorsal artery and venae comitantes, which originate from the subscapular artery and vein. Secondary pedicles are two rows (lateral and medial) of four to six perforating arterial branches and venae comitantes that take origin from the posterior intercostal and lumbar arteries and veins. The length of the major pedicle can be as long as 8 cm, and the arterial diameter can be as large as 2.5 mm. The artery enters the deep surface of the muscle in the posterior axilla, 10 cm inferior to the latissimus muscle insertion into the humerus (55). The motor nerve supply is the thoracodorsal nerve (C6 through C8), and the sensory innervation of the skin is supplied by multiple cutaneous branches of the intercostal nerves. Generally, this is not used as a sensate flap.

The latissimus dorsi is the largest transfer available, with a muscle surface area of 25 cm × 35 cm^2 and skin territory of 30 cm × 40 cm^2 (56). The latissimus dorsi is an expandable muscle because function is preserved by the remaining synergistic shoulder girdle muscles.

This flap is mainly used for coverage of extensive defects (dorsum, palm, multiple fingers, and even large wounds that extend to the forearm). The defects of multiple fingers can be covered together as surgical syndactyly and can be separated later. The fingers can be preserved with proper coverage. If the muscle is too bulky, skin graft can be performed at 3 weeks after trimming the excess superficial layer of the muscle. When necessary, the latissimus dorsi flap can be combined with the lower slips of the serratus anterior muscle for coverage of even more extensive defects at different locations (Figs. 13 and 14).

Rectus Abdominis

The rectus abdominis is a vertically oriented muscle that extends between the costal margin and the pubic region, and it is enclosed by the anterior and posterior rectus sheaths. It is a type 3 muscle (two dominant pedicles) based

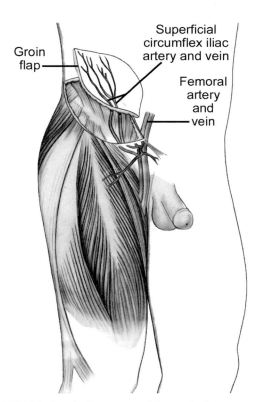

FIGURE 10. Surgical anatomy of the groin flap.

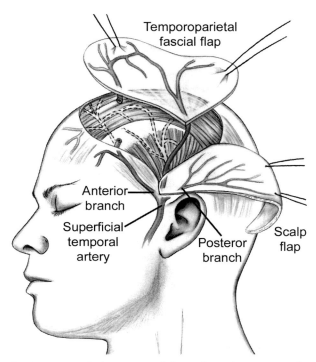

FIGURE 11. Surgical anatomy of the scalp and temporoparietal fascia flap.

on the superior epigastric artery and vein and inferior epigastric artery and vein. The pedicle length is 5 to 7 cm superiorly and 8 to 10 cm inferiorly.

Each of the dominant pedicles supplies just more than one-half of the muscle. There is an anastomosis between these vessels, which are usually sufficient to support the nondominant half, if one of the two pedicles is ligated. Because of the larger size and easier dissection of the inferior epigastric vessel, this is usually used for free tissue transfer. The seventh through twelfth intercostal nerves supply the motor enervation, and the lateral cutaneous nerves from the seventh through twelfth intercostal nerves provide sensation to the skin. The size of the muscle is as large as 25 cm × 6 cm^2, and the skin territory can reach 21 cm × 14 cm^2 (31). It allows coverage of large defects; compared to latissimus dorsi or lateral thigh flaps, there is no need for repositioning of the patient during the operation, which allows two teams to work in parallel, and the long pedicle allows good access to recipient vessels (57). The bulkiness that accompanies this flap is considerable, and it flattens after a period of 3 to 6 months (58). One of the complications of using this flap is the abdominal defect that is caused, which may lead to weakness and, possibly, hernia formation (Fig. 15).

Gracilis

The gracilis muscle is a type 2 muscle (dominant pedicle and several minor pedicles). It is a thin, flat muscle that lies

between the adductor longus and sartorius muscle, anteriorly, and the semimembranosus, posteriorly. The dominant pedicle is the ascending branch of medial circumflex femoral artery and venae comitantes. The length of the pedicle is 6 cm, and the diameter of the artery is 1.6 mm. The minor pedicles are one or two branches of the superficial femoral artery and venae comitantes. Their length is 2 cm, and the diameter is 0.5 mm (59). Motor innervation is the anterior branch of the obturator nerve, which is located between the abductor longus and magnus muscles, and it usually enters the muscle above the level of the dominant vascular pedicle The anterior femoral cutaneous nerve (L2 and L3) provides sensory innervation to the majority of the anterior medial thigh. The size of the muscle is 6 cm × 24 cm^2. The skin territory is 16 cm × 18 cm^2, but the skin over the distal half of the muscle is not reliable when the flap is elevated, based on its dominant vascular pedicle with division of the minor vascular pedicles.

In obese patients, the musculocutaneous flap may be too bulky, thus necessitating the use of a skin graft placed on the muscle. This flap can be used for medium-sized defects, such as those of the dorsum of the hand and first web (Fig. 16).

Omentum

The omentum is a visceral structure that contains fat and blood vessels within a thin membrane. It extends from the stomach to the transverse colon and beyond and covers the anterior peritoneal contents. It has two dominant pedicles: right gastroepiploic artery and vein, with a length of 6 cm

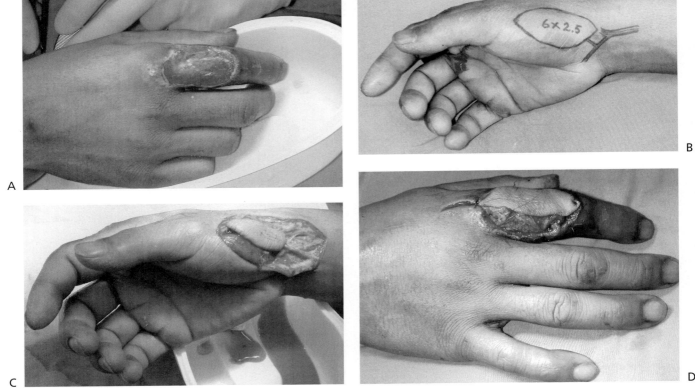

FIGURE 12. A: Injury of the soft tissue dorsal aspect of the proximal phalanx of second finger of the right hand. **B:** Plan of the thenar flap before harvesting. **C:** The flap before detachment of the pedicle. **D:** The flap was inset in the injury area.

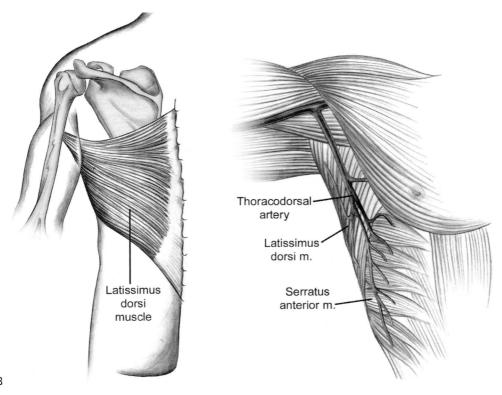

FIGURE 13. A: Latissimus dorsi muscle. **B:** Vascular pedicle to the serratus anterior and latissimus dorsi muscles (m.).

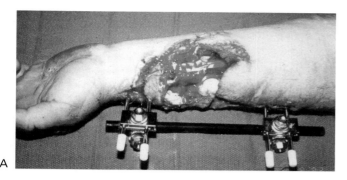

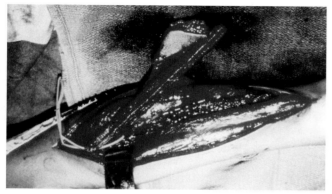

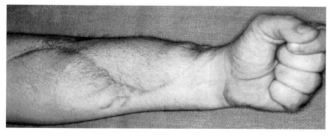

FIGURE 17. A: Trauma of the forearm with bone and soft tissue defect. **B:** Osteoseptocutaneous fibula flap before detaching the pedicle. **C:** The wound after coverage with the skin paddle from the flap.

of bleeding after pinprick. This complication can be caused by arterial spasm, vessel plaque, torsion of the pedicle, pressure on the flap, technical error with injury to the pedicle, a flap that is harvested and that is too large for its blood supply, or small vessel disease (due to smoking or diabetes). Pressure on the pedicle can be caused by tendons or tight skin closure. Management of arterial compromise requires prompt surgical intervention to restore the blood flow (62). Pharmacologic intervention includes vasodilators, calcium blockers, and anticoagulants for flap salvage that presents with arterial insufficiency (63).

Venous outflow obstruction can be suspected, when the flap has a violaceous color, brisk capillary refill, normal or elevated temperature, and production of dark blood after pinprick. Venous insufficiency can occur that is due to torsion of the pedicle, flap edema, hematoma, or tight closure of the tissue over the pedicle. The venous outflow obstruc-

tion can result in extravasation of red blood cells, endothelial breakdown, microvascular collapse, thrombosis in the microcirculation, and, finally, flap death. Given the irreversible nature of the microcirculatory changes in venous congestion that occur even after short periods of time, the surgeon must recognize venous compromise as early as possible. These complications can occur alone or in any combination. The clinical observation and the monitoring of the patient (e.g., with Doppler laser) should alert the surgeon, who has to decide between conservative and operative intervention. Conservative treatment may include drainage of the hematoma by the bedside and release of a few sutures to decrease pressure. In cases of venous congestion, leeches may be helpful if insufficient venous outflow cannot be established, despite a patent venous anastomosis. The leeches inject a salivary component (hirudin) that inhibits platelet aggregation and the coagulation cascade. The flap is decongested initially, as the leech extracts blood, and is further decongested as the bite wound oozes, after the leech detaches (62).

The donor site should be given the same attention as the recipient site during postoperative period. Complications of the donor site include hematoma, seroma, and sensory nerve dysfunction and scar formation.

TREATMENT OF LATE COMPLICATIONS

Occasionally, free flaps, despite early return to the operating room for vascular compromise, do fail. Options for management include the performance of a second free tissue transfer, noting the technical or physiologic details that led to initial failure. Most of the time, free tissue transfers that fail are due to technical errors in judgment, which may include flap harvest, compromise of the pedicle during the harvest, improper microvascular technique during anastomosis, or improper insetting that results in increased tissue tension and edema and tendon adhesions. The next decision that is made by the operating surgeon about the management of this patient is based on several factors. Obviously, if a patient requires a free flap in the first place, a second free flap should be considered. If a decision is made not to redo the flap, it could be left in place using the so-called Crane principle. The Crane principle can be applied to cases in which a local flap or free tissue transfer goes on to necrosis, in part or totally, by performing a biologic dressing or eschar over a wound bed. If there is no infection, then the eschar can be left on the wound bed, with hopes that some healing can occur underneath the eschar. This would be in the form of granulation tissue that may form under the eschar. Ultimately, the eschar could be removed, and, with an appropriate granulation bed, the wound can be skin grafted, thus obviating the need for another free tissue transfer. It is the authors' preference that this is not usually done, because the flap can become a source of sepsis and can further compromise local tissues. Necrotic nonviable flaps should be removed, and a temporary wound dressing, such as a bead pouch or wound hemo-vac, is used. If a second free flap is considered, obvious errors that lead to flap compromise need to be recognized. It may be prudent to obtain an arteriogram, to evaluate coagulation profile, and to research other issues that lead to failure.

AESTHETIC CONSIDERATIONS

Ultimately, providing patients with a functional limb after free tissue transfer is most important. Careful selection of the flap, as well as consideration of donor scar management, can result in a satisfactory aesthetic result. The use of tissue expanders can help by decreasing donor site morbidity, as well as the need for debulking of flaps, which can result in an improved cosmetic result (64).

ENDOSCOPIC HARVESTING

After the introduction of endoscopic techniques in almost every field of surgery, the application of the techniques in reconstructive microsurgery represents the natural evolution of this trend. Less postoperative pain, smaller scars in the donor area, better visualization of the operative field with the magnified video, and better hemostasis are only a few of the advantages of this technique. These advantages have been seen in a series of patients in which latissimus dorsi harvesting was compared in the endoscopic technique and the traditional technique (65). Successful microvascular transplantation of gracilis muscle that is harvested with endoscopic guidance is also described in the literature (66,67).

PREFABRICATIONS

Prefabrication of flaps allows custom flaps to be constructed based on the requirements of a specific defect. The exploration of this new frontier may increase the possibility of reconstructive capabilities and decrease the donor morbidity of classical reconstructions.

Larger flaps than those that are naturally perfused by the pedicle may be transferred after being prefabricated. Examples include pretransfer delay of a cutaneous flap to include a larger skin island and pretransfer expansion of a flap to generate an additional amount of precious specialized tissue. By extending the limits of perfusion, delay allows the transfer of a much larger amount of tissue than would be allowed by the original pedicle. Specific preferred blocks of tissue, which are not naturally perfused by anatomically well-defined axial vessels or by a reliable pedicle that is easy to use for transfer, may be used, such as skin flaps that need to be thin. Flap prefabrication

enables reduction of the donor-site morbidity. Examples include pretransfer expansion of a flap to allow primary closure of the donor site The functional status of the replacement part may be ascertained before transfer by converting a lengthy, multiple-stage posttransfer reconstruction into an elegant, single-step transfer of a finished functional flap.

The current methods of flap prefabrication are based on the following principles of reconstructive surgery: delay or expansion, grafting, and vascular induction that uses staged flap transfer. A pretransfer grafting of flaps may be necessary, when complete graft take is mandatory to the success of the reconstruction, and when posttransfer grafting is neither feasible nor practical. Vascular induction that uses staged flap transfer is based on the concept that a small flap of muscle, fascia, intestine, omentum, or even an arteriovenous bundle or fistula can become a "vascular carrier" and can be induced to provide an alternative blood supply through neovascularization to a larger block of tissue after a relatively short staging period (68).

Recent advances in cell biology may open the door to a new method of prefabrication by inducing the transformation of a flap from one tissue type to another. An application of these advancements can be found in bone and joint reconstruction, which is still most commonly performed with less than ideal alloplastic materials and remains a formidable challenge, despite advances in free tissue transfer. With the possibility of inducing mesenchymal tissue to differentiate into bone, a simple muscle flap may be molded and transformed into a vascularized bone graft of desired shape and size (69,70).

THOROUGH EVALUATION OF MICROSURGERY COST AND OUTCOME

Today, the versatility and vascularity of free tissue transfers have made them indispensable tools for reconstructive surgeons. Although free flap procedures can provide definitive treatment in a single operation, they are still expensive and require specialized practitioners. The cost of microsurgery in the treatment of the spectrum of eligible patients has not been defined. Some groups, however, have assembled cost estimates and have made initial inroads into outcomes and measurements of cost effectiveness (71,72).

Reduction in complication rates would reduce the cost of microsurgical procedures. Currently, efforts are under way to reduce free flap costs at all stages of care by shortening the operating time with the use of new devices, shortening the monitoring time postoperatively, and even exploring in selected patients the possibility of using an outpatient monitoring system (73). There is still a long way to go to achieve this goal; for today, the consensus is that free flap procedures are costly, but they are also effective (74).

REFERENCES

1. Jacobson JH, Suarez SE. Microsurgery and anastomosis of small vessels. *Surg Forum* 1960:243.
2. Bunke CM. Experimental digital amputation and replantation. *Plast Reconstr Surg* 1965;36:62.
3. Kleinert HE, Romero JL. Small blood vessels anastomosis for salvaged of severely injured upper extremity. *J Bone Joint Surg* 1963;45:788.
4. Isenberg JS, Sherman R. Zone of injury: a valid concept in microvascular reconstruction of the traumatized lower limb? *Ann Plastic Surg* 1996;36:270.
5. Levin LS. The reconstructive ladder. An orthoplastic approach. *Orthop Clin North Am* 1993;24:393.
6. Levin LS, Nunley JA. The management of soft-tissue problems associated with calcaneal fractures. *Clin Orthop* 1993;290:151.
7. Levin L. Débridement. *Tech Orthop* 1995;10:104.
8. Kindwall EP, Gottlieb LJ, Larson DL. Hyperbaric oxygen therapy in plastic surgery: a review article. *Plast Reconstr Surg* 1991;88:898.
9. Argenta LC, Morykwas MJ. Vacuum-assisted closure: a new method for wound control and treatment: clinical experience. *Ann Plast Surg* 1997;38:563; discussion, 577.
10. Arnez ZM. Immediate reconstruction of the lower extremity—an update. *Clin Plast Surg* 1991;18:449.
11. Goldberg JA, Alpert BS, Lineaweaver WC, et al. Microvascular reconstruction of the lower extremity in the elderly. *Clin Plast Surg* 1991;18:459.
12. Byrd HS, Cierny GD, Tebbetts JB. The management of open tibial fractures with associated soft-tissue loss: external pin fixation with early flap coverage. *Plast Reconstr Surg* 1981;68:73.
13. Byrd HS, Spicer TE, Cierney GD. Management of open tibial fractures. *Plast Reconstr Surg* 1985;76:719.
14. Godina M. Early microsurgical reconstruction of complex trauma of the extremities. *Plast Reconstr Surg* 1986;78:285.
15. Lister G, Scheker L. Emergency free flaps to the upper extremity. *J Hand Surg* 1988;13:22.
16. Yaremchuk MJ, Brumback RJ, Manson PN, et al. Acute and definitive management of traumatic osteocutaneous defects of the lower extremity. *Plast Reconstr Surg* 1987;80:1.
17. Chen S, Tsai YC, Wei FC, et al. Emergency free flaps to the type IIIC tibial fracture. *Ann Plast Surg* 1990;25:223.
18. McCabe SJ, Breidenbach WC. The role of emergency free flaps for hand trauma. *Hand Clin* 1999;15:275.
19. Dirschl DR, Dahners LE. The mangled extremity: when should it be amputated? *J Am Acad Orthop Surg* 1996;4:182.
20. Lange RH. Limb reconstruction versus amputation decision making in massive lower extremity trauma. *Clin Orthop* 1989;243:92.
21. Hansen ST Jr. The type-IIIC tibial fracture. Salvage or amputation [Editorial]. *J Bone Joint Surg* 1987;69:799.
22. Kuntscher MV, Homann H-H, Levin LS, et al. The concept of fillet flaps: classification, indications, and analysis of their clinical value. *Plast Reconstr Surg* 2001;108:885.
23. Cierny GD, Mader JT. Approach to adult osteomyelitis. *Orthop Rev* 1987;16:259.
24. Mathes SJ, Alpert BS, Chang N. Use of the muscle flap in chronic osteomyelitis: experimental and clinical correlation. *Plast Reconstr Surg* 1982;69:815.
25. Mathes SJ, Feng LJ, Hunt TK. Coverage of the infected wound. *Ann Surg* 1983;198:420.
26. Eshima I, Mathes SJ, Paty P. Comparison of the intracellular bacterial killing activity of leukocytes in musculocutaneous and random-pattern flaps. *Plast Reconstr Surg* 1990;86:541.
27. Bostwick JD, Nahai F, Wallace JG, et al. Sixty latissimus dorsi flaps. *Plast Reconstr Surg* 1979;63:31.
28. Harii K, Yamada A, Ishihara K, et al. A free transfer of both latissimus dorsi and serratus anterior flaps with thoracodorsal vessel anastomoses. *Plast Reconstr Surg* 1982;70:620.
29. Bunkis J, Walton RL, Mathes SJ. The rectus abdominis free flap for lower extremity reconstruction. *Ann Plast Surg* 1983;11:373.
30. Barwick WJ, Goldberg JA, Scully SP, et al. Vascularized tissue transfer for closure of irradiated wounds after soft tissue sarcoma resection. *Ann Surg* 1992;216:591.
31. Mathes SJ, Nahai F. *Reconstructive surgery: principles, anatomy & technique.* New York: Churchill Livingstone, 1997.
32. Yousif NJ, Warren R, Matloub HS, et al. The lateral arm fascial free flap: its anatomy and use in reconstruction. *Plast Reconstr Surg* 1990;86:1138; discussion, 1146.
33. Katsaros J, Schusterman M, Beppu M, et al. The lateral upper arm flap: anatomy and clinical applications. *Ann Plast Surg* 1984;12:489.
34. Chen HC, el-Gammal TA. The lateral arm fascial free flap for resurfacing of the hand and fingers. *Plast Reconstr Surg* 1997;99:454.
35. Muhlbauer W, Herndl E, Stock W. The forearm flap. *Plast Reconstr Surg* 1982;70:336.
36. Song R, Gao Y, Song Y, et al. The forearm flap. *Clin Plast Surg* 1982;9:21.
37. Cormack GC, Duncan MJ, Lamberty BG. The blood supply of the bone component of the compound osteo-cutaneous radial artery forearm flap—an anatomical study. *Br J Plast Surg* 1986;39:173.
38. Masser MR. The preexpanded radial free flap [see comments]. *Plast Reconstr Surg* 1990;86:295; discussion, 302.
39. Barwick WJ, Goodkind DJ, Serafin D. The free scapular flap. *Plast Reconstr Surg* 1982;69:779.
40. Dos Santos LF. The vascular anatomy and dissection of the free scapular flap. *Plast Reconstr Surg* 1984;73:599.
41. Urbaniak JR, Koman LA, Goldner RD, et al. The vascularized cutaneous scapular flap. *Plast Reconstr Surg* 1982;69:772.
42. Roth JH, Urbaniak JR, Koman LA, et al. Free flap coverage of deep tissue defects of the foot. *Foot Ankle* 1982;3:150.
43. Song YG, Chen GZ, Song YL. The free thigh flap: a new free flap concept based on the septocutaneous artery. *Br J Plast Surg* 1984;37:149.
44. Koshima I, Kawada S, Etoh H, et al. Flow-through anterior thigh flaps for one-stage reconstruction of soft-tissue defects and revascularization of ischemic extremities. *Plast Reconstr Surg* 1995;95:252.
45. Man D, Acland RD. The microarterial anatomy of the dorsalis pedis flap and its clinical applications. *Plast Reconstr Surg* 1980;65:419.
46. May JW Jr, Chait LA, Cohen BE, et al. Free neurovascular flap from the first web of the foot in hand reconstruction. *J Hand Surg* 1977;2:387.
47. Chen HC, Buchman MT, Wei FC. Free flaps for soft tissue coverage in the hand and fingers. *Hand Clin* 1999;15:541.

48. Mathes SJ, Buchannan R, Weeks PM. Microvascular joint transplantation with epiphyseal growth. *J Hand Surg* 1980;5:586.

49. Samson MC, Morris SF, Tweed AE. Dorsalis pedis flap donor site: acceptable or not? *Plast Reconstr Surg* 1998;102:1549.

50. Chuang DC, Jeng SF, Chen HT, et al. Experience of 73 free groin flaps. *Br J Plast Surg* 1992;45:81.

51. Abul-Hassan HS, von Drasek Ascher G, Acland RD. Surgical anatomy and blood supply of the fascial layers of the temporal region. *Plast Reconstr Surg* 1986;77:17.

52. Brent B, Upton J, Acland RD, et al. Experience with the temporoparietal fascial free flap. *Plast Reconstr Surg* 1985;76:177.

53. Chowdary RP, Chernofsky MA, Okunski WJ. Free temporoparietal flap in burn reconstruction. *Ann Plast Surg* 1990;25:169.

54. Mathes SJ, Nahai F. Classification of the vascular anatomy of muscles: experimental and clinical correlation. *Plast Reconstr Surg* 1981;67:177.

55. Bartlett SP, May JW Jr, Yaremchuk MJ. The latissimus dorsi muscle: a fresh cadaver study of the primary neurovascular pedicle. *Plast Reconstr Surg* 1981;67:631.

56. Lassen M, Krag C, Nielsen IM. The latissimus dorsi flap. An overview. *Scand J Plast Reconstr Surg* 1985;19:41.

57. Reath DB, Taylor JW. Free rectus abdominis muscle flap: advantages in lower extremity reconstruction. *South Med J* 1989;82:1143.

58. Horch RE, Stark GB. The rectus abdominis free flap as an emergency procedure in extensive upper extremity soft-tissue defects. *Plast Reconstr Surg* 1999;103:1421.

59. Giordano PA, Abbes M, Pequignot JP. Gracilis blood supply: anatomical and clinical re-evaluation. *Br J Plast Surg* 1990;43:266.

60. Prowans P, Deskur Z, Zyluk A, et al. Transplantation of the greater omentum and complication. *Chir Narzadow Ruchu Ortop Pol* 1998;63:529.

61. Bunke H. *Monitoring in microsurgery: transplantation-replantation.* Philadelphia: Lea & Febiger, 1991.

62. Utley DS, Koch RJ, Goode RL. The failing flap in facial plastic and reconstructive surgery: role of the medicinal leech. *Laryngoscope* 1998;108:1129.

63. Pang CY, Forrest CR, Morris SF. Pharmacological augmentation of skin flap viability: a hypothesis to mimic the surgical delay phenomenon or a wishful thought. *Ann Plast Surg* 1989;22:293.

64. Chowdary RP, Murphy RX. Delayed debulking of free muscle flaps for aesthetic contouring debulking of free muscle flaps. *Br J Plast Surg* 1992;45:38.

65. Lin CH, Levin LS. Free flap expansion using balloon-assisted endoscopic technique. *Microsurgery* 1996;17:330.

66. Spiegel JH, Lee C, Trabulsy PP, et al. Endoscopic harvest of the gracilis muscle flap. *Ann Plast Surg* 1998;41:384.

67. Fine NA, Orgill DP, Pribaz JJ. Early clinical experience in endoscopic-assisted muscle flap harvest. *Ann Plast Surg* 1994;33:465–469; discussion, 469.

68. Morrison WA, Dvir E, Doi K, et al. Prefabrication of thin transferable axial-pattern skin flaps: an experimental study in rabbits [see comments]. *Br J Plast Surg* 1990;43:645.

69. Khouri RK, Koudsi B, Reddi H. Tissue transformation into bone in vivo. A potential practical application. *JAMA* 1991;266:1953.

70. Khouri RK, Upton J, Shaw WW. Principles of flap prefabrication. *Clin Plast Surg* 1992;19:763.

71. Kroll SS, Evans GR, Goldberg D, et al. A comparison of resource costs for head and neck reconstruction with free and pectoralis major flaps. *Plast Reconstr Surg* 1997;99:1282.

72. Laughlin RT, Smith KL, Russell RC, et al. Late functional outcome in patients with tibia fractures covered with free muscle flaps. *J Orthop Trauma* 1993;7:123.

73. Kutlu N. Out-patients upper extremity free flaps. *J Reconstr Microsurg* 1998;14:269.

74. Heinz TR, Cowper PR, Levin LS. Microsurgery cost and outcome. *Plast Reconstr Surg* 1999;89:89.

68

RHEUMATOID ARTHRITIS IN THE HAND AND DIGITS

JAMES W. STRICKLAND
DALE DELLACQUA

GENERAL CONSIDERATIONS

The normal anatomy of the hand and digits consists of an intercalated sequence of wrist bones, metacarpals, and phalanges that are joined together by joints that are supported by ligaments that permit motion while ensuring stability during function. Joint movement is achieved through the integrated function of the extrinsic flexor and extensor muscle–tendons and the small intrinsic muscles of the hand. Rheumatoid arthritis is a systemic, immune-mediated inflammatory disorder that alters the synovium around joints and tendons through a proliferation of synovial lining cells, angiogenesis, and increased lymphocytes in perivascular areas (1). This can result in a disruption of the normal skeletal architecture of the wrist and hand and a compromise of the normal delicately balanced function of the muscles and tendons on that skeleton.

The wrist and the metacarpophalangeal (MCP) and proximal interphalangeal (PIP) joints are the parts of the hand anatomy that are most commonly affected by rheumatoid arthritis; the flexor tendon sheaths may also be affected. Involvement of the joints and tendons of the hand may begin with mild synovitis with symptoms that are secondary to increased joint pressure; nerve embarrassment, such as carpal tunnel syndrome; or the mechanical interference, with tendon gliding within covered spaces, as is experienced with trigger finger disorders. Over time, rheumatoid synovium destroys articular cartilage, invades subchondral bone, and attenuates or ruptures the supporting joint capsules and ligaments, thus resulting in instability and deformity. The multiple bones of the wrist and hand form a continuous, intercalated, and mutually dependent series of osseous structures. Breakdown at any part of the bony chain usually results in deformity of the joints that are proximal or distal to the involved joint, particularly when they are also involved in the rheumatoid process. For example, the characteristic ulnar translocation of the rheumatoid wrist results in an obligatory radial deviation of the metacarpals that, in turn, creates forces on the diseased MCP joints that lead to the development of ulnar deviation of the digits (Fig. 1).

The surgeon who deals with rheumatoid conditions of the wrist and hand must have a thorough appreciation for the disease and how it affects the muscles, tendons, and small joints of the hand. The history of a patient's condition, including a discussion of all involved joints, the amount of pain, and the degree of functional impairment, is an important first step in determining the suitability of that patient for surgical intervention. A thorough examination of all upper extremity joints, muscle–tendon strength and integrity, nerve function, and upper extremity vascular status should be carried out during the surgeon's initial examination of a rheumatoid patient. Multiple visits and reassessments are often needed to appreciate the state of the disease and its progression in a given patient.

Surgical efforts to retard the progression or correct functionally compromising deformities can best be approached if one has a strong appreciation for the pathomechanics of the deformities themselves. It must always be borne in mind that rheumatoid arthritis is a progressive disease that involves many joints in the upper and lower extremities and the spine. Consideration for the whole person and his or her overall physical and mental states is extremely important in the assessment of any benefits to be derived from surgery on the hand. Close cooperation between the hand surgeon and the patient's rheumatologist is essential, and patients must be well versed on the realistic expectations of surgery, the rehabilitation that is required to maximize results, the possibility of recurrence, and the potential for additional surgery.

This chapter discusses the pathomechanics of rheumatoid deformities at the MCP joints, the PIP joints, and the thumb and the surgical options for the effective management of those deformities. It is immediately conceded

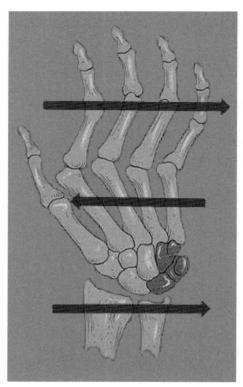

FIGURE 1. Demonstration of the dynamic sequence of skeletal deformity that is often seen in rheumatoid arthritis. Ulnar translocation of the carpus results in radial deviation of the metacarpals, which creates forces that favor ulnar deviation of the digits.

that those individual rheumatoid joint conditions are rarely isolated and that a recognition of the status of adjacent wrist and hand joints often dictates what, if any, operative procedure may be beneficial. When there is widespread rheumatoid disease that involves the wrist and multiple finger joints, the surgeon is well served by a conservative approach that recognizes where reasonable motion can be preserved or reestablished and where fusions may be more appropriate.

There are many factors that must be taken into consideration before electing to recommend surgery for a rheumatoid patient. A thorough review of the state of the patient's rheumatoid disease is essential to avoid so-called tunnel vision on the potential for wrist or hand surgery. Patients who are seriously impaired by involvement of other joints, such as hips, knees, spine, shoulders, or elbows, may have to prioritize their surgical options, and the ability to ambulate may take precedence over upper extremity dysfunction. Patients who are in an exacerbation period of their disease, who are taking high doses of steroids or other compromising antiarthritic medications, who are generally in poor health, or who lack sufficient motivation to endure the rigors of reconstructive hand surgery and the obligatory postsurgical therapy are usually poor candidates for operative intervention.

METACARPOPHALANGEAL JOINTS

Normal Anatomy

The MCP joints of the index, middle, ring, and small fingers are condylar joints that have three basic planes of motion; extension and flexion, radial and ulnar deviation, and a small amount of rotation. The metacarpal heads are wider on the palmar surface than on the dorsal surface, whereas the base of the proximal phalanx has a shallow concavity. Lateral stability of the MCP joints is provided by the collateral ligaments that arise from the radial and ulnar sides of the metacarpal heads, traverse the joint in a slightly diagonal direction, and insert on the bases of the proximal phalanges. Because of the cam configuration of the joint, the collateral ligaments are lax in extension, which permits side-to-side motion, and tight in full flexion, in which little lateral movement can occur.

The palmar plate of the MCP joints is strongly attached to the proximal phalanx, with a looser, membranous attachment to the metacarpal neck. It prevents hyperextension of the joint, forms the floor of the flexor tendon sheath, and is joined by the intermetacarpal ligament that spans between each joint and the sagittal bands from the extensor mechanism. Movement of the MCP joint results from the action of the flexor tendons and the intrinsic muscle–tendons that pass by it. The intrinsic muscles help stabilize the MCP joints during extension, move the fingers from side to side, and serve as strong MCP flexors during the coordinated grasping activities of the hand.

Pathophysiology

The MCP joints are frequently sites of rheumatoid synovitis. The disease affects the support structures around the joint in a manner that produces the characteristic flexion and ulnar deviation deformities that are so commonly seen in the advanced rheumatoid hand. Ultimately, the proximal phalanges sublux or dislocate palmarly, at which point they often come to lie beneath the metacarpal heads (3,4) (Fig. 2). The palmar displacement of the proximal phalanges results from a combination of factors (5), including displacement of the flexor tendons, laxity of the collateral ligaments, attenuation of the dorsoradial support system, and secondary spasm or contraction of the intrinsic muscles. Ulnar deviation of the digits occurs at the MCP joints and also involves several deforming factors in combination (3). Rheumatoid involvement of the wrist leads to ulnar translocation and supination of the carpus, which result in an obligatory radial deviation of the metacarpals and initiate a number of imbalancing forces that favor ulnar deviation of the digits (6,7) (Fig. 3). The normal tendency of the fingers to move into slight ulnar angulation during full flexion, ulnar displacement of the extensor tendons, an increased ulnar approach of the flexor tendons, and an increased ulnar pull of the junctura tendineae have been implicated

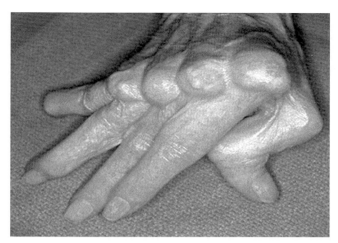

FIGURE 2. Rheumatoid deformities of the metacarpophalangeal joints. Flexion and ulnar deviation of the digits. Severe boutonnière deformity of the thumb.

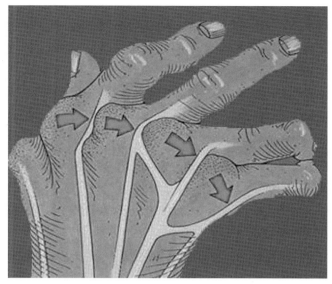

FIGURE 4. Displacement of the extensor tendons into the ulnar valleys between the metacarpal heads.

in the development of ulnar digital deviation (8). The ulnar displacement of the extensor tendons is thought to result from synovitis in the radial extensor triangle and stretching of the radial-sided transverse extensor fibers (sagittal bands) (Fig. 4). When displaced well into the valleys on the ulnar side of the MCP joints, the extensor tendons may lose their ability to extend the fingers, and extension efforts actually

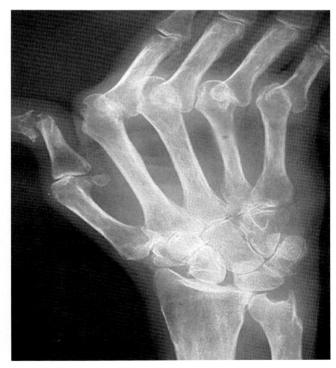

FIGURE 3. X-ray of (supination) severe multilevel rheumatoid deformities. Ulnar translocation and palmar rotation of the carpus, radial deviation of the metacarpals, and dislocation and ulnar deviation of the digits.

accentuate the ulnar deviation deformities (9). Intrinsic muscle tightness, whether primary or secondary, and a weakened dorsoradial support system, including the joint capsule and collateral ligaments, also contribute to the development of the deformity (5).

Chronic invasive synovitis within the MCP joints results in erosion of articular cartilage and bone and, eventually, destruction of the metacarpal heads. The combination of MCP joint laxity, subluxation or dislocation of the proximal phalangeal bases, and joint surface destruction can produce severe deformities with varying degrees of pain and dysfunction. Depending on the sites and intensity of the MCP synovitis, the loss of joint support and dislocation may occur before the articular surfaces of the metacarpal heads erode. Once the MCP joints have dislocated, any further joint erosion is unlikely to occur. Nonetheless, the severe deformities probably preclude any type of surgical restoration, short of joint replacement.

Evaluation

The need to thoroughly understand all aspects of the rheumatoid patient before considering surgery cannot be overemphasized. The status of the disease and how it has affected a particular individual's lifestyle is critical to determining whether operative procedures that are designed to improve hand function may realistically be of long-term value. Focusing on deformities of the MCP joints alone as potential candidates for surgery may totally miss the patient's needs and expectations and may culminate in a disappointed patient. Considerations for any surgery on the rheumatoid patient include the patient's overall health status, and other joints that are involved, so that the surgeon can assess which joints, if any, may benefit from reconstructive surgery. How are the patient's hands needed for ambulation? How well will the patient withstand the surgery, and, above all, how well motivated is the patient for the procedure and the protracted rehabilitation programs that maximize the results of surgery?

The surgeon must also learn if a rheumatoid patient has active and progressive disease that is well controlled medically or is in remission. Although it was once argued that the surgery in the presence of a flare-up or extremely active phase of the disease was contraindicated, that dictum is no longer considered absolute. Some patients who tend to have fairly frequent exacerbations and remissions of their rheumatoid arthritis may fare better if surgery is carried out during a reasonably inactive period, but, for others, finding such a quiet window of opportunity may not be possible.

For the hand with MCP joint deformities, it is extremely important to determine the status of the shoulder, elbow, wrist, and thumb before concluding that replacement of the digital MCPs is the appropriate way to proceed. In particular, the condition of the patient's wrist is critical to the success or failure of procedures that are designed to replace deformed MCP joints and to realign the digits (10). Allowing the wrist to remain ulnarly translocated and supinated and the metacarpals to remain radially deviated inevitably places undue ulnarly angulating forces on the area in which surgery is carried out to rebalance existing MCP joints or joint replacement procedures. In such cases, it is usually best to reposition the wrist and hand and to stabilize it with a radiolunate fusion, as described by Chamay et al. (11). Wrist replacement or wrist fusion may also be needed for the severely involved rheumatoid wrist, and extensor or flexor tendon ruptures may be dealt with concomitantly with MCP joint procedures or before more distal restorative efforts are carried out. Deformities and dysfunction of the PIP joints and thumb should also be addressed, with considerations made with regard to how they might affect the outcome of MCP joint procedures. Patients with flexible, minimally involved PIPs probably achieve less flexion of their MCP arthroplasties than those patients with stiff boutonnière or swan-neck deformities who can deliver all the power and excursion of their flexor tendons to the new implants.

The physical examination of a new patient with rheumatoid arthritis must be extensive and thorough, even if it initially appears that the deformities of the MCP joints represent the patient's most significant problem. Rheumatoid patients have involvement, some of which is obvious and some of which is occult, of many structures and tissues in their upper extremities. Unless one appreciates all areas of pathology and dysfunction, surgically compromising factors may be overlooked. Observing and recording the active and passive range of motion for all upper extremity joints is followed by assessing the strength of muscle groups. Palpation of the wrist and small joints of the hand helps determine the existence a synovitis, and the experienced examiner can learn to distinguish between watery synovial exudates and a chronic, well-organized synovial thickening. Contractures are noted, intrinsic muscle tightness is tested, ulnar deviation of the digits is measured, and tendon ruptures are noted. Evidence of vasculitis or vascular insufficiency should be observed and recorded, and peripheral nerve compromise, such as carpal tunnel embarrassment of the median nerve or posterior interosseous nerve dysfunction, should be completely evaluated. The integrity and quality of the patient's skin should be assessed, because many long-standing rheumatoid patients have thin skin, particularly when they have been taking corticosteroid medications. Areas of bruising often indicate capillary fragility, and any signs of clotting disorders should be noted. Finally, strength should be recorded, and, on some occasions, a simple battery of tests that simulates the patient's activities of daily living can be carried out to determine the level of functional compromise that has resulted from the rheumatoid process.

Radiographs are extremely important in the assessment of the status of a rheumatoid patient's bones and joints. Deformities of the wrist are particularly important because ulnar translocation and supination of the carpus produce radial deviation of the metacarpals and, if left untreated, may be detrimental to the long-term success of MCP arthroplasties. Early erosion of the metacarpal heads is often best seen in the radiologic views, as described by Brewerton (12), and the articular integrity of both sides of the joint should be carefully observed. Subluxation or dislocation of the bases of the proximal phalanges beneath the metacarpal heads can be appreciated by the superimposition of the bones on anterior-posterior radiographs and on oblique or lateral projections. The articular status of the PIP joints should also be carefully assessed radiographically because destroyed or stiffened PIPs affect the outcome of MCP joint procedures. Finally, the joints of the thumb should be studied, and a hyperpronated projection of the carpometacarpal joint (CMC) is particularly important when there is a zigzag collapse pattern.

Classification of Stages

It may be helpful to think of rheumatoid MCP joint involvement in stages and Stirrat's (9) modification of Nalebuff's (13) classification is valuable in making surgical decisions based on the existing pathology:

Early: MCP synovitis with little or no extension lag or ulnar deviation.
Minimal pain.
Moderate: Early erosions of metacarpal heads around collateral ligament origins.
Some extensor tendon displacement, ulnar deviation, or extension lag, or a combination of these.
Minimal pain.

Late: Articular destruction or joint subluxation, or both. Increased extension deficit (may be passively correctable), ulnar deviation, and extensor tendon displacement.

More painful.

Very late: Joint destruction, fixed palmar subluxation or dislocation, severe ulnar deviation, and ulnar and palmar displacement of the extensor tendons.

Often, pain is a factor, and dysfunction is considerable.

It must be recognized that, although this type of staging classification for the rheumatoid MCP joint is useful, it is an oversimplification of the many variations in clinical presentation that this capricious disease may produce. For instance, it is not unusual to see complete dislocation of the MCP joints without significant articular destruction in patients who have experienced a rather florid and rapidly progressive disease process. It is inappropriate to make surgical decisions based solely on the stage of the MCP disease. Many factors, including age, functional needs, general status of the patient, response to medical management, involvement of other joints, and the patient's desires and motivation, contribute to decisions regarding the probable benefits of operative intervention.

Treatment of Rheumatoid Metacarpophalangeal Joint Disease

Conservative Treatment

In the early stages of MCP joint involvement, treatment is centered around medical management and splinting. In recent years, there have been some dramatic advances, including the injectable or infusion biologic agents, in the effective medical control of rheumatoid disease. Hopefully, these encouraging medicinal developments will continue, and realistic control of the destructive sequence of events will greatly reduce deformities and pain in the hands of rheumatoid patients. Splinting may provide some pain relief for patients with rheumatoid MCP joint disease, particularly when used at night and during periods of inflammation. It is not, however, realistic to believe that splints that are applied nightly to correct MCP flexion and ulnar deviation have any significant likelihood of stopping or slowing the progression of deformity.

Operative Treatment: Synovectomy and Soft Tissue Rebalancing

Considerations

The value of MCP joint synovectomy and soft tissue rebalancing procedures is limited to certain clinical situations, and decisions regarding the use of these procedures must be tempered by the understanding that they are more palliative than curative. Surgical experience is extremely important when considering these methods, and the rapid postsurgical return of synovitis or joint imbalance can be disappointing to patient and surgeon alike.

Synovectomy of the MCP joints involves the surgical ablation of much of the chronically inflamed rheumatoid synovium with the hope of arresting or slowing the progression of the disease. The results of the procedures are debatable, and there are no definitive studies that conclusively demonstrate that they alter the natural progression of the MCP joint disease. Some studies even suggest that synovectomy may actually decrease the range of joint motion and, by doing so, may worsen hand function (14). When the possibility of motion loss is combined with the likelihood of recurrence, it is easy to appreciate why rheumatologists and experienced hand surgeons are conservative when considering synovectomy of the MCP joints of the rheumatoid hand.

Synovectomy of the MCP joints should probably be reserved for a relatively few rheumatoid patients with chronic, persistent, well-organized synovitis with few radiologic changes and minimal deformity. Rarely, painful synovitis may be a surgical consideration, and a reasonable period of conservative treatment and observation is appropriate before proceeding with surgery, particularly considering that as many as 30% of patients with rheumatoid arthritis have periods of spontaneous remission or migration of the disease to other joints. Surgeons can develop an appreciation for the nature of MCP synovitis by carefully observing the feel of the synovial swelling over the joints during palpation. Those joints in which the synovitis has produced an abundance of fluid rebound quickly from pressure by the examiner's finger, whereas more organized, chronic synovitis pits when compressed and rebounds slowly. It is the authors' belief that long-standing, organized synovitis is much more amenable to surgical ablation than the watery type of synovitis in which recurrence seems to occur more rapidly.

The decision to proceed with a surgical synovectomy of rheumatoid MCP joints results from serial evaluations of the progression of the disease, a patient's level of MCP discomfort and dysfunction, the response to good medical management, and other factors, including the involvement of the wrist and PIP joints and the general medical and arthritic condition of the patient. Rheumatoid patients who have satisfactory function, minimal MCP pain, and little evidence of increasing deformity over time are probably not good candidates for synovectomy and can actually be made worse by overly aggressive operative intervention.

Some surgeons believe that the addition of soft tissue rebalancing procedures to MCP synovectomy can have a beneficial effect on hand function and slows the development of severe deformities. Procedures that recentralize displaced extensor tendons or that release contracted intrinsic tendons may improve MCP extension and alignment, provided that the joints can easily be corrected passively, and the articular surfaces are reasonably good before surgery (15–18). In the authors' experience, extensor tendon repositioning or selective intrinsic releases, or both, may be used in those few patients

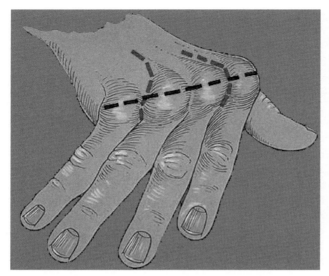

FIGURE 5. Incision options for surgical procedures on the metacarpophalangeal joints: transverse across the metacarpal heads or longitudinal between the index- and middle-finger metacarpophalangeal joints and between the ring- and small-finger metacarpophalangeal joints.

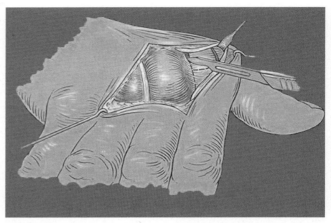

FIGURE 6. Exposure of the metacarpophalangeal joints through a longitudinal incision. Capsular incision with the extensor tendon displaced radially.

who fit the indications for synovectomy and also demonstrate a loss of digital extension secondary to ulnar displacement of the extensor tendons or mild, passively correctable MCP subluxation with demonstrable intrinsic tightness. Attempts to reconstruct and rebalance rheumatoid MCP joints by reefing the radial collateral ligaments or carrying out crossed intrinsic transfers are less predictable and may result in a loss of some of the preexisting joint motion (17,19–22). Recurrence from any of these soft tissue procedures is frequent, given the progressive nature of the rheumatoid disease process and the persistence of multiple deforming forces on the joints. Given the predictable long-term improvement that is afforded by MCP arthroplasty procedures, it may be reasonable to withhold synovectomy and soft tissue surgery in the rheumatoid patient who is relatively pain free and functions satisfactorily in lieu of later arthroplasty (9,16).

Authors' Preferred Technique

To carry out synovectomy and soft tissue rebalancing procedures on multiple rheumatoid MCP joints, the surgeon may elect to use a transverse approach or longitudinal incisions between the index and middle and the ring and small metacarpal heads (Fig. 5). The authors' personal preference is the use of 2- to 3-cm longitudinal incisions. With experience, these incisions can provide excellent exposure of all four MCP joints and heal promptly with minimal scarring. More importantly, they are in the plane of MCP joint flexion and extension, rather than being placed in tension during early exercise programs, as a transverse incision is. Furthermore, longitudinal incisions are not directly over the joints, and there is therefore less risk of joint infection with any wound breakdown after MCP joint surgery.

All soft tissues are carefully reflected off the extensor mechanism that overlies the MCP joints, and great care is taken to preserve the longitudinally oriented veins. Transverse or obliquely directed vessels may be cauterized, and complete visualization of the extensor tendons and their sagittal band extensions can then be achieved. The extensor mechanisms are incised through the ulnar sagittal bands directly along the ulnar sides of the extensor tendons when they are displaced into the ulnar valleys between the metacarpal heads. An elevator is then placed under the extensor tendons and above the joint capsules and is directed across to the radial side of each joint, after which the tendons may be levered into the valleys on the radial sides of the joints. If the extensor tendons remain centralized over the MCP joints, they may be split longitudinally, and the two parts of the tendon may be retracted to each side of each joint. The joint capsules are carefully opened using longitudinal or **H**-shaped incisions (Fig. 6), and the synovium is then removed with a scalpel blade or a small hand surgery rongeur (Fig. 7). Traction on the fingers facilitates the ability to remove synovium from the palmar aspect of the joints and the recesses behind the metacarpal origins of the collateral ligaments. Small bone cysts in the metacarpal heads may be curetted, and bone spicules that result from periarticular erosions may be excised (Fig. 8).

If the intrinsic tendons have been shown to be tight and are contributing to the development of MCP joint flexion and ulnar deviation deformities, release of the ulnar intrinsic tendons should be performed. The radial and ulnar intrinsic tendons may be divided if sufficient tightness persists after release of the ulnar side. It should be remembered that the intrinsics have a bony insertion into the base of the proximal phalanges, where they act as strong MCP joint flexors, and a tendon contribution to the lateral bands of the extensor mechanism, where they assist the extrinsic extensor tendon to extend the PIP joint. The bands then join over the middle phalanx to provide distal interphalangeal (DIP) joint

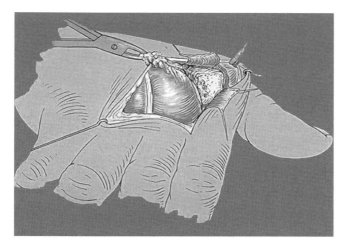

FIGURE 7. Synovectomy of the index finger metacarpophalangeal joint.

extension through a common terminal tendon. For rheumatoid intrinsic tightness, it is usually necessary to divide the intrinsic tendons, including the abductor digiti quinti, proximal to their insertions into the base of the proximal phalanges. This can be accomplished by passing a small hemostat palmarward alongside the metacarpal heads toward the transverse intermetacarpal ligaments. The hemostat is then directed toward the adjacent MCP joint and lifted dorsally to deliver the intrinsic tendons into view. Care must be taken to isolate only the intrinsic tendons to the desired digit and to protect the neurovascular structures that lie deep to the palmar ligaments. The offending tendons are then divided proximal to the base of the proximal phalan-

ges, and intrinsic tightness testing is carried out by passively flexing the PIP joints with the MCP joints held in full extension to demonstrate the completeness of the releases. It is not unusual to have to repeat this process to identify and to divide additional intrinsic muscle–tendons until a thorough release can be confirmed.

Closure is initiated by suturing the joint capsule whenever sufficient capsule can be identified and preserved during the synovectomy and soft tissue procedures. When the extensor tendons have been released from their subluxed or dislocated position into the ulnar valleys beside the MCP joints, they are centralized by reefing the stretched radial sagittal fibers. Imbrication of the sagittal fibers is easily accomplished by placing sutures longitudinally along the radial side of the extensor tendons and then passing the same suture palmarward down to the radial-most edge of the sagittal fibers. A small, straight hemostat is then passed under the transversely oriented suture material to bridge between the two suture placements, and the suture is tied over the hemostat. One or two such imbricating sutures securely maintain the extensor tendon in a centralized position, and the extensor tendon's stability can be checked by passively flexing and extending the MCP joint. Loosely tagging some adjacent areolar tissue to the ulnar side of the extensor tendon serves to help minimize the likelihood of any radial subluxation of the centralized tendon during MCP flexion and to complete a two-layer closure over the joint. The skin is closed with fine sutures, and a bulky compressive dressing with a palmar splint is applied to the forearm, wrist, and hand. The MCP joints are immobilized in full extension, and the PIP joints are usually left free for motion if no procedures have been carried out at that level.

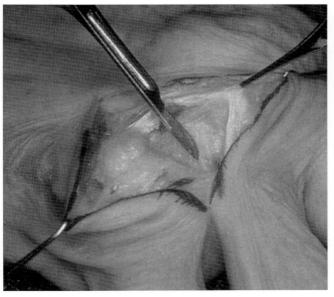

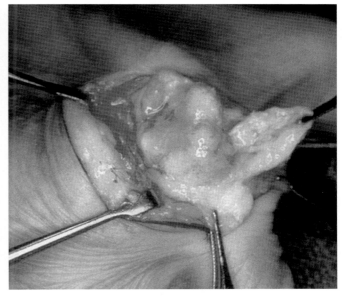

A   B

FIGURE 8. **A:** Intraoperative photograph of metacarpophalangeal joint capsular exposure after releasing the extensor tendon along its ulnar border. **B:** Intraoperative photograph of metacarpophalangeal joint synovitis with the capsule reflected.

Postoperative Rehabilitation

The patient is seen at 7 to 9 days postsurgery, and the bulky dressing is removed. A dynamic split is applied with an outrigger, which connects to digital slings, by rubber bands. The splint is carefully positioned and tensioned to maintain the fingers in full extension and slight radial deviation. MCP flexion is permitted within the splints. The patient's progress is carefully monitored during frequent visits to the hand therapist. If there is any tendency toward extension stiffness, passive flexion exercises are added to the therapy regimen, and dynamic flexion splinting may be initiated. With a vigorous, well-monitored therapy regimen, there should be little likelihood of the loss of MCP flexion. Over time, however, the initial improvement in digit position and relief of pain may well be negated by the continued progression of the rheumatoid disease and the influence of multiple deforming forces.

Complications

Complications of synovectomy and soft tissue reconstruction procedures for the rheumatoid MCP joint include wound breakdown, infection, joint stiffness, and the loss of the tendon or digital repositioning that has been achieved by the procedures. The skin of the hands of patients with long-standing rheumatoid disease, and particularly of those patients who have been extensively managed by steroid medications, is usually quite thin and fragile. It must be protected from excessive manipulation or compression during surgery and must be permitted an adequate time period (usually 2 weeks or more) for healing before sutures are removed. Wound breakdown can occur from devascularization of the skin flaps or from excessive tension on the wounds during the early application of motion stress during exercises. The author believes that this is a particular problem for patients who have had their MCP joints approached through a transverse incision. When it does occur, surgical incision separations should be managed by careful wound hygiene and protection. Exercise programs may have to be curtailed or modified, and secondary wound resuture may be advisable if there is no significant infection. Infections must be managed aggressively with decompression, débridement, sterile dressings, and oral or systemic antibiotics. MCP joint stiffness can be a problem, particularly when the joints are immobilized for too long in extension or when the postsurgical therapy program is not closely monitored and is altered according to the varied performance of the joints in different patients. The impending loss of motion must be rapidly recognized and aggressively treated. Failure to achieve the desired restoration of digital alignment may occur, particularly when the procedures are not adequately protected during the postoperative healing period. When the procedures fail, there is little that can be done to rectify the situation, and repeat surgery or arthroplasty procedures may be the best salvage options.

Operative Treatment: Arthroplasty

Considerations

When the rheumatoid MCP joint surfaces have been destroyed, or the joints have developed severe deformities, consideration should be given to arthroplasty procedures. For many years, surgeons relied on techniques of soft tissue stabilization and interposition when trying to improve advanced arthritic deformities of the MCP joint (23–25). These procedures sometimes produced excellent digit realignment and functional improvement, but their results were unpredictable. Prosthetic replacement procedures for the MCP joint were devised in the late 1950s and early 1960s (26,27), but the biomechanics of these joints were not adequately worked out, and the joints were not well tolerated by the fragile rheumatoid tissues. Swanson (28) and Neibauer and Landry (29) pioneered the development of silicone rubber implants in the 1960s, and, with some design and material improvements, they have remained the most reliable method for MCP replacement (30). Attempts to apply the cemented total-joint replacement concepts that have been so successful for the hip and knee to the rheumatoid MCP joint were ultimately abandoned because of the difficulty in achieving the right biomechanical balance and satisfactory long-term performance (31). The use of metal and polyethylene prostheses or joint replacements that are fabricated from pyrolytic carbon materials have shown early promise for MCP joint restoration, but their indications are currently limited to joints that can be fully extended passively (30). Therefore, these new implants are not applicable to the majority of advanced rheumatoid patients who present in hand surgeons' offices with fixed flexion deformities at their MCP joints.

Silicone rubber implants have been used as interpositional spacers after resection of the metacarpal heads of severely involved rheumatoid MCP joints since the 1970s. They have provided reliability to MCP arthroplasty by replacing techniques of soft tissue reconstruction that were unpredictable and technically demanding. Although there have been modest changes in the design and composition of the silicone materials, the implants and their replacement techniques have not changed greatly since they were first introduced in 1969 (8,32–35). The methods for carrying out silicone rubber replacement arthroplasties are complex and demanding. Attention to detail is critical, and the surgeon must appreciate the fact that the removal of arthritic MCP bone and the insertion of a silicone spacer are only a small part of the success of these arthroplasties. The soft tissue rebalancing procedures that must accompany the implant insertion and a well-designed and implemented postsurgical rehabilitation program are even more critical to the short- and long-term performance of MCP joint replacements. It most instances, the goals of MCP replacement arthroplasty are the improvement of digital extension and alignment while retaining a functionally acceptable range of MCP flexion.

A thorough examination of the status of the shoulder, the elbow, the wrist, the PIP joints, and the thumb is extremely important in decisions regarding MCP joint replacement arthroplasty and any procedures that may be carried out concomitantly. The wrist, in particular, is important because the frequent rheumatoid sequence of ulnar carpal translocation and supination and radial deviation of the metacarpals has been demonstrated to result in substantial forces that favor ulnar deviation of the digits at the MCP joints (Fig. 1). Carrying out interpositional arthroplasty procedures on MCP joints when the metacarpals are radially aligned most assuredly results in a return of ulnar deviation of the digits. Common sense demonstrates that flexible silicone rubber implants whose stems are perpendicular to the body of the implant cannot successfully reposition the digits into colinearity with the forearm bones when there is improper fitting of the implants or angulation of their stems. Forces that are created by wrist and metacarpal malpositioning inevitably accentuate the ulnar angulation of the fingers. Therefore, it is necessary to correct or to reduce the ulnar translocation of the carpus and to straighten the metacarpals before or at the same time as MCP joint arthroplasty. This can best be accomplished by a Chamay radiolunate arthrodesis procedure (11,36) or by total wrist arthrodesis.

Swan-neck or boutonnière deformities of the PIP joints also affect hand performance after MCP joint arthroplasty procedures. Clearly, the best hand function after MCP reconstruction is experienced by those patients with little or no PIP involvement. Fixed hyperextension or flexion deformities of the PIPs compromise the ability to reach around and to grasp an object with full contact between the object and the palmar aspect of the digits. Interestingly, it has been a consistent observation that the MCP joint flexion that is achieved after arthroplasty procedures is better when the PIPs are stiffened than when they are fully flexible, probably because the flexor tendon power and excursion can be concentrated at the MCP level. Some surgeons would consider soft tissue procedures or PIP joint arthrodeses concomitantly with MCP arthroplasties, whereas others would prefer to maximize the recovery from the MCP joint procedures before tending to the PIP joint deformities. In some instances, the surgeon and patient may agree to accept modest PIP deformities and to strive for the best functional recovery from their MCP surgery. The surgical management of thumb deformities can often be addressed at the same time as MCP joint arthroplasties. Considering that boutonnière MCP flexion deformities of the thumb occur much more frequently than zigzag collapse or swan-neck deformities, arthrodesis of the thumb MCP joint is often all that is necessary, and it can easily be combined with digital MCP arthroplasties.

Rheumatoid patients with deformity and dysfunction of the MCP joints are candidates for surgical silicone rubber implant arthroplasty when the joints have reached the late stage. Fixed flexion deformities, with or without articular destruction, usually in combination with ulnar deviation of the digits are often the presentation that leads to consideration for surgery. There are instances when a mild extension loss and digital deviation exists at the MCP joints, and flexion remains functionally adequate. Proceeding with arthroplasties in those individuals might well be inappropriate, considering that their actual functional level is probably quite good. More advanced deformities, often with subluxation or dislocation of the MCP joints, are much more disabling, and, those patients can expect substantial improvement from the MCP repositioning, realignment, and rebalancing that arthroplasty procedures should accomplish. Although pain occasionally enters into the consideration for surgery on the MCP joints, it is surprising how frequently there is little or no discomfort that is associated with these deformities.

Authors' Preferred Technique

Silicone rubber interpositional arthroplasty of the rheumatoid MCP joints is usually carried out on an in-patient basis under regional or general anesthesia. There are several commercially available types of implants, and hand surgeons have their own preferences as to the best type for a particular patient. Although the implant that was designed by Swanson is still the most commonly used (Fig. 9), other prostheses that use different silicone rubber compounds and design modifications have achieved some popularity, and each type has special preparation and placement instruments that are unique to that type of implant. The authors currently use an anatomically neutral, preflexed silicone implant (Neuflex, DePuy Orthopaedics, Warsaw, IN) that is designed to provide improved flexion without an increased incidence of implant failure (Fig. 10A–J).

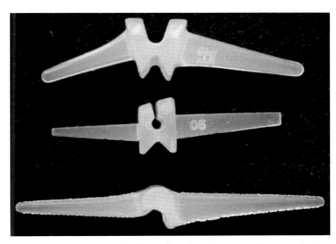

FIGURE 9. Photograph of Neuflex (*top*), Avanta (Avanta Orthopaedics, Inc., San Diego, CA) (*middle*), and Swanson (*bottom*) metacarpophalangeal implants.

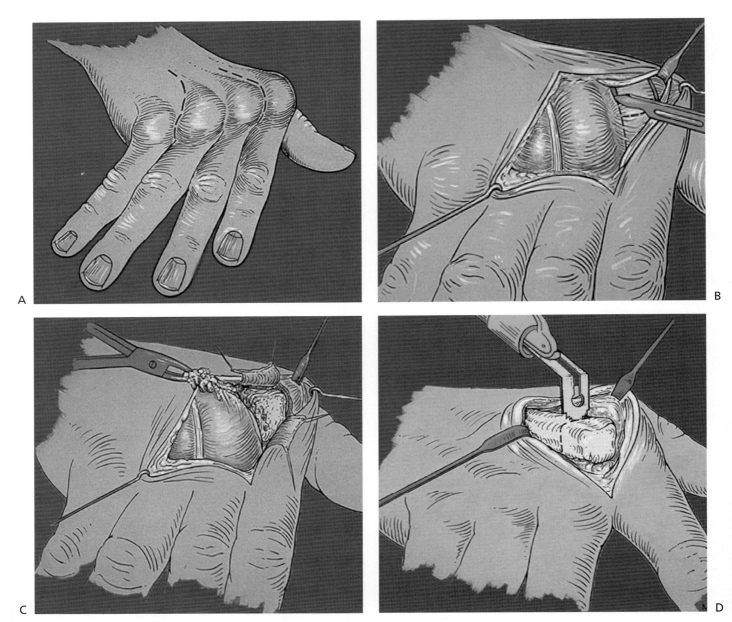

FIGURE 10. A: Authors' preferred incisions for metacarpophalangeal joint replacement surgery by using Neuflex (DePuy Orthopaedics, Warsaw, IN) implants. **B:** Release of the extensor tendon along its ulnar border followed by capsular incision. **C:** Synovectomy of the metacarpophalangeal joint. **D:** Removal of the arthritic metacarpal head by using a sagittal saw. (*continued*)

In general, all silicone arthroplasty procedures use incision and soft tissue exposure methods that are identical to those that are described in the section Operative Treatment: Synovectomy and Soft Tissue Rebalancing of this chapter, and the authors' preference is strongly biased toward longitudinal incisions between the index- and long-finger MCP joints and between the ring- and small-finger MCP joints. The ulnarly displaced extensor tendons are released along their ulnar borders well out on the sagittal fibers of the extensor hoods, although some surgeons prefer to excise the extensor hood on the radial, rather than the contracted,

ulnar side (37). After releasing the displaced extensor tendons, they are carefully separated from the underlying MCP joint capsules and are reflected radially to expose the joint capsules. Incisions into the joint capsules may be longitudinal or H-shaped to provide adequate visualization of the metacarpal heads (Fig. 11A). Before excising the metacarpal heads, the radial collateral ligament is released from the neck of the second metacarpal, so that it may be reconstructed at the end of the procedure in a manner that preserves lateral and rotatory alignment and pinch stability for the index finger. The amount of metacarpal head that is

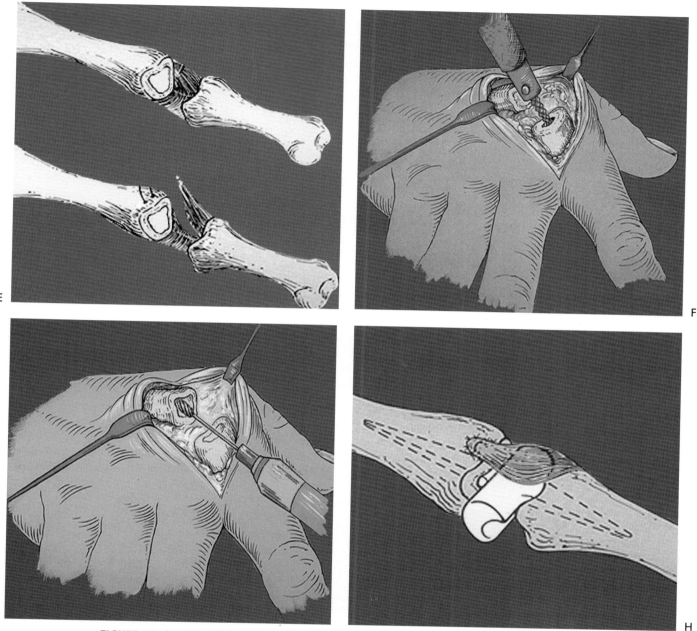

FIGURE 10. (*continued*) **E:** Radial collateral ligament preparation after excision of the metacarpal head. Sutures have been placed in the distal metacarpal for dorsal reattachment of the collateral ligament. **F:** Reaming of the medullary canal of the proximal phalanx in preparation for implant arthroplasty. **G:** Reaming of the medullary canal of the metacarpal using a small power bur. Dorsal repair of the radial collateral ligament preparation after seating of the silicone rubber implant. (*continued*)

resected is determined by the width of the body of the probable implant and, to some extent, by the severity of the fixed flexion deformity of each MCP joint. The cut is made transversely with a sagittal cutting saw and is usually near the juncture of the metacarpal neck and head.

Release of the ulnar intrinsic tendons is recommended by some, particularly when there is substantial preoperative ulnar deviation of the digits (9,28,38), although tight intrinsics are usually relaxed by MCP head excision. The author rarely divides the ulnar intrinsics because of the weakening effect that their loss has on the already weakened rheumatoid hand. There are, however, instances in which the abductor digiti minimi is so contracted that it must be divided to allow realignment of the small finger. Radial collateral ligaments should be preserved whenever possible, and the ulnar collateral is usually released from its phalangeal insertion. Some addi-

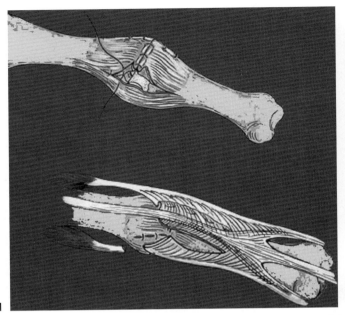

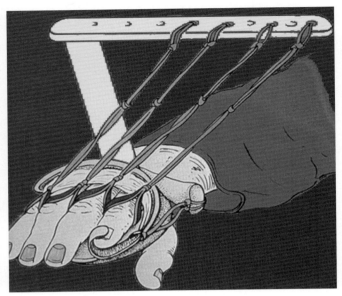

FIGURE 10. (*continued*) **I:** Capsular repair (*above*). Imbrication of the radial expansion of the extensor hood (*below*). **J:** Depiction of extensor-radial deviation dynamic outrigger splint.

tional distance between the distal end of the metacarpal and the base of the proximal phalanx can be achieved by division of the palmar plate. It is sometimes wise to maintain MCP joint balance by transversely removing some of the proximal phalangeal base, rather than excessively excising the distal metacarpal shaft, to achieve sufficient space between the two bones for implant placement. After smoothing the ends of both bones

and removing any remaining hypertrophic synovium, the medullary canals of the opposing metacarpal and phalanx are reamed with the instruments that are provided for each type of implant (Fig. 11B–D), and the trial implants are used to determine the best size for each joint (Fig. 11E,F). The use of power reaming instruments to achieve a satisfactory intramedullary fit for the implant must be carried out with great care, as such

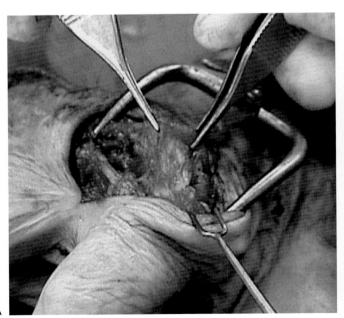

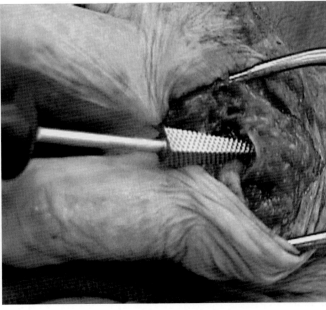

FIGURE 11. A: Exposure and synovectomy of the metacarpophalangeal joint during implant arthroplasty. **B:** Preparation of the medullary canal of the metacarpal by using specialized reamers. (*continued*)

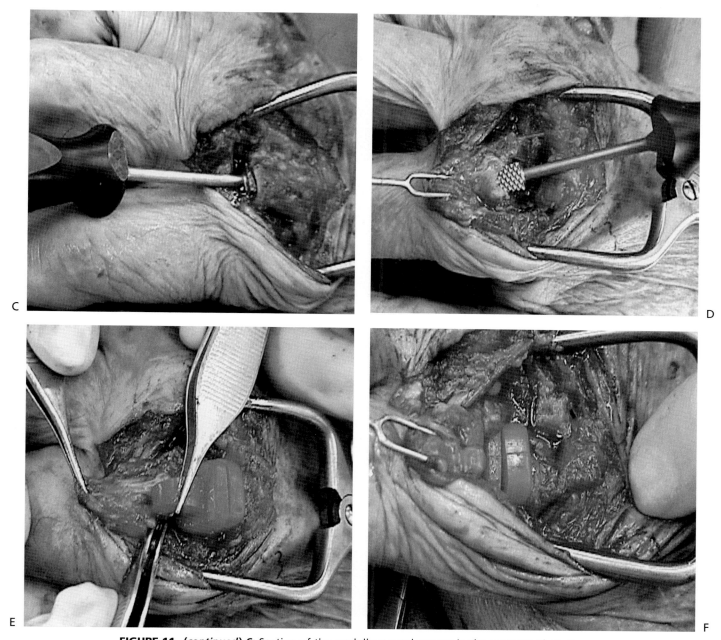

FIGURE 11. (*continued*) C: Seating of the medullary canal reamer in the metacarpal. **D:** Reaming of the proximal phalanx medullary canal. **E:** Seating of the trial-sizing implant. **F:** Completed seating of the trial implant. Note the closed position with the joint in full extension. (*continued*)

efforts run the risk of excessively thinning or even splitting the cortical bone. For the most part, the largest size of the silicone rubber implant for an MCP joint is determined by the proximal stem fit into the metacarpal, with the proximal phalanx rarely dictating the proper prosthesis. The implants must fit snugly with their stems totally within bone, and the joints must passively extend and flex fully after trial implant placement. Any residual intrinsic tightness can be tested at this point, and additional releases may be required. With the trial implants removed, the radial collateral ligament and surrounding portions of the capsule

and palmar plate are mobilized to the base of the proximal phalanx of the index finger. Care must be taken to make this soft tissue preparation sufficiently long, so that it can be repositioned on the dorsoradial aspect of the second metacarpal at the time of closure. Two small holes on the dorsum of the metacarpal are made with a 0.035-in. Kirschner wire that is approximately 5 mm from its transected end, and a 3-0 braided synthetic suture is passed from outside in to inside out, in preparation for the collateral ligament replacement. After implanting the definitive MCP implants, motion is again checked (Fig. 11G–I), and the

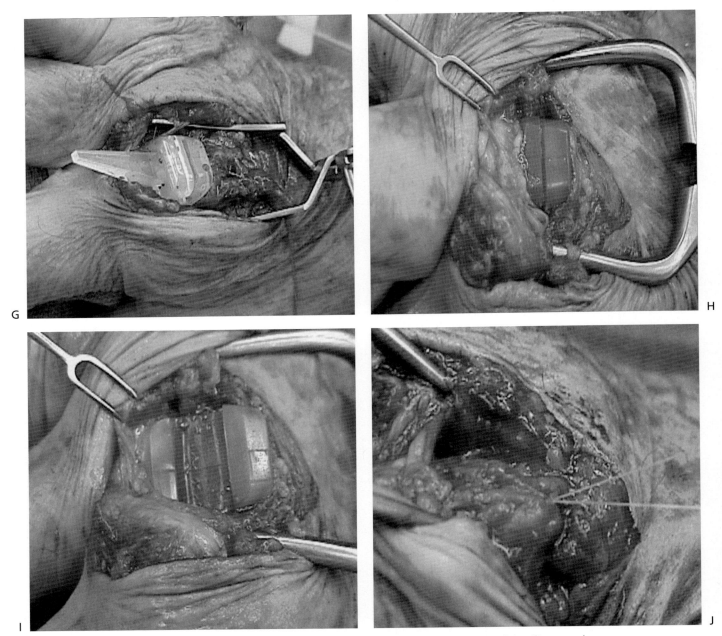

FIGURE 11. (*continued*) **G:** Proximal seating of the implant. **H:** Appearance of the silicone replacement implant in full extension. **I:** Appearance of the implant with the joint in flexion. **J:** Reconstruction of the radiocollateral ligament (index) and capsular closure.

capsule is closed in a proximal ulnar-to-distal radial bias that favors radial deviation of the digit. The extensor tendons are centralized by imbricating the radial sagittal bands (Fig. 11J), and a loose attachment of areolar tissue from the ulnar side of the joint to the extensor tendon completes a two-layer coverage of the implants. The joints are carefully tested through a range of motion, and a roll towel is placed beneath all fingers to maintain their alignment and extension during wound closure. A large compressive dressing positions the MCP joints in full extension and straight alignment at the conclusion of the procedure.

Postoperative Rehabilitation

The postoperative rehabilitation program is extremely important to the success of MCP joint arthroplasty for patients with rheumatoid arthritis. Protocols vary somewhat, but all are designed to influence the healing of soft tissues and the encapsulation of the implants in such a manner that there is a functional balance between motion, alignment, and stability. The patient is seen at 7 to 9 days postsurgery, and the bulky dressing is removed. A dynamic splint is applied with an outrigger that connects to digital slings by rubber bands. The splint is carefully positioned

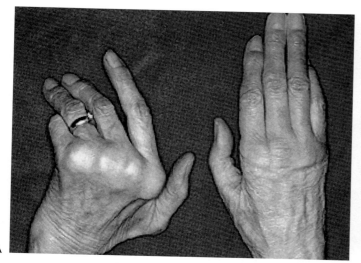
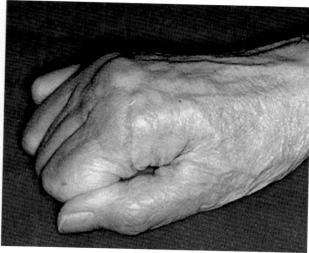

A

B

FIGURE 12. A: Appearance of the left hand before surgery and the right hand after surgery many months after silicone replacement arthroplasty of the metacarpophalangeal joints in a patient. **B:** Postoperative flexion of the same patient's right hand after metacarpophalangeal replacement arthroplasty.

and tensioned to maintain the fingers in full extension and slight radial deviation. MCP flexion is permitted and encouraged within the splints, and the patient's progress is carefully monitored during frequent visits to the hand therapist. A palmar resting pan splint is applied for night use, because it ensures correct positioning of the digits and is less likely to be dislodged during sleep. If there is any tendency toward extension stiffness, passive flexion exercises are added to the therapy regimen, and dynamic flexion splinting may be initiated. Patients who regain extension quickly need therapy adjustments to reduce the likelihood of recurrent ulnar deviation of the digits. Splinting and protected motion are usually continued for 3 months, and a joint-protection program is usually instituted by the therapist at the conclusion of the rehabilitation program. With a vigorous, well-monitored therapy regimen, most rheumatoid patients experience an improvement in digital extension and alignment while maintaining a functional amount of MCP flexion (Fig. 12). Over time, there may be some loss of the improvement in digital position and function that is achieved by implant arthroplasty procedures.

Complications

Complications of implant arthroplasty of the rheumatoid MCP joints may be due to soft tissue problems, implant positioning, or material failure. They include wound breakdown, infection, joint stiffness, implant dislocation, recurrent deformity, and implant fracture. Fortunately, wound breakdown and infection have rarely been seen after these procedures (38). Wound breakdown can occur from devascularization of the skin flaps or from excessive tension on the wounds during the early application of motion stress during exercises, and it is most frequent in thin-skinned rheumatoid patients who have been treated with steroids

for an extended period of time. When it does occur, surgical incision separations should be managed by careful wound hygiene, protection, and, occasionally, secondary closure. Infections must be managed aggressively with decompression, débridement, sterile dressings, and oral or systemic antibiotics. When the joint itself becomes infected, implant removal is almost always required. MCP joint stiffness can be a problem, particularly when the joints are immobilized for too long in extension, or when the postsurgical therapy program is not closely monitored and altered according to the varied performance of the joints in different patients.

Failure to achieve desired MCP flexion after silicone rubber-implant arthroplasty must be rapidly recognized and aggressively treated. The authors' observation has been that thin-skinned patients usually achieve the best recovery of flexion but are more prone to the redevelopment of some ulnar deviation of the digits. Conversely, thicker-skinned patients with no history of steroid use retain better alignment but may have a difficult time achieving as much flexion at their MCP joints. Therefore, it may be prudent to delay the initiation of a motion program for as long as 3 weeks in the patient with thin skin. Recurrent ulnar deviation of the digits may often result from a failure to correct ulnar translocation of the wrist and radial deviation of the metacarpals before or concomitantly with MCP implant arthroplasty (Fig. 13).

The dislocation of the stem of an implant usually occurs in the immediate postoperative period and tends to involve the distal (phalangeal) stem. There is no alternative to returning to the operating room and reinserting the stem, which are combined with an effort to deal with the cause of the displacement. Fracturing of the implants is a definite long-term problem after the use of any of the currently

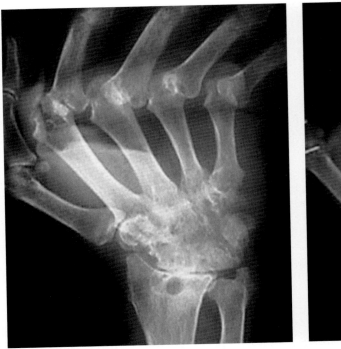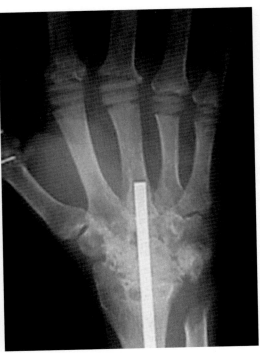

A

B

FIGURE 13. A: Preoperative x-rays of patient with severe, multilevel rheumatoid deformities, including carpal coalition and ulnar translocation, radial deviation of the metacarpals, and dislocation and ulnar deviation of the digits. **B:** Postoperative x-rays of the same patient after wrist fusion by using a pin that was placed down the medullary canal of the third metacarpal, Darrach excision of the distal ulna, and metacarpophalangeal replacement arthroplasties by using silicone rubber implants.

available silicone rubber implants. Some MCP joints continue to perform satisfactorily after implant fracturing, and patients may not even be aware of the subtle changes in position or function. Recurrent MCP joint deformity and a palpable palmar step-off of the proximal phalanx are usually evidence of implant fracture. A fairly simple replacement of the fractured implant can be carried out, with care taken to remove any sharp bone edges and to correct any force imbalances that may have contributed to the failure. Because there is little need to remove additional bone stock, and the fibrous capsule around the previous implant is still in place, the postreplacement rehabilitation program can be considerably less demanding.

INTERPHALANGEAL JOINTS

Normal Anatomy

The normal function of the digits of the hand results from a complex and highly integrated balance of the digital joints and the extrinsic and intrinsic muscle–tendon units that move them. Any disruption of the normal skeletal stability or the integrity of the tendons that insert on elements of that skeleton can result in collapse deformities at the affected joints. The breakdown of one or more components of the

articulated chain of hand and wrist bones can have a profound effect on adjacent joints, often producing an opposite configuration of deformity. Rheumatoid arthritis often produces two different patterns of finger deformity in the fingers. The so-called swan-neck deformity is characterized by PIP joint hyperextension and DIP joint flexion, whereas the boutonnière deformity reverses that deformity with PIP flexion and DIP extension. The swan-neck deformity occurs approximately twice as often as the boutonnière pattern, and adjacent fingers may be affected in opposite ways.

Swan-Neck Deformity

Pathophysiology

The rheumatoid swan-neck deformity is characterized by PIP joint hyperextension and DIP flexion. In addition, flexion deformity at the MCP joint may be part of the deformity and an integral component of the digital imbalance (Fig. 14). Flexible swan-neck deformities may be mainly a cosmetic problem, although snapping or impaired dexterity from the awkward and delayed sequence of digital flexion may compromise function. The inability to flex the PIP joints with severe fixed swan-neck deformities results in a loss of the ability to conform the digits to objects during grasp (39,40).

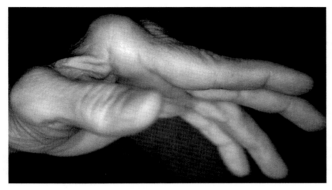

FIGURE 14. Characteristic configuration of the swan-neck deformity with metacarpophalangeal joint flexion, proximal interphalangeal joint hyperextension, and distal interphalangeal joint flexion.

Swan-neck deformity in rheumatoid arthritis is usually a result of PIP joint synovitis, most often with concomitant synovitis of the flexor tendons. The inflammation results in attenuation of the palmar joint housing (the collateral ligaments, the palmar plate, and the insertion of the flexor digitorum superficialis tendon). Periarticular tenosynovitis and PIP synovitis do not act in isolation to cause swan-neck deformity. Flexed postures of the wrist (less frequently) or the MCP joints (most frequently) create a relative shortening of the long digital extensors and an increased extension moment at the PIP joint. Flexor tenosynovitis leads to decreased excursion of the flexor tendons within the digit, which increases their pull at the MCP joint and decreases their efficiency at the PIP joint. All of these factors contribute to an imbalance between the flexor, extensor, and intrinsic systems, which results in hyperextension of the PIP joint and attendant dorsal displacement of the lateral bands, thus weakening their ability to extend the DIP joint (Fig. 15) (39).

Intrinsic muscle–tendon tightness also contributes to the development of swan-neck deformity. In addition, rheumatoid digits commonly develop fixed flexion at the MCP joints. The existence of these codeformities enhances the swan-neck tendency by increasing the extension pull of the intrinsic and extrinsic systems on the PIP. The resultant PIP hyperextension greatly reduces the effective pull of the relatively lengthened lateral bands at the DIP level, thus producing a flexion deficit at that level. Although the swan-neck configuration may be limited to the PIP and DIP joints, a three-joint flexion (MCP), hyperextension (PIP), and flexion (DIP) sequence usually is present. Rheumatoid mallet deformities also can contribute to a hyperextension deformity of the PIP joint. The forces of digital extension concentrate at the PIP joint, as their action on the distal joint is lost as a result of attenuation or rupture of the terminal tendon. Unopposed flexor digitorum profundus action at the DIP joint exacerbates the deformity. With time, dorsal subluxation of the lateral bands becomes fixed,

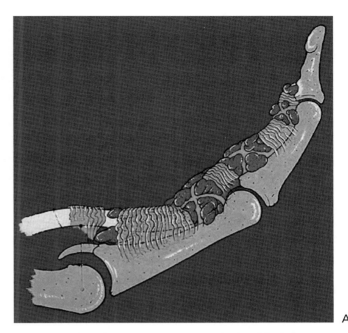

A

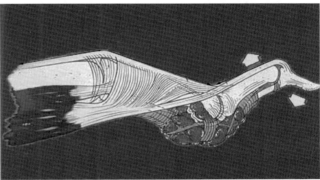

B

FIGURE 15. A: Illustration of florid tenosynovitis of the flexor tendon sheath with bulging in the cruciate synovial spaces between the annular pulleys. **B:** Illustration of the characteristic configuration of the swan-neck deformity with synovitis of the flexor tendon sheath, flexion at the metacarpophalangeal joint, hyperextension at the proximal interphalangeal joint, and flexion at the distal interphalangeal joint.

and the central slip tendon and the triangular ligament shorten. The lateral retinacular ligaments become attenuated, and the dorsal skin and subcutaneous tissue also may contract with long-standing, fixed PIP hyperextension. The PIP joint becomes increasingly fixed, and, with persisting active disease, the articular cartilage of the PIP joint is destroyed. During this sequence, a flexible deformity converts to a rigid one.

Long extensor tendon subluxation, loss of MCP joint cartilage, and volar subluxation and dislocation of the proximal phalanx on the metacarpal head may decrease this effect of relative shortening of the long digital extensors as the disease advances. These effects, which would decrease the tendency of the finger to assume a swan-neck configuration, may mitigate some of the deforming force. Once the PIP joint has collapsed into hyperextension, and the lateral bands sublux dorsally, it is rare to see any significant reversal of the deformity. The multifactorial nature of the deformity must be appreciated if a rational approach to correction is to be developed.

Swan-neck deformities are flexible and passively correctable or fixed. Fixed deformities are divided into those with preservation of some joint space and those with destroyed articular surfaces. This classification has direct implications as to the choice of surgical procedure for the deformity.

Management Considerations

As in any patient with rheumatoid arthritis, the total condition of the patient, the level of motivation, and the degree of dysfunction that is caused by the deformity must be assessed carefully before surgical intervention. Many patients also have significant disease that involves other upper-extremity joints (shoulder, elbow, wrist, and thumb). Consideration of the patient's pain and functional status, as it is affected by each joint, figures into any decision as to the appropriateness of swan-neck surgery. Procedures may have to be prioritized on the basis of the patient's attainable long-term needs and desires. For some rheumatoid patients with advanced deformities and dysfunction, improvement of swan-neck deformities is of less benefit than wrist stabilization, thumb MCP fusion, and MCP arthroplasty of the digits.

Many patients have little or no functional impairment secondary to flexible hyperextension at the PIP level. Despite some snapping as the lateral bands suddenly move palmarward during digital flexion, they do not need corrective measures. Other patients reach a point at which it is difficult to initiate active PIP flexion and experience difficulty grasping objects. In those instances, procedures that mobilize the lateral band and perform tenodesis of the joint to prevent hyperextension are of benefit.

When the deformity is fixed, patients lack the ability to wrap their hands tightly around curved objects, with contact limited to the palmar surface of the hyperextended PIPs. Pain is often present with rigid contractures, and, in appropriate situations, PIP joint mobilization procedures may be helpful, provided that the joint articular surfaces are not badly destroyed. The change in digital posture (hyperextension to flexion) that these procedures produce can be of considerable functional benefit.

For rigid swan-neck deformities with destroyed joint surfaces, arthrodesis of the PIP joint is usually the most practical option. Although there may be some instances in which a flexible implant arthroplasty can be used to improve the deformity, the authors have found those procedures to be generally unreliable in the rheumatoid patient, mainly because of the complex rebalancing of deforming forces that must be used during such reconstructive efforts and the inability to consistently attain stability of rheumatoid PIP joints around an inherently unstable implant.

Evaluation

A detailed history must be taken, and a physical examination must be performed. Instabilities of the cervical spine (especially the atlantoaxial articulation) are frequent in these patients and may represent anesthetic risks, particularly if the patient is to undergo a general anesthetic. Inquiry into recent steroid use should be carried out, as perioperative adjustment of dosage may be required, as well as supplemental steroid administration at the time of surgery.

A complete evaluation of all coexistent deformities is required. To ignore the contributions of the long extensor tendon, the MCP or wrist joints, the intrinsic muscles, or the skin and subcutaneous tissue to the creation of the digital swan-neck deformity is to invite the failure of surgical correction. The PIP deformity cannot be addressed in isolation. Flexor tenosynovitis, which restricts tendon excursion, may be a significant factor in the development of swan-neck deformities. In these instances, tenosynovectomy or a palmar traction lysis of the flexor tendons may be an important addition to the corrective procedure. Long extensor tendon subluxation or dislocation must be recognized in the preoperative evaluation, so that it can be corrected by an extensor tendon realignment procedure. A fixed flexion deformity of the MCP joint relatively tightens the extrinsic digital extensors. In these instances, consideration should be given to an MCP synovectomy or, in the presence of gross joint destruction or dislocation, a flexible implant arthroplasty.

The presence of ulnar subluxation or dislocation of the MCP joint also serves to tighten the intrinsic digital extensors. If a flexible MCP arthroplasty is performed, the surgeon should plan on resection of sufficient bone at the level of the metacarpal head and the base of the proximal phalanx to lengthen relatively the intrinsic and the extrinsic digital extensors. These procedures at the MCP joint alone may improve mild flexible swan-neck deformities, although it is frequently necessary to carry out additional surgery at the PIP level to rebalance or reposition that joint.

Treatment of Rheumatoid Swan-Neck Deformities

Conservative Treatment

In reality, there is little that can be offered conservatively to the rheumatoid patient who is developing a swan-neck configuration to one or more digits. Because the pathomechanics of the disorder are so complex and multifactorial, exercise programs and splinting are rarely successful in slowing the progression of the deformity, particularly when the patient has an aggressive disease with involvement of multiple digital joints. In the early stages of deformity, when the palmar snapping of the lateral bands from their dorsally displaced position during finger flexion is annoying to patients, small digital extension block splints that are designed to permit PIP flexion, but restrict hyperextension, may be helpful.

Operative Treatment

Considerations

Surgical procedures that are designed to stop or to retard the development of rheumatoid swan-neck deformities depend, almost entirely, on the severity of the deformity and the status of the PIP joint and adjacent joints. If the PIP joints can be actively or passively moved to full flexion, then flexor tenosynovectomy with or without concomitant soft tissue rebalancing procedures may improve function and halt, or slow, the progression or the sequence of deformity. Fixed PIP hyperextension that cannot be passively improved or x-ray evidence of articular destruction mitigates for soft tissue or joint procedures that are designed to improve the position or stability of the joints, despite little or no improvement in the actual arc of motion.

Incisions should be planned so that they are not directly over the PIP, where the dorsal tension that is created by joint flexion may compromise healing. In the long-standing fixed deformity, contraction of the dorsal skin and subcutaneous tissue over the PIP may make wound closure difficult after the joint is corrected into a flexed position. In those instances, it is preferable to leave the distal part of the wounds open. These small open wounds can be expected to heal quickly and do not compromise postoperative therapy.

Flexor Tenosynovitis

The prolific synovitis of rheumatoid arthritis can significantly affect finger function, particularly when it occurs in the nonextendable flexor tendon sheaths (Fig. 16). Rheumatoid nodules may form on either of the flexor tendons within the digital canal, and their presence may mechanically impair tendon excursion. Swelling of the palmar aspect of the distal palm and digits is often detected, and palpable crepitus, or triggering, during active finger flexion and extension indicates the presence of synovial involvement of the sheath and tendons. When the excursion of the flexor tendons is sufficiently impaired, there is a loss of digital motion and, ultimately, stiffness of the interdigital joints. Ruptures of flexor tendons that result from chronic synovial invasion within flexor tendon sheaths may occur infrequently. When rheumatoid flexor tenosynovitis has been present for several months, and particularly when there is associated triggering or interdigital joint motion loss, or both, it is appropriate to proceed with a tenosynovectomy and nodule removal of the flexor tendons in the distal palm and digit. It must be noted, however, that division of the first annular pulley, the preferred method of trigger finger decompression in nonrheumatoid patients, is usually contraindicated in most patients with active rheumatoid disease, because such a release increases the flexion and ulnar deviation moment arm of the flexor tendons and

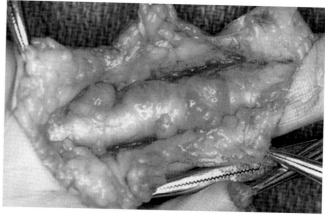

FIGURE 16. Photograph of a digit with severe flexor tenosynovitis.

may cause or accelerate the development of deformity at the MCP joint. The technique that is described by Ferlic and Clayton (41) in which one slip of the flexor digitorum superficialis is excised to decompress the flexor sheath without violating an annular pulley is the preferred technique of most surgeons for tenosynovectomy.

Authors' Preferred Technique of Flexor Tenosynovectomy. Connection of oblique incisions that are centered beneath the involved digit or digits is designed to permit simple zigzag extensions proximally and distally, depending on the amount and extent of the tenosynovitis that is encountered. The offending tenosynovium and any tendon nodules are excised in the palm proximal to the first annular pulley and distally in the cruciate synovial windows between the annular pulleys. The material is best removed sharply with the tip of a scalpel or by stripping it away by using a small rongeur. It is possible to work on both sides of the pulleys without dividing or narrowing them, and tenosynovium beneath the pulleys can be delivered into view by placing proximal traction on the tendons and flexing the finger. Gentle passive manipulation of stiffened interdigital joints may be beneficial once the flexor tendons have been cleaned of diseased synovium and nodules, and a decision is then made as to the necessity of excising one slip of the flexor superficialis. This may be easily accomplished in the C1 cruciate window by a smooth beveled cut that is placed just at the point at which the slip that is being excised rejoins the opposite slip (Fig. 17). There are even occasions when the sheath is so crowded with diseased tendon that excising the entire superficialis is advisable. Active and passive digital motion is commenced rapidly after flexor tenosynovectomy for patients with rheumatoid arthritis. If the procedure has been mainly in the palm, the involved finger is bandaged in a manner that permits active and passive motion immediately after surgery. If the incision involves the digit, the bandage should be removed within 2 days, so that motion exercises can be initiated.

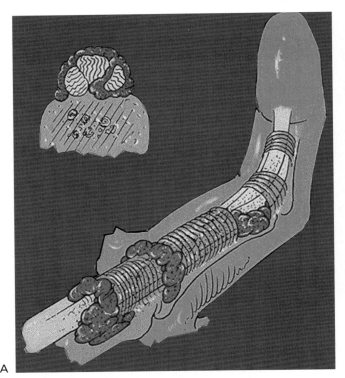

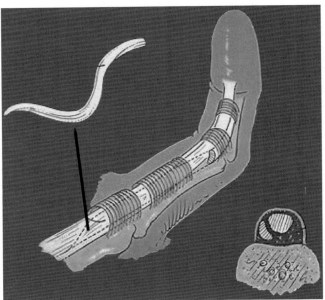

FIGURE 17. A: Rheumatoid tenosynovitis of the flexor tendon sheath. **B:** Tenosynovectomy of the flexor tendon sheath with excision of one slip of the flexor digitorum superficialis.

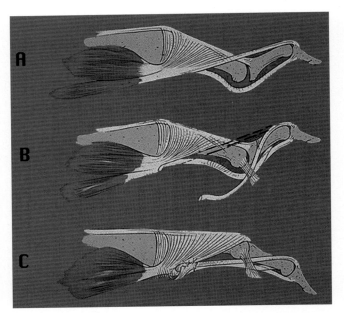

FIGURE 18. Littler (42) tenodesis for swan-neck deformity **(A)** with proximal transection and mobilization of one lateral band, which is then transferred beneath Cleland's ligament **(B)** and attached to the intrinsic tendon or flexor tendon sheath with the PIP joint in flexion **(C)**. Some surgeons prefer to transfer the band to the opposite side of the finger.

Flexible Swan-Neck Deformities

Occasionally, the hand surgeon has the opportunity to see swan-neck deformities at an early stage, when snapping of the centralized extensor lateral bands is the primary problem, and there is little hyperextension at the PIP joint and minimal demonstrable intrinsic tightness. In those cases, extension block splinting may be adequate, or, if surgery is selected, simple mobilization of the lateral bands may be accomplished under digital block anesthesia and provides excellent relief from the mechanical annoyance of snapping and some modest intrinsic decompression, as well.

For flexible deformities, one of several methods of accomplishing a tenodesis of the PIP joint to prevent hyperextension can be effective. The method that is described by Littler (42) recreates the function of the oblique retinacular ligament (ORL) by using a lateral band that is detached near the base of the proximal phalanx and is routed palmar to Cleland's ligaments or completely beneath the flexor sheath to the opposite side of the proximal phalanx where it is anchored to an annular pulley (43) (Fig. 18). A lateral band rerouting procedure that was advocated by Zancolli (44,45) and Tonkin et al. (46) has proven to be simple and effective. This procedure can be used even in the presence of modest joint-space narrowing.

Authors' Preferred Technique for Flexible Swan-Neck Deformities. We prefer the method described by Zancolli (44,45) for performing a simple and effective tenodesis of the rheumatoid PIP joint with a flexible swan-neck hyperextension deformity. A dorsal curvilinear incision around the PIP joint is made 1 to 2 mm dorsal to the mid-lateral line of the finger, from the midpoint of the proximal phalanx to the DIP joint. This approach permits easy access to the dorsally subluxed lateral bands, which then are mobilized. Dissection is carried across the dorsum of the digit and palmarward on one (usually ulnar) lateral side, so that the deflected flap provides exposure of the extensor apparatus, the retaining ligaments, and the flexor tendon sheath. Cleland's ligament is divided to allow access to the palmar aspect of the finger. The fibrous flexor sheath is approached directly, as the neurovascular structures are still safely palmar to the surgical field. Care must be taken to identify the digital artery and nerve when there is severe PIP hyperextension.

The dorsally displaced lateral bands are now identified, and the lateral band to be used as a tenodesis (usually ulnar) is dissected free of its dorsal attachment to the central extensor slip for approximately 1 cm proximal and 1 cm distal to the PIP joint. The mobilized lateral band is then delivered palmar to the axis of rotation of the PIP joint, as the joint is passively flexed. Sufficient proximal and distal release of the lateral band should be carried out, so that it may be displaced down to the level of the flexor sheath at the level of the PIP joint. The mobilized lateral band should not be detached either proximally or distally, and excessive mobilization should be avoided to preserve sufficient tension for the tenodesis to be effective.

The location of the PIP joint is now determined. The collateral ligament, volar plate, and the fibrous flexor sheath (the third annular pulley at this level) are identified and exposed. The digital artery and nerve are retracted in a volar direction. A scalpel is used to create a 1-cm-wide dorsally based flap of flexor sheath at the level of the joint. The sheath flap is opened as far palmarward as possible and is left attached to the volar plate and adjacent PIP joint structures.

The mobilized lateral band is displaced in a palmar direction and is brought to lie under the sheath flap. With the PIP joint held in flexion, the flap of flexor sheath is now replaced in its anatomic position, trapping the lateral band inside. The band now lies within the fibrous flexor sheath, adjacent to the flexor tendons. The base of the sheath prevents subluxation of the lateral band in a dorsal direction and ensures that it remains palmar to the axis of rotation of the PIP joint. The flap of flexor sheath is now repaired anatomically by using two or three sutures of 3-0 or 4-0 braided nonabsorbable sutures (Fig. 19).

The PIP joint is passively flexed, and the mobility of the mobilized lateral band within its new tunnel is confirmed.

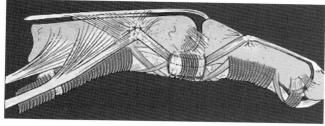

FIGURE 19. Zancolli's method (44,45) of lateral band tenodesis. The lateral band is mobilized and repositioned into the flexor tendon sheath at the level of the proximal interphalangeal joint.

The lateral band is gently grasped proximal to the repaired flexor sheath sling and mild proximally directed traction is exerted on it to demonstrate that the band glides freely. Before wound closure, the resistance to PIP joint extension is gently evaluated. The joint is first allowed to return to its new resting posture, with the finger supported by the surgeon's grasp of the proximal phalanx. Dorsally directed pressure is exerted on the tip of the digital pulp, and the tendency of the PIP to extend past neutral is evaluated. The PIP should extend no farther than 10 to 15 degrees of flexion and, on release of dorsally directed pressure, should return to its new resting posture of approximately 30 to 35 degrees of PIP flexion. If the tension on the displaced lateral band is not sufficient to prevent hyperextension, proximal and distal sutures can be used to tighten it back to the central tendon or the triangular ligament.

Postoperative Management. At 2 weeks postsurgery, a dorsal blocking splint that maintains the PIP in 30 degrees of flexion and permits full composite digital flexion is applied. Daytime splint protection is removed at 6 weeks, and night splinting is continued for 3 months.

Fixed Swan-Neck Deformities

Severe fixed PIP joint hyperextension deformities usually are accompanied by adjacent flexion deformities at the MCP and DIP joints, and patients with these deformities struggle with many common daily activities. In particular, they have difficulty making uniform palmar-digital contact with objects that they are attempting to grasp, because they can only bring pressure against the objects with the palmar aspect of their PIP joints. Because these joints have little motion or are rigidly fixed, tenodesis procedures are of no value, and the goal of most procedures is to attempt to mobilize the joints into a more functional position. If the articular surfaces of the PIP joints are reasonably good, then soft tissue mobilization should provide some long-term value by changing the posture and motion arc of the digits to one of flexion instead of hyperextension. If the joint surfaces are destroyed, arthrodesis of the PIP and, perhaps, the DIP joints is the best method of repositioning the digit for improved contact and function.

For fixed PIP hyperextension deformities without gross joint destruction, most hand surgeons perform a combination of extensor tenolysis, dorsal capsulotomy, partial collateral ligament release, and lateral band mobilization after the techniques that have been described by Nalebuff et al. (47–49) and Gainor and Hummel (50). In these procedures, soft tissue releases are sequentially carried out until the PIP joint can be brought into fully unresisted flexion with the lateral bands displaced palmar to the axis of rotation of the PIP joint. For fixed deformity with gross joint destruction and pain, arthrodesis is the most predictable procedure. PIP joint arthroplasty with flexible implants has usually performed poorly in rheumatoid PIP joints, because

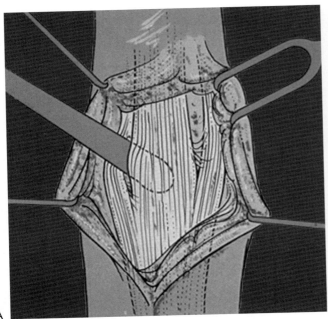
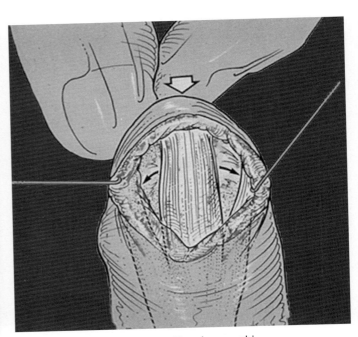

A

B

FIGURE 20. **A:** First stage of mobilization of a fixed swan-neck deformity. Lateral bands are mobilized at the level of the proximal interphalangeal (PIP) joint, and a tenolysis of the extensor tendon is carried out over the proximal phalanx. **B:** Capsulectomy of the PIP joint by division of the dorsal capsule and sequential releases of the radial and ulnar collateral ligaments of the PIP joint.

they often remain unstable, redeform, and fail over time. Newer metal polyethylene or pyrocarbon PIP joint replacements have been developed, but their long-term value in rheumatoid patients with ligamentous laxity and osteoporotic bone has not yet been clearly established.

Authors' Preferred Technique. In the absence of PIP joint pain and gross destruction of the articular cartilage, an extensor tenolysis, dorsal PIP capsular release, and lateral band mobilization constitute our preferred procedure. A curvilinear dorsal incision is made that begins at the midline of the proximal aspect of the proximal phalanx. The incision gently curves radially or ulnarly toward the middle of the incision at the PIP joint. It then curves back toward the midline until the dorsal DIP crease is reached. A radial- or ulnar-based flap of skin, subcutaneous tissue, and fat then is raised across the entire dorsum of the PIP joint and the distal aspect of the proximal phalanx. The dorsal draining veins are included in the flap. Epitenon is left overlying the extensor apparatus and is not included in the flap.

A longitudinal incision is made between each lateral band and the central slip. Proximally, the incision is made between the lateral band and the central extensor tendon; distal to the insertion of the central tendon at the base of the middle phalanx, the incision is through the contracted triangular ligament. Gentle sharp dissection is used to free the undersurface of the lateral bands from the underlying bone and joint capsule. The tenolysis of the central extensor tendon is performed (Fig. 20A). A round-edged elevator is passed underneath the central tendon at the level of the joint and is passed proximally against the undersurface of the central tendon, freeing it from any adhesions and scar. After completion of the tenolysis, an incision is made in the PIP joint on both sides of and beneath the central tendon. A small scalpel blade is passed from dorsal to palmar directly into the joint, parallel to the opposing articular surfaces of the proximal and middle phalanges, and adjacent to the central slip. The dorsal capsulectomy is now complete.

With the finger held in the surgeon's hand, flexion pressure is applied to the PIP joint (Fig. 20B). The scalpel blade then is placed inside the collateral ligaments, parallel to the long axis of the finger. In this manner, it can be used to release the dorsal-most ligament fibers from their bony origin on the proximal phalanx. Small, incremental cuts are placed alternately in the radial and ulnar ligaments until the joint moves easily into full flexion. If there is any rebound tendency for the joint to spring back into extension, additional collateral division should be carried out. Occasionally, in severe fixed deformities, transarticular pinning of the PIP joint for 7 to 10 days may be required to overcome the residual tendency for extension contracture.

As the PIP joint is delivered into full flexion, palmar subluxation of the mobilized lateral bands occurs. The lateral bands now lie volar to the axis of rotation of the PIP joint. No fixation of the lateral bands in this position is required. If the bands appear attenuated and incapable of fully extending the DIP joint, imbricating sutures may be used to shorten and to tighten them distally to the PIP joint.

If the wound closure is difficult or appears to be excessively tight with the PIP joint in flexion, the distal part of the wound over the middle phalanx should be left open, and uncomplicated healing can be expected (Fig. 20). A sterile dressing with a dorsal static extension-block plaster splint is applied to the finger, maintaining the PIP in 45 degrees of flexion and the DIP in full extension.

Postoperative Care. Lateral band mobilization and capsular or collateral ligament–release hyperextension deformity of the PIP joint rarely recurs after this procedure. In fact, some modest amount of extension lag usually results and is quite acceptable to patients who are accustomed to rigid recurvatum of their digits. For that reason, active flexion and extension exercises may begin as soon as pain subsides, usually 1 to 2 weeks postoperatively. If the PIP joints were pinned in flexion after mobilization of the lateral bands, the pins are removed at 7 to 10 days postoperatively, and active range of motion is begun.

Static palmar gutter finger splints are to be used between exercises, and a dorsal block splint is helpful in the rare instances in which the joint has a tendency to return to hyperextension. Dynamic PIP flexion or extension splinting may be used after 3 weeks to improve the arc of motion of the PIP joint.

Complications of Procedures for Rheumatoid Swan-Neck Deformity

Infections or hematomas are managed in the standard fashion. Distal wounds on the digits may safely be left open and are dressed in a sterile fashion, with routine dressing changes until they are healed.

Recurrent deformity should be addressed in a fashion that is similar to that for the initial deformity; that is, an assessment of contributing abnormalities should be undertaken, followed by an evaluation of the flexibility of the deformity. When the disease continues to affect the joint, radiographs help determine the extent of articular destruction and whether there is any hope of preserving joint motion. In the event of severe joint destruction or pain, arthroplasty or arthrodesis is performed.

Results of Treatment of Rheumatoid Swan-Neck Deformity

Tonkin et al. (46) reported their results of a procedure that was similar to that described herein for flexible deformity. They reported successful correction of PIP hyperextension deformity (an average of 16 degrees preoperatively) to 11 degrees of PIP flexion postoperatively. Their patients regained or improved their range of preoperative flexion. Our results are in agreement with those that were reported.

Keifhaber and Strickland (51) reported their results with lateral band release and dorsal capsulotomy for fixed deformity. Although patients initially gained an average of 55 degrees of flexion in the immediate postoperative period, grad-

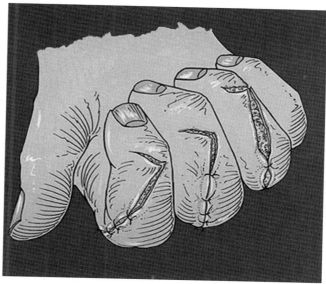

FIGURE 21. Illustration of leaving the distal wounds open after capsulectomy of the PIP joints for long-standing and severe swan-neck deformity.

ual postoperative loss of some of the arc of flexion was the rule (Fig. 8). A mean loss of almost one-third (17 degrees) was seen postoperatively over 3 to 12 months (Fig. 21). The authors recognize that "the long-term loss of flexion may be unavoidable" because of the progression of the underlying rheumatoid disease. The key benefit, however, was that the entire arc of PIP motion shifted into flexion, allowing improved use of the fingers in prehensile and grasping activities.

BOUTONNIÈRE DEFORMITY

Pathophysiology

Boutonnière deformities of the rheumatoid PIP joints represent the exact opposite of the digital configuration that is seen in swan-neck deformities. They are a combination of PIP flexion and DIP hyperextension with or without a concomitant hyperextension deformity at the MCP level. Although swan-neck digital deformities may take origin at any of three digital joints (MCP, PIP, or DIP), boutonnière deformities are always secondary to pathology at the PIP level, with changes at the adjacent joints occurring secondary to the PIP imbalance.

Dorsal synovitis of the rheumatoid PIP joints results in capsular distention and attenuation of the central extensor tendon. Over time, there is a lengthening of the triangular fibers of the extensor mechanism that allows for a palmar displacement of the lateral bands. The lateral bands ultimately migrate below the axis of motion of the PIP joint, where they become PIP flexors rather than extensors. Because of their unrestricted approach to the DIP joint, the lateral bands combine with the shortened ORLs to increase the terminal extension force and to produce hyperextension and decreased

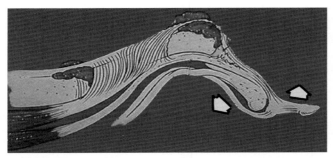

FIGURE 22. Characteristic configuration of rheumatoid boutonnière deformity with metacarpophalangeal joint hyperextension, proximal interphalangeal joint flexion, and distal interphalangeal joint hyperextension, with florid synovitis depicted over the proximal interphalangeal joint.

flexion at that joint (Fig. 22). It is the deformity at the DIP level that distinguishes the boutonnière deformity from other causes of PIP flexion and demonstrates the pathophysiology of the lesion. In their early stages, the deformities are passively correctable, but, with fibrosis of the periarticular joint structures, the deformity becomes fixed and extremely refractory to any reconstruction by soft tissue means.

Management Considerations

Early boutonnière deformities do not greatly compromise digital or hand function and may be largely ignored by patients with rheumatoid arthritis. The involved digits continue to flex well, and, because the PIP joints are passively extensable, they can be pushed straight when grasping objects. Unfortunately, the progression to fixed PIP flexion and DIP extension occurs fairly rapidly in some patients, and the failure to seize the short window of opportunity, when there is a possibility for surgical rebalancing of the deformity, may result in a stiffened digit with minimal reconstructive options. Therefore, the considerations for operative improvement of rheumatoid boutonnière deformities are strongly influenced by the severity of the deformity and whether the PIP joint can be passively corrected. Dynamic extension splinting for these deformities is poorly tolerated and rarely successful, and, even when passive straightening of the PIP joint is achieved, the joints usually have sufficient residual fibrosis that they are refractory to surgical rebalancing.

Evaluation

Evaluation of rheumatoid boutonnière deformities may not be as straightforward as it seems. Observation of the resting configuration of the digit usually gives a strong indication of the underlying pathology. The patient's demonstration of active flexion and extension and the ability to grasp large and small objects assist the assessment of the functional impact of the deformity. Of equal importance is the careful examination of all three digital joints (MCP, PIP, and DIP), and the experienced examiner can usually recognize the quality and

quantity of joint synovitis with a palpating finger. Passive flexion and extension of the joints should also be measured, and it is important to appreciate the amount of resistance to passive manipulation as a reflection of the pericapsular fibrosis that affects each joint. Full passive extension of the PIP joint should be achieved easily if surgical restoration of active extension is to have a reasonable likelihood of success. Finally, the DIP joint should be passively flexed with the PIP joint in full flexion and full extension (if possible) to determine the amount of oblique retinacular tightness and the degree of arthrofibrosis that affects the joint. Full active and passive DIP flexion with no evidence of intrinsic tightness may suggest that a flexed PIP joint is not truly a boutonnière deformity with the characteristic underlying pathology. Armed with the information that results from a thorough evaluation of the status of the digits with these deformities, a rational treatment program can be devised.

Treatment of Boutonnière Deformities

Conservative Treatment

When seen early, when the PIP joint flexion contractures are minimal and easily correctable, a local steroid injection may reduce the amount of synovitis and may slow the progression of the deformity. If the PIP lacks a few degrees of full passive extension, dynamic splinting may return digital balance. When severe fixed deformities are present, exercise programs and dynamic splinting are usually of little or no value.

Operative Treatment

Considerations
Surgical procedures that are designed to stop or retard the development of rheumatoid boutonnière deformities depend on the severity of the deformity. If the PIP joints can be passively moved to full extension, but doing so results in an inability to flex the DIP joint, and, conversely, flexion of the PIP improves DIP flexion, tightness of the ORLs has been established. Some surgeons prefer to address this problem by sectioning the terminal extensor tendon directly over the middle phalanx (52) just distal to the triangular ligament. Doing so does not directly address the tightness of the ORL and it may be more logical to use a simple method, which is described by Zancolli (15), in which the lateral 20% of each side of the terminal extensor tendon that contains the insertion of the ORLs is excised. This procedure effectively releases the tightened ORLs without weakening the effect of the terminal tendon.

In more advanced boutonnière deformities with PIP flexion lags of 30 to 40 degrees and retained passive correction, it may be worth considering one of many techniques for reconstructing the central extensor tendon and increasing the power of PIP extension (53–56). However, the surgeon should realize that rebalancing the boutonnière deformity secondary to the ravages of rheumatoid arthritis

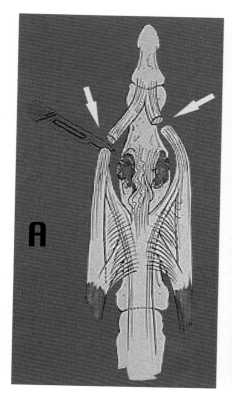
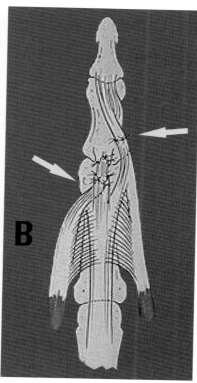

FIGURE 23. A: The technique of Matev (59) by first dividing the lateral bands at different levels (*arrows*) over the proximal interphalangeal joint. **B:** Completion of the Matev repair of the rheumatoid boutonnière deformity by repairing the longer proximal and distal ends of the lateral bands over the middle phalanx and by using the remaining lateral band to tighten and reinforce the central extensor slip at the proximal interphalangeal level.

is much more difficult than repairing the same deformity after trauma. Soft tissues that are rendered fragile, weak, and attenuated by rheumatoid disease are much less amenable to successful restoration, and the compromised status of rheumatoid joints further complicates the possibility of success. Goals for such procedures must be modest, with improved extension and retardation of the progression of the deformity being much more realistic than contemplation of the return of normal digital function.

Fixed flexion deformities of the PIP joint in rheumatoid arthritis are, quite simply, unsalvageable (57,58). Any attempt to release contracted soft tissues and to restore active PIP extension by tendon reconstruction inevitably leads to a rapid return of deformity and stiffness. When the deformities are severe or painful, arthrodesis is the only viable option.

Flexible Boutonnière Deformities

In those digits with a mild active extension lag (less than 30 degrees), full passive PIP extension, and loss of DIP flexion with the PIP extended, a partial excision of the sides of the terminal tendon may improve DIP flexion (15). The procedure may be carried out under digital block anesthesia by using a small longitudinal incision over the distal one-half of the dorsum of the middle phalanx. One-cm longitudinal segments are excised from each side of the terminal tendon, and the amount removed need not exceed 20% of the width of the tendon. These segments should include the insertion of the ORLs and weaken their ability to extend the DIP joint. Confirmation of the adequacy of the release can be determined by passively flex-

ing the DIP joint with the PIP joint held in full extension (intrinsic-intrinsic test). A local lysis of the terminal tendon is usually carried out as well, and active and passive flexion exercises may be commenced almost immediately.

For boutonnière deformities with more than a 30-degree active extension deficit at the PIP joint and full passive extension, extensor tendon reconstruction can be considered, provided that the articular surfaces of the joint are still in good condition. Attention should also be given to returning improved DIP flexion. Most of the many procedures that are designed to accomplish this rebalancing involve a dorsal mobilization of the palmarly displaced lateral bands and some type of restoration or augmentation of the central extensor tendon slip near its insertion into the base of the middle phalanx. Lengthening or partial or complete tenotomy of the terminal tendon is usually added to improve DIP flexion.

Authors' Preferred Technique. Although the authors admit that their results with using any of the procedures that are designed to improve PIP extension and DIP flexion for rheumatoid boutonnière deformities have been disappointing, the method that was described by Matev (59) has probably been the most reliable. In this procedure, the lateral bands are separated and divided at different lengths over the middle phalanx, the longer proximal and distal ends are sutured together to permit improved DIP flexion, and the short proximal end is used as a transfer into the insertion of the central extensor slip to tighten and to reinforce its action on the PIP joint (Fig. 23). The procedure cannot be considered unless the PIP can be fully and easily passively extended, and the joint surfaces are satisfactory.

The dorsum of the finger is approached through a curvilinear incision that is centered around one side of the PIP joint, the extensor apparatus is exposed, and the PIP joint is passively delivered into full extension and held there with an obliquely oriented 0.035-in. Kirschner wire that is passed from distal to proximal through the middle phalanx, across the PIP joint, and into the proximal phalanx. The lateral bands are then identified over the middle phalanx and divided in a manner that leaves one proximal stump approximately 3 mm longer than the opposite stump. The long distal and long proximal stumps are then sutured together in a lengthened state that should improve the ability of the DIP joint to flex. It may be necessary to lyse the distal terminal tendon and gently manipulate the DIP into flexion to assess the appropriate amount of lengthening that is required.

The central extensor tendon is usually found to be markedly attenuated, and it may be shortened by a reefing technique or, preferably, by excising several millimeters of the tendon near its insertion and resuturing it in a shortened state. The shorter, proximal, lateral band stump is then passed beneath and through the central slip and is pulled fairly tight. Several nonabsorbable, buried sutures are then used to secure the lateral band to the central slip insertion. The wound is then closed, and a compressive dressing is applied with the finger in full extension.

Postoperative Care. At 2 weeks postsurgery, the dressing is changed, and the sutures are removed. A small supporting gutter splint is applied, and appropriate pin protection and hygiene are provided. If possible, the pin is kept in place for 6 to 8 weeks, depending on the previously judged quality of the central slip repair and lateral band transfer. Gentle active motion may then be initiated with the PIP joint splinted in extension in between exercise periods. After 4 weeks, splints are designed to allow active and gentle passive DIP flexion. At 3 months postoperatively, passive motion may be added to the exercise regimen. Despite these efforts, some extension lag is expected at the PIP and DIP joints, and the deformity may slowly worsen in the face of an ongoing, progressive disease process.

Fixed Boutonnière Deformities

When the joint contracture does not exceed 50 or 60 degrees, function may not be too severely impaired, and it may be reasonable to accept the deformity without any operative intervention. More severe deformities, significant interference with lifestyle needs, or, in rare instances, pain may create the indication for arthrodesis of the PIP joints. The procedure can be combined with extensor tenotomy over the middle phalanx or DIP fusion, depending on the status of that joint. Arthrodesis of rheumatoid PIP joints is best accomplished by a tension-band wiring technique. The

use of Herbert screws for PIP fixation is sometimes a problem, because the screw threads may sink into the soft rheumatoid bone and may change the position of the fusion into more than the desired amount of extension.

Complications of Procedures for Rheumatoid Boutonnière Deformity

The most notable complication after any of the procedures for the rheumatoid boutonnière deformity is simply the failure of the procedure itself. Techniques that are designed to return PIP extension and DIP flexion in the face of poor quality soft tissues, osteoporotic bone, multiple-level deformities, and the relentless progression of the disease are compromised from the outset. Even those techniques that perform well initially may deteriorate with time. Less common problems include infection, wound breakdown, and nonunion of arthrodesed joints.

Results of Treatment for Rheumatoid Boutonnière Deformity

Keifhaber and Strickland (51) reported their long-term results of various methods of soft tissue repair and arthroplasty of boutonnière deformities, and the results were generally poor. Many others authors emphasized the difficulty of returning satisfactory function by using soft tissue techniques, and arthrodesis appears to be the one consistently reliable procedure for severe fixed PIP and DIP deformities.

THUMB

The thumb serves as the pillar of the hand. Pain and deformity can limit the ability to perform strong pinch and grasp and significantly affect hand function. Although the deformity can be disabling, treatment can be extremely rewarding.

The classification of rheumatoid deformities of the thumb is based on the location of the initial deformity and the secondary compensatory positions of the metacarpal and phalanges. The type 1 deformity (boutonnière deformity) and the type 3 deformity (swan-neck deformity) are the most common. The type 2, type 4 (gamekeeper's injury), and type 5 deformities are uncommon (60).

Pathophysiology

MCP joint flexion with interphalangeal (IP) joint hyperextension is the characteristic appearance of the type 1, or boutonnière, deformity (Fig. 24). The deformity begins with a proliferative synovitis of the MCP joint. The MCP synovitis leads to an attenuation of the extensor pollicis brevis (EPB) with subsequent ulnar and palmar translation of the extensor pollicis longus (EPL). This transfer-of-force

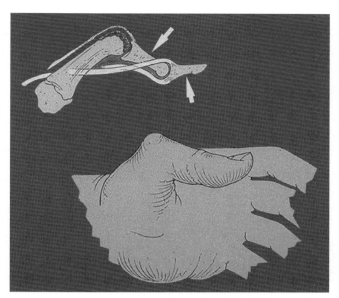

FIGURE 24. The pathomechanics and configuration of the type 1, or boutonnière, deformity of the rheumatoid thumb. Dorsal synovitis of the metacarpophalangeal joint with attenuation of the dorsal support system and palmar subluxation of the wing tendons.

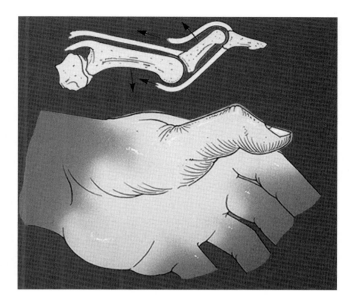

FIGURE 25. Pathomechanics and configuration of the rheumatoid type 3, or swan-neck, deformity of the thumb. Subluxation and destruction of the base of the carpometacarpal joint, followed by adduction of the first metacarpal, hyperextension of the metacarpophalangeal joint, and flexion at the interphalangeal joint.

vector creates a hyperflexion of the MCP, with the EPL displacing palmar to the central axis of the MCP joint. Secondary radial abduction of the thumb metacarpal then compensates for the hyperflexed MCP. With long-standing deformity, passive correction is no longer possible, and fixed contracture of the MCP and IP joints occurs.

MCP joint hyperextension, IP joint flexion, and metacarpal adduction characterize the type 3, or swan-neck, deformity (Fig. 25). This deformity always begins with synovitis and subluxation of the CMC of the thumb. The secondary adduction of the thumb metacarpal leads to an extensor tendon tightening that is combined with the palmar plate laxity, which is produced by efforts to expand the thumb web distance to grasp large objects, producing MCP hyperextension.

Type 4 (gamekeeper's injury) and type 5 deformities are the result of synovitis of the MCP joint, with the type 4 deformity affecting the ulnar collateral ligament, and the type 5 deformity primarily affecting the palmar plate of the MCP joint. The rare type 2 deformity results in a combination of type 1 and 3 deformities and is characterized by MCP flexion IP hyperextension and CMC subluxation.

In considering procedures to restore function to any of the rheumatoid thumb deformities, the status of the wrist and digits must be considered, and any restorative procedures that are planned for those joints should be incorporated into a master strategy for the entire hand. Fortunately, the type I, or boutonnière, configuration is the most common rheumatoid thumb deformity, and it can be dealt with satisfactorily with a repositioning and stabilizing arthrodesis, which can be integrated with almost any other procedures for the rheumatoid hand.

Surgery is recommended to address pain, deformity, and disability. Although many patients function reasonably well with significant deformity, many do not appreciate the subtle alterations in function that result from the deformity and the instability of components of the bones and joints, which comprise the thumb ray.

Evaluation

Careful assessment of the status of the thumb is an important component of any examination of the hand in the rheumatoid patient. The active and passive motion of the CMC and the MCP and IP joints should be carried out, and the joints should be palpated for synovitis and stressed to determine stability. Watching the patient use the thumb for pinch and grasp and measurement of the strength of those functions helps the surgeon appreciate the functional compromise that results from thumb deformities. X-ray evaluations, including hyperpronated studies of the thumb CMC, are also useful in determining the articular integrity and alignment of the thumb joints. Several office visits are sometimes required to understand the patient's functional limitations and expectations.

Treatment of Type 1 Boutonnière Deformities

Conservative Treatment

Splinting to stabilize the position of the thumb may temporarily improve hand function and may relieve pain. Medical management of the synovitis also improves pain and may

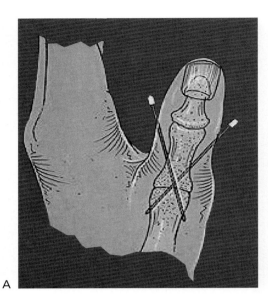
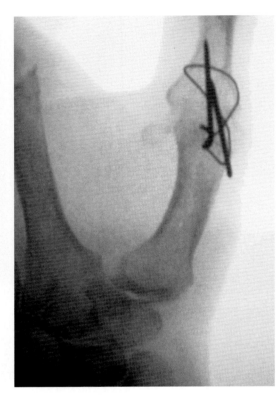

FIGURE 26. A: Drawing of the metacarpophalangeal joint fusion of the rheumatoid thumb by using crossed Kirschner pins. **B:** X-ray of metacarpophalangeal joint fusion of the type 1 boutonnière deformity of the rheumatoid thumb by using a tension-band wire technique.

slow the progression of the deformity (61). Intermittent steroid injections may also be of some benefit in the early stages of thumb joint synovitis and can be used as an adjunct to medical management.

Operative Treatment

Considerations

Surgical treatment of the deformed thumb is dependent on the severity of the joint destruction, the ability to passively correct the deformity, and the patient's expectations. Synovectomy of the MCP joint can be performed early in the proliferative phase and is generally reserved for patients with no deformity and pain that is recalcitrant to splinting and injections. The synovitis typically returns rather rapidly (62) and is an infrequent surgical option. Severely arthritic joints, unstable or dislocated joints with articular defects, and joints that are not passively correctable are treated with a simple fusion of the MCP or IP joint. The fusions of the thumb are generally well tolerated and straightforward. Fusion of the MCP joint of the thumb is particularly beneficial for patients with the type 1, or boutonnière, configuration, and it is well recognized that there is little or no functional loss from fusing the thumb MCP in neutral extension or slight flexion. Fusions are time tested and allow patients a quick return to functional activities, with a low complication rate, minimal postoperative therapy requirements, and a fusion rate that approaches 100% (63). In a classic assessment of the practical benefit of the most common procedures for the rheumatoid hand, Souter (64) rated MCP joint arthrodesis of the thumb as the single most predictable and beneficial procedure.

The moderate- to advanced-stage type 1 deformities (boutonnière) can sometimes be treated with MCP arthroplasty (65). Although MCP arthroplasty can modestly improve the functional range of motion, gains of as much as 20 degrees (66) may not justify the added complications and possible need for revision. When one considers the excellent return of pain-free alignment and stability that predictably results from MCP fusion of the rheumatoid thumb, it is hard to defend an arthroplasty that may not perform as well in any of those parameters (Fig. 26). Type 1, or boutonnière, deformity, type 4 (gamekeeper's) deformity, and type 5 deformity are best managed by MCP fusion by using a tension band technique, power-driven staples, or crossed Kirschner pins. A stable and painless IP joint should not be surgically treated. A fusion of the IP is performed only when the joint is destroyed, unstable, or dislocated. In those instances in which there has been severe erosion or bone loss, bone grafts may have to be used to save length and stability (67).

Author' Preferred Method. The MCP joint is approached from a dorsal midline incision that is centered over the joint and extends proximally and distally by 4 cm. Branches of the radial sensory nerve are protected. The interval between the EPB and the EPL is split. A transverse capsular incision is elevated from the joint to expose the metacarpal head and the base of proximal phalanx. The radial and ulnar collateral ligaments are released, allowing exposure of the joint surface. Cartilage is removed down to subchondral cancellous bone in a proximal convex and distal concave manner. A 0.045-in. Kirschner wire is used to establish a transverse tunnel in the proximal phalanx, 5 mm distal to the joint surface to be fused. The tunnel is easily created with the wire in the dorsal 50% of the bone. A 25-gauge stainless steel wire is passed through the bone holes transversely.

Two 0.045-in. Kirschner wires are then positioned in the metacarpal head and driven retrograde until the proximal phalanx can be easily reduced. The pins are then driven antegrade, with the MCP now positioned in approximately 10 degrees of flexion. The wire is then tensioned in a figure-of-eight pattern. The capsule is repaired over the wire construct. A palm-based thumb spica with an IP-free protective splint is used for 4 to 6 weeks until fusion is radiographically healed.

IP fusion, when necessary, is performed with a transverse incision at the level of the joint. Débridement of the cartilage and exposure of the subchondral bone is performed. Compression is obtained with mini Acutrak or Herbert screws in 5 degrees of flexion. Because of the size of the thumb IP joint, single screw fixation may not be adequate, and a supplementary obliquely oriented transarticular Kirschner pin may be needed to provide additional, temporary stabilization.

Treatment of Type 3 Swan-Neck Deformity

Conservative Treatment

Little can be done to alter the sequence of events that results in the grotesque collapse deformities of the rheumatoid thumb. Splinting, exercise programs, or steroid injections have little effect on the mechanical disruption of the integrated osseous chain of the thumb. Once the CMC loses its stability and subluxes laterally, a predictable and progressive pattern of imbalance produces equal and opposite deformities at the MCP and IP joints.

Operative Treatment

Considerations

Type 3 swan-neck or zigzag collapse deformities of the thumb result in severe functional impairment. The deformity always originates at the CMC, which subluxes laterally to produce an adducted position of the first metacarpal. The resulting imbalance and the patient's functional adjustments to the narrowed first web space lead to hyperextension at the metacarpal phalangeal joint, which in turn weakens the extensor forces at the IP joint, which assumes a flexed position. Surgical treatment must first concentrate on repositioning and stabilizing the CMC and bringing the first metacarpal out into abduction.

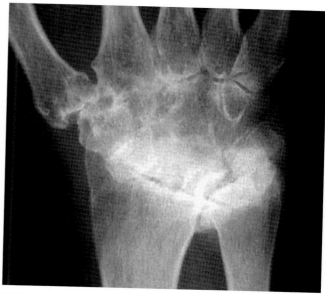

FIGURE 27. Advanced rheumatoid wrist with complete coalition of carpal bones. The borders of the trapezium cannot be delineated, thus making trapezium excision and suspension arthroplasty techniques difficult.

Resection arthroplasty with ligament reconstruction is believed, by some authors, to be suitable for all stages of the deformity (65), but, in actuality, such procedures may be difficult to achieve in rheumatoid patients. Patients with rheumatoid disease, and particularly those who have been managed with long-term steroid medications, usually have lax soft tissues that are difficult to reconstruct. In addition, advanced rheumatoid wrist disease often results in a coalition of the carpus, with all or most of the carpal bones merging into a single osseous unit (Fig. 27). As a result, the soft tissue suspension and interposition procedures that are so effective for osteoarthritis are technically difficult and unreliable for the restoration of the rheumatoid basilar joint. In those patients, the use of a synthetic implant, such as a silicone rubber great-toe prosthesis that is placed between the base of the first metacarpal and the coalesced carpus, may be helpful (Fig. 28). Once the CMC procedure is complete, it is often wise to place crossed pins between the first and second metacarpals to maintain wide abduction of the thumb for the first 4 to 6 weeks after surgery. MCP fusion is necessary only if the joint is destroyed, painful, and unstable or has persistent hyperextension that fails to correct after the first metacarpal has been repositioned.

Authors' Preferred Technique

A curvilinear incision is centered dorsally over the thumb CMC and is extended 4 to 5 cm proximally and distally. The interval between the EPB and the abductor pollicis longus is opened, and the capsule is deflected off of the trapezium, taking great care to protect the radial artery that lies directly over the scaphotrapezoid joint. Because the carpus is often coalesced in the rheumatoid wrist, it is usually difficult to delin-

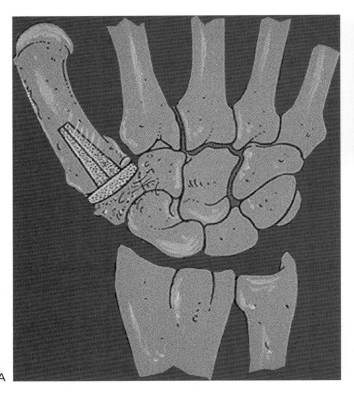

A

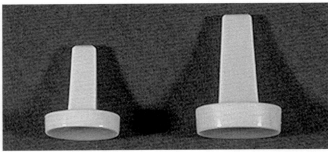

B

FIGURE 28. A: Illustration of placement of a great-toe prosthesis in the interval between the trapezium and the base of the first metacarpal, with its stem in the medullary canal of the first metacarpal. **B:** Two sizes of silicone great-toe implants for carpometacarpal joints in type 3 deformity.

eate the boundaries of the trapezium. The base of the adducted first metacarpal is identified, and a hand osteotome or a 7-mm sagittal saw is then used to remove a wedge-shaped section of the first metacarpal base and the contiguous carpus. The wedge is approximately 1 cm wide laterally and approximately one-half of that width medially. When removed, it permits the first metacarpal to be levered back into abduction. If the space between the carpus and the repositioned metacarpal is not adequate for the insertion of a silicone rubber great-toe implant, additional increments of bone can be excised. At this point, a straight awl is used to widen and to deepen the medullary canal of the first metacarpal, and, after fitting trial implants, the great-toe prosthesis is implanted. It should be mentioned that, when a silicone rubber great-toe prosthesis is not available, the surgeon must resourcefully seek out suitable substitutes, such as an Ashworth-Blatt prosthesis or even the button (19-mm ligament suture button, 904219-Arthrotek) that is used by some orthopedic surgeons for anterior cruciate ligament reconstruction (Fig. 29).

With the first metacarpal maintained in wide abduction and opposition, two 0.045-in. Kirschner pins are driven through the lateral side of the first metacarpal, across the first web space, and into the second metacarpal to maintain the widened web space and first metacarpal position until healing has occurred. The overlying capsular structures are then snugly repaired over the new joint, and components of the palmar-most slip of the abductor pollicis longus (digastric tendon) may be used to further reinforce the repair. Several imbricating stitches are used to tighten the abductor tendon, and the wound is closed in the usual fashion.

At this point, it is necessary to check the thumb MCP joint. If it remains hyperextensible, arthrodesis should be carried out in the fashion that was described earlier in this section. Rarely, the IP joint must be fused as well. Remarkably, a combination of CMC arthroplasty and fusion of the MCP and IP joints can return excellent function to thumbs with these severe collapse configurations (Fig. 30A–C). A well-padded compression dressing that incorporates a supporting splint is applied at the conclusion of the procedure.

Postoperative Care

The patient returns to the office for suture removal at 10 days to 2 weeks postsurgery, and a lighter plastic splint is applied at that time. Pin protection and hygiene instructions are given, and the wide abduction-opposition of the

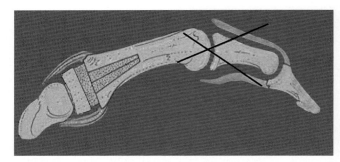

FIGURE 29. Reconstruction of the rheumatoid type 3 swanneck or zigzag collapsed deformity by using an implant at the basilar thumb joint and an arthrodesis of the metacarpophalangeal joint.

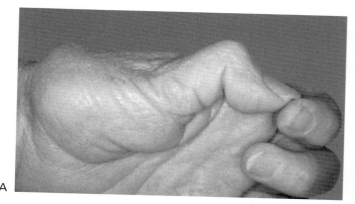

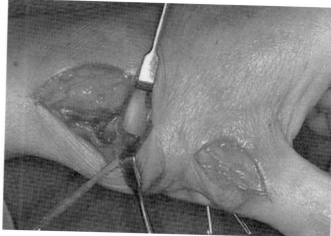

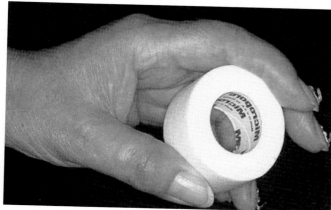

FIGURE 30. A: Photograph of a severe type 3 swan-neck or zig-zag deformity of the rheumatoid thumb. **B:** Appearance of the same thumb during reconstruction by implant arthroplasty at the carpometacarpal joint and fusion of the metacarpophalangeal joint. **C:** The same patient many months after thumb reconstruction with markedly improved position of the thumb and stability that was afforded by the metacarpophalangeal joint arthrodesis.

thumb is maintained by the pins and splint. At 6 to 8 weeks, the pins are removed from the metacarpals, and a gentle, active range of CMC motion is initiated. Strengthening exercises are begun at approximately 3 months.

Complications of Procedures for Rheumatoid Thumb Deformity

Postoperative wound breakdown or infection is always a concern for rheumatoid patients, because of their often-compromised immune systems, the use of steroid medications, and poor tissue resistance. Loss of fixation because of poor purchase of pins or wires in the soft rheumatoid bone can compromise fusions or metacarpal positioning of the type 3–deformity restoration.

REFERENCES

1. Harris ED Jr. Rheumatoid arthritis. Pathophysiology and implications for therapy. *N Engl J Med* 1990;18:1277–1289.
2. Fleming A, Crown JM, Corbett M. Early rheumatoid disease. I. Onset. *Ann Rheum Dis* 1976;35:357–360.
3. Flatt AE. Some pathomechanics of ulnar drift. *Plast Reconstr Surg* 1966;37:295–303.
4. McMaster M. The natural history of the rheumatoid metacarpophalangeal joint. *J Bone Joint Surg* 1972;54:687–697.
5. Zancolli E. *Structural and dynamic bases of hand surgery,* 2nd ed. Philadelphia: JB Lippincott Co, 1979:325–370.
6. Shapiro JS, Heigna S, Nasatir S, et al. The relationship of wrist motion to ulnar phalangeal drift in the rheumatoid patient. *Hand* 1971;3:68–75.
7. Smith RJ, Kaplan EB. Rheumatoid deformities of the metacarpophalangeal joint and fingers. *J Bone Joint Surg* 1967;49:31–47.
8. Hakstian RW, Tubiana R. Ulnar deviation of the fingers. The role of joint structure and function. *J Bone Joint Surg* 1967;49:299–316.
9. Stirrat CR. Metacarpophalangeal joints in rheumatoid arthritis of the hand. *Hand Clin* 1996;12:515–529.
10. Taleisnik J. Rheumatoid synovitis of the volar compartment of the wrist joint: its radiologic signs and its contribution to wrist and hand deformity. *J Hand Surg* 1979;4:526–535.
11. Chamay A, Della SantaD, Vilaseca A. Radiolunate factor of stability for the rheumatoid wrist. *Ann Chir Main* 1983;2:5–17.
12. Brewerton DA. A tangential radiographic projection for demonstrating involvement of the metacarpal heads in rheumatoid arthritis. *Br J Radiol* 1967;40:233–234.
13. Nalebuff EA. Metacarpophalangeal arthroplasty. In: Blair W, ed. *Techniques in hand surgery.* Baltimore: Williams & Wilkins, 1996.
14. Ellison MR, Kelley KJ, Flatt AE. The results of surgical synovectomy of the digits in rheumatoid disease. *J Bone Joint Surg* 1971;53:1041–1060.
15. Zancolli EA. *The structural and dynamic bases of hand surgery,* 2nd ed. Philadelphia: JB Lippincott Co, 1979:305–360.
16. Feldon P, Millender LH, Nalebuff EA. Rheumatoid arthritis

in the hand and wrist. In: Green DP, Hotchkiss RN, ed. *Operative hand surgery*, 3rd ed. New York: Churchill Livingstone, 1993:1587–1690.

17. Flatt AE. *The care of the rheumatoid hand*, 3rd ed. St. Louis: CV Mosby, 1974.

18. Harris C Jr, Riodan DC. Intrinsic contracture in the hands and its surgical treatment. *J Bone Joint Surg* 1954;36:10–20.

19. Straub LR. The rheumatoid hand. *Clin Orthop* 1959;15:127–139.

20. Straub LR. The etiology of finger deformity in the hand affected by rheumatoid arthritis. *Bull Hosp Joint Dis* 1960;21:322–329.

21. Ellison MR, Flatt AE, Kelley KJ. Ulnar drift of the fingers in rheumatoid disease. Treatment by crossed intrinsic tendon transfer. *J Bone Joint Surg* 1971;53:1061–1082.

22. Osler LH, Blair WF, Stevens CM, et al. Crossed intrinsic transfer. *J Hand Surg* 1989;14:963–971.

23. Smith-Peterson MN, Aufranc OE, Larson CB. Useful surgical procedures for rheumatoid arthritis involving joints of the upper extremity. *Arch Surg* 1943;46:764–770.

24. Riodan DC, Fowler SB. Surgical treatment of rheumatoid deformities of the hand. *J Bone Joint Surg* 1958;40:1431–1432(abst).

24a. Smith-Peterson MN, Aufranc OE, Larson CB. Useful surgical procedures for rheumatoid arthritis involving joints of the upper extremity. *Arch Surg* 1943;46:764–770.

25. Vainio K. Surgery of rheumatoid arthritis. *Surg Ann* 1974;6:309–335.

26. Brannon EW, Klein G. Experiences with a finger joint prosthesis. *J Bone Joint Surg* 1959;41:87–102.

27. Flatt AE. Restoration of rheumatoid finger-joint function. Interim report on a trial of prosthetic replacement. *J Bone Joint Surg* 1961;43:753–774.

28. Swanson AB. Flexible implant arthroplasty for arthritic finger joints: rationale, technique, and results of treatment. *J Bone Joint Surg* 1972;54:435–455.

29. Neibauer JJ, Landry RM. Dacron-silicone prostheses for the metacarpophalangeal and interphalangeal joints. *Hand* 1971;3:55–61.

30. Berger RA, Beckenbaugh RD, Linscheid RL. Arthroplasty in the hand and wrist. In: Green DP, Hotchkiss RN, Pederson WC, eds. *Operative hand surgery*, 4th ed. New York: Churchill Livingstone, 1999:147.

31. Steffie AD, Beckenbaugh RD, Lincsheid RL, et al. The development, technique and early clinical results of total joint replacement of the metacarpophalangeal joint of the fingers. *Orthopaedics* 1981;4:175–180.

32. Swanson AB. Finger joint replacement by silicone rubber implants and the concept of implant fixation by encapsulation. International workshop on artificial finger joints. *Ann Rheum Dis* 1969;28[Suppl]:47–55.

33. Madden JW, DeVore G, Arem A. A rational postoperative management program for metacarpophalangeal joint implant arthroplasty. *J Hand Surg* 1977;2:358–366.

34. Nalebuff EA. Metacarpophalangeal surgery in rheumatoid arthritis. *Surg Clin North Am* 1969;49:823–832.

35. Nalebuff EA. The rheumatoid hand. Reflections on metacarpophalangeal arthroplasty. *Clin Orthop* 1984;182:150–159.

36. Linscheid RL, Dobyns JH. Radiolunate arthrodesis. *J Hand Surg* 1985;10:821–829.

37. Beckenbaugh RD, Linscheid RL. Arthroplasty in the hand and wrist: In: Green DP, ed. *Operative hand surgery*, 2nd ed. New York: Churchill Livingstone, 1988;178.

38. Swanson A, Swanson G. Flexible implant resection arthroplasty of the metacarpophalangeal joint. In: Strickland JW, ed. *The hand*. Philadelphia: Lippincott–Raven Publishers, 1998:421–438.

39. Strickland JW, Boyer MI. Swan-neck deformity. In Strickland JW, ed. *The hand*. Philadelphia: Lippincott–Raven Publishers, 1998:459–470.

40. Rizio LR, Belsky MR. Finger deformities in rheumatoid arthritis. *Hand Clin* 1996;12:531–540.

41. Ferlic DC, Clayton ML. Flexor tenosynovectomy in the rheumatoid finger. *J Hand Surg* 1978;3:364–367.

42. Littler JW. Restoration of the oblique retinacular ligament for correcting hyperextension deformity of the proximal interphalangeal joint. In: Tubiana R, ed. *La main rheumatoide*. Paris: Expansion Scientifique Francaise, 1969:155–157.

43. Thompson JS, Littler JW, Upton J. The spiral oblique retinacular ligament (SORL). *J Hand Surg* 1987;3:482–487.

44. Zancolli EA. *Structural and dynamic bases of hand surgery*, 2nd ed. Philadelphia: JB Lippincott Co, 1979:71–73.

45. Zancolli EA, Zancolli E Jr. In: Lamb DW, ed. *The paralyzed hand*. New York: Churchill Livingstone, 1987:163–165.

46. Tonkin MA, Hughes J, Smith KL. Lateral band translocation for swan-neck deformity. *J Hand Surg* 1992;17:260–267.

47. Nalebuff EA. The rheumatoid swan-neck deformity. *Hand Clin*1989;5:203–214.

48. Nalebuff EA, Feldon PG, Millender LH. In: Green DP, ed. *Operative hand surgery*, 2nd ed. New York: Churchill Livingstone, 1988:1724–1736.

49. Nalebuff EA. The rheumatoid swan-neck deformity. *Hand Clin* 1989;5:203–214.

50. Gainor BJ, Hummel GL. Correction of rheumatoid swan-neck deformity by lateral band mobilization. *J Hand Surg* 1985;10:370–376.

51. Kiefhaber TR, Strickland JW. Soft tissue reconstruction for rheumatoid swan-neck and boutonniere deformities: long-term results. *J Hand Surg* 1993;18:984–989.

52. Dolphin JA. Extensor tenotomy for chronic boutonnière deformity of the finger. Report of two cases. *J Bone Joint Surg* 1965;47:161–164.

53. Ferlic DC. Boutonnière deformities in rheumatoid arthritis. *Hand Clin* 1989;5:215–222.

54. Littler JW, Eaton RG. Redistribution of forces in the correction of the boutonnière deformity. *J Bone Joint Surg* 1967;49:1267–1274.

55. Nalebuff EA, Millender LH. Surgical treatment of the boutonnière deformity in rheumatoid arthritis. *Orthop Clin North Am* 1975;6:753–763.

56. Urbaniak JR, Hayes MG. Chronic boutonnière deformity—an anatomic reconstruction. *J Hand Surg* 1981;6:379–383.

57. Souter WA. The problem of boutonnière deformity. *Clin Orthop* 1974;104:116–133.

58. Flatt AE. *Care of the arthritic hand*, 5th ed. St. Louis: CV Mosby, 1995:261.

59. Matev I. Transposition of the lateral slips of the aponeurosis in treatment of long-standing "boutonnière" deformity of the fingers. *Br J Plast Surg* 1964;17:281–286.

60. Nalebuff EA. Diagnosis, classification and management of rheumatoid thumb deformities. *Bull Hosp Joint Dis* 1968;29:119–137.

61. Van der Heide A, Jacobs JW, Bijlsma JW, et al. The effectiveness of early treatment with "second-line" antirheumatic drugs. *Ann Intern Med* 1996;124:699–707.

62. Lipscomb PR. Synovectomy of the distal two joint of the thumb and fingers in rheumatoid arthritis. *J Bone Joint Surg* 1967;49:1135–1140.

63. Stanley JK, Smith EJ, Muirhead AG. Arthrodesis of the metacarpal-phalangeal joint of the thumb: a review of 42 cases. *J Hand Surg* 1989;14:291–293.

64. Souter WA. Planning treatment of the rheumatoid hand. *Hand* 1979;11:3–16.

65. Feldon PG, Terrano AL, Nalebuff EA, et al. In: Green DP, Hotchkiss RN, Pederson WC, eds. *Green's operative hand surgery,* 4th ed. New York: Churchill Livingstone, 1999:1723–1725.

66. Terrano A, Millender L, Nalebuff E. Boutonnière rheumatoid thumb deformity. *J Hand Surg* 1990;15:999–1003.

67. Nalebuff EA, Millender LH. Reconstructive surgery and rehabilitation of the hand. In: Kelley WN, Harris ED, Ruddy S, et al., eds. *Textbook of rheumatology.* Philadelphia: WB Saunders, 1981:1900–1920.

69

RHEUMATOID ARTHRITIS OF THE WRIST

DANIEL B. HERREN
BEAT R. SIMMEN

Rheumatoid arthritis (RA) is the most common systemic inflammatory disease with a world-wide prevalence of approximately 1% and an incidence rate of 0.03% (1). The majority of patients develop RA between the ages of 30 and 60 years. RA is a chronic, systemic autoimmune disease that is characterized by an immunologically caused chronic inflammatory synovitis. Probably driven by a still unknown antigen response, a cascade of immunologic and inflammatory processes are mediated, which finally lead to destruction of joints and soft tissues. Genetics seem to play an important role in the pathogenesis of RA. In monozygotic twins, there is a 30% to 50% chance of that both persons are affected, compared to a 1% rate in the general population (2,3). Besides the possible genetic background of the disease, bacterial and viral infection have been speculated as trigger agents that cause RA (4,5). However, newer studies suggest that osteoclasts mediate focal bone erosion. This may offer a new approach for the treatment of this disease (6).

The onset of RA shows first an acute inflammatory reaction within the synovial membrane, which becomes congested (7). As shown by magnetic resonance imaging (MRI), the degree of synovitis correlates with the edema formation of the periarticular bone (8). Along with this acute inflammation, a complex cell transformation within the synovial cells starts, including cellular and humeral immunologic processes. Becoming chronic, as a process, the inflammation leads to the formation of the so-called rheumatoid pannus, which is a mass of granulation tissue that includes all cell mediators of chronic inflammation surrounded by a matrix of connective tissue (9). This pannus plays an important role in the destruction process of the cartilage of the affected joint and may show tumorlike characteristics.

One of the major areas of current investigation in RA includes the role of cytokines in the pathogenesis. Cytokines are molecules that are synthesized locally and have a strong biological effect in the cell-mediated processes of the disease. The best known cytokines are interleukin-1 (IL-1) and tumor necrosis factor α (TNF-α). Both molecules promote inflammation with stimulation of other inflammatory factors (10). The understanding of the complex mechanism in the action of these cytokines gave the rationale to the development of new drugs that fight the inflammatory process (11,12). These more biological therapies, especially the anti–TNF-α drugs, changed the face of the disease for many patients.

The advances in the understanding of the pathogenesis of RA will open new ways for therapy in the future. Besides the aforementioned anticytokine therapy, anti–T-cell therapy might be another interesting form of biological treatment. Different trials with anti–T-cell antibodies could prove some clinical benefit. Gene therapy, a completely different and new treatment approach, may bring a major revolution in the future (13).

The recognition of the pattern of progression of the disease in general may have important implications in the management of the patient. A prospective study by Masi et al. (14) described three different patterns of articular involvement: a monocyclic form that is seen in 20% of the patients who have a single cycle of disease with remission for at least 1 year, a polycyclic course in 70% of the patients with an intermittent or continuing course, and a progressive pattern in approximately 10% of patients with increasing joint involvement over a long period of time. In addition, different factors were identified as indicators of poor outcome in RA (15–17) (Table 1).

Taking all these factors together, one realizes that RA is a disease with many different faces. Thus, treatment should be individualized for every patient.

NATURAL COURSE OF THE RHEUMATOID WRIST

Adult Rheumatoid Arthritis

The wrist, as one of the main targets in RA (18,19), plays a key role in the chain of the articulations in the upper extremity. The understanding of the pathomechanics and the possible course of the disease allows an individualized management for every patient.

TABLE 1. FACTORS FOR POOR OUTCOME IN RHEUMATOID ARTHRITIS

Female gender	Subcutaneous nodules
Older age	Low education level
Radiologic destruction	Extraarticular disease
High-titer rheumatoid factor	HLA-DR4 positivity

Three main factors play an important role in the pathologic process of wrist deformation: cartilage destruction, synovial expansion, and ligamentous laxity. The cartilaginous thinning is caused by cytochemical effects with degradation and inhibition of new cartilage synthesis (20). The synovial expansion may cause bony erosion, particularly at the sites of vascular penetration of bone, such as in the radial origin of the Testut ligament. These erosions cause sharp bony edges, which might lead to tendon rupture (21). In addition, synovial expansion causes stretching of the retaining extrinsic and intrinsic ligaments of the wrist, thus causing carpal supination and ulnar translation (22,23). The stretching of the scapholunate ligament results in a scapholunate dissociation, whereas more global laxity and instability are responsible for the ulnar translation (24). Force application across the wrist is predominantly caused by muscles which act in palmar and ulnar directions. With ongoing destruction of the rheumatoid wrist, they lose their physiologic moment arms in relation to the center of rotation and become a deforming force (22,25). Youm et al. (26), in describing the carpal height ratio, measured rheumatoid wrists and summarized the aforementioned pathomechanical effects, which create a reduction of the carpal height. Parallel to the processes at the radiocarpal and midcarpal joints, the distal radioulnar joint undergoes pathologic changes, which were first described by Backdahl (27) and subsequently were called the *caput ulnae syndrome*. The ulnar side of the wrist is often the first place of significant synovitis in the rheumatoid wrist. Long-term prognosis, however, is determined by the progression of the disease at the radiocarpal level. Together with progressive ligamentous laxity, a dorsal subluxation of the ulna or, even more frequently, a palmar subluxation of the carpus occurs. An associated supination of the carpus causes a luxation of the extensor carpi ulnaris (ECU), a major stabilizer of the ulnar side of the wrist and the distal ulna. The kinematics of the distal radioulnar joint change with a displacement of the center of rotation. This may cause a radioulnar impingement and a painful block in supination (28). This wrist deformity pattern has an influence in the development of deformities of the distal aspects of the hand. Shapiro et al. (29) associated radial carpal supination together with palmar subluxation with ulnar phalangeal drift (25,30), ulnar carpal translocation with radial phalangeal deviation, and loss of carpal height with swan-neck deformity of the fingers (31).

Disease activity and, thus, deformity pattern vary considerably in RA patients. To typify the different pattern of wrist involvement, Flury et al. (32) and Simmen and Huber (33) described, based on serial radiographs over the

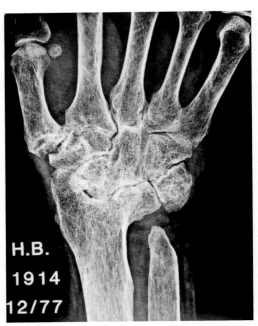

FIGURE 1. Type 1 (ankylosing) rheumatoid wrist with spontaneous fusion of the radiolunate joint.

course of the disease, three distinguished types of destruction. They are classified as type 1, 2, or 3 wrists. Type 1 rheumatoid wrists show a spontaneous tendency for ankylosis (Fig. 1); type 2 wrists show a destruction pattern that resembles the osteoarthritic wrist, with changes remaining relatively stable over time (Fig. 2); and type 3 wrists show a

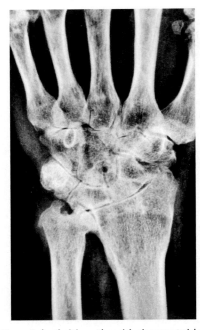

FIGURE 2. Type 2 (arthritic-arthrosis) rheumatoid wrist with a destruction pattern that is similar to osteoarthritic changes. The carpus is still well centered, with destruction of the radiocarpal and the midcarpal joints.

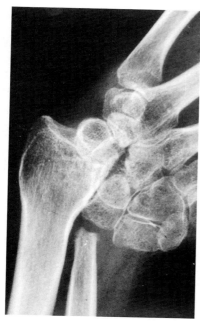

FIGURE 3. A type 3A (ligamentous unstable) rheumatoid wrist that shows complete dislocation of the carpus to the palmar-ulnar side, with preserved bone stock.

disintegration with progressive destruction and loss of alignment. Type 3 is further subdivided into types 3A and 3B: Type 3A (Fig. 3) has more ligamentous destabilization, and type 3B (Fig. 4) shows more bony destruction with, finally, complete loss of the wrist architecture. The classification into the different types of the natural course of the

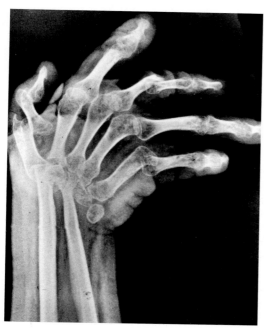

FIGURE 4. The type 3B (bony unstable) rheumatoid wrist with complete bony destruction, loss of bone stock, and dislocation of the carpus.

disease at the wrist level is based on serial radiographs with measurements of carpal height ratio (26) and ulnar translation (34). A change in the carpal height ratio of more than 0.015 or an increase of ulnar translation of more than 1.5 mm per year, or both, classifies a wrist in the type 3 category (32). An extension of this classification, combining the typing and staging of the destruction in the wrist, is presented in the section Classification and Treatment Algorithm of the Rheumatoid Wrist.

Juvenile Rheumatoid Arthritis

Juvenile rheumatoid arthritis (JRA) is the most common connective tissue disease during childhood. Clinically, it may present as a classical polyarthritis, as pauciarthritis with fewer joints involved, or as Still's disease with more systemic symptoms, such as fever and rash. The basic inflammation mechanism and the pathophysiology is similar to RA in adults. In contrast to adults only, in approximately 20% of JRA cases, the rheumatoid factor is positive, and the diagnosis is often given by the clinical symptoms and the radiographic changes (35–38). The knee and the wrist are the two areas in which bony changes most commonly are seen (39). The basic medical treatment of JRA is similar to treatment in adults. It is widely accepted that the treatment in this young patients' group should be aggressive, and the introduction of methotrexate has changed the prognosis dramatically (40,41).

Wrist involvement in JRA occurs in approximately 60% of the patients (37,38). Muscle imbalance, together with the physiologic palmar tilt of the radius and the stretched ligaments, leads to a progressive palmar subluxation of the radiocarpal joint. Spontaneous wrist joint fusion is significantly more common in patients with JRA compared to adults (42). The wrist often gets stiff in palmar flexion and ulnar deviation (37,38,42–46).

Because these patients are young, and their skeletons are often still immature, conservative therapy with splinting and physical therapy plays an important role.

The general surgical approach is similar to that for adult RA. The indication for a surgical treatment depends on the clinical course of the disease. It is generally accepted that wrist synovitis that is persistent to medical treatment for more than 6 months should be addressed surgically (47–50). Pain relief after synovectomy is significant, and recurrent synovitis is uncommon. Radiosynoviorthesis is contraindicated in children (47). Owing to the aforementioned spontaneous wrist fusion pattern, corrective osteotomy with arthrodesis in a more functional position might be needed.

The distal ulna should be addressed more conservatively in children than in adults. In contrast to adults, JRA children develop, because of different epiphyseal growth, most often a shortened ulna. Open physes preclude distal ulnar resection, which would exacerbate the length discrepancy. Hemiresection arthroplasty or a Sauve-Kapandji procedure, combined with a synovectomy of the distal radioulnar joint, is preferred by some (39); ulnar lengthening is preferred by others (51). Some cases require a simultaneous radial corrective osteotomy. During hemiresection types of procedures, the periosteum has to be removed carefully, because children tend to reform new bone.

EPIDEMIOLOGY OF WRIST INVOLVEMENT IN RHEUMATOID ARTHRITIS

The first recognized report on RA goes back to 1800 with an article by Landré-Beauvais. As of 2003, there is still no specific diagnostic marker available, and the diagnosis relies on certain clinical, radiologic, and serologic criteria. The most commonly used criteria for the classification of RA were defined by the American College of Rheumatology. Among the criteria, arthritis of the hand joint, including the wrist, is rated with the highest sensitivity (96.6%) with a specificity of 74.8% (52). Most authors believe that the onset of RA is multifocal or that it starts in the hand (18). Usually, the wrist joint has an early involvement in the course of the disease and is rapidly destroyed once it is hit by the inflammation process (19). It might be expected that 10 years after the onset of the disease 90% of the wrist joints show symptoms compared to 75% of the shoulders and 60% of the elbows (19). There are few data available for the joint that are affected in juvenile arthritis, but it seems that the prognosis for this group of patients, regarding destruction of the wrist joint, is even worse (38).

Soft tissue involvement around the wrist is common. Pulki (53) reported on a series of 500 hospitalized patients. He found synovitis in 32% and tendon ruptures in 7%. It might be speculated, confirmed by clinical experience, that the rate of soft tissue involvement is even higher. Along with flexor tendon synovitis, median nerve compression is observed in as much as 50% of patients (54,55).

EVALUATION OF THE RHEUMATOID WRIST

Clinical Examination

RA is a disease process that affects almost all organ systems in the body and is not limited to the musculoskeletal system. On first examination of a patient who has RA, a complete history and physical are mandatory. It is important to know about conservative therapy, especially current medication. An extensive history allows the physician to learn about the patient's needs, demands, and wishes, which are important factors when talking about indications for surgery. The presence of deformity does not necessarily lead to functional impairment. It is important to recognize the individual activity of the disease in every patient and to find possible points of improvement within the conservative

treatment strategy. RA is a life-long condition, and the disease activity might change over time. Current activity, possible future course, and interaction of joint problems should always be considered (56). Lower extremity treatment in RA treats the ability to walk; treatment of the disease that affects the upper extremity preserves the patient's ability to work and to remain independent.

The physical examination should always check the whole chain of articulations within the limb to be treated. Because the elbow joint places the hand in space, bad function of this joint might endanger the result of interventions at the level of the hand.

When assessing the function of the upper extremity, the following parameters should be checked:

- Localized swelling and tenderness; the extent and the exact anatomic localization should be noted.
- The degree and location of the deformity should be checked; the degree to which the deformity is actively or passively correctable should be distinguished.
- The range of motion, using a goniometer, should be recorded according to the neutral-zero method; at the level of the hand, all joints should be measured, regardless of the planned site of intervention.
- The examination of the wrist differentiates between the radiocarpal, midcarpal, and distal radioulnar joints.
- Often due to marked deformity or pain, or both, the classic instability signs in the wrist might be difficult to check; do not hurt the patient more than necessary during the examination.
- Check for tendon continuity; especially important tendons on wrist level are the radial-sided extensors. Independent function of the superficial and deep flexors must be controlled, as well as independent function of the two extensors in the second and fifth digits.
- Compression neuropathy, especially carpal and cubital tunnel syndrome, should be ruled out; sensibility should be checked using the two-point discrimination method.
- If applicable, strength measurement should be performed; grip strength and key pinch are recorded, using a Jamar dynamometer or a vigorimeter.

Additional Examinations

Radiologic Examination

The type and the extent of the destruction in the wrist are best seen in conventional radiographs, which should always be taken in at least two different planes, preferably in anteroposterior and true lateral views. It is not only the actual destruction that is of interest but also the evolution of the destruction over time. Radiographs that are taken in fixed intervals (depending on the activity of the disease, in 6- to 12-month intervals) give additional important information to optimize surgical treatment strategy (33,57). In the early course of the disease the radiographs should be

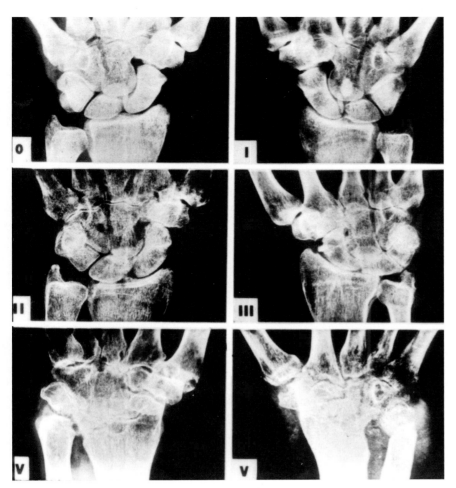

FIGURE 5. Radiologic staging according to Larsen et al. (58). Stages 0 to V in the rheumatoid wrist.

read for supple signs of inflammation and destruction, such as joint effusion and erosions. Among the different radiologic classifications, the staging system that was created by Larsen, Dale, and Eek (LDE) is the most common (58) (Fig. 5). The LDE classification differentiates between six stages of destruction in which stage I represents the least extent of destruction and stage V stands for the final stage, with complete destruction of the wrist joint. Because the LDE classification only describes the extent of the actual destruction, the natural course of the disease and optimal treatment modalities are difficult to assess. The Wrightington group, which centered around the work of Hodgson et al. (59) and Alnot and Fauroux (60), tried to incorporate more practical guidelines in their rheumatoid wrist classification schemes. Despite the more practical approach, both classifications still lack the ability to anticipate future development of wrist destruction. Based on radiologic long-term analysis, Simmen and Huber (33) and Flury et al. (32) proposed a new classification of rheumatoid wrist involvement that considers the type of destruction to the possible future development of the disease, with direct consequences of surgical decisions. Three patterns of destruction are distinguished, based on the morphology of destruction and the course and duration of the disease (for details see the section Natural Course of the Rheumatoid Wrist).

Computed Tomography and Magnetic Resonance Imaging

Computed tomography (CT) and MRI are rarely indicated in the evaluation of a rheumatoid wrist. There is limited additional information that these examinations could provide. If a special hand MRI is not available, most RA patients do not tolerate the uncomfortable position on the examination table. However, MRI has a higher sensitivity and a higher negative predictive value with equal specificity than regular x-ray examination for detecting inflammatory changes (61).

For the following conditions, CT or MRI examination might be considered:

- Evaluation of the amount and extent of synovitis in an unclear diagnosis or in the early stages of the disease (MRI)
- Extent and localization of tenosynovitis and tendon ruptures, especially in the flexor tendons (MRI)
- Assessment of disease activity and monitoring of response to medication (MRI) (62–64)
- Evaluation of the distal radioulnar joint (CT)

Sonography and Three-Phase Bone Scintigraphy

Sonography as a diagnostic tool gets more and more popular, and the introduction of high-resolution transducers with 15 MHz enhanced the diagnostic value. Experienced examiners with linear scanner mode probes achieve the precise detection of erosions and synovitis with a high intra- and interobserver reliability (65). This technology has good potential, especially in early stages of the disease, and might be an important supplement in the armamentarium of diagnostic tools.

Three-phase bone scintigraphy has the advantage of evaluation of the whole body, which might be of importance at the beginning of the disease to sort out the most actively inflammatory joints (61). However, scintigraphic changes are never as specific as they are in the other diagnostic tools and must be seen as a part of a whole examination complex.

Electrophysiology

The incidence of compression neuropathy in patients who have RA is high. Carpal tunnel syndrome in association with flexor tenosynovitis is observed in as much as 60% of the patients (66) (Fig. 6). The second most frequent involvement includes the ulnar nerve at the level of the elbow. Because the regeneration potential of compressed peripheral nerves, especially in older patients, is limited, and the results of nerve decompression generally are good, indications for the decompression procedure should be generous (67). Even in the absence of clinical symptoms,

peripheral nerve damage may be present (68). Shinoda et al. (69) therefore proposed a new grading system for carpal tunnel syndrome, including clinical signs and symptoms rather than electrodiagnostic findings. This grading system facilitates operation indications and helps choose the appropriate surgical procedures.

Besides entrapment neuropathy, myelopathy and spinal cord involvement, especially at the level of the cervical spine, are common in RA (70). Because subjective and objective neurologic symptoms may develop gradually and often are masked by the joint and soft tissue involvement, patients who report bilateral disturbance of sensory motor function in the hand must be evaluated for possible pathology at the level of the cervical spine. Radiologic screening of the cervical spine includes anteroposterior and lateral views, as well as functional radiographs in active flexion and extension. The presence of cranial migration of the dens and instability of the atlantoaxial should be checked (71). If instability is suspected, MRI examination of the cervical spine is indicated, and, besides the classical electrophysiologic measurements, transcranial brain stimulation helps evaluate the central motor pathways (72).

Functional Assessment of the Rheumatoid Wrist and Hand

To evaluate the pretherapeutic state of the hand, disease progression, and outcome of treatment, specific assessment tools of wrist and hand function are needed. Functional instruments should ideally be quantifiable, valid, reliable, and sensitive to change (46). Because not only improvement of single function parameters but also general improvement of health status and quality of life should be measured, specialized tools were developed. In patients with RA, three different approaches to assess the extent to which the hand is affected might be differentiated:

1. Description of the anatomic deviation and disorders. Usually, the deformities are recorded by measuring them with the use of a goniometer, completed with photographic documentation (73). Video-based image analysis might be a newer approach to describe deformity in a more standardized fashion (74).
2. Measurement of functional deterioration. To assess the functional deterioration of a rheumatoid hand, different tests have been described (75–78). These tests have a more generalized approach to measure hand function and allow judgment of hand function in complex deformity patterns. However, limitations in the activities of daily living may be more important for the patient than impairment in a single complex task. Therefore, newer tools to measure hand-related function in the activities of daily living have been introduced. The focus is more on disability than on functional deterioration.
3. Assessment of disability. The tools to measure disability are usually self-administered questionnaires. There

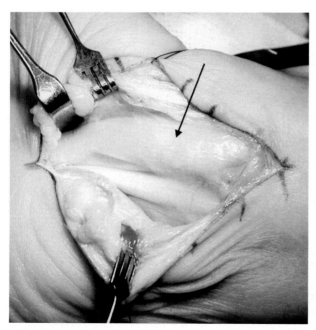

FIGURE 6. Severe compression neuropathy of the median nerve. The arrow points to the pseudoneuroma, which developed owing to flexor tendon synovitis in the carpal tunnel.

are more general assessments of upper extremity function, like the Disabilities of the Arm, Shoulder, and Hand questionnaire, or more hand-related (Michigan hand outcomes questionnaire) (80) and wrist-related (patient-rated wrist evaluation questionnaire) (81) tools. All these questionnaires try to assess function under subjective aspects.

All of these tests must be performed by specialized trained therapists and allow the therapist to judge changes before and after treatment. Ideally, every patient with the diagnosis of RA should be evaluated in a standardized manner before treatment starts.

INVOLVEMENT OF THE SOFT TISSUES AROUND THE WRIST

Flexor Tendons

Tenosynovitis of the flexor tendons at the wrist is a common finding in RA. At the wrist level, it may cause locking, limitation of motion, nerve compression, and, as an end stage, rupture of tendons. Early clinical signs include localized pain, morning stiffness, triggering of single digits, and nocturnal paresthesia due to carpal tunnel syndrome. An unusual presentation might be the so-called trigger wrist, in which synovial nodules within the flexor tendons may cause triggering during the passage underneath the transverse carpal ligament (82). In rheumatoid patients, flexor tendon involvement seems to correlate with a higher disease activity. Gray and Gottlieb (83) observed a significantly higher prevalence of rheumatoid nodules, carpal tunnel syndrome, wrist extensor synovitis, and elbow epicondylitis in patients with active flexor tendon inflammation. Duche et al. (84) distinguished three main groups of synovitis: isolated carpal tenosynovitis (20%), palmodigital tenosynovitis (50%), and diffuse tenosynovitis (30%). Ruptures of flexor tendons are significantly less frequent than extensor tendon ruptures in RA (83,85–87). The two main mechanisms of tendon destruction are invasion of the tendon by the inflammatory synovial mass or attrition on prominent bony spurs, or a combination of both (86–92). Owing to its anatomic localization near the scaphoid, the flexor pollicis longus (FPL) tendon, followed by the profundus to the index finger, is the most common flexor tendon to rupture (93). It is not only a direct bony spur but also the carpal instability in advanced wrist destruction that might cause the tendon attrition (89,91). Next in the order of decreasing frequency of rupture are the profundus tendon to the little finger, for which rupture is caused by an ulnar side bony spur; the superficialis tendon to the index; and the remaining profundus tendons.

Although FPL and also index profundus ruptures often cause little disability in rheumatoid patients, aggressive indication for revision surgery is warranted to prevent further tendon rupture (for reconstructive surgery see the section Tendon Reconstruction) (Fig. 7).

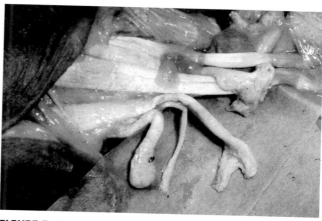

FIGURE 7. Intraoperative finding of multiple extensor ruptures. The aspects of the tendon ends suggest an attrition mechanism.

Extensor Tendons

The anatomy of the extensor tendon compartments of the wrist causes a different clinical picture than the involvement of the flexor tendons. Valeri et al. (94) observed in an extensive MRI study more peritendinous effusion in the flexor compartment, whereas, in the dorsal compartments, higher degrees of tendon fluid collection or pannus within the tendon sheath, or both, was found. The extensor tendons are surrounded by tenosynovium, beginning just before the proximal border of the extensor retinaculum and continuing several centimeters distal to the retinaculum. More distally, the tendons are covered by a peritenon rather than a tenosynovium. These anatomic features defined the localization of tenosynovitis in the extensor compartment. Extensor tenosynovitis often presents as a painless soft tissue mass at the dorsum of the wrist in the area of the retinaculum or, more frequently, distal to it. Pain in the extensor tendons, unlike the flexor tendons, is unusual; in theses cases, an underlying wrist pathology must be excluded. Correlated wrist and finger extension might cause impingement of the tenosynovial mass. Extensor tendon synovitis, especially at the ulnar side of the wrist, can be the first sign of RA in a patient. The tenosynovitis may be limited to one single tendon or a tendon compartment or may be more generalized. Involvement of the first tendon compartment is rare (95). In the initial stages of inflammation, fluid production is increased, followed by synovial thickening with adhesions to the tendons (94). In the further course, the synovium continues to proliferate and creates granulomas that infiltrate the tendons. It results in weakening of the tendon with possible rupture (96). The amount of synovial mass in the extensor compartments does not correlate with the degree of tendon damage, and prediction of possible ruptures is difficult, even when MRI as a diagnostic tool is used (97). The final rupture of an extensor tendon might be the end of a process with synovial infiltration, attrition

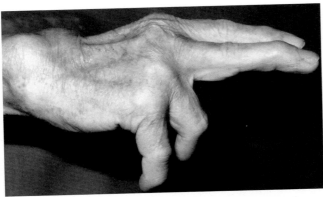

FIGURE 8. Clinical picture of caput ulnae syndrome with ruptures of the extensor tendons to the small and ring fingers.

on bony prominence, and ischemia (95,98–100). Dorsal dislocation of the ulna and persistent tenosynovitis of more than 6 months are additional risk factors (101). Owing to its anatomic course, the tendon of the extensor digiti minimi ruptures first. This rupture might be clinically silent, because the extensor digitorum communis extends all four fingers. Therefore, patients must be checked for independent little finger extension (102). Subsequently, the tendons may rupture from ulnar to radial, whereas index tendon ruptures are rare (Figs. 7 and 8). If a patient is unable to extend all four fingers, as well as the distal end of the thumb, he or she should be evaluated for possible interosseous nerve entrapment at the level of the forearm (103).

OPTIONS FOR NONOPERATIVE TREATMENT

The goals of the treatment of RA are the reduction of inflammation and the preservation of joint function. These goals are achieved best by a combined approach, including medical, surgical, and rehabilitation modalities (104). It is recognized that, after the onset of the disease, only 1 or 2 years are left before irreversible damage to the cartilage occurs (105). Therefore, aggressive medical treatment in early stages of the disease should be used. The decision of which type of basic medication is indicated is based on the clinical, laboratory, and radiologic findings, which define the activity and the prognosis of the disease. Despite this aggressive approach, true remission of the disease, as defined by the American College of Rheumatology (106), remains difficult to achieve. A current classification for antirheumatic drugs distinguishes between symptom-modifying antirheumatic drugs and disease-modifying antirheumatic drugs. Symptom-modifying antirheumatic drugs improve clinical symptoms without modifying the course of the disease in a certain period (e.g., nonsteroidal antiinflammatory drugs); disease-modifying antirheumatic drugs are able to prevent

or even to decrease joint erosions and improve function in association with decreased inflammatory activity (e.g., methotrexate).

Antiinflammatory Agents (Nonsteroidal Antiinflammatory Drugs)

Antiinflammatory agents as potent inhibitors of cyclooxygenase and prostaglandin are an important part of the treatment in RA. These drugs have a positive influence on pain and inflammation but do not inhibit synovial proliferation; thus, they have no influence on the progression of the disease. Newer drugs with selective cox-2 inhibition should have fewer side effects. These drugs are particularly useful in the early phase of the disease, when spontaneous remission is still possible. In the later course of the disease, they have more complementary function.

Corticosteroids

Low-dose corticosteroids combined with nonsteroidal antiinflammatory drugs are particularly useful while waiting for the effect of the so-called second-line drugs or to cut a flare-up of the disease. The long-term complications are significant and increase in dosages larger than 10 mg per day. Local intraarticular or soft tissue injections of glucocorticoids remain an important weapon in well-localized processes. However, in cases of regular local recurrence, surgical treatment should be considered.

Second-Line Drugs

Second-line drugs include slow-acting drugs like antimalarial agents, gold, salazopyrin, D-penicillamine, cyclosporin, and methotrexate. These drug have, using different mechanisms, disease-modifying characters. With the help of these drugs, a good control of disease activity and an improved function may be achieved in approximately 30% of RA patients (107). All of these drugs have significant side effects, and close monitoring of the patients is needed. There is no doubt that the early use of methotrexate may change the course of the disease significantly (108).

Parallel to the better understanding of the pathophysiologic mechanism of RA, new therapeutic approaches were developed. The so-called biological agents target various aspects of the immunosystem that are involved in the pathologic process. In particular, anti–TNF-α and anti–IL-1 antagonists changed the therapy of RA dramatically. Several clinical trials could show that these agents significantly decrease the signs and symptoms of joint inflammation and slow down the progression of radiologic joint damage (12,108–113). Longer clinical follow-up studies are missing, and careful monitoring of patients is needed, because a higher incidence of infection under this medication is reported (113,114).

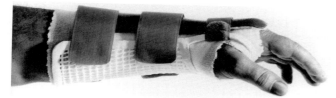

FIGURE 9. Cock-up resting splint with dorsal cover.

Radiosynoviorthesis

Radiosynoviorthesis is a synovectomy with the use of radio-isotopes. The most commonly used isotopes are yttrium 90, rhenium 186, and erbium 169. These isotopes act with β-rays in the absence of α-rays. The choice of which isotope is used depends on the joint that is to be treated and on the activity of the disease. Yttrium, for example, is the agent of choice for hip and knee synovectomy owing to its deep penetration. Rhenium is chosen for middle-sized joints, such as the wrist and the elbow, and erbium is more frequently used in small joints. Radiosynoviorthesis can only be used in closed joint spaces, and, therefore, its use, for example, in the shoulder, where rotator cuff lesions are frequent, is limited. The results of the synoviorthesis depend on the stage of the disease (the earlier the better), the joint that is treated (the knee has better results than the wrist), and the amount of synovitis. To enhance the results of synoviorthesis, a preceding surgical synovectomy may be performed. Usually, a interval of 6 to 8 weeks after surgery is needed to allow the joint capsule to heal. Indications for synoviorthesis decreased parallel to the reduction of synovitis that was observed with the new therapeutic agents.

Role of Physical and Occupational Therapy

In the team approach of fighting RA, physical, and especially occupational, therapists play an important role. The goals of physical and occupational therapy are pain alleviation and maintenance or improvement of mobility and function, as well as maintenance of strength. The traditional, well-established methods of physical therapy can be

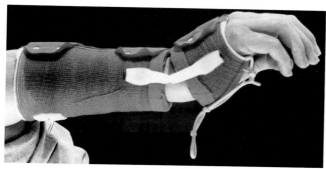

FIGURE 10. Dynamic wrist splint for mobilization in palmar flexion.

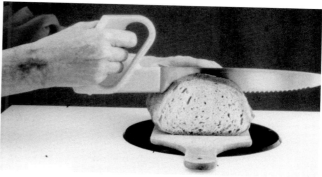

FIGURE 11. Assistive device for cutting bread.

used to achieve theses goals. It is of crucial importance to respect the patient's individual disease pattern and activity, as well as his or her personal needs and preferences. Multijoint involvement forces the therapist to set priorities and to establish a balanced treatment plan. Newer therapy forms, such as aqua jogging, have become more popular.

It is important to document the patient's status on a regular basis, including functional photographs. This documentation helps to judge the efficacy of a therapy and is an important additional source of information when a surgical strategy is chosen.

Splints are an important work horse in occupational therapy and require high technical skills, as well as an understanding of the pathophysiology of the disease. Modern thermoplastic materials offer an almost infinite variety of splints (Figs. 9 and 10).

Preoperative indications for splints are

- Resting splints for painful inflamed joints
- Correction of deformities with static or dynamic splints
- Inhibition or correction of tissue contraction

The postoperative indications for splints include

- Stabilization of the joint in physiologic axes
- Protection of sutured tissues
- Stretching of postoperative contractions
- Training of assistive or resistive joint mobility

Ergonomic instruction helps protect the affected joints. The patients must learn to keep optimal posture in leisure, as well as during activity. The use of assistive devices in the activities of daily living might preserve the patient's independence (Fig. 11).

SURGICAL MANAGEMENT OF THE RHEUMATOID WRIST

Timing of Surgery

The success of surgical reconstruction highly depends on a well-considered strategy in timing the different surgical

TABLE 2. FACTORS THAT INFLUENCE THE INDICATIONS FOR RHEUMATOID ARTHRITIS SURGERY

Concomitant musculoskeletal involvement	Patient's desires
General health condition	Compliance
Disease activity	Social environment
Patient's needs	Medical environment

procedures. The goals of surgical interventions in RA include alleviation of pain, functional improvement, prevention of future deformity, and cosmesis. Table 2 summarizes the factors that might influence the indications for surgical procedures. Whenever possible, surgery should be performed under stable medical conditions; this provides a fitter patient and allows the identification of the most active parts of the local disease (115). The following general rules, based on the work done by Souter (56,115), should serve as a rough guideline when choosing priorities in the surgical sequence (Table 3). To classify surgical interventions in RA, Souter (115) also established a ranking system of operations. Based on the parameters of elimination of pain, improvement of function, preventive value, cosmetic improvement, and hazard of complications, with a maximum score of 20 points, the possible operations are ranked as first-order (more than 15 points), second-order (12 to 15 points), or third-order (less than 12 points) interventions. At the level of the hand and wrist, Table 4 lists the corresponding procedures. It is certainly advised, if there is a choice, to start with a first-order intervention or a so-called winner operation. This gives confidence to the patient, as well as to the referring physician.

Table 4 considers the possible combination of operations within the hand and wrist or within other anatomic regions. As a multijoint disease, rheumatoid patients often require an almost endless number of interventions, and one might be tempted to pack as much as possible into one single procedure. A combination of foot and hand operations may make sense, if there are no crutches needed for the protection of the lower limbs postoperatively. To restore prosupination, ulnar head resection with dorsal wrist synovectomy might be combined with radial head resection and elbow synovectomy. A careful analysis of the needs dur-

TABLE 3. SOME GENERAL RULES FOR RHEUMATOID SURGERY

Lower limb before upper limb
From proximal to distal
Painful joints first
Prophylaxis versus reconstruction versus salvage
Consider combinations: hand and foot, elbow and wrist, wrist and metacarpophalangeal joints
Start with a winner operation (Table 4)

TABLE 4. RANKING OF OPERATIONS ACCORDING TO THE EFFECT THAT CAN BE EXPECTED

Ranking	Operation
First order	Caput ulnae resection
	Dorsal tenosynovectomy
	Arthrodesis of first MCP joint
	Synovectomy of flexor tendons
Second order	Arthroplasty of the MCP joints
	Arthrodesis of the proximal interphalangeal joints
	Correction of swan-neck deformity
	Carpal synovectomy
	Carpal arthrodesis (arthroplasty)
Third order	Synovectomy of MCP joints
	Correction of boutonnière deformity
	Proximal interphalangeal arthroplasty (carpal arthroplasty)

MCP, metacarpophalangeal.
Adapted from Souter W. Planning treatment of the rheumatoid hand. *Hand* 1979;11:3.

ing rehabilitation is important before a combined procedure is proposed.

In general, despite the aggressive medication and the nature of the disease, bone and soft tissue healing are considered to be normal in RA. Whether immunosuppressive medication should be discontinued in the perioperative phase is still controversial. Studies (116,117) and personal experience suggest the continuation of the medication; the possible benefits of discontinuation do not outweigh the risk of a flare-up of the disease.

Prophylactic Surgery

Synovectomy of the Wrist Joint

Before wrist synovectomy is indicated, ideally, a classification of the type of destruction is useful. According to the Schulthess classification (33), types 1 (ankylosis) and 2 (arthritic) wrists may qualify for this procedure, whereas, in type 3 wrists (destabilization), in addition to the synovectomy, bony stabilization is needed. In early stages of the disease, it may be difficult to distinguish these different types.

The removal of synovitis decreases the pressure in the joint and may have some sort of prophylactic effect before the synovial mass has stretched the retaining structures (118). In addition, some denervation effect is supposed (119–123). With the newer second-line drugs, the number of isolated wrist synovectomies is decreasing. The main effect of synovectomy is pain relief but often at the expenses of some wrist motion, especially in flexion (124–128). To diminish this problem, arthroscopic synovectomy might be considered in selected cases of localized synovitis if no extensor tendon or distal ulna treatment is needed (129–132).

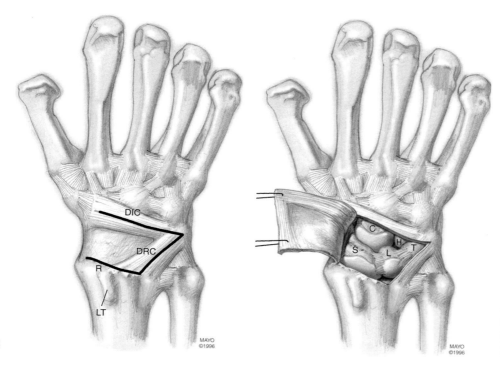

A,B

FIGURE 12. **A:** Dorsal wrist approach with radial-based capsulotomy. Outline of the incision. **B:** Dorsal wrist approach with radial-based capsulotomy after elevation of the capsular flap with good exposure of the radiocarpal and midcarpal joints. C, capitate; DIC, dorsal intercarpal ligament; DRC, dorsal radiocarpal ligament; H, hamate; L, lunate; LT, lunotriquetral; R, radius; S, scaphoid; T, triquetrum. (From Berger RA, Bishop AT. A fibersplitting capsulotomy technique for dorsal exposure of the wrist. *Tech Hand Upper Extrem Surg* 1997;1:2–10, with permission.)

In general, the indications for carpal synovectomy include

- Persistent synovitis that does not respond to adequate medication for more than 6 months
- Persistent pain and localized tenderness without major bony deformation
- Treatment in combination with dorsal tenosynovectomy or treatment of the distal ulna, or both

Technical Aspects

The rheumatoid wrist is approached via a dorsal straight incision that is centered over the axis of the third metacarpal. The subcutaneous tissue dissection is limited on the radial side by the identification and protection of the delicate superficial branches of the radial nerve and on the ulnar border of the wrist by the identification of the superficial branch of the ulnar nerve. The extensor retinaculum is longitudinally divided in the interval between the fifth and sixth extensor compartments. If needed, an extensor synovectomy is performed. The terminal branch of the posterior interosseus nerve is identified on the radial floor of the fourth extensor compartment and is resected for approximately 2 cm. The wrist joint is opened with a longitudinal incision in the axis of the capitate, and two triangular flaps raised from the radius, or it is opened with the approach that was described by Berger (133) (Figs. 12 and 13). This gives access to the radiocarpal and midcarpal joints, and synovectomy can be performed by using special rongeurs. An extension device might help reach all corners of the wrist joint. The capsule is closed preferably with absorbable sutures. Testing the closure on the operation

table, the surgeon must ensure that the closure is not too tight and does not limit flexion. In cases of capsular defects, the distal part of the retinaculum is used as capsular reinforcement. The authors prefer to divide the retinaculum in any case and to protect the tendons distally by placing the distal one-third to the distal one-half of the retinaculum underneath the extensor tendons. There is no need for formal reconstruction of the different extensor compartments, but the sixth compartment, containing the ECU, must be recentered over the distal ulna. Some authors advocate, in cases of beginning ulnar translation, a tendon transfer of the extensor carpi radialis longus to the extensor carpi radialis brevis (125,134,135), a method that the authors do not perform. If needed, subcutaneous drainage is placed, and the skin is closed carefully.

During the rehabilitation process, the wrist is placed in a resting splint in the intrinsic-plus position. Gently, movement might be started after secured skin healing. The aggression in the rehabilitation process should be individualized according to the healing properties of the patient and the preoperative status and intraoperative findings. Wrists that tend to be unstable should be protected longer, whereas stiff wrists may be mobilized more aggressively. All patients need some sort of wrist protection for at least 4 to 6 weeks.

Synovectomy of the Tendons

Extensor Tendons

Similar indications for extensor tendon synovectomy are given as those in the indication list of wrist synovectomy. Per-

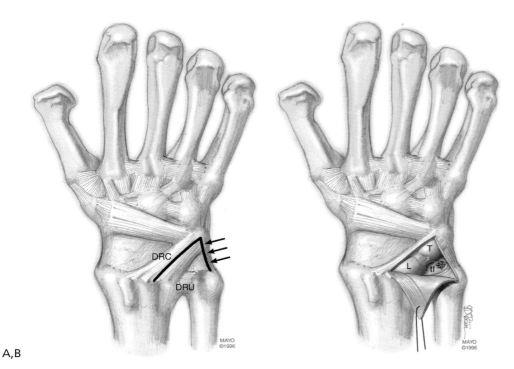

A,B

FIGURE 13. **A:** Dorsal wrist approach with ulnar-based capsulotomy. Outline of the incision. **B:** Dorsal wrist approach with ulnar-based capsulotomy after elevating the capsular flap with good exposure of the distal radioulnar (DRU) joint. DRC, dorsal radiocarpal ligament; L, lunate; T, triquetrum; tf, triangular fibrocartilage. (From Berger RA, Bishop AT. A fiber-splitting capsulotomy technique for dorsal exposure of the wrist. *Tech Hand Upper Extrem Surg* 1997;1:2–10, with permission.)

sistent, even painless, swelling in the extensor compartment after adequate medical treatment indicates a surgical intervention. Clinically, it is almost impossible to select patients with the highest likelihood of tendon rupture. Rarely, isolated extensor tenosynovectomy is performed, because most patients with RA have some sort of involvement of the distal radioulnar joint or the radiocarpal compartment that must be addressed at the same time. In cases of tendon rupture, patients must be informed of the consequences of tendon reconstruction or untreated ruptures (see the section Extensor Tendons in the section Tendon Reconstruction).

Flexor Tendons

The two main indications for isolated flexor tendon synovectomy are carpal tunnel syndrome and revision of tendon ruptures. As outlined in the section Flexor Tendons in the section Involvement of the Soft Tissues around the Wrist, carpal tunnel is frequent in RA, and a generous indication for decompression, together with a tendon revision and synovectomy, is given. In cases of flexor tendon rupture, a revision is almost mandatory to prevent further tendon damage. Decompression of the median nerve with tenosynovectomy is an effective procedure with little morbidity. It is possible to combine dorsal wrist surgery with decompression of the carpal tunnel, because no special requirements in the rehabilitation procedures are needed for the flexor synovectomy.

Technical Aspects. The flexor tendons at wrist level in RA are usually addressed with an open, classical, extended carpal tunnel approach. Endoscopic carpal tunnel release might be reserved for the rare cases of isolated median nerve compression without suspicion of significant flexor synovitis. The

authors prefer an incision that is centered in the extension of the fourth finger in the area of Guyon's canal. Depending on the expansion of the synovitis, the incision might be extended proximal to the wrist crease; in most patients, it is sufficient to approach directly over the carpal tunnel. In the rare cases of simultaneous compression of the ulnar nerve at the wrist level, a decompression of the ulnar nerve in Guyon's canal may be performed simultaneously. After division of the palmar aponeurosis, the transverse carpal ligament is visualized and divided completely on the most ulnar border. This secures a good coverage of the median nerve with the radial site of the divided ligament. A formal neurolysis is not recommended, to avoid scarring within the nerve. Flexor tendon revision and synovectomy can now be performed. Special attention has to be paid to the floor of the carpal tunnel; sharp bony edges should be identified and smoothed with the use of a rongeur. Partial flexor tendon laceration may be débrided. A minimum of 40% to 50% of the tendon must be intact; otherwise, tendon reinforcement might be advocated. Although several possibilities of reconstruction of the transverse carpal ligaments are described, the authors prefer to leave the carpal canal open, and only skin closure is performed. In the rehabilitation process, excessive wrist flexion should be avoided, and the wrist should be protected in a removable night splint in intrinsic-plus position for as long as 6 weeks. Functional use for light daily activities is encouraged.

Treatment of the Distal Radioulnar Joint

The treatment of the distal radioulnar joint has, besides functional and, therefore, reconstructive aspects, a significant prophylactic importance. It is a frequent target of RA destruction.

According to Resnick (136), synovial proliferation is observed in three areas of the distal radioulnar joint: distal to the ulnar head, in the prestyloid recess, and in the recess of the ECU tendon. This is important to recognize when a synovectomy of the distal radioulnar joint is performed. The damage of the synovitis is related to the duration and degree of inflammation, as well as the mechanical stress of the anatomical structure (137). The synovitis invades the triangular fibrocartilage complex and the palmar and dorsal radioulnar ligaments, resulting in destabilization of the distal radioulnar joint. The synovial infiltration of the ECU tendon provokes a palmar subluxation of the tendon with further instability (138). Parallel processes at the dorsal lip of the sigmoid notch enhance this situation (139). The classic caput ulnae syndrome, as described by Backdahl (27), is an end stage of this destruction process and shows a characteristic dorsal prominence of the distal ulna in combination with a local bulge of the synovia and possible signs of tendon rupture. The mobility of the forearm rotation is markedly reduced and painful. Instability of the distal radioulnar joint may produce a painful clicking in prosupination.

However, deformation alone is not necessarily an indication for surgery. Often, a combination of pain and functional impairment, together with the need to prevent further damage, sets the indication for a surgical procedure (140). A more aggressive approach is required in cases of extensor tendon rupture to prevent further damage (141). There is a controversial discussion about the use of local steroids in this area; first, the infiltration often treats only a part of the complex distal radioulnar joint (120), and, second, an already damaged tendon might be weakened further (120,140,142).

The basic principle of the surgical correction of the distal radioulnar joint in RA includes

- Joint and tendon synovectomy
- Partial or total resection of the ulnar head
- Stabilization of the ulnar stump
- Stabilization of the radiocarpal joint if needed

There are only early cases, most often in younger patients, with limited destruction, which might qualify for joint and tenosynovectomy only. In the majority of cases, the distal ulna has to be addressed by complete or partial resection or by fusion of the distal radioulnar joint with a Sauve-Kapandji procedure. Complete resection of the ulnar head was first described by Darrach (143) for treatment of sequelae after distal radius fractures. This concept was later adapted for the rheumatoid hand first by Smith-Peterson et al. (144) and subsequently by many other investigators (27,53,87,120,122,125,140,142,145–156). The general results of the combined approach with synovectomy and ulnar head resection are consistent with good to excellent pain relief and a minimal incidence of recurrent synovitis and symptomatic distal ulnar stump instability (125,127,157,158). However, critical analysis,

especially of higher-demand patients, shows a significant rate of failures and unsatisfactory results, such as instability of the distal ulnar stump (159–161) and a significant increase in ulnar wrist translocation (140,151,162,163). To overcome these problems, different variations of ulnar head resection, such as the Bower's hemiresection-interposition arthroplasty (164) or the matched ulnar resection according to Watson (165), were also proposed for the rheumatoid wrist. These techniques have the advantage of leaving some of the stabilizing structures of the ulnar side of the wrist, although a correction of the carpal subluxation and a complete stabilization of the distal radioulnar joint are difficult to achieve. Greater popularity, especially among the European surgeons, has been noted for the Sauve-Kapandji procedure (166) in which the distal ulnar stump is fused more proximally to the radius with an ulnar pseudarthrosis. This procedure preserves the stabilizing elements on the ulnar aspects of the wrist. Several series reported good results for rheumatoid conditions (60,167–172), although unstable distal ulnar stumps are also reported (170). Different procedures were proposed to prevent or to correct this ulnar stump instability. The most popular are stabilization slings from the ECU or the flexor carpi ulnaris (161,164) or the pronator quadratus interposition transfer (173). Because most distal ulnar stumps tend to be dorsally dislocated, it makes more sense to use flexor carpi ulnaris tenodesis. In addition, once ulnar translation is started, it is unlikely that this process can be stopped with a Sauve-Kapandji operation (174). Those cases need a stabilization on the level of the radiocarpal joint.

Another method to treat a destroyed distal radioulnar joint is ulnar head replacement. It was first described by Swanson (175), who used a silicone cap for better stabilization of the ulnar side of the wrist. Several studies proved unsatisfactory results in the long term (176,177) with these implants, and, therefore, this technique is no longer recommended. Subsequently, different implants have been developed, as a more constrained articulation with two components (178,179) or as a simpler replacement of the distal ulna with a ceramic head (180). These implants were primarily developed as salvage for recurrent instability after failed surgery at the distal ulna. Their long-term results will determine if more generous indications might be justified.

Among all these possibilities, the authors prefer the following surgical approaches to the rheumatoid distal radioulnar joint:

Ulnar head resection is combined with dorsal tenosynovectomy in elderly and less-demanding patients.

The Sauve-Kapandji procedure, if needed, is combined with a flexor carpi ulnaris tenodesis or a pronator transposition in younger, more demanding RA patients.

Type 3 wrists (destabilization), according to the Schulthess classification, need additional stabilization of the radiocarpal joint.

In cases with unsalvageable, functionally unacceptable, recurrent instability of the distal ulna, an ulnar head prosthesis may be considered.

Technical Aspects

In any case, even if only the distal radioulnar joint is addressed, a similar approach to that used for dorsal wrist synovectomy (see the section Synovectomy of the Wrist Joint) is recommend. First, it allows the overview of all extensor compartments, and, second, in RA, the likelihood of future surgery of the radiocarpal joint is high.

After the incision of the dorsal retinaculum in the interval between the fifth and sixth compartments, a tenosynovectomy is performed. The distal radioulnar joint is exposed through a longitudinal incision, starting just proximal to the triangular fibrocartilage. Joint synovectomy is performed, and, in cases with a mainly preserved distal radioulnar joint, bony spurs might be removed. In the indication of ulnar head removal, the distal ulna is resected together with the periosteum as distally as possible, just proximal to the proximal end of the sigmoid notch. The complete removal of the periosteum prevents the so-called carrotlike appearance of the ulnar stump after a longer follow-up. Free forearm rotation with no impingement to the radius must be checked on the operation table. For the Sauve-Kapandji procedure, after completion of the local synovectomy and removal of the cartilage on both joint surfaces, the forearm is held in a neutral position, and a pin is inserted at the side of the later screw, fixing the ulna to the radius. The position of the pin is controlled under fluoroscopy. The distance to create the pseudarthrosis should not be more than 10 to 12 mm and should be placed as distally as possible. The bone segment should be removed together with the periosteum to prevent calcifications. The pin is then replaced by a 2.7-mm cannulated screw. There is no need for bone grafting of the cartilage defect; in contrast, Rothwell et al. (181) described a simplified technique in which the distal radioulnar joint is not formally exposed before screw fixation. The screw must not be placed bicortically; in contrast, a too-long implant may cause extensor tendon irritation in the first extensor compartment. In cases of marked overlength of the ulna, the distal stump might be proximalized before definitive fixation. If needed, a distally based sling of the flexor carpi ulnaris is harvested (caveat: be aware of the proximity of the ulnar nerve), and a tenodesis through a drill hole in the ulna stump is completed. For the ulnar head resection or the Sauve-Kapandji procedure, the capsule is carefully closed by using strong single sutures with absorbable material, which are placed while the assistant reduces the distal ulna to the palmar side. Together with the refixation of the retinaculum, the ECU is recentered.

For rehabilitation, the wrist is protected in a so-called sandwich splint with a dorsal cover. This stabilizes the distal ulna while gentle forearm rotation in this splint is started, as soon as the patients tolerates it. The splint should be worn for 6 weeks. In the case of a Sauve-Kapandji operation, radiographs taken after this time should show bony fusion.

Reconstructive Surgery

Partial Fusion

The expected natural course of the disease at the radiocarpal level has great implications for the decision of which surgical procedure should be performed. Type 1 and 2 wrists have a low probability of undergoing radiocarpal dislocation. Therefore, surgical treatment, including the aforementioned wrist and tendon synovectomy and usually ulnar head resection, gives satisfactory long-term results (57,59,134,146,149, 150,152,155,156,163,182–187). In contrast, type 3 wrists, because of ligamentous or bony destruction, or both, require a procedure that provides realignment and stability. It is important to classify the wrist as early as possible in the course of the disease. It is easier to distinguish the different forms if the destruction is not too advanced. In later stages of the disease, an original type 2 wrist, which is considered stable, might undergo significant carpal collapse and may begin to mimic type 3 (unstable) evolution. Partial fusion of the rheumatoid wrist has, in early stages, a prophylactic character, whereas, in an established deformation pattern, a reconstructive element might be attributed.

The concept of partial fusion in rheumatoid wrists was first described by Chamay et al. (188) and later by Linscheid and Dobyns (189). Chamay et al. (188) applied their observation of spontaneous radiolunate fusion with preserved functional range of motion and long-term stability to the treatment of rheumatoid deformities. The idea of limited fusion in the rheumatoid wrist includes the realignment of the subluxed carpus by reduction of the proximal carpal row combined with long-term stability. In cases of excessive radiocarpal damage, the concept of limited wrist fusion might be expanded to a radioscapholunate fusion (152). A review of the literature shows good clinical results and high patient satisfaction for limited wrist fusion in rheumatoid patients. The range of motion varies postoperatively but, on average, is reported to be in functional range (188–200). It should be noted, however, that most series observed deterioration over time with ongoing destruction of the wrist (189,191,192,194,196,197,199–202) (Fig. 14). Advanced disease stages and already destabilized wrists should therefore be treated by total wrist fusion (191). Because the radiolunate fusion provides stability on the ulnar side of the wrist, it is usually combined with an ulnar head resection. It is possible to perform radiolunate fusion together with a Sauve-Kapandji procedure (Fig. 15). Although there may be a theoretical advantage to that approach, no series so far has shown superior results.

Technical Aspects

The same approach to the wrist is used as described in the section Synovectomy of the Wrist Joint. After the access to

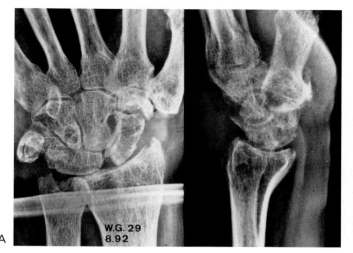

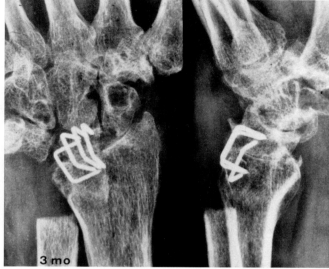

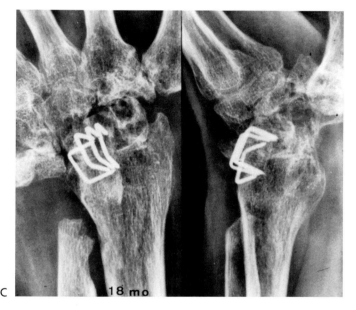

FIGURE 14. A: Initial radiograph of a rheumatoid wrist with ulnar drift of the carpus and destruction of the radiocarpal joint. **B:** Three months after radiolunate fusion. There is already cyst formation in the scaphoid and ongoing destruction of the scaphoradial joint. **C:** Eighteen months after radiolunate fusion. There is a marked carpal collapse and destruction of the midcarpal joint. The wrist was converted in a total wrist fusion.

the carpus, a complete synovectomy is performed. The indication for radiolunate fusion with ulnar translation of the wrist or destruction of the radiolunate fossa with at least some preservation of the radioscaphoid fossa, or both, is confirmed. In the authors' experience, even quite significant cartilage alterations in the scaphoid fossa are clinically well tolerated, and the indication for partial fusion versus total fusion should be generous. In cases of complete destruction of the radiocarpal joint and preservation of the midcarpal joint, radioscapholunate fusion with or without midcarpal arthroplasty (203) might be considered. The remaining cartilage is removed from the radiolunate joint to the subchondral cancellous bone, maintaining the curvature of both articulating elements to allow good matching of the lunate with the radius. The lunate is inset so that the radius covers approximately two-thirds of the lunate. The reduction is held with a preliminary Kirschner wire. Fluoroscopic radiographic examination should be performed to confirm the correct

position of the lunate in all planes. In cases of severe bone deficiency, a bone graft, often harvested from the resected ulnar head, might be used. The internal fixation may be performed with titanium power staples with a dimension of 13 mm × 10 mm (Fig. 16); when good bone quality is present, with a 2-mm mini condylar plate; or by other methods (Fig. 17). The arrangement of the staplers is critical; ideally, two to three staplers should be placed in different converging angles to prevent redislocation (Fig. 18). The wrist capsule is closed in such a way that the implants are completely covered. This is important, especially when a condylar plate is used, to avoid tendon irritation.

Postoperatively, the wrist is immobilized for 6 to 8 weeks, depending on the bone quality, in a splint or a plaster cast. After radiologic evidence of healing, wrist mobilization can be started.

The most common complication in radiolunate fusion is malpositioning of the hardware. Staples or screws can

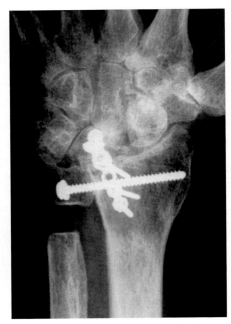

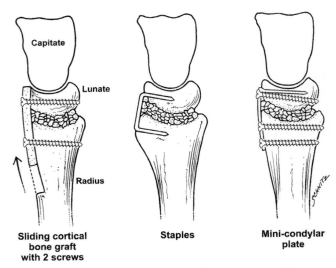

FIGURE 17. Different types of radiolunate fusion fixations. (From Herren DB, Simmen BR. *J Am Soc Surg Hand* 2002;2:21–32, with permission.)

FIGURE 15. Combined radiolunate fusion and Sauve-Kapandji procedure.

penetrate or bridge the midcarpal joint and can cause damage to the cartilage, thus necessitating hardware removal (189,192,198,200). This complication must be considered a technical error, because careful fluoroscopic intraoperative checks can avoid this problem.

The fusion rate in all series is high and consistently exceeds 90%. Despite this high success rate, cases with severely affected bone quality and strong deviating forces may fail to fuse. Good internal fixation, best performed

with staples or a mini plate, and cast immobilization for 6 to 8 weeks are mandatory.

Total Wrist Fusion

There is an ongoing discussion of whether to fuse a destroyed rheumatoid wrist or to indicate a radiocarpal arthroplasty (204). Despite the good clinical results of complex wrist arthroplasty (205–209), the complication rate remains high. In addition, wrist arthroplasty requires good bone stock and a reasonable or reconstructible tendon balance, two conditions that are rarely present in advanced

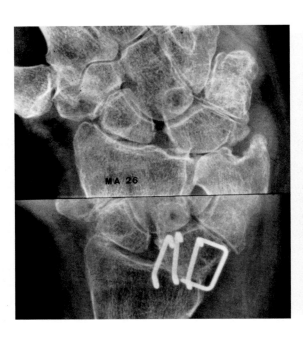

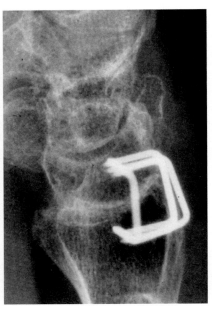

FIGURE 16. Radiolunate fusion with power staplers. There is a correct position of the lunate in both planes.

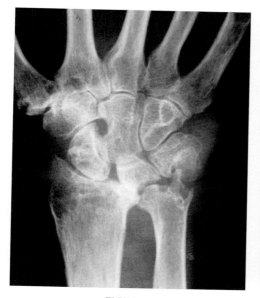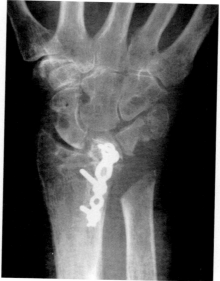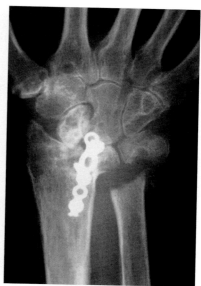

FIGURE 18. Radiolunate fusion with a 2-mm condylar plate. Despite good initial reposition, there was redislocation of the carpus back to initial deformity. Subjectively, there was no pain, and no revision was needed.

rheumatoid destruction. Silicon wrist spacers offer an alternative, although they are only recommended by most investigators in low-demand patients (210–213). A more complete discussion on wrist arthroplasty is found in a separate chapter.

Most wrists with advanced rheumatoid disease require a definitive stabilization by total wrist fusion. A pain-free, stable wrist joint often outweighs the disadvantage of the lack of mobility (154,156,199,204,214–225). Although bilateral wrist fusion is still a subject of controversy (204,226), personal experience and a publication by Rayan et al. (227) effectively show high patient acceptance even for bilateral fusion. However, subjectively, most patients would like to have at least one mobile wrist. Two main concerns dominate the discussion that surrounds wrist arthrodesis: the position of fusion and the surgical technique to obtain secure and stable fixation.

A functional range of motion has been found to consist of 10 degrees of flexion and 35 degrees of extension for most activities of daily living (228). By analyzing different tasks, activities concerning personal care and hygiene were found to be performed in slightly flexed wrist positions. However, besides overall function, wrist position seems to affect grip strength. Flexed wrist posture is associated with decrease of grip strength, whereas there is no difference in strength between neutral (0 degrees) and an extended fusion position (229,230). In patients who have RA, associated elbow and shoulder disease, as well as bilateral hand involvement, has to be taken into consideration when choosing the ideal arthrodesis position. Lateral deviation affects the position and the function of the fingers, especially with coexisting ulnar drift at the metacarpophalangeal (MCP) joint level. Five degrees

to 10 degrees of ulnar deviation are needed to counterbalance an ulnar drift of the fingers (22,137,231). Most investigators prefer a neutral flexion-extension position with mild ulnar deviation for wrist fusion in rheumatoid patients (149,152,153,183,216,227,232,233). In the authors' experience, an individual decision has to be made for every patient. Preoperative evaluation can be performed with splints in different wrist positions. In most cases, a neutral or slightly flexed position for the dominant hand, to facilitate personal care, and a slightly extended position for the nondominant hand combined with 5 to 10 degrees of ulnar deviation are chosen.

Different fixation methods for wrist fusion have been described in the literature. Since the first description by Clayton 1965 (183), which was later popularized by Mannerfelt and Malmsten (232), different investigators have favored the Rush or Steinmann pin technique in the original method or with slight modifications (199,214–219,221–225,234,235). There are some reports of radiocarpal fusion using bone grafts with or without absorbable internal fixation (220,236,237). Bone grafting alone had a longer time to fusion than a combination of bone grafting and internal fixation (215). As an alternative to the pin technique, plate fixation for wrist fusion is popular (238,239), especially in posttraumatic conditions. A comparison between plate and pin fusion techniques in rheumatoid patients showed no significant difference in the clinical results or in the complication rate (240).

However, pin fixation has some significant advantages over the plate fixation in RA. RA is more frequent in women, who, with small wrist sizes, cannot always accommodate the plate, which is often too bulky to be applied. In

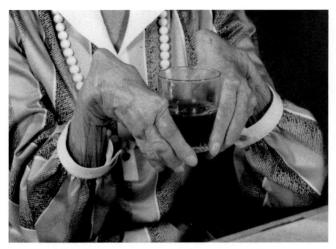

FIGURE 19. Patient with severe dislocation of both wrists.

addition, the soft tissue and skin conditions may not be ideal to cover a plate adequately, and, most often, a secondary removal of the implant is needed. In severe RA, bone quality might be so poor that no screw fixation is possible at all. Rheumatoid patients also have a high fusion rate that tends to require less rigid fixation than osteoarthritic patients. Lastly, pin osteosynthesis is clearly less costly.

Technical Aspects

To perform a total wrist fusion, the wrist is approached in the same way as that previously described for wrist synovectomy or partial fusion. Some of the rheumatoid wrists have

a severe deformation with ulnar and palmar dislocation (Fig. 19). In such circumstances, because of contracted soft tissue, some shortening of the radius is required to allow reduction of the wrist. In RA, wrist fusion is almost always performed together with the removal of the ulnar head. After resection of the radius, the radiocarpal and the midcarpal joints are débrided down to cancellous bone. If the reduction is possible without too much tension on the soft tissues, the pin insertion point in the third metacarpal is prepared. The proximal one-third of the third metacarpal, the interval between the second and third metacarpals, or the intramedullary shaft of the third metacarpal can be chosen (Fig. 20). If the axis is more favorable, the second metacarpal can also be used. When using the proximal one-third insertion technique, an ulnar lateral bone window of approximately 6 by 4 mm is made. A special tapered rasp is then used to open the canal for the pin. The rasp should be directed to the middle of the capitate, perforating the proximal carpal row in the scaphoid or the lunate. A Rush pin that is 2.5 to 3.5 mm in diameter and approximately 15 to 25 cm in length is then bent to accommodate the desired fusion position and is advanced from the metacarpal to the radius. Alternatively, the pin can be placed through a hole that is made in the head of the third metacarpal and is driven proximally in an intramedullary fashion, although this method fixes the angle of fusion to neutral, or it can be driven into the junction of the bases of the second and third metacarpals, allowing some control over the angle of fusion but slightly less rigid fixation. Before final placement of the rod, cancellous bone graft from the ulnar head is placed. If additional rotation stability is required, two or

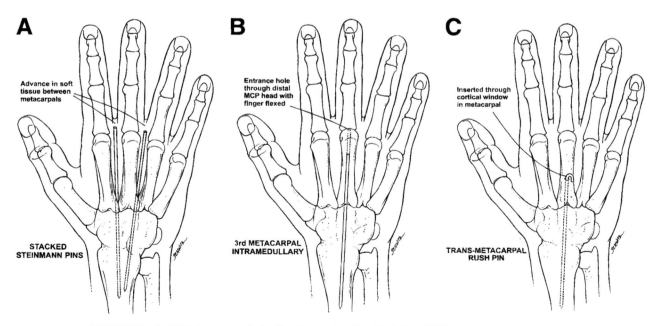

FIGURE 20. A–C: Techniques of pin fixation in total wrist fusion. MCP, metacarpophalangeal. (From Herren DB, Simen BR. *J Am Soc Surg Hand* 2002;2:21–32, with permission.)

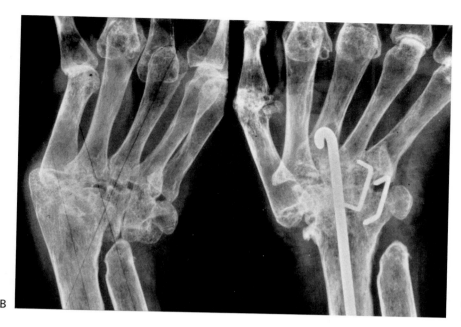

A,B

FIGURE 21. A: Complete dislocation of a rheumatoid wrist type 3. **B:** Final radiograph after completed Rush pin and staple augmentation total wrist fusion.

three titanium staples may be placed to bridge the former radiocarpal joint (Fig. 21). Postoperatively, a splint is applied for 1 to 2 weeks, followed by a cast for 6 to 7 weeks, until radiographic fusion has occurred.

Nonunion is rare in patients who have RA. The average fusion rate in the literature is more than 90% (199,216–219,222,224,225,232,234,235,238,242). In the Rush pin technique, care should be taken at the insertion point of the pin at the metacarpal base. Predrilling of holes before opening the cortex might prevent iatrogenic fractures. In using the Steinmann pin technique, between the metacarpals or in an intramedullary fashion in the third metacarpal, one must ensure good fixation of the pin into the distal radius and a good interference fit of the pin at the metacarpal bases or within the third metacarpal. The most common problem, especially when using the Rush pin technique, is obtaining the desired wrist position. Exact planning and careful prebending of the rod are helpful.

Tendon Reconstruction

Extensor Tendon Reconstruction

As outlined in the section Extensor Tendons in the section Involvement of the Soft Tissues around the Wrist, rupture of extensor tendons is the final stage of a complex pathomechanical process. The best treatment of tendon rupture is prevention with early aggressive treatment of the distal radioulnar joint and the accompanying tenosynovitis.

It is mandatory, when planning extensor tendon reconstruction, to assess wrist and MCP joint function. Any wrist correction or treatment of MCP joint dysfunction, or both, should be best performed together with the tendon reconstruction. No tendon reconstruction can mobilize a subluxed MCP joint, and a secondary procedure that con-

sists of MCP joint reconstruction and extensor tenolysis may not give satisfactory results (95). If there is any doubt about MCP joint function, traction on the distal ends of the tendons for reconstruction demonstrates the quality of MCP joint extension ability. If needed, subluxed extensor tendons should be recentered over the MCP joints at the same time that the extensor reconstruction is performed.

Direct end-to-end repair of ruptured tendon in rheumatoid patients is almost never feasible. The long-standing process of tendon attrition creates a wide zone of destruction within the tendon. Therefore, the most frequently used techniques for extensor tendon repair are tendon transfer and, in selected cases, tendon reconstruction with a free tendon graft (92,98,243–245). With two sites of suture lines, the free tendon graft has the disadvantage of greater possibility of adherence, although Bora et al. (243) reported no differences between free tendon grafts and tendon transfers. As free tendon grafts, the palmaris longus tendon or, in cases of wrist fusion, a graft from the radial wrist extensors might be used. The use of toe extensor tendons in RA must be carefully chosen to avoid secondary morbidity.

Tendon transfers might be performed as end-to-side transfers or end-to-end reconstruction. Table 5 gives an overview of possible transfer settings for the different rupture scenarios. The best tendon for transfer is the extensor indicis proprius (EIP) tendon, followed by the flexor superficialis of the ring and middle fingers. The use of wrist extensor tendons is not advised because the excursion of the wrist motors is significantly less than that of the finger extensor tendons, thus producing incomplete motion. The prognosis of tendon reconstruction is best in single or double tendon rupture, whereas the treatment of multiple ruptures is considered as a salvage procedure (92,246). The rupture of the extensor tendons to the thumb is often an

TABLE 5. POSSIBLE TENDON TRANSFER SETS IN THE DIFFERENT CLINICAL SCENARIOS

Ruptured tendons	Transfer	Alternatives
EDM	EDM to EDC V	No treatment
EDM, EDC V	EDC V to EDC IV	EDC V to EDC IV
		EIP to EDM
EDM, EDC V, EDC IV	EIP to EDM (+ EDC V) EDC IV to EDC III	
EDM, EDC V, EDC IV, EDC III	EIP to EDC IV and V EDC III to EDC II	Flexor digitorum superficialis IV to EDC IV and V EIP to EDC III

EDC, extensor digitorum communis; EDM, extensor digiti minimi; EIP, extensor indicis proprius.

isolated event, which is best treated with a transfer of the EIP to the extensor pollicis longus tendon.

Technical Aspects. The wrist is approached in the same manner as already described. Extensor tendon status is explored after synovectomy. Free gliding of the distal end of the ruptured tendon is confirmed by pulling on the distal stump; otherwise, tenolysis must be performed. Partially attenuated tendons are débrided and reinforced with a free tendon graft if needed (more than 60% to 70% loss). The tendons are prepared for the transfer. The EIP tendon is divided at the level of the index MCP joint with a separate incision. The EIP tendon is on the more ulnar side of the two tendons. The flexor digitorum superficialis tendon of the ring finger is harvested over a Bruner type of incision, proximal to the proximal interphalangeal (PIP) joint. The stumps of the distal end of this tendon are fixed to the palmar plate to prevent swan-neck deformity. The proximal musculotendinous unit is brought through the interosseous membrane to the dorsal aspect of the wrist or over the radial border. The radial routing has the advantage to keep the transferred tendon away from the damaged ulnar wrist compartment, and the pull of the tendon counters ulnar wrist translocation (95). The end-to-side and end-to-end reconstructions are performed by using the weaving technique that was described by Pulvertaft (247). Ideally, three tendon passages, each transposed 90 degrees to the other, are used, secured with several single sutures. To adjust the tension on the transfer is probably the most difficult part of the intervention. As a general rule, the transferred muscle–tendon unit should be slightly overstrained, compared to the neighbor digits. This may be tested best with the teno-desis effect in wrist flexion-extension; in cases of wrist fusion, the tension must be judged according to the sponta-neous position of the fingers. When in doubt, it is better to have too much tension, because stretching in the rehabilita-tion process is almost always possible, whereas spontaneous shortening is never observed. At least one strip of the exten-sor retinaculum should be reconstructed to prevent bow-

stringing, but it must be checked that no interference with the site of tendon weaving occurs.

Postoperatively, the wrist is immobilized in 20 to 30 degrees of extension with the MCP joints in minimal flex-ion; the PIP and distal interphalangeal are left free for immediate mobilization. After 4 weeks, wrist remobiliza-tion may be started. Dynamic splinting is only necessary when a significant flexion loss is observed.

Flexor Tendon Reconstruction
As outlined in the section Involvement of the Soft Tissues around the Wrist, the flexor tendon that ruptures most commonly in RA is the FPL, followed by the profundus tendon of the index finger. Rupture of flexor tendons in the region of the finger pulleys is rare, and most flexor tendons rupture in the carpal canal. Principally, this is a good zone for safe flexor tendon reconstruction with minimal danger of postoperative adhesions. In cases of flexor tendon rup-ture, a surgical revision is mandatory to prevent further ruptures. Before revision surgery and possible tendon reconstruction, the following points should be clarified:

- How much functional loss does the patient have with the ruptures?
- What is the general condition of the wrist and finger joints?
- Is the patient suitable for a possible long rehabilitation process with a unpredictable result?

As an alternative to tendon reconstruction, interphalangeal joint fusion, especially in already arthritic joints, might be indicated with far fewer rehabilitation difficulties. If the indication to flexor tendon reconstruction is given, the fol-lowing reconstruction principles might be recommended (21,85,87,92,93,248):

- Isolated FPL ruptures are reconstructed with a transfer of a superficialis tendon, preferably from the ring finger, depending on the conditions of the other tendons.
- Ruptures of profundus tendons are best transferred with an end-to-side tenodesis to an intact adjacent profundus tendon.
- In cases of rupture of the profundus and superficialis tendons in one finger, a tendon transfer from an intact superficialis is performed.
- Some investigators have recommended bridge grafts (21,85); others, including the authors, prefer tendon transfers (93).
- Isolated superficialis tendon ruptures, which are rare, need no reconstruction.

Technically, the palmar wrist is opened similarly to the technique that was described in the section Flexor Tendons in the section Involvement of the Soft Tissues around the Wrist with an extensile carpal tunnel approach. Tendon transfer or bridging is performed with the same techniques as in extensor tendon reconstruction.

TABLE 6. UNIVERSAL CLASSIFICATION OF TYPING AND STAGING OF INFLAMMATORY WRIST ARTHROPATHY

Universal wrist classification in inflammatory polyarthropathy
Type of disease
  Slow progressive type without significant OA (destructive type)
  Slow progressive type with marked OA changes (reactive type)
  Progressive soft tissue disruption (ligamentous type)
  Progressive bony destruction (mutilans type)
  Spontaneous intercarpal ankylosis (juvenile type)
Stage of disease
  Early, erosions with or without early reducible translation (LDE stages I and II)
  Translation, translocation, volar subluxation, nonreducible, with or without radiocarpal OA (LDE stages III and IV)
  Some or all of the previous characteristics with midcarpal joint loss
  Disorganized wrist, with or without significant bone substance loss
  Intercarpal ankylosis

LDE, Larsen, Dahle, and Eek classification; OA, osteoarthritis.
Adapted from Stanley JK, Lluch A, Herren DB, et al. Universal wrist classification in inflammatory polyarthropathy (*in preparation*).

In rehabilitation, dynamic splinting that is similar to flexor tendon sutures is advocated. A Kleinertlike splint with the wrist in almost neutral position or only slightly flexed for 4 weeks is needed. Tendon transfers, as well as tendon grafts, are more stable than direct tendon sutures and might be treated more aggressively, especially in cases of early limitation in finger motion. Most often, the rehabilitation is prolonged, and flexion or extension loss is possible. Ertel et al. (85), in their series, achieved active motion in 88% of their cases, with an average range of motion in the thumb interphalangeal joint of 23 degrees and an average range of motion in the PIP of the digits of only 55 degrees.

Salvage Procedures

The definition of wrist salvage procedures in RA is quite difficult. Some authors might believe that wrist fusion is already considered as a salvage, because it implies a definitive end in the treatment ladder. However, in the disease course of RA patients, a multitude of interventions is to be expected, and there is no space for experimental procedures. In the wrist, resection interposition arthroplasty might be considered a salvage procedure together with silicone wrist replacement. The latter is described in Chapter 79, Wrist Arthroplasty.

Resection (Interposition) Arthroplasty

The rationale of resection arthroplasty, with or without interposition, includes the removal of destroyed opposing articular surfaces together with the need to preserve some motion. Proximal row carpectomy, which is successfully used for other pathologic wrist conditions, does not work in the rheumatoid wrists (249). The lunate fossa is often destroyed in RA, and the important palmar ligaments are too stretched to stabilize the distal row.

In proper resection arthroplasty, parts of the proximal or distal row, together with the distal radius, are resected, often combined with interposition of some biological material. The most popular biological materials are tendons, fascia, or capsular sheet (250–254). Taleisnik (203) proposed a combined radiocarpal fusion with a midcarpal arthroplasty using a silicone interposition.

All of theses procedures were more or less abandoned in favor of real joint replacement or wrist fusion. Nevertheless, newer attempts to optimize these procedures, together with possible failures of modern implants, may give this approach a revival in the future.

CLASSIFICATION AND TREATMENT ALGORITHM OF THE RHEUMATOID WRIST

A treatment algorithm may always be discussed controversially. A disease, such as RA, with so many different faces may profit from a certain classification. Besides typing and staging wrist involvement in RA, the distribution of certain categories should describe surgical consequences. The classifications that are presented in Tables 6 through 8 are based on the observations of experienced RA surgeons and summarize the ideas of Stanley et al. (255).

TABLE 7. FREQUENCY OF OBSERVED COMBINATIONS

Disease type	Stage of disease				
	I	II	III	IV	V
A: Destructive	Very common in early disease	Very common	Severe disease	Late stage	Rare
B: Reactive	Very common in early disease	Very common	Common	Uncommon	Uncommon
C: Ligamentous	Not commonly seen at this stage	Common	Rare	Common	Never
D: Mutilans	Common	Uncommon	Uncommon	Common	Never
E: Juvenile	Common in early disease	Common	Common	Very rare	Very common

TABLE 8. TREATMENT OPTIONS ACCORDING TO THE TYPE AND THE STAGE OF THE DISEASE IN THE WRIST

Disease type	Stage of disease				
	I	II	III	IV	V
A: Destructive	Synovectomy; soft tissue balancing ± ulnar head surgery	R(S)L fusion; ulnar head surgery	Capitate head replacement + R(S)L fusion; ± ulnar head surgery TWR	TWR or pan-arthrodesis	TWR or pan-arthrodesis
B: Reactive	Synovectomy; soft tissue balancing ± ulnar head surgery	R(S)L fusion; ulnar head surgery	Capitate head replacement + R(S)L fusion; TWR	TWR or pan-arthrodesis	TWR or pan-arthrodesis
C: Ligamentous		R(S)L fusion ± ulnar head surgery	Panarthrodesis	Panarthrodesis	
D: Mutilans	R(S)L fusion ± ulnar head surgery	Panarthrodesis	Panarthrodesis	Panarthrodesis	
E: Juvenile	Synovectomy; soft tissue balancing ± ulnar head surgery	Panarthrodesis	Panarthrodesis	Panarthrodesis	Panarthrodesis

R(S)L, radio(scapho)lunate fusion; TWR, total wrist replacement.

REFERENCES

1. Alaracon G. Epidemiology of rheumatoid arthritis. *Clin North Am* 1995;21:589–604.
2. Evans T, Han J, Singh R, et al. The genotypic distribution of shard-epitope DRB1 alleles suggests a recessive mode of inheritance of rheumatoid arthritis disease-susceptibility gene. *Arthritis Rheum* 1995;38:1754–1761.
3. Seldin M, Amos C, Ward A, et al. The genetic revolution and the assault on rheumatoid arthritis. *Arthritis Rheum* 1999;42:1071–1079.
4. Ottenhoff T, Torres P, De las Aguas J, et al. Evidence for an HLA-DR4–associated immune-response gene for mycobacterium tuberculosis: a clue to the pathogenesis of rheumatoid arthritis? *Lancet* 1986;2:310–312.
5. Philips P. Infectious agents in the pathogenesis of rheumatoid arthritis. *Semi Arthritis Rheum* 1986;16:1–10.
6. Goldring SR. Bone and joint destruction in rheumatoid arthritis: what is really happening? *J Rheumatol Suppl* 2002;65:44–8.
7. Kraan M, Versendaal H, Jonker M, et al. Asymptomatic synovitis precedes clinically manifest arthritis. *Arthritis Rheum* 1998;41:1481–1488.
8. McGonagle D, Conaghan P, O'Connor P, et al. The relationship between synovitis and bone changes in early untreated rheumatoid arthritis: controlled magnetic resonance imaging study. *Arthritis Rheum* 1999;42:1706–1711.
9. Zvaifler N, Firestein G. Pannus and pannocytes: alternative models of joint destruction in rheumatoid arthritis. *Arthritis Rheum* 1994;37:783–789.
10. Arend W, Dayer J. Inhibition of the production and effects of interleukin-1 and tumor necrosis factor in rheumatoid arthritis. *Arthritis Rheum* 1995;38:151–160.
11. Hurlimann D, Forster A, Noll G, et al. Anti-tumor necrosis factor-alpha treatment improves endothelial function in patients with rheumatoid arthritis. *Circulation* 2002;106:2184–2187.
12. Dayer JM. Interleukin 1 or tumor necrosis factor-alpha: which is the real target in rheumatoid arthritis? *J Rheumatol Suppl* 2002;65:10–15.
13. Moreland L, Heck L, Koopmann W. Biologic agents for treating rheumatoid arthritis: concepts and progress. *Arthritis Rheum* 1997;49:397–409.
14. Masi A, Feigenbaum S, Kaplan S. Articular pattern in the early course of rheumatoid arthritis. *Am J Med* 1983;75:16–26.
15. Callaghan L, Pincus T. Formal education level as a significant marker of clinical status in rheumatoid arthritis. *Arthritis Rheum* 1988;31:1346–1357.
16. Ehrhardt C, Mumford P, Venables P, et al. Factors predicting a poor life prognosis in rheumatoid arthritis: an eight year prospective study. *Ann Rheum Dis* 1989;48:7–13.
17. Sheerer Y, Bloch D, Mitchell D, et al. The development of disability in rheumatoid arthritis. *Arthritis Rheum* 1986;29:494–500.
18. Fleming A, Benn RT, Corbett M, et al. Early rheumatoid disease. II. Patterns of joint involvement. *Ann Rheum Dis* 1976;35:361–364.
19. Hamalainen M, Kammonen M, Lehtimaki M. Epidemiology of wrist involvement in rheumatoid arthritis. *Rheumatology* 1992;17:1–7.
20. Cush J, Lipsky P. Celluar basis of rheumatoid inflammation. *Clin Orthop* 1991;265:9–22.
21. Ertel AN. Flexor tendon ruptures in rheumatoid arthritis. *Hand Clin* 1989;5:177–190.
22. Shapiro JS. The wrist in rheumatoid arthritis. *Hand Clin* 1996;12:477–498.
23. Ritt M, Stuart P, Berglund L, et al. Rotational stability of the carpus relative to the forearm. *J Hand Surg* 1995;20:305–311.
24. Viegas S, Pattersson R, Ward K. Extrinsic wrist ligaments in the pathomechanics of ulnar translation. *J Hand Surg* 1995;20:312–318.
25. Shapiro JS. A new factor in the etiology of ulnar drift. *Clin Orthop* 1970;68:32–43.
26. Youm Y, McMurthy RY, Flatt AE, et al. Kinematics of the wrist. I. An experimental study of radial-ulnar deviation and flexion-extension. *J Bone Joint Surg* 1978;60:423–431.
27. Backdahl M. The caput ulna syndrome in rheumatoid arthritis: a study of the morphology, abnormal anatomy and clinical picture. *Acta Rheuma Scand* 1963;[Suppl 5]:1–8.
28. Bogoch ER, Weiler P, McCalden R, et al. Periulnar deformity in the rheumatoid wrist. *Rheumatology* 1992;17:43–51.

29. Shapiro JS, Heijna W, Nasatir S, et al. The relationship of wrist motion to ulnar phalangeal drift in the rheumatoid hand. *Hand* 1971;3:68–75.

30. Pahle JA, Raunio P. The influence of wrist position on finger deviation in the rheumatoid hand: a clinical and radiological study. *J Bone Joint Surg* 1969;51:664–669.

31. Shapiro JS. Wrist involvement in rheumatoid swan neck deformity. *J Hand Surg* 1982;7:484–491.

32. Flury MP, Herren DB, Simmen BR. Rheumatoid arthritis of the wrist. Classification related to the natural course. *Clin Orthop* 1999;366:72–77.

33. Simmen BR, Huber H. The wrist joint in chronic polyarthritis—a new classification based on the type of destruction in relation to the natural course and the consequences for surgical therapy. *Handchir Mikrochir Plast Chir* 1994;26:182–189.

34. Di Benedetto MR, Lubbers LM, Coleman CR. A standardized measurement of ulnar carpal translocation. *J Hand Surg* 1990;15:1009–1010.

35. Laxer RM, Clarke HM. Rheumatic disorders of the hand and wrist in childhood and adolescence. *Hand Clin* 2000;16:659–671.

36. Ansell BM. Juvenile arthritis. *Clin Rheum Dis* 1984;10:657–672.

37. Granberry WM, Mangum GL. The hand in the child with juvenile rheumatoid arthritis. *J Hand Surg* 1980;5:105–113.

38. Chaplin D, Pulkki T, Saarimaa A, et al. Wrist and finger deformities in juvenile rheumatoid arthritis. *Acta Rheumatol Scand* 1969;15:206–223.

39. Simmons B, Nutting J, Bernstein R. Juvenile rheumatoid arthritis. *Hand Clin* 1996;12:573–589.

40. Ravelli A, Viola S, Ramenghi B, et al. Radiologic progression in patients with juvenile chronic arthritis treated with methotrexate. *J Pediatr* 1998;133:262–265.

41. Harel L, Wagner-Weiner L, Poznanski AK, et al. Effects of methotrexate on radiologic progression in juvenile rheumatoid arthritis. *Arthritis Rheum* 1993;36:1370–1374.

42. Maldonado-Cocco JA, Garcia-Morteo O, Spindler AJ, et al. Carpal ankylosis in juvenile rheumatoid arthritis. *Arthritis Rheum* 1980;23:1251–1255.

43. Bjorkengren AG, Pathria MN, Sartoris DJ, et al. Carpal alterations in adult-onset Still disease, juvenile chronic arthritis, and adult-onset rheumatoid arthritis: comparative study. *Radiology* 1987;165:545–548.

44. Findley TW, Halpern D, Easton JK. Wrist subluxation in juvenile rheumatoid arthritis: pathophysiology and management. *Arch Phys Med Rehabil* 1983;64:69–74.

45. Weinberger A, Evans D, Ansell BM. Wrist involvement in juvenile chronic arthritis five years after onset of disease. *Isr J Med Sci* 1982;18:653–654.

46. Rothschild BM, Hanissian AS. Severe generalized (Charcot-like) joint destruction in juvenile rheumatoid arthritis. *Clin Orthop* 1981;155:75–80.

47. Granberry WM, Brewer EJ Jr. Results of synovectomy in children with rheumatoid arthritis. *Clin Orthop* 1974;101:120–126.

48. Goldie IF. Synovectomy in rheumatoid arthritis: a general review and an eight-year follow-up of synovectomy in 50 rheumatoid knee joints. *Semin Arthritis Rheum* 1974;3:219–251.

49. Eyring EJ, Longert A, Bass JC. Synovectomy in juvenile rheumatoid arthritis. Indications and short-term results. *J Bone Joint Surg* 1971;53:638–651.

50. Fink CW, Baum J, Paradies LH, et al. Synovectomy in juvenile rheumatoid arthritis. *Ann Rheum Dis* 1969;28:612–616.

51. Mink van der Molen AB, Hall MA, Evans DM. Ulnar lengthening in juvenile chronic arthritis. *J Hand Surg* 1998;23:438–441.

52. Harris ED. Rheumatoid arthritis pathophysiology and implications on therapy. *N Engl J Med* 1990;322:1277–1289.

53. Pulki T. Rheumatoid deformities of the hand. *Acta Rheumatol Scand* 1961;7:85–88.

54. Gray R, Gottlieb N. Hand flexor tenosynovitis in rheumatoid arthritis. *Arthritis Rheum* 1977;20:1003–1007.

55. Herbison G, Teng C, Martin J, et al. Carpal tunnel syndrome in rheumatoid arthritis. *Am J Phys Med* 1973;52:68.

56. Souter W. Present attitudes on timing of surgical interventions in the treatment of rheumatoid disease. *Ann Chir Gynaecol* 1985;74:19–25.

57. O'Brien ET. Surgical principles and planning for the rheumatoid hand and wrist. *Clin Plast Surg* 1996;23:407–420.

58. Larsen A, Dale K, Eek M. Radiographic evaluation of rheumatoid arthritis and related conditions by standard reference films. *Acta Radiol Diagn* 1977;18:481–491.

59. Hodgson SP, Stanley JK, Muirhead A. The Wrightington classification of rheumatoid wrist x-rays: a guide to surgical management. *J Hand Surg* 1989;14:451–455.

60. Alnot JY, Fauroux L. Synovectomy in the realignment-stabilization of the rheumatoid wrist. Apropos of a series of 104 cases with average follow-up of 5 years. *Rev Rheum Mal Osteoartic* 1992;59:196–206.

61. Hopfner S, Treitl M, Krolak C, et al. Diagnosis of initial changes in the hand of patients with rheumatoid arthritis—comparison between low-field magnetic resonance imaging, 3-phase bone scintigraphy and conventional x-ray. *Nuklearmedizin* 2002;41:135–142.

62. Sugimoto H, Takeda A, Hyodoh K. Early-stage rheumatoid arthritis: prospective study of the effectiveness of MR imaging for diagnosis. *Radiology* 2000;216:569–575.

63. Smith MD. Assessment of disease activity in rheumatoid arthritis using magnetic resonance imaging: quantification of pannus volume in the hands. *Rheumatology (Oxford)* 1999;38:680–681.

64. Jevtic V, Watt I, Rozman B, et al. Prognostic value of contrast enhanced Gd-DTPA MRI for development of bone erosive changes in rheumatoid arthritis. *Br J Rheumatol* 1996;35[Suppl 3]:26–30.

65. Wakefield RJ, Gibbon WW, Conaghan PG, et al. The value of sonography in the detection of bone erosions in patients with rheumatoid arthritis: a comparison with conventional radiography. *Arthritis Rheum* 2000;43:2762–2770.

66. Barnes C, Curry H. Carpal tunnel syndrome in rheumatoid arthritis: a clinical and electrodiagnostic survey. *Ann Rheum Dis* 1970;26:226–230.

67. Sturm T, Kisslinger E, Wessinghage D, et al. Chronic polyarthritis and carpal tunnel syndrome. Results of follow-up. *Z Rheumatol* 1995;54:56–62.

68. Lanzillo B, Pappone N, Crisci C, et al. Subclinical peripheral nerve involvement in patients with rheumatoid arthritis. *Arthritis Rheum* 1998;41:1196–1202.

69. Shinoda J, Hashizume H, McCown C, et al. Carpal tunnel syndrome grading system in rheumatoid arthritis. *J Orthop Sci* 2002;7:188–193.

70. Ono K. Myelopathy hand: new clinical signs of cervical cord damage. *J Bone Joint Surg* 1987;69:215–219.

71. Boden S, Dodge L, Rechtine G, et al. Rheumatoid arthritis of the cervical spine: a twenty year analysis with predictors of paralysis and recovery. *J Bone Joint Surg* 1993;75:1282–1297.

72. Dvorak J, Herdmann J, Theiler R. Magnetic transcranial brain stimulation: painless evaluation of central motor pathways: normal values and clinical application in spinal cord diagnostics: upper extremities. *Spine* 1990;15:155–160.

73. Ansell B. Outcome assessment in rheumatoid arthritis. *Ann Rheum Dis* 1969;28[Suppl 8].

74. Gschwend N. Assessment of the functional gain of various operations in the complex hand. *Rheumatology* 1987;11:80–91.

75. Backman C, Mackie H, Harris J. Arthritis hand function test: development of a standardized assessment tool. *Occup Ther J Res* 1991;11:245–256.

76. Clawson D, Souter W, Carthum C, et al. Functional assessment of the rheumatoid hand. *Clin Orthop* 1971;77:203–210.

77. Dellhag B, Bjelle A. A grip ability test for use in rheumatology practice. *Rheumatology* 1995;22:1559–1565.

78. Evans D, Lawton D. Assessment of hand function. *Clin Rheum Dis* 1984;10:697–725.

79. Reference deleted.

80. Chung K, Pillsbury M, Walters M, et al. Reliability and validity testing of the Michigan Hand Outcomes Questionnaire. *J Hand Surg* 1998;23:575–587.

81. Labi M, Gresham G, Rathey U. Hand function in osteoarthritis. *Arch Phys Med Rehabil* 1982;9:438–440.

82. Carvell JE, Mowat AG, Fuller DJ. Trigger wrist phenomenon in rheumatoid arthritis. *Hand* 1983;15:77–81.

83. Gray RG, Gottlieb NL. Hand flexor tenosynovitis in rheumatoid arthritis. Prevalence, distribution, and associated rheumatic features. *Arthritis Rheum* 1977;20:1003–1008.

84. Duche R, Canovas F, Thaury MN, et al. Tenosynovectomy of the flexors in rheumatoid polyarthritis. Analytic study of short term and long term mobility of the fingers. *Ann Chir Main Memb Super* 1993;12:85–92.

85. Ertel AN, Millender LH, Nalebuff E, et al. Flexor tendon ruptures in patients with rheumatoid arthritis. *J Hand Surg* 1988;13:860–866.

86. Konig A, Konig G. Lesional pattern and clinical symptoms in rheumatoid flexor tendon disease. *Z Rheumatol* 1999;58:277–282.

87. Hallett JP, Motta GR. Tendon ruptures in the hand with particular reference to attrition ruptures in the carpal tunnel. *Hand* 1982;14:283–290.

88. Mannerfelt L, Norman O. Attrition ruptures of flexor tendons in rheumatoid arthritis caused by bony spurs in the carpal tunnel. A clinical and radiological study. *J Bone Joint Surg* 1969;51:270–277.

89. Baer W, Dumont CE. Mechanical wearing down of flexor tendons in rheumatoid arthritis as a result of extreme volar-flexed intercalated segment instability. *Scand J Plast Reconstr Surg Hand Surg* 2002;36:189–191.

90. O'Dwyer KJ, Jefferiss CD. Scaphoid exostosis causing rupture of the flexor pollicis longus. *Acta Orthop Belg* 1994;60:124–126.

91. Zangger P, Simmen BR. Spontaneous ruptures of flexor tendons secondary to extreme DISI deformity of the lunate in a rheumatoid wrist. A case report. *Ann Chir Main Memb Super* 1993;12:250–256.

92. Moore JR, Weiland AJ, Valdata L. Tendon ruptures in the rheumatoid hand: analysis of treatment and functional results in 60 patients. *J Hand Surg* 1987;12:9–14.

93. Ferlic DC. Rheumatoid flexor tenosynovitis and rupture. *Hand Clin* 1996;12:561–572.

94. Valeri G, Ferrara C, Ercolani P, et al. Tendon involvement in rheumatoid arthritis of the wrist: MRI findings. *Skeletal Radiol* 2001;30:138–143.

95. Wilson RL, DeVito MC. Extensor tendon problems in rheumatoid arthritis. *Hand Clin* 1996;12:551–559.

96. Neurath M, Stofft E. Ultrastructural causes of ruptures of hand tendons in patients with rheumatoid arthritis. A transmission and scanning electron microscopic study. *Scand J Plast Reconstr Surg* 1993;27:59–65.

97. Rubens DJ, Blebea JS, Totterman SM, et al. Rheumatoid arthritis: evaluation of wrist extensor tendons with clinical examination versus MR imaging—a preliminary report. *Radiology* 1993;187:831–838.

98. Williamson SC, Feldon P. Extensor tendon ruptures in rheumatoid arthritis. *Hand Clin* 1995;11:449–459.

99. Potter T, Kuhns J. Rheumatoid tenosynovitis. Diagnosis and treatment. *J Bone Joint Surg* 1958;40:1230–1235.

100. Ehrlich G, Peterson L, Sokoloff L. Pathogenesis of rupture of extensor tendons at the wrist in rheumatoid arthritis. *Arthritis Rheum* 1959;2:332–346.

101. Ryu J, Saito S, Honda T, et al. Risk factors and prophylactic tenosynovectomy for extensor tendon ruptures in the rheumatoid hand. *J Hand Surg* 1998;23:658–661.

102. Williamson L, Mowat A, Burge P. Screening for extensor tendon rupture in rheumatoid arthritis. *Rheumatology (Oxford)* 2001;40:420–423.

103. Millender L, Nalebuff E, Holdsworth D. Posterior interosseus nerve syndrome secondary to rheumatoid arthritis. *J Bone Joint Surg* 1973;55:753–757.

104. Massarotti E. Medical aspects of rheumatoid arthritis: diagnosis and treatment. *Hand Clin* 1996;12:463–475.

105. Sharp J, Wolfe F, Mitchell D, et al. The progression of erosion and joint space narrowing scores in rheumatoid arthritis during the first twenty-five years of the disease. *Arthritis Rheum* 1991;34:660–664.

106. Pinals R, Baum J, Bland J, et al. Preliminary criteria for clinical remission in rheumatoid arthritis. *Arthritis Rheum* 1981;24:7–10.

107. Porter D, McInnes I, Hunter J, et al. Outcome of second line therapy in rheumatoid arthritis. *Ann Rheum Dis* 1994;53:812–815.

108. Breedveld FC. Current and future management approaches for rheumatoid arthritis. *Arthritis Res* 2002;4[Suppl 2]:S16–S21.

109. Jobanputra P, Barton P, Bryan S, et al. The effectiveness of infliximab and etanercept for the treatment of rheumatoid arthritis: a systematic review and economic evaluation. *Health Technol Assess* 2002;6:1–110.

110. Abuzakouk M, Feighery C, Jackson J. Tumor necrosis factor blocking agents: a new therapeutic modality for inflammatory disorders. *Br J Biomed Sci* 2002;59:173–179.

111. Bresnihan B. Preventing joint damage as the best measure of biologic drug therapy. *J Rheumatol* 2002;29[Suppl 65]:39–43.

112. Geborek P, Crnkic M, Petersson IF, et al. Etanercept, infliximab, and leflunomide in established rheumatoid arthritis: clinical experience using a structured follow up program in southern Sweden. *Ann Rheum Dis* 2002;61:793–798.

113. Shanahan JC, St. Clair W. Tumor necrosis factor-alpha blockade: a novel therapy for rheumatic disease. *Clin Immunol* 2002;103:231–242.

114. Weisman MH. What are the risks of biologic therapy in rheumatoid arthritis? An update on safety. *J Rheumatol Suppl* 2002;65:33–38.

115. Souter W. Planning treatment of the rheumatoid hand. *Hand* 1979;11:3.

116. Bridges SJ, Lopez-Mendez A, Han K, et al. Should methotrexate be discontinued before elective orthopedic surgery in patients with RA. *J Rheumatol* 1991;19:984–988.

117. Perhala R, Wilke W, Clough J, et al. Infectious complications following large joint replacement in RA patients treated with methotrexate versus those not treated with methotrexate. *Arthritis Rheum* 1991;34:146–152.

118. Tubiana R. Technique of dorsal synovectomy on the rheumatoid wrist. *Ann Chir Main Memb Super* 1990;9:138–145.

119. Millender LH, Nalebuff EA. Preventive surgery—tenosynovectomy and synovectomy. *Orthop Clin North Am* 1975;6:765–792.

120. Clayton ML, Ferlic DC. The wrist in rheumatoid arthritis. *Clin Orthop* 1975;106:192–197.

121. Wilkinson MC. Synovectomy for rheumatoid arthritis. *Clin Orthop* 1974;100:125–142.

122. Nicolle FV, Holt PJ, Calnan JS. Prophylactic synovectomy of the joints of the rheumatoid hand. Clinical trial with 4 to 8-year follow-up. *Ann Rheum Dis* 1971;30:476–480.

123. Kessler I, Vainio K. Posterior (dorsal) synovectomy for rheumatoid involvement of the hand and wrist. A follow-up study of sixty-six procedures. *J Bone Joint Surg* 1966;48:1085–1094.

124. Shott S. Effect of early synovectomy on the course of rheumatoid arthritis. *J Rheumatol* 1993;20:199.

125. Allieu Y, Lussiez B, Asencio G. Long-term results of surgical synovectomies of the rheumatoid wrist. Apropos of 60 cases. *Rev Chir Orthop Reparatrice Appar Mot* 1989;75:172–178.

126. Vahvanen V, Patiala H. Synovectomy of the wrist in rheumatoid arthritis and related diseases. A follow-up study of 97 consecutive cases. *Arch Orthop Trauma Surg* 1984;102:230–237.

127. Thirupathi RG, Ferlic DC, Clayton ML. Dorsal wrist synovectomy in rheumatoid arthritis—a long-term study. *J Hand Surg* 1983;8:848–856.

128. Edstrom B, Lugnegard H, Syk B. Late synovectomy of the hand in rheumatoid arthritis. *Scand J Rheumatol* 1976;5:184–190.

129. Wei N, Delauter SK, Beard S, et al. Office-based arthroscopic synovectomy of the wrist in rheumatoid arthritis. *Arthroscopy* 2001;17:884–887.

130. Adolfsson L, Frisen M. Arthroscopic synovectomy of the rheumatoid wrist. A 3.8 year follow-up. *J Hand Surg* 1997;22:711–713.

131. Adolfsson L, Nylander G. Arthroscopic synovectomy of the rheumatoid wrist. *J Hand Surg* 1993;18:92–96.

132. Roth JH, Poehling GG. Arthroscopic "-ectomy" surgery of the wrist. *Arthroscopy* 1990;6:141–147.

133. Berger RA, Bishop AT. A fiber-splitting capsulotomy technique for dorsal exposure of the wrist. *Tech Hand Upper Extremity Surg* 1997;1:2–10.

134. Alnot JY, Leroux D. Realignment stabilization synovectomy in the rheumatoid wrist. A study of twenty-five cases. *Ann Chir Main* 1985;4:294–305.

135. Chantelot C, Fontaine C, Jardin C, et al. Radiographic course of 39 rheumatoid wrists after synovectomy and stabilization. *Chir Main* 1998;17:236–244.

136. Resnick D. Why the ulnar styloid? *Radiology* 1974;112:29–35.

137. Linscheid RL, Dobyns JH. Rheumatoid arthritis of the wrist. *Orthop Clin North Am* 1971;2:192–197.

138. Spinner M, Kaplan E. Extensor carpi ulnaris: its relationship to the stability of the distal radioulnar joint. *Clin Orthop* 1970;68:124–129.

139. Weiler P, Bogoch ER. Kinematics of the distal radioulnar joint in rheumatoid arthritis: an in vivo study using centrode analysis. *J Hand Surg* 1995;20:937–943.

140. Clawson MC, Stern PJ. The distal radioulnar joint complex in rheumatoid arthritis: an overview. *Hand Clin* 1991;7:373–381.

141. Vaughan-Jackson O. Attrition rupture of tendons in the rheumatoid hand. *J Bone Joint Surg* 1958;40:1431.

142. O'Donovan TM, Ruby LK. The distal radioulnar joint in rheumatoid arthritis. *Hand Clin* 1989;5(2):249–256.

143. Darrach W. Fractures of the lower extremity of the radius: diagnosis and treatment. *JAMA* 1927;89:1683–1685.

144. Smith-Peterson M, Aufranc O, Larson C. Useful surgical procedures for rheumatoid arthritis involving joints of the upper extremity. *Arch Surg* 1943;46:764–770.

145. Brumfield RH Jr, Conaty JP, Mays JD. Surgery of the wrist in rheumatoid arthritis. *Clin Orthop* 1979;142:159–163.

146. Eiken O, Haga T, Salgeback S. Assessment of surgery of the rheumatoid wrist. *Scand J Plast Reconstr Surg* 1975;9:207–215.

147. Fraser KE, Diao E, Peimer CA, et al. Comparative results of resection of the distal ulna in rheumatoid arthritis and post-traumatic conditions. *J Hand Surg* 1999;24:667–670.

148. Gschwend N. The rheumatic hand. *Orthopaedics* 1998;27:167–174.

149. Linscheid RL. Surgery for rheumatoid arthritis—timing and techniques: the upper extremity. *J Bone Joint Surg* 1968;50:605–613.

150. Mannerfelt L. Surgical treatment of the rheumatoid wrist and aspects of the natural course when untreated. *Clin Rheum Dis* 1984;10:549–570.

151. Melone CP Jr, Taras JS. Distal ulna resection, extensor carpi ulnaris tenodesis, and dorsal synovectomy for the rheumatoid wrist. *Hand Clin* 1991;7:335–343.

152. Nalebuff EA, Garrod KJ. Present approach to the severely involved rheumatoid wrist. *Orthop Clin North Am* 1984;15:369–380.

153. Straub LR, Ranawat CS. The wrist in rheumatoid arthritis. Surgical treatment and results. *J Bone Joint Surg* 1969;51:1–20.

154. Taleisnik J. Rheumatoid arthritis of the wrist. *Hand Clin* 1989;5:257–278.

155. Tubiana R, Toth B. Rheumatoid arthritis: clinical types of deformities and management. *Clin Rheum Dis* 1984;10:521–548.

156. Vainio K. Surgery of rheumatoid arthritis. *Surg Ann* 1974;6:309–335.

157. Brumfield RH, Kushner S, Gellman H. Results of dorsal wrist synovectomies in the rheumatoid hand. *J Hand Surg* 1990;15:612–617.

158. Tulipan D, Eaton R, Eberhart R. The Darrach procedure defended: technique redefined and long-term follow-up. *J Hand Surg* 1991;16:438–444.

159. Bieber E, Linscheid RL, Dobyns JH. Failed distal ulna resections. *J Hand Surg* 1988;13:193–200.

160. Kleinman WB, Greenberg JA. Salvage of the failed Darrach procedure. *J Hand Surg* 1995;20:951–958.

161. Tsai TM, Shimizu H, Adkins P. A modified extensor carpi ulnaris tenodesis with the Darrach procedure. *J Hand Surg* 1993;18:697–702.

162. Black R, Boswick JJ, Wiedel J. Dislocation of the wrist in rheumatoid arthritis: the relationship to distal ulnar resection. *Clin Orthop* 1977;124:184–188.

163. Ishikawa H, Hanyu T, Tajima T. Rheumatoid wrists treated with synovectomy of the extensor tendons and the wrist joint combined with a Darrach procedure. *J Hand Surg* 1992;17:1109–1117.

164. Bowers WH. Distal radioulnar joint arthroplasty: the hemiresection-interposition technique. *J Hand Surg* 1985;10:169–178.

165. Watson HK, Ryu JY, Burgess RC. Matched distal ulnar resection. *J Hand Surg* 1986;11:812–817.

166. Sauvée-Kapandji A. Nouvelle technique the traitement chirurgical des luxations recidivantes isolee de l'extremite inferieur du cubitus. *J Chir* 1936;47:589–594.

167. Ferlic DC, Clayton ML. Synovectomy of the hand and wrist. *Ann Chir Gynaecol Suppl* 1985;198:26–30.

168. Milroy P, Coleman S, Iver R. The Sauve-Kapandji procedure: technique and results. *J Hand Surg* 1992;17:411–414.

169. Taleisnik J. The Sauve-Kapandji procedure. *Clin Orthop* 1992;275:110–23.

170. Vincent KA, Szabo RM, Agee JM. The Sauve-Kapandji procedure for reconstruction of the rheumatoid distal radioulnar joint. *J Hand Surg* 1993;18:978–983.

171. Low CK, Chew WY. Results of Sauve-Kapandji procedure. *Singapore Med J* 2002;43:135–137.

172. Chantelot C, Feugas C, Strouck G, et al. Stability of the forearm after resection of the distal ulna and proximal radius in rheumatoid arthritis: report of 11 cases. *Chir Main* 2002;21:1–4.

173. Ruby LK, Ferenz CC, Dell PC. The pronator quadratus interposition transfer: an adjunct to resection arthroplasty of the distal radioulnar joint. *J Hand Surg* 1996;21:60–65.

174. Gainor B, Schaberg J. The rheumatoid wrist after resection of the distal ulna. *J Hand Surg* 1985;10:837–844.

175. Swanson AB. Implant arthroplasty for disabilities of the distal radioulnar joint. Use of a silicone rubber capping implant following resection of the ulnar head. *Orthop Clin North Am* 1973;4:373–382.

176. Sagerman SD, Seiler JG, Fleming LL, et al. Silicone rubber distal ulnar replacement arthroplasty. *J Hand Surg* 1992;17:689–693.

177. McMurtry RY, Paley D, Marks P, et al. A critical analysis of Swanson ulnar head replacement arthroplasty: rheumatoid versus nonrheumatoid. *J Hand Surg* 1990;15:224–231.

178. Scheker LR, Babb BA, Killion PE. Distal ulnar prosthetic replacement. *Orthop Clin North Am* 2001;32:365–376.

179. Kapandji AI. Distal radio-ulnar prosthesis. *Ann Chir Main Memb Super* 1992;11:320–332.

180. van Schoonhoven J, Fernandez DL, Bowers WH, et al. Salvage of failed resection arthroplasties of the distal radioulnar joint using a new ulnar head prosthesis. *J Hand Surg* 2000;25:438–446.

181. Rothwell AG, O'Neill L, Cragg K. Sauve-Kapandji procedure for disorders of the distal radioulnar joint: a simplified technique. *J Hand Surg* 1996;21:771–777.

182. Allieu Y, Brahin B, Asencio G, et al. The surgical treatment of the rheumatoid wrist. Current perspectives. *Ann Chir Main* 1984;3:58–65.

183. Clayton ML. Surgical treatment at the wrist in rheumatoid arthritis. *J Bone Joint Surg* 1965;47:741–750.

184. Kirschner P. Results after arthrodeses of the wrist joint. *Aktuelle Probl Chir Orthop* 1977;2:87–92.

185. Kulick RG, De Fiore JC, Straub LR, et al. Long-term results of dorsal stabilization in the rheumatoid wrist. *J Hand Surg* 1981;6:272–280.

186. Linclau L, Dokter G. Operative treatment of dorsal lesions of the wrist in rheumatoid arthritis. *Acta Orthop Belg* 1988;54:185–188.

187. Osterman AL, Hood J. Synovectomy, arthroplasty, and arthrodesis in the reconstruction of the rheumatoid wrist and hand. *Curr Opin Rheumatol* 1991;3:102–108.

188. Chamay A, Della Santa D, Vilaseca A. Radiolunate arthrodesis. Factor of stability for the rheumatoid wrist. *Ann Chir Main* 1983;2:5–17.

189. Linscheid RL, Dobyns JH. Radiolunate arthrodesis. *J Hand Surg* 1985;10:821–829.

190. Chamay AG. Radiolunate arthrodesis in the rheumatoid wrist. *J Hand Surg* 1986;11:771.

191. Della Santa D, Chamay A. Radiological evolution of the rheumatoid wrist after radio-lunate arthrodesis. *J Hand Surg* 1995;20:146–154.

192. Doets HC, Raven EE. A procedure for stabilizing and preserving mobility in the arthritic wrist. *J Bone Joint Surg* 1999;81:1013–1016.

193. Hagena FW, Siekmann W, Refior HJ. Extension of the "dorsal wrist stabilization" by radio-ulnar arthrodeses in chronic polyarthritis. *Aktuelle Probl Chir Orthop* 1989;37:89–94.

194. Halikis MN, Colello-Abraham K, Taleisnik J. Radiolunate fusion. The forgotten partial arthrodesis. *Clin Orthop* 1997;341:30–35.

195. Hulsbergen-Kruger S, Partecke B. Intercarpal and radiocarpal resection arthroplasty and arthrodesis. *Orthopaedics* 1999;28:899–906.

196. Inoue G, Tamura Y. Radiolunate and radioscapholunate arthrodesis. *Arch Orthop Trauma Surg* 1992;111:333–335.

197. Ishikawa H, Hanyu T, Saito H, et al. Limited arthrodesis for the rheumatoid wrist. *J Hand Surg* 1992;17:1103–1109.

198. Minami A, Kato H, Iwasaki N, et al. Limited wrist fusions: comparison of results 22 and 89 months after surgery. *J Hand Surg* 1999;24:133–137.

199. Rittmeister M, Kandziora F, Rehart S, et al. Radio-lunar Mannerfelt arthrodesis in rheumatoid arthritis. *Handchir Mikrochir Plast Chir* 1999;31:266–273.

200. Stanley JK, Boot DA. Radio-lunate arthrodesis. *J Hand Surg* 1989;14:283–287.

201. Chamay A, Della Santa D. Radiolunate arthrodesis in rheumatoid wrist (21 cases). *Ann Chir Main Memb Super* 1991;10:197–206.

202. Evans DM, Ansell BM, Hall MA. The wrist in juvenile arthritis. *J Hand Surg* 1991;16:293–304.

203. Taleisnik J. Combined radiocarpal arthrodesis and midcarpal (lunocapitate) arthroplasty for treatment of rheumatoid arthritis of the wrist. *J Hand Surg* 1987;12:1–8.

204. Vicar AJ, Burton RI. Surgical management of the rheumatoid wrist—fusion or arthroplasty. *J Hand Surg* 1986;11:790–797.

205. Cobb TK, Beckenbaugh RD. Biaxial total-wrist arthroplasty. *J Hand Surg* 1996;21:1011–1021.

206. Fourastier J, Le Breton L, Alnot Y, et al. Guépar's total radio-carpal prosthesis in the surgery of the rheumatoid wrist. Apropos of 72 cases reviewed. *Rev Chir Orthop Reparatrice Appar Mot* 1996;82:108–115.

207. Menon J. Universal total wrist implant: experience with a carpal component fixed with three screws. *J Arthroplasty* 1998;13:515–523.

208. Meuli HC. Total wrist arthroplasty. Experience with a non-cemented wrist prosthesis. *Clin Orthop* 1997;342:77–83.

209. Adams B. Total wrist arthroplasty. *Semin Arthroplast* 2000;11:72–81.

210. Rossello MI, Costa M, Pizzorno V. Experience of total wrist arthroplasty with Silastic implants plus grommets. *Clin Orthop* 1997;342:64–70.

211. Stanley JK, Tolat AR. Long-term results of Swanson Silastic arthroplasty in the rheumatoid wrist. *J Hand Surg* 1993;18:381–388.

212. McCombe PF, Millroy PJ. Swanson Silastic wrist arthroplasty. A retrospective study of fifteen cases. *J Hand Surg* 1985;10:199–201.

213. Summers B, Hubbard MJ. Wrist joint arthroplasty in rheumatoid arthritis: a comparison between the Meuli and Swanson prostheses. *J Hand Surg* 1984;9:171–176.

214. Barbier O, Saels P, Rombouts JJ, et al. Long-term functional results of wrist arthrodesis in rheumatoid arthritis. *J Hand Surg* 1999;24:27–31.

215. Howard AC, Stanley D, Getty CJ. Wrist arthrodesis in rheumatoid arthritis. A comparison of two methods of fusion. *J Hand Surg* 1993;18:377–380.

216. Kobus RJ, Turner RH. Wrist arthrodesis for treatment of rheumatoid arthritis. *J Hand Surg* 1990;15:541–546.

217. Mikkelsen OA. Arthrodesis of the wrist joint in rheumatoid arthritis. *Hand* 1980;12:149–153.

218. Millender LH, Nalebuff EA. Arthrodesis of the rheumatoid wrist. An evaluation of sixty patients and a description of a different surgical technique. *J Bone Joint Surg* 1973;55:1026–1034.

219. Papaioannou T, Dickson RA. Arthrodesis of the wrist in rheumatoid disease. *Hand* 1982;14:12–16.

220. Pech J, Sosna A, Rybka V, et al. Wrist arthrodesis in rheumatoid arthritis. A new technique using internal fixation. *J Bone Joint Surg* 1996;78:783–786.

221. Rechnagel K. Arthrodesis of the wrist joint. A follow-up study of sixty cases. *Scand J Plast Reconstr Surg* 1971;5:120–123.

222. Skak SV. Arthrodesis of the wrist by the method of Mannerfelt. A follow-up of 19 patients. *Acta Orthop Scand* 1982;53:557–559.

223. Stanley JK, Hullin MG. Wrist arthrodesis as part of composite surgery of the hand. *J Hand Surg* 1986;11:243–244.

224. Vahvanen V, Tallroth K. Arthrodesis of the wrist by internal fixation in rheumatoid arthritis: a follow-up study of forty-five consecutive cases. *J Hand Surg* 1984;9:531–536.

225. Zenz P, Obrovsky M, Schwagerl W. Mannerfelt arthrodesis of the wrist joint in patients with chronic polyarthritis. A retrospective analysis of 24 cases. *Z Orthop Ihre Grenzgeb* 1999;137:512–515.

226. Cooney WP III, Beckenbaugh RD, Linscheid RL. Total wrist arthroplasty. Problems with implant failures. *Clin Orthop* 1984;187:121–128.

227. Rayan GM, Brentlinger A, Purnell D, et al. Functional assessment of bilateral wrist arthrodeses. *J Hand Surg* 1987;12:1020–1024.

228. Brumfield RH, Champoux JA. A biomechanical study of normal functional wrist motion. *Clin Orthop* 1984;187:23–25.

229. Larsson SE. Compression arthrodesis of the wrist. A consecutive series of 23 cases. *Clin Orthop* 1974;99:146–153.

230. Pryce JC. The wrist position between neutral and ulnar deviation that facilitates the maximum power grip strength. *J Biomech* 1980;13:505–511.

231. Hastings DE, Evans JA. Rheumatoid wrist deformities and their relation to ulnar drift. *J Bone Joint Surg* 1975;57:930–934.

232. Mannerfelt L, Malmsten M. Arthrodesis of the wrist in rheumatoid arthritis. A technique without external fixation. *Scand J Plast Reconstr Surg* 1971;5:124–130.

233. Rayan GM. Wrist arthrodesis. *J Hand Surg* 1986;11:356–364.

234. Christodoulou L, Patwardhan MS, Burke FD. Open and closed arthrodesis of the rheumatoid wrist using a modified (Stanley) Steinmann pin. *J Hand Surg* 1999;24:662–666.

235. Lee DH, Carroll RE. Wrist arthrodesis: a combined intra-medullary pin and autogenous iliac crest bone graft technique. *J Hand Surg* 1994;19:733–740.

236. Juutilainen T, Patiala H. Arthrodesis in rheumatoid arthritis using absorbable screws and rods. *Scand J Rheumatol* 1995;24:228–233.

237. Lenoble E, Ovadia H, Goutallier D. Wrist arthrodesis using an embedded iliac crest bone graft. *J Hand Surg* 1993;18:595–600.

238. Hartigan BJ, Nagle DJ, Foley MJ. Wrist arthrodesis with excision of the proximal carpal bones using the AO/ASIF wrist fusion plate and local bone graft. *J Hand Surg* 2001;26:247–251.

239. Hastings H II, Weiss AP, Quenzer D, et al. Arthrodesis of the wrist for post-traumatic disorders. *J Bone Joint Surg* 1996;78:897–902.

240. Rehak DC, Kasper P, Baratz ME, et al. A comparison of plate and pin fixation for arthrodesis of the rheumatoid wrist. *Orthopedics* 2000;23:43–48.

241. Reference deleted.

242. Vahvanen V, Kettunen P. Arthrodesis of the wrist in rheumatoid arthritis. A follow-up study of 62 cases. *Ann Chir Gynaecol* 1977;66:195–202.

243. Bora FW Jr, Osterman AL, Thomas VJ, et al. The treatment of ruptures of multiple extensor tendons at wrist level by a free tendon graft in the rheumatoid patient. *J Hand Surg* 1987;12:1038–1040.

244. Goldner J. Tendon transfers in rheumatoid arthritis. *Orthop Clin North Am* 1974;5:425–444.

245. Nalebuff EA, Patel MR. Flexor digitorum sublimis transfer for multiple extensor tendon ruptures in rheumatoid arthritis. *Plast Reconstr Surg* 1973;52:530–533.

246. Nalebuff E. Surgical treatment of tendon rupture in the rheumatoid hand. *Surg Clin North Am* 1969;49:799–809.

247. Pulvertaft G. Surgery in the treatment of the rheumatoid hand. *Postgrad Med J* 1964;35:113.

248. Walker LG. Flexor pollicis longus rupture in rheumatoid arthritis secondary to attrition on a sesamoid. *J Hand Surg* 1993;18:990–991.

249. Ferlic DC, Clayton ML, Mills M. Proximal row carpectomy: a review of rheumatoid and non-rheumatoid patients. *J Hand Surg* 1991;16:420–424.

250. Koneczny O. Corium-plasty of the wrist joint. *Handchir Mikrochir Plast Chir* 1989;21:79–84.

251. Raunio P. The role of non-prosthetic surgery in the treatment of rheumatoid arthritis by fusions and auto-arthroplasties. Current practice at the Rheumatism Foundation Hospital, Heinola. *Ann Chir Gynaecol Suppl* 1985;198:96–102.

252. Tillmann K, Thabe H. Technique and results of resection and interposition arthroplasty of the wrist in rheumatoid arthritis. *Reconstr Surg Traumatol* 1981;18:84–91.

253. Stellbrink G, Tillmann K. Resection-interposition arthroplasty of the wrist joint in chronic polyarthritis (proceedings). *Z Rheumatol* 1976;35[Suppl 4]:530–534.

254. Boeckx WD, De Lorenzi F, van der Hulst RR, et al. Free fascia temporalis interpositioning as a treatment for wrist ankylosis. *J Reconstr Microsurg* 2002;18:269–274.

255. Stanley JK, Lluch A, Herren DB, et al. Universal wrist classification in inflammatory polyarthropathy *(in preparation)*.

70

CRYSTALLINE ARTHRITIS AND OTHER ARTHRITIDES

YOUSAF ALI

GOUT

Definition and Classification

Gout is a syndrome that is characterized by intermittent, acute swelling of the joints that is due to an inflammatory response to monosodium urate (MSU) crystals. Although the host response to MSU crystals is variable, the disease manifests in only a limited number of ways:

- Acute gouty arthritis
- Accumulation of crystalline-rich aggregates (tophi)
- Renal dysfunction (gouty nephropathy)

Pathogenesis

The development of hyperuricemia that results in clinical events occurs via two discrete mechanisms. Underexcretion of uric acid is the most common metabolic defect and, although not fully understood, occurs because of a genetic abnormality at least in certain patients (1,2). Approximately 85% of patients with gout are underexcretors of uric acid, with a urate clearance of less than 6 mL per minute. This is important to know from a therapeutic standpoint, because drugs can be used to accelerate uric acid loss if the daily tubular excretion is diminished. Occasionally, overproduction of uric acid occurs and is associated with an excess of purine precursors from dietary causes or from abnormal handling of urate. In a small minority of patients, inherited dysregulation of purine metabolism accounts for hyperuricemia. In 1964, a familial disorder of urate overproduction that was combined with neurologic dysfunction and self-mutilation was described and was traced to a deficiency in hypoxanthine guanine phosphoribosyl transferase. This rare disease, which is termed *Lesch-Nyhan syndrome*, results in excessive production of uric acid and juvenile onset of gout (3).

Renal handling of uric acid remains the key factor in the development of hyperuricemia. Hence, classification schemes can be subdivided into the mechanism that is responsible for the elevation of uric acid: overproduction or underexcretion. This scheme is a useful tool for the clinician when attempting to correct the underlying cause and direct therapy (Table 1).

The response of cells (usually polymorphonuclear leukocytes) to the presence of MSU crystals is pivotal in the pathophysiology of acute gouty arthritis. During an attack, an activation of signal transduction pathways occurs that leads to rapid neutrophil influx. Chemotactic factors, such as interleukin-1 (IL-1), IL-6, and tumor necrosis factor (TNF), perpetuate this process and result in the systemic features that are commonly observed (e.g., fever, swelling, leukocytosis) (4).

Epidemiology

Gout is predominantly a disease of middle-aged men. It is rare in children and premenopausal women. The peak age of onset in men is between 40 and 50 years of age and in women is after 60 years of age. Because the prevalence of the disease varies with age and increasing serum urate levels, estimates of prevalence vary widely. In men, it is estimated to occur in 5 to 28 of 1,000 men, and, in women, it occurs in 1 to 6 of 1,000 women (5). The annual incidence is estimated at 1 to 3 of 1,000 and 0.2 of 1,000 in men and women, respectively.

Clinical Significance and Natural History

Gout is characterized by three distinct stages: asymptomatic hyperuricemia, acute intermittent gout and chronic tophaceous gout. The latter stage usually develops after 10 to 15 years of intermittent gout. Although most people with hyperuricemia do not develop gout, data from the Normative Aging Study showed that serum levels of uric acid between 7 and 8 mg per dL had a cumulative incidence of gouty arthritis of 3%. In subjects with levels greater than 9 mg per dL, the 5-year incidence rose to 22% (6). From this study, it appears that not only the age of the subject but

TABLE 1. ACQUIRED CAUSES OF HYPERURICEMIA

Urate overproduction	Urate underproduction
Hypoxanthine guanine phosphoribosyl transferase deficiency	Idiopathic
	Enhanced tubular reabsorption
	Azotemia
5-phospho-α-D-ribosyl pyrophosphate synthetase superactivity	Lead nephropathy (saturnine gout)
	Acidosis
Nutritional (excess dietary purines)	Hyperparathyroidism, hypothyroidism
Fructose administration	Drugs: diuretics, cyclosporin,
Myeloproliferative disorders	nicotinic acid, pyrazinamide,
Lymphoproliferative disorders	low-dose aspirin, ethambutol
Alcohol abuse	
Psoriasis	

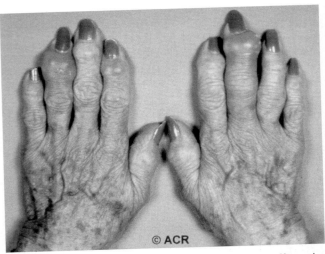

FIGURE 1. Hands of a patient with acute gout that affects the distal interphalangeal joints. (Reprinted from the Clinical Slide Collection on the Rheumatic Diseases, with permission from the American College of Rheumatology.)

also the degree of hyperuricemia seem to be important in predicting the clinical outcome.

The risk of damage outside the musculoskeletal system is not insignificant. Approximately 10% of patients with gout develop uric acid–containing stones, and this may rise to as high as 50% in patients with a serum urate levels that are greater than 13 g per dL. Obesity, hypertension, and hypertriglyceridemia are also often found in patients with gout.

If untreated, subcutaneous tophi can also develop; they have a propensity toward the fingers, wrists, olecranon bursae, and Achilles tendons and occasionally require surgical removal.

Evaluation

> The victim goes to bed and sleeps in good health. About two o'clock in the morning he is awakened by pain in the great toe…the night is passed in torture, sleeplessness, turning of the part affected and perpetual change of posture.

Sydenham's classic description demonstrates the clinical scenario that is typically associated with gout (7). Patients usually develop severe pain in the affected joint, which becomes warm, red, and swollen. Typically, the attacks are monoarticular and begin abruptly. Occasionally, nonarticular structures, such as the olecranon bursa and Achilles tendon, are involved. Generally, most attacks are self-limited and resolve within 7 to 10 days.

Because the solubility of MSU crystals is diminished at lower temperatures, gout has a predilection for acral areas. The joints that are most commonly involved in gout include the first metatarsophalangeal joint (podagra), the insteps, the ankles, the heels, the knees, the wrists, and the elbows. Alcohol ingestion, trauma, or acute medical illness often precedes an attack. The surgical intern should have a high degree of suspicion in the febrile postoperative patient who develops a swollen, painful joint (Fig. 1).

Laboratory Features and Diagnosis

The preferred method for confirming the presence of acute gout is arthrocentesis of fresh synovial fluid. Because differentiation between sepsis and acute gouty arthritis is often difficult, aspiration is essential. The presence of intracellular, negatively birefringent, needle-shaped crystals is diagnostic for gout. Occasionally, uric acid crystals occur extracellularly as innocent bystanders; therefore, if there is any suspicion for septic arthritis, a culture should always be obtained.

The synovial fluid in acute gout is usually inflammatory with a predominance of neutrophils (a leukocyte count of 20,000 to 100,000). The serum uric acid is generally unhelpful during an attack, because this level is often normal. Hematologic indices often confirm acute inflammation, and patients frequently have elevated acute phase reactants (erythrocyte sedimentation rate and platelets). If the patient is being considered for uricosuric therapy, a 24-hour urine uric acid test can be obtained to confirm urinary underexcretion. Assuming the patient's diet is regular, the 24-hour excretion of uric acid should not exceed 800 mg per 24 hours.

Imaging Studies

Patients with gout typically have unremarkable radiographs early in the course of the disease. During an attack, soft tissue swelling is observed. After several years of exposure to uric acid crystals, tophi and erosions can be seen. Tophi appear as soft tissue densities that overlie the joint and can become calcified. The erosions typically have sclerotic margins with overhanging edges. Because of their appearance, they are occasionally referred to as *rat bite erosions*. Compared to rheumatoid arthritis (RA), gout is characterized by preservation of joint space and lack of osteopenia (Fig. 2).

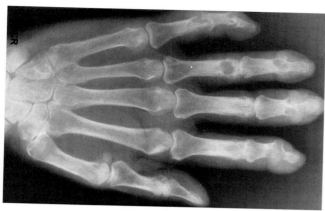

FIGURE 2. Roentgenogram that shows chronic tophaceous gout that results in overhanging edges and rat bite erosions. (Reprinted from the Clinical Slide Collection on the Rheumatic Diseases, with permission from the American College of Rheumatology.)

Treatment

Acute Gout

Patients who are in the midst of an acute attack of gout experience excruciating pain. Therapy should be rapid in onset, safe, and effective. Three choices exist: colchicine, nonsteroidal antiinflammatory drugs (NSAIDs), and corticosteroids (5). NSAIDs are most widely used and have a rapid onset of action but are unfortunately contraindicated in many patients. Indomethacin is frequently prescribed, but other NSAIDs may be equally effective (8).

Colchicine is an alkaloid that is derived from the plant *Colchicum autumnale* and has been used in the treatment of gout for more than two centuries (9). It acts by inhibiting polymerization of microtubules and inhibits neutrophil chemotaxis and phagocytosis. When used early on in the attack, it can be extremely effective. Unfortunately, gastrointestinal upset is the rule, and side effects include increased peristalsis, diarrhea, abdominal pain, and cramping. It is usually given orally at 0.6 mg hourly until significant side effects occur or the patient's symptoms subside. Generally, no more than 6 mg should be given at any one time, and further doses should be avoided for at least 7 days. To avoid the gastrointestinal side effects, colchicine may also be administered via the intravenous route. One milligram should be diluted in normal saline solution and can be repeated to a maximum dose of 3 mg. Because colchicine toxicity is potentially fatal and irreversible, this route should be administered only in patients with normal renal and hepatic function (10). Care should be taken not to allow extravasation of the drug, because a local chemical thrombophlebitis can occur.

In patients in whom colchicine and NSAIDs are contraindicated, systemic corticosteroids may be used. Generally, 20 to 40 mg daily of prednisone or its equivalent can be used for the initial attack, and then the drug can be tapered

off over the next few days. Another option is adrenocorticotrophic hormone, 40 to 80 IU intramuscularly every 6 to 12 hours, although there are few data to show its superiority over traditional therapy (11). Urate-lowering drugs, such as allopurinol, should be avoided in the acute setting, as fluctuations in urate levels can prolong or precipitate an attack.

Intermittent Gout

Because many patients are asymptomatic between attacks, the decision to intervene should be balanced against the daily requirement for urate-lowering medication and lifestyle change. Treatment can be initiated once reversible risk factors, such as alcohol and dehydration, are corrected. Most rheumatologists start hypouricemic therapy if the patient has more than three attacks per year, develops gouty nephropathy, or has asymptomatic hyperuricemia with urate levels greater than 12 mg per dL. If attacks occur despite a urate-lowering drug, the addition of once-daily colchicine should be considered, as it can reduce the frequency of attacks by 75% (12) (Fig. 3).

Chronic Tophaceous Gout

The goal of therapy in tophaceous gout is to allow resorption of tophi, such that erosive or compressive complications can be avoided. Solubilization of urate occurs at levels less than 5 mg per dL and can usually be achieved by allopurinol or uricosuric drugs, such as probenecid. Allopurinol is preferred, as it is effective in overproducers and underexcretors of uric acid. A dosage of 300 mg daily is

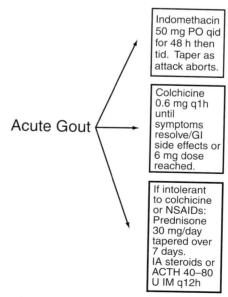

FIGURE 3. Management of acute gout. ACTH, adrenocorticotropic hormone; GI, gastrointestinal; IA, intraarticular; IM, intramuscular; NSAID, nonsteroidal antiinflammatory drug.

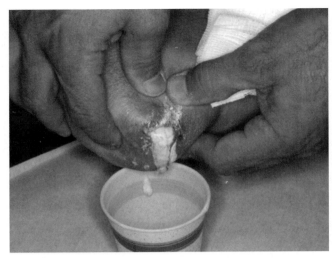

FIGURE 4. Tophaceous gouty material in the olecranon bursa: incorrect management.

usually adequate; however, this should be adjusted in patients with renal insufficiency or in the elderly (Fig. 4).

Surgical Approach to Gout

Generally, the management of gout is nonsurgical. Nevertheless, there are many case reports of tophi that cause compression of important structures and that have responded poorly to conventional therapy. Most commonly, tophi can become troublesome, depending on their location, and occasionally develop secondary infection that requires surgical débridement (13). In 1980, Gelberman et al. (14) described disruption of the extensor mechanism at the proximal interphalangeal (PIP) joint, which required tophectomy and reconstruction of the extensor tendon. Gouty tenosynovitis can present as infection, nerve compression, or digital stiffness (15). Moore described ten patients in whom extensive urate deposition was encountered in the extensor and flexor tendons at the wrist and digital theca. Operative intervention was required to debulk tophaceous deposits, to improve tendon gliding, and to ameliorate pain (16). Surgical intervention is also required when chronic gout results in carpal tunnel syndrome due to compression of the median nerve by tophaceous deposits (17).

CALCIUM PYROPHOSPHATE DIHYDRATE DEPOSITION

Definition and Classification

Calcium pyrophosphate dihydrate (CPPD) is a calcium-containing crystal that can deposit in joints, thus resulting in an acute inflammatory arthritis. This is also termed *pseudogout*. Most patients with CPPD arthritis are elderly, although there are certain metabolic disorders that appear to predispose to the condition. Strong associations have been shown to exist with hyperparathyroidism, hemochromatosis, amyloidosis, hypomagnesemia, and hypophosphatasia.

Pathogenesis

Acute pseudogout is caused by a release of CPPD crystals into the joint. Rapid phagocytosis of crystals by polymorphonuclear leukocytes ensues, and cytokine release activates the inflammatory cascade. Stimulated joint-lining cells secrete proteolytic enzymes, such as collagenase, which result in damage to the articular cartilage. Most patients with CPPD crystals have been shown to have elevated levels of synovial fluid inorganic phosphate. It has therefore been postulated that interaction with calcium-containing crystals occurs and results in CPPD deposition (18).

Epidemiology

Data on articular cartilage calcification (chondrocalcinosis) are derived mostly from radiographic surveys of the knee. Most studies suggest that the disease is predominantly in women, with a peak age of 65 to 75 years of age. The Framingham study showed an overall prevalence of 8% in people older than 63 years of age and as much as 27% in patients older than 85 years of age (19).

Clinical Significance and Natural History

Three presentations are commonly encountered: acute pseudogout, asymptomatic radiographic disease, and chronic arthritis. Acute attacks result in rapid inflammation of the joint and usually respond to aspiration alone. Generally, the pain subsides within 1 to 3 weeks. Polyarticular involvement may occur and usually requires longer therapy. In patients with relapsing disease, joint lavage may be required (20). Patients who develop a more chronic form of the disease generally have knee involvement with chronic stiffness and restricted movement. This occurs with or without superimposed acute attacks. The pattern of joint involvement typically results in severe degenerative changes at the metacarpophalangeal (MCP) joints, wrists, elbows, and shoulders. Unfortunately, a small percentage of elderly women develop a progressive, destructive arthropathy that may resemble Charcot's joints (21).

Evaluation

Acute pseudogout results in rapid swelling, pain, and warmth of the affected joint. The most common areas that are involved are, in descending order, the knee, wrist, MCP joint, hips, shoulders, elbows, and ankles. Compared to gout, the attacks tend to be less severe but are also precipitated by trauma and acute illness. Early morning stiffness, fatigue, and synovitis can accompany a small minority of patients, and the presence of these symptoms may cause confusion with RA. In these cases, it is vital to review all serologic and radiologic data to avoid unnecessary administration of potentially toxic immunosuppressive agents.

Laboratory Features

The diagnosis of pseudogout is confirmed by arthrocentesis. Polymorphonuclear neutrophil excess with intracellular, weakly positively birefringent, rod-shaped crystals are characteristic. Other lab values that are commonly seen include a peripheral leukocytosis and elevated acute phase reactants. Similar to gout, septic arthritis can coexist; thus, a Gram's stain and culture should always be obtained, particularly in the hospitalized patient.

Imaging Studies

Chondrocalcinosis is the term that is given to CPPD crystals when they deposit in cartilage. On radiographs, they are most commonly visualized in the triangular fibrocartilage of the wrist, the knee menisci, and the symphysis pubis. CPPD differs from osteoarthritis (OA) in that isolated patellofemoral or wrist disease is quite common. Calcific deposits are also seen in ligaments, tendons, and the articular capsule. They are usually punctate or linear in distribution and frequently occur parallel to the subchondral bone end plate.

Treatment

In most cases, arthrocentesis of the affected joint is adequate to abort an acute attack. Assuming that synovial fluid cultures are sterile, the author prefers a local corticosteroid injection (e.g., 20 to 40 mg of triamcinolone) that offers additional, more rapid relief of symptoms. Because patients are often hospitalized at the time of the attack, the affected limb should be rested, and topical ice may be helpful. Colchicine and NSAIDs may also be used but are often contraindicated in elderly patients with compromised renal and gastrointestinal function.

Unfortunately, unlike gout, there are no current therapies available to reverse or retard the deposition of CPPD crystals. Oral, daily colchicine can be used as prophylaxis in patients who have more frequent attacks. In patients who are younger than 55 years of age, secondary associated diseases, such as hyperparathyroidism and hemochromatosis, should be excluded.

Surgical Management

Pseudogout is managed medically. Exceptions include the presence of CPPD pseudotumor-causing median nerve compression and carpal tunnel syndrome (22,23). In 1995, Ishida described seven cases of massive focal CPPD deposition (tophaceous pseudogout) that presented as a mass or swelling. Surgical resection and observation under polarized microscope revealed CPPD crystals. The ages of patients ranged from 31 to 86 years of age and involved the temporomandibular, metatarsophalangeal, and hip joints and the cervical spine. Chondroid metaplasia was found in and around the areas of CPPD deposition. Some of these areas showed cellular atypia in chondrocytes that was suggestive of a malignant cartilage tumor (24). Surgeons and pathologists should be able to recognize this rare form of CPPD deposition disease and to identify crystals in the calcified deposits, thus avoiding the misdiagnosis of benign or malignant cartilaginous lesions.

OTHER CRYSTALS

A number of different crystals are identified within joints. Although many occur as innocent bystanders (e.g., cholesterol, oxalate), basic calcium phosphate (BCP) crystals tend to be associated with acute arthritis. There are four major manifestations of BCP crystals (25):

- Acute calcific periarthritis
- Calcific tendonitis
- Large-joint destructive arthropathy [Milwaukee shoulder syndrome (MSS)]
- OA

The true incidence of BCP arthritis is unknown, and, in most cases, the presence of periarticular calcification appears to represent a local process. The most common area to be affected appears to be the shoulder.

Natural History

Acute calcific periarthritis results in sudden onset of severe shoulder pain. Radiographs, although generally unremarkable, can show soft tissue swelling or calcification. Although the mechanism of inflammation is poorly understood, the crystals appear to gain access to the joint via dissolution of deposits in the rotator cuff (26). Due to the severity of the attacks, they are often confused with gout. Attacks can also occur around the small joints of the hands, and, in young women, this is often mistaken for gout (27). The absence of MSU crystals and the presence of calcification on x-rays distinguish it from gout. When the calcium deposits in the tendon sheaths, the syndrome is referred to as *calcific tendonitis*. This may be acute or chronic, depending on the coexistence of inflammation, and is generally diagnosed when calcific deposits are observed.

MSS occurs predominantly in elderly patients who manifest with pain and stiffness of one or both shoulders. Typically, the patients have glenohumeral joint degeneration

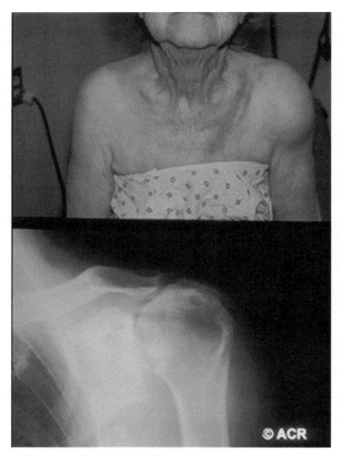

FIGURE 5. Milwaukee shoulder syndrome due to apatite crystals in an elderly patient. Note the radiographic glenohumeral joint destruction and large effusion. (Reprinted from the Clinical Slide Collection on the Rheumatic Diseases, with permission from the American College of Rheumatology.)

with blood-tinged large effusions. Synovial fluid analysis reveals noninflammatory fluid. This type of arthritis is associated with BCP crystals; although the role of BCP crystals is not clear, many investigators feel they are most likely an epiphenomenon. Approximately 50% of patients also have symptomatic knee involvement, with radiologic changes of OA usually involving the lateral compartment (28). Several factors predispose to the development of MSS. These include trauma, overuse, hemodialysis, and recurrent shoulder dislocation (Fig. 5).

The concurrence of OA and BCP crystals has been recognized for some time. Although the true incidence of BCP crystals in degenerative joints is unknown, it is estimated to be between 30% to 60% (29). It is currently a topic of debate whether BCP crystals are causative in OA or are present in the joint owing to cartilage breakdown.

Evaluation

Roentgenograms are the easiest way to detect calcific material in the joint. Unfortunately, soft tissue swelling may be the

only finding in calcific periarthritis, which makes the diagnosis tricky, particularly when arthrocentesis is not performed. Magnetic resonance imaging or arthrography can be useful to detect coexistent cuff tears but are generally not indicated clinically. Calcification often occurs in clumps and can be mistaken for ossification or small avulsion fractures.

Synovial fluid often resembles that of OA, although, occasionally, a chalklike or creamy material can be obtained. Unlike gout or CPPD arthritis, there is no reliable microscopic test. BCP crystals are not birefringent; however, they can be visualized with the addition of alizarin red S stain. Unfortunately, this stain is not widely available and is also associated with frequent false-positive results (30).

Treatment

NSAIDs are used to treat BCP-associated arthritis. Occasionally, needle aspiration is required to hasten recovery. This acts by disrupting deposits and accelerating phagocytosis. If large deposits are present, surgical intervention may be required to facilitate removal of calcium debris.

MSS is more problematic, mostly because the shoulder has undergone a significant amount of destruction by the time that the condition has been recognized. Because most patients are elderly, simple large-volume arthrocentesis and corticosteroid injections can temporize symptoms, but this usually results in progression of the disease. Caporeli et al. (31) were successful in alleviating symptoms by local tidal irrigation followed by methyl prednisone and tranexamic acid injection. Surgical intervention is also considered for refractory pain. Although there are no strict guidelines, some authorities prefer anterior acromioplasty and rotator cuff repair. If humeral head collapse has occurred, a total shoulder replacement and cuff repair are advised (32).

OTHER ARTHRITIDES

Psoriatic Arthritis

The arthritis that is associated with psoriasis is important to recognize, because the hand is commonly involved. Most typically, an inflammatory arthritis occurs in the setting of a negative rheumatoid factor (RF) and obvious skin disease. There are a variety of different presentations, although asymmetric oligoarticular disease is most frequently observed, followed by a pseudorheumatoid pattern, and then axial disease. If untreated, severe destruction of joints can occur, which results in arthritis mutilans.

Pathogenesis

The etiology of psoriatic arthritis is unclear. As with many autoimmune diseases, clinical expression occurs due to a combination of environmental, genetic, and immunologic factors. Initial studies revealed a high concordance rate of

70% in monozygotic twins, compared to 30% in dizygotic twins, which suggests a strong genetic basis for the disease (33). Immunologic studies have shown that patients who express the HLA-A26, -B38, and -DR4 antigens have an increased association with psoriatic arthritis. Because there is incomplete concordance among monozygotic twins, environmental factors must also play a role in disease pathogenesis. Cross reactivity of cutaneous components and bacterial antigens, such as *Streptococcus*, are purported to trigger disease in some individuals (34).

Most authorities believe that psoriasis is an autoreactive inflammatory disorder that is characterized by a T–helper 1 response in the skin (35). Histologic examination reveals an accumulation of T cells in the dermis of patients, which in turn produces inflammatory cytokines, such as IL-1, TNF, and transforming growth factors. Secretion of these intercellular messengers results in recruitment of inflammatory cells into the extravascular spaces of the dermis and subsequent synovial membrane proliferation. It is believed that the process that results in psoriatic skin lesions is similar to that of psoriatic arthritis (36).

Epidemiology

Approximately 7% of patients with psoriasis develop arthritis. The overall prevalence of the disease in the United States is 0.1% (37). The male to female ratio is equal; however, it appears to be uncommon in Asians and African blacks. Women tend to have more symmetric disease, and men have more axial inflammation.

Clinical Significance and Natural History

Approximately 95% of patients with psoriatic arthritis have peripheral joint disease. The most common presentation is that of a patient with known psoriasis who develops large-joint oligoarthritis followed by distal interphalangeal (DIP) involvement. Dactylitis is also common and results in the typical sausage digit, which can be surprisingly transient and involves the whole length of the digit owing to tendon sheath inflammation.

It is still widely accepted that RA has a more aggressive course than psoriatic arthritis. Earlier data are conflicting: Gladman et al. (38), in Toronto, analyzed 220 patients with psoriatic arthritis and showed that at least 10% of patients develop severe disability (American Rheumatism Association functional class IV). A more recent study from Minnesota suggested that psoriatic arthritis is a mild, uncommon disease with no significant increase in mortality (39).

Evaluation

Approximately 70% of patients have psoriasis many years before they develop arthritis. Rarely, the arthritis precedes the skin disease, and, in these cases, a careful cutaneous skin

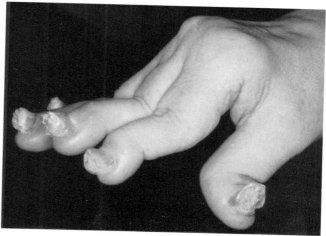

FIGURE 6. Psoriatic arthritis. A patient with characteristic nail-bed changes and rheumatoidlike features with swan-neck deformities.

exam sometimes reveals digital pitting, which is a helpful clue. Often, the pattern of disease (i.e., oligoarticular inflammation without systemic symptoms and a negative RF) should alert the physician to the possibility of psoriatic arthritis or spondyloarthropathy.

Although most patients present with inflammation of fewer than four joints, a symmetric polyarthritis that affects the MCP and PIP joints also occurs, and this is commonly confused with RA. Distinguishing features include the absence of RF in the setting of cutaneous disease. Radiologic exam often reveals bony ankylosis of the DIP joints, which is uncommon in RA (Fig. 6).

Five percent of patients develop telescoping of the digits and severe joint deformity. This is termed *arthritis mutilans*. Layers of redundant skin appear, and the examiner is occasionally able to extend the digit to its original length (Fig. 7).

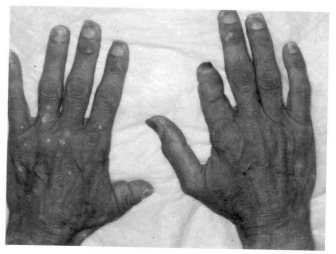

FIGURE 7. The hands of a patient with psoriatic arthritis; note the telescoping of the digits.

Spinal involvement is often asymptomatic and occurs in as much as one-third of patients. Sacroiliitis is usually unilateral and is often found as an incidental finding on pelvic x-rays. Extraarticular manifestations include enthesitis, conjunctivitis, uveitis, and aortic valve insufficiency.

Office Tests

Patients who present with inflammation in the joints deserve a serologic evaluation, including acute phase reactants, such as erythrocyte sedimentation rate and C-reactive protein. Because a pseudorheumatoid picture can occur, and psoriatic plaques can be elusive, the author also obtains an RF routinely. Nevertheless, the clinical picture is often straightforward, and intense immunologic evaluation, such as antinuclear antibodies and complement levels, is rarely helpful. The degree of inflammation in the joints often mirrors that in the serum, and these markers can be a helpful way to measure response to therapy. Because psoriatic arthritis is a clinical diagnosis, there are no definitive tests. The presence of RF should suggest coexistent RA, although this is uncommon.

Imaging Studies

Psoriatic arthritis has a characteristic radiologic appearance. Unlike RA, a fusiform swelling in association with marked joint space loss, ankylosis of the interphalangeal joints, and preservation of bony mineralization are typical. In more aggressive cases, joint erosion occurs at the proximal phalanx with proliferation at the distal phalanx. This is termed the *pencil-in-cup deformity* and is highly suggestive of psoriatic arthritis.

Treatment

The mainstay of medical therapy for psoriatic arthritis is similar to RA, which is described elsewhere. Most rheumatologists start with NSAIDs and then step up to disease-modifying drugs, such as methotrexate. The latter drug is popular because it has a dual beneficial effect on the skin. Given the potential toxicity of immunosuppressive therapy, careful patient assessments should be made, and close liaison between rheumatologists is advised.

Recent advances in biotechnology and research have elucidated some of the pathways that are involved in systemic inflammation. TNF is now well known to be present in increased amounts in the joints and skin. A recent study in which TNF antagonists were administered to 60 patients with psoriatic arthritis resulted in 87% improvement in symptoms at 12 weeks, compared to 23% improvement in placebo-controlled patients (40). Etanercept, which acts by competitive inhibition of the soluble P-75 TNF receptor, has resulted in a dramatic improvement in skin findings and arthritis in some refractory patients (B. Finck, Immunex, *personal communication*).

Surgery

Although surgery is rarely indicated in psoriatic arthritis, it certainly has a role in the patients who are refractory to medical management. Surgery usually involves salvage procedures to relieve pain or to improve position. Zangger et al. (41) described 71 operations in 43 patients with psoriatic arthritis; most patients required DIP or PIP fusion. Although 50% of the patients were lost to follow-up, overall conventional scoring of the procedures showed good to excellent results. Leibovic et al. (42) described conflicting data; they analyzed 224 PIP arthrodeses using Kirschner wires, Herbert screws, tension band wiring, and plates. Nonunion occurred in 31 cases and was highest in psoriatic arthritis. The Herbert screw was associated with the lowest complication rate.

Seronegative Spondyloarthropathies

The seronegative spondyloarthropathies are a discrete group of inflammatory arthritides that are characterized by involvement of the axial skeleton, peripheral joints, and periarticular structures. Ankylosing spondylitis, psoriatic arthritis, Reiter's syndrome, and the enteropathic arthritides all are classified under this framework. These conditions are covered briefly in this section, because hand involvement is relatively rare.

Traditionally, infection has been thought to be the basis of disease, because microbial antigens have been detected in the joints of patients with spondyloarthropathy. When rats that express the HLA-B27 antigen are raised in a germ-free environment, the peripheral arthritis is prevented, thus implicating the need for foreign antigens to precipitate disease (43).

The pattern of joint distribution should give rise to the clinical suspicion of spondyloarthropathy. Most patients have peripheral arthritis, which is oligoarticular and asymmetric; dactylitis is common. Typically, the lower limb is affected, apart from psoriasis, which affects the hand and wrist. Sacroiliitis is common and is frequently seen as an asymptomatic radiologic finding. Enthesopathy remains the hallmark of the disease, and patients with ankylosing spondylitis can develop progressive spinal fusion due to inflammation of the longitudinal ligaments of the spine. Inflammatory bowel disease should be considered in patients who develop peripheral arthritis in the setting of gastrointestinal disturbance. Extraarticular manifestations include aortitis, uveitis, and apical lung fibrosis. Treatment involves antiinflammatory drugs, including NSAIDs, sulfasalazine, and methotrexate. Local corticosteroid injections are useful for refractory enthesitis or monoarticular disease.

Systemic Lupus Erythematosus

Systemic lupus erythematosus (SLE) is the prototypic autoimmune disease that is characterized by end-organ dys-

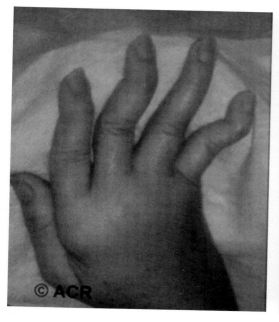
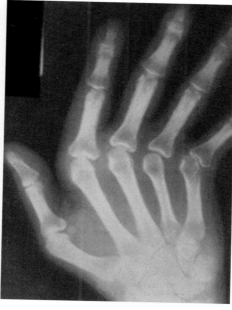

FIGURE 8. Jaccoud's arthritis in a patient with systemic lupus erythematosus. The radiograph shows nonerosive disease. (Reprinted from the Clinical Slide Collection on the Rheumatic Diseases, with permission from the American College of Rheumatology.)

function and is associated with a positive antinuclear antibody (ANA).

Pathogenesis

SLE involves a complex series of inflammatory pathways that result in organ-specific tissue injury. The core disturbance involves defects in B cells and autoantigen-specific T helper cells, thus resulting in a loss of self-tolerance. Autoantibody production ensues, giving rise to immune complex deposition and complement-driven cell damage (44).

There appears to be a strong genetic component to the disease, and SLE occurs concordantly in 25% to 50% of monozygotic twins and 5% of dizygotic twins.

Epidemiology

Peak incidence occurs during childbearing years, and women are predominantly affected in a ratio of 9:1. The estimated prevalence is 1 in 2,000 individuals in the outpatient setting, although this varies depending on the study population (45). In the United States, SLE is three times more common in blacks than whites, although lupus has been found to be quite common in Sweden, a predominantly white population.

Evaluation

The clinical manifestations of SLE are protean and range from constitutional abnormalities to severe end-organ failure. Laboratory evaluation for SLE involves detection of ANA, hematologic abnormalities, and complement deficiencies. The presence of ANA confers a 99% sensitivity but is not specific for SLE. The criteria for SLE and a vast array of symptoms are beyond the scope of this text; how-

ever, arthralgias and arthritis are important to recognize and typically involve the small joints of the hands.

Unlike RA, the arthritis of SLE is typically nonerosive and is occasionally reducible. Soft tissue swelling is common, but large effusions are rare. A deforming type of arthritis, which is called *Jaccoud's arthritis*, involves ulnar deviation of the MCPs, subluxation, and contractures. Tenosynovitis and tendon rupture are also quite common in SLE, and the latter is frequently seen in patients on high-dose steroids (Fig. 8).

Treatment of arthritis includes NSAIDs and antimalarials, and, in refractory disease, methotrexate can be used as a reasonable alternative (46). Surgery is rarely indicated.

Scleroderma

Systemic sclerosis (scleroderma) is a rare connective tissue disorder affecting skin and internal organs. The hallmark of the disease is cutaneous tightening which is caused by an excess of extracellular matrix deposition. There are essentially two forms of scleroderma:

Limited disease: This form of scleroderma involves skin thickening distal to the forearms, with little internal organ damage; pulmonary hypertension can occur and is associated with anticentromere antibodies. Skin calcification is quite common.

Diffuse disease: Fibrotic skin extends proximal to the forearms. Patients with this form of scleroderma are more likely to have renal, cardiac, and pulmonary involvement. Patients have antibodies to Scl-70 (topoisomerase type I) more frequently.

Pathogenesis

Microvascular occlusion and fibrosis occur in the skin and deep organs and ultimately result in end-organ dysfunction.

Immune systemic dysregulation results in the activation of dermal cells and fibroblasts, which then respond by overexpression of the extracellular matrix. Although autoantibodies are found in patients with scleroderma, the humoral system plays a minor role in pathogenesis compared to the overactive T-cell response. Serum complement levels usually remain constant, which suggests a lack of antigen antibody deposition in tissues.

Although anticytokine therapy has received much attention in recent years, data for scleroderma remain disappointing. Cytokines, such as TNF, IL-1, IL-4, IL-6, and IL-10, have all been implicated in disease activation, but, as of 2003, antagonism of these molecules has not resulted in significant clinical improvement (47).

Epidemiology

The incidence of scleroderma is estimated at 19 cases per million per year. The general incidence is higher in women than men, with a ratio of 3:1. The average age of onset is between 45 and 65 years of age (48).

Scleroderma is found with a greater-than-expected incidence in certain occupations. South African miners who are exposed to silica dust have a relative risk of approximately 25% of developing the disease. Cases have also been reported in patients who were exposed to tainted rapeseed oil and L-tryptophan. Genetic factors are thought to play a minimal role in disease contribution; more than one person affected in a family is rare.

Evaluation

For the purpose of this text, only the musculoskeletal manifestations are discussed. Nonspecific arthralgias are extremely common, although, in the early stages, diffuse edema that affects both hands may be the only clue to the disease. As tendon involvement occurs, friction rubs can be auscultated and tend to be associated with a poorer prognosis. Progression of the disease results in joint atrophy and pain over the affected digit due to skin tightening. Swan-neck deformity with underlying osteopenia, osseous resorption of digital tufts, and soft tissue calcinosis is also characteristic of late disease (Fig. 9).

Muscle atrophy and weakness occur as patients become more immobilized; a small minority of patients develop a myositis overlap with elevation of creatine phosphokinase and muscle inflammation on biopsy. In addition to joint symptoms, 90% of patients with scleroderma have Raynaud's phenomenon. This manifests with fingertip ulceration, ischemic demarcation, and, ultimately, autoamputation. Unlike primary Raynaud's phenomenon, the presence of surrounding tissue fibrosis and platelet activation complicates any therapeutic intervention.

Treatment

Arthralgias and tendon inflammation are generally treated with NSAIDs, although the response is often disappoint-

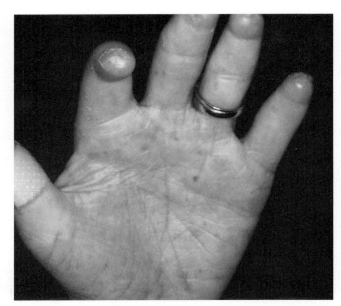

FIGURE 9. The hand of a patient with limited scleroderma and Raynaud's phenomenon. Autoamputation has occurred, resulting in digital shortening. Note the palmar telangiectasias.

ing. Low-dose corticosteroids can be used if symptoms are severe, although higher doses may precipitate renal crisis and should be used with care. A multidisciplinary approach is vital, and early involvement of physical therapy may limit flexion contractures and may improve mobility.

Soft tissue calcinosis may result in ulceration, pain, and infection. Multiple regimens including warfarin, colchicine, and calcium channel antagonists have been used, although, as of 2003, no treatment has been shown to retard this process (49).

Bottomley et al. have used a carbon dioxide laser in several patients with limited scleroderma and superficial calcinosis. At 20 months, 57% of treated areas showed complete resolution with an average healing time of 6 weeks. This option may obviate the need for surgical intervention.

The treatment of Raynaud's phenomenon is covered elsewhere in this text (Chapter 94).

Surgical Treatment

Surgery of the hand poses a difficult problem. Diminished circulation and skin fibrosis result in a hostile environment for the surgeon. Although arthrodesis is generally recommended for severe contraction deformities, complications, including infections and poor wound healing, are common. Arthroplasty and excision of painful calcinosis have been successfully performed in specialized centers. A series by Melone et al. (50) describes 272 hand operations with favorable results; the emphasis is placed on patients with tension-free wounds, judicious skeletal shortening, and healing by secondary intention.

Patients who develop new onset of wrist pain should undergo radiologic evaluation. Several patients have been described in whom osteonecrosis of the lunate bone has developed in the absence of corticosteroids. All patients had limited scleroderma but severe Raynaud's phenomenon. Improvement in symptoms occurred after bone grafting. Osteonecrosis may be an underrecognized cause of bone pain in scleroderma patients (51).

REFERENCES

1. Scott JT, Pollard AC. Uric acid excretion in the relatives of patients with gout. *Ann Rheum Dis* 1970;29:397–400.
2. Emmerson BT, Nagal SL, Duffy DL, et al. Genetic control of the renal clearance of urate: a study of twins. *Ann Rheum Dis* 1992;51:375–377.
3. Wilson JM, Stout JT, Palella TD, et al. A molecular survey of hypoxanthine-guanine phosphoribosyl transferase deficiency in man. *J Clin Invest* 1986;77:188–195.
4. Terkeltaub RA, Ginsburg MH. The inflammatory reaction to crystals. *Rheum Dis Clin North Am* 1988;14:353–364.
5. Cohen MG, Emmerson BT. Crystal arthropathies: gout. In: Klippel JH, Dieppe PA, eds. *Rheumatology*. London: Mosby, 1998:8–14.
6. Campion EW, Glynn RV, DeLabry LO. Asymptomatic hyperuricemia: risks and consequences in the Normative Aging Study. *Am J Med* 1987;82:421–426.
7. Wyngaarden JB, Kelley WN. *Gout and hyperuricemia*. New York: Grune & Stratton, 1976.
8. Arnold MH, Preston SJ, Buchanon WW. Comparison of the natural history of untreated acute gouty arthritis vs. acute gouty arthritis treated with NSAIDs. *Br J Clin Pharmacol* 1988;26:488–489.
9. Hartung EF. History of the use of colchicine and related medications in gout. *Ann Rheum Dis* 1954;13:190–201.
10. Wallace SL, Singer JZ. Systemic toxicity associated with intravenous administration of colchicine–guidelines for use. *J Rheumatol* 1988;15:495–499.
11. Axelrod D, Preston S. Comparison of parenteral ACTH with oral indomethacin in the treatment of acute gout. *Arthritis Rheum* 1988;31:803–805.
12. Paulus HE, Schlosstein LH, Godfrey RC, et al. Prophylactic colchicine therapy of intercritical gout. A placebo controlled study of probenecid-treated patients. *Arthritis Rheum* 1987;17:609–614.
13. Piza-Katzer H, Komorcu F, Reining-Fiesta A. Surgical therapy of pronounced gouty tophi in both hands. Case report. *Handchir Mikrochir Plast Chir* 1997;29:96–100.
14. Gelberman RH, Doty DH, Hamer ML. Tophaceous gout involving the proximal interphalangeal joint. *Clin Orthop* 1980;147:225–227.
15. Abrahamsson SO. Gouty tenosynovitis simulating an infection. A case report. *Acta Orthop Scand* 1987;58:282–283.
16. Moore JR, Weiland AJ. Gouty tenosynovitis in the hand. *J Hand Surg* 1985;10:291–295.
17. Chuang HL, Wong CW. Carpal tunnel syndrome induced by tophaceous deposits on the median nerve: case report. *Neurosurgery* 1994;34:919–920.
18. Cheung HS, Ryan LM. Role of crystal deposition in matrix degradation. In: Woessner FJ, Howell DS, eds. *Joint carti-lage degradation: basic and clinical aspects*. New York: Marcel Dekker Inc, 1995:209.
19. Felson DT, Anderson JJ, Naimark A, et al. The prevalence of chondrocalcinosis in the elderly and its association with knee osteoarthritis: the Framingham study. *J Rheum* 1989;16:1241–1245.
20. Bird HA, Ring EF. Therapeutic value of arthroscopy. *Ann Rheum Dis* 1978;37:78–79.
21. Doherty M, Dieppe P. Clinical aspects of calcium pyrophosphate dihydrate crystal deposition. *Rheum Dis Clin North Am* 1988;14:395–414.
22. Chiu KY, Ng WF, Wong WB, et al. Acute carpal tunnel syndrome caused by pseudogout. *J Hand Surg* 1992;17:299–302.
23. Kuhlmann JN, Fahed I, Mimoun M, et al. Pseudotumoral chondrocalcinosis and carpal tunnel syndrome. Apropos of a case report. *Ann Chir Main* 1988;7:310–313.
24. Ishida T, Dorfman HD, Bullough PG. Tophaceous pseudogout. *Hum Pathol* 1995;26:587–593.
25. Dieppe PA, Doherty M, MacFarlane DG, et al. Apatite associated destructive arthritis. *Br J Rheum* 1984;23:84–91.
26. Faure G, Dalcussi G. Calcific tendonitis: a review. *Ann Rheum Dis* 1983;42[Suppl]:49–53.
27. McCarthy GM, Carrera GF, Ryan LM. Acute calcific periarthritis of the finger joints: a syndrome of women. *J Rheum* 1993;20:1077–1080.
28. Halverson PB, Cheung HS, Mcarty DJ. Milwaukee shoulder syndrome (MSS): description of predisposing factors. *Arthritis Rheum* 1987;30:S131.
29. Gibilisco PA, Schumacher HR, Hollander JL, et al. Synovial fluid crystals in osteoarthritis. *Arthritis Rheum* 1985;28:511–515.
30. Paul H, Reginato AJ, Shumacher HR. Alizarin red S staining as a screening test to detect calcium compounds in synovial fluid. *Arthritis Rheum* 1983;26:191–200.
31. Caporeli R, Rossi S, Montecucco C. Tidal irrigation in Milwaukee shoulder syndrome. *J Rheumatol* 1994;21:1781–1782.
32. Neer CS, Craig EV, Fukada H. Cuff tear arthropathy. *J Bone Joint Surg* 1983;69:1232–1244.
33. Elder JT, Naiv RP, Voorhees JJ. Epidemiology and genetics of psoriasis. *J Invest Dermatol* 1994;102:24S–27S.
34. Gladman DD, Farewell VT. The role of HLA antigens as indicators of disease progression in psoriatic arthritis. *Arthritis Rheum* 1995;38:845–850.
35. Griffiths CE, Voorhees JJ. Psoriasis, T cells and autoimmunity. *J R Soc Med* 1996;89:315–319.
36. Panayi GS. Immunology of psoriasis and psoriatic arthritis. *Baillieres Clin Rheumatol* 1994;8:419–427.
37. Cuellar ML, Silveira LH, Espinoza LR. Recent developments in psoriatic arthritis. *Curr Opin Rheumatol* 1994;6:378–384.
38. Gladman DD, Shuckett R, Russell ML, et al. Psoriatic arthritis: an analysis of 220 patients. *Q J Med* 1987;62:127–141.
39. Shbeeb M, Uramoto KM, Gibson LE, et al. The epidemiology of psoriatic arthritis in Olmsted County, Minnesota, USA, 1982–1991. *J Rheumatol* 2000;27:1247–1250.
40. Mease PJ, Goffe BS, Metz J, et al. Etanercept in the treatment of psoriatic arthritis and psoriasis: a randomized trial. *Lancet* 2000;356:385–390.

41. Zangger P, Esufali ZH, Gladman DD, et al. Type and outcome of reconstructive surgery for different patterns of psoriatic arthritis. *J Rheumatol* 2000;27:967–974.

42. Leibovic SJ, Strickland JW. Arthrodesis of the proximal interphalangeal joint of the finger: comparison of the use of the Herbert screw with other fixation methods. *J Hand Surg* 1994;19:181–188.

43. Taurog JD, Richardson JA, Croft JT, et al. The germfree state prevents development of gut and joint inflammatory disease in HLA B-27 transgenic rats. *J Exp Med* 1994;180:2359–2364.

44. Hohan C, Datta SK. Lupus. Key pathogenic mechanisms and contributing factors. *Clin Immunol Immunopathol* 1996;77:209–220.

45. Hochberg MC. Systemic lupus erythematosus. *Rheum Dis Clin North Am* 1990;16:617–639.

46. Wilson K, Abeles M. A 2 year, open-ended trial of methotrexate in systemic lupus erythematosus. *J Rheumatol* 1994;21:1674–1677.

47. Black CM, Denton CP. Scleroderma. In: Brennan FM, Feldman M, eds. *Role of cytokines in autoimmunity.* Austin, TX: RG Landes Co, 1996;8:153–174.

48. Medsger TA Jr. Epidemiology of systemic sclerosis. *Clin Dermatol* 1994;12:207–216.

49. Hussman J, Russell RC, Kucan JD, et al. Soft tissue calcifications: differential diagnosis and therapeutic approaches. *Ann Plast Surg* 1995;34:138–147.

50. Melone CP Jr, McLoughlin JC, Beldner S. Surgical management of the hand in scleroderma. *Br J Dermatol* 1996;135:302–304.

51. Matsumoto AK, Moore R, Alli P, et al. Three cases of osteonecrosis of the lunate bone of the wrist in scleroderma. *Curr Opin Rheumatol* 1999;11:514–520.

71

OSTEOARTHRITIS OF THE HAND AND DIGITS: DISTAL AND PROXIMAL INTERPHALANGEAL JOINTS

THOMAS W. KIESLER

The most common form of arthritis, osteoarthritis (OA), is a condition that is characterized by articular cartilage deterioration. Involvement in the hand is seen most commonly at the thumb carpometacarpal joint and at the interphalangeal (IP) joints. The cartilage changes are manifested by joint enlargement, pain, swelling, stiffness, contracture, and angular deformity. Nonoperative therapy is the cornerstone of treatment. In recalcitrant cases, however, surgical treatment is appropriate to provide pain relief and joint stability. IP joint débridement, mucous cyst excision, arthroplasty, and arthrodesis are the mainstays of surgical treatment.

SURGICAL ANATOMY AND BIOMECHANICS

The proximal interphalangeal joint (PIPJ) and the distal interphalangeal joint (DIPJ) are simple diarthroidal ginglymus (hinge) joints, which essentially allow motion in only one plane. Primary lateral stability is achieved by the strong radial and ulnar collateral ligaments. The bony architecture of the opposing proximal and distal bones provides secondary constraint (1). The biconvex distal surface articulates with the reciprocal proximal biconcave condylar surface. The central intercondylar ridge of the proximal bone interlocks with the distal central ridge. The bony and ligamentous anatomy together impart the necessary stability for pinch activities.

Besides stability, the PIPJ and DIPJ allow a wide range of motion for gripping activities. The normal sagittal plane arcs of range of motion at the PIPJ and the DIPJ are 0 to 105 degrees and 0 to 85 degrees, respectively. Functional arcs of motion, however, are only 36 to 86 degrees (with an average of 60 degrees) and 20 to 61 degrees (with an average of 39 degrees) at the PIPJ and the DIPJ, respectively (2). The value of the PIPJ to overall hand function is clearly evident by the fact that it contributes 85% of intrinsic digital flexion and 30% of the overall combined flexion of the finger (3).

PATHOPHYSIOLOGY

Classic OA is a noninflammatory primary cartilage disease that is characterized by progressive articular cartilage deterioration and reactive new bone formation. A less common type of OA, erosive or inflammatory OA, involves the DIPJs and PIPJs of postmenopausal women. It has a more abrupt onset and more swelling and tenderness than classic OA (4). Posttraumatic OA is another subset of OA that has a clearly defined etiology: traumatic intraarticular cartilage disruption. Regardless of the type of OA, the pathogenesis is similar. Age, systemic factors, genetics, and trauma can predispose one to the development of OA. However, the specific joint that is affected and the severity of the disease are usually dictated by local biomechanical factors (5).

Articular cartilage is composed of water, collagen, proteoglycan, and chondrocytes. The biochemical changes that are seen in the cartilage of aging joints are increased water content, decreased protein content, increased collagen stiffness, and decreased proteoglycan mass, size, and proportion. Chondrocytes become larger, acquire increased lysosomal activity, and fail to reproduce. The combined overall effect of these changes is a loss of cartilage strength and elasticity (6). However, changes that are found in cartilage from symptomatic older osteoarthritic patients are different than those that are seen in the cartilage of older asymptomatic patients.

Pathophysiologically, the initiating event in cartilage degradation that leads to OA has been theorized to be mechanical stress that leads to altered chondrocyte metabolism, production of matrix metalloproteinases, and disruption of collagen matrix properties (7). As a process, therefore, OA is biochemically mediated. It is the local mechanical factors, however, that most likely initiate and perpetuate the process; the process begins with cartilage microfracture and fibrillation and ends in complete bone eburnation (5).

As the articular cartilage degenerates, the subchondral bone reacts to the abnormal load by cyst formation, sclero-

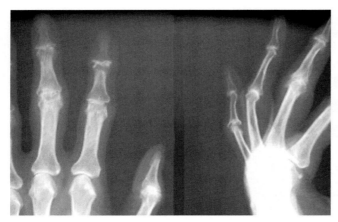

FIGURE 1. Interphalangeal joint osteoarthritis with osteophyte formation, subchondral sclerosis, and cyst formation.

sis, and marginal osteophyte formation (Fig. 1). Most commonly, the narrowing and wear of the joint space are asymmetric, thus resulting in an angular deformity. Joint stability and mechanics can be adversely affected, further altering the stresses across the joint and perpetuating the osteoarthritic process. Joint enlargement, joint incongruity, and pericapsular contracture result in loss of motion in the flexion-extension arc.

The pathophysiology of mucous cysts, small ganglion cysts at the DIPJ, is much less well understood. Although not considered a clear etiologic factor in the production of the mucous cyst, OA has been reported to be an associated finding in nearly 80% to 100% of cases (8,9). Kleinert et al. (10) have suggested that the lesion arose from the joint capsule in the vicinity of a dorsal osteophyte, as they found a definite pedicle that led to the joint capsule of the DIPJ in all cases that were reported. As the cyst fills with fluid and enlarges, it can place pressure on the germinal matrix of the

nail bed and can cause longitudinal grooving of the nail plate. Large cysts can cause thinning of the overlying skin.

INCIDENCE

OA is considered a universal problem of humans. There appears to be a heritable component in its distribution within the population (11). It is seen in at least one joint by the age of 75 years and has become the second most common cause of disability in adults in the United States (7). Evaluation of the prevalence of OA among 17 specific populations showed quite a wide variation, with Alaskan Eskimos who are older than 40 years of age having the lowest prevalence for both men (22%) and women (24%). The mean prevalence of the entire study group for persons 35 years of age and older was found to be 60% for men and women (11). The symptoms that are associated with classic OA often begin in the fifth to sixth decade of life. Women are more often affected than men of the same age.

EVALUATION

History and Physical Examination

Clinically, the most common patient complaint is the insidious onset of joint pain and stiffness that interferes with function of the digit or hand, making pinch and grip activities difficult. The joint symptoms are initially activity related but may progress to the extent that they are noticed at rest and at night. In some cases, however, cosmetic concerns may be the sole reason that a patient presents to the surgeon's office. Patients may complain of a "crooked," malaligned joint (Fig. 2) or may give a history of having noticed painless periarticular joint enlargement; Heberdens's nodes (Fig. 3) and Bouchard's nodes are noted at the DIPJ and the PIPJ, respectively. Inspection of the osteoarthritic DIPJ usually shows some degree of Heberden's nodes along the radial and ulnar aspects of the joint. Angular deformity can range from minimal to quite dramatic.

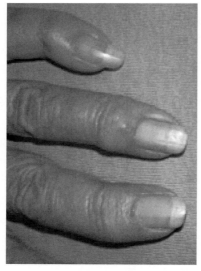

FIGURE 2. Malaligned osteoarthritic interphalangeal joints.

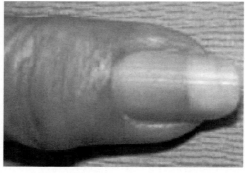

FIGURE 3. Large Heberden's node around an osteoarthritic distal interphalangeal joint.

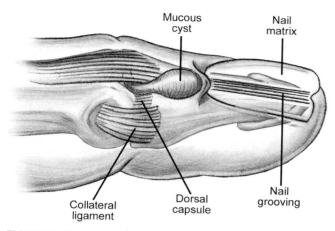

FIGURE 4. Mucous cyst that is adjacent to an osteoarthritic joint. Nail plate grooving may result if the cyst places pressure on the germinal matrix.

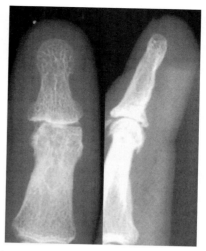

FIGURE 6. Asymmetric joint space narrowing at the proximal interphalangeal joint.

Large mucous cysts that are adjacent to the joint can cause longitudinal grooving of the nail plate (Fig. 4).

Similarly, the PIPJ usually shows some sign of enlargement. Cyst formation is less likely but is not uncommon (Fig. 5). More chronic PIPJ OA oftentimes shows some degree of angular deformity. Palpation of the joint line at the PIPJ or DIPJ elicits tenderness and may demonstrate an effusion. Radial and ulnar deviation stresses may demonstrate varying degrees of instability, depending on the severity of the disease. In chronic cases, range of motion is generally diminished compared to the unaffected joints and occasionally displays a coarse crepitus. Pinch and grip strength are often decreased due to discomfort or instability, or both.

Diagnostic Studies

Plain radiographs are generally all that is needed to confirm the diagnosis of an osteoarthritic joint. Dedicated, true, orthogonal posteroanterior, lateral, and oblique

views are required to accurately evaluate the joint line. Magnified views are sometimes helpful to identify subtle abnormalities in small digits. Asymmetric joint space narrowing (Fig. 6) is the earliest radiographic finding, followed later by marginal osteophyte formation (Fig. 7). Subchondral cyst formation, broadening of the base of the phalanx, and subchondral sclerosis are the hallmark findings of advanced OA at the DIPJ and the PIPJ (Fig. 8) (12).

Radiographs that demonstrate more symmetric joint space narrowing, erosions, and considerable destruction may indicate an inflammatory disease process, such as rheumatoid arthritis, psoriatic arthritis, gout, or Reiter's syndrome. In this case, laboratory tests, including erythrocyte sedimentation rate, rheumatoid factor, uric acid level, and complete blood count, should be obtained to further evaluate such a process.

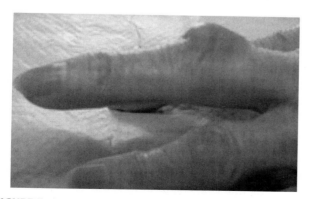

FIGURE 5. Large proximal interphalangeal joint periarticular cyst in an osteoarthritic joint. Note the angular deformity and joint space loss.

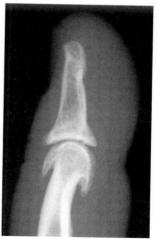

FIGURE 7. Volar and dorsal osteophyte formation at the thumb interphalangeal joint.

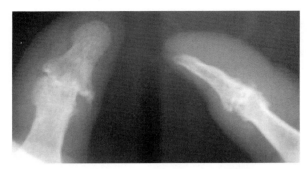

FIGURE 8. Findings of advanced osteoarthritic interphalangeal joint: angular deformity, broadening of the base of the phalanx, and cyst formation.

NONOPERATIVE TREATMENT

The natural history of OA is usually benign. Because there is currently no medical therapy for the underlying disease process in OA, treatment is symptomatic only. Consequently, patient education is crucial. Treatment can be appropriately administered only if the surgeon accurately comprehends the patient's pain level and the disparity between the patient's current level of activity and the desired level of activity. After confirmation that an inflammatory arthropathy is not present, the patient can generally be assured that, although pain control may at times be a formidable task, complete disability, as is sometimes seen in RA, is unusual. A thorough explanation of the status of the joint disease and the treatment options, along with their respective risks and benefits, educates the patient and allows him or her to actively participate in his or her care plan. Nonoperative means are nearly always used first.

The primary goal of nonoperative treatment is pain relief. The resulting increased function of the affected hand is usually a result of adequate pain control. Initially, symptomatic treatment includes controlling exposure to provocative activities that produce pain, swelling, and stiffness. This includes modification of work and leisure activities. Completely eliminating these activities is most important during acute flare-ups. Formal hand therapy can be used to instruct patients on joint protection techniques, especially in tip-to-tip pulp pinch and lateral key pinch (13). Therapy is also useful to teach techniques for edema control and the use of adaptive devices, as well as gentle range-of-motion and strengthening exercises. Preservation of motion may aid in the maintenance of hand function. Splinting can be used to immobilize a tender joint during a flare-up, to provide rest at night or after activities, or to provide support and protection during activities.

Medical treatment includes analgesic use, which is usually adequate if symptoms are mild and episodic. Acetaminophen use has been shown to be as effective as nonsteroidal antiinflammatory drug (NSAID) treatment (14). NSAID use is popular and can decrease symptoms. The side effects that are reported with prolonged use, especially in elderly patients, demand judicious use of these drugs. NSAID use is contraindicated in patients with recent or active peptic ulcer disease, bleeding diathesis, congestive heart failure, renal insufficiency, or current anticoagulation use.

If symptoms persist, intraarticular steroid injections may be administered. First introduced in 1954, intraarticular steroids can give temporary symptomatic relief during acute flare-ups but unfortunately cannot reverse the osteoarthritic process (15). Because of its relatively low solubility, triamcinolone preparations deliver the best long-term results (16). Because the steroid is administered locally, the systemic complications that are seen with oral steroids are rare. However, local complications can include subcutaneous fat atrophy and depigmentation. Joint sepsis can occur from improper technique. Some feel that repeated injections can lead to further joint destruction by inhibiting production of chondroitin sulfate (12) or could cause attenuation of the central tendon at the PIPJ, leading to a boutonnière deformity (16).

SURGICAL MANAGEMENT: DISTAL INTERPHALANGEAL JOINT

Mucous Cyst Excision

Mucous cyst excision is indicated in cysts that have created longitudinal grooving of the nail plate and in large cysts that have caused significant thinning of the overlying skin and risk rupture. Ruptured cysts create a direct path from the skin into the joint, setting the stage for bacterial contamination and the development of septic arthritis. Simple incision and drainage or aspiration have not been shown to effectively eradicate these lesions and may even promote infection of the cyst.

Early surgical techniques relied on radical cyst excision with skin grafting (8,17). Later techniques recommended cyst excision combined with special attention to osteophyte excision, joint débridement, and wound closure by local rotation flap or simple repair (9,10). Kleinert et al. (10) had no recurrences at 12- to 18-month follow-up, whereas Eaton et al. (9) reported only one recurrence in 50 cases, with follow-up ranging from 6 months to 10 years. All nail plate deformities resolved within 6 months. Both studies reported recovery of preoperative range of motion and no complications. Moreover, both studies clearly demonstrate that concomitant osteophyte excision and joint débridement are the critical adjuncts to cyst excision to minimize cyst recurrence.

Preoperatively, patients must thoroughly understand that mucous cyst excision and joint débridement do nothing to treat the underlying disease process of OA. Any expectations that this procedure alone can ameliorate the remainder of their joint symptoms or halt the osteoarthritic disease process must be dispelled.

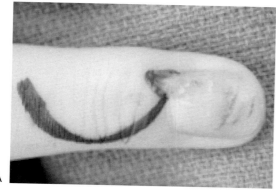

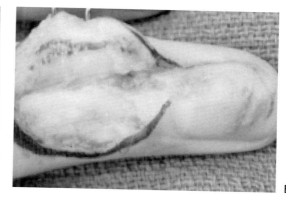

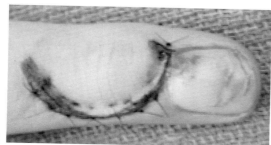

FIGURE 9. A: Preferred rotation flap skin incision for mucous cyst excision in cases in which the skin is severely thinned or in which the cyst obliterates the eponychial fold. Note that the excised cyst has been triangulated. **B:** Elevated rotation flap that exposes the base of the nail plate, the terminal extensor tendon insertion, and the distal interphalangeal joint. **C:** The flap is sutured into place after rotation into the defect.

Author's Preferred Technique

After obtaining adequate general or local anesthetic, the affected upper extremity is placed outstretched on an arm board and is sterilely prepped and draped. The extremity or digit is exsanguinated, and a pneumatic brachial or digital elastic drain tourniquet is set. The incision that the author chooses depends on whether primary wound closure is likely to be possible. Rotation flap coverage should be considered in situations in which the cyst is extremely large and the overlying skin is extremely thinned or in which the cyst involves the eponychium and its excision leaves a defect with exposed nail bed. If any or both of these situations are present, the author uses a small rotation flap technique that has been described by Atasoy (18). This incision allows for access to the radial and ulnar aspects of the DIPJ and allows adequate wound coverage (Fig. 9A). The cyst and overlying skin are triangulated and excised sharply down to the paratenon and germinal matrix. The full-thickness flap is developed and raised off the paratenon for later rotation and insetting (Fig. 9B).

If excision of the cyst does not likely require flap coverage, the author uses one of the standard approaches to the DIPJ (Fig. 10). The author's preference is the Y-shaped incision. This incision usually allows placement of one of the distal arms directly over the cyst and again allows reliable access to the radial and ulnar aspects of the joint for débridement. Irrespective of the initial incision used, full-thickness skin flaps are raised by using an atraumatic technique to expose the terminal tendon and its margins. As the dissection continues distally, the cyst wall is encountered. The plane between the overlying skin and the cyst is devel-

oped, and the cyst is dissected free from the surrounding tissues. Care is taken to avoid damaging the germinal matrix at the distal extent of the incision. A longitudinal incision is made along the radial and ulnar margins of the terminal tendon, extending from the joint capsule proximally. The cyst and its stalk are traced to their origin in the joint capsule at the interval between the collateral ligaments and the terminal tendon. With the collateral ligaments protected, the cyst, its stalk, and the adjacent dorsal capsule are excised. A blunt elevator is used to retract the terminal tendon, and the joint is thoroughly inspected. All marginal osteophytes and remaining dorsal capsule around the joint

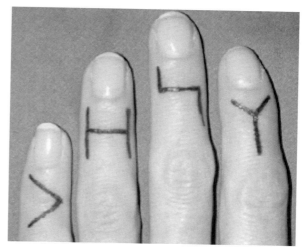

FIGURE 10. Standard approaches to the distal interphalangeal joint for mucus cyst excision, arthrodesis, or arthroplasty.

are removed with a small rongeur. Intraoperative fluoroscopy may be advantageous to confirm adequate débridement. The tourniquet is released, and hemostasis is obtained. The wound is irrigated, and the skin is sutured with 4-0 nonabsorbable sutures. If a local flap was used, it is rotated into position to cover the defect (Fig. 9C). A bulky finger dressing is applied, maintaining full extension at the DIPJ with a gutter splint.

Postoperatively, the dressing and sutures are removed at 10 to 14 days. Edema control and scar massage are initiated, as are active, active assist, and gentle passive range-of-motion exercises. A gutter splint is fashioned for wear between exercise periods if any extensor lag is present. Strengthening exercises may be started at 3 to 4 weeks postoperatively.

Distal Interphalangeal Joint Arthrodesis

Arthrodesis is the most common form of surgical treatment for OA of the DIPJ once nonoperative management is no longer effective. The patient's functional needs must be carefully assessed. DIPJ arthrodesis is indicated when pain, instability, or malalignment has become so severe that it interferes with function of the digit or hand, especially with pinch activities. Arthrodesis improves appearance, corrects deformity and instability, and, as a result of pain relief, increases strength and function. The trade-off, cessation of joint range of motion at the DIPJ, is generally not considered to be a severe functional limitation. An alternative to arthrodesis, DIPJ arthroplasty, is considered in persons whose vocation or avocation specifically requires maintenance of DIPJ flexion.

The goal of any arthrodesis is a stable bony union in a proper position within a reasonable period of time (19). Many techniques of varying complexity have been described for IP arthrodeses (DIPJ and PIPJ), each similar in that the remaining articular cartilage and subchondral bone are removed, and the joint is placed in the desired position and is held in this position until union is achieved. Moreover, common to each of the techniques is the tenet that careful preparation of the bone ends is critical. The bone ends are prepared in a "cup and cone" configuration (20) or with flat bony cuts (21) by using an oscillating saw or rongeur. The techniques differ in the shape of skin incision, the approach to the joint, the bone surface preparation, the bone fixation, and the use of bone graft. Although bone graft has been proposed as an internal structural support (19,22), supplemental graft is generally not required in the osteoarthritic patient. Severe deformity rarely, however, may mandate its use to correct malalignment.

Fixation options for DIPJ arthrodesis include a single Kirschner wire (K-wire) (23), crossed K-wires (24), external dynamic compression (25), an interosseous wire loop (21,26), a combination interosseous wire and intramedullary fixation (27), and compression screws (28–30).

Comparisons of the fixation techniques for DIPJ fusion have been performed (31,32). Engel et al. (31) found compression screw fixation to afford quicker return to work and significantly less lengthy immobilization time when compared to K-wires alone. Nonunion occurred in three cases in each treatment group. Time to union was equal. Wyrsch et al. (32) evaluated the biomechanical characteristics of the Herbert screw (Zimmer, Warsaw, IN) and tension-band wire fusion techniques in a cadaveric study. The Herbert screw was found to have superior anteroposterior bending strength, greater torsional rigidity, and similar lateral bending strength, all characteristics that may be clinically important in small joint arthrodesis.

The complications that are associated with DIPJ fusion have been reviewed by Stern and Fulton (33). They evaluated 185 DIPJ and thumb IP joint arthrodeses using crossed K-wires, the Herbert screw, or combination of K-wire and interosseous wire fixation. The highest overall complication rate occurred in the psoriatic arthritis cohort (44%). Patients who were surgically treated for an osteoarthritic joint had the second lowest overall rate of complications (21%), just slightly greater than chronic posttraumatic arthritis (17%). Of the 61 patients with OA, major complications included nonunions (eight), malunions (three), deep infection (one), and osteomyelitis (one). Nonunion rate among the three techniques was not statistically significant, 11% to 12%. Minor complications included dorsal skin necrosis (4%), cold intolerance (3%), paresthesias (3%), permanent PIPJ stiffness (3%), and superficial wound infection (2%).

Author's Preferred Technique

A Y-shaped dorsal incision is made, centered at the DIPJ. The terminal extensor tendon is identified. Using an atraumatic technique, full-thickness skin flaps are raised and retracted with stay sutures. The terminal extensor tendon is transversely incised just proximal to the DIPJ level. Sharp subperiosteal dissection is used to elevate the margins of the capsule, while osteophytes are removed with a small rongeur. Care must be taken not to damage the proximal extent of the germinal matrix that is located at the extensor tendon insertion. The collateral ligaments are released from their proximal attachments radially and ulnarly. The joint is hyperflexed, allowing access and complete visualization of the bony surfaces. A small oscillating saw or rongeur is used to remove all remaining cartilage and subchondral bone from the opposing surfaces down to cancellous bone. Whether the fusion is to be in slight flexion or in a neutral position, meticulous mating of the bony surfaces is critical for the appropriate coronal, sagittal, and rotational alignment. Once alignment is finalized, fixation is applied.

The desired position of fusion dictates the type of fixation. For fusions in slight flexion (usually as much as 20 degrees), the author recommends K-wire fixation. Place

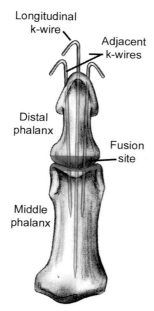

FIGURE 11. Distal interphalangeal joint arthrodesis using Kirschner wires (k-wires).

two to three 0.035-in. K-wires antegrade through the base of the distal phalanx, exiting at the tip pulp, just inferior to the nail plate. Place the first wire longitudinally, and confirm with fluoroscopy that it is centered within the distal phalanx. Place the remaining wires at an angle through an adjacent starting hole. Reduce the bony surfaces accurately, and drive the longitudinal wire retrograde into the middle phalanx (Fig. 11). Adjust rotational alignment, and, with compression maintained at the fusion site, drive the remaining wires across the fusion site into the middle phalanx. The wires should cross within the middle phalanx, not at the fusion site. Confirm accurate alignment and bony opposition visually and radiographically. Ensure that no distraction exists at the fusion site. The tourniquet is released, and hemostasis is obtained. The extensor mechanism and skin are closed separately. A well-padded finger dressing is placed. The wires may be cut beneath the skin or left above the skin level and capped.

Internal screw fixation, Herbert screw, or Acutak screw (Acumed, Beaverton, OR) is the implant of choice when fusion in neutral position is chosen. However, adequate bone stock and sufficient cross-sectional area to contain the screw must be present (33). Care must be taken to choose a screw with a distal thread diameter that is small enough not to violate or fracture the distal phalanx. Mini screws may be required in small phalanges.

The author has found it helpful to make a pilot hole in the distal and middle phalanges with a K-wire before using the Herbert hand drill. This helps prevent accidental cortical penetration and nailbed injury and assists in obtaining accurate provisional alignment. Under radiographic control, a 0.035-in. K-wire is placed just palmar to the nail and

is advanced retrograde from the tip of the distal phalanx into the base. After ensuring that the wire is well centered within the distal phalanx in anteroposterior and lateral planes, the fusion site is reduced, and the wire is driven into the middle phalanx, creating the pilot hole. The K-wire is removed. A small stab incision is made in the fingertip at the site of K-wire insertion. The main Herbert drill (smaller) is placed retrograde through the pilot hole in the distal phalanx. Similarly, the drill is passed retrograde through the middle phalanx. The small Herbert drill is removed. The larger Herbert drill is then placed retrograde through the tip of the distal phalanx only.

A Herbert screw of appropriate size to extend from the distal phalanx tuft to the cortical isthmus of the middle phalanx is chosen. The screw is advanced retrograde to a depth that completely buries the trailing threads in the distal phalanx. The leading threads should stop at a point just proximal to the middle phalanx neck. Appropriate rotational alignment is confirmed by comparing the plane of the adjacent nail plates to that of the fused digit. Coaptation at the fusion site should be confirmed radiographically and by direct vision (Fig. 12). The tourniquet is released, and hemostasis is obtained. The extensor mechanism and skin are closed separately with nonabsorbable sutures. A bulky finger dressing is applied.

Postoperatively, sutures are removed at 10 to 14 days. Aggressive active, active assist, and passive range of motion of the PIPJ and the metacarpophalangeal (MCP) joint are started. The arthrodesis site is protected with an Orthoplast gutter splint. Appropriate edema control is initiated. Union is monitored radiographically. If K-wires are used, they can usually be removed by 6 to 10 weeks after surgery. Strengthening is then initiated.

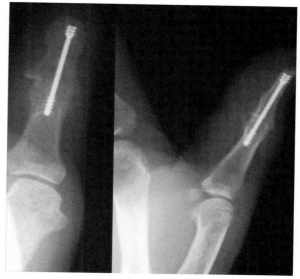

FIGURE 12. Intraoperative radiograph of thumb interphalangeal joint fusion that shows accurate coaptation of the bony surfaces after placement of the internal screw fixation.

Distal Interphalangeal Joint Arthroplasty

An alternative to arthrodesis, DIPJ arthroplasty, can also be used to eliminate pain at the arthritic DIPJ. Its advantage over arthrodesis is the maintenance of some degree of motion at the DIPJ for pinch and grip activities. Postoperatively, range of motion has been reported to average 30 to 40 degrees, with an average extensor lag of 12 degrees (34–36). DIPJ arthrodesis sacrifices the fine fingertip control that is modulated by the action of the flexor digitorum profundus (37). DIPJ arthroplasty is usually, however, only rarely used. Most authors agree that DIPJ arthroplasty is indicated for patients whose occupations or avocations mandate the maintenance of some degree of DIPJ motion to perform fine manipulative activities (34, 35,38). To be considered, however, sufficient bone stock must be present, and the flexor-extensor mechanism must be intact and functional. Relative indications include patients with severe OA involvement in multiple digits of the same hand or patients with an adjacent PIPJ fusion on the same digit (35,37).

The advantage of retained motion must be weighed against the potential complications of DIPJ arthroplasty. Postoperative lateral instability, long-term implant survival, pinch power, skin erosion, and implant breakage from repetitive stress are areas of concern. Wilgus (37) found lateral stability to be satisfactory in all 38 DIPJ arthroplasties at an average follow-up of 10 years. Forty-three percent were stable to lateral stress, 52% showed some instability with a definite end point, and one implant was judged to be grossly unstable. Seventy-one percent were found to have improved power. One implant eroded through the skin, one was removed for infection, and one was found to be broken postoperatively at 30 months. Similarly, Brown (34) reviewed his short-term results in 21 arthroplasties with an average follow-up of 26 months. He judged all implants to be stable. One implant required removal owing to skin erosion; however, no implant breakage was reported.

Operative Techniques

An approach to the DIPJ for implant arthroplasty requires adequate exposure for accurate preparation of the bony surfaces, osteophyte removal, and implant placement. Unlike the PIPJ, the anatomy of the DIPJ does not allow direct complete joint access without transection of the terminal extensor tendon (34,36,37) or detachment of one of the collateral ligaments (Fig. 13), (35,38). As a result, both approaches require a period of strict immobilization postoperatively to allow for healing of the periarticular tissues before starting range-of-motion exercises.

Author's Preferred Technique

A Y-shaped dorsal skin incision is used. Full-thickness skin flaps are raised radially and ulnarly, using an atraumatic technique. Care is taken not to damage the germinal matrix distally. A longitudinal incision is made along the radial and ulnar margins of the terminal extensor tendon. The tendon is gently freed from the middle phalanx by using a small elevator. The author prefers to approach the DIPJ by incising the terminal extensor tendon 5 mm proximal to the joint (36,37). This approach not only spares the insertion of the terminal tendon, it preserves the stability of the joint by not violating the integrity of the collateral ligaments. The tendon is reflected distally, and marginal osteophytes are débrided. A small oscillating saw is then used to remove the head of the middle phalanx distal to the collateral ligament insertions (Fig. 14). This cut must be perpendicular to the long axis of the phalanx in the sagittal and coronal planes. Awls are used to identify the intramedullary canals proximally and distally. Radiographic confirmation that the awls are well centered within the canals is advised. The canals are enlarged with broaches to allow for the appropriate

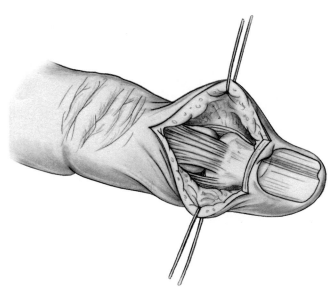

FIGURE 13. Arthroplasty approach to the distal interphalangeal joint requires takedown of the terminal extensor tendon or one of the collateral ligaments.

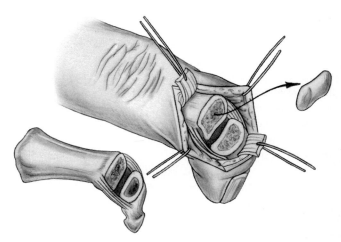

FIGURE 14. After terminal tenotomy, the head of the middle phalanx is removed just distal to the collateral ligament origin.

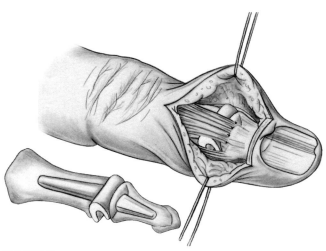

FIGURE 15. With the prosthetic implant in position, the extensor tendon is repaired with nonabsorbable suture.

implant. If necessary, a power bur may be used to allow acceptance of the implant. Care must be taken not to violate the volar or dorsal cortices. The trial prosthesis is inserted. The implant should fit flush with the bone ends, without buckling. Once accurate fit is confirmed, the permanent prosthesis is inserted by using a no-touch technique. With the joint in full extension, the terminal tendon is repaired by using 4-0 nonabsorbable suture (Fig. 15). While maintaining the joint in full extension, lateral stability of the implant is assessed. Under radiographic control, a 0.035-in. K-wire is passed retrograde from the tip of the distal phalanx into the volar portion of the flexor sheath to maintain extension at the joint. Care must be taken to avoid the implant. The tourniquet is released, and hemostasis is obtained. The skin is closed, and a bulky finger dressing with a volar gutter extension splint is applied.

Postoperatively, the bulky dressing and sutures are removed at 2 weeks. Edema control is initiated. The DIPJ is supported continuously in full extension with a volar gutter splint, such as that used for treatment of a mallet injury (39). Most critical at this juncture is initiation of active, active assist, and passive range-of-motion exercises to the PIPJ and the MCP joint. The K-wire is removed at 4 weeks; however, immobilization at the DIPJ is maintained full time for another 4 weeks (8 weeks total) with the gutter splint (36,37). At 8 weeks, gradual active motion is initiated. If an extensor lag is noted during this time, a short period of full-time splinting is restarted. Resistive exercises with putty can usually be started at 10 to 12 weeks (40). Night splinting is continued for a total of 3 to 4 months.

SURGICAL MANAGEMENT: PROXIMAL INTERPHALANGEAL JOINT

Similar to DIPJ OA, surgical management of the end-stage osteoarthritic PIPJ is indicated when all nonoperative treat-

ments have proven ineffective in providing pain relief in activities of daily living or occupational pursuits. If there is persistent unrelenting pain, gross malalignment, loss of motion, and complete cartilage loss, surgical treatment should be considered. The goal of surgery is to provide pain relief and to improve function and appearance. Definitive surgical treatment at the PIPJ, however, is the least well defined in the management of the osteoarthritic hand (41). Although arthrodesis and joint arthroplasty are the currently acceptable treatment options, determining which procedure is most appropriate is still an unsolved issue. The ideal surgical procedure for the osteoarthritic PIPJ would provide stability for lateral and key pinch in the radial digits and should maintain or attempt to restore the flexion arc in the ulnar digits for gripping activities.

Literature abounds that describes the numerous techniques and results of PIPJ arthrodesis that provide excellent stability, albeit at the cost of eliminating motion (19–21,28,42–62). Similarly, the evolution and results of several motion-sparing PIPJ arthroplasty techniques have been well chronicled. These include perichondral resurfacing arthroplasty (63,64) and tendon or capsule interposition (65), silicone flexible implant (66,67), and prosthetic replacement (68–76). Studies that directly compare arthrodesis to arthroplasty and those that assess treatment solely in the osteoarthritic PIPJ are rare. As a result, interpretation of the individual series is difficult, and treatment recommendations are often based on extrapolations to the osteoarthritic patient from the rheumatoid and posttraumatic arthritic populations.

There is general agreement that lateral stability for pinch activities is of paramount importance at the index finger PIPJ. Although in most cases, arthrodesis of the index PIPJ is the most appropriate surgical procedure to accomplish this goal (77), Millender and Nalebuff (78) believed that arthroplasty was also appropriate in the index finger if the joint is well aligned with good collateral ligaments. In a 1987 review of their results, Stern and Ho (16) cautioned against the use of silicone implants in the PIPJs of the radial digits owing to concern that stresses on the radial collateral ligament during key pinch may lead to implant failure. As a result, they recommended against implant arthroplasty and favored PIPJ arthrodesis in all of the following circumstances of PIPJ OA: (a) index finger OA, (b) a young, active patient, (c) loss of bone stock with or without angulation in the coronal plane, (d) preoperative motion of less than 30 degrees, and (e) failed implant arthroplasty.

In an effort to clarify treatment recommendations, Pellagrini and Burton (41) reviewed their series of 43 procedures at the PIPJ, 83% of which were osteoarthritic, treated with arthrodesis, silicone interposition arthroplasty, or cemented arthroplasty. At an average follow-up of 4 years, silicone implants demonstrated a mean active range of motion of 56 degrees, an extensor lag of 3 degrees, and periarticular erosions in 27% of cases. At 2-year follow-up, the mean range of motion of the Biomeric arthroplasties was 66.4

degrees. However, 71% required revision due to mechanical failure of the elastomer hinge. When compared with arthrodesis in the radial digits, grip and pinch strength in the arthroplasty patients was less likely to equal or to exceed the contralateral hand. They recommended against the use of implant arthroplasty in the radial digits, and proposed arthrodesis in 30 to 40 degrees of flexion for the index finger PIPJ (and occasionally in the long finger PIPJ if it is also used predominantly for pinch activities) as the procedure of choice. Silicone implant arthroplasty was recommended only for the ulnar digits of older patients.

Although arthrodesis is generally well tolerated in the radial digits, arthrodesis of the PIPJ in the ulnar digits severely impairs the hand's ability to grip and can limit motion in adjacent digits owing to the quadraegia effect. Therefore, motion-preserving procedures should be given strong consideration, especially in the ulnar digits. However, before embarking on surgical treatment of the osteoarthritic PIPJ, one must be cautious and must consider the patient's age and functional, vocational, and recreational needs, as well as which digit is involved. It is mandatory that all pertinent factors and their ramifications be discussed with the patient.

Proximal Interphalangeal Joint Arthrodesis

PIPJ arthrodesis is recommended for end-stage OA of the index PIPJ and in the ulnar digits when the need for stability outweighs that of range of motion. Early techniques relied on the use of bone pegs to provide stability until fusion occurred (19,22). Later, K-wires alone were used in conjunction with various bone preparation techniques: straight cuts (42), chevron bone cuts (43), cup and cone (20,44,45), convex-concave (46), or tenon (47). Concerns about distraction at the arthrodesis site with K-wires alone led to use of compression clamp K-wire fixation (25,48) or intraosseous wiring alone (21) or in combination with K-wires (26,49). Lister (26) reported a nonunion rate of 9% when using intraosseous wiring that was supplemented with K-wire fixation. In 1980, Allende and Engelem (50) reported on another internal fixation compression technique, tension band wiring, which was originally described by Segmuller (51). The tension band principle, conversion of the dorsal tension forces into palmar compressive forces at the bone ends, has proven effective in PIPJ arthrodesis. Given the stability of the construct, postoperative splinting is short-term, and early range of motion of adjacent digits is possible, theoretically preventing stiffness. Nonunion rates range from only 0% to 5% (50,52–55). Other minor complications of tension band wiring for PIPJ arthrodesis, which were reported by Stern et al. (55), include prominent hardware that requires removal (9%) and superficial infections (10).

Kovach et al. (79) performed an *in vitro* biomechanical analysis that compared crossed K-wires, intraosseous wiring, and tension band wiring at the PIPJ. They found tension band wiring to be superior in strength in anteroposterior bending and torsion. No significant difference was detected with regard to lateral bending. Ijsselstein et al. (56) retrospectively evaluated the clinical results of a series of patients who were treated with percutaneous K-wires or tension band wiring. Combining the results at the MCP joint, the PIPJ, and the DIPJ, they reported a 15% rearthrodesis rate and an infection rate of 18% in the K-wire group, compared to a 5% rearthrodesis rate and a 2% infection rate in the tension band wiring group. They believed that the disadvantages of longer operating time, more extensive dissection, and the possibility of hardware irritation were far outweighed by the stability and lower complication rates of tension band wiring.

Compression screw fixation for small joint arthrodesis was first introduced in 1984 by Faithfull and Herbert (28), who postulated that the compression that was afforded by the screw would decrease nonunion rates even further. They reported a 100% fusion rate at all joints in the digit. Similarly, a high fusion rate was reported by Ayres et al. (52) (98%) and Katzman et al. (57) (100%), with average time to union at the PIPJ being 6 and 8.1 weeks, respectively. Ayres et al. (52) reported that two (4%) of the Herbert screws were removed owing to painful prominence, and fracture of the dorsal cortical bridge occurred in four patients (7%). They believe that these complications (which occurred early in the series) are avoidable if one pays careful attention to detail in preparing the entrance hole at the proximal phalanx, not attempting to change rotational alignment as the distal threads engage, and ensuring that the screw is fully seated. Finally, Leibovic and Strickland (58) evaluated 224 PIPJ arthrodeses that were performed for various diagnoses and were secured with a number of different techniques. Average time to radiographic union, as judged by the presence of trabeculae crossing the fusion site, was most rapid with the Herbert screw (9 weeks) as compared to K-wire (10 weeks) and tension-band wire (11 weeks). Nonunion occurred in 21% of K-wire fusions and 4.5% of tension band fusions and was nonexistent in Herbert screw fusions. No nonunions were seen in the subset of osteoarthritic patients, and no cortical fractures occurred with placement of the screw. They emphasized making the dorsal starting hole well proximal from the arthrodesis site and then overdrilling the hole before screw insertion to avoid fracture.

Internal fixation with plates and screws (59,60) and external fixation devices (61,62) are reserved for special situations in which there has been extraordinary bone loss. Because this is generally not the case in the osteoarthritic PIPJ, these methods are rarely used in primary fusion.

Author's Preferred Technique

The author prefers the tension band technique for PIPJ arthrodesis. A dorsal curvilinear incision is made, centered at the PIPJ. Full-thickness skin flaps are raised. The central slip is incised in the midline distally through its insertion. Alternatively, the joint may be approached via a Chamay incision, creating a distally based flap of central tendon (80). The extensor tendon is reflected along with the joint capsule, protecting the lateral bands. The collateral ligaments are released from their attachments at the proximal phalanx, and the joint is hyperflexed. Osteophytes are removed with a rongeur. The articular surfaces are resected with an oscillating saw. The desired amount of flexion must be chosen before making the cuts. The index and middle fingers are best served with a fusion angle of 15 to 30 degrees to optimize their position for pinching activities. The ulnar digits, which are more involved in gripping activities, are more functional in 30 to 45 degrees of flexion (81). Both surfaces are cut, each at a slight angle, the sum of which produces the total amount of flexion required for the digit involved. Precise cuts are required to ensure that no angular or rotational malalignment exists.

Two parallel K-wires (0.035 or 0.045 in., depending on the size of the joint) are driven retrograde from the cut surface of the proximal phalanx to exit the dorsal shaft. The arthrodesis site is compressed with the surgeon's fingers, and one of the K-wires is driven antegrade. The K-wires are advanced distally along the intramedullary canal or, for added fixation, are angled volarly to exit the volar cortex of the middle phalanx (81). After the first wire is advanced, rotational alignment and coaptation at the arthrodesis site are assessed. Small adjustments are made before fixing the final position with the second K-wire. Next, a 0.035-in. K-wire is driven transversely across the middle phalanx 1 cm distal to the arthrodesis site. This drill hole must be positioned dorsal to the axis of rotation. A strand of 25- or 26-gauge wire is passed through the hole distally and then around the base of the pins proximally in a figure-of-eight fashion. The wire is tightened with a needle driver in the standard fashion, compressing the arthrodesis site. The wires are bent slightly, cut close to the bone, and are rotated toward the bone surface to minimize irritation (Fig. 16). The wire is similarly cut and is positioned close to the surface of the bone. The extensor mechanism and skin are closed separately with nonabsorbable sutures. The digit is placed into a sterile bulky safe position dressing.

Postoperatively, the dressing can be changed within 5 to 7 days. The stability of the tension band construct allows adjacent joints to be mobilized immediately. Edema control measures are instituted. A custom-molded gutter splint is applied to the PIPJ. Sutures are removed at 10 to 14 days. The splint is continued until stress testing no longer elicits pain. Resistive exercises are started at approximately 8 to 12 weeks after surgery, after clinical union is achieved.

Proximal Interphalangeal Joint Arthroplasty

Many arthroplasty techniques have been proposed to preserve motion and function at the PIPJ as an alternative to arthrodesis. Resection arthroplasty and palmar plate interposition with or without flexor digitorum superficialis tenodesis and perichondral grafting are biologic arthroplasty

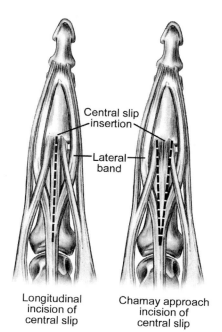

FIGURE 16. Approaches to the proximal interphalangeal joint: longitudinal central tendon splitting and the Chamay approach, in which the triangular distally based flap of the central tendon is raised and reflected distally.

techniques that use autogenous tissue (63–65). Carroll and Taber (65) reported on 30 patients who were treated with palmar plate interposition, of whom only 16 had satisfactory results. Lateral stability was problematic. Ostegaard and Weilby (63) combined palmar plate advancement with flexor digitorum superficialis tenodesis. They reported adequate stability and range of motion in three patients, one with OA. Seradge et al. (64) reported on 20 patients who underwent resurfacing arthroplasty of the PIPJ using the perichondrium of the sixth or seventh rib. They felt that their results were less than acceptable and recommended avoiding the procedure in arthropathies that resulted from healed pyarthrosis, in systemic diseases with joint involvement, in patients who require concomitant tendon reconstruction, or in patients who are older than 40 years of age.

Prosthetic replacement has been extensively used at the PIPJ. Early prosthetic replacement with constrained hinged metal-metal or metal-plastic designs (82–84) met with considerable complications that were related to subsidence, cortical protrusion, loosening, implant failure, and metallosis. Swanson developed the silicone rubber flexible implant and began implanting the prosthesis in 1966. Since that time, it has been the most popular replacement material at the PIPJ and is considered by many to be the gold standard for PIPJ arthroplasty. In 1985, Swanson et al. (66) reviewed 424 joints, 153 of which were osteoarthritic, with an average follow-up of 5.14 years. Overall, 98.3% of patients had complete pain relief. Postoperatively, range of motion improved in all diagnoses, with 68% of the osteoarthritic

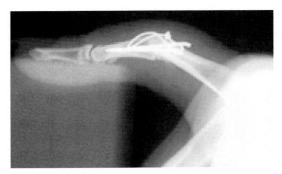

FIGURE 17. Proximal interphalangeal joint arthrodesis, using a tension band technique.

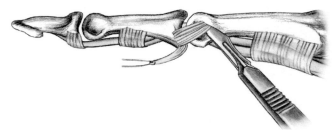

FIGURE 19. After palmar plate release and collateral ligament recession from the proximal attachment, the joint is hyperextended into the "shotgun" position, exposing the joint surfaces.

joints having greater than 40 degrees of motion. Complications included implant fracture (5.19%), ulnar deviation (lateral instability) greater than 5 to 10 degrees (3.7%), infection (0.36%), and implant dislocation (0.36%). The revision rate was 10.9%. Survivorship of the Swanson implant has been studied by Iselin and Conti (67) in posttraumatic arthritis. They found the arthroplasty to be quite durable, and it was successful in 91% of joints at 2 years, 87% at 5 and 7 years, and 81% at 9 years.

Concerns about clinical instability, particulate synovitis, bone remodeling, and implant fracture have prompted development of prostheses that are anchored to the bone itself: the osseointegrated titanium-silicone implant (68) and the unconstrained cemented surface replacement arthroplasty (69). Moller et al. (68) reported that osseous integration of the prosthesis occurred in 41 of 44 fixtures. The prosthesis was abandoned in its current design, how-

ever, owing to an unacceptably high (18%) rate of silastic spacer fracture. Linscheid et al. (69) recently reviewed their results of using a cemented surface replacement arthroplasty at the PIPJ in 47 patients, 24 of whom had OA. At an average follow-up of 4.5 years, average postoperative range of motion measured 14 to 61 degrees (an arc of 47 degrees), a gain of 12 degrees compared to preoperative measurements. The average extension deficit was 14 degrees. The best results occurred in those patients with OA. Instability was seen in only five joints, all with bone and capsular loss that was associated with rheumatoid or posttraumatic arthritis, none with OA. Specifically, prosthetic replacement of the index PIPJ finger was believed to tolerate well the lateral stresses that were associated with pinch. There was no evidence of radiographic loosening. Overall, complications were seen in 19 of 66 joints.

Operative Techniques

Implant arthroplasty at the PIPJ can be performed from a lateral, dorsal, or volar approach (66,69,75,76). The lateral approach alleviates the need to violate the extensor mechanism; however, one collateral ligament and the

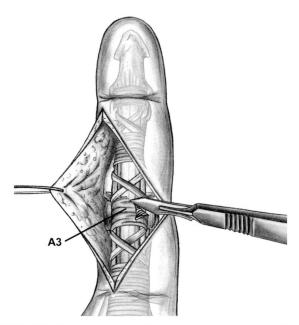

FIGURE 18. Volar approach to the proximal interphalangeal joint for replacement arthroplasty. The flexor sheath is reflected, allowing visualization of the flexor tendons. A3, third annular pulley.

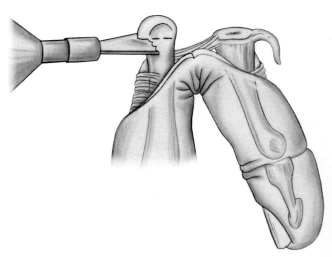

FIGURE 20. The head of the proximal phalanx is removed by using an oscillating saw. The collateral ligaments are spared.

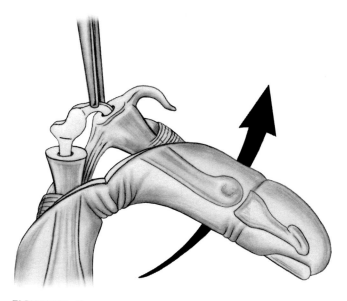

FIGURE 21. Permanent proximal interphalangeal joint implant insertion.

volar plate must be detached (69). Lindscheid et al. (69) believed the lateral approach posed difficulties in preparing the intramedullary canals and obtaining consistent alignment of the components and subsequently abandoned its use. The dorsal approach involves a longitudinal split of the central tendon (66), proximal central tendon release, central tendon insertion detachment (69), or development of a distally based flap of central tendon (80). Depending on the extent of violation of the extensor tendon mechanism, initiation of postoperative range-of-motion exercises may need to be delayed. Although the volar approach requires release of the volar plate and collateral ligaments, it spares the flexor and extensor tendon mechanisms. This allows for immediate active range-of-

motion exercises (75,76). The need for collateral ligament repair is controversial (75,76,85).

Author's Preferred Technique

The author prefers the volar approach that was described by Schneider (75) for flexible silicone arthroplasty of the osteoarthritic PIPJ. The preferred anesthetic is an intermetacarpal nerve block and intravenous sedation. This allows for intraoperative assessment of range of motion. A wrist tourniquet is inflated after exsanguination. A volar Bruner incision is made, centered at the PIPJ. The radial and ulnar neurovascular bundles are identified, and a full-thickness skin flap is raised off the flexor sheath and is retracted with a suture. The flexor sheath is incised transversely just distal to the second annular pulley and just proximal to the fourth annular pulley and is reflected laterally (Fig. 17). A small elastic drain is used to retract the flexor tendons.

The palmar plate is released from the proximal phalanx, and the collateral ligaments are recessed from their proximal attachment (Fig. 18). The joint is "shotgunned" open with hyperextension, exposing the joint surfaces (Fig. 19). Osteophytes are removed with a rongeur. An oscillating saw is used to resect the proximal phalanx condyles perpendicular to long axis of the bone, removing only enough bone to allow for the thickness of the implant (Fig. 20). The base of the middle phalanx is not resected. The intramedullary canals are entered with the awl, and each is enlarged with broaches until the appropriate size is obtained. Care must be taken to ensure that the broaches are placed squarely within the canal to prevent rotational malalignment. The trial implant is placed, and active range of motion and stability are assessed. The permanent implant is inserted (Fig. 21). Radiographs are obtained to ensure proper alignment and placement of the implant (Fig. 22). The collateral ligaments are not repaired unless there is considerable instabil-

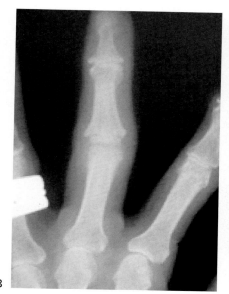

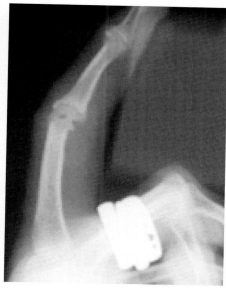

A,B

FIGURE 22. Posteroanterior **(A)** and lateral **(B)** postoperative radiographs of proximal interphalangeal joint arthroplasty.

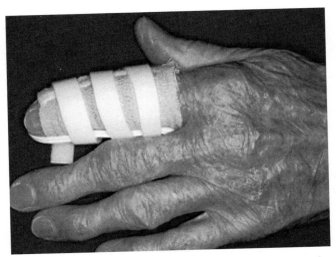

FIGURE 23. Postoperative extension gutter splint. Note the edema control.

ity. If needed, they can be reattached through drill holes in the proximal phalanx. The reflected portion of the flexor sheath is transposed deep to the flexor tendons and is reattached in such a manner as to resurface the volar portion of the joint. The tourniquet is released, and hemostasis is obtained. The skin is closed with 4-0 nonabsorbable suture. A bulky dressing with dorsal blocking splint is applied.

Postoperatively, the patient returns in 2 to 3 days for dressing change. A gutter splint is fashioned, holding the digit in full extension (Fig. 23). The lateral sides of the splint may be made higher to prevent medial and lateral stresses to the joint. Active and passive range-of-motion exercises are performed four times per day (Fig. 24). The splint is worn between exercise periods and at night. At 5 to 7 days postoperatively, dorsal taping or dynamic flexion

splinting may be initiated if passive flexion is less than 70 degrees, provided that there is no extensor lag that is greater than 30 degrees. Sutures are removed at 2 weeks. At 3 weeks, exercises are increased to each hour, provided that there is no extensor lag that is greater than 25 degrees. Gentle strengthening is initiated at 8 weeks, beginning with a soft ball and progressing to putty. The patient should be weaned from the splint, and the splint should be discontinued by 12 weeks (86).

REFERENCES

1. Kiefahber TR, Stern PJ, Grood ES. Lateral stability of the proximal interphalangeal joint. *J Hand Surg* 1986;11:661–669.
2. Hume MC, Gellman H, McKellop H, et al. Functional range of motion of the joints of the hand. *J Hand Surg* 1990;15A(2):240–243.
3. Littler JW, Herndon JH, Thompson JS. Examination of the hand. In: *Reconstructive plastic surgery,* vol. 6, 2nd ed. Converse JM, ed. Philadelphia: WB Saunders, 1977:2971–2974.
4. Belhorn LR, Hess EV. Erosive osteoarthritis. *Semin Arthritis Rheum* 1993;22:298–306.
5. Dieppe P. Osteoarthritis and related disorders. In: Klippel JH, Dieppe P, ed. *Rheumatology,* 2nd ed. London: Mosby, 1988:8:11–12.
6. Miller MD. *Review of orthopaedics.* Philadelphia: Lippincott Williams & Wilkins, 1992.
7. Fife RS. Osteoarthritis; epidemiology, pathology, and pathogenesis. In: Klippel JH, ed. *Primer on rheumatic diseases,* 11th ed. Atlanta: Arthritis Foundation, 1997:216–218.
8. Constant E, Royer JR, Pollard RJ, et al. Mucous cysts of the fingers. *Plast Reconstr Surg* 1969;43:241–246.

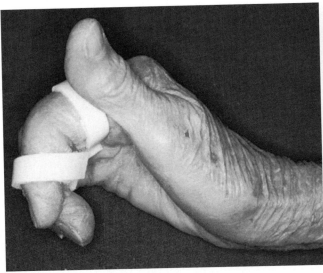

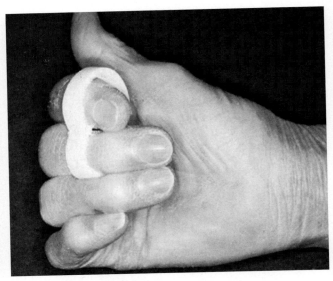

A

FIGURE 24. A,B: Postoperative active range-of-motion exercises for proximal interphalangeal joint arthroplasty.

9. Eaton RG, Dobranski AI, Littler JW. Marginal osteophyte excision in treatment of mucous cysts. *J Bone Joint Surg* 1973;55A:570–574.

10. Kleinert HE, Kutz JE, Fishman JH, et al. Etiology of the so-called mucous cyst of the finger. *J Bone Joint Surg* 1972;54:1455–1458.

11. Peyron JG. Epidemiologic and etiologic approach to osteoarthritis. *Semin Arthritis Rheum* 1979;8:288–306.

12. Swanson AB, Swanson G. Osteoarthritis of the hand. *J Hand Surg* 1983;8:669–675.

13. Linscheid RL, Dobyns J, Beckenbaugh R, et al. *Mayo Clin Proc* 1979;54:227–240.

14. Bradley JD, Brandt KD, Katz BP, et al. Comparison of an anti-inflammatory dose of ibuprofen, an analgesic dose of ibuprofen and acetaminophen in the treatment of patients with osteoarthritis of the knee. *N Engl J Med* 1991;325:87–91.

15. McGrath MH. Local steroid therapy of the hand. *J Hand Surg* 1984;9:915–921.

16. Stern PJ, Ho S. Osteoarthritis of the proximal interphalangeal joint. *Hand Clin* 1987;3:405–412.

17. Bourns HK, Sanerkin NG. Mucoid lesions of the fingers and toes. Clinical features and pathogenesis. *Br J Surg* 1963;50:860–866.

18. Atasoy E, O'Neill WL. Local flap coverage about the hand. *Atlas Hand Clin* 1998;3:179–234.

19. Moberg E. Arthrodesis of finger joints. *Surg Clin North Am* 1960;40:465–470.

20. Carroll RE, Hill NA. Small joint arthrodesis in hand reconstruction. *J Bone Joint Surg* 1969;51:19–12.

21. Robertson DC. The fusion of interphalangeal joints. *Can J Surg* 1964;7:433–437.

22. Potenza AD. Brief note: a technique for arthrodesis of finger joints. *J Bone Joint Surg* 1973;55:1534–1536.

23. Nemethi CE. Phalangeal fractures treated by open reduction and Kirschner wire fixation. *Indust Med* 1954;23:148.

24. Bunnell S. Joints. In: Boyes J, ed. *Surgery of the hand*, 4th ed. Philadelphia: JB Lippincott Co, 1948:320–324.

25. Braun RM, Rhoades CE. Dynamic compression for small bone arthrodesis. *J Hand Surg* 1985;10:340–343.

26. Lister G. Intraosseous wiring of the digital skeleton. *J Hand Surg* 1978;3:427–435.

27. Zavitsanos G, Watkins F, Britton E, et al. Distal interphalangeal arthrodesis using intramedullary and interosseous fixation. *Hand Surg* 1999;4:51–55.

28. Faithfull DK, Herbert TJ. Small joint fusions of the hand using the Herbert bone screw. *J Hand Surg* 1984;9:167–168.

29. Bednar MS. Distal interphalangeal joint fusion. *Atlas Hand Clin* 1988;3:1–16.

30. Teoh LC, Yeo SJ, Singh I. Interphalangeal joint arthrodesis with oblique placement of an AO lag screw. *J Hand Surg* 1994;19:208–211.

31. Engel J, Tsur H, Farin I. A comparison between K-wire and compression screw fixation after arthrodesis of the distal interphalangeal joint. *Plast Reconstr Surg* 1977;60:611–614.

32. Wyrsch B, Dawson J, Aufranc S, et al. Distal interphalangeal joint arthrodesis comparing tension band wire and Herbert screw: a biomechanical and dimensional analysis. *J Hand Surg* 1996;21:438–443.

33. Stern P, Fulton D. Distal interphalangeal joint arthrodesis: an analysis of complications. *J Hand Surg* 1992;17:1139–1145.

34. Brown LG. Distal interphalangeal joint flexible implant arthroplasty. *J Hand Surg* 1989;14:653–656.

35. Culver JE, Fleegler EJ. Osteoarthritis of the distal interphalangeal joint. *Hand Clin* 1987;3:385–401.

36. Zimmerman NB, Suhey PV, Clark GL, et al. Silicone interpositional arthroplasty of the distal interphalangeal joint. *J Hand Surg* 1989;14:882–887.

37. Wilgus EF. Distal interphalangeal joint silicone interpositional arthroplasty of the hand. *Clin Orthop* 1997;342:38–41.

38. Snow JW, Boyes JG, Greider JL. Implant arthroplasty of the distal interphalangeal joint of the finger for osteoarthritis. *Plast Reconstr Surg* 1977;60:558–560.

39. Swanson AB, Leonard JB, Swanson G. Implant resection arthroplasty of the finger joints. *Hand Clin* 1986;2:107–117.

40. Schwartz DA, Peimer CA. Distal interphalangeal joint implant arthroplasty in a musician. *J Hand Ther* 1998;11:49–52.

41. Pellagrini VD, Burton RI. Osteoarthritis of the proximal interphalangeal joint of the hand: arthroplasty or fusion? *J Hand Surg* 1990;15:194–208.

42. Burton RI, Margles SW, Lunseth PA. Small joint arthrodesis in the hand. *J Hand Surg* 1986;11:678–682.

43. Pribyl CR, Omer GE, McGinty L. Effectiveness of the chevron arthrodesis in small joints of the hand. *J Hand Surg* 1996;21:1052–1058.

44. Das GA, Belskey MR. Arthrodesis of the proximal interphalangeal joint with K-wire technique. In: Blair WF, ed. *Hand surgery techniques*. Baltimore: Williams & Wilkins, 1996:816–823.

45. McGlynn JT. Smith RA, Bogumill GP. Arthrodesis of the small joint of the hand: a rapid and effective technique. *J Hand Surg* 1988;13:595–599.

46. Watson HK, Shaffer, SR. Concave-convex arthrodesis in joints of the hand. *Plast Reconstr Surg* 1970;46:368–371.

47. Lewis RC, Nordyke MD, Tenny JR. The tenon method of small joint arthrodesis in the hand. *J Hand Surg* 1986;11:567–569.

48. Breitbart AS, Blat PM, Staffenberg DA, et al. An experimental study of small-joint compression arthrodesis. *Ann Plastic Surg* 1997;39:47–52.

49. McGrath JC, Vigil DV, Cohen MJ. A modified approach to cup-and-cone arthrodesis of the small joints of the hand. *Contemp Orthop* 1996;32:335–339.

50. Allende BT, Engelem JC. Tension-band arthrodesis in the finger joints. *J Hand Surg* 1980;5:269–271.

51. Segmuller G. *Surgical stabilization of the skeleton of the hand.* Bern: Hans Huber Publishers, 1977.

52. Ayres JR, Goldstrohm GL, Miller GJ, et al. Proximal interphalangeal joint arthrodesis with the Herbert screw. *J Hand Surg* 1988;13:600–603.

53. Khuri MS. Tension band arthrodesis in the hand. *J Hand Surg* 1986;11:41–45.

54. Uhl RL, Schneider LH. Tension band arthrodesis of the finger joints: a retrospective review of 76 consecutive cases. *J Hand Surg* 1992;17:518–522.

55. Stern PJ, Gates NT, Jones TB. Tension band arthrodesis of small joints in the hand. *J Hand Surg* 1993;18:194–197

56. Ijsselstein CB, van Egmond, DB, Kovius SE, et al. Results of small-joint arthrodesis: comparison of Kirschner wire fixation with tension band wire technique. *J Hand Surg* 1992;17:952–956.

57. Katzman SS, Gibeault JD, Dickson K, et al. Use of a Herbert screw for interphalangeal arthrodesis. *Clinical Orthop* 1993;296:127–132.

58. Leibovic SJ, Strickland JW. Arthrodesis of the proximal interphalangeal joint of the finger: comparison of the use of the Herbert screw with other fixation methods. *J Hand Surg* 1994;19:181–188.

59. Wright CS, McMurtry RY. AO arthrodesis in the hand. *J Hand Surg* 1983;9:932–935.

60. Kleinert JM, Gateley D. Proximal interphalangeal joint fusion: special situations. *Atlas Hand Clin* 1998;3:31–39.

61. Bishop AT. Small joint arthrodesis. *Hand Clin* 1993;9:683–689.

62. Seitz WH, Sellman DC, Scarcella JB, et al. Compression arthrodesis of the small joints of the hand. *Clinical Orthop* 1994;304:116–121.

63. Ostgaard SE, Weilby A. Resection arthroplasty of the proximal interphalangeal joint. *J Hand Surg* 1993;18:613–615.

64. Seradge H, Kutz JA, Kleinert HA. Perichondral resurfacing arthroplasty in the hand. *J Hand Surg* 1984;9:880–886.

65. Carroll RE, Taber TH. Digital arthroplasty of the proximal interphalangeal joint. *J Bone Joint Surg* 1954;36:912–920.

66. Swanson AB, Maupin BK, Gajjar NV, et al. Flexible implant arthroplasty in the proximal interphalangeal joint of the hand. *J Hand Surg* 1985;10:796–805.

67. Iselin F, Conti E. Long-term results of proximal interphalangeal joint resection arthroplasties with a silicone implant. *J Hand Surg* 1995;20:S95–S97.

68. Moller K, Sollerman C, Geijer M, et al. Early results with osseointegrated proximal interphalangeal joint prostheses. *J Hand Surg* 1999;24:267–274.

69. Lindscheid RL, Murray PM, Vidal MA, et el. Development of a surface replacement arthroplasty for proximal interphalangeal joints. *J Hand Surg* 1997;22:286–298.

70. Neibauer JJ, Landry RM. Dacron-silicone prosthesis for the metacarpophalangeal and interphalangeal joints. *Hand* 1971;3:55–61.

71. Hage JJ, Yoe EPD, Zevering JP, et al. Proximal interphalangeal joint silicone arthroplasty for posttraumatic arthritis. *J Hand Surg* 1999;24:73–77

72. Doi K, Kuwata N, Kawai S. Alumina ceramic finger implants: a preliminary biomaterial and clinical evaluation. *J Hand Surg* 1984;9:740–749.

73. Ashworth CR, Hansraij KK, Todd AO, et al. Swanson proximal interphalangeal joint arthroplasty in patients with rheumatoid arthritis. *Clinical Orthop* 1997;342:34–37.

74. Dryer RF, Blair WF, Shurr DG, et al. Proximal interphalangeal joint arthroplasty. *Clinical Orthop* 1984;185:187–194.

75. Schneider LW. Proximal interphalangeal joint arthroplasty: the volar approach. *Semin Arthroplast* 1999;2:139–147.

76. Lin HH, Wyrick JD, Stern PJ. Proximal interphalangeal silicone replacement arthroplasty: clinical results using the anterior approach. *J Hand Surg* 1995;20:123–132.

77. Amadio PC, Wood MB. Alternative reconstructive procedures of the proximal interphalangeal joint. In: Morrey BF, ed. *Reconstructive surgery of the joints*, 2nd ed. New York: Churchill Livingstone, 1996:279–286.

78. Millender LH, Nalebuff EA. Commentary on osteoarthritis of the proximal interphalangeal joint. *Hand Clin* 1987;3:405–412.

79. Kovach JC, Werner FW. Palmer AK, et al. Biomechanical analysis of internal fixation techniques for proximal interphalangeal joint arthrodesis. *J Hand Surg* 1986;11:562–566.

80. Chamay A. A distally based dorsal and triangular tendinous flap for direct access to the proximal interphalangeal joint. *Ann Chir Main* 1988;7:179–183.

81. Leibovic S. Arthrodesis of the proximal interphalangeal joint of the finger using tension band wiring or Herbert screws. *Atlas Hand Clin* 1998;3:17–30.

82. Brannon EW, Klein G. Experiences with a finger-joint prosthesis. *J Bone Joint Surg* 1959;41:87–102.

83. Flatt AE. Restoration of rheumatoid finger-joint function: interim report on trial of prosthetic replacement. *J Bone Joint Surg* 1961;43:753–774.

84. Condamine JL, Benoit JY, Comtet JJ, et al. Proposed digital arthroplasty critical study of the preliminary results. *Ann Chir Main* 1988;7:282–232.

85. KirkpatrickWH, Kozin SH, Uhl RL. Early motion after arthroplasty. *Hand Clin* 1996;12:73–86.

86. Cannon N, ed. *Diagnosis and treatment manual for physicians and therapists,* 3rd ed. Indianapolis: The Hand Rehabilitation Center of Indiana, 1991.

72

OSTEOARTHRITIS OF THE HAND AND DIGITS: METACARPOPHALANGEAL AND CARPOMETACARPAL JOINTS

DAVID R. STEINBERG

SURGICAL ANATOMY AND BIOMECHANICS

Metacarpophalangeal Joint

The metacarpophalangeal (MCP) joint is a condyloid joint. The metacarpal head is narrow dorsally and widens palmarly. This leads to greater bony stability between the base of the proximal phalanx and the metacarpal head when the joint flexes beyond 70 degrees. Further joint stability is provided by components of the capsule. Weakest is the membranous dorsal capsule, which is loosely reinforced by the extensor tendon. The palmar plate has a thick fibrocartilaginous attachment to the proximal phalanx and a thinner membranous origin from the metacarpal neck. It forms the floor of the flexor tendon sheath and is attached to the extensor hood through the sagittal bands. Laterally, the palmar plate is contiguous with the deep transverse intermetacarpal ligament, which links adjacent MCP joints. The true collateral ligaments, as well as the accessory collateral ligaments that attach the palmar plate to the collateral, provide medial and lateral stability.

The asymmetry of the metacarpal head produces a cam effect, which causes the collateral ligaments to tighten when the joint is flexed. When the joint is extended, these structures allow approximately 15 degrees of radial and ulnar deviation and a small arc of rotation. The normal MCP joint describes an arc of motion from 20 degrees' hyperextension to 90 to 100 degrees' flexion.

Carpometacarpal Joint

All four carpometacarpal (CMC) joints in the hand are relatively stable due to thick intermetacarpal and palmar and dorsal CMC ligaments. Small medial and lateral facets create some degree of osseous stability between the bases of adjacent metacarpals. Additional stability is provided in the index and long fingers by the inherent bony support created by the irregular distal articular contours of the trapezium, trapezoid, and capitate. In contrast, the articulations of the ring and small finger metacarpals with the hamate allow flexion, extension, and a small amount of rotation. The radial facet of the hamate is transversely oriented, allowing 10 degrees of flexion-extension of the ring metacarpal. The small finger metacarpal articulates with the obliquely oriented ulnar facet of the hamate and describes an arc of motion between 20 and 30 degrees. Secondary dynamic support is provided to the CMC joints by the broad insertions of the flexor carpi radialis, the extensor carpi radialis longus (ECRL), the extensor carpi radialis brevis (ECRB), and the extensor carpi ulnaris (ECU) onto the index, long, and small finger metacarpal bases, respectively. Additional forces are transmitted to the fifth CMC joint by the flexor carpi ulnaris, which inserts onto the metacarpal base (via the pisometacarpal ligament) and the hypothenar muscles.

PATHOPHYSIOLOGY

Progressive deterioration of articular cartilage is the hallmark of osteoarthritis (OA). This leads to narrowing of the joint space, subchondral sclerosis, and inflammation of the synovium. Subsequently, marginal osteophytes develop. More severe cartilage destruction, invasive synovitis, and significant periarticular erosions characterize a more aggressive form of OA known as *erosive* or *inflammatory* OA (1,2).

OA of the hand may occur in 15% to 28% of patients older than the age of 45 years (3). It usually develops during the fifth and sixth decades, with women affected as much as ten times more than men. Degenerative changes in the hand may be present in up to 80% of the elderly, with the greatest predilection for the distal interphalangeal joints of the fingers and CMC joint of the thumb (4).

Metacarpophalangeal Joint

It is generally believed that the MCP joints of the hand are rarely affected by primary OA. However, there are some reports that indicate a certain degree of MCP involvement in patients with some form of OA. In one large study, 12% to

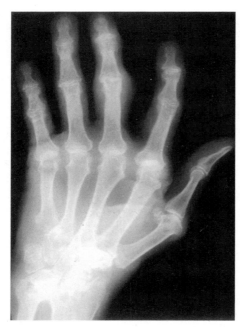

FIGURE 1. X-ray of hand of 72-year-old woman with degenerative changes suggestive of erosive osteoarthritis. Metacarpophalangeal involvement is confined to index finger. The wrist and multiple interphalangeal joints are also affected.

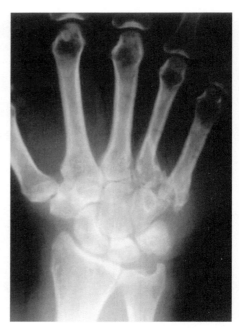

FIGURE 2. X-ray of hand that has developed intraarticular malunion of fifth carpometacarpal joint, with prominent dorsoulnar osteophyte.

25% of individuals with generalized osteoarthrosis complained of symptoms at the MCP joint (3). Ehrlich (2) reported a series of patients with inflammatory OA (which he equated with erosive OA) in whom degenerative changes occurred in the MCP joints. In these cases, the disease pattern was symmetric and involved the radial side of the hand more frequently (12% index, 7% long, 2% ring and small fingers) (Fig. 1). Most cases of OA of the MCP joint develop secondary to intraarticular fracture or ligamentous instability. The MCP joint is prone to infection from penetrating trauma such as a human bite. Degenerative changes may then develop secondary to sepsis of this joint. Hemochromatosis (5), acromegaly, and calcium pyrophosphate disease also may lead to arthritis in the MCP joint.

Carpometacarpal Joint

OA occurring at the index or long finger CMC joints is referred to as a *carpal boss*. Dorsal osteophytes develop on one or both sides of the joint: at the base of the metacarpal and the distal edge of the capitate or trapezoid. A small ganglion sometimes arises from the arthritic joint. Posttraumatic OA is most likely to develop in the small finger CMC joint. When there is involvement of the ring finger, which is rare, it is almost always associated with concomitant fifth CMC joint disease. Ligamentous instability after dislocation may result in degenerative changes in these joints. The fifth CMC joint is prone to fracture-dislocation (reverse Bennett's fracture). Intraarticular malunion of the metacarpal base in this relatively mobile joint may lead to secondary arthritis (Fig. 2).

Most cases of OA of the hand develop insidiously and slowly progress over a few years before stabilizing at varying degrees of severity. Erosive OA presents acutely; it remains active from a few months to a few years before becoming quiescent (1). Severe joint destruction and finger deformity can occur during this active phase.

EVALUATION: CLINICAL

Metacarpophalangeal Joint

Patients initially notice mild to moderate pain. Early in the disease process, this may be the only presenting symptom. As arthritis progresses, swelling, stiffness, and occasional ulnar drift occur. Synovitis and an effusion may be evident directly over the joint; more subtle swelling may manifest as loss of the dorsal concavity between adjacent metacarpal heads. Patients have difficulty making a tight fist and generating a strong grip, which limits their ability to grasp objects. Full extension also may be compromised. Some individuals demonstrate snapping or locking of the MCP joint. This condition can be classified into two groups: spontaneous and degenerative (6). Spontaneous locking occurs in patients younger than 50 years old with normal radiographs; the index finger is most commonly affected. Degenerative locking occurs in the older patient with OA when the collateral ligament (usually radial), accessory collateral ligament, or interosseous tendon catches on a marginal osteophyte (7). The long and ring fingers are more often involved in this group.

Patients with erosive or inflammatory OA present with signs of acute inflammation-erythema, warmth, swelling, and pain, which eventually evolve into a quiescent stage. In most cases of erosive OA, and, certainly, in posttraumatic arthritis, only one or two MCP joints are significantly affected. Some patients with nontraumatic arthritis also demonstrate involvement of interphalangeal joints, with Heberden's and Bouchard's nodes. Others present primarily with MCP and wrist disease, with sparing of more distal joints (8).

A thorough history may reveal previous trauma to the joint, familial predisposition to arthritis, and other joint or systemic complaints. Other causes of painful, stiff, or popping digits that must be considered in the differential diagnosis of OA of the MCP joint include trigger finger, extensor tendon subluxation, and rheumatoid arthritis (RA). The patient with multiple trigger digits may complain of morning stiffness, with the fingers in a semiflexed position, pain between the mid-palm and proximal interphalangeal joint, and catching of the fingers. Physical examination may reveal flexor tendon nodules and tenderness proximal to the MCP joint in the palm, with absence of MCP swelling and dorsal tenderness. Extensor tendon subluxation over the metacarpal head causes snapping, with pain centered over the MCP joint. This usually occurs in association with RA, after penetrating trauma that severs a junctura tendinum (9), or after blunt trauma that causes rupture of a sagittal band. Subluxation of the extensor tendon is evident on examination. RA tends to involve all MCP joints, often with greater changes in the ulnar digits. Other distinguishing features of this disease include boutonnière and swan-neck deformities, rheumatoid nodules, frequent involvement of the distal ulna, and more widespread joint and soft tissue disease.

Carpometacarpal Joint

Patients with a carpal boss present with tender swelling over the dorsum of the hand. The onset is gradual, with no antecedent trauma. Pain may be exacerbated by activities requiring frequent wrist flexion and extension, which is caused by tendinitis of the ECRL and ECRB tendons as they pass over the dorsal osteophyte. The mass is firm, nonmobile, and smaller than 5 to 10 mm in diameter. There may be an associated small ganglion in 30% of cases (10). Fusi et al. (11) described a stress test of the CMC joint, in which the MCP joints of the index and long fingers are held in flexion while the metacarpals are simultaneously distracted and rotated. This reportedly reproduces pain in the arthritic CMC joint. Care should be taken when interpreting results of this maneuver, as it can cause discomfort in an asymptomatic joint. The carpal boss is accentuated with maximal wrist flexion and may be confused with the more common dorsal wrist ganglion. The examiner may mistakenly believe he or she is palpating a mobile cyst, when actually he or she is feeling an inflamed wrist extensor tendon slip medially or laterally over the osteophyte. Care-

ful localization of the mass aids in diagnosis, as the boss is palpable over the CMC joints, whereas the wrist ganglion arises more proximally from the scapholunate interval. Attempted aspiration will yield no fluid and result in increased patient discomfort and physician frustration.

OA of the small finger CMC joint causes ulnar hand pain that is aggravated when attempting power grip. Decreased ability to flex this joint interferes with formation of the metacarpal arch for gripping objects and cupping the palm; inability to flatten the palm adversely affects hand function. Swelling, tenderness, and crepitus are more easily appreciated dorsally. Severe degenerative changes may cause intrinsic atrophy and hand weakness from irritation and entrapment of the deep motor branch of the ulnar nerve, which passes over the palmar aspect of these joints. The author has treated one such case; a similar ulnar motor neuropathy in association with acute injury has also been described (12).

EVALUATION: IMAGING STUDIES

Metacarpophalangeal Joint

Degenerative changes of the MCP joint are seen on four standard radiographic views of the hand—posteroanterior, lateral, radial, and ulnar obliques. Joint space narrowing, subchondral sclerosis, intraarticular malunion, and angular deformity are evident on posteroanterior and lateral radiographs. Oblique views aid in identifying subtle intraarticular changes as well as the peripheral osteophytes responsible for locking of the MCP joint (Fig. 3). Posner et al. (13)

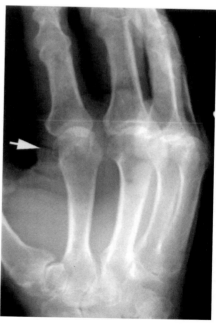

FIGURE 3. Oblique x-ray of index metacarpophalangeal joint demonstrating prominent radial osteophyte (*arrow*) that caused intermittent locking.

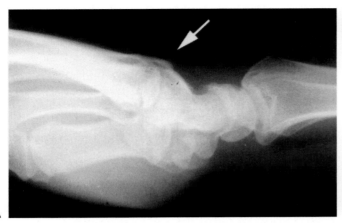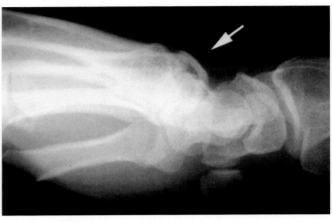

A   B

FIGURE 4. A: Lateral x-ray of patient with symptomatic carpal boss (*arrow*). **B:** Thirty-degree supinated lateral x-ray of same patient more accurately demonstrates osteophyte bridging the carpometacarpal joint (*arrow*).

have recommended arthrotomography as an additional diagnostic test for the locked MCP joint, although the author has no experience with this technique. Magnetic resonance imaging currently plays a limited role in the evaluation of OA of MCP joint. Although it can demonstrate the pathology of a locked MCP joint and synovitis, magnetic resonance imaging rarely assists in diagnosis or surgical planning.

Carpometacarpal Joint

OA of the CMC joint is more difficult to detect on standard radiographs. A prominent carpal boss may be visible on a lateral view (Fig. 4). A lateral view with the hand and forearm supinated 30 degrees is the best projection for visualizing small osteophytes. Results of this technique reportedly can be improved by additionally placing the hand in 20 to 30 degrees of ulnar deviation (10). Sixty-three percent of patients will have bony anomalies present on x-ray, ranging from a separate ossicle (*os styloideum*) to complete bridging between the metacarpal and carpal bones (11). The CMC joints of the ring and small fingers are best viewed on an anteroposterior radiograph with the forearm pronated 30 degrees (14).

EVALUATION-ANCILLARY STUDIES

The diagnosis of OA in the hand usually can be made with a careful history, thorough physical examination, and radiographic evaluation. Other studies may be indicated if rheumatoid disease or crystalline-induced arthropathy are being considered in the differential diagnosis. Synovial fluid may be aspirated from the MCP joint and examined for cell count and crystals. A routine autoimmune panel (including erythrocyte sedimentation rate, complement levels, rheumatoid factor, and antinuclear antibodies) may

assist in the diagnosis of certain systemic disorders. If any uncertainty about the diagnosis remains, then consultation with a rheumatologist may be indicated.

NONOPERATIVE TREATMENT

The goals of OA management include reduction of pain, control of inflammation, and restoration of function. The symptoms of OA can be reduced with a combination of rest, intermittent splinting, and oral nonsteroidal antiinflammatory drugs. Patients can benefit from the ministrations of a hand therapist. In addition to fabricating splints, the therapist can provide treatments to minimize inflammation and adaptive devices to assist with hand function.

Some authors have advocated nonsurgical treatment of the locked MCP joint (13,15). The joint is distended with local anesthetic to elevate the entrapped collateral ligament, followed by gentle manipulation. This technique has been successful in 6 of 13 patients reported in two series (13,15). Closed manipulation without joint distention is not effective (7,16). Some authors do not believe manipulation is indicated (6,16), although only one case of fracture has been reported as a complication of closed treatment (17).

Judicious use of intraarticular corticosteroids may reduce pain and inflammation when these initial measures are ineffective. Caution must be exercised, as excessive steroid administration into joints or around tendons may lead to progressive cartilage deterioration (18) or tendon rupture (19). Most reported experiences with intraarticular corticosteroids have been in larger joints. The earliest published reports described 50% to 90% reduction in symptoms with injections of hydrocortisone (20,21). Some relief was noted within 24 hours, with an average duration of 2 to 3 weeks. Stolzer et al. (22) found that 92% of patients obtained a minimum of 1 to 4 weeks of symptomatic relief from intraarticular corticosteroid injections in the hand.

A variety of new pharmacologic agents for treating OA have recently been added to the physician's armamentarium, including intraarticular hyaluronic acid substitutes and glucosamine/chondroitin sulfate. Early clinical experience in large joints (e.g., the knee) has demonstrated some degree of symptom remission (23). The efficacy of these medications in the treatment of hand arthritis has not yet been established.

Author's Preferred Treatment

Nonsteroidal antiinflammatory drugs and rest constitute the first line of treatment for hand OA.

The individual should modify activities at home or work to minimize motion of involved joints. Custom-fabricated thermoplastic splints can immobilize the hand and wrist in an appropriate position. A hand-based splint should hold affected MCP joints in 60 degrees of flexion. CMC arthritis is best immobilized in a forearm-based splint with the wrist in 20 to 30 degrees of extension. The exact wearing schedule should be customized to the individual patient's needs.

If this treatment is ineffective after a few weeks, or if the patient presents with more advanced symptoms, then referral to a hand therapist is indicated. Hand therapists can offer paraffin treatment and other modalities to decrease inflammation and instruct the patient in joint mobilization exercises. The therapist can also provide the patient with simple adaptive aids to improve hand function for activities of daily living.

Intraarticular steroid injections may alleviate symptoms when the preceding measures have failed. One to 2 cc of betamethasone sodium phosphate mixed with 1% plain lidocaine in a 1:1 ratio is administered through a 25-gauge needle. Intraarticular injections are performed for MCP and ulnar CMC joints. For a symptomatic carpal boss, a peritendinous injection is given to treat ECRL/ECRB tendinitis. A better response is seen when the patient is splinted almost continuously for 2 to 3 weeks in conjunction with the injection. Patients with other inflammatory conditions, such as de Quervain's tenosynovitis (24) or flexor tenosynovitis (trigger finger), have benefited from this combined approach. A repeat steroid injection in conjunction with splint immobilization has been successful in cases in which injection alone was insufficient.

SURGICAL MANAGEMENT: METACARPOPHALANGEAL JOINT

Surgical intervention is indicated for a symptomatic locking MCP joint. Of 52 cases of MCP locking described in the literature, 29 were due to OA (7,13,15). Ten percent of locked MCP joints recovered spontaneously after 1 to 2 weeks of observation. Patients with a persistently locked MCP joint who fail closed manipulation are good candi-

dates for surgical release. Débridement of the palmar or radial osteophyte and release of the involved soft tissues lead to satisfactory resolution of symptoms.

Patients with severe arthritis that has not responded to an appropriate period of conservative management should be offered operative intervention. Reconstructive options for significant degenerative disease include implant arthroplasty, soft tissue arthroplasty, and arthrodesis. Experience with any of these techniques for OA is limited: Implant arthroplasty is much more commonly performed for RA (refer to Chapter 67 for more complete discussion), whereas the latter two procedures are more often reserved for salvage of a failed implant.

The first replacement arthroplasty for the MCP joint was developed by Flatt in the 1960s (25). This hinged, metallic prosthesis never gained widespread use due to problems with insertion, fracture, loosening, and skin necrosis. Swanson (26) and Niebauer and Landry (27) independently developed a flexible stemmed silicone implant. By design, the Swanson implant acts as a spacer that provides immediate stability, with secondary support developing during encapsulation of the silicone. MCP motion occurs through a combination of flexion-extension of the hinge mechanism and pistoning of the implant stems within the medullary canals. In general, the patient may expect an arc of motion from 40 to 60 degrees, with an extensor lag averaging 10 to 20 degrees (28–32). In OA, this procedure can eliminate pain and improve function, with some patients able to return to manual labor (33). Modifications of this prosthesis include newer implant designs (NeuFlex implant, DePuy, Warsaw, IN) that reportedly allow greater motion with less strain, as well as the addition of titanium grommets to the stems to improve implant durability (Fig. 5).

Due to concerns regarding inherent design limitations, implant breakage, and potential synovitis of the silicone devices, some surgeons have attempted total joint replacement for the MCP joint. Steffee et al. (34) developed a prosthesis consisting of a metal phalangeal replacement that articulated with a polyethylene metacarpal component. This product never gained widespread acceptance due to problems with loosening and implant failure (35). Semiconstrained surface replacements for the MCP joint better simulate normal joint motion and require less bone resection and soft tissue disruption. The osteoarthritic joint with minimal bone loss and preservation of soft tissue restraints may be an ideal indication for these implants. Some of these are being studied in clinical trials—preliminary results are encouraging, although joint instability has been a problem in certain cases (35–37). In addition, unconstrained implants of pyrolytic carbon, which possess excellent wear properties and some degree of bony appositional growth, have become available. Because dislocation is an inherent risk with this design, preservation of the collateral ligaments and careful soft tissue repair is essential (Fig. 6). Currently, silicone

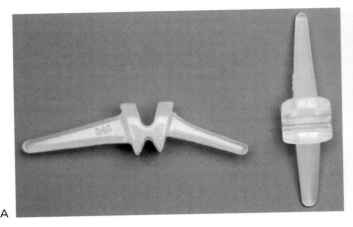

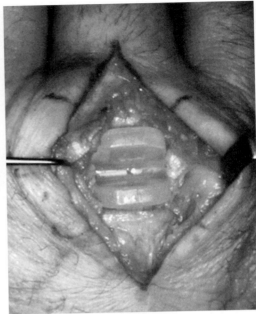

FIGURE 5. Use of a NeuFlex (DePuy, Warsaw, IN) silicone implant **(A)** in a patient with an isolated metacarpophalangeal joint arthrosis **(B)**.

implant arthroplasty remains the procedure of choice for reconstruction of the arthritic MCP joint.

Author's Preferred Technique: Locked Metacarpophalangeal Joint

A palmar approach to the locked MCP joint is the most versatile, allowing access to both radial and ulnar pathology. A more lateral approach can be used in the index finger if the surgeon is convinced that the radiovolar osteophyte is

the cause of locking. The digital neurovascular bundles are protected as the flexor tendon sheath is exposed. The A1 pulley is released, and the flexor tendons gently retracted to expose the palmar plate. A longitudinal incision is made on the side of pathology between the palmar plate and accessory collateral ligament. The underlying osteophyte is exposed and resected with a rongeur. The opposite side of the joint may similarly be exposed if indicated. Skin is closed in routine fashion. A soft dressing is applied and immediate motion encouraged.

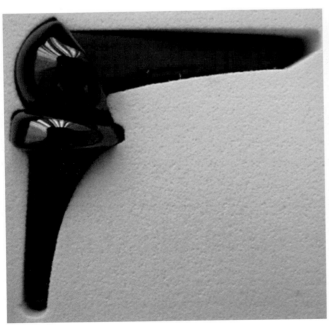

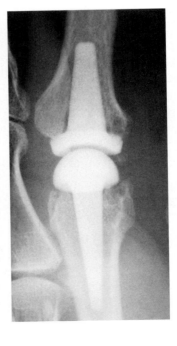

FIGURE 6. The pyrolytic carbon metacarpophalangeal implant **(A)** requires careful insertion in the osteoarthritic patient, as noted on the anteroposterior radiograph **(B)**.

Author's Preferred Technique: Metacarpophalangeal Joint Silicone Arthroplasty

The basic principles and surgical techniques in MCP joint silicone arthroplasty for OA are similar to those used in the rheumatoid hand. If a single MCP joint is involved, as is often the case in degenerative or posttraumatic arthritis, the surgeon may prefer a gently curving longitudinal dorsal incision instead of the standard transverse incision used when replacing all four joints. If the extensor mechanism is intact, without the tendon subluxation and sagittal band attenuation seen in RA, then the central tendon is incised longitudinally. The capsule is incised longitudinally to expose the base of the proximal phalanx and the metacarpal neck. Any contracted soft tissues must be meticulously released at this time; the collateral ligaments should be elevated from their origin. Bone resection and canal preparation are identical to that for RA. A trial implant is first placed to check soft tissue balance. The actual prosthesis is inserted with smooth forceps using a "no-touch" technique. The extensor tendon is repaired with a running nonabsorbable braided suture. Skin is closed with interrupted sutures over a Penrose drain. Intraoperative radiographs confirm implant placement and joint reduction. A bulky dressing is applied, with the fingers supported in full extension with a volar forearm-based splint out to the fingertips. Postoperative therapy begins within 1 week of surgery. A dynamic extension splint is used during waking hours for 6 weeks. Gentle active flexion within this splint is encouraged. A static resting splint is fabricated for nighttime use. The patient may be required to use this for 3 months. The surgeon and therapist should follow the patient closely; any tendency toward pronation of the index finger must be managed with appropriate splint modifications (38).

SURGICAL MANAGEMENT: CARPOMETACARPAL JOINT

Surgical resection is indicated for the painful carpal boss that has been unresponsive to conservative measures. Excision of any associated ganglion as well as the dorsal osteophyte is necessary to minimize recurrence and ensure a successful outcome. Long-term relief has been reported in 94% of cases (11). More diffuse degenerative changes in the radial CMC joints, often secondary to ligament instability, may require arthrodesis. Satisfactory results can be expected in more than 90% of patients, with a nonunion rate of less than 5% (39).

When nonoperative treatment fails to control symptoms in the arthritic fifth CMC joint, surgical intervention should be considered. Open reduction of chronically dislocated CMC joints occasionally can yield satisfactory results (14,40,41). This procedure should not be performed unless there is absolutely no evidence of articular damage, either radiographically or intraoperatively. A few authors have recommended arthroplasty of this joint. In 16 patients with symptomatic malunions of ulnar CMC fracture dislocations, 15 were successfully treated with partial resection arthroplasty (42). Silicone interposition arthroplasty, which can restore 15 to 30 degrees of CMC motion, has not received much attention in the literature (43).

The most commonly recommended operation for posttraumatic arthritis or instability of the fifth CMC joint has been arthrodesis. This leads to diminution or complete resolution of pain and improvement in grip strength (44). The fourth and fifth CMC joints must be fused in 20 to 30 degrees of flexion to maintain the distal metacarpal arch. Some authors believe that arthrodesis of these mobile joints leads to decreased motion and concomitant development of tight grip (42). However, mobility of the fifth ray is preserved by compensatory motion that occurs at the triquetral hamate joint (44).

Author's Preferred Technique: Carpal Boss

The osteophyte is approached through a dorsal transverse incision. Major longitudinal vessels and cutaneous nerves should be preserved. The index CMC joint is approached between ECRL and ECRB tendons. For exposure of the long finger CMC joint, the ECRL/ECRB tendons are retracted radially and the digital extensors ulnarly. In some cases, the insertion of the wrist extensor may require subperiosteal elevation to enhance joint exposure. Any associated ganglion, including its stalk and capsular origin, is excised. A longitudinal incision is made in the joint capsule to expose the metacarpal base and distal carpal bone. The dorsal osteophytes on one or both or these should be excised with a rongeur or sharp osteotome down to normal articular cartilage. This should result in a slight concave configuration of the joint (Fig. 7). The capsule, periosteum, and wrist extensor insertions are reapproximated. Skin is closed in routine fashion. The wrist is immobilized in 15 to 20 degrees of extension for 4 weeks, followed by intermittent splinting for an additional 2 weeks.

Author's Preferred Technique: Fifth Carpometacarpal Arthritis

Small dorsoradial osteophytes formed from malunions of fifth CMC fracture/dislocations can be treated effectively with resection arthroplasty. The technique is similar to carpal boss excision. A transverse incision is made directly over the joint. Major longitudinal vessels and cutaneous branches of ulnar sensory nerve should be preserved. Transverse or longitudinal capsulotomy allows visualization of the joint; subperiosteal elevation of ECU insertion may be required. Arthritic spurs on both sides of the joint are excised with a rongeur until normal articular cartilage is

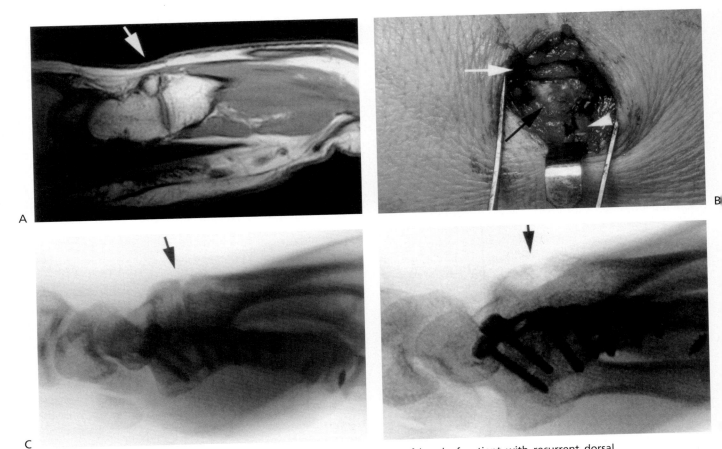

FIGURE 7. A: Sagittal magnetic resonance imaging of hand of patient with recurrent dorsal pain 1 year after carpal boss excision demonstrates recurrent osteophyte with *os styloideum.* (*arrow*). **B:** Intraoperative view of carpal boss of third carpometacarpal (CMC) joint approached between radial wrist extensors (*white arrow*) and digital extensors (under retractor). Bridging osteophyte (*black arrow*) obscures joint line (*arrowhead*). **C:** Preoperative lateral x-ray illustrates third CMC joint before resection (*arrow*). **D:** Postoperative lateral x-ray illustrates concave appearance of CMC joint after adequate resection of carpal boss (*arrow*).

encountered. The capsule, periosteum, and ECU insertion are reapproximated. Skin is closed in routine fashion. The author prefers to immobilize the wrist for 2 weeks, followed by gradual mobilization, although others have recommended a more aggressive exercise program (42).

CMC arthrodesis is indicated for more extensive arthritis or failed resection arthroplasty. A more extensile approach is required, using either a longitudinal incision or a lazy-S that incorporates a previous transverse scar. The joint is visualized through a longitudinal capsulotomy with mobilization of ECU insertion. Both articular surfaces of the CMC joint are curetted down to subchondral bone. A trough perpendicular to the joint is created dorsally in the hamate and fifth metacarpal base. A corticocancellous graft is fashioned to fit into the trough, and cancellous chips are inserted into the joint. The joint must be immobilized in 20 to 30 degrees of flexion. The author prefers to stabilize the arthrodesis with 0.045-in. Kirschner wires, although this is not necessarily required if the inlay graft provides absolute stability (44). Capsule and skin are closed in rou-

tine fashion. Wrist and ulnar two digits are immobilized in a forearm-based ulnar gutter splint or cast until there is radiographic evidence of fusion, which usually occurs by 8 weeks. Kirschner wires may be removed at this time.

COMPLICATIONS

Corticosteroid injections for OA of the hand and digits are usually well tolerated with minimal side effects. Complications that are mainly cosmetic include local depigmentation in dark-skinned individuals and subcutaneous fat necrosis. Infection, a potentially devastating development, is rare, occurring in 0.001% to 0.072% of joints after intraarticular injection (45,46). Multiple corticosteroid injections may lead to cartilage degeneration, thus accelerating the progression of OA (18,47,48). A similar deleterious effect of corticosteroids may occur in tendons. Anecdotal clinical reports [reviewed by Stefanich (49)] and a series of experimental studies (19,50–53) have documented tendon ruptures and decreased tensile strength of tendons and ligaments when exposed to corticosteroids. When tendon rupture does occur, there is usually enough segmental degeneration that grafting or tendon transfer is required to restore function.

Although phalangeal fracture is a potential risk of closed manipulation of a locked MCP joint, there is only one reported case in the literature (17). This can be prevented by first insufflating the joint and then applying only gentle manipulation. The surgeon should realize that manipulation frequently fails and should not hesitate to consider open reduction early in the course of treatment.

Less than 10% of patients have recurrent or residual pain after carpal boss excision. This may be due to inadequate resection, particularly if symptoms recur within the first few months after surgery (11). If symptoms persist after an intraarticular lidocaine injection, then the physician should look for another source of dorsal hand pain. If symptoms are temporarily eliminated, and a trial of conservative therapy is ineffective, then a more thorough surgical excision of the joint should be performed. The other cause of persistent pain in both the radial and ulnar CMC joints is more diffuse OA. Diagnosis is aided by preoperative tomograms or computed tomography scans. If these imaging studies or intraoperative inspection reveals significant degenerative changes of joint, then CMC arthrodesis should be performed.

MCP arthroplasties are more prone to failure in the patient with posttraumatic arthritis due to the increased demands they place on an otherwise normal hand. Swanson (26) does not believe that implant fracture is synonymous with failure; many patients continue to experience satisfactory hand function if encapsulation of the implant has occurred. An arthroplasty can be revised if failure is due to loosening or dislocation, with careful attention to prosthesis stabilization and soft tissue rebalancing.

Resection arthroplasty can salvage an implant that has failed due to infection or after multiple surgeries. Bunnell (54) covered a reshaped metacarpal head with fascia lata; most of his patients obtained 70 degrees of flexion. Weilby (55) stabilized the joint after bony resection by suturing the proximal edge of the palmar plate to the dorsal metacarpal head. Vainio (56) developed a resection/interposition arthroplasty in which a transected extensor tendon was interposed into the joint and attached to the palmar plate.

As motion is so crucial to the function of the MCP joint, fusion is poorly tolerated. In certain instances, however, this may be the only alternative available. Arthrodesis is most reasonably considered for the index finger, which primarily must function with the thumb to provide stable pinch. The ulnar three digits are less able to produce tight grip when their MCP joints are fused. The accepted positions for MCP arthrodesis describe a gentle cascade from radial to ulnar: 25 degrees' flexion in the index finger, increasing in increments of 5 degrees to reach 40 degrees' flexion in the small finger.

The approach to the MCP joint is identical to that for arthroplasty. Excision of the collateral ligaments allows maximal joint exposure. The bony surfaces are denuded down to subchondral bone using commercially available cup and cone reamers. The most successful methods of fixation include tension-band wiring and dorsal plating using 2.0 mm or 2.7 mm mini plates, with fusion rates from 96% to 100% (57,58). The extensor tendon is repaired with a running nonabsorbable braided suture. Skin is closed with interrupted nylon sutures. The hand is immobilized for 1 week, followed by custom splinting of the MCP joint. Early interphalangeal joint motion is encouraged. The patient is gradually weaned from the splint. Immobilization is discontinued when there is radiographic evidence of fusion.

REFERENCES

1. Marmor L, Peter JB. Osteoarthritis of the hand. *CORR* 1969;64:164–173.
2. Ehrlich GE. Inflammatory osteoarthritis—I. The clinical syndrome. *J Chron Dis* 1972;25:317–328.
3. Lawrence JS. Generalized osteoarthrosis in a population sample. *Am J Epidemiol* 1969;90:381–389.
4. Caspi D, Flusser G, Farber I, et al. Clinical, radiographic, demographic, and occupational aspects of hand osteoarthritis in the elderly. *Semin Arthritis Rheum* 2001;30:321–331.
5. Schumacher HR Jr. Arthropathy in hemochromatosis. *Hosp Pract* 1998;33:81–86, 89–90.
6. Harvey FJ. Locking of the metacarpo-phalangeal joints. *J Bone Joint Surg* 1974;56B:156–159.
7. Rankin EA, Uwagie-Ero S. Locking of the metacarpophalangeal joint. *J Hand Surg* 1986;11A:868–871.
8. Kellgren JH, Lawrence JS, Bier F. Genetic factors in generalized osteoarthrosis. *Ann Rheum Dis* 1963;22:237–255.
9. Saldana MJ, McGuire RA. Chronic painful subluxation of the metacarpal phalangeal joint extensor tendons. *J Hand Surg* 1986;11A:420–423.
10. Cuono CB, Watson HK. The carpal boss: surgical treatment and etiological considerations. *Plast Reconstr Surg* 1979;63:88–93.
11. Fusi S, Watson HK, Cuono CB. The carpal boss—a 20 year review of operative management. *J Hand Surg* 1995;20B:405–408.
12. Peterson P, Sacks S. Fracture-dislocation of the base of the fifth metacarpal associated with injury to the deep motor branch of the ulnar nerve: a case report. *J Hand Surg* 1986;11A:525–528.
13. Posner MA, Langa V, Green SM. The locked metacarpophalangeal joint: diagnosis and treatment. *J Hand Surg* 1986;11A:249–253.
14. Bora FW Jr, Didizian NH. The treatment of injuries to the carpometacarpal joint of the little finger. *J Bone Joint Surg* 1974;56A:1459–1463.
15. Guly HR, Azam MA. Locked finger treated by manipulation. *J Bone Joint Surg* 1982;64B:73–75.
16. Aston JN. Locked middle finger. *J Bone Joint Surg* 1960;42B:75–79.

17. Langenskiold A. Habitual locking of the metacarpophalangeal joint by the collateral ligament, a rare cause of trigger finger. *Acta Chir Scand* 1949;99:73–78.

18. Mankin HJ, Conger KA. The acute effects of intra-articular hydrocortisone on articular cartilage in rabbits. *J Bone Joint Surgery* 1966;48A:1383.

19. Balasubramanian P, Prathap K. The effect of injection of hydrocortisone into rabbit calcaneal tendons. *J Bone Joint Surgery* 1972;54B:729.

20. Hollander JL, Brown EM Jr, Jessar RA, Brown CY. Hydrocortisone and cortisone injected into arthritic joints. *JAMA* 1951;147:1629.

21. Hollander JL, Brown EM Jr, Jessar RA, et al. Local antirheumatic effectiveness of higher esters and analogues of hydrocortisone. *Ann Rheum Dis* 1954;13:297.

22. Stolzer BL, Eisenbeis CH, Barr JH Jr, et al. Intraarticular injections of adrenocorticosteroids in patients with arthritis. *Penn Med* 1962;65:911.

23. Brief AA, Maurer SG, DiCesare PE. Use of glucosamine and chondroitin sulfate in the management of osteoarthritis. *J Am Acad Orthop Surg* 2001;9:71–78.

24. Witt J, Pess G, Gelberman RH. Treatment of de Quervain tenosynovitis. A prospective study of the results of injection of steroids and immobilization in a splint. *J Bone Joint Surg [Am]* 1991;73:219–222.

25. Flatt AE. *The care of the rheumatoid hand.* St. Louis: Mosby, 1968.

26. Swanson AB. Silicone rubber implants for replacement of arthritic or destroyed joints in the hand. *Surg Clin North Am* 1968;48:1003–1013.

27. Niebauer J, Landry R. Dacron-silicon prosthesis for the metacarpophalangeal and interphalangeal joints. *Hand* 1989;3:55–61.

28. Swanson AB. Flexible implant arthroplasty for arthritic finger joints. *J Bone Joint Surg [Am]* 1972;54-A:435–455.

29. Beckenbaugh RD, Dobyns JH, Linscheid RL. Review and analysis of silicone-rubber metacarpophalangeal implants. *J Bone Joint Surg* 1976;58A:483–487.

30. Blair WF, Shurr DG, Buckwalter JA. Metacarpophalangeal joint implant arthroplasty with a silastic spacer. *J Bone Joint Surg* 1984;66A:365–370.

31. Adams BD, Blair WF, Shurr DG. Schultz metacarpophalangeal arthroplasty: a long-term follow-up study. *J Hand Surg* 1990;15A:641–645.

32. Foliart DE. Swanson silicone finger joint implants: a review of the literature regarding long-term complications. *J Hand Surg* 1995;20A:445–449.

33. Millender LH, Nalebuff EA. Metacarpophalangeal joint arthroplasty utilizing the silicone rubber prosthesis. *Orthop Clin* 1973;4:349–371.

34. Steffee AD, Beckenbaugh RD, Linscheid RL, Dobyns JH. The development, technique, and early clinical results of total joint replacement for the metacarpophalangeal joint in the finger. *Orthopedics* 1981;4:175–180.

35. Beckenbaugh RD. Preliminary experience with a noncemented nonconstrained total joint arthroplasty for the metacarpophalangeal joints. *Orthopedics* 1983;6:962–965.

36. Cook SD, Beckenbaugh RD, Redondo J, et al. Long-term follow-up of pyrolytic carbon metacarpophalangeal implants. *J Bone Joint Surg* 1999;81:635–648.

37. Linscheid RL. Implant arthroplasty of the hand: retrospective and prospective considerations. *J Hand Surg* 2000;25A:796–816.

38. DeVore GL, Muhleman CA, Sasarita SG. Management of pronation deformity in metacarpophalangeal joint implant arthroplasty. *J Hand Surg* 1986;11A:859–861.

39. Joseph RB, Linscheid RL, Dobyns JH, Bryan RS. Chronic sprains of the carpometacarpal joints. *J Hand Surg* 1981;6A:172–180.

40. Waugh RL, Yancey AG. Carpometacarpal dislocations. *J Bone Joint Surg* 1948;30A:397–404.

41. Hagstrom P. Fracture dislocation in the ulnar carpometacarpal joints. *Scand J Plast Reconstr Surg* 1975;9:249–251.

42. Black DM, Watson HK, Vender MI. Arthroplasty of the ulnar carpometacarpal joints. *J Hand Surg* 1987;12A:1071–1074.

43. Green WL, Kilgore ES Jr. Treatment of fifth digit carpometacarpal arthritis with Silastic prosthesis. *J Hand Surg* 1981;6A.

44. Clendenin MB, Smith RJ. Fifth metacarpal/hamate arthrodesis for posttraumatic osteoarthritis. *J Hand Surg* 1984;9A:374–378.

45. Hollander JL. Intrasynovial corticosteroid therapy in arthritis. *Maryland Med J* 1970;19:62.

46. Gray RG, Tenebaum J, Gottlieb NL. Local corticosteroid injection treatment in rheumatic disorders. *Semin Arthritis Rheum* 1981;21:92.

47. Salter RB, Gross A, Hall JH. Hydrocortisone arthropathy-an experimental investigation. *CMAJ* 1967;97:374.

48. Moskowitz RW, Davis W, Sammarco J, et al. Experimentally induced corticosteroid arthropathy. *Arthritis Rheum* 1970;13:236.

49. Stefanich RJ. Intraarticular corticosteroids in treatment of osteoarthritis. *Orthop Rev* 1986;15:27–33.

50. Wrenn RN, Goldner JL, Markee JL. An experimental study of the effect of cortisone on the healing process and tensile strength of tendons. *J Bone Joint Surg* 1954;36A:588.

51. Ketchum LD. Effects of triamcinolone on tendon healing and function. *Plast Reconstr Surg* 1971;47:471.

52. Noyes FR, Grood ES, Nussbaum NS, Cooper SM. Effect of intra-articular corticosteroids on ligament properties. *Clin Orthop* 1977;123:197.

53. Wiggins ME, Fadale PD, Ehrlich MG, Walsh WR. Healing characteristics of type I collagenous structure treated with corticosteroids. *Am J Sports Med* 1994;22:279–288.

54. Bunnell S. *Surgery of the hand.* Philadelphia: JB Lippincott, 1964:298–350.

55. Weilby A. Resection arthroplasty of the metacarpophalangeal joint using interposition of the volar plate. *Scand J Plast Reconstr Surg* 1977;11:239–242.

56. Vainio K. Vainio arthroplasty of the metacarpophalangeal joints in rheumatoid arthritis. *J Hand Surg* 1989;14A:367–368.

57. Allende BT, Engelem JC. Tension-band arthrodesis in the finger joints. *J Hand Surg* 1980;5A:269–272.

58. Wright CS, McMurty RY. AO arthrodesis in the hand. *J Hand Surg* 1983;9A:932–935.

73

OSTEOARTHRITIS OF THE HAND AND DIGITS: THUMB

MICHAEL S. BEDNAR

SURGICAL ANATOMY AND BIOMECHANICS

Motion at the thumb carpometacarpal (CMC) joint occurs through the reciprocal concave surfaces of the proximal thumb metacarpal and the distal articular surface of the trapezium. Because of the lack of bony congruity, the stability of the joint is dependent on ligamentous restraint.

The intracapsular palmar oblique ligament, or beak ligament, attaches to the apex of the thumb metacarpal. It has been shown to tighten in pronation of the thumb, as occurs during forceful lateral pinch, and, in this position, is the primary stabilizer against dorsal translation of the metacarpal on the trapezium (1). Loss of this ligamentous support moves the ligamentous pivot point for metacarpal flexion distally. This increases the translation of the metacarpal on the trapezium and increases shear forces between the articular surfaces. In a cadaver study simulating acute dorsal CMC dislocation, other authors have demonstrated that the dorsoradial ligament is the primary stabilizer against dorsal translation (2). In addition, a recent study has identified 16 ligaments stabilizing the trapezium and the trapeziometacarpal joint (3). The dorsoradial and deep anterior oblique (beak) ligaments stabilize the CMC joint. The deep anterior beak ligament allows pronation during palmar abduction. The dorsal trapezio–second metacarpal, volar trapezio–second metacarpal, and volar trapezio–third metacarpal ligaments function as tension bands and prevent instability from cantilever forces (Fig. 1).

The dorsal expansion of the abductor pollicis longus (APL) is the major stabilizer of the thumb in supination. Because pinch rarely places the thumb in supination, it is less important than the palmar beak ligament in joint stability. The anterior capsular recess is between these two structures, deep to the thenar muscle. It provides an excellent surgical window to the joint that does not disturb joint stability. The anterior beak ligament, a superficial capsular ligament, is oriented from proximal dorsal to distal palmar along the anterior and posterior surfaces of the joint cap-

sule. It does not stabilize the thumb metacarpal in flexion or discourage dorsal metacarpal translation.

In the pathologic condition, chondromalacia of the palmar compartment of the thumb CMC joint is associated with degeneration of the palmar beak ligament. The ligament detaches from its normal position congruent with the joint surface. This effectively moves the attachment of the stabilizing beak ligament distally, compromising its mechanical efficiency in checking dorsal migration of the metacarpal on the trapezium during dynamic flexion-adduction of the thumb (4). Female specimens were more likely to have this type of destruction. These specimens were also more likely to show eburnation in the palmar joint surface of the metacarpal. In patients with less severe arthritis on x-ray, the eburnation was only on the most palmar perimeter of the joint (5). Patients with more severe radiographic changes were noted to have increased dorsal extension of the eburnation. Chondromalacia most commonly occurs in the dorsal compartment. It corresponds to a noncontact area during lateral pinch and is not associated with degenerative change of the palmar beak ligament. This pattern predominates in men. It appears to be secondary to poor joint nutrition from inadequate surface contact and represents the normal aging process.

A predictable pattern of articular degeneration occurs at the CMC joint. Metacarpal surface degeneration originates at the palmar, peripheral margin adjacent to the palmar beak ligament attachment. In the flexion-adduction position (pinch position), the compression force is concentrated on the palmar articular surface. The joint compression force at the trapeziometacarpal surfaces has been shown to be 12 times greater than the force generated at the tips of the thumb and index finger in lateral pinch (6). With thumb motion, there is axial rotation, which subjects the articular surfaces to shear force. The magnitude of the shear force is proportional to the amount of pinch force exerted. As the disease progresses, the region progresses dorsally toward the center of the metacarpal joint surface. Articular cartilage loss and eburnation of the trapezium occur more centrally

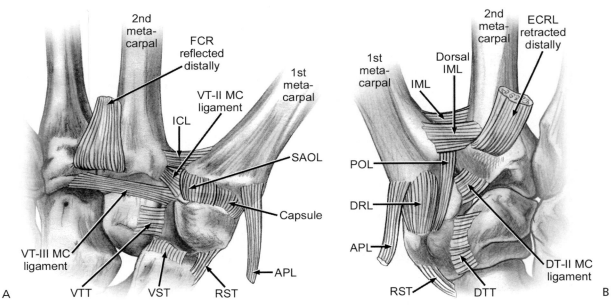

FIGURE 1. **A:** Deep volar ligaments of the carpometacarpal joint. **B:** Dorsal ligaments of the carpometacarpal joint. APL, abductor pollicis longus; DRL, dorsoradial ligament; DT-II MC, dorsal trapezio–second metacarpal; DTT, dorsal trapeziotrapezoidal ligament; ECRL, extensor carpi radialis longus; FCR, flexor carpi radialis; ICL, intercarpal ligament; IML, intermetacarpal ligament; POL, posterior oblique ligament; RST, radial scaphotrapezial ligament; SAOL, superficial anterior oblique ligament (beak ligament); VST, volar scaphotrapezial ligament; VT-II MC, volar trapezio–second metacarpal; VT-III MC, volar trapezio–third metacarpal; VTT, volar trapeziotrapezoidal ligament.

on the palmar side of the joint. As the disease progresses, the cartilage loss enlarges concentrically.

PATHOPHYSIOLOGY

Degeneration of the thumb CMC joint occurs in a predictable pattern. Initially, ligamentous laxity and repetitive loading may predispose certain individuals to synovitis of the joint. This occurs more frequently in young women and is believed to be related to the development of osteoarthritis in later years (7). This hypothesis is further supported by the observation that ligament reconstruction in the palmar beak ligament in young women with symptomatic hypermobile joints leads to less synovitis and fewer degenerative changes (8).

As the disease progresses, the joint surfaces become degenerated, and osteophytes are formed. Later in the disease progression, dorsoradial subluxation of the thumb metacarpal on the trapezium occurs. An adduction contracture of the thumb metacarpal may occur via the adduction force of the adductor pollicis muscle and the subluxation force of the APL muscle insertion into the base of the thumb metacarpal. Inability to abduct via the CMC joint leads to a hyperextension deformity of the metacarpophalangeal (MCP) joint and, occasionally, instability of the MCP ulnar collateral ligament. In later stages of the process, degeneration of the scaphotrapezial (ST) joint also occurs. Although the trapezium articulates with the thumb and index metacarpals and trapezoid,

only the CMC and ST joints lie along the compression axis of the thumb and are most commonly involved in "pantrapezial arthritis" (9).

Radiographic evidence of basal joint degeneration will ultimately develop in approximately 1 in 4 women and 1 in 12 men (10). Women outnumber men by a ratio of 10 to 15:1 in published series of joint reconstructions. There appears to be a correlation between the development of thumb CMC degeneration and hereditary and environmental factors. There is a poorly understood correlation between women and their female children and the development of generalized primary degenerative arthritis. Racial differences have been noted in postmortem specimens. There is a significantly higher incidence of joint eburnation and chondromalacia in Caucasian as compared to Japanese and Chinese hands (11–13), which is thought to be related to flattening of the Asian joint (14).

However, there is a poor correlation between radiographic and clinical disease (15). Likewise, it is noted that clinical symptoms may abate as the joint destruction becomes more marked. Therefore, treatment of the arthritic joint should be based on clinical and not radiographic parameters.

EVALUATION

Clinical

The typical patient presenting with thumb CMC arthritis is a postmenopausal woman complaining of thumb or radial-sided hand and wrist pain without traumatic onset, progressively worsening over a few months to a few years. Pain is exacerbated with pinching and grasping activities such as turning a key in a lock, handwriting, holding a heavy book, sewing, and pulling on pants or hose. Patients state the pain is either at the CMC joint or in the thenar eminence. Patients often note the pain is episodic and relieved with rest or nonsteroidal antiinflammatory drugs (NSAIDs). Some patients describe the inability to perform activities as related to loss of strength or dexterity. Patients often are referred for the diagnosis of carpal tunnel syndrome, de Quervain's stenosing tenosynovitis, or trigger thumb.

Findings on clinical examination are dependent on the stage of the disease. The thumb appears normal in early disease, but the adduction contracture and dorsal subluxation of the thumb metacarpal base are readily apparent in advanced disease. Enlargement of the CMC joint is secondary to inflammation and osteophyte formation.

Fingertip palpation of the individual joints is important in establishing the diagnosis. The CMC joint is best palpated dorsal to the insertion of the APL tendon. The scaphotrapeziotrapezoid (STT) joint is best palpated palmarly over the distal pole of the scaphoid. Just proximal to this region are the ridge of the trapezium and the flexor carpi radialis (FCR) tunnel. Patients with FCR tendinitis have pain at this location. The tendons of the first dorsal compartment should be palpated, and a Finkelstein test should be performed to examine for de Quervain's stenosing tenosynovitis. Palpation of the palmar thumb MCP joint with active flexion of the interphalangeal (IP) joint tests for trigger thumb.

Range of motion of the CMC, MCP, and IP joints of both thumbs should be measured. The loss of CMC abduction and extension relates to the adduction contracture of the first ray. Hyperextension of the MP joint relative to the contralateral side should be determined passively, as well as during active pinch.

Laxity of the thumb CMC joint is determined clinically (16). The patient's hand is grasped by the examiner's hand, and the base of the thumb metacarpal is grasped between the thumb and index fingers of the examiner's other hand. The ulnar three fingers of the examiner's hand grasp the patient's proximal and distal phalanges. The thumb metacarpal is translated radial-ulnar as well as dorsal-palmar and compared to the contralateral side. This maneuver produces pain in the inflamed joint and crepitus in the arthritic joint. In the crank test, axial loading of the thumb is combined with passive flexion-extension of the metacarpal. The grind test combines axial loading with rotation of the thumb metacarpal through a flexed MCP joint. Both tests produce pain and crepitus in the diseased joint.

Finally, all patients with thumb CMC arthritis should be examined for carpal tunnel syndrome. The overall prevalence of both conditions in patients undergoing basal joint reconstruction is 26% to 29% (17). In specific high-risk population—namely, women, diabetics, and workers' compensation patients—the prevalence is between 46% and 80%.

Imaging Studies

Standard x-rays of the thumb CMC joint include pronated anteroposterior, oblique, and true lateral views. The pronated anteroposterior view (Robert view) is done by hyperpronating the forearm and internally rotating the shoulder to allow the dorsal surface of the thumb to lie on the x-ray plate. It shows all four trapezial facets. The oblique and lateral x-rays show the severity of CMC disease and the palmar beak.

CMC joint stress views assess the degree of joint subluxation (18). A 30-degree posteroanterior view is done of both thumbs from the carpus to the tip. The patient is instructed to press the opposing thumb tips firmly together as the film is exposed. Radial subluxation of the thumb metacarpal is measured. A lateral pinch is done to assess dorsal subluxation. A lateral x-ray is taken while the patient performs a key pinch.

Eaton and Glickel have staged the pathologic changes observed on x-ray (19). In stage I, x-rays are normal or show widening of the CMC joint, indicating synovitis. Stress views usually show CMC joint subluxation. In stage II, the joint space is narrowed, and osteophytes and loose bodies are smaller than 2 mm. In stage III, the joint space is further narrowed, subchondral sclerosis is present, osteophytes and loose bodies are greater than 2 mm, and there are no abnormalities of the ST joint. In stage IV, there are degenerative changes of the CMC and ST joints.

Although x-ray studies are helpful in staging the patient's disease, treatment of the patient is dependent on the patient's signs and symptoms.

NONOPERATIVE TREATMENT

All patients diagnosed with thumb CMC arthritis should be treated initially with conservative care. Patients are encouraged to modify their activities by using larger pens and increasing the grips on their golf clubs. All patients are fitted with a custom-made thumb spica splint with the IP joint free. Hand-based splints (Fig. 2) are less restrictive and better tolerated than forearm-based splints, but forearm-based splints provide better immobilization. Patients are told initially to wear the splint on a near–full-time basis until symptoms resolve (usually 3 to 4 weeks) and then to wear it for symptom exacerbation. Splinting combined with NSAID medication decreases synovitis and joint effusion. If symptoms persist, an injection of cortisone into the CMC joint provides transient relief. Although not a cure for the problem, the temporary symptom relief provided by the injection may help the patient decide if surgical reconstruction is indicated.

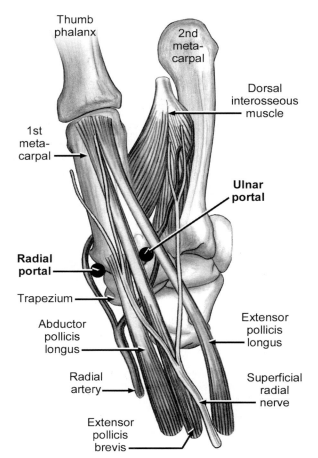

FIGURE 2. Portals and surface anatomy for thumb carpometa-carpal arthritis. The first radial portal is radial to the abductor pol-licis longus tendon, and the first ulnar portal is between the extensor pollicis brevis and extensor pollicis longus tendons. Note proximity of the radial artery to the first ulnar portal.

There are few reports of conservative care of thumb CMC arthritis. Swigart et al. reported that 76% of patients with stage I or II disease and 54% of patients with stage III or IV disease obtained sufficient symptomatic relief to allow continued activities with intermittent splint use (20). Other authors have stated that a majority of patients can be treated with conservative care (21).

Author's Preferred Treatment

All patients presenting with thumb CMC arthritis are splinted and treated with NSAIDs for at least 1 month. Many patients state that intermittent splinting is enough to relieve symptoms and that they desire no further treatment. When splinting does not provide adequate relief, the thumb CMC joint is injected with corticosteroids. Nearly all patients experience temporary relief after the injection. Patients are told that if their symptoms return and cannot be managed with splinting or conservative care keeps them from participating in activities they enjoy, surgical recon-struction should be performed.

SURGICAL MANAGEMENT: STAGE I

The indication for surgery of the degenerative thumb CMC joint is failure of conservative care to provide sufficient symp-tom relief to allow the patient to participate in activities.

The type of surgical procedure is related to the stage of the disease. In symptomatic stage I disease, a reconstruction of the volar ligament, as described by Eaton and Littler, is indicated (18). The authors state that there are no clear objective criteria that define the need for surgical intervention in early basal joint disease. However, long-term follow-up by these authors has confirmed the durability of the procedure and its propen-sity to minimize the progression of degenerative changes (22).

Volar ligament reconstruction is only indicated when there is no eburnation and only the earliest changes of chondromalacia in the contact areas of the palmar joint sur-faces. The joint surfaces may be examined directly during the procedure, but if eburnation is noted, the procedure must be abandoned or converted into an arthroplasty. Arthroscopic evaluation of the joint surface provides a less invasive method of examining the joint surfaces and the integrity of the beak ligament when the preoperative deci-sion is made not to proceed to arthroplasty (23). Although thermal shrinkage of capsular tissue shows some promise for improving stability in the shoulder joint, its effective-ness in stabilizing the thumb CMC joint is unknown.

Technique

Thumb Carpometacarpal Arthroscopy

With the patient supine, a pneumatic tourniquet is applied to the upper arm, and a countertraction strap is placed around the arm and operating table. The arm is prepped and exsanguinated. A single fingertrap is used to apply 5 to 7 lbs of vertical traction to the thumb. Two arthroscopic portals are used (Fig. 2). The first radial portal is located just anterior to the APL tendon. It is the preferred portal for viewing the dorsoradial, posterior oblique, and ulnar collateral ligaments. The first ulnar portal is just ulnar to the extensor pollicis brevis (EPB) tendon. It is the preferred portal for viewing the beak ligament.

A 20-gauge needle is first inserted into the joint to gauge the angle of entry. The joint is injected with 1 to 2 cc of saline. A 3-mm longitudinal incision is made over each portal, with care taken not to injure sensory nerve branches or the radial artery. A 1.9-mm trocar is inserted into each portal, aiming slightly distally. A short-barrel 1.9-mm arthroscope is inserted into one portal, and a probe or 2.0-mm full-radius side shaver is inserted into the other. The shaver is used to remove synovitis to allow inspection of the joint surfaces and capsular ligaments.

Palmar Ligament Reconstruction

An incision is made over the thumb metacarpal at the inser-tion of the thenar muscles, curving proximally and ulnarly to the FCR tendon. Care is taken to preserve sensory nerve branches and the branch of the radial artery in the area. The thenar muscles are elevated from the metacarpal shaft and dissected radially to ulnarly until the base of the metacarpal and the palmar capsule of the CMC joint are exposed. Often, the tendinous slip of the APL into the thenar muscles must be detached. The joint capsule between the beak ligament and the APL metacarpal insertion is incised along the trapezium and reflected distally to expose the joint surface for inspection. Supination of the thumb allows visualization of the metacarpal beak.

A drill hole is made through the thumb metacarpal base for passage of the FCR tendon (Fig. 3). Progressively larger gouges are passed from dorsal to palmar, entering the cortex 4 to 5 mm distal to the articular surface and perpendicular to the thumbnail. Eaton and Littler recommend placing the hole parallel to the joint surface, whereas Pellegrini recommends an oblique line so as to exit the palmar cortex adjacent to the articular margin of the metacarpal beak. A 28-gauge stainless steel wire is passed through the hole to facilitate passage of the FCR tendon.

One-half of the FCR tendon is harvested through two short transverse incisions. The most proximal incision is at the musculotendinous junction, usually 8 to 10 cm above the wrist flexion crease. The ulnar half of the tendon is cut proximally. Due to the rotation of the tendon, this half becomes the radial half at the wrist. The tendon is split distal to the FCR tunnel through the trapezial ridge. The tendon is passed through the drill hole in the metacarpal and sutured under tension to the dorsal metacarpal periosteum. During tensioning, the metacarpal is pronated, abducted, and reduced palmarly, relative to the trapezium. The remaining tendon is passed deep to the APL tendon near its insertion. Final tension is established as the tendon is passed deep to the other half of the FCR tendon. The graft is looped around the tendon and sutured back to itself. The joint capsule is closed, the thenar muscles are reattached to the metacarpal, and the skin is closed. The patient is placed into a thumb spica cast in thumb abduction and pronation for 4 weeks.

Patients begin active range of motion of the IP and MCP joints at 4 weeks postoperatively. At 2 months postoperatively, active mobilization of the CMC joint is started along with thenar strengthening exercises. Patients begin strengthening for pinch and grip at 3 months postoperatively.

SURGICAL MANAGEMENT: STAGES II TO IV

The majority of patients in these stages are surgically treated with either a trapeziectomy and ligament reconstruction or a trapezial-metacarpal fusion. Some authors have recommended osteotomy of the thumb metacarpal to change the contact point of the diseased articular surface. However, long-term studies are not yet available for these procedures. The use of a silicone implant after trapeziectomy in osteoarthritis is contraindicated due to the development of silicone synovitis and bone erosion. Other metallic and metallic polyethylene implants have been introduced but currently do not have the proven success of either trapeziectomy and ligament reconstruction or fusion procedures.

Trapeziectomy alone was first described by Gervis in 1949 (24). The major complication was proximal migration of the thumb, presenting a cosmetic and functional problem. In some studies, patients complained of weakness and instability after the procedure (25,26). However, one recent report states that the pain relief is comparable to that obtained with more involved procedures (27). Currently, the procedure is indicated in very low-demand elderly patients and patients after a failed infected implant arthroplasty (28).

Fascial arthroplasty of the CMC joint was described by Froimson in 1970 (29). After trapeziectomy, the FCR was transected and rolled into an "anchovy" to reduce thumb shortening and improve pinch strength. Froimson later recommended a hemiresection in patients with stage III disease to prevent further shortening (30).

Ligament reconstruction with tendon interposition (LRTI) arthroplasty was described by Burton and Pellegrini in 1986 (31) (Fig. 4). The FCR tendon is passed through a

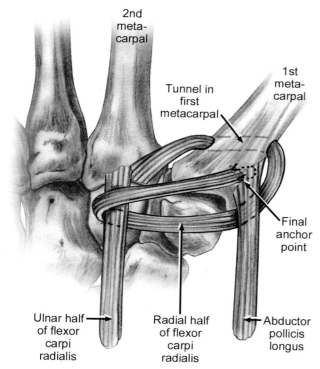

FIGURE 3. Technique of volar thumb carpometacarpal ligament reconstruction. Half of the flexor carpi radialis tendon is passed through a drill hole in the base of the thumb metacarpal. After exiting the dorsal metacarpal, the tendon is passed dorsal to the abductor pollicis longus and through the remaining flexor carpi radialis before being sewn to the palmar carpometacarpal capsule and abductor pollicis longus tendon.

(Figure labels: 2nd metacarpal; 1st metacarpal; Tunnel in first metacarpal; Final anchor point; Ulnar half of flexor carpi radialis; Radial half of flexor carpi radialis; Abductor pollicis longus)

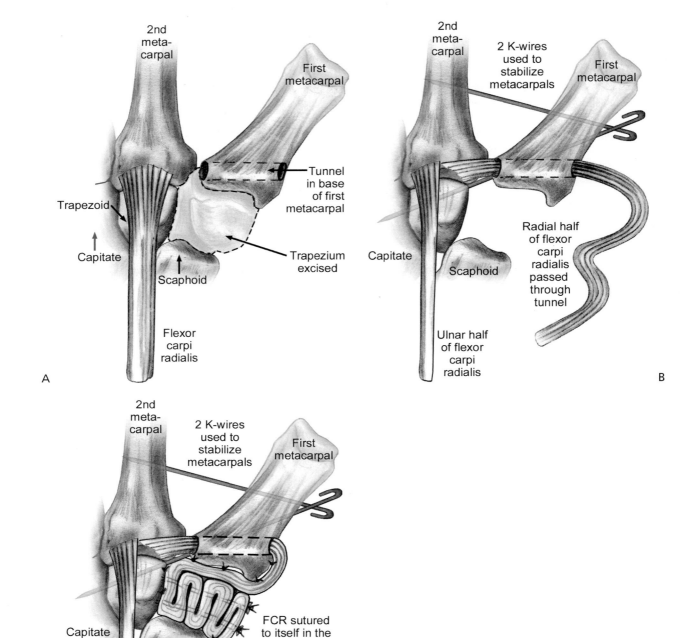

FIGURE 4. Technique of ligament reconstruction with tendon interposition. **A:** After trapeziectomy, a drill hole is made from proximal palmar to distal dorsal through the thumb metacarpal. **B:** The entire flexor carpi radialis (FCR) is harvested proximally and passed through the drill hole. **C:** The remaining FCR is made into an "anchovy" and sewn to the FCR tendon before entering the drill hole in the thumb metacarpal. K-wires, Kirschner wires.

drill hole in the thumb metacarpal to reconstruct the beak ligament. The remaining FCR tendon is placed into the space left by the trapeziectomy to act as a fascial arthroplasty. Although it was initially described only in stage IV, currently, a complete trapeziectomy is performed in all stages to simplify the procedure.

Burton and Pellegrini followed their patients at 2-, 6-, and 9.4-year intervals (31,32). Pinch and grip strengths were shown to improve between 2 and 6 years. At 9.4 years, there was an overall 92.5% increase in grip and a 50% increase in pinch compared to preoperative values. Subjectively, at 9.4 years, 95% of patients reported excellent pain relief. In the same time, loss of arthroplasty space was 11% to 13% of immediate postoperative values.

Thompson reported on his "suspensionplasty" in 1986 (33). After a trapeziectomy, a dorsal slip of the APL tendon is detached proximally; passed through the dorsal cortex of the thumb metacarpal, out of the articular surface of the proximal metacarpal, and through a drill hole in the base of the index metacarpal; and weaved into the extensor carpi radialis longus tendon. Early results are equivalent to the LRTI, but no long-term studies have been reported. The suspensionplasty is an excellent alternative to the LRTI when the FCR is unable to be used secondary to severe fraying or degeneration from the disease process or inadvertent laceration during trapeziectomy. LRTI can also be used in revision procedures in which the FCR is no longer available.

Weilby reported his series of arthroplasties in 1988 (34). After a trapeziectomy, one-half of the FCR is harvested proximally. The tendon is weaved between the APL and the remaining FCR tendons. Grip strength postoperatively was 80% of normal, and there was no appreciable degradation over time.

The alternative to arthroplasty in stage II, III, and early stage IV is arthrodesis of the trapeziometacarpal joint. Bamberger reported a series of 39 fusions in 37 patients (35). There were five delayed unions and three nonunions. Twenty-four patients were seen at an average of 4 years of follow-up. Subjectively, 18 patients had good to excellent results and few functional complaints. There was a 72% reduction in adduction/abduction and a 61% reduction in flexion/extension, but the loss of motion did not appear to affect function. As measured by x-ray, the joint fused in 20 to 50 degrees of palmar abduction and 12 to 48 degrees of extension. Two of 12 patients had progression of preexisting ST joint degenerative changes. They noted no increase in MCP joint range of motion. The authors state that arthrodesis should not only be used for posttraumatic arthritis in the young person, but also for older patients with primary osteoarthritis isolated to the CMC joint.

Technique

Ligament Reconstruction with Tendon Interposition

With the patient supine, an upper arm tourniquet is applied, and the arm is prepped and draped. The arm table is positioned to allow fluoroscopy during the procedure. The arm is exsanguinated, and the tourniquet is inflated.

The trapezium may be approached palmarly or dorsally. The palmar approach is the same as described for the palmar ligament reconstruction (see above). The advantages of this approach are that the incision is made palmar to the branches of the dorsal sensory branch of the radial nerve and the FCR tendon is fully visualized during removal of the trapezium. The disadvantages are that the radial artery is not visualized during excision of the trapezium and that some patients may develop a tender, hypertrophic scar in the glabrous skin of the thenar eminence.

The dorsal approach has been popularized by Burton and Pellegrini (25). An inverted-Y incision is made in line with the EPB tendon. The palmar limb is placed in the wrist flexion crease, and the dorsal limb toward the pulse of the radial artery is placed in the snuffbox. The branches of the dorsal sensory branch of the radial nerve are identified and protected throughout the case. After the EPB tendon is transected from its insertion and retracted, a subperiosteal capsular incision is made deep to its course. Full-thickness flaps are raised to expose the entire trapezium. A minimal bony resection of the metacarpal articular surface is performed, with more bone taken dorsally than palmarly. The trapezium is excised, taking care to protect the FCR tendon. The FCR tendon is freed of adhesion to its insertion into the index metacarpal. One-half of the FCR is harvested through a series of short incisions. The tendon is divided at its musculotendinous junctions and passed into the trapezial fossa. Two nonabsorbable sutures are placed into the deep capsule for later use. A drill hole is then made into the base of the thumb metacarpal perpendicular to the plane of the thumbnail. A Kirschner wire (K-wire) is placed longitudinally into the dorsoradial corner of the metacarpal intramedullary canal. The wire exits the metacarpal head distally so as to prevent MCP joint hyperextension. The FCR tendon is passed into the medullary canal of the metacarpal and through the hole in the dorsal cortex. The tendon is sutured to the dorsal cortex while the thumb is reduced. Excessive traction on the thumb will lead to lengthening of the tendinous restraint, thereby leading to proximal migration of the thumb. The tendon is sutured to itself in the trapezial fossa. The remaining tendon is rolled on itself and sewn to the capsule via the previously placed deep sutures. The capsule is repaired. The K-wire is advanced across the space and into the scaphoid. The EPB tendon is sewn to the proximal metacarpal to augment abduction and extension and eliminate a metacarpophalangeal hyperextension force.

Postoperatively, the thumb is immobilized with a short arm thumb spica cast or splint for 1 month. Patients begin immediate range-of-motion exercises of the IP joint. The immobilization is discontinued at 1 month and active range-of-motion exercises of the MP and CMC joints are initiated. During the third month, strengthening and resistive exercises are begun. The patient may resume full activity at 3 months postoperatively. Grip and pinch strength and incisional tenderness are expected to improve for up to 1 year.

Author's Preferred Method

A variety of modifications have been made to the original procedure. The palmar exposure is preferred because it improves visualization of the FCR tendon and protects the sensory nerve branches. The entire FCR tendon is used rather than half. The benefits are that it is easier to harvest the entire tendon and that the development of tendinitis at the insertion of the FCR tendon is less common. On rare occurrences, loss of the FCR leads to slight ulnar deviation with wrist flexion. The majority of the subchondral bone of the proximal metacarpal is removed during placement of the drill hole for the FCR tendon. Therefore, removal of the articular surface is not necessary. The FCR tendon may be more firmly attached to the metacarpal when sewn via a suture anchor rather than to the periosteum. The drill hole in the dorsal cortex for the FCR tendon should exit 1 cm from the proximal extent of the metacarpal. The suture anchor can be placed proximal or distal to the hole. Finally, the thumb is immobilized with only a splint and not a K-wire.

Suspensionplasty

The dorsal approach and trapeziectomy, as described for the LRTI, are performed. Drill holes are then made in the thumb and index metacarpal bases. The thumb metacarpal hole is made in the dorsoradial cortex 1 cm distal to and directly in line with the APL insertion. The hole exits the articular surface through its center. A second drill hole is made in the trapezial facet of the index metacarpal, exiting dorsal and ulnar at the insertion of the extensor carpi radialis brevis (ECRB). This second drill hole can be made more distally if the surgeon opts to suspend the metacarpal more distally.

The entire dorsal slip of the APL is transected at the musculotendinous junction. All adhesions to its bony insertion are dissected. The tendon is turned 180 degrees and inserted through the thumb and then the index metacarpal holes. Care must be taken to remove osteophytes from the index and thumb metacarpal bases. Tension is applied to the APL tendon, and it is weaved and sewn to the ECRB tendon. A K-wire is placed down the shaft of the metacarpal into the scaphoid. Interposition material, such as tendon or fascia lata, may be placed into the trapezial fossa.

Postoperatively, a thumb spica splint is applied for 5 to 6 weeks. The splint and pin are removed and range-of-motion exercises are begun. Power grip and pinch activities are not recommended until 12 weeks postoperatively.

Author's Preferred Method

Although the author favors the modification of LRTI for the surgical treatment of thumb CMC arthritis, suspensionplasty is the author's first choice when the FCR tendon is no longer available. In revising a failed LRTI, the FCR tendon may be ruptured, stretched, infected, or incompetent. Substitution of the APL for the FCR works equally well in suspending the thumb. Pelligrini has noted that excessive traction on the APL during suspensionplasty creates an overly tight ligament and produces painful impingement with the index metacarpal (25).

Trapeziometacarpal Fusion

A dorsal approach as described for the LRTI is used. The ideal position for the fusion is 30 to 40 degrees of abduction, 15 to 20 degrees of extension, and pronation to allow tip-to-tip pinch of the thumb and fingers (approximately 10 degrees). Stern suggests that the position for fusion is appropriate when the distal phalanx of the thumb rests on the middle phalanx of the index finger of a fully clenched fist (35). The articular surface and subchondral bone may be excised in a cup and cone fashion, or parallel cuts may be made in the trapezium and metacarpal to cancellous bone. House recommends inserting a K-wire between the thumb and index metacarpals after positioning the thumb CMC joint and before performing the parallel cuts with an oscillating saw. Fixation may be accomplished with a variety of methods. When K-wires are used, two 0.045-in. wires are inserted into the medullary canal, one exiting radially and one ulnarly. The bony surfaces are opposed, and one wire is advanced. The pronation of the thumb is checked, and the second wire is advanced into the trapezium. The K-wire may be supplemented with a staple. When plates are used, the pin of the condylar blade plate is inserted into the trapezium between the APL and abductor pollicis brevis. The arthrodesis site is compressed, and screws are placed into the metacarpal shaft. Supplemental bone graft from the distal radius should be used in all fusions.

Postoperatively, a forearm-based thumb spica cast with the IP joint free is applied until trabecular bone traverses the arthrodesis site. Once the fusion is complete, the pins are removed, and the patient may begin full activities.

Author's Preferred Method

The primary indications for trapeziometacarpal arthrodesis are reconstruction of stage III or early stage IV degenerative disease in a young manual laborer and stabilization of the thumb during reconstruction of the tetraplegic's hand. As with any arthrodesis, preparation of the bony surfaces to adequately expose cancellous bone is the most important consideration. With cup and cone preparation, care must be taken to remove all subchondral bone while preserving the contour of the bony surfaces to provide bony apposition. Parallel osteotomy cuts will ensure cancellous bone and bone contact surfaces, but it will shorten the thumb ray more than the cup and cone method. Despite this disadvantage, the author still prefers parallel osteotomies for trapeziometacarpal fusion.

No one method of fixation has been shown to be superior in reducing nonunions or delayed unions. Therefore, choice of fixation should be dependent on the surgeon's level of comfort with the various techniques.

Complications

The most common complication after surgical treatment of the arthritic thumb CMC joint is persistent pain. Although long-term studies show high levels of patient satisfaction regarding pain relief, many patients may complain of thumb pain after surgery for the first 3 to 6 months. Pain that persists past this point deserves more careful evaluation.

Persistent pain is evaluated by considering each of the structures within the operative site. A hypertrophy scar or cutaneous neuroma is a frequent cause of pain. Patients complain of a burning pain or hypersensitivity over the incision. On occasion, patients may develop complex regional pain syndromes from irritation of these sensory branches. Once the diagnosis is considered, early aggressive desensitization of the region is initiated in a therapy program. If this fails to relieve symptoms, intervention via a pain management consult should be pursued.

Persistent pain from the thumb metacarpal may be secondary to proximal migration of the metacarpal or arthritic degeneration between the thumb and index metacarpals. Proximal migration of the thumb metacarpal is less likely to occur when a ligament reconstruction is performed versus when the trapezium is simply removed. When significant proximal migration occurs with LRTI, the integrity of the ligament reconstruction must be questioned. Magnetic resonance imaging may be helpful in determining if the FCR tendon is intact. During revision surgery, assessment of the ligament reconstruction may be difficult secondary to scarring. The surgeon must be prepared to do a secondary reconstruction with another source of tendon.

Pain between the thumb and index proximal metacarpals is a difficult problem to treat. Care is taken during the reconstruction not to overtighten the repair, especially when performing a suspensionplasty. Patients may require a prolonged period of postoperative immobilization to allow the symptoms to resolve.

The other major complication is failure to address the associated hyperextension of the MCP joint. Secondary MCP hyperextension can be a source of pain and may lead to poor outcomes (36,37). Treatment of the MCP joint is based on the amount of hyperextension. When hyperextension is 30 degrees or less and painless, no treatment is required. When pain is present, the joint should be pinned in neutral, and the EPB should be transferred from the proximal phalanx to the metacarpal. When hyperextension is greater than 30 degrees, the MCP is fused, or a palmar capsulodesis is performed. Arthrodesis is favored for joints with ulnar collateral ligament instability and arthritic changes and with normal joints with little passive flexion. When a palmar capsulodesis is performed, the palmar plate is imbricated in pants-over-vest fashion, and the EPB tendon is detached from the proximal phalanx and sewn to the metacarpal. The joint is held with a K-wire for 6 weeks.

The complications of wound dehiscence and infection are more common when the procedure is done for rheumatoid arthritis than when it is done for osteoarthritis. In rheumatoid patients, delayed wound healing may be attributable to systemic corticosteroids, cytotoxic agents, and antimetabolites like cyclophosphamide (Cytoxan), hydroxychloroquine (Plaquenil), and methotrexate sodium (Methotrexate). The effects of methotrexate sodium can be reversed by holding the medication for 10 to 14 days preoperatively and administrating folic acid daily. Consideration should be given to meticulous hemostasis and delay in removing sutures from the wound.

Infection is more likely to occur in the immunocompromised patient. If infection of the tendinous arthroplasty occurs, the tendon should be removed, the bone should be curetted to bleeding bone, and the patient should be placed on appropriate antibiotics. In many instances, no further ligament reconstruction is required.

SUMMARY

Osteoarthritis of the thumb CMC joint is most commonly due to laxity of the palmar beak ligament with degeneration of the palmar metacarpal and central trapezial joint surfaces. Degenerative changes occur most commonly in Caucasian women. When conservative care is insufficient to relieve symptoms, surgical reconstruction of the beak ligament is indicated. In patients with arthritic changes, the entire trapezium is excised at the time of ligament reconstruction. Long-term results of the procedures report that 90% to 95% of patients achieve good to excellent results after surgery.

REFERENCES

1. Pellegrini VD Jr, Olcott CW, Hollenberg G. Contact patterns in the trapeziometacarpal joint: the role of the palmar beak ligament. *J Hand Surg [Am]* 1993;18:238–244.
2. Strauch RJ, Behrman MJ, Rosenwasser MP. Acute dislocation of the carpometacarpal joint of the thumb: an anatomic and cadaver study. *J Hand Surg [Am]* 1994;19:93–98.
3. Bettinger PC, Linscheid RL, Berger RA, et al. An anatomic study of the stabilizing ligaments of the trapezium and trapeziometacarpal joint. *J Hand Surg [Am]* 1999;24:786–798.
4. Doerschuk SH, Hicks DG, Pellegrini VD. Histopathology of the palmar beak ligament in trapeziometacarpal osteoarthritis. *J Hand Surg [Am]* 1999;24:496–504.
5. Pellegrini VD Jr. Osteoarthritis of the thumb trapeziometacarpal joint: a study of the pathophysiology of articular cartilage degeneration. II. Articular wear patterns in the osteoarthritis joint. *J Hand Surg [Am]* 1991;16:975–982.
6. Cooney W, Chao E. Biomechanical analysis of static forces in the thumb during hand function. *J Bone Joint Surg* 1977;59:27–36.
7. Eaton RG, Littler JW. Ligament reconstruction for the painful thumb carpometacarpal joint. *J Bone Joint Surg [Am]* 1973;55:1655–1666.

8. Eaton RG, Lane L, Littler JW, et al. Ligament reconstruction for the painful thumb carpometacarpal joint: a long-term assessment. *J Hand Surg [Am]* 1984;9:692–698.

9. North ER, Eaton RG. Degenerative joint disease of the trapezium: a comparative radiographic and anatomic study. *J Hand Surg [Am]* 1983;8:160–167.

10. Armstrong AL, Hunter JB, Davis TRC. The prevalence of degenerative arthritis of the base of the thumb in post-menopausal women. *J Hand Surg [Br]* 1994;19:340–341.

11. Pellegrini VD Jr. Osteoarthritis of the thumb trapeziometacarpal joint: a study of the pathophysiology of articular cartilage degeneration. I. Anatomy and pathology of the aging joint. *J Hand Surg [Am]* 1991;16:967–974.

12. Fujisawa K. Arthrosis of the carpometacarpal joint of the thumb (the third report)—a comparative radiographic and anatomical study. *J Jpn Soc Surg Hand* 1988;5:412.

13. Kihara H. Anatomical study of the normal and degenerative articular surfaces on the first carpometacarpal joint. *J Jpn Orthop Assoc* 1992;66:228.

14. Pellegrini VD Jr. Primary idiopathic osteoarthritis in the upper extremity: report of the 1992 Sterling Bunnell Traveling Fellow. *J Hand Surg [Am]* 1993;18:1093–1094.

15. Aune S. Osteoarthritis in the first carpometacarpal joint. *Acta Chir Scand* 1955;109:449.

16. Barron OA, Glickel SZ, Eaton RG. Basal joint arthritis of the thumb. *J Am Acad Orthop Surg* 2000;8:314–323.

17. Florack T, Miller R, Pellegrini VD Jr, et al. The prevalence of carpal tunnel syndrome in patients with basal joint arthritis of the thumb. *J Hand Surg [Am]* 1992;17:624–630.

18. Eaton RG, Littler JW. Ligament reconstruction for the painful thumb carpometacarpal joint. *J Bone Joint Surg* 1973;55A:1655–1666.

19. Eaton RG, Glickel SZ. Trapeziometacarpal osteoarthritis: staging as a rationale for treatment. *Hand Clin* 1987;3:455–471.

20. Swigart CR, Eaton RG, Glickel SZ, et al. Splinting in the treatment of arthritis of the first carpometacarpal joint. *J Hand Surg [Am]* 1999;24:86–91.

21. Wolock BS, Moore JR, Weiland AJ. Arthritis of the basal joint of the thumb: a critical analysis of treatment options. *J Arthroplasty* 1989;4:65–78.

22. Eaton RG, Lane LB, Littler JW, et al. Ligament reconstruction for the painful thumb carpometacarpal joint: a long-term assessment. *J Hand Surg [Am]* 1984;9:692–699.

23. Berger RA. A technique for arthroscopic evaluation of the first carpometacarpal joint. *J Hand Surg [Am]* 1997;22:1077–1080.

24. Gervis WH. Excision of the trapezium for osteoarthritis of the trapeziometacarpal joint. *J Bone Joint Surg* 1949;31B:537–539.

25. Pellegrini VD Jr. The basal articulations of the thumb: pain, instability, and osteoarthritis. In: Peimer CA, ed. *Surgery of the hand and upper extremity*, vol. 1. New York: McGraw-Hill, 1996:1019–1039.

26. Murley AHG. Excision of the trapezium in osteoarthritis of the first carpometacarpal joint. *J Bone Joint Surg* 1960;42B:502–507.

27. Varley GW, Calvey J, Hunter JB, et al. Excision of the trapezium for osteoarthritis at the base of the thumb. *J Bone Joint Surg* 1994;76B:964–968.

28. Weilby A, Sondorf J. Results following removal of silicone trapezium metacarpal implants. *J Hand Surg [Am]* 1978;3:154.

29. Froimson AI. Tendon arthroplasty of the trapeziometacarpal joint. *Clin Orthop* 1970;70:191–199.

30. Froimson AI. Tendon interposition arthroplasty of carpometacarpal joint of the thumb. *Hand Clin* 1987;3:489–505.

31. Burton RI, Pellegrini VD Jr. Surgical Management of basal joint arthritis of the thumb. Part II. Ligament reconstruction with tendon interposition arthroplasty. *J Hand Surg [Am]* 1986;11:324–332.

32. Tomaino M, Pellegrini VD Jr, Burton RI. Long-term followup of ligament reconstruction with tendon interposition arthroplasty of basal joint arthritis of the thumb. *J Bone Joint Surg* 1994;77A:346–355.

33. Thompson J. Surgical management of trapeziometacarpal arthrosis. *Adv Orthop Surg* 1986;10:105.

34. Weilby A. Tendon interposition arthroplasty of the first carpo-metacarpal joint. *J Hand Surg [Br]* 1988;13:421–425.

35. Bamberger HB, Stern P, Keifhaber TR, et al. Trapeziometacarpal joint arthrodesis: a functional evaluation. *J Hand Surg [Am]* 1992:17:605–611.

36. Blank J, Feldon P. Thumb metacarpophalangeal joint stabilization during carpometacarpal joint surgery. *Atlas Hand Clin* 1997;2:217–225.

37. Eaton RG, Floyd WE III. Thumb metacarpophalangeal capsulodesis: an adjunct procedure to basal joint arthroplasty for collapse deformity of the first ray. *J Hand Surg [Am]* 1998;13:449–453.

74

PRINCIPLES OF LIMITED WRIST ARTHRODESIS

ARNOLD-PETER C. WEISS

Osteoarthritis of the wrist is a common malady that is seen in multiple age groups. Rheumatoid arthritis of the wrist is far less common, although it is seen frequently in patients with advanced disease. In both conditions, if the degenerative changes have spread throughout the carpus and radiocarpal joint, treatment is generally directed to arthrodesis of the entire wrist, thus providing a stable, pain-free wrist, or total wrist arthroplasty, which eliminates pain but allows some functional arc of motion (1–4). In certain patients, the arthritis pattern only affects a few of the intercarpal wrist joints or a portion of the radiocarpal joint, if it has not gotten to the stage in which it affects all of the joints throughout the wrist (5). In these patients, limited arthrodesis of the wrist can provide a pain-free, stable wrist construct and still can preserve some motion through the intact joints (6–9). The basic understanding of how to evaluate patients clinically and radiographically to stage the most appropriate type of procedure and highlights of the technical caveats of undertaking limited wrist arthrodesis are detailed in this chapter.

BASIC PRINCIPLES

Surgical treatment for the reconstruction of the wrist via intercarpal or radiocarpal arthrodesis hinges on the ability to eliminate motion by arthrodesis of the offending joints or by undertaking surgical elimination of the offending joints to reduce pain. The ultimate goal is to try to preserve as much motion as possible while simultaneously eliminating pain that is related to the joints that have focal arthritis. A careful radiographic evaluation of each of the joints that provides motion to the wrist is essential, and the surgeon needs to understand the different arthrodesis options that are available, given the particular radiographic pattern that is present.

Expected motion outcome after limited wrist arthrodesis is relatively predictable based on experimental cadaver studies of simulated arthrodesis and long-term follow-up studies of specific arthrodeses that were performed for various

problems (10–15). Overall, any fusion that involves the midcarpal joint generally allows a postoperative range of motion from one-half to two-thirds of normal. Arthrodesis that involves the radiocarpal joint and that preserves motion through the midcarpal joint generally provides a postoperative range of motion of one-third to one-half of normal motion. These postoperative motion expectations should be discussed with the patient to select the treatment option that is ideal for the patient's particular situation and to place reasonable expectations on what can be expected from the surgery on a long-term basis. Surgical treatment options that maintain the most congruent, normal joint articulation that is possible provide the most predictable long-term outcomes with respect to pain relief and maintenance of motion (5,9).

ANALYSIS OF RADIOGRAPHS

In general, well-performed posteroanterior and lateral radiographs of the wrist provide sufficient information to accurately gauge which limited arthrodesis would be the most appropriate for any specific patient. Occasionally, with significant osseous overlap or osteophyte formation, a computed tomography scan of the wrist may provide additional information that can help differentiate between two close surgical options. The most important three joints to examine on standard radiographs are the radioscaphoid, the radiolunate, and the head of the capitate in its articulation with the proximal row (Fig. 1). Radioscaphoid arthritis is one of the earliest types of arthritis and is seen in numerous conditions, including scaphoid nonunion and long-term scapholunate ligament disruption (9,16). Frequently, the entire radioscaphoid joint becomes involved, and significant pain and deformity are noted. For successful treatment at this stage, elimination of the entire scaphoid or, in some cases, fusion of the scaphoid to the radius is required to eliminate pain. The radiolunate joint is one of the last areas of the wrist to see degenerative changes. It is frequently

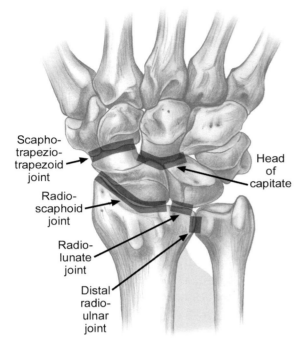

FIGURE 1. Careful radiographic assessment should be undertaken. The main joints to examine are the radioscaphoid, the radiolunate, and the head of the capitate. Secondary joints are the scaphotrapeziotrapezoid joint and the distal radioulnar joint.

Scapho-trapezio-trapezoid joint

Radio-scaphoid joint

Radio-lunate joint

Distal radio-ulnar joint

Head of capitate

used for many surgical reconstructive procedures and becomes the main articulation in patients who undergo four-corner arthrodesis, capitolunate arthrodesis, and proximal row carpectomy. Except in cases of posttraumatic arthritis after distal radius fractures, it is unlikely to see significant degenerative changes in the radiolunate joint, therefore allowing its frequent use to maintain motion in many patients (17–19). The head of the capitate is the

main articulation for the midcarpal joint. It is of importance in a proximal row carpectomy, in which it is one of the main articulating surfaces with the radiolunate joint, and it should also be examined carefully to determine whether fusion of the capitate within the arthrodesis is required (20). Frequently, in moderate to severe stages of degenerative change in the wrist, the capitate head shows deterioration and loss of articular congruity. In these patients, treatment should be directed at incorporating the head of the capitate within the fusion mass, thus eliminating any potential pain from abnormal motion at this joint.

SURGICAL EXPOSURES

Skin exposure can use a limited dorsal transverse incision or a more extensile longitudinal or T-shaped incision to expose the retinaculum and, ultimately, the dorsal wrist. With patients who have specific focal areas of arthritis that require a small area of local fusion [e.g., the scaphotrapeziotrapezoid (STT) joint], a limited dorsal transverse incision can provide adequate exposure without significant soft tissue dissection (21–25). Additional advantages of limited dorsal transverse incisions include their excellent appearance postoperatively and the relatively limited soft tissue dissection, whereas disadvantages include a difficulty in extending the incision for exposure in the event of unforeseen surgical issues. For small, as well as large, fusion areas, a longitudinal or T-shaped incision can be used for the skin surfaces with multiple different incisions that are being used to extend through the retinaculum and capsule to the carpus. The extensor pollicis longus (EPL) tendon can be transposed out of the third dorsal compartment, and an interval between the second and fourth compartments is opened, exposing the dorsal carpus (Fig. 2) (3). Longitudi-

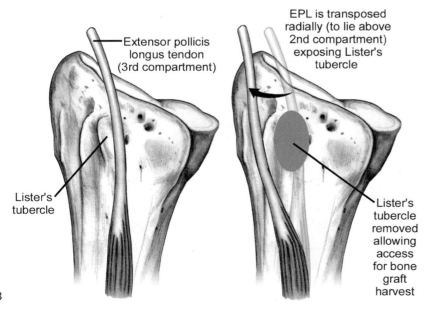

Extensor pollicis longus tendon (3rd compartment)

EPL is transposed radially (to lie above 2nd compartment) exposing Lister's tubercle

Lister's tubercle

Lister's tubercle removed allowing access for bone graft harvest

FIGURE 2. A,B: Dorsal exposure of the wrist allows release of the third compartment from which the extensor pollicis longus (EPL) tendon can be transposed radially, exposing Lister's tubercle. Removal of Lister's tubercle allows access to the distal radius for bone graft harvest. During layered closure, the EPL tendon is left transposed radially, therefore lying over the second compartment distally.

A,B

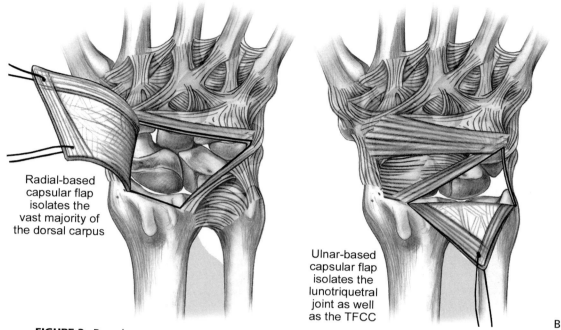

FIGURE 3. Dorsal exposure to the deep structures of the wrist can use ligament-sparing techniques. Two flaps can be fashioned, one that isolates the vast majority of the dorsal carpus **(A)** and a second on the ulnar base **(B)** that is a triangular form that can access the lunotriquetral joint, as well as the triangular fibrocartilage complex (TFCC).

Labels in figure:
- Radial-based capsular flap isolates the vast majority of the dorsal carpus
- Ulnar-based capsular flap isolates the lunotriquetral joint as well as the TFCC
- A
- B

nal capsular incisions do disrupt the transverse intercarpal and radiocarpal ligaments, potentially resulting in greater postoperative scar formation even with anatomic reapproximation. Alternatively, a ligament-sparing dorsal exposure can provide excellent visualization of the entire carpus, while maintaining capsular incisions in line with the dorsal wrist ligaments and allowing easier closure and the likelihood of less postoperative scar formation (Fig. 3) (26–28). Lister's tubercle is almost always removed to provide a flat surface from which a distal radius bone graft can be obtained to be used during the arthrodesis itself.

TECHNICAL TIPS

- Maintain precise capsular incisions by using a no. 15 blade, which maintains the integrity of the capsule and allows a careful and strong repair during closure. The use of dissecting scissors to explore the capsule can shred some of the soft tissues, thus resulting in the inability to get excellent suture "bites" during closure.
- Attempt to preserve all of the extrinsic and intrinsic ligaments of the wrist that are not affected directly by the procedure itself. Many of the extrinsic ligaments of the wrist are required for long-term stability of limited wrist arthrodesis. The radioscaphocapitate (RSL) ligament and the long radiolunate ligament provide antitranslational stability to the carpus after four-corner arthrodesis with scaphoid excision for degenerative changes that are

seen in scaphoid nonunion advanced collapse and scapholunate advanced collapse (27,28). In addition, the intrinsic ligaments can provide additional stability to the fusion mass in the immediate postoperative period, if their sacrifice is not required by the procedure that is selected.

- Careful attention to the sensory branches of the radial and ulnar nerves is essential during exposure of the dorsal wrist, regardless of the technique that is used. Injury to these nerves, especially the sensory branch of the radial nerve, can impart significant postoperative discomfort and dysesthesias in the patient and can make an otherwise successful limited wrist arthrodesis less than satisfactory. The sensory branch of the radial nerve fibers is extremely sensitive to any type of traction trauma, and a careful "no-touch" technique should be attempted to prevent dysesthetic symptoms postoperatively.
- Limited denervation of the carpus is also helpful in eliminating postoperative pain. The distal branches of the posterior interosseous nerve can be easily seen in the floor of the fourth compartment, and, generally, a 1-cm segment can be resected, providing some denervation to the proximal carpus itself.
- In general, transposition of the EPL tendon is desirable to avoid any secondary problems from the distal radius bone graft site, which generally goes through Lister's tubercle (3). By transposing the EPL tendon radially, leaving it transposed on closure, and removing Lister's tubercle, excellent quality bone graft can be obtained,

and no possibility of EPL impingement on a roughened Lister's tubercle occurs postoperatively.
■ Be certain that any hardware that is used for fixation during the arthrodesis does not impinge dorsally or volarly during clinical range of motion. One should check this intraoperatively with range of motion as well as by using mini fluoroscopic examination to ensure that no hardware penetration has occurred volarly. The use of mini fluoroscopic examination intraoperatively with motion ensures that impingement does not occur in joints that are not being fused.

LIMITED WRIST ARTHRODESIS

Limited wrist arthrodesis involves the local fusion of a portion of the carpus while maintaining motion through another area of the carpus that is not affected by the arthritis itself (8). After radiographic examination for the area of focal arthritis, surgical treatment can be undertaken to fuse the joints that are affected by the degenerative changes themselves, while allowing motion to occur at the remaining wrist joints that are unaffected by arthritis. Because the wrist has complex articulations that provide its overall function, some motion is always lost owing to partial wrist arthrodesis. However, the maintenance of perfect congruity of the remaining joints that provide motion can provide long-term pain relief and the lack of further secondary degenerative changes. Although iliac crest cancellous bone grafting is certainly appropriate, most limited wrist arthrodeses can be safely performed by using cancellous bone graft that is taken from the distal radius and by salvaging some cancellous bone from any individual carpal bones that are excised. Bone graft substitutes are probably not, in and of themselves, able to predictably obtain a successful arthrodesis at this juncture without some significant cancellous bone graft being placed, as well. Undoubtedly, the use of bone growth factors and other stimulatory compounds will increase in the future and may eventually eliminate the need for cancellous bone grafting to achieve stable, limited wrist arthrodesis.

Basic Arthrodesis Principles

■ Take down at least one-half of the joint surfaces that are involved in the arthrodesis, leaving a small portion of the volar joint intact to preserve carpal spacing and to maintain appropriate carpal reduction (Fig. 4).
■ Denude all degenerative surfaces down to good cancellous bone graft, removing any hard, subchondral bone that might inhibit predictable arthrodesis.
■ Use high-quality autogenous cancellous bone graft, which should be packed very tightly into the spaces that are being fused to provide some intrinsic stability and maximum osteogenic potential.
■ Use the most rigid fixation method possible for the arthrodesis that is being undertaken to allow earlier

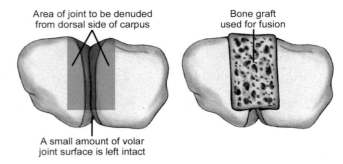

FIGURE 4. Denudation of cartilage and hard subchondral bone should be taken down to the cancellous level at the site that is being fused. Good-quality autogenous graft is then packed into the interstices. A portion of the volar joint is maintained to allow maintenance of carpal spacing.

range of motion and decreased overall stiffness during the postoperative period.
■ During the postoperative period, and especially when undertaking therapy, sequential radiographs can provide valuable information regarding fusion rate, as well as any potential problems of inappropriate motion at the arthrodesis site.
■ Always attempt to reduce any carpal bones that are out of position (e.g., the lunate in a dorsal intercalated segment instability alignment) to their normal position before provisional fixation and ultimate stable fixation (Fig. 5). Frequently, one can use a 0.062-in. Kirschner wire as a joystick to reduce the lunate, which is the bone that is affected most often, into its normal alignment, thus reconstituting carpal height and preventing secondary impingement due to a malpositioned arthrodesis.

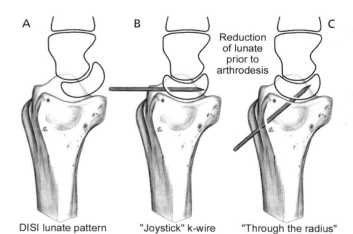

FIGURE 5. Any abnormal alignment of the carpus needs to be reduced before arthrodesis. The most frequent abnormal alignment involves the lunate in a distal intercalated segment instability (DISI) pattern **(A)**. One can use a free Kirschner wire (k-wire) as a joystick to move the lunate out of DISI **(B)**. Alternatively, one can use a "through-the-radius" technique **(C)** with flexion of the wrist, which brings the lunate out of DISI, and then can pin, in that position, the lunate via the dorsal distal radius. When the hand is then brought back into extension, the lunate is generally reduced.

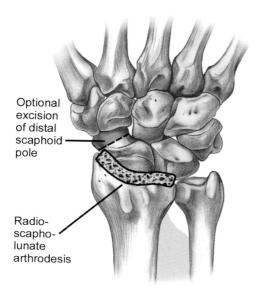

FIGURE 6. Radioscapholunate arthrodesis with optional excision of the pole of the distal scaphoid.

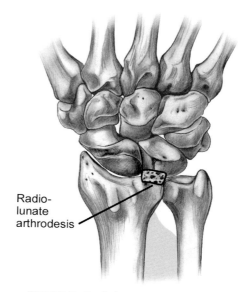

FIGURE 7. Radiolunate arthrodesis.

Radioscapholunate Arthrodesis

Patients who have severe distal radius fractures, subsequent degenerative joint disease throughout the radiocarpal joint that involves the entire joint surface, and yet a well-maintained midcarpal joint are ideal candidates for an RSL arthrodesis (17–19) (Fig. 6). Rigid fixation of the scaphoid, lunate, and radius can be provided by using powered staples or a Spider plate (Kinetikos Medical Inc., San Diego, CA) to provide the best possible rigid fixation. Without excision of the distal scaphoid pole, one can expect approximately one-third of the normal motion to occur, but this can be increased to approximately one-half of normal motion with excision of the distal one-half of the scaphoid.

Radiolunate Arthrodesis

Radiolunate arthrodesis is most commonly performed in rheumatoid arthritis to prevent ulnar translation of the carpus and to maintain overall alignment of the carpus and metacarpals with the forearm axis (29–32) (Fig. 7). Long-term results have shown some degradation of the radiolunate arthrodesis with subsequent translation, but successful outcomes can be obtained for relatively long periods of time. The use of radiolunate fusions in osteoarthritic patients is far less common, although, in certain cases in which extrinsic ligament disruption has occurred, this particular arthrodesis may provide some overall support. Fixation can be generally obtained with powered staples, individual screws, or a mini Spider plate.

Scaphotrapeziotrapezoid Arthrodesis

Although far less common than the thumb carpometacarpal arthritis, degenerative changes at the STT joint can cause

focal pain (21–25) (Fig. 8). The use of a small transverse incision, with distal radius autogenous bone graft, generally provides adequate exposure. Fixation can be obtained with multiple Kirschner wires or a mini Spider plate, and the overall predictability of fusion rate is high. Radial styloidectomy should always be performed to prevent secondary impingement problems and radial-sided wrist pain. Average range of motion is approximately two-thirds of normal.

Scaphocapitate Arthrodesis

Scaphocapitate arthrodesis is usually performed for scapholunate instability problems (33,34) (Fig. 9). Its over-

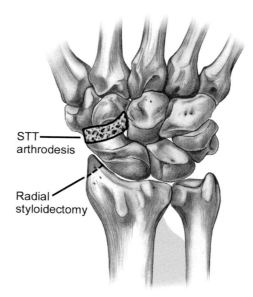

FIGURE 8. Scaphotrapeziotrapezoid (STT) arthrodesis, which should be accompanied by a radial styloidectomy.

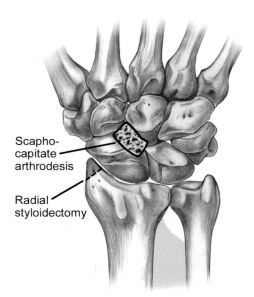

FIGURE 9. Scaphocapitate arthrodesis, which should be accompanied by a radial styloidectomy.

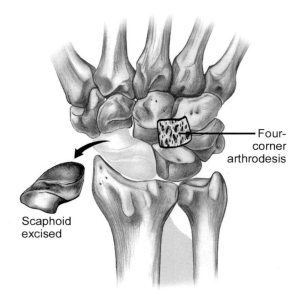

FIGURE 10. Four-corner arthrodesis, which should be accompanied by scaphoid excision in patients who have radioscaphoid arthritis (generally those with scapholunate advanced collapse or scaphoid nonunion advanced collapse wrist). For patients with midcarpal instability, an *in situ* four-corner arthrodesis can be performed, leaving the scaphoid intact.

all mechanical characteristics are similar to those seen with an STT arthrodesis. The procedure is rarely used for arthritic changes. Fixation can be obtained by multiple methods by using multiple Kirschner wires, powered staples, or mini Spider plate fixation.

Four-Corner Arthrodesis

Four-corner arthrodesis, which involves the capitate, lunate, hamate, and triquetrum, is most commonly performed as a reconstruction for wrists with scapholunate advanced collapse or scaphoid nonunion advanced collapse (9,35–37) (Fig. 10). One must ensure that full reduction of the lunate is undertaken before arthrodesis to prevent any dorsal impingement on wrist extension. A large Kirschner wire joystick is generally used to accomplish lunate reduction. Provisional fixation with a few Kirschner wires is generally required. Overall fixation can use multiple Kirschner wires, powered staples, headless screws, or a Spider plate. The use of a Spider plate for fixation of four-corner fusion is ideal, because it provides immediate rigid fixation, circumferential compression, and a lack of any potential impingement problems and eliminates sensory nerve irritation during the postoperative period. One can expect approximately 50% to 60% of the normal motion. Motion generally plateaus at 6 to 9 months postsurgery.

Scapholunocapitate Arthrodesis

Scapholunocapitate arthrodesis is commonly used for large scapholunate ligament tears that involve significant diastasis of the scaphoid and lunate yet without the presence of degenerative changes at the radioscaphoid joint (37,38)

(Fig. 11). Excellent pain relief can be obtained with this procedure, although motion loss can, on occasion, be significant. A radial styloidectomy is almost always performed to decrease overall impingement potential with wrist motion. During radial styloidectomy, care must be undertaken to preserve the extrinsic-stabilizing ligaments of the wrist. Postoperative motion range of one-third to one-half of normal wrist motion can be expected.

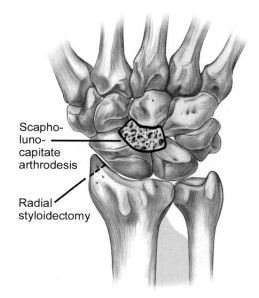

FIGURE 11. Scapholunocapitate arthrodesis. Radial styloidectomy should generally be performed with this procedure.

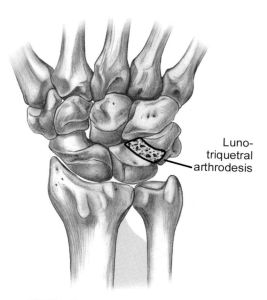

FIGURE 12. Lunotriquetral arthrodesis.

Luno-
triquetral
arthrodesis

Lunotriquetral Arthrodesis

Lunotriquetral arthrodesis is most commonly used in patients who have lunotriquetral instability that is marked by pain and a volar intercalated segment instability deformity of the lunate (Fig. 12). Although the procedure can provide adequate pain relief and can stabilize the interval, the rate of successful arthrodesis is lower than the success rate that is seen with a four-corner arthrodesis. This finding is probably due to the small surface area of the joint being fused. Recently, it has been believed that soft tissue reconstruction procedures have provided better overall outcome

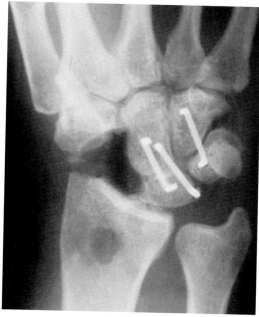

FIGURE 14. Multiple staples are used to obtain arthrodesis in a four-corner fusion. (Reprinted with permission of Arnold-Peter C. Weiss.)

with less loss of motion. Postoperative range of motion is approximately one-half of normal (39,40).

FIXATION METHODS

Kirschner Wires

Kirschner wires are the most common method of orthopedic fixation (Fig. 13). They are inexpensive and easy to use and provide adequate fixation. Disadvantages include the requirement for prolonged cast immobilization, the need for removal, and problems related to the

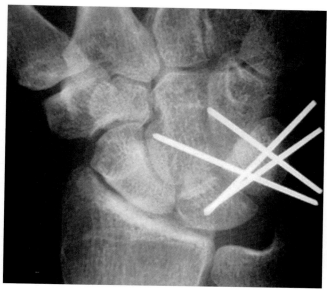

FIGURE 13. Multiple Kirschner wires are used to obtain arthrodesis in a four-corner fusion. (Reprinted with permission of Arnold-Peter C. Weiss.)

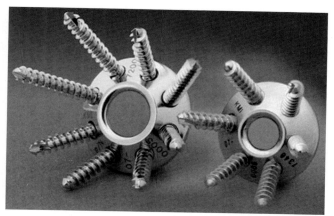

FIGURE 15. Spider and mini Spider plates that are specially designed for limited intercarpal arthrodesis. These plates can be used for nearly all of the intercarpal arthrodeses that have been described. (Reprinted with permission of Arnold-Peter C. Weiss.)

sensory branch nerve fibers that frequently impinge on the pins themselves. There is a risk for pin protrusion and pin tract infection. Initial stability is relatively good, and fusion rates are quite acceptable with this technique (41,42).

Staples

Standard staples, which are implanted with manual or power-driven devices, provide limited compression but do provide some stability (Fig. 14). Because these protrude, leaving a portion of the staple on the dorsal aspect of the carpus, they can easily impinge in wrist extension, and care must be taken to ensure that no impingement occurs. They are relatively easy to use, although their application in a multiplanar fashion can be challenging. Newer staples that provide a memory compression force may provide

more optimal outcomes, although impingement problems are still an issue.

Headless Screws

Headless screws can provide good and stable compression across an arthrodesis site. A downside to this fixation method is that the screw generally needs to go through the joint surface, where range of motion occurs. Most often, more than one screw is required, and it can be challenging to place these screws in a nonparallel fashion. Nevertheless, with meticulous technique, excellent stability can be achieved in selected fusions.

Specialized Plates

Specialized plates have been recently designed that provide for the ability of rigid fixation of the carpal bones (Fig. 15). The Spider and mini Spider plates (Kinetikos Medical Inc.,

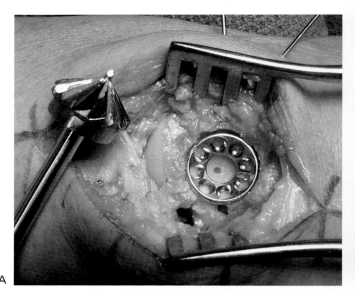

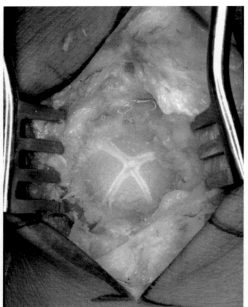

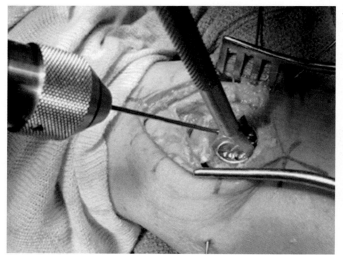

FIGURE 16. After provisional fixation and exposure of the joints that are to be fused, a rasp is used to form the recessed cone into the carpal bones **(A)**. Exposure of the joints is identified after rasping **(B)**, and an additional portion of the joint should be taken down to allow the bone graft to be placed deeper within the joint surfaces. After ensuring that there is no protrusion of the Spider or mini Spider plate, a specially designed plate holder and drill guide is used to start placing screws **(C)**. (*continued*)

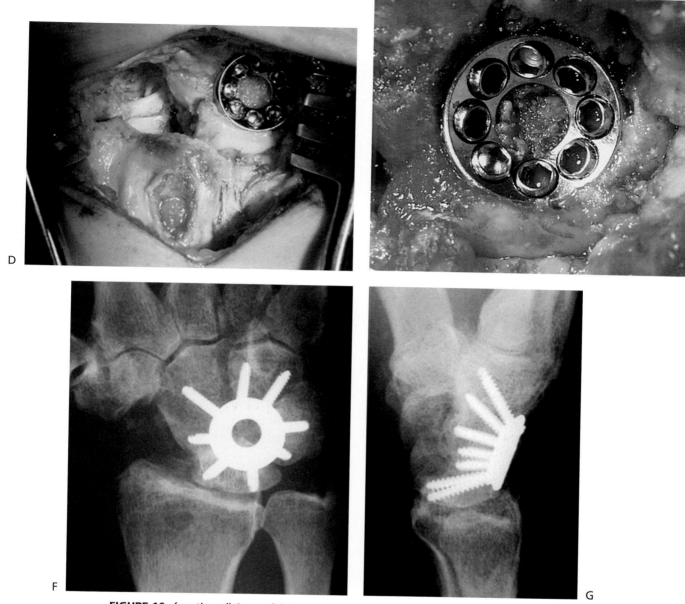

FIGURE 16. *(continued)* Successful placement of the Spider or mini Spider plate **(D)** allows a verification of range of motion in which no instability between the bones that are being fused should be seen. In addition, the extrinsic ligaments are easily visualized in this illustration and are found to be intact. **E:** A close-up of the Spider plate with its accompanying screws, followed by graft packing through the central hole. Posteroanterior **(F)** and lateral **(G)** radiographs demonstrate excellent fixation of a four-corner arthrodesis with the Spider plate.

San Diego, CA) were first introduced 3 years ago with an innovative design. The technique for providing a fusion by using this plate as well as the ability to recess the plate within the carpal bones that are being fused was originally described by the author. The plate allows for complete recessed application (so that no portion of the plate protrudes dorsally, thus eliminating potential impingement), rigid fixation with cancellous screws in the carpal bones that are being fused, the placement of autogenous bone graft through the center of the plate at the site of the fusion, and circumferential com-

pression of the bones that are being fused when screw tightening occurs (Fig. 16). The plates are available in eight- and six-hole versions. The eight-hole version is ideally suited to four-corner and RSL arthrodeses, whereas the six-hole version is suited to scapholunocapitate, STT, and scaphocapitate fusions. The plates provide enough rigid fixation to allow earlier range of motion, compared to alternative forms of fixation. Fusion rates from two studies that involved limited wrist fusions reported a 100% fusion rate with the use of these plates (37).

REFERENCES

1. Abbott LC, Saunders JB, Bost FC. Arthrodesis of the wrist with the use of grafts of cancellous bone. *J Bone Joint Surg* 1942;24:883–898.

2. Hastings H II, Weiss AP, Quenzer D, et al. Arthrodesis of the wrist for post-traumatic disorders. *J Bone Joint Surg* 1996;78A:897–902.

3. Weiss APC, Hastings H II. Wrist arthrodesis for traumatic conditions: a study of plate and local bone graft application. *J Hand Surg* 1995;20:50–56.

4. Weiss APC, Wiedeman G Jr, Quenzer D, et al. Upper extremity function after wrist arthrodesis. *J Hand Surg* 1995;20.

5. Watson HK, Ryu J. Evolution of arthritis of the wrist. *Clin Orthop* 1986;201:57–67.

6. Hastings DE, Silver RL. Intercarpal arthrodesis in the management of chronic carpal instability after trauma. *J Hand Surg* 1984;9:834–840.

7. Minami A, Kato H, Iwasaki N, et al. Limited wrist fusions: comparison of results 22 and 89 months after surgery. *J Hand Surg* 1999;24:133–137.

8. Siegel JM, Ruby LK. A critical look at intercarpal arthrodesis: review of the literature. *J Hand Surg* 1996;21:717–723.

9. Watson HK, Goodman ML, Johnson TR. Limited wrist arthrodesis. Part II: intercarpal and radiocarpal combinations. *J Hand Surg* 1981;6:223–233.

10. Douglas DP, Peimer CA, Koniuch MP. Motion of the wrist after simulated limited intercarpal arthrodeses: an experimental study. *J Bone Joint Surg* 1987;69:1413–1418.

11. Gellman H, Kauffman D, Lenihan M, et al. An in vitro analysis of wrist motion: the effect of limited intercarpal arthrodesis and the contributions of the radiocarpal and midcarpal joints. *J Hand Surg* 1988;13:378–383.

12. Iwasaki N, Genda E, Barrance PJ, et al. Biomechanical analysis of limited intercarpal fusion for the treatment of Kienböck's disease: a three-dimensional theoretical study. *J Orthop Res* 1998;16:256–263.

13. Palmer AK, Werner FW, Murphy D, et al. Functional wrist motion: a biomechanical study. *J Hand Surg* 1985;10:39–46.

14. Rozing PM, Kauer JM. Partial arthrodesis of the wrist. An investigation in cadavers. *Acta Orthop Scand* 1984;55:66–68.

15. Short WH, Werner FW, Fortino MD, et al. Distribution of pressures and forces on the wrist after simulated intercarpal fusion and Kienböck's disease. *J Hand Surg* 1992;17:443–449.

16. Kirschenbaum D, Schneider LH, Kirkpatrick WH, et al. Scaphoid excision and capitolunate arthrodesis for radioscaphoid arthritis. *J Hand Surg* 1993;18:780–785.

17. Bach AW, Almquist EE, Newman DM. Proximal row fusion as a solution for radiocarpal arthritis. *J Hand Surg* 1991;16:424–431.

18. Inoue G, Tamura Y. Radiolunate and radioscapholunate arthrodesis. *Arch Orthop Trauma Surg* 1992;111:333–335.

19. Nagy L, Büchler U. Long term results of radioscapholunate fusion following fractures of the distal radius. *J Hand Surg* 1997;22:705–710.

20. Imbriglia JE, Broudy AS, Hagberg WC, et al. Proximal row carpectomy: clinical evaluation. *J Hand Surg* 1990;15:426–430.

21. Crosby EB, Linscheid RL, Dobyns JH. Scaphotrapezium trapezoidal arthrosis. *J Hand Surg* 1978;3:223–234.

22. Eckenrode JF, Louis DS, Greene TL. Scaphoid-trapezium-trapezoid fusion in the treatment of chronic scapholunate instability. *J Hand Surg* 1986;11:497–502.

23. Frykman EB, Ekenstam FA, Wadin K. Triscaphoid arthrodesis and its complications. *J Hand Surg* 1988;13:844–848.

24. Kleinman WB. Long-term study of chronic scapho-lunate instability treated by scapho-trapezio-trapezoid arthrodesis. *J Hand Surg* 1989;14:429–445.

25. Watson HK, Hempton. Limited wrist arthrodesis. I. The triscaphoid joint. *J Hand Surg* 1980;5:320–327.

26. Berger RA, Bishop AT, Bettinger PC. New dorsal capsulotomy for the surgical exposure of the wrist. *Ann Plast Surg* 1995;35:54–59.

27. Berger RA, Landsmeer JM. The palmar radiocarpal ligaments: a study of adult and fetal human wrist joints. *J Hand Surg* 1990;15:847–854.

28. Siegel DB, Gelberman RH. Radial styloidectomy: an anatomical study with special reference to radiocarpal intracapsular ligamentous morphology. *J Hand Surg* 1991;16:40–44.

29. Chamay A, Della Santa D. Radiolunate arthrodesis in rheumatoid wrist (21 cases). *Ann Chir Main Super* 1991;10:197–206.

30. Chamay A, Della Santa D, Vilaseca A. Radiolunate arthrodesis. Factor of stability for the rheumatoid wrist. *Ann Chir Main* 1983;2:5–17.

31. Halikis MN, Colello-Abraham K, Taleisnik J. Radiolunate fusion. The forgotten partial arthrodesis. *Clin Orthop* 1997;341:30–35.

32. Linscheid RL, Dobyns JH. Radiolunate arthrodesis. *J Hand Surg* 1985;10:821–829.

33. Moy JO, Peimer CA. Scaphocapitate fusion in the treatment of Kienböck's disease. *Hand Clin* 1993;9:501–504.

34. Pisano SM, Peimer CA, Wheeler DR, et al. Scaphocapitate intercarpal arthrodesis. *J Hand Surg* 1991;16:328–333.

35. Krakauer JD, Bishop AT, Cooney WP. Surgical treatment of scapholunate advanced collapse. *J Hand Surg* 1994;9:358–365.

36. Lanz U, Krimmer H, Sauerbier M. Advanced carpal collapse: treatment by limited wrist fusion. In: Büchler U, ed. *Wrist instability.* London: Martin Dunitz Ltd., 1996:139–145.

37. Weiss AP. Limited wrist arthrodesis using a specialized plate. *Trans Am Soc Surg Hand* Chicago, IL, 2003.

38. Rotman MB, Manske PR, Pruitt DL, et al. Scaphocapitolunate arthrodesis. *J Hand Surg* 1993;18:26–33.

39. Sennwald GR, Fischer M, Mondi P. Lunotriquetral arthrodesis. A controversial procedure. *J Hand Surg* 1995;20:755–760.

40. Ritt MJ, Linscheid RL, Cooney WP III, et al. The lunotriquetral joint: kinematic effects of sequential ligament sectioning, ligament repair, and arthrodesis. *J Hand Surg* 1998;23:432–445.

41. Larsen CF, Jacoby RA, McCabe SJ. Nonunion rates of limited carpal arthrodesis: a meta-analysis of the literature. *J Hand Surg* 1997;22:66–73.

42. McAuliffe JA, Dell PL, Jaffe R. Complications of intercarpal arthrodesis. *J Hand Surg* 1993;18:1121–1128.

SCAPHOTRAPEZIOTRAPEZOID AND SCAPHOCAPITATE FUSIONS

PETER D. BURGE

Scaphocapitate (SC) fusion was first described by Sutro in 1946 for scaphoid nonunion (1). Seven cases in which both poles of the fractured scaphoid were fused to the capitate were reported by Helfet (2). Peterson and Lipscomb (3) described scaphotrapezial fusion in three cases of degenerative arthritis and one case of scaphotrapeziotrapezoid (STT) fusion for traumatic arthritis with scaphoid subluxation. They reasoned that because individuals with congenital carpal fusions have wrists that are functionally normal, surgically created fusions should be compatible with good function. However, this assumption ignores subtle developmental changes in articular surface shape and ligament anatomy that may compensate for congenital absence of motion at an intercarpal joint; the normal wrist may behave differently after surgical intercarpal fusion in adult life. STT fusion in 13 patients was described by Watson and Hempton in 1980 (4). Although enthusiasm has been tempered in recent years by better understanding of complication rates and by concern that restriction of motion of the scaphoid may lead to abnormal loading of articular cartilage and premature degenerative arthritis, STT and SC fusions remain useful techniques for certain wrist disorders.

ANATOMY

The scaphoid has a concave oval facet articulating with the radial surface of the head of the capitate and a convex distal surface that in 80% of wrists is divided by a central ridge, giving separate facets that articulate with the trapezium and trapezoid (5). The trapezoid has flat radial and ulnar surfaces that articulate with the trapezium and capitate, respectively; it is bound tightly by ligaments to these bones. The slightly concave proximal surface articulates with the distal pole of the scaphoid. The flat radial surface of the distal capitate articulates with the trapezoid and is continuous with the convex lateral surface of the capitate head, which articulates with the scaphoid (Fig. 1).

The scaphotrapezial ligament runs distally from the radiopalmar aspect of the scaphoid distal pole to insert along the trapezial ridge and to the radial aspect of the trapezium.

The SC ligament arises between the trapezoid and capitate facets of the scaphoid on its palmar surface and attaches to the palmar surface of the waist of the capitate (Fig. 2). The capitate–trapezium ligament passes from the radiopalmar aspect of the trapezium into the palmar waist of the capitate and is not attached to the trapezoid. It may serve to support the distal pole of the scaphoid, and it reinforces the palmar aspect of the STT joint capsule (6). The trapeziotrapezoid and trapezoid–capitate joints appear to allow virtually no movement.

BIOMECHANICS

The bones of the distal carpal row are linked to each other and to the bases of the index and middle metacarpals by stout ligaments that permit very little movement; for practical purposes, the distal row may be regarded as a fixed unit that is firmly joined to the metacarpals. The proximal row is mobile and lacks tendon or muscle attachments—it is "a prisoner of circumstance," and the positions of its bones are determined by their shape, by the ligaments that hold them to each other and to the adjacent rows, and by externally applied forces. Carpal instabilities are abnormal motions of the bones of the proximal row, either singly or in combination.

The proximal row flexes during radial deviation of the wrist and extends during ulnar deviation. Put simply, the scaphoid flexes during radial deviation so as to accommodate to the decreasing space between the distal row and the radius. In ulnar deviation, the helicoidal slope of the triquetrohamate joint drives the triquetrum into extension, and this motion is transmitted to the lunate and thence to the scaphoid through the lunotriquetral and scapholunate interosseous ligaments. In scapholunate instability (and its bony analogue scaphoid nonunion), the excessive flexion of the scaphoid leads to carpal collapse, and to excessive load-

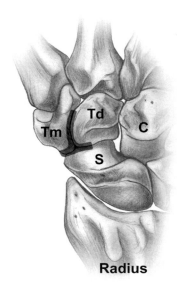

FIGURE 1. The scaphotrapeziotrapezoid joint forms an inverted T. The trapezoid–capitate and trapeziotrapezoid joints are relatively immobile. C, capitate; S, scaphoid; Td, trapezoid; Tm, trapezium.

ing and loss of articular congruity in the elliptical radio-scaphoid joint. The end stage is the scapholunate advanced collapse pattern of degenerative arthritis (7). A primary aim of both STT and SC fusions is prevention or correction of excessive scaphoid flexion.

STT motion is a simple rotational movement about a single axis that passes through the radiopalmar aspect of the

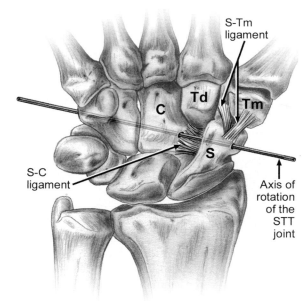

FIGURE 2. The axis of rotation of the scaphotrapeziotrapezoid (STT) joint passes through the waist of the capitate (C) and the radiopalmar aspect of the distal scaphoid (S). S-C, scaphocapitate; S-Tm, scaphoid-trapezium; Td, trapezoid; Tm, trapezium. (From Moritomo H, Viegas SF, Elder K, et al. The scaphotrapeziotrapezoidal joint. Part 2: a kinematic study. *J Hand Surg [Am]* 2000;25:911–920, with permission.)

distal scaphoid and the waist of the capitate (Fig. 2) (6) and is essentially the same in both flexion/extension and radial/ulnar deviation of the wrist. This rather simple pattern of motion contrasts with the complex behavior of the scaphoid with respect to the radius during radial/ulnar deviation and flexion/extension of the wrist. Because the trapezium–trapezoid and trapezoid–capitate joints are immobile, fusion of the scaphoid to the trapezoid has bio-mechanical effects very similar to those of SC fusion.

STT fusion alters loading and contact areas in the radio-scaphoid joint (8). STT motion is crucial to the adaptive positioning of the scaphoid during radial and ulnar deviation of the wrist. An appreciation of the way that STT and SC fusions alter the motion, loading, and congruity of the radio-carpal joint, especially with respect to the scaphoid and its relationship with the radius, is fundamental to understanding the rationale of these procedures and their effect on the wrist. The normal pattern of motion of the scaphoid allows it to remain congruent with the radius in the face of the constantly changing relationship between the distal carpal row and the elliptical scaphoid fossa of the radius. This adaptive mechanism is lost when motion of the scaphoid is restricted by its fusion to the distal row. The flexion–extension component of scaphoid movement decreases, and the scaphoid rotation axis approaches the axis of the capitate, causing it to behave like a bone of the distal row. The loss of scaphoid flexion during radial deviation of the wrist increases stress in the radioscaphoid joint during radial deviation, and there is corresponding stress on the scapholunate ligaments in ulnar deviation because the scaphoid is unable to extend (9). Simulated STT and SC fusions increased loading in the radio-scaphoid joint (Fig. 3) (8,10). These kinematic changes have

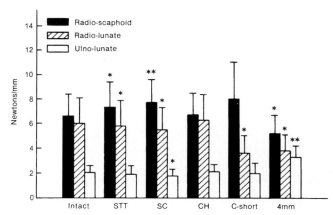

FIGURE 3. Average peak pressures at the radioscaphoid, radio-lunate, and ulnolunate joints in intact wrists and after simulating the following operations: scaphotrapeziotrapezoid (STT) fusion, scaphocapitate (SC) fusion, capitate–hamate (CH) fusion, capitate shortening (C-short) plus CH fusion, and ulnar lengthening/radial shortening (4 mm). *, $p < .05$; **, $p < .005$ compared with intact (Tukey test). (From Horii E, Garcia-Elias M, Bishop AT, et al. Effect on force transmission across the carpus in procedures used to treat Kienböck's disease. *J Hand Surg [Am]* 1990;15:393–400, with permission.)

given rise to concern that STT and SC fusions predispose to degenerative arthritis in the radioscaphoid joint. Radioscaphoid impingement has been observed after STT fusion, and routine radial styloidectomy has been advocated (11).

The effect of STT fusion and SC fusion on wrist motion was simulated in cadaver wrists by fixation with two Herbert screws (9). STT fusion reduced the range of flexion–extension by 22 degrees, and SC fusion reduced it by 18 degrees. Radial deviation and ulnar deviation were reduced by 20 degrees and 26 degrees, respectively. Clinically, stiffness due to preexisting disease or to immobilization after surgery may further restrict motion after intercarpal fusion. The average range of motion in the flexion/extension plane in 13 reports of STT fusion was 62% of normal (12). SC fusion reduced wrist extension on average by 28 degrees, flexion by 40 degrees, radial deviation by 14 degrees, and ulnar deviation by 14 degrees (13). The range of motion reached a plateau after approximately 6 months (13) and strength after approximately 1 year.

The arc and range of wrist motion are affected by the position of fusion of the scaphoid with respect to the distal carpal row. Radioscaphoid angle and wrist motion were measured in cadaver wrists before and after simulated STT and SC fusions with the scaphoid in extended, neutral, and flexed positions with respect to the long axis of the radius (14). Radial deviation and wrist extension increased as the scaphoid became more flexed; ulnar deviation and flexion increased as the scaphoid became more extended. The optimum radioscaphoid angle for maximum wrist motion was 41 degrees to 60 degrees for STT fusion and 30 degrees to 57 degrees for SC fusion.

INDICATIONS

The specific indication for STT fusion is degenerative arthritis of the STT joint (Table 1). SC fusion has been advocated for isolated SC arthritis (13) and for resistant scaphoid nonunion (1,2). Both STT fusion and SC fusion have been advocated for chronic static scapholunate instability and for Kienböck's disease; for these two indications, SC fusion is probably equivalent functionally to STT fusion because fusion of the scaphoid to the trapezoid effectively links the scaphoid rigidly to the capitate through the relatively immobile trapezoid–capitate joint.

Degenerative Arthritis

Causes of STT arthritis include previous trauma and calcium pyrophosphate deposition disease, but most cases are

TABLE 1. INDICATIONS FOR SCAPHOTRAPEZIOTRAPEZOID FUSION

Isolated scaphotrapeziotrapezoid degenerative arthritis
Scapholunate instability
Kienböck's disease

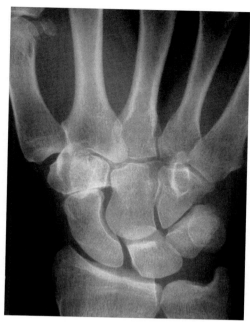

FIGURE 4. Degenerative arthritis of the scaphotrapeziotrapezoid joint.

idiopathic (Fig. 4). Scaphotrapezial arthropathy was present on radiographs of 44% of 160 wrists that showed chondrocalcinosis of the triangular fibrocartilage and in 14% of age- and sex-matched controls without chondrocalcinosis (15). The prevalence of isolated STT osteoarthritis was 2% of 143 postmenopausal females with distal radial fractures (16). The STT arthritis that accompanies advanced trapeziometacarpal arthritis is best treated by trapezial excision arthroplasty with or without ligament reconstruction.

Many cases of isolated STT arthritis respond to nonoperative treatment with splintage, activity modification, and steroid injection. Fusion is reserved for the minority of cases that fail to respond to these measures. Relief of pain is generally good (17,18).

Excision arthroplasty by removal of the distal pole of the scaphoid (19) is an alternative to STT fusion. Advantages include shorter immobilization and recovery times and probably also a lower complication rate. However, excision of the distal pole of the scaphoid resulted in a dorsiflexion intercalated segment instability pattern of carpal malalignment in 12 of 21 wrists (19). Although malalignment appeared to cause no symptoms, its long-term consequence is unknown.

Kienböck's Disease

Management of Kienböck's disease has centered on techniques that reduce loading of the lunate. Biomechanical studies using pressure-sensitive film (20) and theoretical models (21) have shown that both STT fusion and SC fusion reduce loading of the radiolunate joint but at the expense of overloading adjacent joints, particularly the radioscaphoid joint (Fig. 3) (10). Radial shortening, however, produced a 45% reduction in loading, with only moderate changes in force at the radioscaphoid joint.

Alignment of the scaphoid influences the unloading effect of STT fusion. A neutral or extended position unloads the radiolunate joint regardless of the condition of the lunate (20); the load is shifted to the radioscaphoid joint. However, fusion in a flexed position does not affect lunate load.

The lack of controlled studies hampers the comparison of the results of different procedures in a condition such as Kienböck's disease for which the symptoms are variable and correlate poorly with the radiographic appearance. However, STT fusion and SC fusion have been used with apparent benefit in Kienböck's disease (22–26). STT fusion combined with lunate excision and replacement with rolled tendon gave good relief of pain but less satisfactory range of motion in 12 of 15 wrists at an average of 57 months (27). Stage IIIB was believed to be the specific indication for this procedure, which corrected the flexed posture of the scaphoid. However, progressive radioscaphoid osteoarthritis was the chief cause of poor results and required total wrist fusion in two cases. SC fusion gave good pain relief in 10 of 11 patients at an average of 3 years after SC fusion; the lunate was left *in situ* (25).

The potential for inducing radioscaphoid degenerative arthritis remains a concern with regard to STT and SC fusions. As joint-leveling procedures such as radial shortening are probably more effective in unloading the radiolunate joint and do not greatly increase radioscaphoid loading (10,28), these procedures are preferred over STT fusion and SC fusion in the ulnar minus wrist. Other reasons for preferring radial shortening osteotomy to limited carpal fusion include its simplicity, lower potential for reducing wrist motion, lower complication rate, and more rapid rehabilitation. However, STT fusion or SC fusion may have a place in cases with neutral or positive ulnar variance.

Scapholunate Instability

STT fusion was first used in the treatment of chronic rotatory subluxation of the scaphoid by Peterson and Lipscomb in 1967 (3). Several subsequent studies have suggested that fusion of the STT joint maintains the height of the radial side of the carpus and prevents the scaphoid flexion and rotatory subluxation that lead to pain and weakness in chronic static scapholunate instability (29–31). However, carpal mechanics remain abnormal, and the load-sharing function of the lunate is not restored. Using pressure-sensitive film, Viegas et al. (8) showed that excessive scaphoid loading after simulated perilunate instability was exaggerated by STT and SC fusions (Fig. 5). It may be noted that the effect of fusions on scaphoid loading was much greater in wrists after simulated perilunate instability (Fig. 5) (8) than in normal wrists (Fig. 3) (10).

STT fusion does not close the scapholunate diastasis; indeed, the scapholunate interval may open farther during

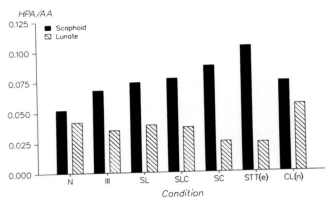

FIGURE 5. Histogram comparing overall scaphoid and lunate high-pressure contact areas as a ratio of the available joints surface area (HPA/AA) for wrists in the normal and the destabilized state as well as for destabilized wrists after various types of intercarpal fusion. CL(n), capitate lunate fusion with the lunate in a neutral posture relative to the capitate; III, stage III perilunate instability; N, normal; SC, scaphocapitate fusion; SL, scapholunate fusion; SLC, scapholunocapitate fusion; STT(e), scaphotrapeziotrapezoid fusion with the scaphoid vertically orientated. (From Viegas SF, Patterson RM, Peterson PD, et al. Evaluation of the biomechanical efficacy of limited intercarpal fusions for the treatment of scapho-lunate dissociation. *J Hand Surg [Am]* 1990;15:120–128, with permission.)

ulnar deviation as the STT fusion mass, capitate, and hamate rotate with the hand into ulnar deviation, and this may be associated with persistent ulnar translation of the carpus. In flexion, the proximal pole of the scaphoid may shift dorsally, where it may impinge on the dorsal rim of the distal radius. Despite these abnormal motion patterns, good medium-term results have been reported, with little evidence of degenerative arthritis at an average follow-up of 56 months. Poor results were associated with failure to correct the flexed posture of the scaphoid. Whether the adverse load-shifting effects of STT and SC fusions lead to degenerative arthritis is a question that will be answered only by longer-term follow-up studies (32).

CONTRAINDICATIONS

Degenerative arthritis of the radioscaphoid joint is a definite contraindication to STT fusion. The radiographic signs may be subtle and include loss of articular cartilage height, subchondral sclerosis, and "beaking" of the radial styloid. These changes may progress rapidly after STT fusion, despite correct alignment of the scaphoid.

OPERATIVE TECHNIQUE

The technical principles set out by Watson and Hempton (4) have been amplified in the light of experience, especially in view of the relatively high complication rate encountered in some studies (33,34) (see Complications). They can be summarized as follows:

- Protection of dorsal sensory nerve branches
- Maintenance of intercarpal distances
- Correct scaphoid alignment
- Preparation of healthy cancellous bone surfaces
- Use of bone graft (usually from the distal radius)
- Stable fixation with buried implants
- Protection by cast or splint until union

Scaphotrapeziotrapezoid Fusion

A transverse incision, as recommended by Watson and Hempton (4), with a second, more proximal transverse incision for

harvesting bone graft from the dorsum of the distal radius, has cosmetic advantages over a longitudinal approach, although the latter may be necessitated by previous wrist surgery. Branches of the superficial radial nerve are sought and protected. The dorsal branch of the radial artery is mobilized and retracted, with any small carpal branches coagulated and divided. Retracting the tendons of the first and second dorsal compartments to either side, a longitudinal incision is made in the capsule of the scaphotrapezial joint (Fig. 6). The joint is identified as an inverted T, and the capsule is reflected off the bones to expose the joint surfaces fully.

At this stage, any excessive flexion of the scaphoid can be corrected, and provisional fixation with Kirschner wires is achieved. It is advisable to check the alignment with intraoperative radiographs, using radiographs of the opposite

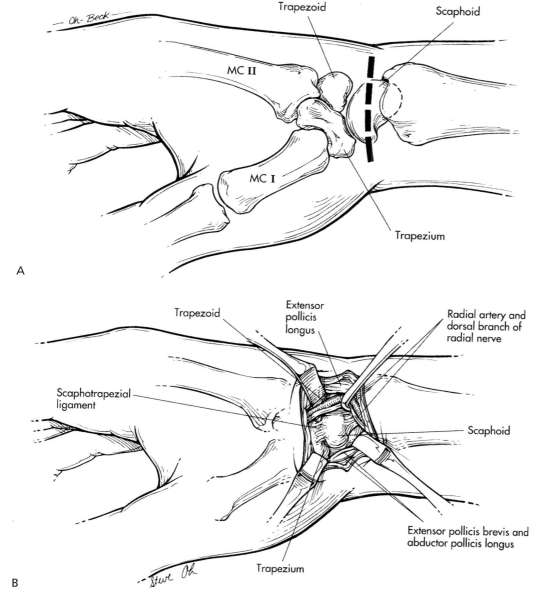

FIGURE 6. A,B: Transverse approach to the scaphotrapeziotrapezoid joint. MC, metacarpal. (From Ruby LK. Arthrotomy. In: Cooney WP, Linscheid RL, Dobyns JH, eds. *The wrist. Diagnosis and operative treatment.* St. Louis: Mosby, 1998, with permission.)

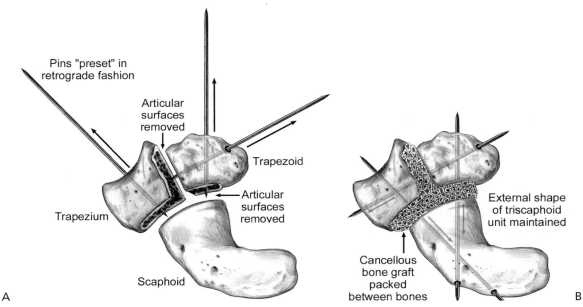

FIGURE 7. A: Articular surfaces are removed and three pins have been "preset" in retrograde fashion. **B:** Cancellous bone graft had been packed between the bones, the external shape of the three-bone unit is maintained, and the pins are driven across the arthrodesis sites. (From Watson HK, Hempton RF. Limited wrist arthrodeses. I. The triscaphoid joint. *J Hand Surg [Am]* 1980;5:320–327, with permission.)

wrist for comparison if necessary. Alignment of the scaphoid must avoid excessive flexion. The optimum position of the fused scaphoid—i.e., the position that maximized wrist motion in simulated fusions of cadaver wrists—was a radioscaphoid angle between 41 degrees and 60 degrees (14). Failure to ensure correct alignment of the scaphoid has been associated with persistent pain (33).

The dorsal 70% of the articular surfaces of the STT joint is then excised to expose cancellous bone. Leaving the palmar 30% of the articular surfaces intact maintains the appropriate intercarpal distances; if the entire surface is removed, the handle of a small elevator can be used to maintain the correct intercarpal separation as the pins are inserted (Fig. 7) (4). Cancellous bone taken from the distal radius in the vicinity of Lister's tubercle, via a separate transverse incision if necessary, is then packed between the prepared surfaces. A radial styloidectomy may be performed if desired (11). No more than 3 to 4 mm of the styloid should be removed to avoid damage to radiocarpal ligaments and the consequent risk of ulnar translation of the carpus (35,36).

Alternative bone grafting techniques include the dowel method (37), using a precision tube saw to prepare the graft bed (centered on the junction of scaphoid, trapezium, and trapezoid) and a slightly larger saw to obtain, from the iliac crest, a matching dowel graft that fits tightly into the bed. A similar method can be used with distal radial graft (38). The iliac crest tends to provide a stronger graft, but the lower morbidity of the distal radial donor site is preferred by patients.

For fixation, Kirschner wires have the virtue of simplicity but require later removal. Three or four wires are required;

they should cross the joints to be fused (4), and it may be helpful to pin the scaphoid to the capitate; however, pins should not cross other joints. The decision to bury the tips subcutaneously or leave them percutaneously is influenced by the consequences of infection of pin tracks that traverse the joint spaces of the wrist—septic arthritis is a potentially disastrous result of pin track sepsis. For this reason, the author buries subcutaneously the ends of all pins that cross the synovial cavity of the wrist joint and accepts the need to remove them in due course.

Passage of pins and screws through any but the dorsal incision entails risks to the superficial radial nerve branches and to the dorsal branch of the radial artery. The author makes an incision large enough to permit blunt dissection down to the joint capsule, as for a wrist arthroscopy portal, and uses an appropriately sized drill guide to protect the soft tissues. The anatomic study of Steinberg et al. (39) is helpful in planning the placement of wires. An equal degree of care is required when removing them.

Alternative methods of fixation include screws and staples (Fig. 8). Screws can generally be left in place indefinitely; unlike Kirschner wires, there is no pressure to remove them, and this can be an advantage if union is slow (Fig. 9). The use of screws is influenced by considerations of access; it may be difficult to achieve the correct angle of attack through the dorsal incision, necessitating a separate radial incision or stab incisions, with the inherent risk to the superficial radial nerve and the dorsal branch of the radial artery. Staples have the advantage that they can be inserted directly through the dorsal approach, avoiding any

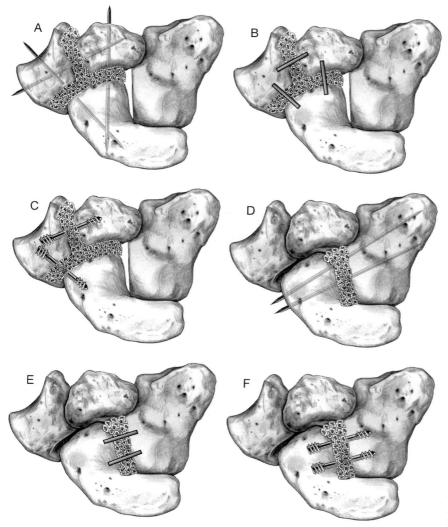

FIGURE 8. Fixation techniques for scaphotrapeziotrapezoid and scaphocapitate fusions. **A,D:** Kirschner wires. **B,E:** Staples. **C,F:** Herbert screws.

risk to dorsal sensory nerves, although the literature contains little about their use in STT and SC fusions.

Most authors recommend immobilization for 8 to 12 weeks. The extent of the cast varies from a simple short arm cast to a long arm cast including the metacarpophalangeal joints of the index and middle fingers (4). A long cast for an initial period of 4 to 6 weeks and a short cast thereafter is a reasonable regimen. Thereafter, graduated progression is made through active range-of-motion exercises and subsequent strengthening exercises, with the maximum range of motion reached at approximately 6 months postoperatively.

Scaphocapitate Fusion

SC fusion can be performed through a transverse or longitudinal skin incision. The joint capsule is opened in the interval between the third and fourth dorsal compartments, protecting superficial radial nerve branches. The adjacent surfaces of the capitate and scaphoid are prepared as for STT fusion (see Scaphotrapeziotrapezoid Fusion), preserving the palmar 30%

of the surfaces to maintain the correct intercarpal relationship. Kirschner wires are driven from the radial surface of the scaphoid into the capitate, with the scaphoid having been positioned at approximately 45 degrees to the long axis of the wrist (Fig. 10). Alternatively, headless screws such as the Herbert and Acutrak screws may be placed across the SC joint. Staples may also be used. Cancellous bone graft from the distal radius is packed into the prepared bone surfaces. The wound is closed, and the limb is immobilized for 8 to 12 weeks, as for STT fusion. However, if secure screw fixation is achieved, the period of immobilization may be shortened.

Results

A review of the literature on intercarpal arthrodesis (12) identified 258 patients in 13 reports of STT fusion, which was performed for a variety of disorders. The average follow-up period was 38 months. Using strict criteria for definition of postoperative pain, 49% of wrists were painful at final follow-up. In this study, any complaint related to pain was recorded as posi-

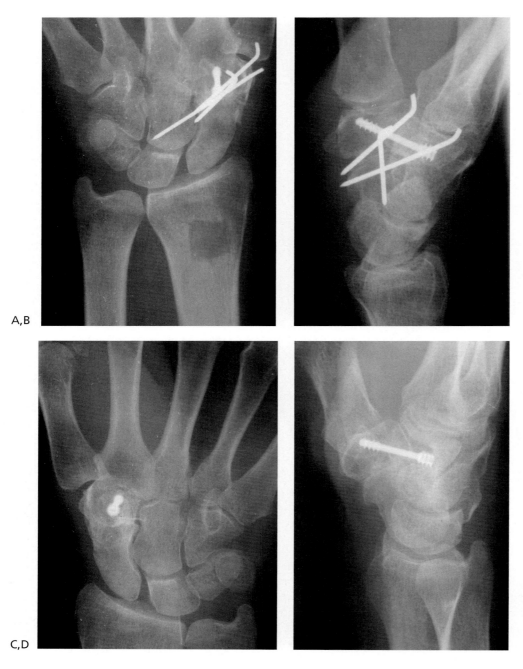

A,B

C,D

FIGURE 9. A,B: Fusion of the scaphotrapeziotrapezoid joint with Kirschner wires, supplemented by a Herbert screw passed between the trapezium and trapezoid. **C,D:** The appearance after 2 years.

tive, but not all cases with mild postoperative pain had poor results. The average range of motion was 62% of the normal flexion/extension arc, and the average grip strength was 74% of normal. Several studies reported cases of radioscaphoid arthrosis developing after STT fusion. Approximately one-third of 258 patients required further operations to treat complications or persistent pain. These procedures included bone grafting, total wrist arthrodesis, proximal row carpectomy, and radial styloidectomy. The results in cases of STT arthrosis were similar to the results in other disorders. The reviewers agreed with Tomaino et al. (40) that postoperative function was more dependent on pain relief than on residual movement. The

short average follow-up in the reviewed papers (36 months) emphasizes the paucity of long-term data on which advice to patients can be based.

Data on the results of SC fusion are more limited. Seven of 17 patients (13) had persistent pain with heavy use. The average loss of flexion/extension was 68 degrees, and grip strength averaged 74% of the unoperated side. SC fusion for Kienböck's disease using two lag screws (25) gave complete pain relief in 10 of 11 patients at an average of 36 months with a 64-degree arc of flexion/extension and grip strength 72% of the unoperated side. Two patients required second operations to achieve union.

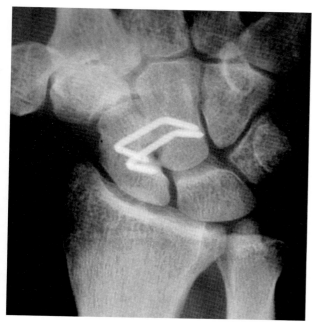

FIGURE 10. An anteroposterior radiograph demonstrates successful scaphocapitate fusion using power staples.

COMPLICATIONS

The complication rate of STT fusion has remained significantly higher than other wrist procedures (33,34,41–43). A review of 13 papers that described 258 patients (12) found a complication rate averaging 43% in those studies in which it was reported, including 13% nonunion. Kleinman and Carroll (33) had 52% complications in 47 wrists. In another series, it was 53% of 40 cases (34). Complications included pin track infection, osteomyelitis, radial styloid impingement, nonunion, and dorsal sensory nerve problems (Table 2). Attention to details of operative technique and to positioning of the scaphoid can do much to minimize the risk of complications. The optimum position of the fused scaphoid—i.e., the position that maximizes wrist motion—is a radioscaphoid angle between 41 degrees and 60 degrees (14). Ulnar translation of the lunotriquetral unit occurred in two of 47 cases treated by Kleinman and Carroll (33). Both were associated with ulnar-sided wrist pain and required total wrist fusion.

TABLE 2. COMPLICATIONS OF SCAPHOTRAPEZIOTRAPEZOID FUSION

Nonunion
Pin track sepsis
Septic arthritis
Osteomyelitis
Radial styloid impingement
Dorsal sensory nerve impairment
Radioscaphoid arthrosis

Radial styloid impingement was reported in 31 of 91 patients at an average of 23 months after STT fusion (11). Impingement was characterized by radial wrist pain on flexion or by limited radial deviation; the symptoms were relieved by radial styloidectomy. These authors recommended routine partial radial styloidectomy at the time of STT fusion.

Complications of SC fusion included nonunion in 2 of 17 patients (13).

REFERENCES

1. Sutro CJ. Treatment of nonunion of the carpal navicular bone. *Surgery* 1946;46:536–540.
2. Helfet AJ. A new operation for ununited fracture of the scaphoid. *J Bone Joint Surg (Br)* 1952;34:329.
3. Peterson HA, Lipscomb PR. Intercarpal arthrodesis. *Arch Surg* 1967;95:127–134.
4. Watson HK, Hempton RF. Limited wrist arthrodeses. I. The triscaphoid joint. *J Hand Surg (Am)* 1980;5:320–327.
5. Moritomo H, Viegas SF, Nakamura K, et al. The scapho-trapezio-trapezoidal joint. Part 1: an anatomic and radiographic study. *J Hand Surg (Am)* 2000;25A:899–910.
6. Moritomo H, Viegas SF, Elder K, et al. The scaphotrapezio-trapezoidal joint. Part 2: a kinematic study. *J Hand Surg (Am)* 2000;25A:911–920.
7. Watson HK, Ballet FL. The SLAC wrist: scapholunate advanced collapse pattern of degenerative arthritis. *J Hand Surg (Am)* 1984;9A:358–365.
8. Viegas SF, Patterson RM, Peterson PD, et al. Evaluation of the biomechanical efficacy of limited intercarpal fusions for the treatment of scapho-lunate dissociation. *J Hand Surg (Am)* 1990;15A:120–128.
9. Garcia-Elias M, Cooney WP, An KN, et al. Wrist kinematics after limited intercarpal arthrodesis. *J Hand Surg (Am)* 1989;14A:791–799.
10. Horii E, Garcia-Elias M, Bishop AT, et al. Effect on force transmission across the carpus in procedures used to treat Kienbock's disease. *J Hand Surg (Am)* 1990;15A:393–400.
11. Rogers WD, Watson HK. Radial styloid impingement after triscaphe arthrodesis. *J Hand Surg (Am)* 1989;14A:297–301.
12. Siegel JM, Ruby LK. A critical look at intercarpal arthrodesis: review of the literature. *J Hand Surg (Am)* 1996;21A:717–723.
13. Pisano SM, Peimer CA, Wheeler DR, et al. Scaphocapitate intercarpal arthrodesis. *J Hand Surg (Am)* 1991;16A:328–333.
14. Minamikawa Y, Peimer CA, Yamaguchi T, et al. Ideal scaphoid angle for intercarpal arthrodesis. *J Hand Surg (Am)* 1992;17A:370–375.
15. Donich AS, Lektrakul N, Liu CC, et al. Calcium pyrophosphate dihydrate crystal deposition disease of the wrist: trapezioscaphoid joint abnormality. *J Rheumatol* 2000;27:2628–2634.
16. Armstrong AL, Hunter JB, Davis TR. The prevalence of degenerative arthritis of the base of the thumb in postmenopausal women. *J Hand Surg (Br)* 1994;19B:340–341.
17. Rogers WD, Watson HK. Degenerative arthritis at the triscaphe joint. *J Hand Surg (Am)* 1990;15A:232–235.

18. Srinivasan VB, Matthews JP. Results of scaphotrapeziotrapezoid fusion for isolated idiopathic arthritis. *J Hand Surg (Br)* 1996;21B:378–380.

19. Garcia-Elias M, Lluch AL, Farreres A, et al. Resection of the distal scaphoid for scaphotrapeziotrapezoid osteoarthritis. *J Hand Surg (Br)* 1999;24B:448–452.

20. Short WH, Werner FW, Fortino MD, et al. Distribution of pressures and forces on the wrist after simulated intercarpal fusion and Kienbock's disease. *J Hand Surg (Br)* 1992;17A:443–449.

21. Iwasaki N, Genda E, Barrance PJ, et al. Biomechanical analysis of limited intercarpal fusion for the treatment of Kienbock's disease: a three-dimensional theoretical study. *J Orthop Res* 1998;16:256–263.

22. Voche P, Bour C, Merle M. Scapho-trapezio-trapezoid arthrodesis in the treatment of Kienbock's disease: a study of 16 cases. *J Hand Surg (Am)* 1992;17B:5–11.

23. Allieu Y, Chammas M, Lussiez B, et al. Surgical treatment of Kienbock disease by scapho-trapezo-trapezoidal arthrodesis. Report of 11 cases. *Ann Chir Main Memb Super* 1991;10:22–29.

24. Watson HK, Monacelli DM, Milford RS, et al. Treatment of Kienbock's disease with scaphotrapezio-trapezoid arthrodesis. *J Hand Surg (Am)* 1996;21A:9–15.

25. Sennwald GR, Ufenast H. Scaphocapitate arthrodesis for the treatment of Kienbock's disease. *J Hand Surg (Am)* 1995;20A:506–510.

26. Moy OJ, Peimer CA. Scaphocapitate fusion in the treatment of Kienbock's disease. *Hand Clin* 1993;9:501–504.

27. Minami A, Kimura T, Suzuki K. Long-term results of Kienbock's disease treated by triscaphe arthrodesis and excisional arthroplasty with a coiled palmaris longus tendon. *J Hand Surg (Am)* 1994;19A:219–228.

28. Werner FW, Palmer AK. Biomechanical evaluation of operative procedures to treat Kienbock's disease. *Hand Clin* 1993;9:431–443.

29. Kleinman WB. Long-term study of chronic scapho-lunate instability treated by scapho-trapezio-trapezoid arthrodesis. *J Hand Surg (Am)* 1989;14A:429–445.

30. Watson HK, Ryu J, Akelman E. Limited triscaphoid intercarpal arthrodesis for rotatory subluxation of the scaphoid. *J Bone Joint Surg* 1986;68A:345–349.

31. Eckenrode JF, Louis DS, Greene TL. Scaphoid-trapezium-trapezoid fusion in the treatment of chronic scapholunate instability. *Clin Orthop* 1986;11:497–502.

32. Mih AD. Limited wrist fusion. *Hand Clin* 1997;13:615–625.

33. Kleinman WB, Carroll CT. Scapho-trapezio-trapezoid arthrodesis for treatment of chronic static and dynamic scapho-lunate instability: a 10-year perspective on pitfalls and complications. *J Hand Surg (Am)* 1990;15A:408–414.

34. Ishida O, Tsai TM. Complications and results of scapho-trapezio-trapezoid arthrodesis. *Clin Orthop* 1993;125–130.

35. Siegel DB, Gelberman RH. Radial styloidectomy: an anatomical study with special reference to radiocarpal intracapsular ligamentous morphology. *J Hand Surg (Am)* 1991;16A:40–44.

36. Nakamura T, Cooney WP III, Lui W, et al. Radial styloidectomy: a biomechanical study on stability of the wrist joint. *J Hand Surg (Am)* 2001;26A:85–93.

37. Sandow MJ, Wai YL, Hayes MG. Intercarpal arthrodesis by dowel bone grafting. *J Hand Surg (Br)* 1992;17B:463–466.

38. Thurston AJ, Stanley JK. Dowel fusion of the scapho-trapezio-trapezoid joint: a description of a new technique. *Hand Surg* 1999; 4:125–129.

39. Steinberg BD, Plancher KD, Idler RS. Percutaneous Kirschner wire fixation through the snuff box: an anatomic study. *J Hand Surg (Am)* 1995;20A:57–62.

40. Tomaino MM, Miller RJ, Burton RI. Outcome assessment following limited wrist fusion: objective wrist scoring versus patient satisfaction. *Contemp Orthop* 1994;28:403–410.

41. Frykman EB, Af Ekenstam F, Wadin K. Triscaphoid arthrodesis and its complications. *J Hand Surg (Am)* 1988;13A:844-849.

42. McAuliffe JA, Dell PC, Jaffe R. Complications of intercarpal arthrodesis. *J Hand Surg (Am)* 1993;18A:1121–1128.

43. Fortin PT, Louis DS. Long-term follow-up of scaphoid-trapezium-trapezoid arthrodesis. *J Hand Surg (Am)* 1993;18A:675–681.

76

FOUR-CORNER FUSION

MARK S. COHEN

Stability of the wrist is provided by the tight-fitting anatomic design of the individual carpal bones and the ligamentous interconnections that control movement of one bone relative to another. Wrist instability results from soft tissue or bony disruption, leading to pathologic carpal orientation. As the bones lose their alignment, they assume a collapsed position, with dissipation of the normal stored potential energy within the wrist (1,2). Motion and load-bearing capacity are lost. Pain occurs secondary to abnormal shear forces, synovitis, and ultimately cartilage degeneration.

The most common form of carpal instability occurs between the scaphoid and lunate. When load-bearing potential of the scapholunate interosseous ligament is lost, the scaphoid collapses into a flexed posture and the triquetrum and lunate extend. Scapholunate dissociation significantly alters articular contact areas and stress patterns within the carpus. Experimentally, only 5 degrees of pathologic flexion of the scaphoid results in a 45% reduction in the radioscaphoid contact area (3). In this setting, arthritic changes begin at the radial styloid articulation with the scaphoid and progress to the proximal radioscaphoid joint. Degeneration then moves to the midcarpal capitolunate joint. This is termed *scapholunate advanced collapse* (SLAC) arthritis (4). This is the final common pathway for a variety of degenerative disorders of the wrist, the most common being scapholunate dissociation. It is also seen in scaphoid nonunion, avascular necrosis of the scaphoid, rheumatoid arthritis, and calcium pyrophosphate deposition disease (pseudogout) (5).

As a result of its concentric design, the radiolunate joint is unloaded and preserved regardless of the etiology or stage of SLAC degeneration. Four-corner fusion of the midcarpal joint (lunate, triquetrum, capitate, and hamate) with scaphoid excision is based on maintenance of this relationship. Successful arthrodesis results in isolated radiocarpal motion with force transmission through the radiolunate articulation and the triangular fibrocartilage complex.

EVALUATION

Patients with advanced wrist arthritis typically present with measurable limitation of motion and function. Pain is variable and is usually aggravated by loading activities. Interestingly, although wrist degeneration has certainly been present for some time (months to years), patients often report a relatively recent onset of symptoms. On examination, soft tissue swelling on the dorsoradial aspect of the wrist is not uncommon. Discomfort can be localized to the radioscaphoid joint both dorsally and radially in the majority of cases. A scaphoid shift test, consisting of palmar pressure applied to the distal scaphoid as the wrist is brought into radial deviation, may reproduce symptoms and elicit crepitation in advanced cases (6). Provocative maneuvers on the ulnar aspect of the wrist are usually negative.

Plain radiographs are most commonly all that is necessary to confirm the diagnosis of SLAC arthritis. A static dissociation between the scaphoid and lunate or a displaced fracture of the scaphoid is typically obvious. Whereas sclerosis and joint space narrowing are easily identified in advanced cases, articular cartilage loss is typically greater than that appreciated on standard radiographic projections (Fig. 1) (7). Conservative treatment measures include activity modification, short-term splintage of the wrist, antiinflammatory medication, and intraarticular cortisone injections. Once advanced carpal degeneration is present, the wrist can be treated only by salvage procedures and there is no urgency for surgical intervention.

SURGICAL MANAGEMENT

The two most common motion-preserving surgical procedures for SLAC wrist arthritis are scaphoid excision and four-corner fusion and proximal row carpectomy (PRC). Proponents of PRC cite technical ease, early mobilization, and the lack of nonunion risk as advantages (8–12). Potential disadvantages of PRC include shortening of the carpus, with associated weakness and incongruity between the capitate and the lunate fossa of the distal radius. Ulnar midcarpal fusion was introduced to relieve pain and restore wrist stability and height while providing more physiologic motion through the preserved radiolunate and ulnocarpal joints (4,13). This is a more technically demanding procedure that typically requires a longer period of postoperative immobilization.

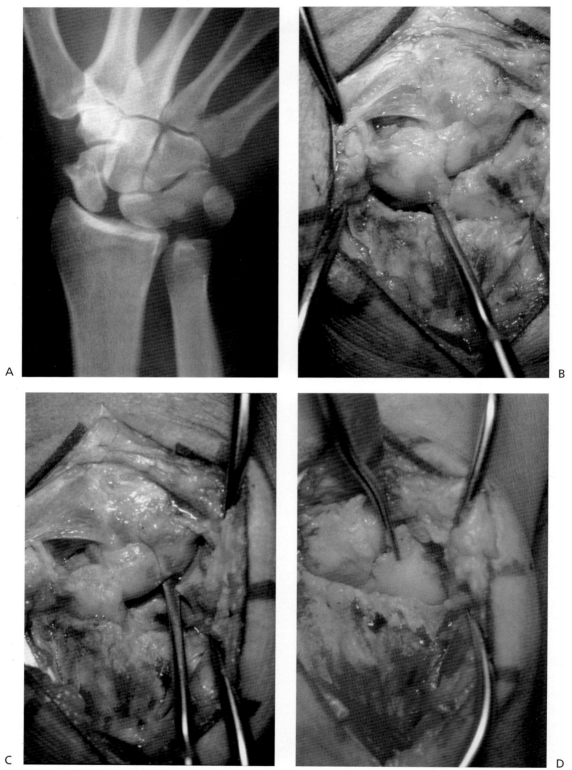

FIGURE 1. A: Anteroposterior view of the wrist in a patient presenting with wrist pain revealing scapholunate dissociation. The patient had palpable radioscaphoid synovitis with crepitation during a scaphoid shift maneuver. Note the apparent lack of radiographic degenerative changes. **B:** Intraoperative view of the proximal pole of the scaphoid (left above elevator) revealing advanced articular loss. **C:** Retractor allowing visualization of midcarpal joint revealing arthrosis of the capitate and hamate as well. Articular changes are often well in advance of those appreciated radiographically. **D:** Note maintenance of the radiolunate joint (tip of forceps) in scapholunate advanced collapse arthritis.

TABLE 1. FOUR-CORNER FUSION: SUMMARY OF REPORTED MOTION AND STRENGTH[a]

Number of cases	Follow-up (mo)	Average extension (degrees)	Average flexion (degrees)	Average[b] flexion–extension arc (%)	Grip strength[b] (%)
100	48	32	42	53	81
24	23	25	23	—	70
23	41	27	27	—	79
20	24	39	43	65	78
18	36	26	34	54	67
17	27	36	31	47	74
Avg. of all reported cases		31	36	54	77

[a]Includes articles with 15 or more patients.
[b]Percentage of opposite, unaffected wrist.
Reprinted with permission from Cohen MS, Kozin SH. Degenerative arthritis of the wrist: proximal row carpectomy versus scaphoid excision and four-corner fusion. *J Hand Surg [Am]* 2001;26:94–104.

Multiple authors have reported successful pain relief with preserved motion and strength after both procedures. A review of the larger series in the literature reveals comparable results in terms of motion and strength (4,14–26). Combining these reports, PRC results in an average flexion–extension arc of approximately 60% of the opposite wrist versus 54% after four-corner fusion (Tables 1 and 2). Average reported grip strength versus the opposite side is 79% after PRC and 77% after four-corner fusion.

There are few reports specifically comparing these two surgical options for the treatment of SLAC arthritis. Wyrick et al. retrospectively compared 17 four-corner fusions with 11 PRC procedures (15). Motion and grip strength were greater in the PRC group. However, due to study limitations, the authors were unable to prove the superiority of one procedure over the other. Tomaino et al. compared nine four-corner patients with 15 patients treated with PRC (14). Although grip strength was similar between groups, range of motion was superior after PRC. Unfortunately, 20% of the PRC patients were not satisfied with their surgical result (versus none of the four-corner group). These authors recommend PRC in the absence of capitate arthrosis. Krakauer et al. compared 23 patients treated with four-corner fusion with 12 PRC patients (24). Wrist motion was greater after PRC, whereas grip strength was superior after four-bone fusion. Pain relief, however, appeared less reliable after PRC, with three of 12 (25%) patients reporting persistent severe pain versus three of 23 (13%) four-corner fusion patients.

Cohen and Kozin compared the largest series of two cohort populations from separate institutions performing exclusively four-corner fusion or PRC for SLAC arthritis (27). Patient groups were matched with respect to age, sex, dominance, stage of arthritis, and preoperative measures of pain and function. Evaluations completed by independent examiners revealed remarkably similar outcomes at a 2-year follow-up. Both procedures resulted in approximately an 80-degree flexion–extension arc measuring nearly 60% of the contralateral wrist. Grip strength was slightly greater after four-corner fusion, averaging 79% of the opposite side

TABLE 2. PROXIMAL ROW CARPECTOMY: SUMMARY OF REPORTED MOTION AND STRENGTH[a]

Number of cases	Follow-up (mo)	Average extension (degrees)	Average flexion (degrees)	Average[b] flexion–extension arc (%)	Grip strength[b] (%)
27	48	84 (extension + flexion)		—	80
24	36–120	46	38	59	—
23	72	37	37	61	79
22	120	48	48	63	81
18	157	40	36	63	83
17	42	35	28	52	67
15	72	40	37	64	77
15	30	39	43	—	84
Avg. of all reported cases		41	38	60	79

[a]Includes articles with 15 or more patients.
[b]Percentage of opposite, unaffected wrist.
Reprinted with permission from Cohen MS, Kozin SH. Degenerative arthritis of the wrist: proximal row carpectomy versus scaphoid excision and four-corner fusion. *J Hand Surg [Am]* 2001;26:94–104.

in these patients versus 71% after PRC ($p > .05$). Four-corner fusion did result in a greater radial-ulnar deviation arc, predominantly due to limited radial deviation after PRC (averaging only 7 degrees). This loss of radial deviation has been reported previously after PRC with or without radial styloidectomy (12,19–22,25,26). Pain and function significantly improved in both groups from preoperative levels using a variety of measures, with little difference between the two procedures.

The indication for four-corner fusion most commonly involves radioscaphoid degeneration with or without midcarpal involvement. In advanced cases of scapholunate dissociation or scaphoid nonunion, there is typically little question regarding the degree of arthrosis, and preoperative planning is straightforward. In some cases, direct inspection of the radioscaphoid joint articular cartilage is required to determine the need for salvage surgery. Once advanced scaphoid fossa degeneration exists, four-corner fusion is a viable option in symptomatic patients who fail conservative measures. Other less common indications for midcarpal fusion include midcarpal instability without radioscaphoid arthrosis (28), avascular necrosis of the scaphoid with collapse, and failed scaphocapitate or scaphotrapezial–trapezoid fusion. Contraindications include radiolunate arthrosis and ulnar translocation of the carpus.

TECHNIQUE

The surgical procedure is typically performed under regional anesthesia. A dorsal longitudinal incision is centered over the proximal carpal row. The wrist joint is entered though the third dorsal compartment, with resection of the posterior interosseous nerve, which lies on the floor of the fourth compartment. The joint capsule is opened and subperiosteally dissected radially and ulnarly. Deep retractors and longitudinal traction help expose the individual carpal articulations. Most commonly, the scaphoid is identified and excised. In nonunion, one can choose to retain the proximal scaphoid pole, which is typically spared from arthrosis with the lunate (29). This increases the surface area of the resultant radiocarpal articulation. It does, however, theoretically increase the chance of late degeneration between the proximal scaphoid pole and the radius, as this joint is not concentric and can be placed under shear if not perfectly reduced.

In scapholunate dissociation, scaphoid resection is facilitated by transecting the bone in the mid-waist perpendicular to its axis. Threaded Steinmann pins are placed into the distal and proximal poles and used as joysticks. Care is taken not to violate the palmar extrinsic radiocarpal ligaments, especially the more ulnar long radiolunate ligament. This is required to stabilize the carpus after fusion. A limited radial styloidectomy can be performed in individuals with large osteophytes to improve visualization.

Reduction of the collapse deformity to realign the midcarpal joint is critical to the success of the procedure. The lunotriquetral relationship can be first reduced by aligning the distal concavity of the two bones from the midcarpal joint. This is secured with 0.045 Kirschner wires. An additional wire can be placed into the lunate and used as a joystick for the proximal carpal row during removal of the cartilage (Fig. 2). The fusion surfaces between the lunate, capitate, hamate, and triquetrum are then denuded down to cancellous bone with a low-speed bur, rongeurs, and curettes. Of note, the lunate often has thick subchondral bone, and it is frequently not possible to denude this surface down to a soft cancellous level. Fine Kirschner wire holes can be placed in the lunate concavity to facilitate vascular ingrowth and union.

Pure cancellous bone graft can be obtained from the excised scaphoid, although this provides only marginal material. Additional autograft is available from the distal radius just proximal to Lister's tubercle (30). The graft can be compressed in a syringe and meticulously packed into the fusion sites. Wrist distraction is then released, and the proximal carpal row is reduced. Care is taken to flex the lunate and palmarly and ulnarly translate the capitate. A slight overreduction (volarflexed intercalated instability) is preferred. With compression maintained across the midcarpus, the reduction can be stabilized with either multiple Kirschner wires or cannulated screws. Wires are placed retrograde from the capitate and hamate into the lunate. It is often helpful to introduce these pins from the second and fourth web spaces, respectively, to begin palmar enough to obtain adequate purchase in the lunate. One additional pin is placed from the triquetrum into the capitate (Fig. 2). Cannulated screws are typically placed antegrade from the lunate and triquetrum into the distal carpal row (Fig. 3). Wrist flexion and extension are tested on the table and greater extension than flexion should be confirmed. The remaining bone graft is applied dorsally across the fusion site. The longitudinal capsulotomy is loosely approximated—but not repaired—to the radius, and the extensor pollicis longus is left outside the repaired retinaculum.

An alternative method of fixation involves the use of a conical plate designed in 1999 to specifically stabilize the midcarpal joint after arthrodesis (Kinetikos Medical, San Diego, CA). This plate is recessed beneath the dorsal articular margin of the carpus after provisional wire stabilization of the reduced midcarpal relationship (Fig. 4). A conical rasp is used to create a recess for the plate, which has eight holes. This allows two screws to be placed into each carpal bone in optimal circumstances. Care must be taken to follow similar principles for arthrodesis when using plate fixation. The fusion surfaces must still be denuded of articular cartilage (at least half of the anteroposterior depth of the joints) and the autograft meticulously packed to optimize healing. The screws are tightened sequentially to obtain stability and circumferential compression. Additional graft can be added

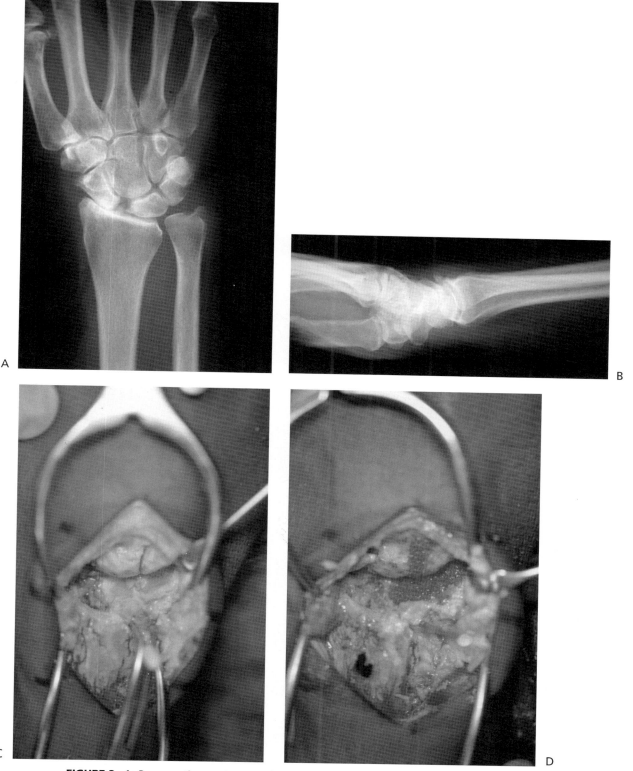

FIGURE 2. **A:** Preoperative posteroanterior and **(B)** lateral radiographs depicting scapholunate advanced collapse arthritis. Note the scapholunate gap, radioscaphoid narrowing, and the extended posture of the lunate on the lateral film. **C:** Intraoperative photograph taken with traction after preparation of the midcarpal articular surfaces for fusion. Note the Kirschner wire in the lunate that is used as a joystick. **D:** Bone graft obtained from the distal radius (note defect) has been meticulously packed into the fusion surfaces. (*continued*)

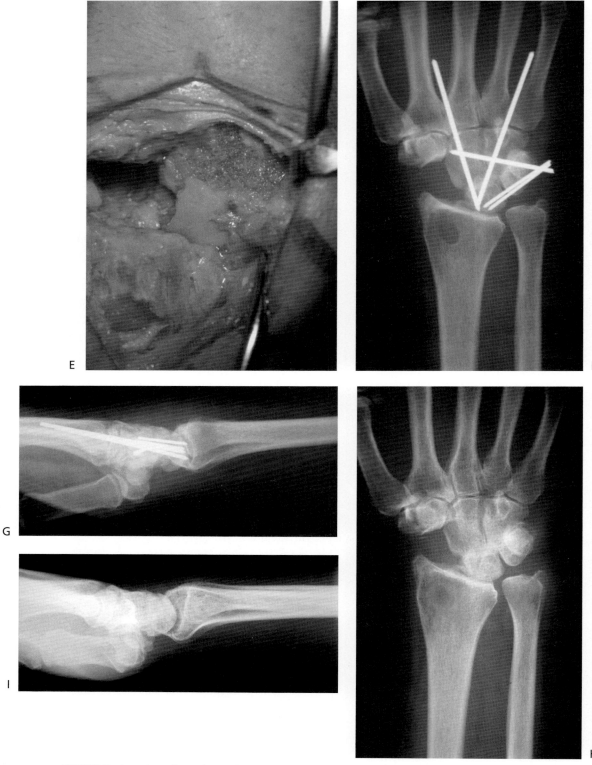

E

F

G

I

H

FIGURE 2. (*continued*) **E:** The midcarpal joint has been reduced and pinned with additional autograft packed dorsally. **F:** Postoperative posteroanterior and (**G**) lateral views revealing scaphoid excision and four-corner pin fixation. Note the position of the retrograde midcarpal pins into the lunate. Mid-axis placement is facilitated by starting these in the second and fourth web spaces, respectively. **H:** Final posteroanterior and (**I**) lateral radiographs depicting consolidation of four-corner arthrodesis.

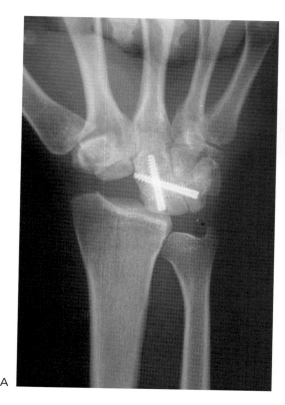

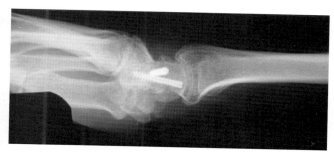

A

B

FIGURE 3. A: Posteroanterior and **(B)** lateral radiographs of four-corner arthrodesis accomplished with cannulated screws. These are placed antegrade with the wrist maximally flexed. Screw fixation allows for more rapid rehabilitation.

to the center of the four-bone articulation after fixation through the central plate opening.

After surgery, patients are placed in a compressive dressing with an internal short arm splint. Digital motion is encouraged immediately after the regional block wears off. At 10 to 14 days postoperatively, a short arm cast is applied in those individuals treated with pins alone. These are typically removed at approximately 8 weeks postoperatively, at

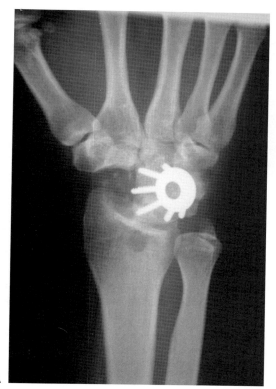

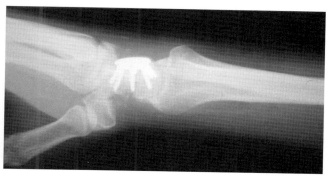

A

B

FIGURE 4. A: Posteroanterior and **(B)** lateral radiographs of a four-corner fusion performed with a conical plate. This provides stable fixation without violation of the articulating surfaces of the lunate and triquetrum.

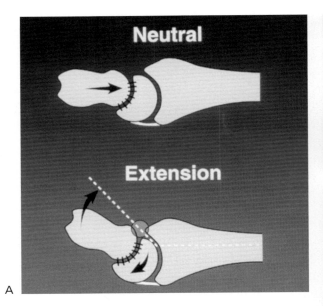

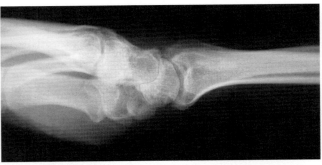

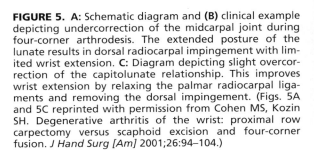

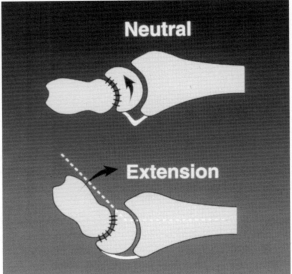

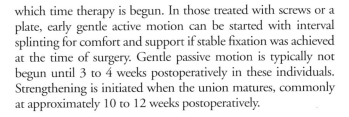

FIGURE 5. A: Schematic diagram and **(B)** clinical example depicting undercorrection of the midcarpal joint during four-corner arthrodesis. The extended posture of the lunate results in dorsal radiocarpal impingement with limited wrist extension. **C**: Diagram depicting slight overcorrection of the capitolunate relationship. This improves wrist extension by relaxing the palmar radiocarpal ligaments and removing the dorsal impingement. (Figs. 5A and 5C reprinted with permission from Cohen MS, Kozin SH. Degenerative arthritis of the wrist: proximal row carpectomy versus scaphoid excision and four-corner fusion. *J Hand Surg [Am]* 2001;26:94–104.)

which time therapy is begun. In those treated with screws or a plate, early gentle active motion can be started with interval splinting for comfort and support if stable fixation was achieved at the time of surgery. Gentle passive motion is typically not begun until 3 to 4 weeks postoperatively in these individuals. Strengthening is initiated when the union matures, commonly at approximately 10 to 12 weeks postoperatively.

TREATMENT ALGORITHM

Individuals with SLAC wrist arthritis who fail conservative treatment measures are candidates for four-bone fusion. Once cartilage loss occurs at the radioscaphoid articulation, either a PRC or midcarpal fusion is a motion-preserving option. A PRC is contraindicated in the presence of advanced arthrosis of the capitate head. The four-corner fusion can be used in either situation. As previously stated, contraindications include radiolunate degeneration and ulnar translocation of the carpus.

COMPLICATIONS

The most common complication after four-corner fusion is dorsal radiocarpal impingement in wrist extension

(14,16). This occurs secondary to inadequate reduction of the capitolunate relationship (Fig. 5). Care must be taken to not leave the lunate in an extended posture (dorsiflexed intercalated segment instability) at the time of fixation. This markedly limits postoperative wrist extension and can lead to impingement. It is recommended to actually overreduce the midcarpal joint into a slight volarflexed intercalated instability pattern to avoid this complication (27). This results in increased wrist extension [which is more important than flexion functionally (31)] without an equal loss of wrist flexion. Flexion of the lunate relaxes the intact palmar radiolunate ligaments, augmenting wrist extension (Fig. 5). In turn, flexion appears less limited by the dorsal capsule and remaining dorsal extrinsic ligaments, neither of which is repaired to the distal radius after exposure and arthrodesis.

Nonunion of four-corner arthrodesis is relatively rare. Originally, the midcarpal fusion technique was limited to the capitolunate articulation. However, the triquetrum and hamate were subsequently added to increase the fusion surface area and improve healing rates. When nonunion occurs, it can be related to technical errors, patient variables (e.g., tobacco use), or a combination of factors (Fig. 6). If pins were originally used, repeat fusion is probably best accomplished with fresh autograft and screws or plate fixation.

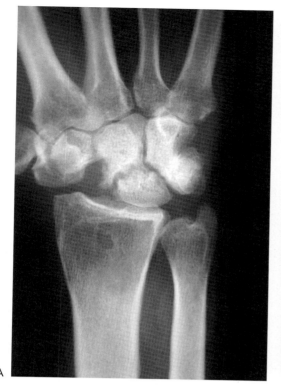

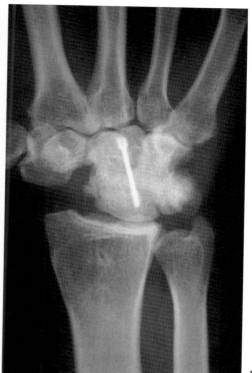

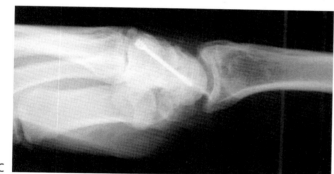

A

B

C

FIGURE 6. A: Posteroanterior radiograph depicting established nonunion of midcarpal fusion. **B:** Final posteroanterior and **(C)** lateral views after revision arthrodesis with autograft and internal screw fixation. Note the loss of correction with incomplete midcarpal reduction due to the nonunion. (Reprinted with permission from Cohen MS, Kozin SH. Degenerative arthritis of the wrist: proximal row carpectomy versus scaphoid excision and four-corner fusion. *J Hand Surg [Am]* 2001;26:94–104.)

CONCLUSION

Scaphoid excision with four-corner fusion is a reliable treatment method for individuals with SLAC arthritis who have failed conservative care. After successful arthrodesis, one can expect maintenance of approximately 60% to 80% of wrist motion and 75% to 80% of grip strength with predictable pain relief. Results are contingent, however, on adherence to the technical principles of the procedure. These include adequate bony preparation, meticulous placement of autograft, and proper reduction of the midcarpal relationship.

REFERENCES

1. Cohen MS. Ligament injuries and instability patterns of the wrist. In: TR Light, ed. *Hand surgery update*, 2nd ed. Rosemont, Ill: American Society for Surgery of the Hand and American Academy of Orthopaedic Surgeons, 1999:97–106.
2. Zdravkovic V, Jacob HA, Sennwald GR. Physical equilibrium of the normal wrist and its relation to clinically defined "instability." *J Hand Surg [Br]* 1995;20:159–164.
3. Burgess RC. The effect of rotatory subluxation of the scaphoid on radioscaphoid contact. *J Hand Surg [Am]* 1987;12:771–774.
4. Watson HK, Ballett FL. The SLAC wrist: scapholunate advanced collapse pattern of degenerative arthritis. *J Hand Surg [Am]* 1984;9:358–365.
5. Chen C, Chandnani VP, Kang HS, et al. Scapholunate advanced collapse: a common wrist abnormality in calcium pyrophosphate dihydrate crystal deposition disease. *Radiology* 1990;177:459–461.
6. Watson HK, Ashmead D, Makhouf MV. Examination of the scaphoid bone. *J Hand Surg [Am]* 1988;13:657–660.
7. Peh WC, Patterson RM, Viegas SF, et al. Radiographic-anatomic correlation at different wrist articulations. *J Hand Surg [Am]* 1999;24:777–780.

8. Ferlic DC, Clayton ML, Mills MF. Proximal row carpectomy: review of rheumatoid and nonrheumatoid wrists. *J Hand Surg [Am]* 1991;16:420–424.

9. Inglis AE, Jones EC. Proximal-row carpectomy for diseases of the proximal row. *J Bone Joint Surg Am* 1977;59:460–463.

10. Inoue G, Miura T. Proximal row carpectomy in perilunate dislocations and lunatomalacia. *Acta Orthop Scand* 1990;61:449–452.

11. Neviaser RJ. On resection of the proximal carpal row. *Clin Orthop Rel Res* 1986;202:12–15.

12. Salomon GD, Eaton RG. Proximal row carpectomy with partial capitate resection. *J Hand Surg [Am]* 1996;21:2–8.

13. Watson HK, Goodman ML, Johnson TR. Limited wrist arthrodesis. Part II: intercarpal and radiocarpal combinations. *J Hand Surg [Am]* 1981;6:223–233.

14. Tomaino MM, Miller RJ, Cole I, et al. Scapholunate advanced collapse wrist: proximal row carpectomy or limited wrist arthrodesis with scaphoid excision. *J Hand Surg [Am]* 1994;19:134–142.

15. Wyrick JD, Stern PJ, Kiefhaber TR. Motion-preserving procedures in the treatment of scapholunate advanced collapse wrist: proximal row carpectomy versus four-corner arthrodesis. *J Hand Surg [Am]* 1995;20:965–970.

16. Ashmead D, Watson HK, Damon C, et al. Scapholunate advanced collapse wrist salvage. *J Hand Surg [Am]* 1994;19:741–750.

17. Culp RW, McGuigan FX, Turner MA, et al. Proximal row carpectomy: a multicenter study. *J Hand Surg [Am]* 1993;18:19–25.

18. Gill DRJ, Ireland DCR. Limited wrist arthrodesis for the salvage of SLAC wrist. *J Hand Surg [Br]* 1997;22:4:461–465.

19. Green DP. Proximal row carpectomy. *Hand Clin* 1987;3:163–168.

20. Imbriglia JE, Broudy AS, Hagberg WC, et al. Proximal row carpectomy: clinical evaluation. *J Hand Surg [Am]* 1990;15:426–430.

21. Jebson PJ, Hayes E, Engber WD. *Proximal row carpectomy: a minimum 10-year follow-up.* Presented at the American Society for Surgery of the Hand, 52nd Annual Meeting, Denver, 1997.

22. Jorgensen EC. Proximal row carpectomy. *J Bone Joint Surg Am* 1969;51:1104–1111.

23. Kirschenbaum O, Schneider LH, Kirkpatrick WH. Scaphoid excision and capitolunate arthrodesis for radioscaphoid arthritis. *J Hand Surg [Am]* 1993;18:780–785.

24. Krakauer JD, Bishop AT, Cooney WP. Surgical treatment of scapholunate advanced collapse. *J Hand Surg [Am]* 1994;19:751–759.

25. Neviaser RJ. Proximal row carpectomy for posttraumatic disorders of the carpus. *J Hand Surg [Am]* 1983;8:301–305.

26. Tomaino MM, Delsignore J, Burton RI. Long-term results following proximal row carpectomy. *J Hand Surg [Am]* 1994;19:694–703.

27. Cohen MS, Kozin SH. Degenerative arthritis of the wrist: proximal row carpectomy versus scaphoid excision and four-corner fusion. *J Hand Surg [Am]* 2001;26:94–104.

28. Lichtman DM, Bruckner JD, Culp RW, et al. Palmar midcarpal instability: results of surgical reconstruction. *J Hand Surg [Am]* 1993;18:307–315.

29. Viegas SF. Limited arthrodesis for scaphoid nonunion. *J Hand Surg [Am]* 1994;19:127–133.

30. Bruno RJ, Cohen MS, Berzins A, et al. Bone graft harvesting from the distal radius, olecranon and iliac crest: a quantitative analysis. *J Hand Surg [Am]* 2001;26:135–141.

31. Palmer AK, Werner FW, Murphy D, et al. Functional wrist motion: a biochemical study. *J Hand Surg [Am]* 1985;10:39–46.

77

RADIOCARPAL AND TOTAL WRIST ARTHRODESIS

HERMANN KRIMMER

In cases of severe arthritic damage to the radiocarpal or midcarpal joint where reconstructive procedures are excluded, salvage procedures are required. The principle of this treatment strategy consists of eliminating the destroyed articular surfaces by fusion. Total wrist fusion is the procedure with the longest history and is the most common treatment. Recently, motion-sparing procedures have become more popular. *Limited wrist fusion* is defined by fusing only the damaged or unstable areas while motion is maintained in the uninjured or stable regions of the joints. In cases of arthritic changes to the radiocarpal joint due, for example, to intraarticular fractures of the radius, the midcarpal joint may be preserved by limiting the fusion to the radioscapholunate joint, thereby maintaining useful mobility. The benefit of limited wrist fusion is well documented, and whenever suitable, this class of operation is preferred (1,2). However, in progressive stages of arthrosis involving the radiocarpal and midcarpal joint or in combination with severe malalignment of the carpus, total wrist fusion may be the best option.

RADIOCARPAL ARTHRODESIS

Clinical Significance

The fundamental principle in the management of distal radial fractures consists of anatomic reduction of the fracture, thus restoring the congruity of the damaged articular surfaces. There has been significant progress made recently in the treatment of intraarticular fractures. Techniques such as arthroscopically assisted reduction and fixation by buttress plate design, which maintain reduction precisely and minimize the risk of secondary dislocation and posttraumatic arthrosis, have been shown to dramatically improve results. Despite efforts to achieve anatomic reductions in severely displaced comminuted fractures, residual displacement or chondrocyte death may compromise results, leading to posttraumatic degenerative disease (3).

Under these conditions, both the radiolunate and the radioscaphoid joints are involved, in contrast to the midcarpal joint, which is nearly always preserved. If significant

shortening of the distal radius results, an additional factor of ulna impaction syndrome may result. The distal radioulnar joint may also be affected; if symptomatic, additional treatment may be necessary (Fig. 1).

Indications

Painful posttraumatic arthrosis of the radiocarpal joint is a common indication for further treatment. From the clinical point of view, patients often describe pain at the radial site of the wrist, often increasing with activity. Occasional swelling is noticed. Function is limited due to reduced grip strength, pain, and restriction of mobility. The goal for any treatment is a stable joint with maximally reduced pain and preferably with mobility, which is of great benefit from a functional point of view. The initial examination evaluates the painful area by palpating and checking the function of the wrist joint and comparing this with the radiologic findings. Additionally, grip strength should be recorded with a standard dynamometer as well as the arc of motion. Standard posteroanterior and lateral radiography usually reveals the damaged radiocarpal area. If in case of intraarticular incongruity, where reconstructive procedures such as correction osteotomy of the radius are contemplated, a computed tomography scan of the joint surface of the radius may prove helpful. It allows more accurate visualization of the subchondral bone architecture (Fig. 2). Finally, arthroscopy allows the most precise assessment of the joint surfaces.

The principle of radiocarpal arthrodesis was introduced by the discovery of spontaneous radiolunate fusion that resulted in a painless and functional wrist. Radiolunate arthrodesis as a surgical procedure was first reported by Chamay et al. to treat ulnar shift of the carpus in patients with rheumatoid arthritis (4). It has rarely been performed in patients with posttraumatic deformities of the wrist, and the results have not been clearly differentiated from rheumatoid cases (5). In nonrheumatoid patients, radiocarpal arthrodesis is indicated primarily for intraarticular malunion involving the radiolunate and occasionally the radioscaphoid joint. Another indication may be instability

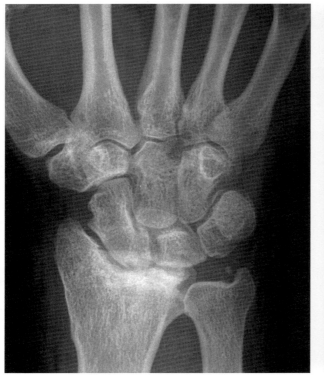 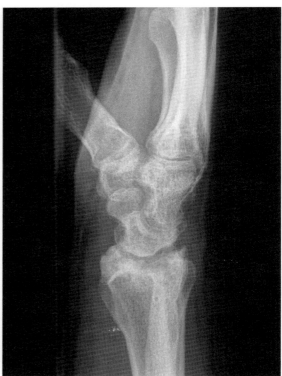

FIGURE 1. Posteroanterior **(A)** and lateral **(B)** x-rays after intraarticular comminuted fracture of the radius in a 21-year-old man. Radiocarpal arthrosis and dorsal intercalated segment instability position of the lunate are evident.

of the entire carpus due to severe damage to the extrinsic radiocarpal ligaments.

Alternative Treatment Options

Nonoperative

Nonoperative treatment methods are limited to immobilization, drug medication, or special pain therapy. Placing

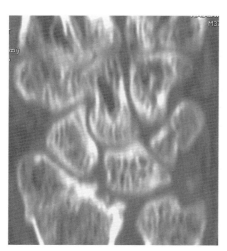

FIGURE 2. Computed tomographic scan demonstrating damaged cartilage at the radiolunate and radioscaphoid fossa.

the involved wrist in a supportive splint may improve function by reduction or loss of mobility, thereby limiting pain. Antiinflammatory or pain drugs alone or in combination with immobilization are suitable to modulate pain. It is well recognized, however, that conservative measures in the face of symptomatic wrists with arthrosis fall short of successful outcomes over the long term.

Operative

Wrist Denervation

Wilhelm first described the concept of eliminating pain in degenerative affections of the wrist joint by division of articular branches of sensory nerves (6). In 2001, he published his long-term experience with this procedure (7). One hundred eighty-seven patients were evaluated, and it was found that after 1.2 years, good and excellent results could be obtained in 81%. After 2.2 years, this percentage slightly decreased to 77.8%; after an average of 10.5 years, good results persisted in 62.5%. Similar results were found concerning grip strength, in which the initial improvement deteriorated with time. However, there was no differentiation according to the severity of the initial problem. In summary, wrist denervation represents a viable alternative for initial treatment. However, in severe cases, the improvements are limited and symptoms may rapidly recur.

Modified Proximal Row Carpectomy (Die-Punch Technique)

Although proximal row carpectomy is considered an acceptable treatment for radioscaphoid arthrosis, it is not suitable in cases of radiolunate arthrosis. Foucher described a technique in which the lunate is fused in an "inset" manner in the lunate fascia, described as a *die-punch technique* (8). Resecting the scaphoid and triquetrum results in maintenance of mobility. In a series of four cases, significant improvement of mobility and grip strength resulted. However, no long-term results of larger cohorts have been reported.

RADIOCARPAL ARTHRODESIS

Total wrist arthrodesis represents the ultimate salvage technique for painful wrist arthrosis. It sacrifices mobility completely, and outcome studies using self-reporting scoring systems have revealed significant disability from the patient's point of view. Additionally, in several cases, the lack of elasticity of the wrist joint may exacerbate pain in other areas around the wrist. Finally, total wrist fusion does not guarantee a pain-free result. However, in progressive stages of arthrosis with damage to the midcarpal joint and lack of extrinsic ligamentous support or in situations of failed partial arthrodesis, total wrist arthrodesis represents the most reliable procedure (9).

Surgical Technique

Regional or general anesthesia is required. I begin the procedure under tourniquet control through a slightly oblique incision on the dorsum of the wrist. The branches of the superficial radial nerve and dorsal ulnar nerve and the dorsal veins are preserved, and the retinaculum is identified. The third extensor compartment is incised, and the retinaculum is subperiosteally elevated to the radial and ulnar side, opening the second and fourth compartments (Fig. 3). At

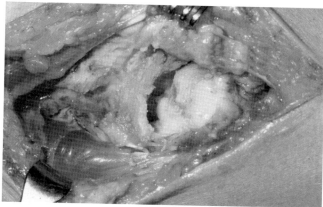

FIGURE 4. Destroyed articular surfaces of the radioscaphoid and radiolunate joint.

the radial border of the fourth compartment, the posterior interosseous nerve is excised. The radiocarpal joint is entered through a transverse incision of the joint capsule. To better visualize the joint, the dorsal rim of the radius may be trimmed with an oscillating saw. Typically, obvious destruction of the radiolunate and radioscaphoid joint surfaces is seen, sometimes in combination with rupture of the scapholunate ligament (Fig. 4). Under these conditions, radioscapholunate arthrodesis is performed. Only in the case of preserved scapholunate ligament and radioscaphoid cartilage might radiolunate arthrodesis be considered an alternative (10). With a slightly curved rongeur, the cartilage and subchondral bone are removed from the scaphoid and lunate fossae of the radius (Fig. 5). By hyperflexing the wrist, the lunate and scaphoid are prepared in the same way to expose cancellous bone. At the ulnar border of the radius, three 1.6-mm Kirschner wires are inserted such that only thin tips are visible through the deteriorated distal radius. One Kirschner wire should fix the scaphoid in the long axis, and the others should secure the lunate. The position of the lunate should be in neutral extension or

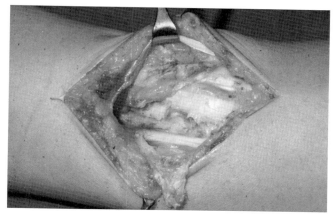

FIGURE 3. Slight oblique incision at the dorsum of the wrist opening the third and fourth extensor compartments.

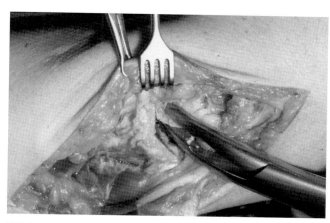

FIGURE 5. Decortication of the radius, the scaphoid, and the lunate with a rongeur.

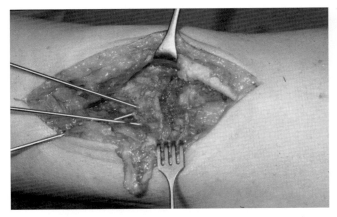

FIGURE 6. The radiocarpal space is filled with cancellous bone. After realignment of the carpus, the Kirschner wires are inserted.

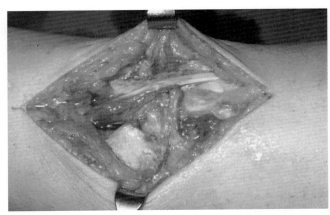

FIGURE 8. The extensor retinaculum is closed, leaving the extensor pollicis longus tendon subcutaneously.

recentered if ulnar translocation is present. Cancellous bone from the iliac crest is packed into the space between lunate, scaphoid, and radius, and the Kirschner wires are advanced into the scaphoid and lunate. Care is taken to avoid overadvancing the wires into the midcarpal joint. (Fig. 6). To improve wrist mobility, Garcia Elias recommends excision of the distal pole of the scaphoid (10a).

Care must be taken to be certain that the Kirschner wires are not advanced into the carpal tunnel to avoid the risk of injuring nerve or tendon structures. After verifying proper placement of the hardware and position of the bones, the Kirschner wires are bent and cut down directly to the radial cortex to avoid any disturbance of the extensor tendons (Fig. 7). The retinaculum is reattached, leaving the extensor pollicis longus tendon subcutaneously (extraretinacular) (Fig. 8).

In cases of an ulnar plus condition due to radial shortening, the radiocarpal space may be overcorrected, thereby balancing the carpus and the ulna in a more neutral variance, preventing ulna impaction. If, however, a damaged distal radioulnar joint is present, shortening or resection of the ulna head may be considered.

Postoperatively, the extremity is immobilized in a fore-based thumb spica cast for 8 weeks. Patients are instructed in active finger range-of-motion exercises on the first postoperative day. After radiographic confirmation with bony consolidation, the midcarpal joint is included in active and passive physiotherapy. Kirschner wire removal is optional (Fig. 9).

Modifications

In an attempt to optimize postoperative range of motion and midcarpal stability, the capsulotomy may be modified to conform to the ligament-splitting technique (11). Although cancellous bone graft has been the historical choice and remains a viable source of good bone, alternatives have been developed. Included are autogenous sources from the olecranon and proximal tibial metaphysis, allograft cancellous bone, and a number of bone substitutes. Fixation alternatives include staples, interosseous headless screws, and plate fixation. Surgeons are encouraged to use the techniques that they are most familiar with and that have yielded the best results in their hands.

Complications

Major complications of radiocarpal arthrodesis include pseudarthrosis, tendon adherence, and insufficient pain relief (12). With the use of Kirschner wires and cancellous bone of the iliac crest, we have achieved a high union rate of 94% (13). We regard the use of plates for this procedure as unnecessary, as the union rate is even less and the complication rate with regard to tendon adherence is higher (12). Rigid fixation with the use of compression screws in a cannulated design proved to be difficult because of the thin cortices of the carpal bones. When the Kirschner wires are inserted at the ulnar border of the radius and countersunk into the cortex, the risk of tendon adherence is minimized and removal remains an option. Insufficient pain relief has to be localized and treated separately. In our experience,

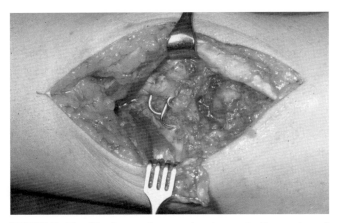

FIGURE 7. The Kirschner wires are bent near to the cortex of the radius.

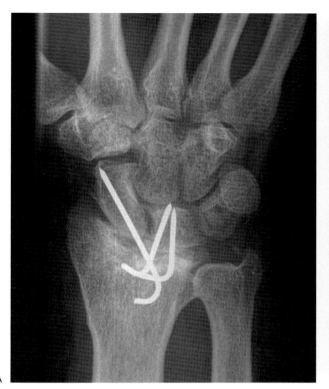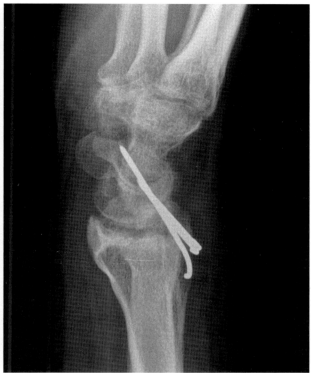

A   B

FIGURE 9. A,B: On postoperative x-ray, the distal part of the scaphoid is resected (see Fig. 1 for the preoperative x-rays). **A:** Posteroanterior view. **B:** Lateral view.

residual pain is most commonly found around the distal radioulnar joint.

Clinical Results

Two reports are available of uniform groups dealing with radiolunate and radiocarpal arthrodesis used for treatment of posttraumatic conditions. In 1991, Sturzenegger and Buchler presented their results of 14 patients who underwent radioscapholunate arthrodesis due to painful radiocarpal arthrosis after comminuted fractures of the distal radius (14). Stabilization was achieved in the majority by means of a 3.5-mm AO T-plate and corticocancellous bone graft from the iliac crest. In addition to the radioscapholunate arthrodesis, nine patients underwent supplementary procedures to the distal radioulnar joint. Average follow-up was 23.8 months. They reported significant pain relief, with 7 out of 14 patients pain-free, four suffering slight discomfort, and three reporting pain during daily activities. No patient complained of pain at rest. Range of motion was reported as an average 30 degrees of extension and 17 degrees of flexion, with grip strength averaging 49.4% relative to the unaffected side.

To evaluate long-term results, Nagy and Buchler reassessed these patients, with an average follow-up period of 8 years (12). Five patients were reoperated on to convert to a total wrist fusion because of symptomatic nonunion or early progressive arthritis of remaining joint surfaces. Two

wrists were still symptomatic. Ultimately, satisfactory results of radioscapholunate fusions were maintained in seven cases. It was found that outcomes were worse with an increasing number of prearthrodesis operations. The high nonunion rate was attributed to technical factors.

In 1996, Saffar reported a series of 11 patients with symptomatic distal radial intraarticular malunions limited to the radiolunate joint (10). All were treated by radiolunate arthrodesis. For fixation, a sliding graft technique from the distal radius or corticocancellous graft harvested from the iliac crest with fixation by two screws was used. Average follow-up was 28.5 months, and union was achieved in 10 out of 11 cases. Pain decreased from continuous or present at light work to absent or slight in all cases. The range of motion averaged 33 degrees of flexion, 39 degrees of extension, 17 degrees of radial deviation, and 29 degrees of ulnar deviation. The average postoperative strength was 57% of the contralateral uninjured side. With an increased number of patients, Saffar confirmed these results in 2001 (15).

Our results of radiocarpal arthrodesis after comminuted fractures of the distal radius were published by Beyermann et al. (13). Eighteen patients were reexamined, and the follow-up ranged from 6 to 66 months. Nonunion occurred in one case, which was successfully treated by a second bone graft. Radiologic examination revealed bony consolidation in all cases at follow-up, and there were no major signs of degenerative arthrosis in the midcarpal joint. Post-

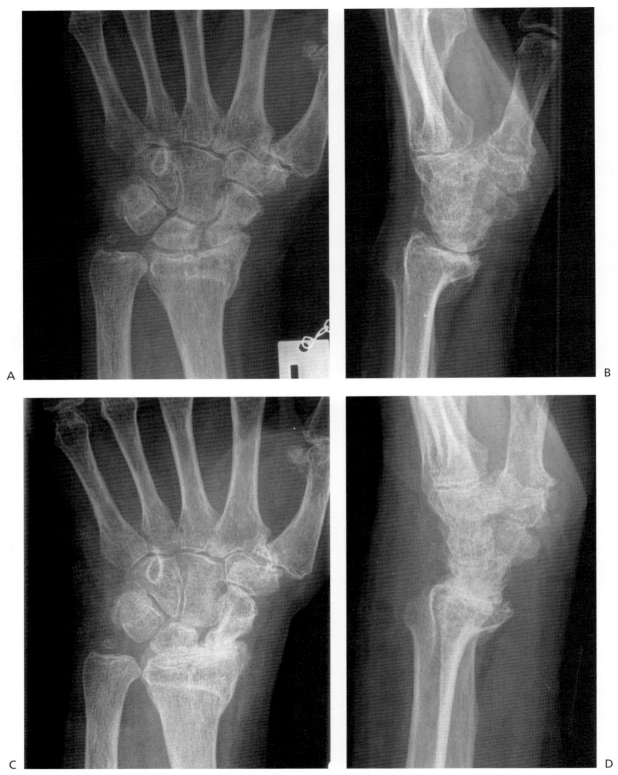

FIGURE 10. A,B: Eleven months after intraarticular fracture of the radius with arthrosis of the radiocarpal joint and palmar dislocation of the entire carpus. **C,D:** Treatment by radioscapholunate fusion and realignment of the carpus.

operative wrist motion averaged 24 degrees of extension, 23 degrees of flexion, 9 degrees of radial deviation, and 16 degrees of ulnar deviation. Average grip strength improved from 31.9 to 51.1 kPa. Pain relief based on a visual analog scale was significant, with 30 points less on average, demonstrating minimal pain at rest (6 points) and slight pain during activity (33 points) postoperatively. The Disabilities of the Arm, Shoulder, and Hand (DASH) score showed 25.7 points on average, reflecting some residual disability but at a significantly lower level than total wrist arthrodesis (Fig. 10).

Radioscapholunate fusion is the preferred treatment in destroyed radiocarpal joints. It provides significant pain relief and improvement of grip strength by maintaining motion. Preferably, cancellous bone from the iliac crest should be used to balance exactly the variance between radius and ulna to prevent ulna impaction syndrome and to achieve a high union rate. If additional damage of the distal radioulnar joint is present, procedures should be considered to resect the ulna (16,17). Radiolunate fusion may be considered as an alternative only when the scapholunate ligament and the radioscaphoid joint are not injured and one can anticipate an improved final arc of motion (10,13). Resecting the distal pole of the scaphoid as part of a radioscapholunate arthrodesis may improve motion but remains to be proved in a large series of patients.

TOTAL WRIST ARTHRODESIS

Clinical Significance and Indication

A stable and sufficiently pain-free wrist remains the goal for surgical treatments of posttraumatic degenerative arthrosis. Historically, total wrist fusion has been regarded as the most predictable treatment concept, with the belief that it results in complete pain relief and only limited functional disability (16,18). However, the medical literature only infrequently documents the result of total wrist fusion in a way that addresses the patient's subjective impression after total wrist arthrodesis. Recently, several reports have been published demonstrating significant disability using the DASH self-reporting scoring system (19,20). The results were similar at different institutions, and the superiority of motion-sparing procedures could be documented (1,2). If no articular cartilage with congruent joint mobility is available and motion-sparing procedures are excluded, one has to keep in mind that wrist fusion is well established historically and typically results in significant pain relief and overall upper extremity functional improvement.

Technical Aspects

Many techniques have been described to accomplish total wrist arthrodesis. The use of large Steinmann pins was preferably performed in rheumatoid cases. Under posttraumatic

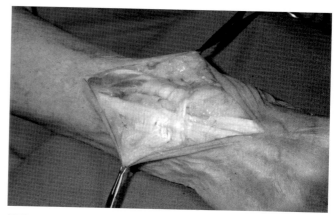

FIGURE 11. Straight incision over the dorsum of the wrist exposing the extensor retinaculum.

conditions, the application of rigid plating techniques allows early recovery without external constraints and leads to a high union rate. Standard compression plates do not contour to the curvature of the carpus. This typically leads to irritation of the extensor tendons and may restrict wrist position. The Synthes wrist fusion plate avoids many of the potential complications of plate irritation due to the low profile of the plate in the distal region over the metacarpals. Another advantage is the precontoured shape, which provides compression over the carpus and results in slight extension of 15 to 20 degrees of the fused wrist without need for any plate manipulation. The source and type of bone graft have varied among different techniques, most favoring corticocancellous bone from the iliac crest. Weiss and Hastings demonstrated that with the use of a low-profile preshaped plate technique, a 100% fusion rate could be achieved with local bone graft from the radius, avoiding a second incision at the iliac crest (21). Patients presenting with large osseous defects or with poor-quality bone should still be considered as candidates for augmentation of their arthrodesis with bone graft from the iliac crest. Controversy remains regard-

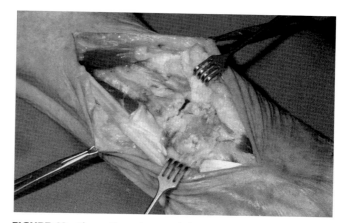

FIGURE 12. The retinaculum and the wrist capsule are subperiosteally detached.

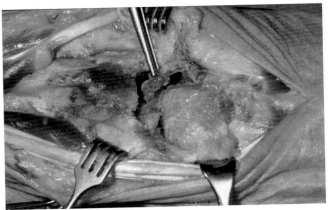

FIGURE 13. The dorsal rim of the radius is resected and the carpus decorticated.

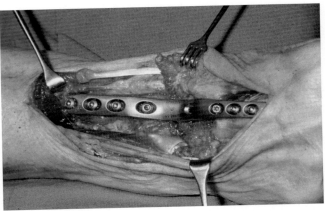

FIGURE 15. The AO wrist fusion plate in place.

ing the necessity of inclusion of the third carpometacarpal joint in the fusion (22,23). I believe that because the Synthes plate is not routinely necessary, the third carpometacarpal should be included in the fusion to improve stability and to prevent painful secondary changes.

Surgical Technique

Under tourniquet control, a straight incision is created over the dorsum of the wrist, starting at the proximal part of the third metacarpal and ending at the distal fourth of the forearm. The subcutaneous nerves and veins are preserved, and the retinaculum is identified (Fig. 11). The third extensor compartment is incised, the tendon is reflected radially, and the retinaculum is subperiosteally detached to the radial and ulnar side, opening the second and fourth compartment. At the radial border of the fourth compartment, the posterior interosseous nerve is excised. The wrist capsule is opened by creating two flaps based proximally at the radial side and distally at the ulnar side, opening the wrist like a window (Fig. 12). This guarantees suturing the capsule over the plate as a deep layer to protect the tendons.

The dorsal rim of the radius is resected, and the dorsal carpus is decorticated (Fig. 13). The intercarpal joints are decorticated to exposed cancellous bone, including the radiolunate, the radioscaphoid, and the capitolunate joints. The third carpometacarpal joint is identified, and the dorsal aspect is removed with a rongeur. The AO wrist fusion system consists of three plates. A long version is appropriate for larger hands and the short version for smaller hands. The long and shorter precontoured versions require removal of the dorsal cortex of the distal radius. A straight version provides stabilization for interposition of corticocancellous bone graft for replacement of large carpal defects caused by trauma or tumor.

The joints to be fused are packed with cancellous bone graft either from local source or iliac crest, and the appropriate plate is positioned over the third metacarpal (Fig. 14). The first screw is placed in the third metacarpal using the middle hole and making certain that the screw passes directly dorsal to palmar in the sagittal plane between the ulnar and radial margins of the third metacarpal. The plate then is aligned over the dorsal aspect of the radius, and one 3.5-mm screw is inserted. The position of the plate and

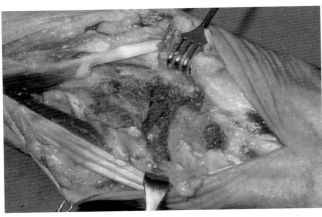

FIGURE 14. The carpal joints are packed with cancellous bone graft.

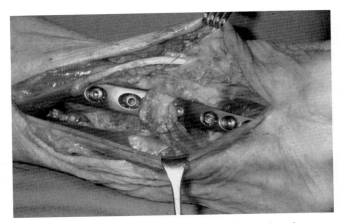

FIGURE 16. The wrist capsule is sutured over the plate.

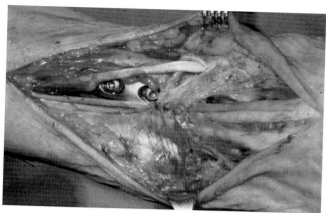

FIGURE 17. The retinaculum is closed, leaving the extensor pollicis longus subcutaneously.

wrist is verified clinically and radiographically. If no changes have to be made, the plate is fixed distally with the 2.7-mm screws. Proximally, one or two screws can be placed in compression with the low-contact dynamic compression plate drill guide. Finally, a 2.7-mm screw is inserted into the capitate (Fig. 15).

The dorsal wrist capsule is closed over the plate and the retinaculum sutured, leaving the extensor pollicis longus tendon in a subcutaneous extraretinacular course (Figs. 16 and 17). A protective splint is worn for 4 to 6 weeks until union is achieved. Active range of motion of the digits to prevent adherence of the extensor or flexor tendons is started from the first postoperative day, in addition to elbow and shoulder range-of-motion exercises.

Complications

Three major problems have been identified as inherent to total wrist arthrodesis: occurrence of nonunion at the wrist or carpometacarpal joint; adherence of tendons with restricted mobility; and persisting pain in the distal radioulnar joint. Nonunion has been shown to be a frequent complication, occurring in up to 19% and requiring repeated surgery (24). With the change to compression plates, the incidence of nonunion has decreased significantly to rates below 8% (19,25). The use of the low-profile and contoured AO plate has made it possible to achieve a 100%

union rate using local bone graft (21). To prevent restriction of mobility of the fingers, physiotherapy immediately after the operation is mandatory. Tendon adherence and irritation frequently occurred with the regular plates, requiring removal of the plate combined with tenolysis. Due to the low-profile design in the distal part and precontoured shape, removal of the AO plate is optional and necessary only in rare cases, with a rate of 4% in our own series (19). Problems around the ulnar head caused by damage of the distal radioulnar joint, painful instability, or ulna plus variance are best treated by hemiresection arthroplasty (16). In cases of persisting painful instability after a salvage procedure at the ulna head, we have solved the problem by implanting an ulna head prosthesis in three cases (26).

Clinical Results

Overall, the satisfaction rate of total wrist arthrodesis is reported as high. Advantages such as pain relief and improved grip strength are attributed to total wrist fusion, but the disadvantages such as functional impairment, social limitations, and postoperative quality of life must be considered individually (27,28). One report using the DASH self-reporting scoring system found significant disability and functional impairment in patients with total wrist arthrodesis, with a ranking of 51 points (20). In a study of 64 patients after total wrist arthrodesis, we found similar results, with the DASH scores averaging 46 points. However, the vast majority of the patients were satisfied and would have undergone the procedure earlier if they had known the final result (19). In our comparative study of total wrist arthrodesis (41 patients) versus four-bone fusion (97 patients) for treatment of posttraumatic carpal collapse, the overall satisfaction rate was similar in both groups (84% and 86%, respectively). The traditional wrist score, however, as well as the DASH score revealed significant superiority of the four-bone fusion based on similar pain relief and functional benefit due to the preserved mobility (1). In progressive radiocarpal and midcarpal arthrosis, inflammatory arthritis, complete loss of carpal ligamentous support with dislocation of the carpus, as well as failed previous operative treatments or failed motion-preserving procedures, total wrist arthrodesis still represents the most reliable surgical option (Fig. 18).

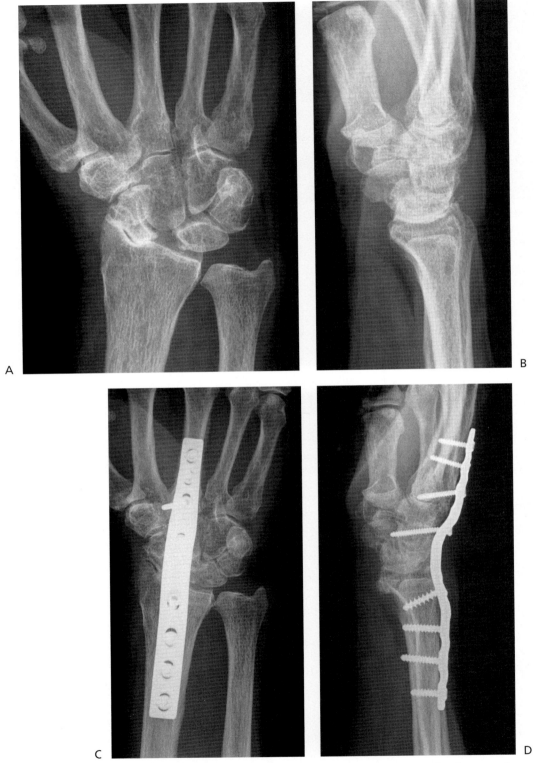

FIGURE 18. A,B: Scapholunate advanced collapse wrist with progressive carpal collapse and ulnar translocation. **C,D:** Treatment by total wrist arthrodesis with the AO wrist fusion plate.

REFERENCES

1. Krimmer H, Wiemer P, Kalb K. Comparative outcome assessment of the wrist joint—mediocarpal partial arthrodesis and total arthrodesis. *Handchir Mikrochir Plast Chir* 2000;32:369–374.
2. Watson HK, Weinzweig J, Guidera PM, et al. One thousand intercarpal arthrodeses. *J Hand Surg [Br]* 1999;24:307–315.
3. Knirk JL, Jupiter JB. Intra-articular fractures of the distal end of the radius in young adults. *J Bone Joint Surg Am* 1986;68:647–659.
4. Chamay A, Della SD, Vilaseca A. Radiolunate arthrodesis. Factor of stability for the rheumatoid wrist. *Ann Chir Main* 1983;2:5–17.
5. Linscheid RL, Dobyns JH. Radiolunate arthrodesis. *J Hand Surg [Am]* 1985;10:821–829.
6. Wilhelm A. Die Denervation der Handwurzel. *Hefte Unfallheilkd* 1965;109–114.
7. Berger RA. Partial denervation of the wrist: a new approach. *Tech Hand Upper Extremity Surg* 1998;2:25–35
8. Foucher G. L'operation dite "die punch" dans les sequelles de fractures articulaires du radius. *Ann Chir Main Memb Super* 1995;14:100–102.
9. Hastings H, Weiss AP, Quenzer D, et al. Arthrodesis of the wrist for post-traumatic disorders. *J Bone Joint Surg Am* 1996;78:897–902.
10. Saffar P. Radio-lunate arthrodesis for distal radial intraarticular malunion. *J Hand Surg [Br]* 1996;21:14–20.
10a. Garcia-Elias M, Lluch A. Partial excision of scaphoid: is it ever indicated? *Hand Clin* 2001;17:687–695.
11. Berger RA, Bishop AT. A fiber-splitting capsulotomy technique for dorsal exposure of the wrist. *Tech Hand Upper Extremity Surg* 1997;1:2–10.
12. Nagy L, Buchler U. Long-term results of radioscapholunate fusion following fractures of the distal radius. *J Hand Surg [Br]* 1997;22:705–710.
13. Beyermann K, Prommersberger KJ, Lanz U. Radioscapholunate fusion following comminuted fractures of the distal radius. *Eur J Trauma* 2001;26:169–175.
14. Sturzenegger M, Buchler U. Radio-scapho-lunate partial wrist arthrodesis following comminuted fractures of the distal radius. *Ann Chir Main Memb Super* 1991;10:207–216.
15. Saffar P. Radiolunate arthrodesis. In: Watson HK, Weinzweig J, eds. *The wrist.* Philadelphia: Lippincott Williams & Wilkins, 2001:867–974.
16. Bowers WH. Distal radioulnar joint arthroplasty: the hemiresection-interposition technique. *J Hand Surg [Am]* 1985;10:169–178.
17. Kapandji IA. The Kapandji-Sauve operation. Its techniques and indications in non-rheumatoid diseases. *Ann Chir Main* 1986;5:181–193.
18. Hastings H, Weiss AP, Strickland JW. Arthrodesis of the wrist. Indication, technique and functional consequences for the hand and wrist. *Orthopade* 1993;22:86–91.
19. Kalb K, Ludwig A, Tauscher A, et al. Treatment outcome after surgical arthrodesis. *Handchir Mikrochir Plast Chir* 1999;31:253–259.
20. Sauerbier M, Kluge S, Bickert B, et al. Subjective and objective outcomes after total wrist arthrodesis in patients with radiocarpal arthrosis or Kienböck's disease. *Chir Main* 2000;19:223–231.
21. Weiss AP, Hastings H. Wrist arthrodesis for traumatic conditions: a study of plate and local bone graft application. *J Hand Surg [Am]* 1995;20:50–56.
22. O'Bierne J, Boyer MI, Axelrod TS. Wrist arthrodesis using a dynamic compression plate. *J Bone Joint Surg Br* 1995;77:700–704.
23. Bolano LE, Green DP. Wrist arthrodesis in post-traumatic arthritis: a comparison of two methods. *J Hand Surg [Am]* 1993;18:786–791.
24. Clendenin MB, Green DP. Arthrodesis of the wrist-complications and their management. *J Hand Surg [Am]* 1981;6:253–257.
25. Sauerbier M, Kania NM, Kluge S, et al. [Initial results of treatment with the new AO wrist joint arthrodesis plate]. *Handchir Mikrochir Plast Chir* 1999;31:260–265.
26. van Schoonhoven J, Fernandez DL, Bowers WH, et al. Salvage of failed resection arthroplasties of the distal radioulnar joint using a new ulnar head prosthesis. *J Hand Surg [Am]* 2000;25:438–446.
27. Field J, Herbert TJ, Prosser R. Total wrist fusion. A functional assessment. *J Hand Surg [Br]* 1996;21:429–433.
28. Nagy L, Buchler U. Is panarthrodesis the gold standard in wrist joint surgery? *Handchir Mikrochir Plast Chir* 1998;30:291–297.

78

PROXIMAL ROW CARPECTOMY

JOSEPH E. IMBRIGLIA

SURGERY ANATOMY AND BIOMECHANICS

The wrist joint is a complex articulation that allows flexion, extension, radial and ulnar deviation, as well as rotation. This multidirectional motion is achieved by motion at both the radiocarpal and intercarpal joints. All reconstructive procedures available for salvage of the wrist joint result in the loss of some of the normal articulations and therefore the loss of some motion. Intercarpal fusions eliminate motion between the capitate, lunate, and scaphoid. Radiocarpal fusions eliminate motion between the radius, scaphoid, and lunate. Preservation of an arc of motion of approximately 60 degrees has been found to allow patients to perform the majority of activities of daily living and to perform most jobs, even those requiring power grip (1). Proximal row carpectomy (PRC), which requires removal of the scaphoid, lunate, and triquetrum, also dramatically alters the mechanics of the wrist joint. In the normal wrist joint, approximately 60% of motion occurs at the radiocarpal joint, and 40% of motion occurs at the intercarpal joints (2). The combination of motion at the radiocarpal and intercarpal joints results in a total flexion/extension arc of 170 to 175 degrees. A PRC converts the multiarticulated wrist joint to a simple hinged type of joint or ball-and-socket joint. Motion between the capitate and radius appears to be translational and rotational, which helps to dissipate some load on the radius (3). There are obvious changes in the normal anatomy when a PRC is performed. After removal of the bones, the capitate articulates with the lunate fossa of the radius. The capitate has a smaller radius of curvature than the lunate and a smaller radius of curvature than the lunate fossa of the radius. This results in a loose hinge type of motion as well as increased pressure between the capitate and lunate fossa. Long-term x-ray studies after PRC show a slow increase in the radius curvature of the capitate and a decrease in the radius curvature of the lunate fossa of the radius as the capitate conforms to the distal radius (3).

PATHOPHYSIOLOGY

PRC has been an alternative salvage procedure for wrist arthritis for more than 40 years (4–10). The procedure is performed for posttraumatic arthritic conditions in which the scaphoradial articulation is arthritic. In early scaphoradial arthritis in which the arthritis is limited to the distal pole of the scaphoid and radial styloid, a radial styloidectomy may be the procedure of choice (Fig. 1). Radioscaphoid arthritis can occur in scapholunate advanced collapse due to scapholunate ligament tears or scaphoradial arthritis due to scaphoid nonunion. Once the arthritis has progressed to the area between the proximal pole of the scaphoid and the radius, it is too late to do a radial styloidectomy (Fig. 2). At this point, the physician must decide on a reconstructive procedure. The choices at this point are (a) scaphoid excision and intercarpal arthrodesis; (b) PRC; (c) complete wrist arthrodesis; and (d) excision of the scaphoid with artificial implant for the scaphoid. However, there is no tested and reliable prosthesis for the scaphoid that can be used (11). From a practical point of view, our choices most often come down to scaphoid excision and four-bone fusion or PRC. If the stage II scaphoradial arthritis goes untreated, most often the arthritis progresses to the area between the capitate and lunate. If there is marked arthritis between the capitate and lunate, as well as arthritis between the scaphoid and radius (Fig. 3), PRC is no longer indicated. In this situation, one can perform a scaphoid excision and four-bone fusion (Fig. 4). If there is arthritis involving the entire proximal radiocarpal joint as well as the intercarpal joints (Fig. 5), a wrist fusion is indicated. In my practice, I have done both proximal row carpectomies and scaphoid excision with four-bone fusion for grade II arthritis between the scaphoid and radius. We have found that, in general, proximal row carpectomies recover faster and have a slightly greater range of motion than scaphoid excisions with four-bone fusion (3,12). The endurance and power of a PRC, however, are not as great as the endurance and power in most patients with scaphoid excision and four-bone fusion. For the average patient who does not do heavy work, I believe PRC is the preferred procedure. If the patient must do heavy work or work that requires repetitive use and endurance, an intercarpal fusion and scaphoid excision may be indicated. The long-term results of PRC have been docu-

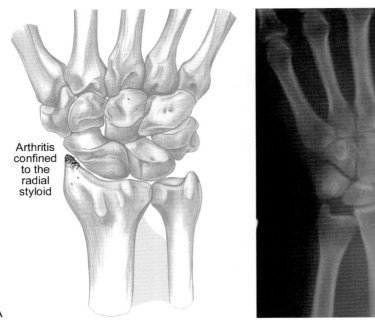

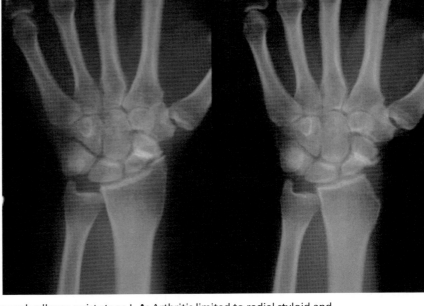

Arthritis confined to the radial styloid

A

B

FIGURE 1. Scapholunate advanced collapse wrist stage I. **A:** Arthritis limited to radial styloid and scaphoid. **B:** Radiograph depicts scaphoid nonunion with arthritis changes limited to the radial styloid. Treatment is radial styloidectomy.

mented (13). Clinically, patients get good pain relief and regain an arc of motion of approximately 60 degrees, with grip strength of 80% of normal. Long-term x-ray studies show that at least half of patients develop some joint space narrowing between the capitate and the radius (14). How many of these completely deteriorate is unknown, but clinically, few patients require reoperation for up to 10 years after the procedure.

CLINICAL EVALUATION

In each patient, it is important to differentiate the causes of the arthritis that brought the patient to the office. The common causes of the posttraumatic arthritis that require reconstructive surgery are (a) scapholunate dissociations with secondary scapholunate advanced collapse; (b) scaphoid nonunions with secondary arthritis between the scaphoid

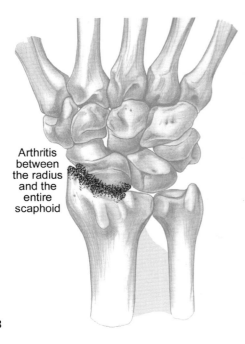

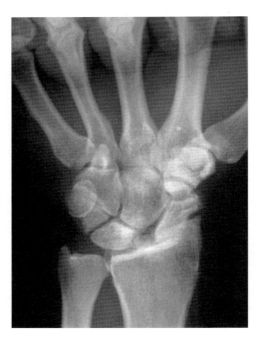

Arthritis between the radius and the entire scaphoid

A,B

FIGURE 2. Scapholunate advanced collapse wrist stage II. **A:** Arthritis between the entire scaphoid and radius. **B:** Radiograph depicts these degenerative changes between the scaphoid and radius. The proximal capitate surface is not damaged.

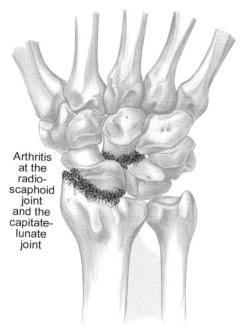

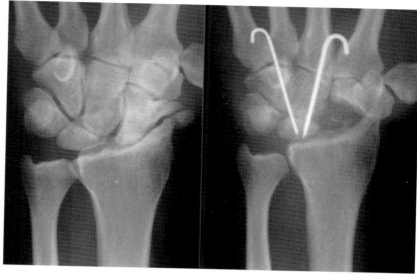

Arthritis at the radio-scaphoid joint and the capitate-lunate joint

A

B

FIGURE 3. Scapholunate advanced collapse wrist stage III. **A,B:** Arthritis at the radioscaphoid joint and the capitolunate joint. Treatment is capitolunate fusion with excision of the scaphoid.

and the radius; (c) Kienböck's disease with collapse; and (d) failed previous operations, including failed scaphoid and lunate prostheses. If there is no history of significant injury, one must be sure that the cause of the arthritis is not inflammatory in nature. Proximal row carpectomies are not indicated when the source of the arthritis is inflammatory.

A number of series have shown that proximal row carpectomies have a much higher failure rate in inflammatory arthropathy (3,14). This should be self-evident as an inflammatory arthropathy involving the wrist joint would affect the cartilage of both the capitate and the distal radius. PRC can work only if the lunate fossa of the radius and the

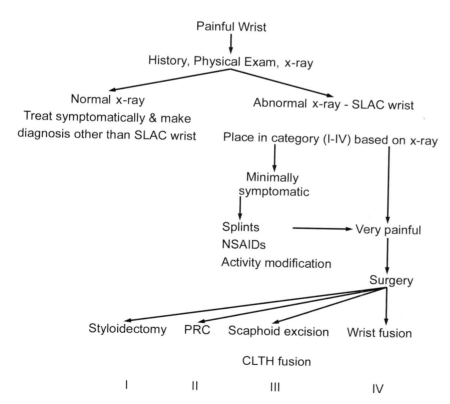

FIGURE 4. Evaluation and management algorithm. CLTH, capitolunotriquetralhamate fusion; NSAIDs, nonsteroidal antiinflammatory drugs; PRC, proximal row carpectomy; SLAC, scapholunate advanced collapse. Roman numerals signify stage of arthritis.

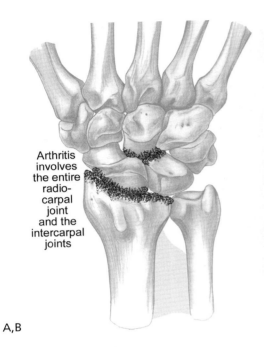

Arthritis involves the entire radio-carpal joint and the intercarpal joints

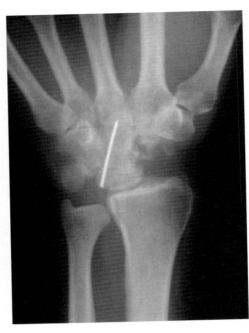

A,B

FIGURE 5. Scapholunate advanced collapse wrist stage IV. **A,B:** Arthritis at the radioscapholunate joint and intercarpal joint. Treatment is wrist fusion.

capitate are disease free. Also important in the history is the patient's occupation. Laborers who perform heavy work may not be able to return to their previous occupations because of loss of grip strength and endurance. Most patients with light to medium jobs can return to their previous employment after PRC. After being sure of the history and excluding inflammatory arthropathy, a physical examination is done. As in all problems about the hand, range of motion of the wrist is measured as well as grip strength and pinch strength. In general, one can tell the patient about his or her eventual motion after PRC based on the preoperative motion. The greater the preoperative range of motion, the greater the postoperative range of motion after PRC. A very stiff wrist preoperatively will often result in limited motion after PRC. In addition to range of motion, grip strength and pinch strength should be recorded. We always record grip strength as a percentage of the uninvolved side. On physical examination, it is also important to measure the supination and pronation of the forearm and be sure there is no history of previous injury to the distal radioulnar joint. This obviously would affect the ultimate outcome. X-rays are obtained in the office, and we commonly get a posteroanterior, a lateral, a supinated view, and radial and ulnar deviation views. These five views are enough to establish a diagnosis and also help in defining the etiology of the problem. One should be able to differentiate an inflammatory arthropathy from a posttraumatic arthritis based on plain x-ray films. Computed tomography scans and magnetic resonance imaging of the wrist are usually unnecessary in establishing the diagnosis. The most difficult area to evaluate for the presence of arthritis is the joint between the capitate and the lunate. On x-ray, it is obvious if there is arthritis between the scaphoid and

radius, but the capitate's surface is often difficult to evaluate. The condition of the capitate's surface will determine whether a PRC can be done or whether the patient will require scaphoid excision and four-bone fusion. If I am not sure of the condition of the capitate's proximal surface, I will tell the patient that I will inspect the capitate when I do the arthrotomy of the wrist. If the capitate's surface is intact, a PRC will be done. If the capitate's surface has been destroyed, a scaphoid excision and four-bone fusion should be done. The other option for this problem would be to do an arthroscopy preoperatively to determine the exact condition of the capitate. I personally do not believe this is necessary and simply adds another procedure to the patient's care.

NONOPERATIVE TREATMENT

When the diagnosis of scapholunate advanced collapse wrist is made, the condition is explained to the patient and the patient is given the options of treatment. If the pain is not severe, splinting and nonsteroidal antiinflammatory drugs can be ordered. This combination of immobilization and antiinflammatory drugs may offer some subjective decrease in symptoms. Likewise, a local steroid injection can be given in an attempt to get symptomatic relief of the pain. The decision to perform surgery is based almost entirely on the patient's complaint of pain. Therefore, if nonsurgical techniques help the patient, I follow the patient every 3 to 4 months and do what is necessary for pain relief. Once the conservative measures no longer relieve pain, surgery becomes the only option.

SURGICAL MANAGEMENT

Once it has been established that the patient's pain is significant enough to warrant surgery and that the x-ray changes are consistent with significant degeneration between the scaphoid and radius along with preservation of the proximal capitate surface, a PRC can be considered. The combination of pain, loss of motion, and grip strength combined with x-ray changes is the indication for PRC. As stated previously, the other surgical options are scaphoid excision and four-bone intercarpal fusion. Using the standard technique described in Surgical Technique, a number of authors have contributed series of patients in whom PRC provided at least 80% good results. Jorgensen (5), Green (8), and Neviaser (7) all had series of patients in whom PRC was performed. In each of these series there were at least 80% good results. Poor results were more common if PRCs were done in a patient with inflammatory arthritis, or if at operation, changes were seen on the proximal capitate surface. Poor results also appear to be more common in patients with Kienböck's disease (Sotereanos, *personal communication*). If a PRC is done in a patient with scapholunate advanced collapse II wrist (arthritic changes confined to the joint between the radius and scaphoid) and if there is no evidence of inflammatory arthropathy, the results are quite reliable (Fig. 6).

Surgical Technique

A dorsal longitudinal incision is performed, often incorporating existing scars. The extensor retinaculum is divided over the fourth compartment. The extensor digitorum communis is retracted to the ulnar side. The extensor pollicis longus and wrist extensors are retracted to the radial side. The posterior interosseous nerve is routinely resected. The wrist capsule is opened longitudinally to allow inspection of the lunate fossa and the articular surface of the capitate. The capsular incision is extended transversely to either side to facilitate exposure of

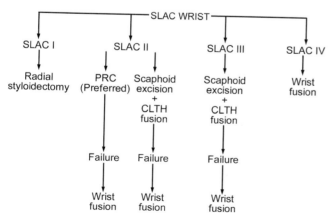

FIGURE 6. Surgical treatment algorithm. CLTH, capitolunotriquetralhamate fusion; PRC, proximal row carpectomy; SLAC, scapholunate advanced collapse.

the scaphoid. The scaphoid is then osteotomized in its midportion. After osteotomy of the scaphoid, the proximal pole of the scaphoid is removed. Once the proximal pole of the scaphoid is removed, the lunate is grasped with a towel clip and is excised. The triquetrum can then be removed in a similar fashion. Finally, the distal pole of the scaphoid is removed sharply. Often, it is necessary to rongeur out the most distal portions of the scaphoid. After the proximal row of bones is removed, the capitate settles into the lunate fossa (Figs. 7 and 8). Passive flexion/extension of the hand is done in neutral and slight radial deviation to detect impingement of the trapezium and the radial styloid. Some patients do require radial styloidectomy because of impingement (8). In general, I prefer not to remove the radial styloid, as there is the potential to disrupt the palmar radiocarpal ligaments and allow ulnar translation of the capitate. Once the bone work is done, the wound is irrigated and capsular closure is performed. A drain is placed in the wound, which is closed with nylon sutures. The patient is immobilized in a well-padded plaster splint for 2 weeks. At 2 weeks, the sutures are removed, the patient is placed in a removable splint, and motion is started. Most of these exercises are done at home. The patient may see a therapist once a week for approximately 4 weeks.

Results

Twenty-seven patients were in our original series of patients who underwent PRC (3). Twenty-six of these patients had satisfactory pain relief at 4 years postoperatively, and none required medication or splints. Of the 19 patients who performed manual labor, 16 returned to work. Two patients required reoperation, both for excision of the radial styloid. One patient in the original series of 27 had persistent pain and required a wrist fusion. There were no cases of carpal subluxation, infection, or reflex sympathetic dystrophy. Twenty-four patients were able to resume their previous activities or a new occupation within 4 1/2 months of surgery. Postoperative range of motion correlated with preoperative motion. All patients maintained or increased flexion and extension. The total arc of motion was increased from 65 degrees of flexion/extension to 84 degrees postoperatively. The average ulnar deviation was 23 degrees postoperatively. There was uniform loss of radial deviation. Grip strength in the original series of patients, as measured by the Jamar dynamometer, improved to an average value of 80% of the contralateral side (range of 50% to 90%). Only three patients, all heavy laborers, were unable to return to their former occupation. These 26 patients were reviewed again at an average of 10 years postoperatively (14). The clinical results held up quite well; however, in 12 of the 26 patients, there were some signs of degeneration on x-ray between the capitate and the radius. In our original studies, we had noted that the radius of curvature of the capitate increases with time. There is also evidence that the compression of the capitate causes deformation of the distal

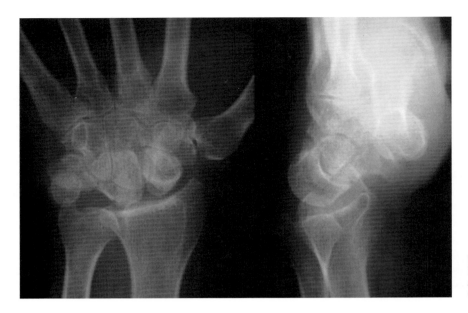

FIGURE 7. Preoperative radiograph of scapholunate advanced collapse wrist grade II. Arthritis at the scaphoradial articulation. Capitate proximal surface is not arthritic.

radius. In 12 patients at 10 years postoperatively, degenerative changes were seen between the capitate and radius.

Clinical results did not appear to deteriorate in conjunction with x-ray results. Results in other large series have been consistent with our results. As long as the stated preoperative criteria are used, the majority of patients can expect good pain relief, a total arc of flexion/extension of 85 degrees, and 80% of grip strength compared with the contralateral side.

Complications

As in any orthopedic procedure involving joints, the critical complications of infection, nerve injury, or dislocation must be avoided. These three complications are unusual after PRC and rarely a source of failure of the procedure. Proximal row carpectomies are generally performed on an outpatient basis. The patient is given intraoperative antibiotics. In our series of well over 100 patients, we have had no postoperative infection using this regimen. In reviewing the literature, it also appears that postoperative infection after PRC is an unusual complication. If there were a postoperative infection and further cartilage destruction, the patient might require a formal wrist arthrodesis. In such a large procedure, one might also expect that there would be some incidence of acute carpal tunnel syndrome after the procedure. This, however, is also extremely unusual and is probably due to the fact that by definition some areas of the transverse carpal liga-

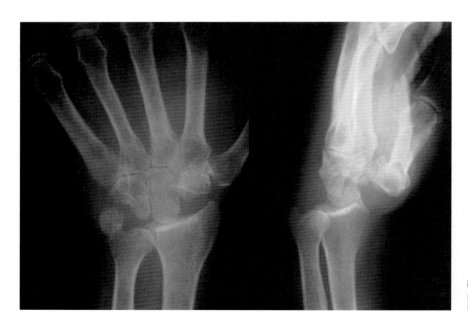

FIGURE 8. Postoperative radiograph after proximal row carpectomy. The capitate articulates with the lunate fossa of the radius.

ment are opened in excising the three carpal bones. Also, by decreasing the overall length of the wrist, some pressure is taken off the carpal canal area. Again, in more than 100 cases, we have not had any acute carpal tunnel syndromes that have required surgical release postoperatively. Finally, the question of postoperative dislocation in PRC is interesting. One would expect that with the removal of the entire proximal row the newly reconstructed joint would be very unstable. Because of this, some authors have actually recommended pinning of the joint. Pinning of the newly reconstructed joint is not necessary. As long as the volar carpal ligaments are left intact, the capitate will not dislocate on the radius. The capitate will shift to the ulnar side but will stabilize in the lunate fossa of the radius. I have been referred one patient with subluxation of the capitate to the ulnar side of the wrist after PRC. This patient had a very large radial styloidectomy. The large radial styloidectomy disrupted the palmar radiocarpal ligaments, resulting in ulnar translocation of the carpus. This patient eventually required wrist fusion. In general, I do not recommend doing a styloidectomy, and if styloidectomy is performed, it should be rather small.

Postoperative infection, postoperative nerve injury, and postoperative dislocation are unusual after PRC. The big problem after PRC is unexplained wrist pain. Wrist pain after PRC could be explained if x-ray and anatomic criteria were not closely adhered to. If on the x-ray there is damage to the capitate surface and PRC is still performed, the cause of the pain and failure of the procedure is the degenerative changes on the capitate. In this situation, wrist fusion is the recommended procedure. Some patients have pain after PRC despite what appears to be adequate articular surfaces on both the capitate and the radius. I would estimate that 5% to 10% of patients fit this category after PRC. In this situation, I would give any patient a full year for recovery before proceeding with any other operative procedure. The average recovery time after PRC is 5 to 6 months.

REFERENCES

1. Palmer AK, Werner FW, Murphy D, et al. Functional wrist motion: a biomechanical study. *J Hand Surg [Am]* 1985;10:39–46.
2. Sarjafian SK, Melamed JL, Goshgarian GM. Study of wrist motion in flexion and extension. *Clin Orthop* 1977;126:153–159.
3. Imbriglia JE, Broudy AS, Hagberg WC, et al. Proximal row carpectomy: clinical evaluation. *J Hand Surg [Am]* 1990;15:426–430.
4. Crabbe WA. Excision of the proximal row of the carpus. *J Bone Joint Surg [Br]* 1964;46:708–711.
5. Jorgensen EC. Proximal row carpectomy: an end result of twenty-two cases. *J Bone Joint Surg [Am]* 1969;51:1104–1111.
6. Inglis AE, Jones EC. Proximal row carpectomy for diseases of the proximal row. *J Bone Joint Surg [Am]* 1977;59:460–463.
7. Neviaser RJ. On resection of the proximal row. *Clin Orthop* 1986;202:12–15.
8. Green DP. Proximal row carpectomy. *Hand Clin* 1987;3:163–168.
9. White GM, Clark GL, Elias LS. Proximal row carpectomy for posttraumatic disorders of the wrist. *J Hand Surg [Am]* 1988;13:310.
10. Stamm TT. Excision of the proximal row of the carpus. *Proc R Soc Med* 1944:38:74–75.
11. Smith RJ, Atkinson RE, Jupiter JB. Silicone synovitis of the wrist. *J Hand Surg [Am]* 1985;1:47–60.
12. Hagberg WC, Imbriglia JE, McKernan DJ, et al. *Biomechanical analysis of fit of the capitate in the lunate fossa after proximal row carpectomies.* Baltimore: American Society for Surgery of the Hand, 1988.
13. Tomaino MM, Delsignove J, Burton RI. Long term results following proximal row carpectomy. *J Hand Surg [Am]* 1994;19:694–703.
14. Imbriglia JE. Proximal row carpectomy. *Atlas Hand Clin* 2000;5:101–109.

79

WRIST ARTHROPLASTY

LEONARD S. BODELL
LISA LEONARD

SURGICAL ANATOMY AND BIOMECHANICS

The wrist has been called the "keystone" of the hand (1–4). Linscheid (5) and other investigators (6,7) have observed that "the wrist is the most complex joint in the body" (8–10). The wrist is also a common site for pathology and is frequently involved in patients with rheumatoid arthritis (RA) (11).

The pivotal role of the wrist lies in its ability to transmit forces from the forearm to the hand and vice versa (4,5,12–15). Simultaneously, it allows for precise hand positioning in space to optimize finger function (16–22).

Motion of the hand relative to the forearm occurs in three main planes: flexion-extension motion (FEM), radioulnar deviation (RUD), and pronation-supination (5–7,23–30). To meet the complex functional requirements of the wrist while maintaining stability, it is necessary to surround the joint with large circumferential muscles, which is impractical, or to use a multijoint design (5). The wrist itself has evolved into two main joints: the radiocarpal (RC) and the midcarpal (MC). Further complexity is added by the fragmentation of the carpus into eight components (Fig. 1) and by the close proximity of the distal radioulnar joint (DRUJ) (8,31–38).

The anatomic area that is relevant to consideration stretches from the distal border of the pronator quadratus to the carpometacarpal joints and was well described by Vesalius in the sixteenth century (39,40).

Anatomy

The DRUJ is an articulation between the sigmoid notch of the distal radius and the distal ulna. In conjunction with the proximal radioulnar joint and the interosseous membrane, the DRUJ allows for forearm rotation (pronation-supination). Distal to the DRUJ, attached between the sigmoid notch and the fovea of the distal ulna, is the triangular fibrocartilage complex (TFC). The distal articular surface of the radius comprises two fossae for articulation with the scaphoid on the radial side and the lunate on the

ulnar side. The articular surface of the distal radius has a 10- to 12-degree palmar tilt in the sagittal plane and 20 to 25 degrees of ulnar inclination in the coronal plane (41). As is noted later in this chapter, these last two anatomic features are incorporated into the designs of several of the newer total wrist arthroplasties (TWAs).

The eight bones of the carpus form two rows. The proximal row consists of the scaphoid, the lunate, and the triquetrum. The pisiform, volar to the triquetrum, is a sesamoid bone within the substance of the flexor carpi ulnaris and does not form part of the carpal articulation. The distal row is comprised of the trapezium, the trapezoid, the capitate, and the hamate. When viewed axially, the carpal bones form an arch, much like a Roman aqueduct, which resists anterior-posterior loading (Fig. 2). This shape has developed to allow for the passage and protection of the carpal tunnel contents (41).

The bones of the wrist possess little intrinsic stability. Static stabilization is largely achieved through a complex series of ligaments. These can broadly be classified into extrinsic and intrinsic ligaments (42). The extrinsic ligaments pass between the bones of the forearm and the carpus, whereas the intrinsic ligaments pass solely between carpal bones. Several of these ligaments are pertinent to TWA. The volar extrinsic ligaments are an important group (43). The radioscaphocapitate (RSC) ligament originates on the palmar surface of the radial styloid and has two components that pass to the tuberosity of the scaphoid and the capitate, respectively. Distally, the RSC ligament interdigitates with the ulnocapitate (UC) ligament. The UC ligament arises proximally from the volar surface of the TFC. Together, these two ligaments constitute the distal, reversed V-shaped ligament. These superficial volar ligaments, along with the volar wrist capsule, should be retained, if at all possible, during arthroplasty surgery to avoid postoperative instability. This can be extremely difficult in the contracted rheumatoid patient who may require a considerable surgical release to achieve soft tissue balancing.

Deep to these ligaments, one finds the deep extrinsic ligaments: short radiolunate, ulnolunate, and ulnotriquetral.

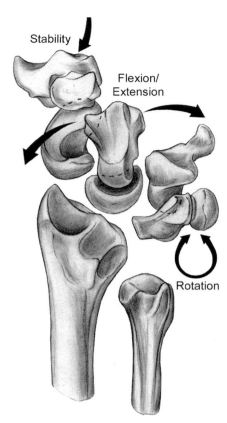

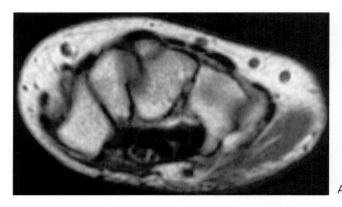

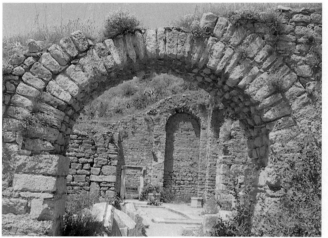

FIGURE 1. Drawing of carpus with distal radius and ulna in three-dimensional perspective with the bones disengaged. The drawing shows the complexity of the shapes of the carpal bones that create static and dynamic stability, while allowing for a large ellipsoidal-shaped range-of-motion envelope. This is due to presence of an instant center of rotation (instant screw axis) rather than a constant center of rotation, which is associated with nonorthogonal axes of motion.

FIGURE 2. **A:** Transverse view of magnetic resonance image of the carpus through the proximal row. Note the arch configuration that resembles Roman aqueduct and passageway construction, as seen in **(B).** This imparts increased structural stability, especially to anterior-posterior loads.

The former, the short radiolunate ligament, aids in stabilizing the lunate from excess extension in the sagittal plane. The latter two ligaments and the UC help stabilize the DRUJ and are known as the *ulnocarpal complex* (44,45). Appreciation of these structures should lead to the careful execution of volar capsular dissection during TWA (Fig. 3).

The main dorsal extrinsic ligament is the radiolunotriquetral ligament (41). It runs obliquely from the dorsomedial edge of the radius as a deep and superficial layer. It inserts onto the lunate and the dorsal ridge of the triquetrum. A short radioscaphoid ligament has also been described (42). The intrinsic dorsal ligaments comprise the scaphoid-trapezium-trapezoid and the dorsal intercarpal. The latter arises from the dorsal rim of the triquetrum and, at that point, is indistinguishable from the radiolunotriquetral. It crosses to the radial side of the carpus and attaches to the trapezium, the trapezoid, and the dorsal scaphoid ridge (Fig. 3). Surgical exposures that attempt to preserve these ligaments can be useful when performing arthroplasty surgery (46).

Other ligaments that should be preserved at operation include the intrinsic interosseous ligaments of the distal

carpal row and the ligaments that cross the carpometacarpal joints (CMCs). The stabilizing function of these structures is frequently also reinforced with local arthrodeses of all but the fourth and fifth CMCs.

Kinematics

The motion of the hand relative to the forearm is primarily composed of FEM and RUD, which occur at the RC and MC joints, and rotation that occurs at the DRUJ. Several authors, including investigators at the Mayo Clinic (6,7,14,15,25,45–50), have demonstrated that a small amount of rotation also occurs in the wrist joint itself. The mean maximum range of FEM in the normal adult is 133 degrees (27,51–53). Owing to different measurement methods, controversy exists as to whether the RC or MC contributes the most to FEM (9). The mean maximum range of RUD in the normal adult is 57 degrees. This is a complex motion that does not occur wholly within the coronal plane. Rotation at the wrist joint has been measured at 7 degrees (51).

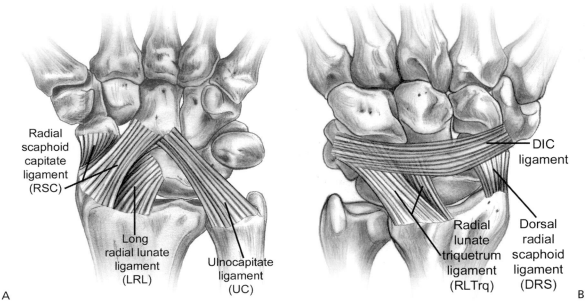

FIGURE 3. Anterior **(A)** and posterior **(B)** views of the wrist with detail of the extrinsic and intrinsic ligaments. DIC, dorsal intercarpal.

There has been a great deal of controversy surrounding the position of the axes of rotation of the wrist. Historically, a single center of rotation was assumed, located in the head of the capitate. This was based on pioneering work by Youm et al. (23). Current investigators, including Patterson et al. (9,54), have shown that the situation is considerably more complex, with a mobile instantaneous axis for each bone and each motion.

Clinically, it is important to consider the functional range of motion (ROM) of the wrist. Without exception, investigators have demonstrated that normal individuals are capable of performing most activities of daily living within a range that is significantly smaller than the extremes that were previously mentioned. Sugimoto et al. (55), in 1977, and later Brumfield and Champoux (56), Palmer et al. (51), Ryu et al. (52), and Nelson (57) have shown that a dorsiflexion of 40 degrees, a palmar flexion of less than 40 degrees, and a combined RUD of less than 40 degrees are sufficient for essentially unrestricted daily activities. The requirements of a patient with RA or bilateral posttraumatic arthritis may well differ from these values but have not been evaluated. Currently, a compromise between motion and stability is often required for patients who undergo TWA surgery.

The magnitude of loads that are transmitted across the wrist during use has not been well studied but has been estimated, by Brand et al. (58), to be on the order of 500 kg. Approximately 80% of the applied load is transmitted to the radius (9,59).

Carpal kinematics is still an unresolved field of investigation. In 1941, MacConaill (7) began to look critically at the problem and proposed a subdivision of the carpus. The scaphoid was singled out as a structural link. He also described

the carpus as a screw-vice or clamp, which would have its individual components (the carpal bones) pushed together and locked in place in certain configurations, thus affording stability to the wrist, based on the anatomy of the carpal bones. As the lunate and triquetrum were considered together, and the bones of the distal row (except for the trapezium) were considered together, this was essentially a row concept. Earlier, Navarro (60) conceptualized the carpus as vertical columns that allow for FEM, as well as rotation. Taleisnik (42) later modified this conceptualization, such that the central or flexion-extension column consisted of the lunate and the entire distal row. The scaphoid was the lateral (or mobile) column, continuing its singular role as was noted by MacConaill. The triquetrum was the medial (or rotation) column. According to Taleisnik (61), this conceptualization of the carpus could account for the motions of the wrist, including the propensity for the synchronous motions of flexion-ulnar-deviation and extension-radial-deviation, the so-called dart thrower's motion. Craigen and Stanley (62), in 1995, and Ferris et al. (63), in 2000, demonstrated two types of motion patterns in volunteers, thus leading them to the conclusion that the wrist functioned more as a row or as a column across a spectrum. The findings were related to relative motion changes on posteroanterior and lateral x-rays, respectively, of the scaphoid or lunate. Although both studies identified a pattern of scaphoid translation, their interpretations were opposite. Ryu (59) has proposed the *four-unit concept* in which the four bones of the distal row are considered as one unit. The scaphoid, lunate, and triquetrum are viewed as moving independently (64) and as constituting the other three units. In this manner, Ryu believes he can account for the various collapse patterns, as well as normal kinematics, especially the differential FEM that is noted between the capitate and lunate and that is not explainable with the columnar theory.

Pathology

As of 2003, wrist arthroplasty has primarily been performed in patients with RA. There are several reasons for this. Eventually, as much as 80% of this group has significant wrist pain and is functionally impaired by disease in this area (11,65–69). This functional impairment often occurs as a result of the loss of a stable platform from which the hand can work. In addition, these patients frequently place low functional demands on their prostheses (3,5,70–73).

RA of the wrist is often progressive and destructive. The basis for this is direct enzymatic joint damage that results from synovitis (74) and direct synovial invasion of the ligaments (75–78). Different patterns of deformity and destruction have been observed. In each individual case, thought must be given as to which structures have been damaged. This allows rational preoperative planning of the most appropriate surgical interventions. A knowledge of common disease patterns helps ensure that relevant copathologies are addressed.

Some disease patterns appear to relate to whether the soft tissues or cartilage and bone are primarily affected. Clayton (70), in 1965, and later Nalebuff and Garrod (79), in 1984, described *stiff* and *loose* types of rheumatoid patients. According to these authors, the stiff patients had relatively more rapid and early cartilage and bone involvement, which resulted in early ankylosis, than the loose type.

A commonly observed pattern of changes begins with involvement of the sixth dorsal compartment and the DRUJ (17). In this case, synovial invasion occurs around the ulnar styloid and the TFC, with attenuation of volar and dorsal capsular structures caused by a joint effusion that results in capsular stretching. There is often also damage to the floor of the extensor carpi ulnaris (ECU) tendon (80). This can lead to volar subluxation of the tendon and dorsal displacement and instability of the ulna relative to the carpus and radius (81,82). A progressive complex develops that includes loss of carpal height, extrinsic muscle imbalance, and ulnar and palmar translation of the carpus. There can develop erosion around the scaphoid at the synovial reflection (83). Cartilage destruction occurs from enzymatic action and compression (84). Flexion of the proximal row and compensatory extension of the distal row then occur with supination of the carpus (Fig. 4) (85,86). Elongation of the moment arm of the extensor carpi radialis longus (ECRL) can promote radial deviation of the wrist and metacarpals (87). Ulnar deviation of the fingers also occurs, and this is thought to have multiple causes (88). Some of these causes include the ulnar and palmar translation of the carpus, a volar descent of the fourth and fifth metacarpals (88), intrinsic muscle spasm, ulnar translation of the digital tendons (89,90), muscle inhibition of the ECU (87,91,92), a flexed posture of the scaphoid and lunate, and a relative increase in the influence of the flexor carpi radi-

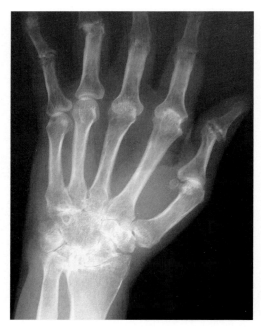

FIGURE 4. X-ray of a typical deformity of the wrist with cartilage, bone, and ligament destruction that is the result of the effects of chronic synovitis.

alis. The resultant radial deviation is believed by Shapiro et al. (87,93) to cause ulnar drift via a zigzag collapse.

The mechanics of the collapse pattern in biarticular, bimuscular systems were described by Landsmeer (94) in 1960 and were used by Stack and Vaughan-Jackson (95) as the basis to explain the observations that were put forth by Shapiro (87) in 1968 and 1970, as well as Pahle and Raunio (96). Hastings and Evans (97), using a standardized x-ray technique, believed that ulnar translation, as measured by migration of the lunate, and not radial deviation, best correlated to ulnar deviation of the fingers.

Straub and Ranawat (98) and, later, Taleisnik (99) have described a pattern of volar synovitis, which is less commonly seen and more difficult to appreciate than the dorsal synovitis that was discussed previously. Mannerfelt and Norman (100) described a syndrome of rupture of the flexor pollicis longus that was associated with scalloping and erosion of a flexed scaphoid.

The caput ulnae syndrome was described by Backdahl (101). It involves persistent synovitis of the DRUJ, volar subluxation or rupture of the ECU, and supination of the carpus due to functional weakening or disruption of the TFC, with relative dorsal prominence of the distal ulna (Fig. 5A).

Rupture of finger extensors was noted in 1948 by Vaughan-Jackson (102). In 1972, Freiberg and Weinstein (103) described the scalloped appearance of the DRUJ as a risk factor for extensor tendon rupture (Fig. 5B). Ryu et al. (104) further clarified the risk factors for extensor tendon rupture in 1998 as persistent extensor tenosynovitis, dorsal prominence of the distal ulna, and scalloping of the DRUJ.

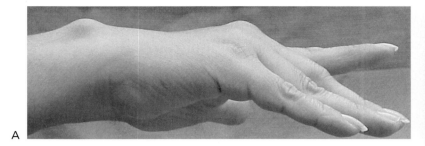

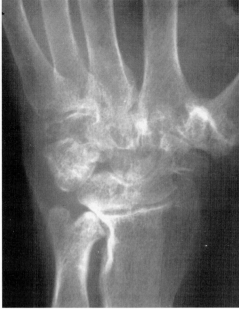

FIGURE 5. A,B: A patient with dorsal prominence of the distal ulna with associated extensor tendon ruptures. This condition is known as *caput ulnae syndrome*, as described by Backdahl (101).

When interosseous ligament attenuation is a dominant pathologic feature, the pattern of collapse may look similar to that of scapholunate advanced collapse. An x-ray that demonstrates radiolunate cartilage changes (Fig. 6) or a clinical exam and history that are suggestive of rheumatoid or other inflammatory disease assist the examiner in the differential diagnosis.

Occasionally, patients with posttraumatic arthritis are considered for TWA. The pathomechanics and pathophysiology of this condition have been well described in earlier chapters of this textbook (see Chapters 16, 18–30) and are not discussed further here.

Degenerative joint disease (DJD) of the wrist and calcium pyrophosphate deposition disorder are relatively common but seldom cause sufficient wrist pain to warrant invasive treatment. Patterson et al. reported, in 1993, a 58% incidence of cartilage erosion with exposed subchondral bone. There was a 27% bilateralism at the same location in 169 paired cadaver wrists (105) (Fig. 7).

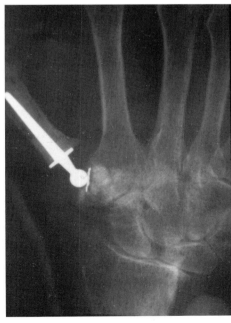

FIGURE 6. X-ray of a patient with scapholunate dissociation secondary to rheumatoid arthritis. Note the evidence of radiolunate arthritic changes.

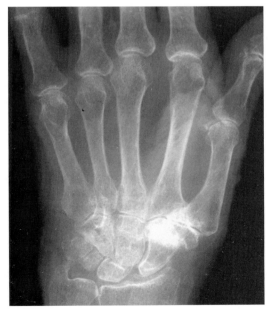

FIGURE 7. X-ray of octogenarian with a diagnosis of calcium pyrophosphate deposition disease. There were minimal symptoms of wrist pain. The presenting complaint was symptoms of carpal tunnel syndrome.

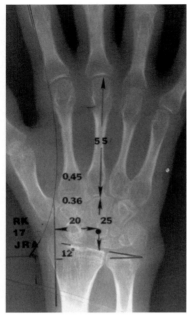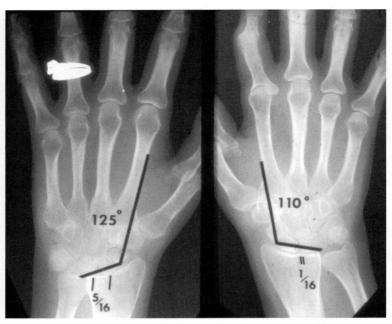

FIGURE 8. A: X-ray showing various methods of measuring the aspects of carpal instability and collapse. (Courtesy of Dr. Ronald Linscheid.) **B:** The method of Shapiro for measuring radial deviation.

There are many other causes of destructive wrist pathology. An exhaustive list was published by Martel (85) in 1964 and was reviewed by Dobyns (106) in 1998. Among the disorders to consider are: ankylosing spondylitis, gout, Reiter's syndrome, psoriatic arthritis, lupus, Jaccoud's arthritis, lipoid dermatoarthritis, tuberculosis, sarcoidosis, villonodular synovitis, ulcerative colitis, Whipple's disease, regional enteritis, viral arthritis, and bypass arthritis.

CLINICAL EVALUATION AND IMAGING

It is always important to obtain a full history at the start of any evaluation. Specific questions should also aim to elicit patient concerns regarding joint pathology that is situated outside the wrist in the upper and lower extremities. This can be particularly important in patients with inflammatory arthropathies in whom multiple joints can be involved and for whom the timing of surgery at each site is often critical (106). The functional aims of the patient should be established.

A thorough clinical examination, including observation of resting postures and joint swelling, should follow. Gentle palpation should reveal any local tenderness and specific abnormal motion, such as at the DRUJ. The passive and active ranges of motion should be recorded, and extensor or flexor lags should be noted as possible signs of tendon rupture. The presence of tendon deficiencies, particularly of the radial wrist extensors, is often considered a contraindication to TWA (82). It should be recalled that pain inhibition of the extensor tendons might give the impression of

complete tendon rupture. Occasionally, these musculotendinous units recover with aggressive postoperative rehabilitation programs. Often, however, extensor activity may be so severely compromised that it results in an unbalanced flexion stance and failure of the implant arthroplasty in these cases. Signs of concomitant nerve compression should not be missed.

Sometimes it is useful to obtain a hand therapist's formal assessment of the patient's overall functional capacity (107–110). This may help clarify which treatment options should be chosen.

Imaging studies should be standardized within a clinic (111–116). This allows for comparison across time and

TABLE 1. SIMMEN HUBER CLASSIFICATION OF THE RHEUMATOID WRIST

Group 1: Rheumatoid arthritis; ankylosis	Commonly seen in juvenile rheumatoid arthritis, due to rapid destruction of joint surfaces in otherwise stable joints.
Group 2: Rheumatoid arthritis; OA	Inflammatory destruction is seen along with changes of secondary OA. There is an equilibrium between rheumatoid arthritis inflammation and OA stabilization effects.
Group 3: Rheumatoid arthritis (disintegration)	Loss of radiocarpal or intercarpal integrity, alignment, and stability. Mutilans; predominant destruction of ligamentous structures.

OA, osteoarthritis.
Note: Grouping of rheumatoid arthritis patterns of the wrist per Simmen Huber. The concept was to classify the *type* of destruction rather than the *extent* of destruction, based on serial x-ray reviews.

promotes better assessment of disease progression. A baseline study should consist of posteroanterior and lateral radiographs in the neutral position (106). Hastings and Evans (97) have shown the value of standard views in more accurately assessing radial deviation. Additional views may occasionally add useful information.

Measurements of carpal height, ulnar translation, scapholunate dissociation, and radial rotation can be used on serial films to evaluate disease pattern type (24,117–121) (Fig. 8). Simmen and Huber (122), as well as Zangger et al. (123), have shown the value of serial x-ray evaluations in determining disease types. Such series demonstrate disease progression and can act as a useful guide to the early course of the disease in RA. This may, in turn, allow stable and unstable forms to be differentiated and thus may aid timely intervention (Table 1). In 1999, Flury et al. (3), correlated three radiologic parameters to identify stable and unstable patterns of disease progression. The three parame-

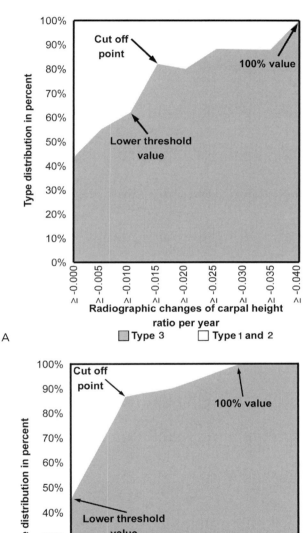

A

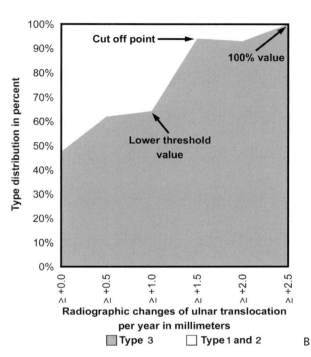

B

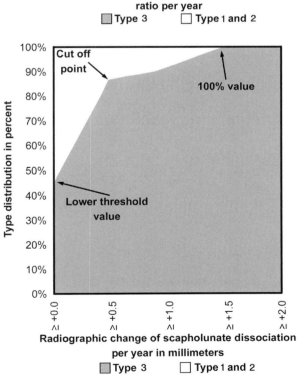

C

FIGURE 9. A: Distribution in stable and unstable pattern types in relation to change per year in carpal height ratio. B: Distribution in stable and unstable pattern types in relation to change per year in ulnar translocation. C: Distribution in stable and unstable pattern types in relation to change per year of scapholunate dissociation.

TABLE 2. COMBINED GROUPS OF THE SIGNIFICANT INDICES AND THEIR MEANING

Message	Group	Change per year
100% Unstable wrists (type 3)	All measured indices are greater than the cutoff point	CHR >−0.015 mm UT >+1.5 mm SLD >+0.5 mm
100% Stable wrists (types 1 and 2)	All measured indices are lower than the lower threshold value	CHR <0 mm UT <+1 mm SLDn = 0 mm

CHR, carpal height ratio; SLD, scapholunate dissociation; UT, ulnar translocation.
From Flury MP, Herren DB, Simmen BR. Rheumatoid arthritis of the wrist, classification related to natural course. *Clin Orthop* 1999;366:72–77, with permission.

ters that were used were carpal height, ulnar translocation, and scapholunate dissociation. There was no correlation with radial rotation. A per-year change of carpal height ratio that is greater than or equal to 0.015, an ulnar translation that is greater than or equal to 1.5 mm, and a scapholunate dissociation that is greater than or equal to 0.5 mm together yielded a 100% certainty of the diagnosis that a patient has an unstable disease progression pattern (Fig. 9; Table 2). Larsen et al. (124) published a classic paper describing six radiographic stages of rheumatoid disease. Alnot and Fauroux (125) modified this to include a description of deformities in the wrist (Table 3). These classifications, along with the Wrightington classification that was published in 1989 (126) (Table 4), have been used by one of the authors of this chapter to produce an algorithm, which includes the indications for TWA, for the management of various wrist disorders (Fig. 10).

Occasionally, when TWA is considered, the more detailed information that is obtained with computerized tomography and magnetic resonance imaging can be helpful. The state of the remaining bone stock can be assessed, and a more accurate assessment of deformities can be made (Fig. 11). In addi-

TABLE 3. ALNOT-FAUROUX CLASSIFICATION OF THE RHEUMATOID WRIST

Stage 0	No radiologic alterations
Stage I	Swelling of periarticular synovial tissue Demineralization Beginning of narrowing of joint lines
Stage II	Minimal narrowing of joint lines Marginal erosions Tendency to radial inclination Subluxation or luxation of DRUJ
Stage III	Narrowing of joint lines (still visible) RC and mediocarpal erosions Instability in frontal plane Luxation of DRUJ
Stage IV	Ankylosis of one or more RC or mediocarpal joint lines Luxation of DRUJ
IVa	Unstable
IVb	Stable by radiolunate ankylosis or impaction
Stage V	Disappearance or destruction of all joint lines Luxation of DRUJ
Va	Unstable with dislocation
Vb	Stable with spontaneous RC ankylosis

DRUJ, distal radioulnar joint; RC, radiocarpal.
Note: Classification outline of Alnot-Fauroux, using the method of Larsen and modified depending on the findings of carpal instability.

tion, true tendon ruptures can be differentiated from musculotendinous units that are inhibited from functioning but may have the potential to be retrained.

NONOPERATIVE TREATMENT

The aims of nonsurgical management are to prevent further damage, to decrease pain, to maintain functional ROM, and to maintain or to improve function (see Chapter 7). Functional splinting (107,109), pharmaceuticals, naturoceuticals (herbal medications), and local injections may all have a role in the management of patients with

TABLE 4. WRIGHTINGTON CLASSIFICATION OF THE RHEUMATOID WRIST

Grade	Description	Suggested treatment
I	Wrist architecture is preserved Mild rotatory subluxation of the scaphoid Periarticular osteoporosis Early cyst formation	Synovectomy Tendon balancing
II	Ulnar translocation Marked volar flexion of the lunate Grossly flexed scaphoid Radiolunate joint destruction or derangement	Darrach procedure or modification Wrist balancing procedures Alternative treatment: radiolunate fusion plus Darrach procedure
III	Gross bony architecture of the radius is preserved Joints between the carpal bones are arthritic Radioscaphoid joint is eroded Volar subluxation of the carpus	Arthroplasty Total wrist fusion
IV	Loss of a large amount of bone stock from the distal radius	Total wrist fusion

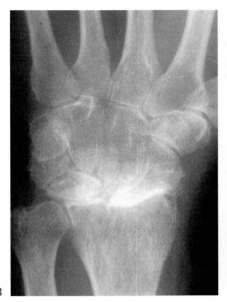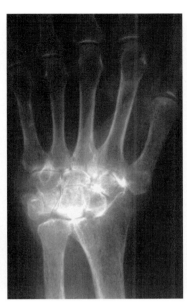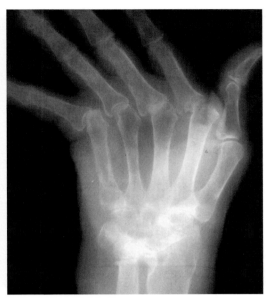

A,B   C

FIGURE 10. Stable patterns of disease seen in figures **A** and **B**, demonstrating Simmen groups 1 and 2. **C:** Simmen group 3 shows a disintegrative pattern.

wrist pain (70,73,127–130). Such conservative measures should always be exhausted before any surgical intervention is undertaken.

ALTERNATIVE SURGERY TO TOTAL WRIST ARTHROPLASTY

The aim of surgery must be to attempt to meet each individual patient's overall requirements as closely as possible. Each available surgical option therefore needs careful consideration. Further details regarding these options are to be found elsewhere in this text (see Chapters 69, 70, 74, 77,

78), but a few of the more relevant procedures are briefly considered here.

In stage II of RA, as defined by Millender and Nalebuff (127), the patient presents with local areas of disease activity with overall good medical control. At this stage, there is often minimal bone or ligament involvement.

Preventative synovectomies and tenosynovectomies are recommended (Fig. 12) (66,81,127,131–133). The literature is replete with reports that confirm the long-term benefits of these procedures at the wrist level (66,133–140). In cases in which progressive joint destruction was observed postsurgery, many of the patients did well even after 12 years (22,66,133,141–143). With arthroscopic synovecto-

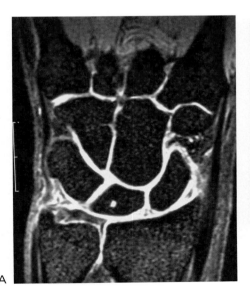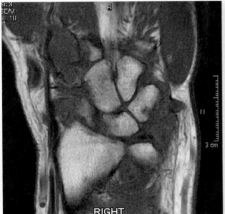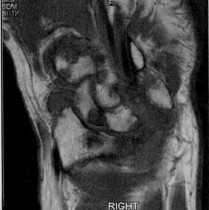

A   B

FIGURE 11. A: Three-dimensional reconstruction of a computed tomography scan of the wrist, showing details of available bone stock. **B:** Thin section fat suppression magnetic resonance image showing bone and articular surface details.

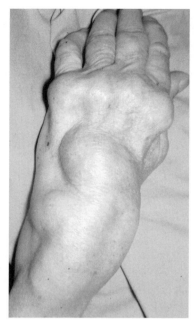

FIGURE 12. Stage II rheumatoid arthritis. The patient has undergone more than 6 months of medical treatment for his rheumatoid arthritis. He has persistent synovitis and tenosynovitis of the hand and wrist. Minimal bony changes were evident on x-rays.

mies added to the armamentarium of the hand surgeon, postoperative recovery time can be reduced (144–148). With this technique, the indications for synovectomy may expand to include more severe radiologic stages in the future (L. S. Bodell, *unpublished data*).

In RA, the DRUJ may be the primary source of functional disability (101,102,149). In this case, many options have been reported in the literature (150).

The *Darrach procedure* is typically used to treat painful, disrupted DRUJs in patients with RA (151–158). The results are noted to be better than those reported for posttraumatic disorders (159–165). In more severe cases, the instability (166,167) may be accompanied by cartilage damage (103,104), synovitis (101,103,104), alteration of tendon collagen (168,169), and tendon ruptures (101,170–173). In some of these cases, it is appropriate to supplement the resection with tendon weaves (174–180), tendon transfers (70,181–184), or radiolunate fusions (3,22,122,185–187).

Progressive radiocarpal instability may occur after a Darrach-type resection (150,161,181,182,188–192). This has led some authors to question the appropriateness of this procedure and to develop alternatives. Bowers (193) and Watson et al. (194), for instance, have described a partial resection of the distal ulna with preservation of the TFC attachment, when possible, and creation of a surface on the distal ulna for firm reattachment of the ulnar sling mechanism (22). Feldon et al. (195) described the "wafer" procedure; its applicability in rheumatoid patients is limited at best, as the problem is generally instability, not impaction (196). Failures of all these methods can be found in the literature (164,192,197,198), with varying measures used for salvage (Fig. 13).

The *Sauve-Kapandji procedure* has also been reported as an alternative to the Darrach operation (199–202), and increasing interest is noted for its application in patients with RA (203–205) (Fig. 14). Some authors have reported that this procedure lessens the tendency for further ulnar drift (203).

DRUJ replacements of the silicone (206–211) and the newer ceramic ball and uHead Ulnar Implant System (Avanta Orthopaedics, San Diego, CA) designs (211–214) are considered later in this chapter.

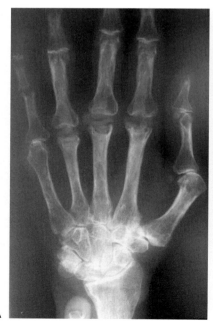

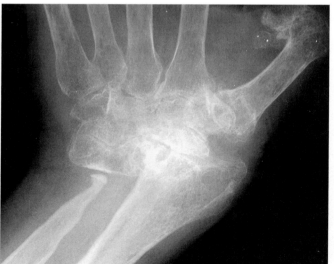

A

B

FIGURE 13. Patients who had a Darrach operation. **A:** No progressive ulnar translation. **B:** Progressive ulnar translation, which demonstrates that ulnar translation is more likely a function of the underlying disease pattern than of the Darrach procedure itself.

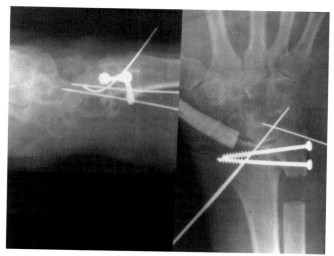

FIGURE 14. Patient with rheumatoid arthritis who was treated with a Sauve-Kapandji operation.

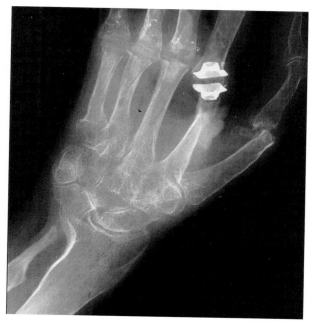

FIGURE 15. Patient with radiolunate fusion, a long-term stable wrist, and satisfactory pain relief.

Proximal row carpectomy is discussed in Chapter 78. It remains a proven alternative to TWA as a motion preserving procedure. There is no support, however, in the literature or in the authors' limited experiences for the use of this operation in patients with RA (215–217).

Distraction arthroplasty was thought to be an alternative for some high-demand patients with degenerative wrist conditions, whose alternative options are TWA or total wrist arthrodesis. Fitzgerald et al. (218) reviewed their experience of 14 patients. Six patients had osteoarthritis (OA), three had scaphoid nonunion advanced collapse (SNAC) of the wrist, and two had silicone synovitis. The remainder had spastic contractures. Three were converted to arthrodesis (one OA, one silicone synovitis, one scaphoid nonunion advanced collapse). Average ROM was 41 degrees of extension and 38 degrees of flexion. Dynamic power was more than one-half of the opposite site. Satisfaction was reported to be high. Historically, this group has demonstrated an unacceptably rapid and high rate of loosening with TWA. Owing to ligamentous laxity, this procedure is less useful in patients with RA.

Denervation procedures, which are covered in detail in Chapter 80, may have a role in the management of selected patients with painful wrists in whom more aggressive or potentially debilitating procedures are otherwise not indicated. The authors were unable to identify literature in support of this procedure in patients with wrist pain that is secondary to inflammatory arthritis (219–224).

Limited wrist arthrodesis (225,226), especially radiolunate arthrodesis, has proven an excellent choice for some patients. In Phoenix, Arizona, this procedure is performed in patients with wrists that fall into Simmen group 3, Wrightington grade II, or Alnot-Fauroux stages II and III. The authors' experience is that more than 75% of these patients have significant pain relief and maintain their functional status without progressive ulnar translation,

even after 5 years (Fig. 15). Progressive cartilage loss and carpal collapse do occur with little difference noted between the treated wrist and the opposite, nonoperated side over the long term (227–232).

Total wrist arthrodesis is discussed in detail in Chapter 77. It has well-documented predictability (233–240), especially with newer plate systems and grafting techniques (241–254). Multiple authors have advocated total wrist arthrodesis in the management of rheumatoid patients with significant pain and cartilage destruction (255–268). It is considered by many to be the gold standard for management of advanced, symptomatic arthritis of the wrist (260,268).

Clendenin and Green (269) have reported on many of the complications and shortcomings of this operation, including nonunions, fractures of the bone grafts, and donor site morbidity. Other authors have opined additional complications with the procedure (270–275). Inherent in the success of this operation is a total loss of wrist motion. In patients with RA, who may require bilateral procedures, this can be functionally limiting. The loss of the tenodesis effect can also impair the residual function of the rheumatoid hand. The importance of preserving CMC motion for the functional outcome of patients with RA is pointed out by Vahvanen and Tallroth (268).

When comparing arthrodesis to arthroplasty, patients who have had both procedures generally prefer arthroplasty (1,276,277). Kobus and Turner (262) reported that all of their patients who were unsatisfied with arthrodesis had had an arthroplasty on the other side. Personal experience has shown that patients who require bilateral wrist surgery do not wish to have an arthrodesis performed on the other

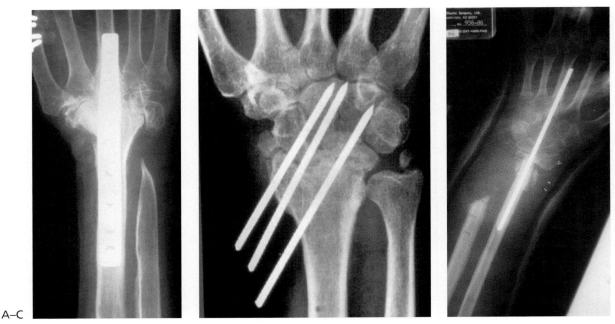

A–C

FIGURE 16. Types of arthrodesis. **A:** Compression plating. **B:** Oblique Steinmann pins. (Courtesy of Dr. Len Ruby.) **C:** Axial pinning.

side if an arthroplasty is performed first. However, good results, even with bilateral arthrodesis in RA patients, have been reported (278,279). An exhaustive treatise on wrist arthrodesis is recommended for the reader's review (280) (Fig. 16).

Biologic, or interposition, arthroplasties—using a variety of materials from platinum plates and chromicized pig bladder to fascia lata, silicone, and perichondrium—are reported in the global literature (281–284). Murphy (285), in 1913, advocated the use of fascia lata and was perhaps the first person to promote this type of operation in the twentieth century. Many of the reports present small series with only a few years of follow-up.

Albright and Chase (286) introduced the concept of a palmar shelf arthroplasty. They emphasized sufficient radial resection to release soft tissue tension, rebalancing of the tendons, and preservation of the carpal surface to minimize the risk of ankylosis postsurgery. A volar bone shelf was created to help prevent recurrent palmar translation of the carpus and hand, especially in the presence of recurrent synovitis. In their nine patients, the results were good to excellent in six, and fair in three. In a longer-term study that was published in 1989 by Gellman et al. (287), they were able to reconfirm the initial observations of Albright and Chase. With time, however, the quality of the results diminished, with pain recurring in 84% of the 63 patients at an 83-month follow-up.

In 1981, Tillmann and Thabe (288) reported on their experience with 49 patients (60 joints), from 1968 to 1977, with a technique that used dorsal retinaculum or volar capsule for interposition. Minimal bone was resected and a small volar shelf was created, per the method of Albright and Chase (286). Over a period of 5 years, postoperative motion and stability were maintained. Pain relief was achieved. They felt that the need for walking aids was only a relative contraindication to the procedure.

With a mean follow-up of 6.8 years, Kulick et al. (289) found that their dorsal stabilization procedure demonstrated excellent pain relief in 85 rheumatoid wrists in 62 patients. However, all patients experienced a decrease in ROM. Eight of their patients developed spontaneous arthrodesis.

Ryu et al. (290) described a technique that the senior author had used for 17 years. It involves creating a cancellous concavity within the radius and a cancellous convexity of the scaphoid and lunate with a flap of capsule or retinaculum that is interposed between the two (22). The 7-year follow-up study, published in 1985, demonstrated excellent resolution of pain, restoration of alignment, and stability, with overall improved function. Sixty-seven percent (19 of 23 patients who were reviewed) went on to spontaneous arthrodesis of the lunate or scaphoid to the radius. Although Jackson and Simpson (291), using silicone sheeting as interpositional material, recommended interpositional arthroplasty for middle-stage disease, most other authors suggest that an interpositional arthroplasty can be used even in the presence of an unstable or disintegrative type of RA (292,293). Additional studies by Eaton et al. (294) and Biyani and Simison (295) further confirm the usefulness of biologic arthroplasties in traumatic and rheumatoid conditions (Fig. 17).

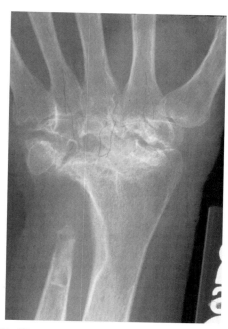

FIGURE 17. Fibrous arthroplasty with a stable, pain-free result at 10 years postsurgery.

TOTAL WRIST ARTHROPLASTY

Early History

It is recorded that Ambroise Paré, in 1536, performed the first joint excision, of an elbow in a patient with destructive infection (281–283). Arguably, Orred performed the first wrist joint resection in 1773 (281–283,296,297). In the nineteenth century, resection arthroplasty of the wrist was commonly performed, with the patient being encouraged to proceed with early motion to avoid ankylosis.

Ritt et al. (283) have published a detailed history of arthroplasty of the wrist. They note that the use of interpositional materials was first recorded in 1840 by John Murray Carnochan. Péan is reported to have used platinum plate in the wrist as early as 1894. The authors have already commented on the early twentieth century work of Murphy (285), who used fascia lata as an interpositional material.

The first TWA is attributed to Themistocles Gluck in 1890. He used an ivory ball-and-socket design with stems for the metacarpals, as well as the radius and ulna (281–283,298). Other than infection (his first patients all had joint destruction from tuberculosis), the implants functioned well. In 1921, he reported on his favorable long-term results (299).

Interpositional arthroplasty lost favor in the early 1900s and did not appear in the literature until interest was reignited in the 1960s by the work of Paul Lipscomb (300). At the same time, Swanson (301) and Niebauer introduced the concept of a silicone interpositional spacer that could offer immediate stability and a foundation on which the reparative fibrous tissue could grow without inhibiting later

motion (281,283). Swanson first started using these silicone implants for the RC joint in 1967 (17) and reported his experience in 1982 and 1984 (19,20).

The onset of the use of metal implants began in 1969, with the Gschwind-Scheier-Bahler implant of Gschwind and Scheier (302). Since then, many implants have been developed with various clinical results (303,304). These are reviewed in detail in the following section. This review shows the main problems with prostheses to date: soft tissue balancing, stability, and loosening, particularly of the distal components. Newer designs have gone some way toward addressing these problems, but the ideal wrist replacement geometry and fixation remain to be elucidated.

Implant Review

A systematic review of the published literature was undertaken to compile this section of the chapter. Although every attempt was made to be as inclusive as possible, some implants may have been unintentionally excluded. To any inventors and investigators who may be excluded, the authors apologize.

Flexible Hinge Spacer

Design, Description, and Philosophy
These implants were developed in 1967. The design is of a flexible, silicone, hinged, intramedullary stemmed, one-piece implant, which is to be used as an adjunct to resection arthroplasty techniques of the RC joint. The purpose was to use the implant as a means of maintaining joint space and alignment while providing some stability during the process of fibrous tissue encapsulation (301). It was hoped that this would decrease the percentage of ankylosis that occurs with resection and some interposition procedures.

The implant has a barrel-shaped midsection, which is flattened on the dorsal and volar surfaces. A Dacron reinforcement in the core provides axial stability and resistance to torque. The original material was medical-grade silicone (conventional silicone elastomer), which was converted to a high-performance elastomer (HP 100, Dow Corning, Midland, MI) in 1974. Other modifications have taken place, including a widening of the barrel hinge in the radioulnar plane, shortening of the distal stem, and widening of both stems (WS design). In 1984, titanium grommets were included for the purpose of protecting the midsection barrel stem interface from shear force and sharp bone edges (Fig. 18). There are five sizes.

Indications and Contraindications
The original indications were stated as RA, DJD, or post-traumatic disabilities, which resulted in

Instability due to subluxation or dislocation of the RC joint

Severe deviation of the wrist that causes musculotendinous imbalance of the digits

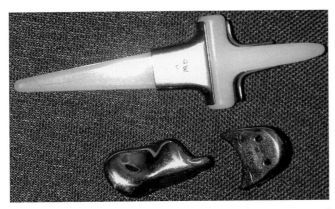

FIGURE 18. Photo of WS configuration with grommets of Swanson silicone radiocarpal spacer implant. Improved results were reported in more recent literature that detailed use of grommets. Titanium scaphoid and lunate implants replaced their silicone counterparts but have found only selective use.

Stiffness or fusion of the wrist in a nonfunctional position (not expressly specified)

Stiffness of a wrist when movement is required for hand function.

The operation was not recommended for people performing heavy manual labor.

Operative Technique

The technique is well described in multiple articles and texts (18–20,40,65,80,277,305–307). A tourniquet is used. A dorsal midline incision is made with careful elevation of skin flaps. The dorsal veins and the dorsal radial and dorsal ulnar sensory nerves are protected throughout the procedure. Originally, the retinaculum was described as being reflected off the ulnar side of the wrist. The authors' approach has been to reflect the retinaculum off the radial side. This has allowed us to advance the retinaculum radially on closure to elevate the ulnar side of the carpus and to help correct the supination collapse pattern. With this approach, it is still possible to split the retinaculum transversely and use one-half for capsular supplementation and one-half to create a pulley for the ECU to hold it in a dorsal position. Another option the authors have used is a Z-lengthening. The distal one-half of the retinaculum is elevated at the level of the sixth compartment. The proximal one-half is elevated off the first or second compartment. This permits one-half to be placed under the tendons to strengthen the dorsal capsule at closure or to lengthen the retinaculum. Tenosynovectomies are performed. The authors open the capsule by using a transverse incision, thus detaching it from the radius, and reflecting it distally via longitudinal radial and ulnar incisions. With the wrist hyperflexed, the lunate, the proximal one-half of the scaphoid, the triquetrum, and the proximal convexity of the capitate are removed. The distal face of the radius is excised at 90 degrees to the long axis of the radius. One to 2

cm of bone is generally removed, depending on the amount of bone loss from disease, soft tissue contractures, and the size of the patient. If the carpus is subluxed volarly and proximally, a careful dissection, to identify what remains of the proximal carpal bones, is essential. Diligence to preserve the volar capsule and to protect the median nerve is critical. A separate capsular incision is often necessary to expose the distal ulna and to allow for a Darrach procedure, or other desired procedure, to be completed. A sharp bone awl is used to locate the third metacarpal canal via the capitate. This is carefully enlarged by using a bur. In patients with RA, reaming of the radius is usually easily achieved, although a starter awl is often needed to get through the subchondral bone. The size of the implant is set most often by the distal bone array. If the grommets are to be used, some additional shaping of the volar radial opening and the capitate is required. Preparation of the distal canal is made first, as this sets the size and avoids leaving a thin cortical shelf of distal radius that might collapse under the vigorous pressure of distal reaming. Proper fit is suggested by a flush seating of the barrel proximally and distally. No buckling should be accepted during flexion to 60 degrees. All contractures of soft tissue are released. Lluch and Proubasta (308) and Lluch (309) recommend intercarpal arthrodesis to decrease the incidence of subsidence. As is noted throughout this chapter, maximum preservation of the carpus and even surgical enhancement to promote intercarpal arthrodesis are technical themes that are generally gaining in popularity for all types of implant arthroplasties.

Capsular reconstruction is accomplished dorsally by using drill holes that are placed into the dorsal radial cortical rim before implant placement. Tension is set to create neutral axial alignment and to block excess volar flexion capacity. The dorsal ulnar capsule is closed. A flap of volar capsule can be used to stabilize the distal ulna, or the surgeon can incorporate tendon weaves. Supplemental capsular reconstruction is accomplished by placing one-half of the retinaculum underneath the extensor tendons. The ECU is placed dorsally, and, if necessary, a separate retinacular pulley can be created to maintain its dorsal position. Routine careful skin closure is used.

Postoperative rehabilitation with an experienced hand therapist is recommended. Postsurgical goals, as outlined by Swanson, are 60 degrees of combined dorsiflexion and palmar flexion, with 10 degrees of radial and ulnar deviation.

Results

In 1984, Swanson et al. (20) reported on their early results. These consisted of experience with 181 implants in 139 patients with a mean follow-up time of 4 years. Overall, they reported excellent tolerance by the host to the implant. Twenty-five wrists (out of 181) were revised. Nine were revised for fracture (5%), four for tendon imbalance, and five for recurrent synovitis. Three wrists were converted to an arthrodesis. Although the majority of patients had

RA, the report did not subdivide the failures by preoperative diagnosis.

Four years earlier, in 1980, Goodmann et al. (277) reported their results from using 37 silicone arthroplasties. All of their patients had a diagnosis of RA. There was an 8% implant fracture rate, with time to fracture averaging 11.6 months. Patients with an arthrodesis on the opposite side preferred the implant side. The best results were found in patients with relatively good ROM and alignment preoperatively. Their conclusions, at that time, were that, for most patients with RA, a wrist arthroplasty (with silicone implant) was preferable to wrist fusion.

In 1986, Brase and Millender (310) reported a longer-term study of this same group of patients. At that time, there was a 20% implant fracture rate. Eleven of these cases had been revised to another silicone spacer, and two of these cases had refractured by the date of publication preparation. Their conclusions at that stage were that indications for silicone wrist arthroplasty should only include low-demand patients with a moderate amount of preserved motion, adequate bone stock, and good alignment. There are several other reports from a number of countries that report their experience with the Swanson flexible hinge (281,305–307,311–319). Fracture rates from 12% to 65% were noted when using the HP 100 material (in contrast to a fracture rate as high as 75% of implants long term with conventional silicone elastomer) (305,310,313–323). Several authors alluded to cystic changes and evidence of particulate synovitis (64,310,320,321,324–327), particularly with the HP 100. Most reported subsidence of the implant and bone resorption (317,320). One group noted 100% subsidence (320), whereas another group correlated bone resorption to recurrence of pain (321).

Rossello et al. (328) and Capone (329) have reviewed their experiences with the Swanson spacer and grommets. In both studies, fractures only occurred with dislocation of the grommet. Increased bone formation around the implant was noted. There was still a 20% incidence of carpal collapse over a 5-year period. This was felt to be correlated to initial severity of the disease.

Summary

The authors' personal experience has been that many patients with flexible hinge spacer implants *in situ* continue to function well for many years if they are low-demand patients. They are often unaware of implant fractures or carpal collapse (Fig. 19). Overall, there still seems to be a limited role for the Swanson silicone hinge spacer. The ideal patient for such an implant would be a low-demand patient who is older than 60 years of age and has quiescent systemic disease. He or she should have significant pain but adequate bone stock for the proper placement of the implant and the grommets. There should be reasonable wrist alignment in the axial and sagittal planes (Simmen groups 1 and 2). Tendon balance and continuity must exist or must be reconstructible. The presence of an arthrodesis in the contralateral wrist or the limitation of other upper extremity joint function, or both, would be likely to encourage the choice of an arthroplasty.

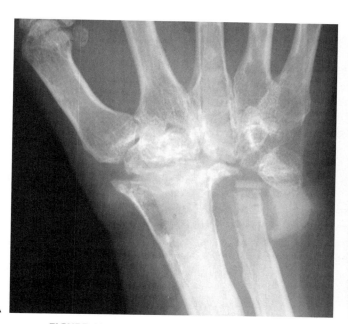
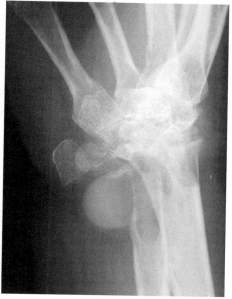

A

B

FIGURE 19. A,B: X-rays taken 27 years after surgery for placement of a Swanson radiocarpal and distal ulnar implant. The patient continued to have excellent alignment and a satisfactory range of motion of a total of 40 degrees of flexion and extension. She presented with ulnar pain that was associated with fracture and displacement of the ulnar head implant.

Clearly the Swanson implant is not indicated in an active patient (20,315,320–322). It is not recommended in the presence of irreparable tendon ruptures or in the case of pathology that is limited to one wrist (e.g., posttraumatic arthrosis).

Total Wrist Arthroplasty Designs

The authors next consider implants that are made of rigid materials, such as cobalt-chrome, titanium, and pyrolytic carbon, with metal or ultrahigh-molecular-weight polyethylene (UHMWPE) articulations. A number of these devices have been manufactured since the 1970s. Groups that represent different concepts are considered. Within a group, the earliest prostheses are evaluated first, so that developments with time can be appreciated.

Individual Carpal Bone Implants

Silicone scaphoid and lunate implants have been available since the early 1970s (330). They have, for example, been used in the management of scaphoid nonunions, scapholunate advanced collapse wrist deformities, and Kienböck's disease. With the material change to HP 100 and increased reports of particulate synovitis (325–327,331,332), these designs came into ill repute. In addition, silicone is not able to bear or to distribute loads well, and these implants were unable to prevent progressive collapse of the carpus (333).

Titanium implants for individual scaphoid and lunate replacement, as well as a combined scapholunate unit, have now been available since the 1980s (Fig. 18). Swanson et al. (334) has continued to report favorable results in the hands that they have treated. Their use has generally been limited. Concerns regarding titanium wear against cartilage (335), implant loosening, and carpal instability have precluded a more universal acceptance of these prostheses.

The early European experience with pyrolytic carbon carpal replacements has been favorable (336). There has been no evidence of reactive synovitis or opposing cartilage wear with these implants. The indications for the use of these prostheses require further clarification. Long-term clinical results are awaited.

Ball-and-Socket Designs

Ball-and-socket implants have a single center of rotation and 3 degrees of freedom. No translation is permitted. There is little resistance to axial torque between the articulating surfaces, and little, if any, ability to transmit such loads from the hand to the forearm (13,14,48).

Gschwind-Scheier-Bahler Wrist

Gschwind and Scheier introduced the Gschwind-Scheier-Bahler wrist in 1969. The design consisted of a constrained ball and socket. They published the 6-month follow-up results of their first seven cases in 1973 (302). The authors

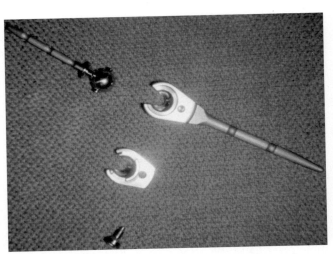

FIGURE 20. Gschwind-Scheier-Bahler prosthesis. An early concept for total wrist arthroplasty designs consisted of a constrained ball-and-socket configuration.

were unable to locate any longer-term studies or reports from other centers. Kapandji (14) made a brief reference to its design. Meuli (337) noted in a 1980 paper that it was no longer being used in its original configuration (Fig. 20).

Meuli Wrist Prosthesis

Design, Description, and Philosophy. The Meuli wrist prosthesis is one of the earliest designs and one that is used the most internationally. The original design was intended to be nonconstrained, with impingement limited to the extremes of motion. There was no axial offset of the stems, and the ball was composed of polyester (Fig. 21). Experience with this prosthesis revealed problems with progressive soft tissue imbalance and tissue reactions, with six patients out of the first 41 developing problems from the polyester (337). The prosthesis was redesigned with a slightly volar and ulnar offset to the axis and a polyethylene ball. In 1986, a third-generation Meuli wrist prosthesis (MWP III) implant was released onto the market, which is still in use. The body of this prosthesis was made from Protasul 100, which is a titanium 6–aluminium 7–niobium–wrought alloy. The surface was corundum blast finished. The ball was fixed to the proximal component and was titanium nitride coated. This articulated with a relatively deep UHMWPE Chirulen socket distally. There are two sizes for the left and the right sides, and the prosthesis can be inserted cemented or uncemented (338–340).

Meuli's design was based on the observations of Youm et al. (4,23) that the center of motion of the wrist was fairly constant and located in the head of the capitate. His design aims to recreate the lunocapitate articulation, which he deemed to be most simply represented by the ball and socket (340). Allowing movement in all planes would also alleviate rotational errors during insertion and would decrease torque stresses that are transmitted from the implant stems to the bone. In addition, as a fixed ful-

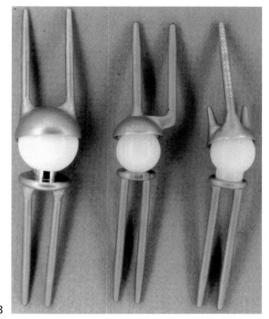
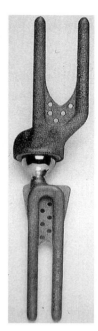

A,B

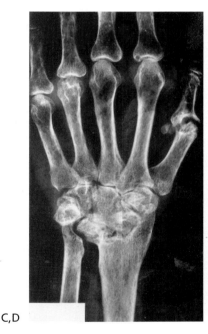
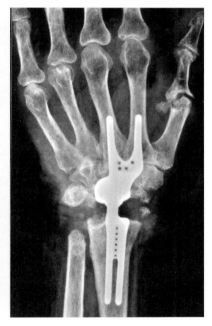

C,D

FIGURE 21. A: Examples of the Meuli wrist prosthesis through generations one through three. **B:** The newest design has an offset to better place the center of rotation of the implant and incorporates a cementless option. Trunion has been eliminated and has been replaced with a metal ball and polymer cup. **C,D:** X-rays of the third generation Meuli wrist prosthesis. Note the preservation of carpus for secure distal component fixation. Destruction of the distal radius does not conflict with good proximal component fixation.

crum implant that was made of rigid materials, it was possible to reestablish carpal height. The plan was for a nonconstrained design that limited impingement to the extremes of motion. Linscheid and Beckenbaugh (341) voiced initial concerns about the ball-and-socket design, as they viewed the wrist as essentially a biaxial joint. It was feared that the rotary axis of the prosthesis would not be able to transmit twisting motions to the forearm. This did not appear to be a significant problem in the clinical setting, and the theoretic reduction of stress transmission at the bone–cement interface was believed to be potentially beneficial (342–344).

Indications and Contraindications. Meuli mainly used his prosthesis in symptomatic rheumatoid patients. Contraindications include patients who undertake heavy work or who require the use of walking aids. Extensor tendon deficits, particularly of the wrist motors, and poor bone stock also prohibit the use of this prosthesis.

Surgical Technique. The surgical procedure is similar in most respects to that already described for the silicone hinge spacer that was designed by Swanson. Minimal bony resection of the radius is important. Early reports recommended resection of the entire scaphoid, lunate, and triquetrum, as well the proximal one-half of the capitate and hamate. This left fixation of the distal components essentially in the weak metacarpal shafts. Meuli now emphasizes the importance of an adequate carpus for primary bony fixation and support of the distal component. Current techniques attempt to preserve one-half of the scaphoid and as much triquetrum as possible so that it is stable and does not cause impingement. The capitate is also preserved, removing only enough to eliminate the proximal convex surface. Solid bone on the palmar side of the carpus is also preserved for additional implant support. The carpal component should be positioned with a 15-degree dorsal inclination within the capitate (340), and guide wires can often assist in the proper positioning of the stemmed components.

Results. Follow-up studies of the early prosthesis designs have been published by Meuli (303,308,345–347) and workers from the Mayo Clinic (341–344,348). These early to mid-term follow-up studies revealed problems primarily with soft tissue balancing. Flexion and ulnar deviation deformity occurred in six of the first 26 implants at the Mayo Clinic with the original design. With the offset design, there were eight such problems in the next 75 cases that were reported (344). Loosening did not appear to be a significant problem. The longest follow-up of these prostheses was published in 1984 by Cooney et al. (349). They reviewed the Mayo Clinic experience with 140 implants. There was an 8.6% dislocation rate. Imbalance, with recurrent ulnar deviation and flexion, occurred in 12.1% of implants. Loosening occurred in 2.9% of cases, but a progressive pattern of volar displacement of the proximal carpal component with associated dorsal tilting of the metacarpal prongs was noted in some cases. This was often associated with carpal tunnel syndrome or flexor tendon rupture, or both, or inflammation. In some cases, this was attributed to component malpositioning at the time of surgery. Subsequently, with the newer design, this pattern has also been associated with the prostheses behaving in a constrained manner with applied loads (350). For example, when gripping an object tightly, no translation is possible, and the forces are transferred to the bone–prosthesis interface. Failure occurs at the point at which this interface is weakest (351).

Two papers were identified from the investigator that dealt specifically with the MWP III implant. In 1995, a multicenter study was published that reviewed the results of 50 implants (338). Meuli's personal series (339) was published in 1997. Both studies included a large percentage of posttraumatic arthritic patients (26.7% in the multicenter report). In both reports, there were significant revision rates, the primary reason for which was distal component loosening. This was often associated with initial malpositioning of the implant. If malpositioning occurred, more than 80% of these cases showed loosening. Prosthesis constraint may also be involved in these cases as the pattern observed is similar to that discussed previously. In addition,

the deeper cup of the MWP III implant renders it inherently more constrained. Two cases were fixed solidly in the carpus but showed intrametacarpal loosening, one with stem fracture. This finding has led to the recommendation to fuse the second and third CMCs as part of the operative technique. Similar findings were reported in a third publication by Goth and Konigsberger (351).

Summary. Proper patient selection and adherence to surgical and mechanical principles impact greatly on the observed outcomes with this prosthesis. Malpositioning, particularly of the distal component, almost certainly results in loosening. This problem can be exacerbated by excessive bony resection at the time of surgery and inadequate carpal bone stock.

It appears, from a review of patients with excellent and good results, that the presence of a deficiency in the radius, as is seen in the Wrightington grade IV and in some Alnot-Fauroux stages IV and V, is not a contraindication to this prosthesis. In the author's opinion, this may be the single best indication for this implant. Other designs, yet to be discussed in this chapter, frequently require better radial bone stock for proximal component fixation.

Hamas Implant

In 1979, Hamas (352) published a report that outlined a mathematic method of determining the normal location of the axes of motion on standard radiographs so as to assist in the design and surgical placement of a TWA. This method helped advance the evolution of implant design. His resultant prosthesis was a single-stemmed ball-and-socket implant. The carpal component stem was set into the third metacarpal with a volar and ulnar offset of the socket. The proximal component was similarly offset. This not only precentered the implant but also tended to shift the hand radially, creating a less than ideal cosmetic effect. Problems were noted with distal component loosening, dorsal erosion through the metacarpal, and palmar impingement into the carpal tunnel, as with the Meuli prosthesis (353). Again, these were attributed to malpositioning on insertion. This implant is no longer available (Fig. 22).

Loda Implant

Designed in Argentina, the Loda wrist implant was originally another offset ball and socket. More constrained than the Meuli prosthesis, the components tended to impinge, with the neck of the distal ball impacting against the rim of the cylindrical cup (4). This could result in dislocation. Carpal excision was 2 cm or more, with distal component fixation occurring in the third metacarpal. Antirotation fins were included to aid in alignment of the distal component. Design revisions included a modification to allow for distal fixation within the carpus. A follow-up series was not available for review or comment. Dr. Loda is no longer actively developing his design (*personal communication,* 2001) (Fig. 23).

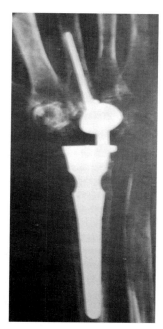

FIGURE 22. Hamas precentered total wrist arthroplasty. Developmental concepts helped advance the understanding of total wrist arthroplasty failures and influence later implant designs.

Trispherical Prosthesis

Design, Description, and Philosophy. This is a semiconstrained implant, with a ball-and-socket articulation that is traversed by a fixed axle. It is designed to provide 15 degrees of combined radial and ulnar deviation, 90 degrees of flexion, 80 degrees of extension, and 10 degrees of axial rotation. The components are manufactured from titanium with an UHMWPE bearing surface. The fixation point of the distal component is in the third metacarpal, with a short stem for antirotation fitting into the second metacarpal base (Fig. 24). The radial component articulating surface is offset towards the ulna to aid in center-of-rotation alignment. This component also recreates the 12-degree palmar tilt of the native distal radius.

Results. Follow-up results have only been published by the developing group. Initial reports considered the results of 22 arthroplasties in 20 patients with RA. The best results were obtained with a 40% to 60% restoration of carpal

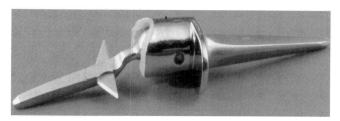

FIGURE 23. The Loda total wrist arthroplasty uses a ball-and-socket construct with distal fins for fixation and alignments.

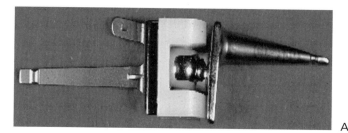

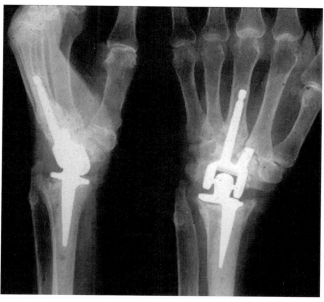

FIGURE 24. A: Example of the trispherical implant with antirotation stem and axle to add stability to what is essentially a ball-and-socket articulation. **B:** X-rays of trispherical total wrist arthroplasty. (Courtesy of Dr. Alan Inglis.)

height and seating of the radial component such that the center of rotation was volar to the medullary canal axis (354,355). This is in marked contradistinction to other ball-and-socket designs in which balanced alignment in the radioulnar plane is a better predictor of good results. The authors' opinion was that the implant's soft constraints against excess radial and ulnar deviation, as well as the mobile center of rotation, could account for this difference.

In 1990, the group reported further follow-up results (356). This report included 35 implants with a follow-up of as long as 11 years (with a mean of 108 months). Pain relief was excellent in 30 of the 35 wrists. They had one case of frank loosening of the distal component, although seven implants demonstrated lucency around the metacarpal stems. They had undertaken one revision for persistent pain. There were six cases of postoperative extensor tendon attrition, all of whom had preoperative tendon ruptures that were reconstructed with tendon transfers. This represented a 40% attrition rate in such patients (6 of 15).

In 1995, Kraay and Figgie (357) calculated a 93% survivorship at 10 and 12 years in 65 consecutive trispherical total wrist procedures. However, the same group, from the

Hospital for Special Surgery (HSS), reported less favorable results in 1997 (358). At this point, they noted a 9% revision rate at an average of 8.7 years (with a range from 3 to 18 years) in 87 implants. Of the 87 implants, one had been revised for sepsis, and five were revised for metacarpal loosening with dorsal cortical perforation. Two patients had developed extensor tendon ruptures without a prior history of tendon attrition. One patient had radial component loosening secondary to incorrect placement. In 1999, O'Flynn et al. (359) presented a case report of a failure of the hinge mechanism with severe synovitis that was associated with titanium wear debris.

Summary. The present recommendations of the investigators include modifications of the published surgical technique (360). They now advocate fusion of the third CMC and insertion of the metacarpal stem beyond one-half the length of the bone. Despite these changes in surgical technique, the authors believe that distal component loosening may continue to be a clinical problem with this design. Poor distal fixation and constrained articulation remain significant mechanical concerns with this design.

Universal Joint Designs

Universal joint design implants incorporate articulations that result in motion with 2 degrees of freedom. There are varying amounts of constraint, depending on the specific implant arrangement. The general trend, as is observed from the presentation below, is toward an ellipsoidal design.

Volz Wrist

Design, Description, and Philosophy. Although no longer in general usage, discussion of the Volz implant is appropriate. It was one of the earliest implants and was also the first to attempt to recreate the biaxial motion of the wrist (304). Volz developed the implant in 1973. The articulation is toroidal, that is, it has two radii of curvature. One radius of curvature has an axis that is orientated in the FEM plane and the other radius has an axis in the RUD plane. Both axes were somewhat radially placed compared to the normal wrist. Essentially, no axial rotation or translation in the radioulnar plane is allowed. The implant allowed for 90 degrees of combined flexion and extension and 50 degrees of RUD. The initial design had two distal prongs for insertion into the second and third metacarpals. In 1977, this design was modified to a single distal prong, which was inserted into the third metacarpal. This stem was also offset dorsally to attempt to improve the alignment of the axes of rotation (Fig. 25).

Surgical Technique. The surgical technique for the Volz implant was similar to previously described techniques. The proximal carpal row was completely excised with the capitate resection at the level of the lesser multangular. Distal fixation

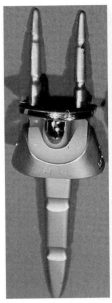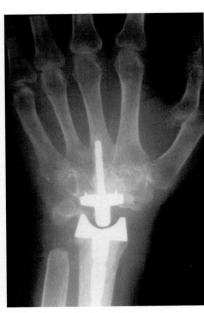

A,B

FIGURE 25. A: Example of the Volz wrist implant, which is a transition from a ball-and-socket design to a biaxial-universal type of articulation. The original design was not precentered in the radioulnar plane. **B:** X-ray of a single stem configuration.

was primarily in the metacarpals. In 1984, a full description of the surgical technique was offered (361). It involved a radial elevation of the retinaculum and noted the requirement to gain full extension of the wrist on the table with a trial implant *in situ*. If this requirement was not satisfied, additional soft tissue or bone resection was recommended.

Results. Volz developed the implant in 1973 and first reported on 17 prostheses (304). The longest follow-up in this study was 13 months. Ulnar deviation was noted in the majority of RA patients but not in those patients with a diagnosis of posttraumatic arthritis. Good results were reported in a preliminary report by Lamberta et al. (362). In a multicenter review that was published in 1977, Volz (363) reported 33% postoperative ulnar deviation, mostly in the RA population. He supposed that the radial displacement of the axes of rotation gave advantage to the ulnar-side wrist flexors and extensors. He recommended flexor carpi ulnaris tenotomy along with release of the palmaris longus.

Several studies with longer follow-up times report progressive deterioration (312,344,364–367). Dennis et al. (365) found 79% of implants had radiographic signs of bone resorption beneath the collar of the radial component. They also documented a 24% rate of loosening and settling of the distal component into the carpus. In addition, 28% were judged to be imbalanced, although this was a much more prominent problem with the original double-pronged prosthesis. Overall, they reported five dislocations in 30 prostheses (17%). Two were early, two were traumatic, and one was chronic. Some problems with flexor tendon inflammation and carpal tunnel syndrome were also encountered.

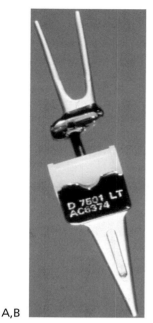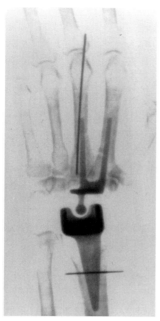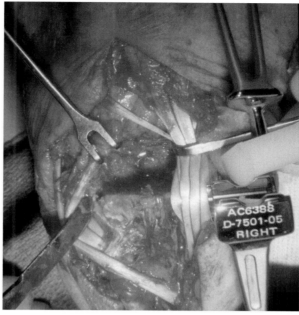

A,B   C

FIGURE 26. **A:** Example of the Weber-Mayo implant. Two areas of articulation to reproduce radioulnar deviation at the metacarpal-poly interface, and flexion-extension motion at the poly-radial component interface. The large size of the radial component and poly resulted in volar impingement and flexor tendon erosions. **B:** X-ray of the implant device. The axes of implant were precentered to reproduce the center of rotation of wrist. **C:** Clinical appearance before insertion at surgery. Note that bone resection was required.

Weber-Mayo Total Wrist Arthroplasty

The Weber-Mayo total wrist arthroplasty implant was devised in the late 1970s and early 1980s. There were two sites of motion (Fig. 26). RUD occurred between the metallic metacarpal component and the polyethylene cylinder. Proximally, the polyethylene cylinder articulated with the radial component allowing for flexion and extension. The concept was to design an implant that would accurately reproduce the center of rotation (as it was understood to exist at the time). This was accomplished by offsetting the radial and metacarpal components toward the ulna. The metacarpal stem was also displaced in a palmar direction. To unload the fixation interfaces, the device was constructed so as to dislocate at the extremes of motion.

Problems with the implant included dislocation in the immediate postoperative period that was due to distraction of the components from swelling. The radial component also proved to be too large in some patients, thus resulting in flexor tendon erosion. Unusually, the best results were reported in patients with OA. The longest surviving implant lasted for 18 years in an active mechanic (Dr. Ed Weber, *personal communication*, 2001).

Guépar Prosthesis

Design, Description, and Philosophy. The Guépar implant was remarkable in two respects. First, it was the earliest design to use a minimally constrained elliptical geometry to mimic the RC articulation. Second, it addressed the funda-mental problem of distal component fixation in a new way. It comprised a high-density polyethylene radial component with ulnar articular offset. The metal distal component was mounted, by using a microscrew, onto a plate that was screwed into the distal carpus and the second and third metacarpals. It was cemented in place (368).

Indications. The device was only implanted into patients with wrists that were "destroyed and dislocated in both planes" (Alnot-Fauroux stages IV and V; interpretation of the authors). All of the patients had RA. By the time of their review of cases extending to 10 years, the investigators concluded that "TWA be reserved for old patients."

Results. The original report was of 45 arthroplasties that were performed between 1979 and 1986 (369). The review was of 32 implants in 28 patients, with an average follow-up of 2.5 years (with a range from 1.0 to 7.5 years). There were nine poor results: five were stiff, and four were loose or dislocated. Two cases had been revised for progressive subsidence of the carpal component, and 18 (56%) had radiologic loosening.

In 1996, Fourastier et al. (370) reported on 72 Guépar TWAs in 64 patients. The longest follow-up was 10 years. Eleven wrists had been revised (15%). By this stage, problems had been encountered with radial component loosening, which was conjectured to be occurring secondary to polyethylene wear. A "constant and evolving" process of bone resorption from beneath the carpal component also occurred, with

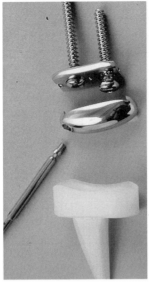 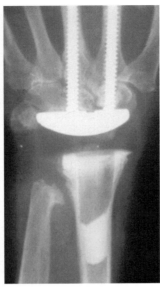

A,B

FIGURE 27. A: Example of an unarticulated Guépar wrist implant with component parts. The microscrew proved a problem with loosening. Distal component fixation in metacarpals led to loosening and osteolysis according to the investigators. **B:** Anteroposterior x-ray of the Guépar implant.

frequent loosening of the microscrew holding the two distal components together. Micromotion between these two parts was proposed as a possible cause of this loosening. They alluded to the need to reconsider the concept of metacarpal fixation (Fig. 27).

Clayton-Ferlic-Volz Prosthesis

In 1988, the original investigators of the Volz implant completely redeveloped their design with the intent of reducing the incidence of imbalance, loosening, and bone resorption that was seen with their earlier implants (371). The new concept was much less constrained than the original, using an elliptical articular surface. This was similar in shape to the Guépar prostheses except that the convex surface was on the radial component rather than the metacarpal component (Fig. 28). The articular surfaces were offset to facilitate wrist balance. Cementless fixation was an option, as the surface was sandblasted. Modular elements were available to optimize the press fit of the radial component. Significant bone resection (2 cm) was still required in most cases. The design still depended mostly on fixation within the third metacarpal for distal component support.

In 1995, Ferlic and Clayton (371) reported the results of 15 of these implants in nine patients between 1988 and 1993. There were four failures due to distal prosthesis loosening and imbalance. Marketing was discontinued in 1993.

Cardan-Type Implant

In 1982, Kapandji (372) published a paper that discussed the biomechanics of the wrist with regard to possible wrist prosthesis designs. He asserted that the wrist is best represented as a universal joint with two axes of motion and two degrees of freedom. Although the overall geometry of the RC joint is condylar (biconvex surface), he felt that a sellar (concave-convex surface or negative toroid) design was more appropriate for a wrist implant. The basis was the need for a low fit coefficient with the condylar design (e.g., Guépar) to permit the desired motion envelope. As condylar and sellar geometries constitute universal joints, he believed that they would be interchangeable in the context of prosthesis design. The advantage of the sellar design, as he saw it, was that it would allow for a higher surface contact area during certain motions, particularly axial rotation (Fig. 29). This, in turn, was considered to allow more efficient load transmission from the hand to the forearm. Designs with less contact would rely more

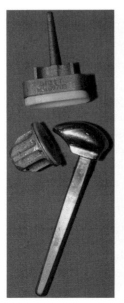 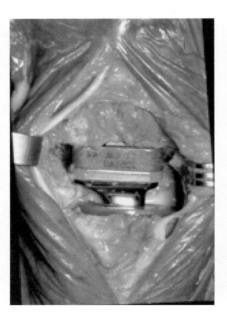 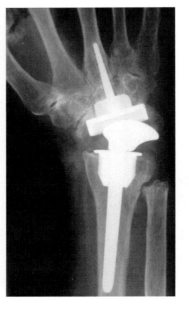

A–C

FIGURE 28. A: Example of the Clayton-Ferlic-Volz prosthesis. It had a modular design, with a cementless option, but required significant bone resection (usually more than 2 cm) **(B)** and had the major distribution of the distal component fixation within the third metacarpal **(C)**.

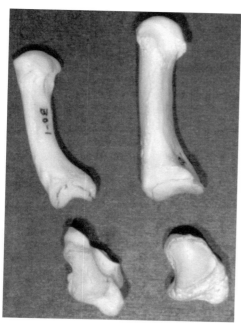

FIGURE 29. Skeletons of a chimpanzee **(left)** and a human **(right)** carpometacarpal thumb joint that show the smaller radius of curvature of the chimpanzee thumb, which is associated with greater inherent stability, which is necessitated by the fact that it is surrounded by smaller muscles, and the chimpanzee's requirement for stability over dexterity and range of motion. (Courtesy of Dr. Mary Marzke.)

heavily on the soft tissue constraints of the wrist to transmit torque loads (as is noted in the normal wrist). These soft tissues are often weakened in patients who undergo wrist arthroplasty and are not able to withstand such loading repetitively. Failure of these soft tissues could result in progressive soft tissue imbalance and dislocations. Another theoretical advantage was that the articulation would feel more normal to the patient and would facilitate improved grasp.

One possible disadvantage of this articulation has been highlighted by Roux et al. (48). He noted that similar designs might generate stress at the bone implant interface and promote implant loosening. Prototype designs were presented. Two drawings were shown, one of which had an additional component for the DRUJ.

Gagey et al. (373) performed a force analysis study on 25 cadavers in 1986. He used this to develop a graphic model of the wrist. A two-component prosthesis with a toroidal articulation was then tested (not the Kapandji design). This showed similar force patterns to the normal wrist when an equivalent ROM was produced. One male patient was mentioned who had received this implant. He had been followed for 1 year, and the result was described as "satisfactory" up to that point. No further clinical data are available, as far as the authors have been able to establish.

Taleisnik Implant

Taleisnik discussed prerequisites that he felt were vital for a successful TWA design in his textbook *The Wrist* (374). He

felt that the approximate overall center of rotation of an implant should be ulnar and palmar to the central axis of the radius to align it with the perceived center of rotation of the normal wrist. The design should be "self-centering" to allow it to find its own balance and should allow reproduction of the "dart thrower's" or "ballistic" motion pattern of the wrist, as previously described by himself. There should be minimal shear loads at the cement–bone or implant–bone interface. He advocated a ROM that was reduced to less than 50% of normal to increase stability and durability. As for all orthopedic procedures, there must be an option for salvage in the event of surgical failure. This usually means conversion to an arthrodesis, which is facilitated by minimizing initial bone resection.

His proposed design contained an articulation that was ovoid rather than ellipsoidal. This was in an attempt to create similar radii for FEM and RUD by bringing their axes of motion closer together. A theoretical advantage of this design is, again, potentially increased contact surface area during motion. The distal component was planned to be metal, and the proximal component was polyethylene. The articulations were offset as he had recommended. As with many other prostheses, the distal component fixation relied primarily on the stem within the third metacarpal, which, as the authors have seen, has often proven inadequate (Fig. 30). No clinical follow-up data using such a prosthesis were identified.

Biaxial Prosthesis

Design, Description, and Philosophy. The biaxial prosthesis was developed between 1978 and 1982 at the Mayo

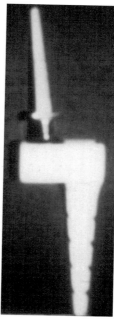

FIGURE 30. Example of Taleisnik total wrist arthroplasty implant. Like the Guépar implant, it used a polyethylene radial component. It was self-centering for improved balance. Distal component fixation is primarily in the metacarpals.

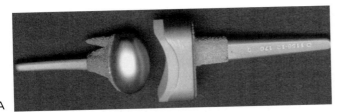

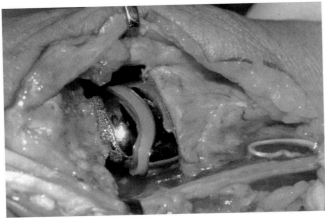

FIGURE 31. A,B: Biaxial total wrist arthroplasty. Note the ellipsoidal articulating surfaces and the nonconstrained design. Fixation of distal component with original surgical technique was primarily within the third metacarpal.

Clinic (344). The design again comprised elliptical articulating surfaces with minimal constraint. The prosthesis stems have porous-coated surfaces. The radial element is a metal-backed concave polyethylene. The articulating surface has ulnar and palmar offset (Fig. 31). The distal component has a single long stem for insertion into the third metacarpal and a small stud that is inserted in the trapezoid to increase rotational stability. The articular surface is a convex metal ellipse. There were originally three sizes. Modifications to the size of the stud and the metacarpal stem have taken place over the years. Long-stemmed and multipronged implants were created in an attempt to address the high incidence of loosening of the distal component, as well as the need for a revision prosthesis. In such cases, there is often severe deficiency of carpal bone stock (Fig. 32). Design changes and modification of the fixation of the distal component are currently under review.

Operative Technique. The biaxial prosthesis surgery has been fully outlined in texts (312), and the essential features are reviewed in a paper by Cobb and Beckenbaugh that was published in 1996 (375). Some differentiating features are summarized.

The retinaculum is opened over the fourth dorsal compartment. Fourth compartment tendons are retracted ulnarward, with radial retraction of the extensor pollicis longus, the ECRL, and the extensor carpi radialis brevis (ECRB). Beckenbaugh removes Lister's tubercle. He recommends always removing the distal ulna just proximal to the sigmoid notch. The distal ulna should be exposed subperiosteally, with a 1-mm flap of capsule and soft tissue left on the radial rim. The authors have found that some patients with posttraumatic DJD develop discomfort at the resection site from convergence of the stump of the distal ulna against the radius. To avoid this, the authors have often not performed a distal ulna resection if neither pain nor pathology at the DRUJ can be demonstrated. This is only possible if the necessary resection of the distal radius does not interfere with DRUJ function and the sigmoid

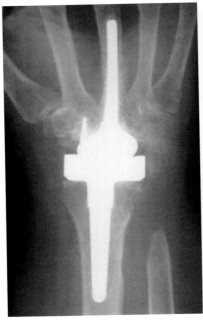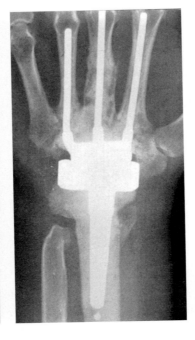

FIGURE 32. Revision components of the biaxial total wrist arthroplasty. The longer stems **(A)** and the multipronged design **(B)** help compensate for carpal bone deficiency.

notch. The standard approach has been to remove sufficient carpus to fit the largest implant possible, thus removing the entire proximal pole of the scaphoid and significant parts of the capitate and hamate. Modifications of this technique, in which a smaller size implant is templated and more carpus is preserved (distal scaphoid, and most of capitate and hamate), allow for fixation of the implant in the carpus and the stem to just pass across the third CMC. Van Leeuwen, as reported by Beckenbaugh (350), now prefers this approach. The authors have also added fusion of the second and third CMCs and intercarpal fusion to the authors' technique not only for the biaxial prosthesis, but also for all of the authors' wrist implants.

The group has developed a postoperative program based on the intraoperative clinical tightness of the fit of the implant. With a tight fit, motion can be started as soon as wound healing permits with limited use of a removable splint. With a loose fit, a short arm cast may be used for as long as 6 weeks. With a so-called normal fit, the wrist is splinted for 2 weeks before initiating protective ROM. Splinting is carried out for an additional 4 weeks, or as deemed necessary by repeat assessment of joint stability. Although a dynamic splinting protocol is uncommonly necessary, one has been published by Johnson et al. (376).

Results. An early report first emerged in 1990 (377) and was followed by a minimum 5-year follow-up study in 1996 (374). As with other TWAs, complete pain relief was documented in 75% of patients. Of 46 implants in living patients, with a mean follow-up of 6.5 years, there were noted to be 11 failures (24%) that required reoperation. Eight of these failures were due to carpal component loosening, one had dislocated, and one was significantly imbalanced. Twenty cases (43%) had radiographic evidence of subsidence of the distal component. Evidence of subsidence at 1 year postsurgery was correlated to subsequent failure. Resting stance was considered abnormal in 21 cases. Grip strength increased from 4.1 kg preoperatively to 5.9 kg at the latest follow-up.

Lirette and Kinnard reported on 15 implants (378). All patients had RA. Mean follow-up was 54 months. All of the patients were rated as good to excellent by the HSS scoring system (Table 5). Four implants (26.7%) had radiologic evidence of loosening. There was one dislocation.

The Wrightington group reviewed a series of 26 patients, mainly with a diagnosis of RA (379). The follow-up was 24 to 62 months. Sixty-nine percent were rated as good or excellent using the HSS scoring system. Radiolucencies were observed around three carpal and two radial components. There was one immediate postoperative dislocation, which was treated uneventfully with closed reduction and 8 weeks of immobilization. The authors felt that continuation of the use of the biaxial prostheses in selected cases was warranted. Publications that consider the results of revision surgery after biaxial TWA, as well as revision

TABLE 5. HOSPITAL FOR SPECIAL SURGERY WRIST SCORING SYSTEM

	Points
Pain level on the visual analogue scale	50
None (0)	
Slight (1–3)	45
Moderate (4–6)	25
Severe (7–10)	0
Function	
Stable arc >40 degrees	30
Stable arc >20 degrees	25
Stable neutral	20
Unstable for power use	10
Unstable	0
Range of motion	
Flexion (1 point for each 5 degrees)	Maximum = 10
Extension (1 point for each 5 degrees)	Maximum = 10
Total	
All points	100

Note: The Hospital for Special Surgery scoring system is used to evaluate wrist implant arthroplasty results. An excellent score is 90 to 100 points, a good score is 80 to 89 points, a fair score is 70 to 79 points, and a poor score is less than 70 points.

from other primary designs that use the revision biaxial components, are available (311,312,350,377,380,381).

Summary. Beckenbaugh discussed his experiences with this prosthesis at the American Society for Surgery of the Hand conference in 2000. He estimated that a 20% revision rate should be anticipated at 5 years postsurgery when using this prosthesis. Most of these show evidence of distal element loosening. He has several patients who still have functioning implants 20 years after surgery. Grip strength has been improved, carpal height has been increased, and hand to forearm balance has been enhanced. Overall, the mid-term results with this prosthesis are an improvement on anything that has been previously reported but are still far from satisfactory.

Menon Prosthesis

Design, Description, and Philosophy. The Menon prosthesis was designed by the late Jay Menon in the middle 1980s (Fig. 33). Its most important feature lies in its method of addressing the problem of distal component loosening. This was done by returning to the concept of screw fixation, which was first seen in the Guépar prosthesis. In addition, the Menon prosthesis can be inserted with minimal bone resection, thus allowing a greater hold in the residual carpus, particularly the capitate rather than in the metacarpals. Another design feature that is emphasized is the carpal base plate. This plate supports the second to fifth rays and facilitates axial load transmission. The articular surface of the radial component is inclined at 20 degrees to the long axis, thus simulating the normal anatomy. Menon felt this feature would encourage less bone resection and facilitate rebalancing. This component no longer has the central

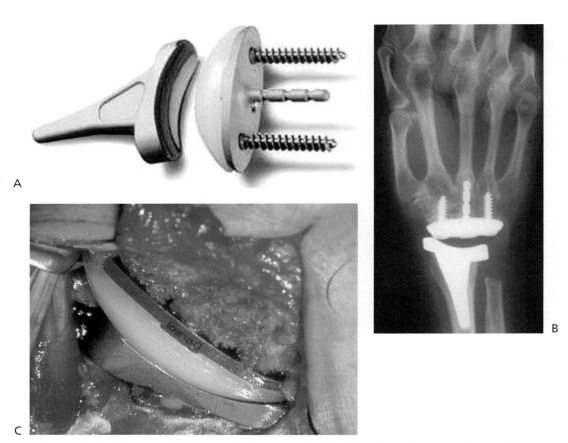

FIGURE 33. A: Menon-KMI-Universal wrist prosthesis (Kinetikos Medical, Inc., San Diego, CA). Note the incline of the radial component to mimic normal anatomy. **B:** In the author's experience, resection of the distal ulna is the most often required. **C:** The convex polyethylene surface has not shown itself to be a problem, even long term. No evidence of distal component loosening has yet been reported. Note the bone graft to secure intercarpal fusion.

stem mesh, as initially described (382,383). The implant is manufactured from a titanium alloy. The central plastic component is convex and ellipsoid and slides onto the distal plate once it has been screwed in place. Different sizes of polyethylene are available to adjust the soft tissue tension preoperatively. Owing to U.S. Food and Drug Administration (FDA) requirements, the original fixation configuration of the distal component, using three screws, was converted to two screws and a fixed central peg. The prosthesis can be inserted with or without cement. However, it is recommended that the radial component, as presently configured, be cemented.

The Universal2 (Kinetikos Medical, Inc., San Diego, CA), now available, represents the efforts of Dr. Brian Adams. He has made changes in the original design to improve stability and ease of insertion. The authors have had the opportunity to insert this implant on several occasions, including in a revision of a chronically dislocated original design of the Menon prosthesis (Fig. 34).

The modifications in the design now allow for the distal and radial components to be inserted without the use of cement. The ulnar inclination has been decreased to 14

degrees. The shape of the ellipsoid surfaces has been altered to decrease the tendency for point contact. An additional lip on the radial component facet increases the anterior-posterior stability of the articulated implant. A bevel on the ulnar side of the radial component now allows for the option, in selected cases, of preserving the ulnar head. New preparation guides allow for more accurate and reproducible bone cuts and insertion of the implant.

Surgical Technique. The surgical approach is similar to those techniques described previously. Menon (382,383) preferred a step-cut exposure for the extensor retinaculum. There are templates and jigs that assist the surgeon in making accurate bone cuts, which are much improved for the Universal2. Minimal carpal resection is undertaken. The aim is to produce a bony edge that is perpendicular to the long axis of the metacarpals just through the base of the capitate. Adams has suggested passing a small Steinmann pin transversely across the carpus before using the oscillating saw (*personal communication*). This reduces the incidence of shattering of the bones and allows improved control of the carpal resection. Part of the scaphoid and tri-

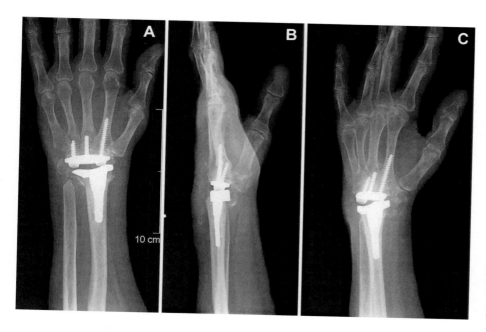

FIGURE 34. Postsurgical view of revision of a failed total wrist arthroplasty using the Universal2 implant. Anteroposterior **(A)**, lateral **(B)**, and oblique views **(C)**.

quetrum should remain after the resection. Intercarpal fusion is a fundamental part of the surgical technique. Bone grafting to restore carpal height or to add bone stock for the carpal component fixation can be accomplished with corticocancellous graft, if indicated. The central peg is inserted in line with the third metacarpal shaft by using image intensification. A radial screw is inserted into the scaphoid through the trapezoid and across the second CMC. An ulnar screw crosses the residual triquetrum and passes into the hamate.

The indications of this implant, according to Dr. Adams, include patients with RA, traumatic arthritis, scapholunate advanced collapse wrist, and OA. It is believed that this implant is potentially indicated for revision of a failed implant. Sufficient bone stock, and soft tissue supports (intact extensor tendons) are required. The use of templates assists in preoperative planning of proper size. Precautions include not having the carpal component extending more than 2 mm over the margins of the carpus at the level of the osteotomy. The radial component should not extend beyond the radial styloid. The angle that is formed by the ulnar portion of its collar should lie near the edge of the sigmoid notch. Fluoroscopy has been helpful for the authors, and its use is recommended.

Dr. Adams has been influential in the design of a sophisticated set of instrumentation to assist in bone preparation. One key, as noted previously, is temporary Kirschner wire fixation of the carpus, if it is unstable, to facilitate bone resection. The other recommendation is the need to excise the lunate before use of the carpal guide. Also, as per Dr. Adams' surgical technique manual, by using a bone awl, a hole can be made through the articular surface of the radius approximately 5 mm below its dorsal rim and just radial to Lister's tubercle. Efforts should be made not to cross the fourth CMC with the ulnar screw.

Results. In 1998, Menon (383) reviewed the results of 37 implants in 31 patients. The follow-up time was 48 to 120 months with a mean of 6.7 years. It is not clear how many of these prostheses used the original configuration of three screws for distal fixation. Eighty-eight percent had excellent pain relief. There were no cases of distal component loosening. There were two cases of radial component loosening that occurred without cement. They were successfully treated by reimplantation with cement. There were five dislocations (14%). Open reduction was required for three of the five cases. This was followed by application of an external fixator for 6 weeks. One patient underwent a closed reduction, and the last patient was revised to an arthrodesis. There was a good long-term outcome in all of these cases. Sollerman et al. (384) have also reported no evidence of distal component loosening with this implant in their first 12 cases.

A multicenter review was presented by Adams (385) at the International Federation of Societies for Surgery of the Hand meeting in 2001. He recorded a 9% incidence of dislocation that occurred in a series of 53 patients. A recent publication by Divelbiss et al. (386) confirms the positive experiences of Sollerman and Adams with this prosthesis. The major issue of concern remains prosthesis dislocation, which leads the authors to recommend that the implant is contraindicated in certain patients with loose type RA and severe bone loss. One patient, who was identified after publication, is showing signs of carpal component loosening. However, this does not appear to be a significant overall problem with this implant or with the newer Universal2.

Summary. Dislocation seemed to be the major clinical problem with this minimally constrained implant and this needed to be addressed (387). The Universal2, with its improved preparation guides and design modifications, appears in early experience to have lessened these concerns

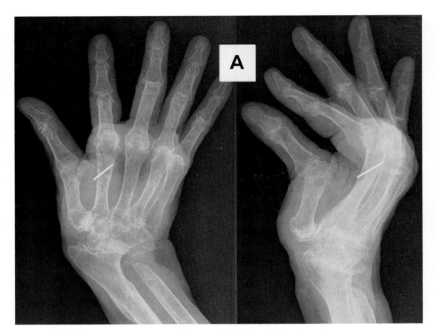

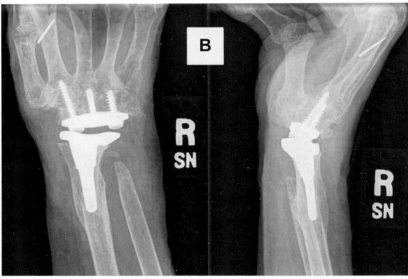

FIGURE 35. A: Preoperative view that demonstrates a patient with severe rheumatoid arthritis that was complicated by a healed distal radial fracture that was associated with a severe deformity. **B:** A 6-month postsurgical view of the patient that demonstrated stable functioning range of motion with excellent axial alignment.

(Fig. 35). Certain other possible disadvantages of this prosthesis are perceived. The plastic component is convex. In spite of some concern in the literature (388), no undue wear of the polyethylene has been observed unless there was initial malalignment of the components (Leonard Sheldon Bodell, personal experience of 17 patients with prototypes of the implant). In the authors' experience, the inclination of the radial cut has not been uniformly advantageous. It has not been found to facilitate soft tissue balancing; indeed, a higher percentage of cases that used this implant have required formal flexor carpi ulnaris lengthening than has been the authors' experience with other prostheses. Again, one sees this concern having been addressed by Adams with the new design. It is possible, however, that it is preferable to obtain soft tissue balancing in this way in

these patients and to aim to restore carpal height rather than resorting to excessive bony resection when tissues have contracted. Another possible disadvantage is that the obliquity of the radial cut almost always mandates some resection of the distal ulna. This is no longer the case when using the Universal2 (Fig. 36). In patients with DJD or posttraumatic arthritis in whom the DRUJ is asymptomatic, it may be optimal to leave this joint undisturbed. Some surgeons have not found this to be the case (Dr. Brian Adams, *personal communication*).

Despite these reservations, the results for this prosthesis as of 2003 are far better than any other design. Marc Garcia-Elias (*personal communication*, 2001) commented that this implant might be considered as the gold standard of TWAs as treatment moves into the twenty-first century.

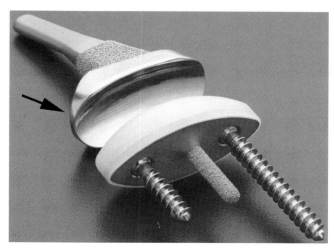

FIGURE 36. The Universal2 implant, with the ulnar side *(arrow)* of the radial component redesigned to allow for preservation, when indicated, of the ulnar head.

RWS Prosthesis

The RWS prosthesis design consists of a semiconstrained three-element device (Fig. 37). There is a radial component of variable thickness UHMWPE, which sits into a metal tray. The radial articular surface is offset in a volar and ulnar direction. The configuration encourages preservation of the radial styloid and, thus, the RSC ligament. It incorporates a resection that is perpendicular to the long axis of

the radius (thus differing from the Menon prosthesis). The metacarpal component has a single stem, which is fixed into the third metacarpal. There is an additional screw, which passes into the second metacarpal. The base of this component rests on the capitate, rather than across the entire remaining distal carpus. The metal is Vitallium.

The mechanics of this articulation seem to have similarities with the Volz and biaxial implants in some ways. A narrow convex element moves within a somewhat crescentic concave element, rather like the Volz implant. There appears to be a higher contact surface area, however, compared to the Volz, which may increase stability. The implant allows for almost 100 degrees of FEM, 40 degrees of RUD, and minimal axial rotation. At the extremes of these ranges, the mechanism impinges on itself to resist further movement. This again is designed to add stability to the construct, hopefully to reduce dislocation rates. These features are reminiscent of the biaxial joint, with a soft block to allow axial torque transmission yet minimize risk of dislocation.

Rozing (389,390) has reported a follow-up of 1 to 6 years with 18 of his implants. All but one had mild or no pain. Three cases of carpal tunnel syndrome developed after 1 year but were not attributed to volar implant impingement or particulate synovitis. One patient was converted to an arthrodesis for unspecified reasons. There was one radial and one carpal revision due to implant loosening. The authors question the present usefulness of TWA in patients with DJD or posttraumatic arthritis.

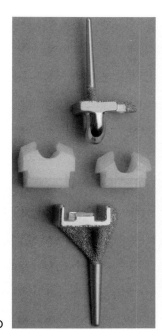
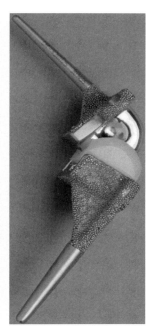
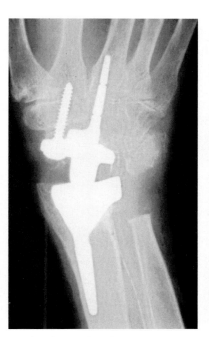
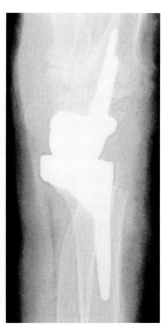

D

FIGURE 37. A–D: Rozing implant. Articulation for this implant has greater constraints than for some other implants in present usage. Technique can preserve the sigmoid notch and can allow for retention of distal ulna, in cases in which it is appropriate to do so. This implant has similar articulation kinematics to the Volz implant but with end point blocks to discourage dislocation. (Courtesy of Dr. P. M. Rozing.)

Anatomic Physiologic Wrist Prosthesis

This anatomic physiologic wrist prosthesis is a cementless design of cobalt-chrome with a hydroxyapatite coating. The articulation is elliptical with titanium nitrite–coated metal-to-metal surfaces. The radial component's articular surface has a 10-degree slope toward the ulna. The carpal component has a central stem for fixation via the capitate into the third metacarpal. Smaller prongs on either side of this central stem fix into the residual carpus. These stems are inserted perpendicular to the shaft of the third metacarpal. This base is attached to a mobile bearing surface that is inclined 10 degrees toward the radius. This arrangement is designed to approximate the proximal carpal row and the radiocarpal articulation (Fig. 38).

The designers published an 18-month follow-up of 30 patients with RA who had undergone TWA with this implant (391). Carpal height measurements, as calculated by Youm and Flatt (4), were improved from 0.31 to 0.52. There was no radiographic evidence of loosening at that early stage. Two patients experienced dislocations, one of which was of the carpal component. Early results are promising, but follow-up is short. It must be remembered that, although many complications occur in the first year, often due to technical issues, deterioration of results, consequent to previously unappreciated problems of the material or the design features of the implant, may not occur for several years.

Osseointegration Swedish Design

In 1997, Lundborg and Branemark (392) presented their early experiences with their wrist arthroplasty designs. This paper also included a discussion of the principles and viability of osseous integration in relation to wrist arthroplasty. This represented a continuation of earlier published work on osseointegration (393) and their experience with uncemented finger implants (394,395).

The wrist implants were individually designed for each of the six patients who were reported. The joint configuration was of a modified ball and socket. An adaptation was made for replacement of the distal ulna in three cases with instability. The follow-up times for this small series ranged from 4.0 to 6.5 years. All of the patients achieved satisfactory pain relief and maintenance of a functional ROM. There were no clinical cases of loosening, and no bony resorption was visible on the radiographs; however, some scattered lytic zones can sometimes be seen around some of the titanium screws.

The authors have had the opportunity to review one of Lundborg's patients with him (*personal communication*). This patient had his surgery 9 years before the discussion. Review of the 9-year postoperative radiographs (Fig. 39) continues to show excellent fixation proximately and distally. This is in spite of severe osteopenia and loss of bone stock, a condition of the underlying disease. The patient was functioning well.

Lundborg's group has shown that osseointegration can succeed even in patients with poor bone stock or inflammatory arthritis. Such fixation techniques seem to hold promise, in combination with other strategies, for improving prosthesis fixation in the future. This implant concept may

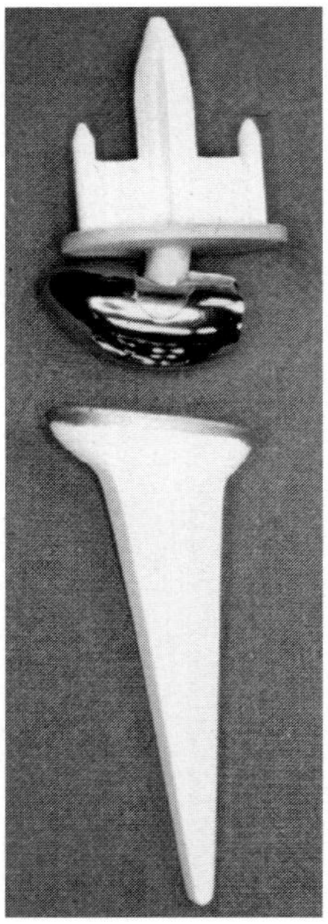

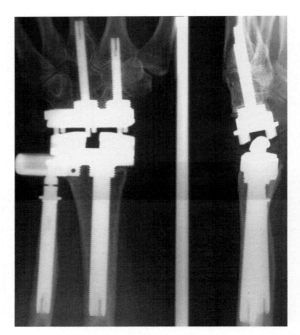

FIGURE 38. New-generation prosthesis design that uses a titanium metal-on-metal articulation construct. Fixation is distally within the carpus if bone can be preserved. The question of whether the radial design causes the center of rotation to be shifted distally remains.

FIGURE 39. X-ray of a 9-year follow-up of patient with osseointegrated Swedish design total wrist arthroplasty. Note that, in spite of poor bone quality, there is no evident implant loosening. (Courtesy of Dr. Göran Lundborg.)

prove suitable as a revision or as a salvage in advanced cases of Simmen group 3.

House Wrist Prosthesis

Menon makes reference to the House wrist prosthesis (382). No published reports were found for review.

The design features a double articulation. A polyethylene interface snap fits over the spherical head of the carpal component. RUD is intended to occur between the head of the carpal component and the polyethylene. FEM is intended to occur at the junction of the polyethylene and the radial component. There is the potential to incorporate and reconstruct the DRUJ. There is an ulnar offset to the radial component's articular surface. The carpal component has a long stem for the third metacarpal, a shorter stem for the second metacarpal, and an ulnar-sided stud (Fig. 40). Potential complications with this construct would seem to be loosening of the distal component with dorsal metacarpal perforation and assembly of the construct during implantation.

Avanta Prosthesis

The Avanta prosthesis is still under development and is a cooperative effort between several clinicians (A. Gupta, W. Cooney, and L. S. Bodell) and Avanta Orthopaedics (San Diego, CA). The implant incorporates a carpal base plate

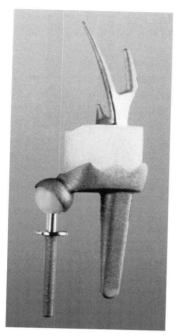

FIGURE 40. House prosthesis. This prosthesis has a complex design, with option for reconstruction of distal radioulnar joint, and two articulating interfaces for radioulnar deviation and flexion-extension motion. (From Menon J. Total wrist arthroplasty. In: Watson HK, Weinzweig J, ed. *The wrist.* Philadelphia: Lippincott Williams & Wilkins, 2001, with permission.)

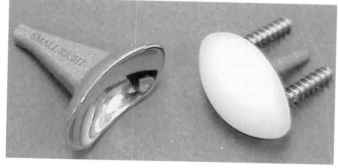

A

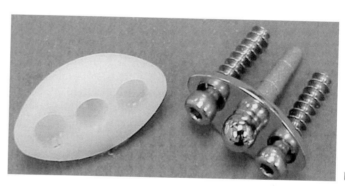

B

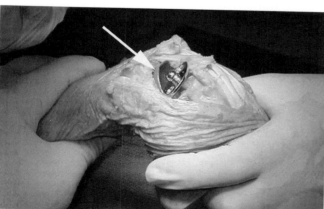

C

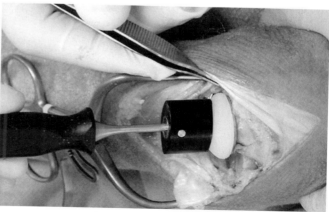

D

FIGURE 41. A: The Avanta implant assembled. **B:** The implant, showing the articulation of the polyethylene insert to the carpal plate that allows for rotation. **C,D:** Intraoperative photo of impaction of the polyethylene component, with the radial component (*arrow*) sitting inside the radial cortical shell as opposed to sitting on the radius, as in other components.

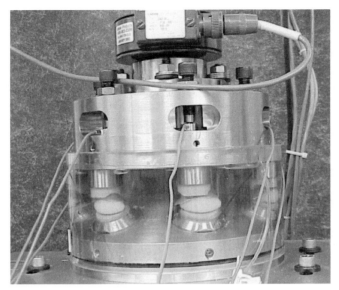

FIGURE 42. Apparatus that was used during the laboratory testing of the Avanta implant in which the data were used during the Food and Drug Administration application review.

to transmit axial load through the entire distal carpus. Fixation is primarily within the capitate and distal carpus. There is a semiconstrained, ellipsoid articulation, which allows for a stable ROM without impingement throughout an arc of full FEM and RUD. The configuration allows for a high-contact surface area throughout this range. A second articulation between the carpal base plate and the polyethylene insert is incorporated. This is designed to allow a soft block to axial rotation, which permits the transfer of torque from the hand to the forearm. The radial component is designed to require minimal bony resection, which allows the implant to sit "inside" and be enveloped by the radial cortical rim. This is a unique feature that is not noted in other radial components to the best of the authors' knowl-

edge. A cementless option is anticipated (Fig. 41). The clinical experience with this implant is still short term, and the numbers are limited. Placement of the implant is relatively straightforward and is facilitated by a simple array of preparation guides and reamers. Data on the laboratory testing of wear, stress loading, and failure modes were reviewed by the FDA during their application review of this device, which was cleared for marketing (FDA 510k#K021859) (Fig. 42).

Giachino Device

Still undergoing initial evaluation (Dr. Giachino, *personal communication*), this device perhaps most closely represents the concept of surface replacement for a TWA (Fig. 43).

The entire proximal carpal row is removed, including the convexity of the capitate. A modified Suave-Kapandji procedure is performed as part of the procedure. Short screws fixate only the carpus. Axial loads are transmitted along the entire distal carpal array and onto the radius and ulna.

Applications for this design might prove to be advanced DJD, posttraumatic arthritis or ankylosing forms of RA without substantial bone loss. It certainly represents a departure from the design concepts of devices as of 2003, and the results of clinical trials are keenly awaited.

Total Modular Wrist Implant Arthroplasty

Designed by Peter Hubach, the total modular wrist (TMW) implant has a distal metal tray that is fixed with long screws into the second and third metacarpals. The polyethylene tray fits onto this carpal element and is concave. The radial component is offset and has a metal convex articulation that matches the carpal element. The original stem of this component is small, but there is now a long-stem alternative (7.5 cm; available since October, 2002) (Fig. 44). An option to replace a damaged DRUJ with a

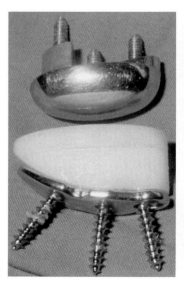
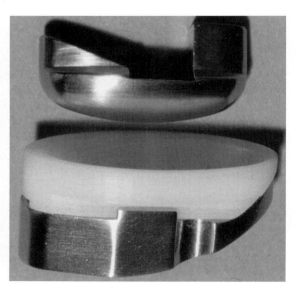

FIGURE 43. Giachino implant, which uses the entire surfaces for load transfer. Fixed with screws and designed similar to a resurfacing implant, this implant may be effective in patients with good bone stock such as in degenerative joint disease, posttrauma, and ankylosing spondylitis. **A:** An earlier design. **B:** A new configuration.

A,B

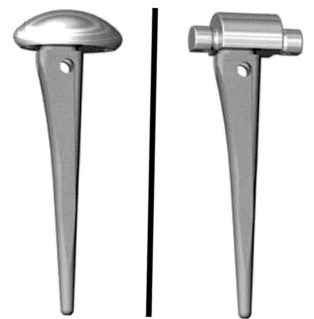

FIGURE 44. Total modular wrist implant 1: Dr. Peter Hubach's total modular long-stem implant.

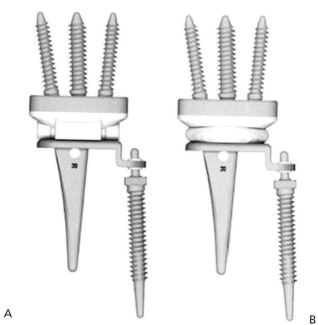

A B

FIGURE 46. Total modular system with constrained design **(A)** and unconstrained design **(B)**.

ball-and-socket articulation is available. A revision design with three distal screws is available (Fig. 45) and is now being used as the standard configuration for all total wrist implantations with the TMW. There are two sizes of polyethylene inlays with four thicknesses to help set proper tension. At this time, the TMW system is arguably the most complete system that is generally available and that also

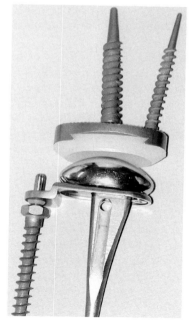

FIGURE 45. Modular design from the Netherlands. It seems to require significant bone resection for insertion and has the option for distal ulna and multiple distal prongs for revision surgery.

contains an excellent cutting guide system to allow for accurate bone cuts (Fig. 46). There exists polyethylene size variation and stem length variation. Standard unconstrained and constrained designs are available. The latter is for patients with marked ulnar deviation, for the loose RA group, and for some revisions. Bone grafting is recommended for revisions and for patients with associated poor or insufficient bone stock. In such cases, Hubach recommends the long-stem radial component. With a diversity of design configurations and size ranges, the TMW offers the hand surgeon a system that is capable of addressing many levels of disease severity and type. Negative results may rest on the demands that are placed on the metacarpal screws, which result in screw loosening and breakout. There is potential difficulty in inserting screws across the CMCs and into the metacarpal medullary canals of three rays (as the authors have experienced in doing revisions with the biaxial prosthesis). Loss of motion at the fourth CMC might prove a detriment to restoration of grip and dexterity, especially in the nonrheumatoid patient.

Results. Hubach (396), in a multicenter study to gain clinical experience, has implanted more than 50 TMW prostheses. Between July, 1999, and December, 2001, the TMW prosthesis was implanted in 30 patients (Fig. 47). The data have been accepted for publication (396). Four of the patients had surgery for revision of failed implants (three Guépar and one Swanson). Postoperative ROM averaged 31 degrees of dorsiflexion and 32 degrees of plantar flexion. Although pronation and supination were generally improved to 88 degrees and 82 degrees, specific indications and issues that referenced the optional ulnar screw device

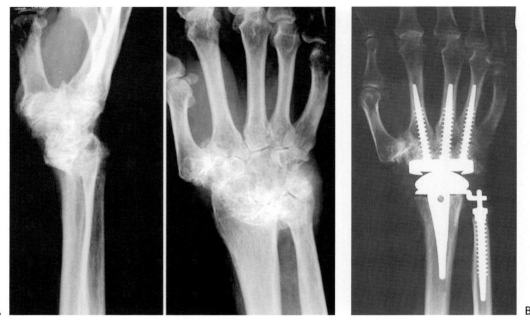

FIGURE 47. Preoperative **(A)** and postoperative **(B)** x-rays, courtesy of Dr. Hubach, of the Hubach prosthesis. Note that the length of the screws is fixated into the second, third, and fourth metacarpals.

were not noted. There were five patients with progressive ulnar deviation, requiring three operations (release of the ECU and flexor carpi ulnaris). One patient needed reoperation to insert a thicker (+4) insert owing to progressive laxity, presumably from implant settling.

Radiolucency occurred at the ulnar screw in two cases and at the second and third MC screws in two patients. Radial component lucency occurred in two patients, which has led Dr. Hubach to use the long stem in all revision cases.

Dr. Hubach's indications are similar to those reported elsewhere and in this chapter. He believes in arthroplasty for patients with RA, in whom both wrists are functionally affected, and for patients with noninflammatory arthritis in whom functional restoration of balance and ROM are needed.

The results from the multiple centers in Holland and Finland (Tiuasanen, Sipole) are positive.

The authors believe that the TMW adds greatly to the potentially successful implants that are becoming available to the hand surgical community. The range of choices makes this system a likely choice for some difficult revision wrist surgeries.

Distal Radioulnar Joint

A thorough discussion of the pathology and treatment options regarding the DRUJ is presented in other chapters of this text (Chapters 16 through 20). Only few pertinent comments regarding replacement of this joint are included in this chapter.

In patients with RA, the DRUJ is often involved, and resection of the distal ulna is well tolerated, as discussed previously. This sort of resection is included in the surgical technique for most of the implants that were discussed previously. In patients with posttraumatic arthritis and DJD of the radiocarpal and MC joints, the DRUJ is often intact and uninvolved. When symptoms in these patients warrant a consideration of wrist arthroplasty, only a limited number of the implants that were discussed previously are possible methods of treatment if the DRUJ is to be retained unaltered. An alternative approach would be to use one of the implants that incorporates or formally replaces the DRUJ.

In patients with isolated DRUJ pathology, several replacements are available. These are now briefly discussed.

A silicone ulnar head arthroplasty has been available since the 1970s (206). As a spacer, it was thought to be useful in some rheumatoid patients (207). It was also reported to decrease the incidence of postresection tendon rupture, a complication that was reported by Newmeyer and Green (191) and Pring and Williams (208). In the mid- to long-term period, problems arose with stem-head junction fractures, particulate synovitis, and bone erosion under the implant collar (209). These problems have led to the discontinuation of its use in most centers (210,211).

Tim Herbert, in 1995, at the Australian Hand Society meeting, presented his early experience with *a metal stem–ceramic ulnar head replacement*. It was designed for primary and revision surgery. Results were encouraging, although there were a few cases of subchondral lucency. van Schoonhoven et al. (212,213) also reported positively regarding this implant. Contraindications included insufficient bone stock to achieve stable fixation and inadequate soft tissue remnants to allow for stabilization of the construct. The latter was felt to be a potential problem in some patients with RA.

The uHead is a metal implant, using a cobalt-chrome modular design, with suture holes for soft tissue reconstruction. It has been recently introduced by the investigators at the Mayo Clinic (214). Biomechanically, the developers have shown the implant's ability to prevent convergence of the ulnar stump against the radius during loading. Convergence is believed to be a major reason for painful symptoms after a Darrach-type procedure. The authors have no experience using these implants in concert with any of the available TWA designs.

AUTHORS' PREFERRED SURGICAL TECHNIQUE

The operation is generally performed under a general anesthetic with the patient supine. One of the authors prefers to use an operating theatre that is equipped with laminar flow. Intravenous antibiotics are given preoperatively and for three doses postoperatively. A carefully padded tourniquet is used with elevation of the arm before inflation. The skin is prepared and draped in a standard fashion, using impervious drapes.

The authors perform a longitudinal dorsal incision that is centered over the third metacarpal. The proximal extension should be sufficient to allow for atraumatic retraction of the skin edges and still to gain easy access to the dorsum of the wrist. The skin flaps are carefully elevated from the extensor retinaculum with preservation of the dorsal sensory nerves. The authors raise the retinaculum from its radial side at the junction of the first and second compartments. This allows the retinaculum to be advanced, if required, during the closure to aid in pronating the carpus. On occasion, the authors open the retinaculum with a transverse step-cut incision. This allows for lengthening of the retinaculum, supplementation of the joint capsule upon closure, or creation of a pulley to resist volar subluxation of the ECU tendon, or a combination of these (Fig. 48).

A tenosynovectomy is now carried out, with further assessment of the extensor tendons being performed. In cases of DJD or posttraumatic arthritis in which there is a good capsule with identifiable ligaments and in which the distal ulna is to be preserved, it is possible to expose the radiocarpal joint by using a ligament-sparing incision (46). In RA, or when the distal ulna is to be exposed, a broad distally based capsular flap is raised. This is elevated as far proximally as possible to facilitate secure reattachment at closure. Synovectomies of the RC, MC, and DRUJ are carried out as indicated. The ulnar head is exposed subperiosteally, and the chosen distal ulna procedure is performed.

Attention is now directed to the distal radius and carpus, which have already been exposed. Lister's tubercle is rongeured flush with the rest of the distal radius. Axial traction is now applied to assess the necessary level of bone resection, the tension of the soft tissues, and the degree of palmar and proximal subluxation of the carpus relative to the radius. Soft tissue contractures should be released in preference to resection of greater amounts of bone. Preservation of the maximum amount of bone stock is necessary to support distal carpal, rather than just metacarpal, fixa-

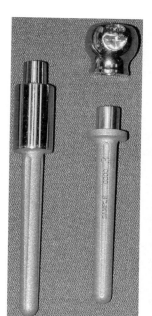
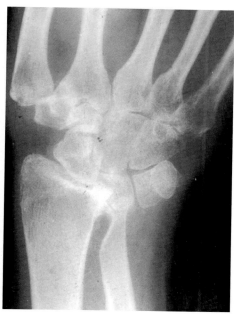
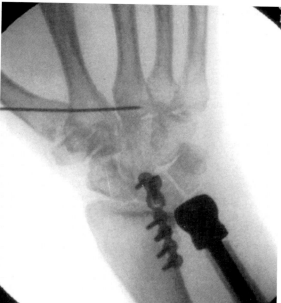

A

B,C

FIGURE 48. A: uHead arthroplasty. Note the suture holes for repair of the triangular fibrocartilage complex and the extensor carpi ulnaris subsheath. It is still unclear whether this is beneficial or causes added shear. **B,C:** Pre- and postoperative example of the uHead in a patient with rheumatoid arthritis who also had a radiolunate fusion.

tion. Anterior capsuloligamentous repair is sometimes necessary. This is most important when using nonconstrained implant designs. It is sometimes necessary to lengthen tendons, particularly the flexor carpi ulnaris, when there is marked volar flexion and ulnar translation. Preparation of the bones should follow the specific technique that is described for the various implant designs. Proper alignment and seating are critical and may be assisted by fluoroscopy during the procedure. Three or four drill holes are made along the dorsal rim of the distal radius through which sutures are passed before implant insertion. This is to facilitate capsular closure.

Soft tissue tensioning is reassessed while the trial components are in place. Soft tissue balancing is critical for success, regardless of the implant that is being used. Stability, centering balance, ROM, pattern of motion, and implant articulation contact area during motion are examined. The authors specifically check for impingement, asymmetric motion, and ease of dislocation in various positions. With the trials in place, the carpal bones are prepared for intercarpal fusion. If desired, cancellous, or corticocancellous bone is made available. Tendon lengthening, or decision for tendon transfers is finalized at this point. The volar capsule can be repaired if necessary before insertion of the real implant. The definitive components are then inserted as recommended by the manufacturer. Most designs allow for insertion of the radial component first. After the implant has been inserted, and tension has been reduced, balance and stability during the ROM are again reassessed. The authors consider the correct tension to have been achieved when the implant can be distracted a few millimeters with light traction. The authors aim for a resting posture of neutral RUD and neutral to 10 degrees of volar flexion. ROM throughout a functional arc should be possible without catching, clunking, or hinging of the joint. A secure dorsal capsular closure is obtained. This adds to implant stability and, with selective advancement, may also facilitate balance. Closure of the retinaculum should include supplementation of a deficient capsule, if necessary, to assure coverage of the components. At least one-half of the retinaculum should cover the extensor tendons to prevent bowstringing. A pulley mechanism should also be created to maintain the ECU dorsal to the distal ulna. Final soft tissue balancing procedures are carried out as necessary. Inability to achieved the desired soft tissue balance and the necessity to remove excessive bone, thus leaving little for implant fixation, are intraoperative indications for the consideration of scrubbing the TWA and proceeding with an arthrodesis.

The goals of the postoperative regime are primarily to prevent perioperative dislocations and to allow for soft tissue healing. Postoperative protocols differ from one implant to another and should be individualized for each patient based on the intraoperative assessments of balance, stability, and soft tissue quality and whether tendon reconstructions or transfers were performed. The less constrained designs generally demand 4 weeks or more of immobilization. Menon

suggests the use of a long arm splint in supination. Gentle active-assisted and passive ROM programs are started between postoperative weeks 1 and 4 in most cases. Night splints are continued as necessary, often for 3 months or more. The authors aim for a final range of flexion and extension of between of 30 and 40 degrees in either direction.

WRIST ARTHROPLASTY COMPLICATIONS

Infection

Infection is the most feared complication for any joint or rheumatoid reconstruction surgeon. In a review of the literature of the available implants for which clinical studies have been reported, deep infection rates were low (1% to 5%). Menon (383) reported one of the highest rates of deep infection at 5% (2 of 37 cases). These two cases were associated with use of high-dose prednisone and immunosuppression. Several cases of superficial infection have been reported. Most of these cases were successfully treated without removal of the implant or long-term sequelae. One case occurred after a dog bite (390).

Some published studies have implicated the use of corticosteroids and immunosuppressive agents in RA patients with the development of deep joint infections (397). In contrast, Garner et al. (398) were unable to find a significant difference in the deep infection rate in matched sets of orthopedic patients with and without a diagnosis of RA. An increased rate of failure of primary wound healing was demonstrated in patients with RA and in those patients who were on corticosteroids. However, these were not related to any long-term complications. Kasdan and June (399) and Sany et al. (400) again found no increase in the incidence of infection after surgery in patients on methotrexate compared to a similar group that was not on the drug. Constitutional deficits, such as the impaired phagocytic capacity of leukocytes, are postulated to be less than normal in RA patients (401).

Extreme care is the fundamental principle to be observed when operating on patients with RA or similar systemic illnesses. Standard joint replacement protocols, such as minimizing operating room traffic and the use of prophylactic antibiotics, should be observed. Atraumatic handling of the skin and soft tissues and meticulous hemostasis to avoid the formation of hematomas are essential. The authors no longer delay surgery if cessation of disease-modifying drugs is the only indication to do so, but consultation with specialists in rheumatology and infectious diseases is often helpful when any doubt exists.

Soft Tissue Imbalance

Soft tissue imbalance is a frequent postoperative complication after TWA. As well as difficulties in the correction of abnormalities at the time of surgery, a progressive disease, such as RA, may exacerbate these problems in the mid- to long-term period. One definition, which is used by Volz, is "the inability to bring the wrist volitionally to the neutral position" (402). The causes of this are legion but may be conveniently considered under the headings of tendon, bone, soft tissues, and control mechanisms. Each interrelates to the other.

Tendons may be malpositioned or their composition or environment may be altered by disease. They may be elongated, contracted, worn by attrition, or ruptured. These factors alter the sum of the force vectors that act on or across the wrist (403). This leads to an imbalanced position if the changes cannot be compensated for by higher-control mechanisms. Malpositioning is commonly seen with volar subluxation of the ECU, particularly in patients with RA. Synovitis is not only painful and mechanically limiting to tendon function, but it also alters the material properties of the tendons. Straub (98) and Taleisnik (99) have emphasized the important role of volar synovitis, and its effect on the flexor tendons, in addition to the more obviously accessible extensors. Elongated or contracted tendons must be reefed or formally lengthened, as necessary. Occasionally, the imbalance cannot be corrected by these means, and a formal tendon transfer may be required. An example of this would be the transfer of the ECRL to the ECU, with pronounced radial deviation of the metacarpals (Clayton procedure) (183,184). Rupture of the ECRL and ECRB have been shown to be particularly relevant to the results of TWA, and many would consider their absence to be a contraindication to arthroplasty (Dr. Alan Inglis, *personal communication*). Ruptures of the extensor tendons are commonly encountered in patients with RA and should be carefully repaired and protected postoperatively to avoid malfunctioning of the prosthesis.

The bony architecture may be altered by disease or surgery. Chronic changes in carpal height and orientation result in soft tissue contractures. Bony alterations also affect the relative moment arms of the tendons that cross the wrist (59,402–404). In the normal wrist, subtle changes in these moment arms occur during wrist motion. For instance, the scaphoid profile changes with wrist motion. This alters the anterior-posterior dimension of the wrist at that level and, consequently, the relative moment arms of the ECRL, ECRB, and flexor carpi radialis. Changing this relationship alters the relative balance of power generation that is possible in various positions by the flexors and extensors. Broadly, the resulting effect is a relative extensor weakness (405). Many similar changes must occur in the process of replacing a complex, multijointed system with something that is geometrically much simpler. The aim should be to use a prosthesis with intrinsic mechanical characteristics that mimic the normal kinematic pattern as closely as possible. It is not currently clear which of the prostheses that were discussed previously does this. This is partly because the authors do not have a complete description, as

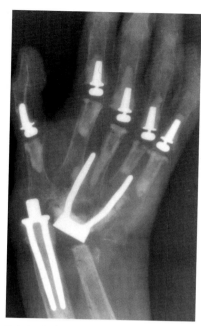

FIGURE 49. Original design by Meuli. Note the unbalanced moment arms, which result in ulnar deviation and dislocation of the components.

yet, of the normal kinematic pattern of wrist motion. Early designs, such as the original Meuli (303) and Volz (304) prostheses, did not possess the required mechanical characteristics. This resulted in a significant number of postoperatively imbalanced wrists (Fig. 49). Hamas (352) more accurately located the perceived center of rotation of the wrist on preoperative radiographs. This not only led to the development of his precentered prosthesis but was also, in part, the stimulus for development of many of the offset prostheses that have been marketed since that time. Hamas also clearly identified another problem that the surgeon faces: implant positioning. In an ideal world, this correct position should place the axes of motion of the prosthesis at the location at which the axes of motion of the patient's normal wrist would have been in health. In practical terms, it is usual to aim to restore carpal height and static alignment. The altered anatomy often precludes accurate identification of the center of rotation.

All or some of the soft tissues of the wrist can be contracted, attenuated, or absent at the time of surgery. Volar capsule contractures are particularly common in RA patients and should be carefully addressed. Reconstruction of the volar RSC ligament may help overcome an ulnar translation tendency. Preservation of the dorsal radiolunotriquetral ligament complex during the exposure and the repair at closure can decrease supination imbalance.

Higher motor control of wrist function is poorly understood. Volz et al. (402) have outlined an analysis of the relationship of the muscle–tendon units that cross the wrist in their review article on the biomechanics of the wrist (Fig.

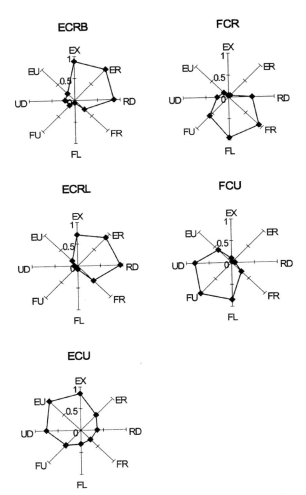

FIGURE 50. Plots of the muscle–tendon units that cross the wrist and their areas of function. Note the much more ubiquitous and seemingly important role of the extensor carpi ulnaris (ECU). Clinically, surgeons have long known of the need to reposition the ECU during total wrist arthroplasty. These studies help define the mechanical basis for this practice. ECRB, extensor carpi radialis brevis; ECRL, extensor carpi radialis longus; EU, extension/ulnar deviation; EX, extension; FCR, flexor carpi radialis; FCU, flexor carpi ulnaris; FL, flexion; FR, flexion/radial deviation; FU, flexion/ulnar deviation; RD, radial deviation; UD, ulnar deviation.

50). These observations have been refined by recent work by Yi-Wen et al. (406) (Fig. 51). They have demonstrated functional positions in which each wrist motor is most active. There is an intricate interplay between agonists and antagonists. In practical terms, the authors know that pain can have a profound inhibitory effect on the function of musculotendinous units around the wrist (92,407). Most TWA procedures provide excellent pain relief, and these units can sometimes then be rerecruited with aggressive physiotherapy.

Dislocation

Early and late dislocations continue to occur despite improvements in implant design (Fig. 52). Provided that care has been taken with soft tissue balancing, tensioning, and implant alignment in the operating room, early dislocations are usually due to a failure to protect the healing soft tissue. Late dislocations may occur secondary to progressive soft tissue imbalance, as discussed previously. Sometimes, the problem is related to progressive bone destruction by the underlying disease (391). Intercarpal fusion may reduce the frequency with which this occurs. Other cases may be related to the intrinsic geometry of the implant chosen. Earlier implants had a radially displaced center of rotation and a resultant high dislocation rate (344,347,361). Of the newer implants, the less constrained implant designs generally have higher dislocation rates. For instance, the biaxial prosthesis has been reported as having a 6% dislocation rate (4 of 64 implants) (375,380). Reported rates for the Menon prosthesis include 14% (5 of 37 implants) (383) and 9% (5 of 53 implants) (385). Such intrinsically unstable designs rely heavily on scrupulous attention to soft tissue repair and balancing to avoid this dislocation. In addition, incorrect placement at the time of surgery becomes relatively more important. Inadvertent removal of excess bone results in inadequate restoration of carpal height. Rotational misalignment can decrease the contact area of the articulating surfaces in certain positions, thus leading to point contact and instability. Inherently, more constrained joint designs are less dependent on these extrinsic elements for stability. Conversely, they are more prone to loosening, because forces are transmitted to the bone–implant or bone–cement interface. As in other joints, several prosthetic options may ultimately need to be available to cover the needs of a variety of circumstances that are presented to the surgeon.

Treatment of dislocations is related to timing and etiology. Early dislocations can often be treated successfully by a closed reduction that is followed by 4 to 6 weeks of immobilization (379,382,383). Posttraumatic dislocations may be amenable to similar management (379). Mid-term dislocations (4 weeks or more) usually require an open reduction that is followed by a period of additional stabilization in a cast or with an external fixator (383). Predisposing causes should be sought and corrected, if necessary. Late dislocations (months to years) are often related to component loosening from progressive disease (391). These frequently require salvage by revision arthroplasty or fusion.

Implant Failure

Implant fractures were frequently observed with the silicone hinged spacer (Fig. 53). More than 65% of implants were noted to be fractured in long-term studies (320). With the advent of HP 100 and the use of grommets, the incidence of fracture has been significantly decreased (328,329).

Few reports of rigid implant failures were noted. Meuli (339) documented one stem fracture of the distal component in his original construct and one in a patient with the

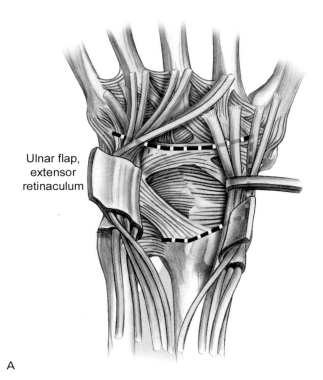

Ulnar flap, extensor retinaculum

A

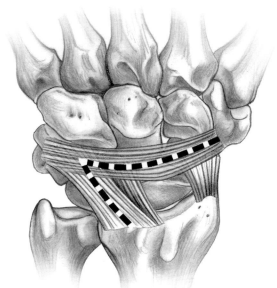

Ligament preserving surgical exposure

B

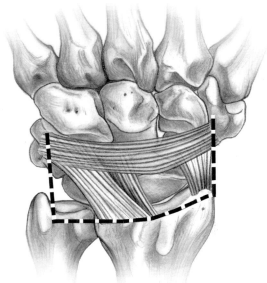

Distal flap surgical exposure

C

FIGURE 51. A: Ulnar-based or step-cut retinacular flap option. **B:** Schematic of ligament-sparing capsular exposure. **C:** Schematic of distally based capsulotomy.

MWP III design. O'Flynn et al. (359) have reported a failure of the axle mechanism of a trispherical implant.

Loosening

Loosening of the silicone wrist spacer has frequently been reported and is thought to relate to silicone synovitis (408). This is secondary to wear debris that forms by attrition of the implant against the bone.

Aseptic loosening that is associated with polyethylene wear debris is a well-recognized problem in lower extremity weight-bearing total joint arthroplasties (409–411). Polyethylene wear from a TWA articulation has not been noted to be a significant problem as of 2003. Several cases were noted with the Guépar implant (369,370), but this was clearly caused by third-body wear from particles that formed by loosening of the microscrew. Transmitted loads are thought to be of a different magnitude to those that are seen in the lower limb, such that each cycle of motion results in less stress on the polyethylene. Even in the long term, wear is unlikely to produce a significant amount of particulate debris unless the construct and motion pattern result in point loading of parts of the polyethylene. This could conceivably occur with misalignment of some of the less constrained prostheses. This is discussed by Menon (382,383) with particular reference to the perioperative placement of his radial component. Better templates and instrumentation should help avoid this eventuality. With a potential increase in use of

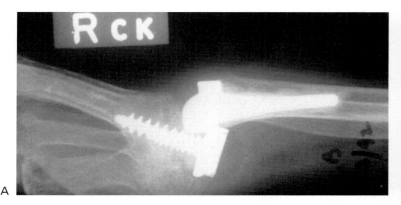

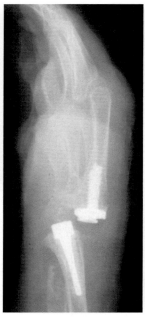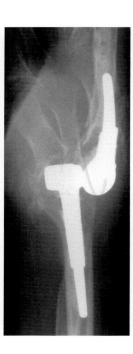

B,C

FIGURE 52. A: Volar dislocation that is associated with initial malalignment. **B,C:** Dorsal dislocations in the nonconstrained types of implants.

TWA in patients who perform heavy-load activities, such wear may become a more common issue for the wrist surgeon to have to manage (Fig. 54).

As of 2003, the majority of the problems that are seen with loosening of TWAs have been mechanical in nature. As such, they relate to the quality of the host bone, the nature of the implant construct, the orientation of implantation, the fixation interface strength, and the postoperative loading pattern. The majority of the observed loosening has been of the carpal component (Fig. 55). Recognition of the motion that is present at the second and third CMCs led initially to the use of a single stemmed component and to formal fusion of the second and third CMCs (347,349,358,361). Arguably, Alnot (369) first recognized the inadequacy of fixing the distal components in the med-

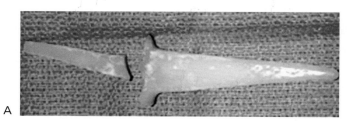

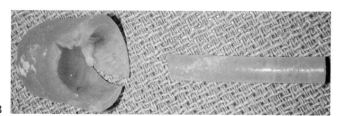

FIGURE 53. A,B: Silicone implant fractures.

ullary canal of the metacarpals as opposed to within the carpus (370). Most surgeons now endeavor to achieve fixation primarily in the carpus (338,339,350). The new generation of prostheses is designed to maximize this concept (339,382,383). The surgical technique for these implants now includes a formal intercarpal fusion of the remaining carpal bones with supplementary bone grafting, if necessary, to provide a solid base for carpal component fixation. The inefficiency of implant designs to transmit axial load effectively across the entire carpus (22) was first considered by Menon (383). His distal component base plate covers the entire residual carpus from the second to fifth ray (scaphoid-trapezoid to triquetrum-hamate). It also covers the entire depth of the bones at that point, from dorsal to volar. This design was based on the force distribution pattern that was demonstrated by Viegas et al. (38).

Whether cement should be used in TWA is arguably less of an issue. Evidence would support the use of cement in RA to block possible wear products from migrating into the implant–bone interface (412) and to support the often weakened bone. An uncemented prosthesis may be of more interest in the future if TWA results improve and if younger patients begin to be considered for surgery.

Fractures of the Radius

Fractures of the radius occur rarely. Dawson (413) reported on four such cases. He noted an increased time to union in these cases, which he attributed to the small residual bony contact area and the presence of cement. Similar to periprosthetic fractures elsewhere in the body, the management of radial fractures that are associated with wrist implants is difficult. A revision with long-

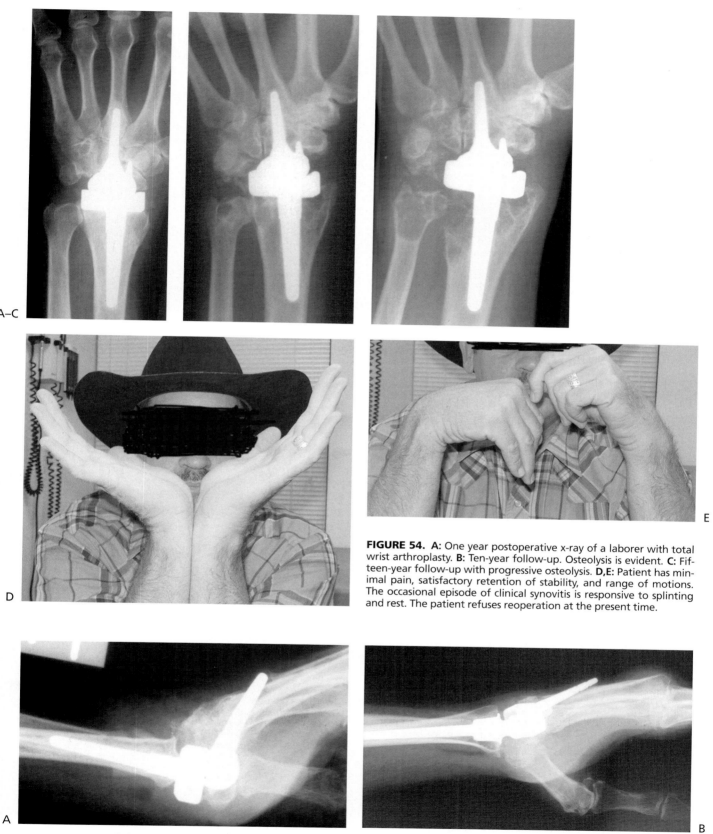

FIGURE 54. **A:** One year postoperative x-ray of a laborer with total wrist arthroplasty. **B:** Ten-year follow-up. Osteolysis is evident. **C:** Fifteen-year follow-up with progressive osteolysis. **D,E:** Patient has minimal pain, satisfactory retention of stability, and range of motions. The occasional episode of clinical synovitis is responsive to splinting and rest. The patient refuses reoperation at the present time.

FIGURE 55. Example of mechanical loosening, which typically involves the distal component. **A:** Biaxial wrist. **B:** Clayton-Ferlic-Volz wrist.

stem custom-designed implants is an option, but this takes manufacturing time and can be expensive. An arthrodesis can be associated with many complications, not the least of which is the possibility of multiple surgeries becoming necessary to achieve a solid fusion (see the following discussion).

Revision and Salvage

If a TWA fails, the options available include implant exchange, conversion to a resection arthroplasty, or conversion to an arthrodesis.

Ferlic et al. (414) documented the inconsistent results of resection arthroplasty after implant failure and removal. Rettig and Beckenbaugh (381) reported on the Mayo Clinic experience using the biaxial implant to replace various failed primary TWA implants. The majority of patients had a satisfactory clinical result with 8 out of 13 patients completely pain free at 31 months. Two of the patients required a second revision, and another patient was converted to an arthrodesis. Two additional revised wrists were noted to be loose on the radiographs.

In 1996, Cobb and Beckenbaugh noted that "revision total wrist arthroplasty has a high incidence of complications. Loosening is a significant problem" (380). They suggested the use of a long-stem or modified multipronged distal component biaxial design for revisions (Fig. 55). This was believed to be particularly indicated if deficient bone stock was noted. Two out of ten patients so treated ultimately went on to an arthrodesis. Two others showed radiographic lucency. The authors' experience with the three-prong configuration is that it is difficult to insert and results in a flattened palm with altered grasp patterns. Beckenbaugh (350) has reported that these implants have held up over time, and most patients are satisfied. Hubach (396) has conveyed his 2-year experience with seven revision arthroplasties, noting good results. Similar positive outcomes might be reasonably anticipated by using a version of the osseointegration technique.

A number of publications have addressed the issue of the success of arthrodesis after a failed arthroplasty. Beer and Turner (415) reported on 13 arthrodeses that were performed after failure of eight silicone and five metal-plastic implants. In total, there were 17 complications with five pseudoarthroses. Tricortical iliac crest bone grafts were used with Steinmann pin fixation, a modification of the technique that was described by Ferlic (414) for wrist arthroplasty salvage. In their conclusions, Beer and Turner recommended a more rigid construct, such as a plate, to attempt to improve the fusion rate. Carlson and Simmons (416) preferred the use of frozen allograft femoral head as graft material, but likewise used Steinmann pin fixation. They concluded that an arthrodesis gave more reliable results than an implant exchange.

Absolute Contraindications to Total Wrist Arthroplasty

The list of absolute contraindications to TWA should include

The presence of active infection
An uncooperative patient or someone who is unwilling to accept arthrodesis as a surgical alternative
A patient with a neurologically nonfunctioning hand
A patient with rupture of the radial wrist extensors

Relative Contraindications to Total Wrist Arthroplasty

The list of relative contraindications to TWA includes

Immunosuppression
Multiple extensor digitorum communis ruptures
Requirement to use a walking aid with that hand postoperatively
Poor bone stock
Active inflammatory disease
Systemic lupus erythematosus (ligament laxity)
Vascular insufficiency or vasculitis
Patients who already have a pain-free, functioning arthrodesis
Young patients
Heavy manual laborers

These lists will change as the results of TWA improve.

INDICATIONS FOR TOTAL WRIST ARTHROPLASTY AND AN ALGORITHM FOR TREATMENT

The decision to perform a TWA must be based on a complete assessment of the individual patient. This assessment should include factors such as the age of the patient, the type of disease process that is involved, the occupational and functional requirements of the person, and whether the patient is willing, or able, to tolerate possible complications (417). The best option is often still not easy to ascertain. There is even controversy as to the most favorable position to perform an arthrodesis, and this can be particularly difficult in patients with systemic inflammatory conditions, such as RA (418–420). In these patients, the present, and future, function of surrounding joints also becomes important, as well as the joints of the other arm.

Bearing these considerations in mind, and considering what has been presented in this chapter so far, it becomes necessary to consider what role wrist arthroplasty has in the overall management of wrist pathology. In the past, it was frequently regarded as a salvage procedure for patients with RA. This should no longer be the case. Even the silastic wrist spacer, with its most limited indications discussed previously, requires

TABLE 6. WRIST DISEASE CLASSIFICATION AND TREATMENT ALGORITHM

Group	Description	Treatment options[a,b]
Group 1	Osteoarthritis, posttraumatic arthrosis, Kienböck's disease, calcium pyrophosphate deposition disease, gout	
1A	Unicompartmental local arthrosis	See relevant treatment for specific process
1B	Progressive unicompartmental arthrosis	Proximal row carpectomy, scaphotrapezi-otrapezoid, scaphocapitate, RSL fusion
1C	Multicompartmental arthrosis; joint lines preserved	Capitate lunate fusion, four-corner fusion
	Collapse patterns evident	TWF, TWA
1D	Loss of carpal alignment and loss of joint line distinction	*TWA*
	Diffuse RC or intercarpal arthrosis	TWF
Group 2	Rheumatoid arthritis, stable pattern	
2A	Synovitis, minimal periarticular erosion or cyst formation, minimal RC cartilage loss	*Synovectomy*
2B	Moderate cartilage loss in RC joint; minimal singular plane derangement	*Synovectomy* RL or RSL fusion for pain symptoms
2C	Multilevel cartilage loss, modest loss of carpal height, mild uniplanar laxity (sagittal plane)	*TWA* Taleisnik procedure TWF
2D	Progress of bone and joint destruction, mild palmar subluxation, no gross axial deformation	*TWA* TWF
Group 3	Rheumatoid arthritis, disintegrative pattern	
3A	Synovitis, loss of carpal height ratio; ulnar translocation; scapholunate dissociation	*Synovectomy plus RL fusion*
3B	Loss of cartilage space, primarily RC; joint lines preserved; early biplanar instability	*Synovectomy plus RL or RSL fusion* TWA
3Ca	Loss of joint definition, collapse of carpal height, carpal translocations and subluxations	*Wrist fusion, leave carpometacarpal joint free*
	Unstable, no evident ankylosis of carpals or RC joint	TWA or biologic arthroplasty
3Cb	Same as group 3Ca, but stabilized (with deformity) via carpal or radiocarpal ankylosis	*Wrist fusion* TWA Biologic arthroplasty
3Da	Severe loss of bone stock, collapse and deformity	*TWF* *Biologic arthroplasty[c]*
3Db	Same as group 3Da, but with stabilizing ankylosis	*TWF* Biologic arthroplasty TWA in select circumstances

RC, radiocarpal; RL, radiolunate; RSL, radioscapholunate; TWA, total wrist arthroplasty; TWF, total wrist fusion.
[a]Italics indicate authors' preferred surgical treatment within each subgroup.
[b]In all group 2 and 3 patients, resection arthroplasty of the distal ulna with or without stabilization is typically indicated and should be performed in presence of a caput ulnae syndrome.
[c]Either total wrist fusion or biologic arthroplasty can be preferred in select situations.

adequate bone stock to achieve satisfactory functional outcomes (421). Increasingly, surgeons are regarding TWA as an active treatment option. When used in a timely fashion in conjunction with other surgical options and aggressive medical management protocols, the aim is to alter disease progression and to improve outcome (379,383,422,423). The difficulty with this approach in the rheumatoid patient is the early prediction of patients who inevitably deteriorate sufficiently to require surgical intervention. This is despite an extensive literature on the subject of different disease patterns and stages in RA (1,122,125–128,132,276). In addition, there is currently no consistent evidence that aggressive medical or surgical intervention alters the natural history of RA (66,132,135,424).

Despite these caveats the authors have devised a treatment algorithm, which combines the schemes of Millender and Nalebuff (127), Simmen and Huber (122), Alnot and Fauroux (125), and Wrightington (126). It is hoped that

this proves useful in establishing a baseline of deliberation when addressing the potential surgical needs of patients as regards the wrist.

The algorithm summary can be seen in Table 6 and in the manuscript by Lehman et al. (425), which has already been recently accepted for publication and reviews the rheumatoid wrist. Patients with primary OA, posttraumatic arthritis, or noninflammatory conditions, such as calcium pyrophosphate deposition disorder, are classified as group 1. This group is subclassified into sections A, B, C, and D. In the presence of unicompartmental local arthrosis they become 1A. With more diffuse unicompartmental involvement, the authors have distinguished group 1B. In both of these circumstances, the relevant treatment options are discussed elsewhere in this text. With multicompartmental involvement, the staging is group 1C (Fig. 56A). Here, in selected situations, TWA is an option for consideration.

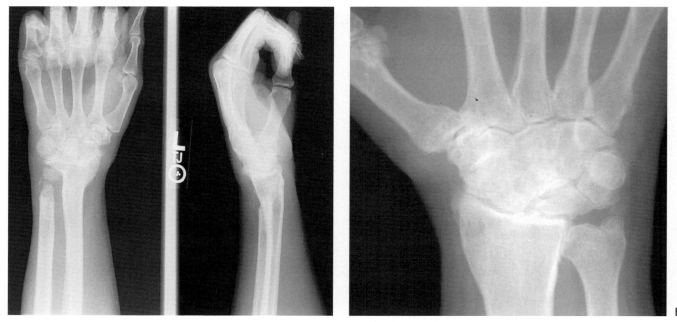

FIGURE 56. Example of an x-ray that demonstrates group 1C **(A)** and group 1D **(B)** of the treatment algorithm.

With progressive loss of carpal alignment and joint space, the authors distinguish group 1D. These are patients who are most likely to benefit from TWA, as the alternative is total wrist fusion. Individual considerations, such as the necessity to preserve motion for their vocational or avocational pursuits, then become important (Fig. 56B).

For patients with an underlying diagnosis of RA or similar systemic inflammatory disease, the authors have elected to divide them into group 2 (stable) and group 3 (unstable, or disintegrative). In group 2, the patients can be further classified into four categories. Group 2A may be defined as synovitis with minimal periarticular erosion or cyst formation and minimal RC cartilage loss. Treatment for group 2A is a synovectomy. In group 2B, the patient exhibits moderate cartilage loss in the RC joint and a minimal single-plane derangement (Fig. 57A). The recommended

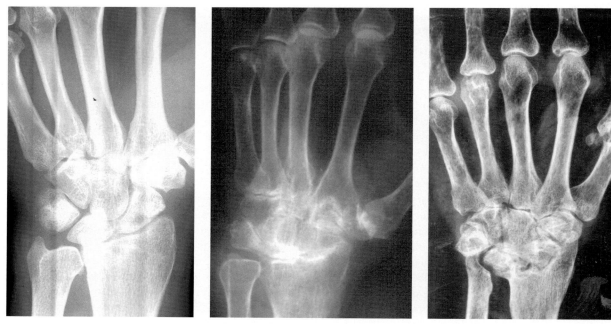

FIGURE 57. X-rays demonstrating group 2B **(A)**, group 2C **(B)**, and group 2D **(C)** of the treatment algorithm.

treatment is a synovectomy with a radiolunate or radio-scapholunate fusion. In group 2C, there is multilevel cartilage loss (RC and MC), with modest loss of carpal height and mild uniplanar laxity (usually in the sagittal plane) (Fig. 57B). At this stage, the authors would recommend TWA. With progressive bone and joint destruction and some palmar subluxation, but without gross deformity in axial alignment, the staging is group 2D (Fig. 57C). Again, in this setting, TWA is a viable alternative to a fusion. In group 3, there are also several subgroups. Group 3A is defined as synovitis that is associated with sufficient changes on serial radiographs to show a loss of carpal

height, scapholunate dissociation, or ulnar translation. These changes have been described in detail by Flury et al. (3). With improvements in preemptive diagnosis techniques, it is hoped that the diagnosis of this pattern of deterioration can be made even sooner. In this circumstance, synovectomy that is performed with a prophylactic radiolunate fusion is to be considered. If recognized early, and if the wrist is stable postsynovectomy, tendon balancing (transfer) is an option. In group 3B, there is loss of cartilage, but joint lines are still visible (Fig. 58A). Early biplanar instability may be present, but the disease is primarily confined to the RC joint. Synovectomy and radiolunate or

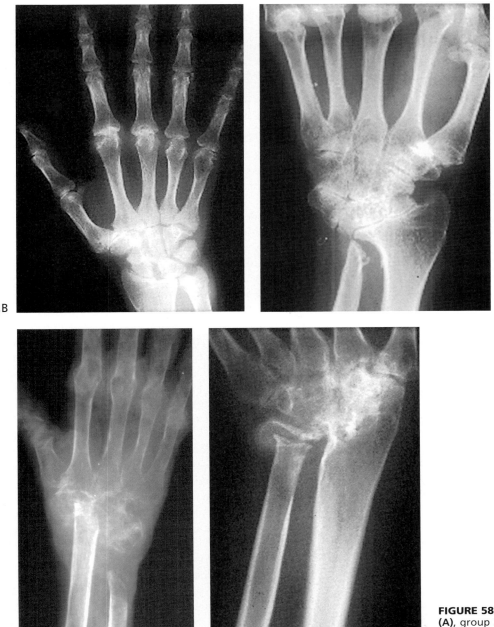

A,B

C,D

FIGURE 58. X-rays demonstrating group 3B **(A)**, group 3C **(B)**, group 3Da **(C)**, and group 3Db **(D)** of the treatment algorithm.

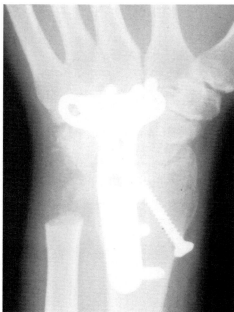

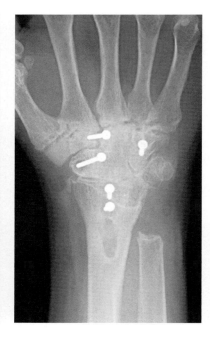

A,B

FIGURE 59. Fusion of the carpus to the radius with preservation of the carpometa-carpal joints to allow for flexion-extension motion. This is useful in patients with rheumatoid arthritis to compensate for some digit range-of-motion limitations. **A:** Plate fixation. **B:** Inlay sliding graft. (Courtesy of Dr. Philippe Kopolov.)

radioscapholunate fusion is the authors' recommendation. In some circumstances at this stage, an aggressive approach of performing a TWA while there is still adequate bone stock could be considered. This would correspond to the "treatment rather than salvage" approach to wrist surgery that was discussed previously and espoused by Menon (382,383) and Sorbie (422). In group 3C (Fig. 58B), one sees a loss of joint-line definition with collapse of carpal height, carpal translocations, and subluxations. In a subgroup 3C, which is similar to those of the Alnot-Fauroux classification, with instability, the authors recommend fusion. If it seems appropriate, attempt to preserve CMC motion and integrity (268). TWA is an option in selected patients, as would be biologic arthroplasties. In subgroup 3Cb in which some stability is achieved by local ankylosis, but with shortening and deformity, a TWA is feasible. Fusion of the entire carpus to the radius is the alternative (Fig. 59). In group 3D (Fig. 58C,D), there is severe loss of bone stock, deformity, and collapse. These patients would correspond to those previously classified as Simmen group 3 and Wrightington grade IV. Total fusion or, in selected patients, a biologic arthroplasty is indicated. In special circumstances, and when using implants that are best designed to deal with this configuration, TWA might eventually have a clinical place in this group. As with group 3C, it is possible to subdivide this group into unstable (3Da) and stable (3Db), as was done in stage V of the Alnot-Fauroux classification. In group 3Da, there is no ankylosis. Fusion crossing the CMCs by using fusion plates or intramedullary fixation with additional bone graft, as determined by the surgeon, is the preferred approach. In group 3Db, with ankylosis, consideration of TWA in selected circumstances would be reasonable.

THE FUTURE

With the success of the more recent designs, it would seem that implant-bone-cement fixation is a relatively solved problem. Dislocations still occur in the more unconstrained designs. Several of the implants require more than 2 cm of bone resection or are technically difficult to insert, especially in the presence of marked carpal volar subluxation with volar radial erosion. The authors are loath to predict what tomorrow will bring, lest the authors' lack of vision be known. The consensus and direction of designs do seem to give some view as to where things might be going. Improved materials that are biocompatible and highly tissue tolerant will become more readily available. Designs will surface, creating the best-fit configurations for stability, balance, and restoration of functional ROM, while maximizing load distribution from the hand to the radius and forearm. As with other joint replacements, a family of implants may evolve to address more specifically the challenges and demands of each individual patient. True surface replacements for the posttraumatic, constrained osseointegration designs to offer motion to patients that would otherwise require salvage total wrist fusions are but two ends of a large potential spectrum.

The authors should enlarge on the works of Meyerdierks et al. (426), Garcia-Elias et al. (427), Viegas et al. (428), Short et al. (429), and Buchanan et al. (430) on wrist kinematics with arthrodeses, so as to apply that knowledge to efforts to effectively simplify wrist motion with efficient arthroplasty designs. Tolbert et al. (431) looked at the kinematics of the normal and prosthetic wrists, reviewing the Swanson, Meuli, Volz, and Hamas designs and noting the lack of conformation to the normal of the designs that were studied. Similar evaluations on the newer generation of implants, and those implants that still only exist on computer screens, will help explain and predict their performance.

Better research tools to define the three-dimensional kinematics of the wrist and to aid with computer designing programs of best-fit configurations are now being evaluated and developed (432).

At the end of the day, it will be the severity of the patient's disease and deformity that will determine most directly the quality of the end result. Perhaps most importantly, therefore, there will need to be better ways to identify and predict disease patterns earlier, so as to guide the rheumatologist and the hand and wrist surgeon in specific, rather than empiric, treatment protocols, to include prophylactic as well as interventional disease-altering medical and surgical options to the patient.

REFERENCES

1. Vicar AJ, Burton RI. Surgical management of the rheumatoid wrist—fusion or arthroplasty. *J Hand Surg* 1986;11:790–797.
2. Rosen A, Weiland AJ. Rheumatoid arthritis of the wrist and hand. *Rheum Dis Clin North Am* 1998;24:101–128.
3. Flury MP, Herren DB, Simmen BR. Rheumatoid arthritis of the wrist, classification related to natural course. *Clin Orthop* 1999;366:72–77.
4. Youm Y, Flatt AE. Design of a total wrist prosthesis. *Ann Biomed Eng* 1984;12:247–262.
5. Linscheid RL. Kinematics considerations of the wrist. *Clin Orthop* 1986;202:27–39.
6. Cyriax EF. On the rotatory movements of the wrist. *J Anat* 1925;60:199–201.
7. MacConaill MA. The mechanical anatomy of the carpus and its bearings on some surgical problems. *J Anat* 1941;75:166–175.
8. Patterson RM, Viegas SF, et al. Quantification of anatomic, geometric and load transfer characteristics of the wrist joint. *Semin Arthroplast* 1995;6:13–19.
9. Patterson RM, Viegas SF. Kinematics of the wrist. In: Watson HK, Weinzweig J, eds. *The wrist.* Philadelphia: Lippincott Williams & Wilkins, 2001.
10. Arkless R. Rheumatoid wrists: cineradiography. *Radiology* 1967;88:543–549.
11. Gschwind N. *Surgical treatment of rheumatoid arthritis.* New York: Thieme Medical Publishers, 1980.
12. Kaplan E. *Functional and surgical anatomy of the hand,* 2nd ed. Philadelphia: JB Lippincott Co, 1965.
13. Kapandji IA. La rotation du pouce sur son axe longitudinal lors carpienne. *Rev Chir Orthop* 1972;58:273–289.
14. Kapandji IA. Etude du carpe au scanner a trois dimensions sous contraintes de pronosupination. *Ann Chir Main* 1991;10:36–47.
15. Ritt MJ, Stuart PR, et al. Rotational stability of the carpus relative to the forearm. *J Hand Surg* 1995;20:305–311.
16. Flatt AE. *The care of the arthritic hand,* 4th ed. St. Louis: CV Mosby, 1983.
17. Flatt AE. *The care of the arthritic hand,* 5th ed. St. Louis: CV Mosby, 1995.
18. Swanson AB. Flexible implant arthroplasty for arthritic disabilities of the radiocarpal joint. A silicone rubber intramedullary stemmed flexible hinge implant for the wrist joint. *Orthop Clin North Am* 1973;4:383–394.
19. Swanson AB, de Groot Swanson G. Flexible implant arthroplasty of the radiocarpal joint—surgical technique and long-term results. In: Inglis A, ed. *AAOS symposium on total joint reconstruction of the upper extremity.* St. Louis: CV Mosby, 1982:301–316.
20. Swanson AB, de Groot Swanson G, Maupin BK. Flexible implant arthroplasty of the radiocarpal joint: surgical technique and long-term study. *Clin Orthop* 1984;187:94–106.
21. Watson HK. Editorial comment. In: Watson HK, Weinzweig J, eds. *The wrist.* Philadelphia: Lippincott Williams & Wilkins, 2001.
22. Watson HK, Weinzweig J. Principles of rheumatoid arthritis. In: Watson HK, Weinzweig J, eds. *The wrist.* Philadelphia: Lippincott Williams & Wilkins, 2001.
23. Youm Y, McMurtry RY, et al. Kinematics of the wrist. *J Bone Joint Surg* 1978;60:423–431.
24. Peh WC, Viegas S, et al. Radiographic-anatomic correlation at different wrist articulation. *J Hand Surg* 1999;24:777–780.
25. Fick R. *Anatomie und Mechanik der Gelenke.* Jena: Gustav Fisher, 1911:357.
26. Brumfield RH Jr, Nickel VL, Nickel E. Joint motion in wrist flexion and extension. *South Med J* 1966;59:909–910.
27. Brumbaugh RB, Crowinshield RD, Blair WF, et al. An in-vivo study of normal wrist kinematics. *J Biomech Eng* 1982;104:176–181.
28. Andrews JG, Youm YA. A biomechanical investigation of wrist kinematics. *J Biomech* 1979;12:83–93.
29. Wright RD. A detailed study of movement of the wrist joint. *J Anat* 1935;70:137.
30. Sarrafian S, Melamed JL, Goshgarian GM. Study of wrist motion in flexion and extension. *Clin Orthop* 1977;126:153–159.
31. Hollingshead WH. *Anatomy for surgeons,* vol. 3, 2nd ed. New York: Harper & Row, 1964.
32. Lewis OJ, Hamshere RJ, Bucknill TM. The anatomy of the wrist joint. *J Anat* 1970;106:539–552.
33. Kauer JM. The interdependence of carpal articulation chains. *Acta Anat* 1974;88:481–501.
34. Landsmeer JM. *Atlas of anatomy of the hand.* New York: Churchill Livingstone, 1976.
35. Johnston HM. Varying positions of the carpal bones in the different movements at the wrist. *J Anat Phys* 1907;41:109.
36. Berger RA, Garcia-Elias M. General anatomy of the wrist. In: An KN, Berger RA, Cooney WP, eds. *Biomechanics of the wrist joint.* New York: Springer-Verlag, 1991:1–21.
37. Schuind F, Linscheid RL, An KN, et al. A normal database of posteroanterior roentgenographic measurements of the wrist. *J Bone Joint Surg* 1992;14:1418–1429.
38. Viegas SF, Tencer AF, Cantrell J, et al. Load transfer characteristics of the wrist. Part I. The normal joint. *J Hand Surg* 1987;12:971–978.
39. Dobyns JH, Linscheid RL. A short history of the wrist joint. *Hand Clin* 1997;13:1–12.

40. Bednar JM. Wrist joint arthroplasties. In: Peimer CA, ed. *Surgery of the hand and upper extremity,* vol. 1. New York: McGraw-Hill, 1996:771–794.

41. Garcia-Elias M. Anatomy of the wrist. In: Watson HK, Weinzweig J, eds. *The wrist.* Philadelphia: Lippincott Williams & Wilkins, 2001.

42. Taleisnik J. The ligaments of the wrist. *J Hand Surg* 1976;1:110–118.

43. Siegel DB, Gelberman RH. Radial styloidectomy: an anatomical study with special reference to radiocarpal intracapsular ligamentous morphology. *J Hand Surg* 1991;16:40–44.

44. Garcia-Elias M, Domènech-Mateu JM. The articular disc of the wrist. Limits and relations. *Acta Anat* 1987;128:51–54.

45. Mayfield JK, Johnson RP, Kilcoyne RF. The ligaments of the human wrist and their functional significance. *Anat Rec* 1976;186:417–428.

46. Berger RA, Bishop AT, Bettinger PC. New dorsal capsulotomy for the surgical exposure of the wrist. *Ann Plast Surg* 1995;35:54–59.

47. Berger RA, Crowninshield RD, Flatt AE. The three-dimensional rotational behavior of the carpal bones. *Clin Orthop* 1982;167:303–310.

48. Roux JL, Micaleff JP, Allieu Y. Biomechanical considerations for wrist arthroplasty. In: Simmen BR, Allieu Y, Lluch A, et al., eds. *Hand arthroplasties.* London: Martin Dunitz Ltd, 2000:183–199

49. Ruby LK, Cooney WP III, et al. Relative motion of selected carpal bones: a kinematic analysis of the normal wrist. *J Hand Surg* 1988;13:1–10.

50. Kapandji IA. *The physiology of the joint. Upper limb,* vol. 1, 5th ed. New York: Churchill Livingstone 1982:138–149.

51. Palmer AK, Werner FW, et al. Functional wrist motion: a biomechanical study. *J Hand Surg* 1985;10:39–46.

52. Ryu J, Cooney WP III, et al. Functional ranges of motion of the wrist joint. *J Hand Surg* 1991;16:409–419.

53. Rawes ML, Richardson JB, Dias JJ. A new technique for the assessment of wrist movement using a biaxial flexion extension electrogoniometer. *J Hand Surg* 1996;21:600–603.

54. Patterson RM, Nicodemus CL, Viegas SF, et al. Normal wrist kinematics and the analysis of the effect of various dynamic external fixators for treatment of distal radius fractures. *Hand Clin* 1997;13:129–142.

55. Sugimoto A, Hara Y, Findley TW, et al. A useful method for measuring daily physical activity by a three-direction monitor. *Scand J Rehabil Med* 1977;29:37–42.

56. Brumfield RH, Champoux JA. A biomechanical study of normal function wrist motion. *Clin Orthop* 1984;187:23–25.

57. Nelson DL. Functional wrist motion. *Hand Clin* 1997;13:83–92.

58. Brand PW, Beach RB, Thompson DE. Relative tension and potential excursion of muscles in the forearm and hand. *J Hand Surg* 1981;6:209–219.

59. Ryu J. Biomechanics of the wrist. In: Watson HK, Weinzweig J, eds. *The wrist.* Philadelphia: Lippincott Williams & Wilkins, 2001.

60. Navarro A. Anatomia y fisiologia del carpo. *Ann Inst Clin Quir Cir Exp Montevideo* 1935.

61. Taleisnik J. *The wrist.* New York: Churchill Livingstone, 1985.

62. Craigen MA, Stanley JK. Wrist kinematics: row, column or both? *J Hand Surg* 1995;20:165–170.

63. Ferris BD, Stanton J, Zamora J. Kinematics of the wrist. *J Bone Joint Surg* 2000;82:242–245.

64. Kobayashi M, Berger RA, Linscheid RL, et al. Intercarpal kinematics during wrist motion. *Hand Clin* 1997;13:143–149.

65. Gschwind N. Le poignet rhumatismal ou les implants articulaires dans le poignet et la main rhumatismale. In: *Vonferences d'enseignement de la SOFCOT.* Paris: Expansion Scientifique Francaise, 1979:13–26.

66. Thirupathi RG, Ferlic DC, Clayton ML. Dorsal wrist synovectomy in rheumatoid arthritis—a long-term study. *J Hand Surg* 1983;8:848–856.

67. Hendrix RW, Urban MA, Schroeder JL, et al. Carpal predominance in rheumatoid arthritis. *Radiology* 1987;164:212–219.

68. Allieu Y, Lussiez B, Ascencio G. The long-term results of synovectomy of the rheumatoid wrist: a report of 60 cases. *Fr J Orthop Surg* 1989;3:188–194.

69. Allieu Y, Lussiez B, Asencio G. Resultats a long terme des synovectomies chirurgicales du poignet rhumatoide. *Rev Chir Orthop* 1989;75:172–178.

70. Clayton ML. Surgical treatment at the wrist in rheumatoid arthritis. *J Bone Joint Surg* 1965;47:741–750.

71. Linscheid RL, Dobyns JH. Rheumatoid arthritis of the wrist. *Orthop Clin North Am* 1971;2:649–665.

72. Shapiro JS. The wrist in rheumatoid arthritis. *Hand Clin* 1996;12:477–498.

73. Gupta A, Wolff TW. The rheumatoid wrist—clinical problems. *Prob Plast Reconstr Surg* 1992;2:263–279.

74. Huh YM, Suh JS, Jeong EK, et al. Role of the inflamed synovii volume of the wrist in defining remission of rheumatoid arthritis with gadolinium-enhanced 3D-SPGR MR imaging. *J Magn Reson Imaging* 1999;10:202–208.

75. Resnick D, Gmelich JT. Bone fragmentation in the rheumatoid wrist: radiographic and pathologic considerations. *Radiology* 1975;114:315–321.

76. Resnick D. Rheumatoid arthritis of the wrist—the compartmental approach. *Med Radiogr Photogr* 1976;52:50–88.

77. Short CL, Bauer W, Reynolds WE. *Rheumatoid arthritis, a definition of the disease and clinical description based on a numerical study of 293 patients and controls.* Cambridge, MA: Harvard University Press, 1957.

78. Van Vugt RM, van Jaarsveld CH, et al. Patterns of disease progression in the rheumatoid wrist: a long-term follow-up. *J Rheumatol* 1999;26:1467–1473.

79. Nalebuff EA, Garrod KJ. Present approach to the severely involved rheumatoid wrist. *Orthop Clin North Am* 1984;15:369–380.

80. Pirela-Cruz MA, Firoozbakhsh K, Moneim MS. Ulna translocation of the carpus in rheumatoid arthritis: an analysis of five determination methods. *J Hand Surg* 1993;18:299–306.

81. Feldon P, Terrono AL, Nalebuff EA. Rheumatoid arthritis of the hand and wrist. In: Green DP, ed. *Operative hand surgery,* 4th ed. New York: Churchill Livingstone, 1999:1651–1739.

82. Ruby LK, Cassidy C. Evaluation and treatment of the rheumatoid wrist. In: Watson HK, Weinzweig J, eds. *The wrist.* Philadelphia: Lippincott Williams & Wilkins, 2001.

83. Mannerfelt L. Surgical treatment of the rheumatoid wrist and aspects of the natural course when untreated. *Clin Rheum Dis* 1984;10:549–570.

84. Cush JJ, Lipsky PE. Cellular basis for rheumatoid inflammation. *Clin Orthop* 1991;265:9–22.

85. Martel WM. The pattern of rheumatoid arthritis in the hand and wrist. *Radiol Clin North Am* 1964;2:221–234.

86. Kauer JM. The collateral ligament function in the wrist joint. Paper presented at: Proceedings of the 112th Meeting of Anatomy Association, 1977.

87. Shapiro JS. A new factor in the etiology of ulnar drift. *Clin Orthop* 1970;68:32–43.

88. Zancolli E. *Structural and dynamic basis of hand surgery.* Philadelphia: JB Lippincott Co, 1972.

89. Brewerton DA. Hand deformities in rheumatoid disease. *Ann Rheum Dis* 1957;16:183–197.

90. Brewerton DA. The rheumatoid hand. *Proc R Soc Med* 1966;59:11–13.

91. Backhouse KM. The mechanics of normal digital control in the hand and analysis of the ulna drift of rheumatoid arthritis. *Ann R Coll Surg England* 1968;43:154–173.

92. Backdahl M, Carlsoo S. Distribution of activity in muscles acting on the wrist. *Acta Morphol Neerl Scand* 1961;4:136.

93. Shapiro JS, Heigna W, Nasatir S. The relationship of wrist motion to ulna phalangeal drift in the rheumatoid patients. *Hand* 1971;3:68–75.

94. Landsmeer JM. Studies in the anatomy of articulation. II. Patterns of movement of bimuscular, biarticular systems. *Acta Morphol Neerl Scand* 1960;3:304–321.

95. Stack HG, Vaughan-Jackson OJ. The zig-zag deformity in the rheumatoid hand. *Hand* 1971;3:62–67.

96. Pahle JA, Raunio P. The influence of wrist position on finger deviation in the rheumatoid hand. *J Bone Joint Surg* 1969;51:664–676.

97. Hastings DE, Evans JA. Rheumatoid wrist deformities and their relation to ulna drift. *J Bone Joint Surg* 1975;57:930–934.

98. Straub LR, Ranawat CS. The wrist in rheumatoid arthritis. *J Bone Joint Surg* 1969;51:1–20.

99. Taleisnik J. Rheumatoid synovitis of the volar compartment of the wrist joint: its radiological signs and its contribution to wrist and hand deformity. *J Hand Surg* 1979;4:526–535.

100. Mannerfelt L, Norman O. Attrition ruptures of flexor tendons in rheumatoid arthritis caused by boney spurs in the carpal canal. A clinical and radiological study. *J Bone Joint Surg* 1969;12:9–14.

101. Backdahl M. The caput ulnae syndrome in rheumatoid arthritis. *Acta Rheum Scand* 1963;[Suppl 5]:1–75.

102. Vaughan-Jackson OJ. Rupture of extensor tendons by attrition at the inferior radioulnar joint. Report of two cases. *J Bone Joint Surg* 1948;30:528–530.

103. Freiberg RA, Weinstein A. The scallop sign and spontaneous rupture of finger extensor tendons in rheumatoid arthritics. *Clin Orthop* 1972;83:128–130.

104. Ryu J, Saito S, et al. Risk factors and prophylactic tenosynovectomy for extensor tendon ruptures in the rheumatoid hand. *J Hand Surg* 1998;23:658–661.

105. Viegas SF, Patterson RM, et al. Wrist anatomy: incidence, distribution, and correlation anatomic variations, tears, and arthrosis. *J Hand Surg* 1993;18:463–475.

106. Dobyns JH. Clinical evaluation of the arthritic wrist. In: Dobyns JH, ed. *The wrist: diagnosis and operative treatment.* St. Louis: Mosby, 1998.

107. Jebsen RH, Taylor N, et al. An objective and standardized test of hand function. *Arch Phys Med Rehab* 1969;50:311–319.

108. Dell PC, et al. Management of rheumatoid arthritis of the wrist. *J Hand Ther* 1996;9:157–164.

109. Sollerman C, Ejeskar A. Sollerman hand function test. *Scand J Plast Reconstr Hand Surg* 1995;29:167–176.

110. Boozer J. Splinting the arthritic hand. *J Hand Ther* 1993;6:46–48.

111. Genant HK, Jiang Y, Peterfy C, et al. Assessment of rheumatoid arthritis using a modified scoring method on digitized and original radiographs. *Arthritis Rheum* 1998;41:1583–1590.

112. Helliwell PS, Hetthen J. Joint symmetry in early and late rheumatoid and psoriatic arthritis. *Arthritis Rheum* 2000;43:865–871.

113. Sharp JT, Gardner JC, Bennett EM. Computer-based methods for measuring joint space and estimating erosion volume in the finger and wrist joint of patients with rheumatoid arthritis. *Arthritis Rheum* 2000;43:1378–1386.

114. Van der Heijde D. How to read radiographs according to the Sharp/van der Heijde method. *J Rheumatol* 1999;26:743–745.

115. Van der Heijde D, Dankert T, et al. Reliability and sensitivity to change of a simplification of the Sharp/van der Heijde radiological assessment in rheumatoid arthritis. *Rheumatology* 1999;38:941–947.

116. Larsen A. How to apply Larsen score in evaluating radiographs of rheumatoid arthritis in long-term studies? *J Rheumatol* 1995;22:1974–1975.

117. Trenham D, Masi A. Carpo-metacarpal ratio, a new quantitative measure of radiologic progression of wrist involvement in rheumatoid arthritis. *Arthritis Rheum* 1976;19:939–944.

118. ZdravlpvocV, Sennwald G. A new radiographic method of measuring carpal collapse. *J Bone Joint Surg* 1997;79:167–169.

119. Dibenedetto MR, Lubbers LM, Coleman CR. A standardized measurement of ulnar carpal translocation. *J Hand Surg* 1990;15:1009–1010.

120. Nattrass GR, King GJ, McMurtry RY, et al. An alternative method for determination of the carpal height ratio. *J Bone Joint Surg* 1994;76:88–94.

121. Shapiro JS. The wrist in rheumatoid arthritis. *Hand Clin* 1996;12:477–498.

122. Simmen BR, Huber H. The rheumatoid wrist: classification related to the type of the natural course and its consequences for surgical therapy. In: Simmen BR, Hagena FW, eds. *The wrist in rheumatoid arthritis. Rheumatology*, vol. 17. Basel, Switzerland: Karger, 1992:13–25.

123. Zangger P, Kachura JR, Bogoch ER. The Simmen Classification of wrist destruction in rheumatoid arthritis. *J Hand Surg* 1999;24B:400–404.

124. Larsen A, Dale K, Eek M. Radiographic evaluation of rheumatoid arthritis and related conditions by standard reference films. *Acta Radiol Diagn (Stockh)* 1977;18:481–491.

125. Alnot JY, Fauroux L. Synovectomy realignment stabilization in the rheumatoid wrist. In: Simmen BR, Hagena FW, eds. *The wrist in rheumatoid arthritis. Rheumatology*, vol. 17. Basel, Switzerland: Karger, 1992:72–86.

126. Hodgson SP, Stanley JK, Muirhead A. The Wrightington classification of rheumatoid wrist x-rays; a guide to surgical management. *J Hand Surg* 1989;14:451–455.

127. Millender LH, Nalebuff EA. Preventive surgery-tenosynovectomy and synovectomy. *Orthop Clin North Am* 1975;6:765–792.

128. O'Brien ET. Surgical principles and planning for the rheumatoid hand and wrist. *Clin Plast Surg* 1996;23:407–420.

129. Terrona AL, Feldon PG, et al. Evaluation and treatment of the rheumatoid wrist. *J Bone Joint Surg* 1995;77:1116–1128.

130. Inglis AE. Rheumatoid arthritis in the hand. *Am J Surg* 1965;109:368–374.

131. Linscheid RL. Surgery for rheumatoid arthritis-timing and technique: the upper extremity. *J Bone Joint Surg* 1968:50:605–613.

132. Hindley CJ, Stanley JK. The rheumatoid wrist. Patterns of disease progression. *J Hand Surg* 1991;16:275–279.

133. Vahvanen V, Pätiälä H. Synovectomy of the wrist in rheumatoid arthritis and related diseases. *Arch Orthop Trauma Surg* 1984;102:230–237.

134. Aschan W, Moberg E. A long-term study on the effect of early synovectomy in rheumatoid arthritis. *Bull Hosp Joint Dis* 1984;44:106–121.

135. Brumfield RH, Kuschner SH, et al. Results of dorsal wrist synovectomies in the rheumatoid hand. *J Hand Surg* 1990;15:733–735.

136. Ferlic DC, Clayton ML. Synovectomy of the hand and wrist. *Ann Chir Gynaecol* 1985;198:26–30.

137. Henderson ED, Lipscomb PR. Surgical treatment of rheumatoid hand. *JAMA* 1961;175:431–436.

138. Millender LH, Nalebuff EA, et al. Dorsal tenosynovectomy and tendon transfer in the rheumatoid hand. *J Bone Joint Surg* 1974;56:601–610.

139. Namba H. Clinical results of synovectomy for rheumatoid wrist compared with the opposite side. *J Jpn Orthop Assoc* 1981;55:527–541.

140. Wynn Parry CB, Stanley JK. Review article: synovectomy of the hand. *Br J Rheumatol* 1993;32:1089–1095.

141. Bohler N, Lack N, et al. Late results of synovectomy of wrist, MP, and PIP joints. Multicenter study. *Clin Rheumatol* 1985;4:23–25.

142. Kessler I, Vainio K. Posterior (dorsal) synovectomy for rheumatoid involvement of the hand and wrist. A follow-up study of sixty-six procedures. *J Bone Joint Surg* 1966;48:1085–1094.

143. McEwen C, et al. Multicenter evaluation of synovectomy in the treatment of rheumatoid arthritis. *Arthritis Rheum* 1977;20:765–771.

144. Whipple TL, Marotta JJ, et al. Techniques of wrist arthroscopy. *J Arthroscop Relat Surg* 1986;2:244–252.

145. Wilkes LL. Arthroscopic synovectomy in the rheumatoid metacarpophalangeal joint. *J Med Assoc Ga* 1987;76:638–639.

146. Adolfsson L, Nylander G. Arthroscopic synovectomy of the rheumatoid wrist. *J Hand Surg* 1993;18:92–96.

147. Atik TL, Baratz ME. The role of arthroscopy in wrist arthritis. *Hand Clin* 1999;15:489–494.

148. Osterman AL. Wrist arthroscopy: operative procedures. In: Green DP, ed. *Green's operative hand surgery,* 4th ed. New York: Churchill Livingstone, 1999:207–222.

149. Blank JE, Cassidy C. The distal radioulnar joint in rheumatoid arthritis. *Hand Clin* 1996;12:499–513.

150. Lichtman DM, Ganocy TK, Kim DC. The indications for and techniques and outcomes of ablative procedures of the distal ulna. The Darrach resection, hemiresection, matched

151. Smith-Petersen MN, Aufranc OE, Larson CB. Useful surgical procedures for rheumatoid arthritis involving joints of the upper extremity. *Arch Surg* 1943;36:764–770.

152. Albert SM, Wohl MA, Rechtman AM. Treatment of the disrupted radio-ulnar joint. *J Bone Joint Surg* 1963;45:1373–1381.

153. Boyd HB, Stone MM. Resection of the distal end of the ulna. *J Bone Joint Surg* 1944;26:313–321.

154. Cracchiolo A III, Marmer L. Resection of the distal ulna in rheumatoid arthritis. *Arthritis Rheum* 1969;12:415.

155. Darrach W. Anterior dislocation of the head of the ulna. *Ann Surg* 1912;56:802–803.

156. Darrach W, Kirby D. Derangements of the inferior radio-ulnar articulation. *Med Rec* 1915;87:708.

157. Darrow JC, Linscheid RL, Dobyns JH, et al. Distal ulnar recession for disorder of the distal radioulnar joint. *J Hand Surg* 1985;10:482–491.

158. Dingman PV. Resection of the distal end of the ulnar (Darrach operation). An end result study of twenty-four cases. *J Bone Joint Surg* 1952;34:893–900.

159. Fraser KE, Diao E, et al. Comparative results of resection of the ulna in rheumatoid arthritis and post-traumatic conditions. *J Hand Surg* 1999;24:667–670.

160. Gainor BJ, Schaberg J. The rheumatoid wrist after resection of the distal ulna. *J Hand Surg* 1985;10:837–844.

161. Ishikawa H, Hanyu T, Tajima T. Rheumatoid wrists treated with synovectomy of the extensor tendons and the wrist joint combined with a Darrach procedure. *J Hand Surg* 1992;17:1109–1117.

162. McKee M, Richards RR. Dynamic radio-ulnar convergence after the Darrach procedure. *J Bone Joint Surg* 1996;78:413–418.

163. Mikic Z, Helal B. The value of the Darrach procedure in the surgical treatment of rheumatoid arthritis. *Clin Orthop* 1977;127:175–185.

164. Bieber EJ, Linscheid RL, et al. Failed distal ulna resections. *J Hand Surg* 1988;13:193–200.

165. Moller M. Forty-eight cases of caput ulnae syndrome treated by synovectomy and resection of the distal end of the ulna. *Acta Orthop Scand* 1973;44:278–282.

166. Spinner M, Kaplan EB. Extensor carpi ulnaris: its relationship to the stability of the distal radio-ulnar joint. *Clin Orthop* 1970;68:124–129.

167. Weiler PJ, Bogoch ER. Kinematics of the distal radioulnar joint in rheumatoid arthritis: an in vivo study using centrode analysis. *J Hand Surg* 1995;20:937–943.

168. Breault-Janicki MJ, Small CF, et al. Mechanical properties of wrist extensor tendons are altered by the presence of rheumatoid arthritis. *J Orthop Res* 1998;16:472–474.

169. Neurath MF, Stofft E. Ultrastructural causes of rupture of hand tendons in patients with rheumatoid arthritis. *Scand J Plast Reconstr Surg Hand Surg* 1992;27:59–65.

170. Straub LR, Wilson EM Jr. Spontaneous rupture of extensor tendons in the hand associated with rheumatoid arthritis. *J Bone Joint Surg* 1956;38:1208–1217.

171. Vaughan-Jackson OJ. Rheumatoid hand deformities considered in the light of tendon imbalance. I. *J Bone Joint Surg* 1962;44:764–775.

resection, and Sauve-Kapandji procedure. *Hand Clin* 1998;14:265–277.

172. Shannon FT, Barton NJ. Surgery for rupture of extensor tendons in rheumatoid arthritis. *Hand* 1976;8:279–286.

173. Wilson RL, DeVito MC. Extensor tendon problems in rheumatoid arthritis. *Hand Clin* 1996;12:551–559.

174. Breen TF, Jupiter JB. Extensor carpi ulnaris and flexor carpi ulnaris tenodesis of the unstable distal ulna. *J Hand Surg* 1989;14:612–617.

175. Goldner JL, Hayes MG. Stabilization of the remaining ulna using one-half of the extensor carpi ulnaris tendon after resection of the distal ulna. *Orthop Trans* 1979;3:330–331.

176. Leslie BM, Carlson G, Ruby L. Results of extensor carpi ulnaris tenodesis in the rheumatoid wrist undergoing a distal ulnar excision. *J Hand Surg* 1990;15:547–551.

177. Melone CP Jr, Taras JS. Distal ulna resection, extensor carpi ulnaris tenodesis, and dorsal synovectomy for the rheumatoid wrist. *Hand Clin* 1991;7:335–343.

178. Ruby LK, Ferenz CC, Dell PC. The pronator quadratus interposition transfer: an adjunct to resection arthroplasty of the distal radioulnar joint. *J Hand Surg* 1996;21:60–65.

179. Tsai TM, Stilwell JH. Repair of chronic subluxation of the distal radioulnar joint (ulna dorsal) using flexor carpi ulnaris tendon. *J Hand Surg* 1984;9:289–294.

180. Tsai TM, Shimizu H, Adkins P. A modified extensor carpi ulnaris tenodesis with the Darrach procedure. *J Hand Surg* 1993;18:697–702.

181. Rana NA, Taylor AR. Excision of the distal end of the ulna in rheumatoid arthritis. *J Bone Joint Surg* 1973;55:96–105.

182. Viegas SF, Pogue DJ, et al. Effects of radioulnar instability on the radiocarpal joint: a biomechanical study. *J Hand Surg* 1990;15:728–732.

183. Boyce TH, Youm Y, et al. Clinical and experimental studies on the effect of extensor carpi radialis longus transfer in the rheumatoid hand. *Hand Surg* 1978;3:390–394.

184. Clayton ML, Ferlic DC. Tendon transfer for radial rotation of the wrist in rheumatoid arthritis. *Clin Orthop* 1974;100:176–185.

185. DellaSanta D, Chamay A. Aspects clinique, radiologique et cinematique du poignet rhumatoide apres resection de la tete du cubitus. *Med Hyg* 1980;38:1046–1057.

186. Alnot JY, Leroux D. La synovectomie reaxation-stablision du poignet rhumatoide. *Ann Chir Main* 1985;4:294–305.

187. Allieu Y. Evolution de nos indication chirugicales dans le traitement du poignet rhumatoide. *Ann Chir Main* 1997;16:179–197.

188. Black M, Boswick JA, Wiedel J. Dislocation of the wrist in rheumatoid arthritis, the relationship to distal ulna resection. *Clin Orthop* 1977;124:184–188.

189. Jensen CM. Synovectomy with resection of distal ulna in rheumatoid arthritis of the wrist. *Acta Orthop Scand* 1983;54:754–759.

190. Nanchahal J, Sykes PJ, Williams RL. Excision of the distal ulna in rheumatoid arthritis: Is the price too high? *J Hand Surg* 1996;21:189–196.

191. Newmeyer WL, Green DP. Rupture of digital extensor tendons following distal ulnar resection. *J Bone Joint Surg* 1982;64:178–182.

192. Goncalves D. Correction of disorders of the distal radioulnar joint by artificial pseudarthrosis of the ulna. *J Bone Joint Surg* 1974;56:462–464.

193. Bowers WH. Distal radioulnar joint arthroplasty: the hemiresection-interposition technique. *J Hand Surg* 1985;10:169–178.

194. Watson HK, Ryu J, Burgess RC. Matched distal ulna resection. *J Hand Surg* 1986;11:812–817.

195. Feldon P, Terrono AL, Belsky MR. The "wafer" procedure. *Clin Orthop* 1992;275:124–129.

196. Resnick D. Rheumatoid arthritis of the wrist: why the ulna styloid? *Radiology* 1974;112:29–35.

197. Gonzalez del Pino J, Fernandez DL. Salvage procedure for failed Bower's hemiresection interposition technique in the distal radioulnar joint. *J Hand Surg* 1998;23:749–753.

198. Kleinman WB, Greenberg JA. Salvage of the failed Darrach procedure. *J Hand Surg* 1995;20:951–958.

199. Sauvé L, Kapandji M. Nouvelle technique de traitment chirurgicval des luxations recidivantes isolees de l'extremite inferieure du cubitus. *J Chir (Paris)* 1936;47:589–594.

200. Taleisnik J. The Suave-Kapandji procedure. *Clin Orthop* 1992;275:110–123.

201. Millroy P, Coleman S, Ivers R. The Sauve-Kapandji operation. Technique and results. *J Hand Surg* 1992;17:411–414.

202. Rothwell AG, O'Neill L, Cragg K. Sauve-Kapandji procedure for disorders of the distal radioulnar joint. A simplified technique. *J Hand Surg* 1996;21:771–777.

203. Tran Van F, Obry CH, et al. Rehabilitation du poignet dorsal rhumatoide par l'intervention de Sauve-Kapandji associee a une synovectomie-reaxation-stabilisation. *Ann Chir Main* 1993;12:115–123.

204. Vincent KA, Szabo RM, Agee JM. The Sauve-Kapandji procedure for reconstruction of the rheumatoid distal radioulnar joint. *J Hand Surg* 1993;18:978–983.

205. Fujita S, Masada K, Hashimoto H, et al. *Modified Sauvé-Kapandji procedure for rheumatoid patients. Proceedings of the 8th Congress of the IFSSH, Istanbul, Turkey, 2001.* Istanbul, Turkey: 2001:473–477.

206. Swanson AB. The ulna head syndrome and its treatment by implant resection arthroplasty. *J Bone Joint Surg* 1972;54:906.

207. McMurtry RY, Paley D, et al. A critical analysis of Swanson ulnar head replacement arthroplasty: rheumatoid versus nonrheumatoid. *J Hand Surg* 1990;15:224–231.

208. Pring DJ, Williams DJ. Closed rupture of extensor digitorum communis tendon following excision of distal ulna. *J Hand Surg* 1986;11:451–452.

209. White RE Jr. Resection of the distal ulna with and without implant arthroplasty in rheumatoid arthritis. *J Hand Surg* 1986;11:514–518.

210. Sagerman SD, Seiler JG, Fleming LL, et al. Silicone rubber distal ulnar replacement arthroplasty. *J Hand Surg* 1992;17:689–693.

211. Stanley D, Herbert TJ. The Swanson ulnar head prosthesis for post-traumatic disorders of the distal radioulnar joint. *J Hand Surg* 1992;17:682–688.

212. van Schoonhoven J, Neustadt B, Fernandez DL. Salvage of failed resection arthroplasties of the distal radioulnar joint using a new ulnar head prosthesis. *J Hand Surg* 2000;25:438–446.

213. van Schoonhoven J, Herbert TJ, Fernandez DL, et al. *The ulna head prosthesis-indications and limitations. Proceedings of the 8th Congress of the IFSSH, Istanbul, Turkey, 2001.* Istanbul, Turkey: 2001:210–214.

214. Berger RA. Prevention of convergence of DRUJ with uHead prosthesis. Paper presented at: AAHS; January, 2001.

215. Stamm TT. Excision of the proximal row of the carpus. *Proc R Soc Med* 1944;38:74–75.

216. Ferlic DC, Clayton ML, Mills MF. Proximal row carpectomy: review of rheumatoid and non-rheumatoid wrists. *J Hand Surg* 1991;16:420–424.

217. Culp RW, McGuigan FX, et al. Proximal row carpectomy: a multicenter study. *J Hand Surg* 1993;18:19–25.

218. Fitzgerald JP, Peimer CA, Smith RJ. Distraction resection arthroplasty of the wrist. *J Hand Surg* 1989;14:774–781.

219. Buck-Gramcko D. Denervation of the wrist joint. *J Hand Surg* 1977;2:54–61.

220. Buck-Gramcko D. Wrist denervation procedures in the treatment of Kienböck's disease. *Hand Clin* 1993;9:517–520.

221. Ekerot L, Holmberg J, Eiken O. Denervation of the wrist. *Scand J Plast Reconstr Surg* 1983;17:155–157.

222. Foucher G, Pretz P, Erhard L, et al. La denervation articulaire, une reponse simple a des problemes complexes de chirurgie de la main. *Chirurgie* 1998;123:183–188.

223. Ishida O, Tsai TM, Atasoy E. Long-term results of denervation of the wrist joint for chronic wrist pain. *J Hand Surg* 1993;18:76–80.

224. Rostlund T, Somnier F, Axelsson R. Denervation of the wrist joint—an alternative in conditions of chronic pain. *Acta Orthop Scand* 1980;51:609–616.

225. Chamay A, DellaSanta D, Vilaseca A. Radiolunate arthrodesis factor of stability for the rheumatoid wrist. *Ann Chir Main* 1983;2:5–17.

226. Campbell CJ, Keokarn T. Total and subtotal arthrodesis of the wrist. *J Bone Joint Surg* 1964;46:1520–1533.

227. DellaSanta D, Chamay A. Radiological evolution of the rheumatoid wrist after radio-lunate arthrodesis. *J Hand Surg* 1995;20:146–154.

228. Doets HC, Raven EE. Radiolunate arthrodesis. A procedure for stabilising and preserving mobility in the arthritic wrist. *J Bone Joint Surg* 1999;81:1013–1016.

229. Ishikawa H, Hanyu T, et al. Limited arthrodesis for the rheumatoid wrist. *J Hand Surg* 1992;17:1103–1109.

230. Linscheid RL, Dobyns JH. Radiolunate arthrodesis. *J Hand Surg* 1985;10:821–829.

231. Stanley JK, Boot DA. Radio-lunate arthrodesis. *J Hand Surg* 1989;14:283–287.

232. Taleisnik J. Combined radiocarpal arthrodesis and midcarpal (lunocapitate) arthritis of the wrist. *J Hand Surg* 1987;12:1–8.

233. Ely LW. Study of the joint tuberculosis. *Surg Gynecol Obstet* 1910;10:561–572.

234. Evans DL. Wedge arthrodesis of the wrist. *J Bone Joint Surg* 1955;37:126–134.

235. Haddad RJ Jr, Riordan DC. Arthrodesis of the wrist. A surgical technique. *J Bone Joint Surg* 1967;49:950–954.

236. Herbert JJ, Paillot J. Techniques et indications de l'arthrodese radio-carpo-metacarpienne par greffon. *J Chir* 1950;66:658–663.

237. Liebolt FL. Surgical fusion of the wrist joint. *Surg Gynecol Obstet* 1938;66:1008–1023.

238. Louis DS, Hankin FM. Arthrodesis of the wrist: past and present. *J Hand Surg* 1986;11:787–789.

239. Ross WT. Arthrodesis of the wrist joint. An analysis of 48 operations. *S Afr Med J* 1950;24:755–757.

240. Smith-Petersen MN. A new approach to the wrist joint. *J Bone Joint Surg* 1940;22:122–124.

241. Stein I. Gill turnabout radial graft for wrist arthrodesis. *Surg Gynecol Obstet* 1958;106:231–232.

242. Field J, Herbert TJ. Total wrist fusion. *J Hand Surg* 1982;21:429–433.

243. Larsson SE. Compression arthrodesis of the wrist. *Clin Orthop* 1974;99:146–153.

244. Lee DH, Carroll RE. Wrist arthrodesis: a combined intramedullary pin and autogenous iliac bone graft technique. *J Hand Surg* 1994;19:733–740.

245. Lenoble E, Ovvadia H. Wrist arthrodesis using an embedded iliac crest bone graft. *J Hand Surg* 1993;18:595–600.

246. Louis DS, Hankin FM, Bowers WH. Capitate-radius arthrodesis: an alternative method of radiocarpal arthrodesis. *J Hand Surg* 1984;9:365–369.

247. Manetta P, Tavani L. Arthrodesis of the wrist with a compression plate. *Ital J Orthop Traumatol* 1975;1:219–224.

248. Martini AK. Handgelenkarthrodese Technik und Ergebnisse. *Orthopaedics* 1999;28:907–912.

249. Pech J, Sosna A. Artrodeza zapesti vlastni metodou. *Acta Chir Orthop Trauma Cechosl* 1993;60:187–195.

250. Salenius P. Arthrodesis of the carpal joint. *Acta Orthop Scand* 1966;37:288–296.

251. Shayfer SS, Toledano B, Ruby LK. Wrist arthrodesis: an alternative technique. *Orthopedics* 1998;21:1139–1143.

252. Sorial R, Tonkin MA, Gschwind C. Wrist arthrodesis using a sliding radial graft and plate fixation. *J Hand Surg* 1994;19:217–220.

253. Viegas SF, Rimoldi R, Patterson R. Modified technique of intramedullary fixation for wrist arthrodesis. *J Hand Surg* 1989;14:618–623.

254. Wood MB. Wrist arthrodesis using dorsal radial bone graft. *J Hand Surg* 1987;12:208–212.

255. Barbier O, Saels P, et al. Long-term functional results of wrist arthrodesis in rheumatoid arthritis. *J Hand Surg* 1999;24:27–31.

256. Bracey DJ, McMurtry RY, Walton D. Arthrodesis in the rheumatoid hand using the AO technique. *Orthop Rev* 1980;9:65–69.

257. Campbell RD Jr, Straub LR. Surgical considerations for rheumatoid disease in the forearm and wrist. *Am J Surg* 1965;109:361–367.

258. Carroll RE, Dick HM. Arthrodesis of the wrist for rheumatoid arthritis. *J Bone Joint Surg* 1971;53:1365–1369.

259. Clayton ML, Ferlic DC. Arthrodesis of the arthritic wrist. *Clin Orthop* 1984;187:89–93.

260. Dupont M, Vainio K. Arthrodesis of the wrist in rheumatoid arthritis. A study of 140 cases. *Ann Chir Gynaecol Fenniae* 1968;57:513–519.

261. Howard AC, Stanley JD, Getty CJ. Wrist arthrodesis in rheumatoid arthritis. *J Hand Surg* 1993;18:377–380.

262. Kobus RJ, Turner RH. Wrist arthrodesis for treatment of rheumatoid arthritis. *J Hand Surg* 1990;15:541–546.

263. Mannerfelt L, Malmsten M. Arthrodesis of the wrist in rheumatoid arthritis. A technique without external fixation. *Scand J Plast Reconstr Surg* 1971;5:124–130.

264. Millender LH, Nalebuff EA. Arthrodesis of the rheumatoid wrist. An evaluation of sixty patients and a description of a different surgical technique. *J Bone Joint Surg* 1973;55:1026–1034.

265. Millender LH, Terrono AL, Feldon PF. Arthrodesis of the rheumatic wrist. In: Gelberman RH, ed. *Master techniques in orthopaedic surgery: the wrist*. New York: Raven Press, 1994:287–300.

266. Papaioannou T, Dickson RA. Arthrodesis of the wrist in rheumatoid disease. *Hand* 1982;14:12–16.

267. Skak SV. Arthrodesis of the wrist by the method of Mannerfelt: a follow-up of 19 patients. *Acta Orthop Scand* 1982;52:557–559.

268. Vahvanen V, Tallroth K. Arthrodesis of the wrist by internal fixation in rheumatoid arthritis: a follow-up study of forty-five consecutive cases. *J Hand Surg* 1984;9:531–536.

269. Clendenin MB, Green DP. Arthrodesis of the wrist—complications and their management. *J Hand Surg* 1981;6:253–257.

270. Baeten Y, DeSmet L, Fabry G. Acute anterior forearm compartment syndrome following wrist arthrodesis. *Acta Orthop Belg* 1999;65:239–241.

271. Belt EA, Kaarela K, et al. Does wrist fusion cause destruction of the first carpometacarpal joint in rheumatoid arthritis? 18 patients followed 2–6 years. *Acta Orthop Scand* 1997;68:352–354.

272. Craigen MA, Stanley JK. Distal ulnar instability following arthrodesis in men. *J Hand Surg* 1995;20:155–158.

273. Trumble TE, Easterling KJ, Smith RJ. Ulnocarpal abutment after wrist arthrodesis. *J Hand Surg* 1988;13:11–15.

274. Zachary SV, Stern PJ. Complication following AO/ASIF wrist arthrodesis. *J Hand Surg* 1995;20:339–344.

275. Ekerot L, Jonsson K, Eiken O. Median nerve compression complicating arthrodesis of the rheumatoid wrist. *Scand J Plast Reconstr Surg* 1983;17:257–262.

276. Murray PM. Current status of wrist arthrodesis and wrist arthroplasty. *Clin Plast Surg* 1996;23:385–394.

277. Goodmann MJ, Millender LH, et al. Arthroplasty of the rheumatoid wrist silicone rubber: an early evaluation. *J Hand Surg* 1980;5:114–121.

278. Rayan GM, Brentlinger A, et al. Functional assessment of bilateral wrist arthrodesis. *J Hand Surg* 1987;12:1020–1024.

279. Weiss AP, Wiedeman G, et al. Upper extremity function after wrist arthrodesis. *J Hand Surg* 1995;20:813–817.

280. van Gemert Jan GW. Arthrodesis of the wrist: a clinical, radiographic and ergonomic study of 66 cases. *Acta Orthop Scand Suppl* 1984;55:vi–147.

281. Bodell LS, Champagne LP, Schofield KA. Small joint arthroplasty: the journey is not yet complete. *Orthop Today* 2000;1:57.

282. McElfresh E. History of arthroplasty. In: Petty W, ed. *Total joint replacement*. Philadelphia: WB Saunders, 1991.

283. Ritt MJ, Stuart PR, Naggar L, et al. The early history of arthroplasty of the wrist. *J Hand Surg* 1994;19:778–782.

284. Seradge H, Kuts JA, Kleinert HE, et al. Perichondral resurfacing arthroplasty in the hand. *J Hand Surg* 1984;9:880–886.

285. Murphy JB. Arthroplasty. *Ann Surg* 1913;57:593.

286. Albright JA, Chase RA. Palmar-shelf arthroplasty of the wrist in rheumatoid arthritis. *J Bone Joint Surg* 1970;52:896–906.

287. Gellman H, Rankin G, Brumfield R Jr, et al. Palmar shelf arthroplasty in the rheumatoid wrist. Result of long-term follow-up. *J Bone Joint Surg* 1989;7:223–227.

288. Tillmann K, Thabe H. Technique and results of resection and interposition arthroplasty of the wrist in rheumatoid arthritis. *Reconstr Surg Traumatol* 1981;18:84–91.

289. Kulick RG, DeFiore JC, et al. Long-term results of dorsal stabilization in the rheumatoid wrist. *J Hand Surg* 1981;6:272–280.

290. Ryu J, Watson HK, Burgess RC. Rheumatoid wrist reconstruction utilizing a fibrous nonunion and radiocarpal arthrodesis. *J Hand Surg* 1985;10:830–836.

291. Jackson IT, Simpson RG. Interpositional arthroplasty of the wrist in rheumatoid arthritis. *Hand* 1979;11:169–175.

292. Allende B. Wrist arthroplasty in rheumatoid arthritis. *Clin Orthop* 1973;90:133–136.

293. Pastacaldi P, Engkvist O. Perichondrial wrist arthroplasty in rheumatoid patients. *Hand* 1979;11:184–190.

294. Eaton RG, Akelman E, Eaton BH. Fascial implant arthroplasty for treatment of radioscaphoid degenerative disease. *J Hand Surg* 1989;14:766–774.

295. Biyani A, Simison AJ. Fibrous stabilization of the rheumatoid wrist. *J Hand Surg* 1995;20:143–145.

296. Orred. First report of joint resection of wrist (1773). Referenced in Spillmann E. Resections. In: Asselin P, Masson G, eds. *Dictionnaire encyclopedique des sciences medicales*, vol. 82. Paris, 1876:433.

297. Spillmann E. Resections. In: Asselin P, Masson G, eds. *Dictionnaire encyclopedique des sciences medicales*, vol. 82. Paris, 1876:433.

298. Gluck T. Die Invaginationsmethode der Osteo-und Arthroplastik. *Berlin Klin Wochenschr* 1890;33:752–757.

299. Gluck T. Uber Osteoplastik. *Arch Klin Chir* 1922;117:13–21.

300. Lipscomb PR. Surgery for rheumatoid arthritis, timing and techniques: summary. *J Bone Joint Surg* 1968;50:614.

301. Swanson AB. Flexible implant arthroplasty for arthritic finger joints. Rationale, technique, and results of treatment. *J Bone Joint Surg* 1972;54:435.

302. Gschwind N, Scheier H. Die GSB. *Handgelenksprothese Orthop* 1973;2:46–47.

303. Meuli HC. Reconstructive surgery of the wrist joint. *Hand* 1972;4:88–90.

304. Volz RG. The development of a total wrist arthroplasty. *Clin Orthop* 1976;116:209–214.

305. Allieu Y, Asencio G, et al. Premiers resultats de l'arthroplastie du poignet par implants de Swanson. A propos de 25 cas. *Ann Chir Main* 1982;1:307–308.

306. Davis RF, Weiland AJ, Dowling SV. Swanson implant arthroplasty of the wrist in rheumatoid patients. *Clin Orthop* 1982;166:132–137.

307. Fatti JF, Palmer AK, Mosher JF. The long-term results of Swanson silicone rubber interpositional wrist arthroplasty. *J Hand Surg* 1986;11:166–175.

308. Lluch A, Proubasta I. Les implants radi-carpiens de Swanson. Résultats à long terme. *Main* 1998;3:176–184.

309. Lluch A. Flexible hinged silicone. In: Simmen BR, Allieu Y, Lluch A, et al., eds. *Hand arthroplasties*. London: Martin Dunitz Ltd, 2000.

310. Brase DW, Millender LH. Failure of silicone rubber wrist arthroplasty in rheumatoid arthritis. *J Hand Surg* 1986;11:175–183.

311. Carlson JR, Simmons BR. Total wrist arthroplasty. *J Am Acad Orthop Surg* 1998;6:308–315.

312. Berger RA, Beckenbaugh RD, Linscheid RL. Arthroplasty in the hand and wrist. In: Green DP, Hotchkiss RN, Pederson WC, eds. *Green's operative hand surgery*, 4th ed. New York: Churchill Livingstone, 1999:172–192.

313. Cimino PM, Riordan D, et al. Wrist arthroplasty: a retrospective study. *Orthopedics* 1987;10:337–341.

314. Costi J, Krishnan J, Pearcy M. Total wrist arthroplasty: a quantitative review of the last 30 years. *J Rheumatol* 1998;25:451–458.

315. Gellman H, Hontas R, Brumfield RH, et al. Total wrist arthroplasty in rheumatoid arthritis. A long term clinic review. *Clin Orthop* 1997;342:71–76.

316. Kleinert JM, Lister GD. Silicone implants. *Hand Clin* 1986;2:271–290.

317. Nylen S, Sollerman C, et al. Swanson implant arthroplasty of the wrist in rheumatoid arthritis. *J Hand Surg* 1984;9:295–299.

318. Schernberg F, Gerard Y, et al. Arthroplastie du poignet rhumatoide par implant de silicone. *Ann Chir Main* 1983;2:18–26.

319. McCombe PF, Millroy PJ. Swanson silastic wrist arthroplasty. A retrospective study of fifteen cases. *J Hand Surg* 1985;10:199–201.

320. Comstock CP, Louis DS, Eckenrode JF. Silicone wrist implant: long-term follow-up study. *J Hand Surg* 1988;13:201–205.

321. Fatti JF, Palmer AK, et al. Long-term results of Swanson interpositional wrist arthroplasty: part II. *J Hand Surg* 1991;16:432–437.

322. Jolly SL, Ferlic DC, et al. Swanson silicone arthroplasty of the wrist in rheumatoid arthritis: a long-term follow-up. *J Hand Surg* 1992;17:142–149.

323. Lundkvist L, Barfred T. Total wrist arthroplasty: experience with Swanson flexible silicone implants, 1982–1988. *Scand J Plast Reconstr Hand Surg* 1992;26:97–100.

324. Peimer C, Medige J, et al. Reactive synovitis after silicone arthroplasty. *J Hand Surg* 1986;11:624–638.

325. Smith RJ, Atkinson RE, Jupiter JB. Silicone synovitis of the wrist. *J Hand Surg* 1985;10:47–60.

326. Khoo CT. Silicone synovitis. The current role of silicone elastomer implants in joint reconstruction. *J Hand Surg* 1993;18:679–686.

327. Haloua JP, Collin JP, Schernberg F, et al. Arthroplasties du poignet rhumatoide par implant de Swanson. Résultats et complications à long terme. *Ann Chir Main* 1989;8:124–134.

328. Rosello MI, Costa M, Pizzorno V. Experience of total wrist arthroplasty with silastic implants plus grommets. *Clin Orthop* 1997;342:64–70.

329. Capone RA Jr. The titanium grommet in flexible implant arthroplasty of the radiocarpal joint: a long-term review of 44 cases. *Plast Reconstr Surg* 1995;96:667–672.

330. Swanson AB. Silicone rubber implants for the replacement of the carpal scaphoid and lunate bones. *Orthop Clin North Am* 1970;1:299–309.

331. Carter PR, Benton LJ, Dysert PA. Silicone rubber carpal implants: a study of the incidences of late osseous complications. *J Hand Surg* 1986;11:639–644.

332. Kleinert WB, Stern PJ, Kiefhaber TR. Complications of scaphoid silicone arthroplasty *J Bone Joint Surg* 1985;67:422–427.

333. Weinzweig J, Watson HK. Scapholunate advanced collapse wrist reconstruction. In: Watson HK, Weinzweig J, eds. *The wrist*. Philadelphia: Lippincott Williams & Wilkins, 2001.

334. Swanson AB, de Groot Swanson G, DeHeer DH, et al. Carpal bone titanium implant arthroplasty—10 year experience. *Clin Orthop* 1997;342:46–58.

335. Haynes DR, Rogers SD, et al. The differences in toxicity and release of bone-resorbing mediators induced by titanium and cobalt-chromium-alloy wear particles. *J Bone Joint Surg* 1993;75:825–834.

336. Pequignot JP, Lussiez B, Allieu Y. *A proximal scaphoid implant which allows adaptive mobility. Proceedings of the 8th Congress of the IFSSH, Istanbul, Turkey, 2001*. Istanbul, Turkey: 2001:227–231.

337. Meuli HC. Arthroplasty of the wrist. *Clin Orthop* 1980;149:118–125.

338. Meuli HC, Fernandez DL. Uncemented total wrist arthroplasty. *J Hand Surg* 1995;20:115–122.

339. Meuli HC. Total wrist arthroplasty experience with a noncemented wrist prosthesis. *Clin Orthop* 1997;342:77–83.

340. Meuli HC. Meuli prostheses. In: Simmen BR, Allieu Y, Lluch A, et al., eds. *Hand arthroplasties*. London: Martin Dunitz Ltd, 2001:202–207.

341. Linscheid RL, Beckenbaugh RD. Total arthroplasty of the wrist to relieve pain and increase motion. *Geriatrics* 1976;31:48–52.

342. Beckenbaugh RD. New concepts in arthroplasty of the hand and wrist. *Arch Surg* 1977;112:1094–1098.

343. Beckenbaugh RD, Linscheid RL. Total wrist arthroplasty. Preliminary report. *J Hand Surg* 1977;2:237–244.

344. Beckenbaugh RD. Implant arthroplasty in the rheumatoid hand and wrist: current state of the art in the United States. *J Hand Surg* 1983;8:675–678.

345. Meuli HC. Arthroplastie du poignet. *Ann Chir* 1973;27:527–530.

346. Meuli HC. Les portheses totales du poignet. In: *Monographnie du GEM. Le poignet*. Paris: Expansion Scientifique Francaise, 1983:245–250.

347. Meuli HC. Meuli total wrist arthroplasty. *Clin Orthop* 1984;187:107–111.

348. Beckenbaugh RD. Total joint arthroplasty. The wrist. *Mayo Clin Proc* 1979;54:513–515.

349. Cooney WP, Beckenbaugh RD, Linscheid RL. Total wrist arthroplasty: problems with implant failures. *Clin Orthop* 1984;187:121–128.

350. Beckenbaugh RD. Biax prostheses. In: Simmen BR, Allieu Y, Lluch A, et al., eds. *Hand arthroplasties*. London: Martin Dunitz Ltd, 2001:209–213.

351. Goth D, Konigsberger H. Erste ehrfahrungen mit der zementfreien Totalendoprosthese des Hangelenkesnach Meuli. *Handchir Mikrochir Pastische Chir* 1993;25:256–261.

352. Hamas RS. A quantitative approach to total wrist arthroplasty: development of a precentered total wrist prosthesis. *Orthopedics* 1979;2:245–255.

353. Siemionow M, Lister GD. Tendon ruptures and median nerve damage after Hamas total wrist arthroplasty. *J Hand Surg* 1987;12:374–377.

354. Figgie HE III, Ranawat CS, et al. Preliminary results of total wrist arthroplasty in rheumatoid arthritis using the trispherical total wrist arthroplasty. *J Arthroplasty* 1988;3:9–15.

355. Figgie HE III, Inglis AE, et al. A critical analysis of alignment factors influencing functional results following trispherical total wrist arthroplasty. *J Arthroplasty* 1986;1:183–195.

356. Figgie MP, Ranawat CS, Inglis AE, et al. Trispherical total wrist arthroplasty in rheumatoid arthritis. *J Hand Surg* 1990;15:217–223.

357. Kraay MJ, Figgie MP. Wrist arthroplasty with the trispherical total wrist prosthesis. *Semin Arthroplasty* 1995;6:37–43.

358. Lorei MP, Figgie MP, et al. Failed total wrist arthroplasty. Analysis of failures and results of operative management. *Clin Orthop* 1997;342:84–93.

359. O'Flynn HM, Rosen A, Weiland AJ. Failure of the hinge mechanism of a trispherical total wrist arthroplasty: a case report and review of the literature. *J Hand Surg* 1999;24:156–160.

360. Ranawat CS, Green NA, et al. Spherical tri-axial total wrist replacement. In: Inglis A, ed. *AAOS symposium on total joint of the upper extremity.* St. Louis: CV Mosby, 1982:265–272.

361. Volz RG. Total wrist arthroplasty: a clinical review. *Clin Orthop* 1984;187:112–120.

362. Lamberta FJ, Ferlic DC, Clayton ML. Volz total wrist arthroplasty in rheumatoid arthritis: a preliminary report. *J Hand Surg* 1980;5:245–280.

363. Volz RG. Total wrist arthroplasty. A new approach to wrist disability. *Clin Orthop* 1977;128:180–189.

364. Volz RG. Total wrist arthroplasty. A review of 100 patients. *Orthop Trans* 1979;3:268.

365. Dennis DA, Ferlic DC, Clayton ML. Volz total wrist arthroplasty in rheumatoid arthritis: a long-term review. *J Hand Surg* 1986;11:483–490.

366. Menon J. Total wrist replacement using the modified Volz prosthesis. *J Bone Joint Surg* 1987;69:998–1006.

367. Bosco JA III, Bynum DK, Bowers WH. Long-term outcome of Volz total wrist arthroplasties. *J Arthroplasty* 1994;9:25–31.

368. Alnot JY. Les arthroplasties du poignet. In: *Monographie du GEM. Le poignet.* Paris: Expansion Scientifique Française, 1983:251–256.

369. Alnot JY. L'arthroplastie totale Guepar de poignet dans la polyarthrite rhumatoide. *Acta Ortho Belg* 1988;54:178–184.

370. Fourastier J, LeBreton L, Alnot Y, et al. La prothese total radio-carpeinne guepar dans la chirurgie du poignet rhumatoide. *Rev Chir Orthop* 1996;82:108–115.

371. Ferlic DC, Clayton ML. Results of CFV total wrist arthroplasty: review and early report. *Orthopedics* 1995;18:1167–1171.

372. Kapandji IA. Principes et experimentation d'une nouvelle famille de protheses de poignet de type cardan. *Ann Chir Main* 1982;1:155–167.

373. Gagey O, Lanoy JK, et al. Prothese totale radio-carpienne. Etude prealable. *Rev Chir Orthop* 1986;72:165–171.

374. Taleisnik J. Treatment: bone and joint procedures. In: Taleisnik J, ed. *The wrist.* New York: Churchill Livingstone, 1985.

375. Cobb TK, Beckenbaugh RD. Biaxial total-wrist arthroplasty. *J Hand Surg* 1996;21:1011–1021.

376. Johnson BM, Flynn MJ, Beckenbaugh RD. A dynamic splint for use after total wrist arthroplasty. *Am J Occup Ther* 1981;35:179–184.

377. Beckenbaugh RD, Brown ML. Early experience with biaxial total wrist arthroplasty. Paper presented at: the 45th Annual Meeting of the ASSH; September, 1990; Toronto, Canada.

378. Lirette R, Kinnard P. Biaxial total wrist arthroplasty in rheumatoid arthritis. *Can J Surg* 1995;38:51–53.

379. Courtman NH, Sochart DH, Trail IA, et al. Biaxial wrist replacement. *J Hand Surg* 1999;24:32–34.

380. Cobb TK, Beckenbaugh RD. Biaxial long-stemmed multipronged distal components for revision/bone deficit total-wrist arthroplasty. *J Hand Surg* 1996;21:764–770.

381. Rettig ME, Beckenbaugh RD. Revision total wrist arthroplasty. *J Hand Surg* 1993;18:798–804.

382. Menon J. Total wrist arthroplasty. In: Watson HK, Weinzweig J, ed. *The wrist.* Philadelphia: Lippincott Williams & Wilkins, 2001.

383. Menon J. Universal total wrist implant: experience with a carpal component fixed with three screws. *J Arthroplasty* 1998;13:515–523.

384. Sollerman C, Boeckstyn M, Bodell LS. Wrist arthroplasty in rheumatoid arthritis using the Menon universal wrist implant. Poster presented at: EFSSH; June, 2000; Barcelona.

385. Adams BD. Wrist arthroplasty using the universal wrist prosthesis. Paper presented at: the 8th Congress of the IFSSH; June, 2000; Istanbul, Turkey. Adams BD. Total wrist arthroplasty. Semin Arthroplasty 2001;11:72–81.

386. Divelbiss BJ, Sollerman C, Adams BD. Early results of the universal total wrist arthroplasty in rheumatoid arthritis. *J Hand Surg* 2002;27:195–204.

387. Adams BD. Total wrist arthroplasty. *Semin Arthroplasty* 2000;11:72–81.

388. Silby TF, Unsworth A. Wear of cross-linked polyethylene against itself. *J Biomed Eng* 1991;13:217–220.

389. Rozing PM. Prothesen van de bovenste extremiteit. *Ned Tijdschr Geneeskd Mei* 1998;142:1256–1261.

390. Rozing PM. Total wrist arthroplasty. *Surg Tech Orthop Trauma* 2000;55:1–6.

391. Radmer S, Andresen R, Sparmann M. Wrist arthroplasty with a new generation of prostheses in patients with rheumatoid arthritis. *J Hand Surg* 1999;24:935–943.

392. Lundborg G, Branemark PI. Anchorage of wrist joint prostheses to bone using the osseointegration principle. *J Hand Surg* 1997;22:84–89.

393. Albrektson T, Branemark PI, et al. Osseointegrated titanium implants: requirements for ensuring a long-lasting direct bone-to-implant anchorage in man. *Acta Orthop Scand* 1981;52:155–170.

394. Lundborg G, Branemark PI, Carlsson I. Metacarpophalangeal joint arthroplasty based on the osseointegration concept. *J Hand Surg* 1993;18:693–703.

395. Moller K, Sollerman C, Geijer M, et al. Osseointegrated silicone implants. 18 patients with 57 MCP joints followed for 2 years. *Acta Orthop Scand* 1999;70:109–115.

396. Hubach P. TMW prosthesis prospective review. *Acta Orthop Scand* 2003 *(in press)*.

397. Shapiro RF, Resnick D, Castles JJ, et al. Fistulizations of rheumatoid joints. Spectrum of identifiable syndromes. *Ann Rheum Dis* 1975;34:489–498.

398. Garner RW, Mowat AG, Hazleman BL. Wound healing after operations on patients with rheumatoid arthritis. *J Bone Joint Surg* 1973;55:134–144.

399. Kasdan ML, June L. Postoperative results of rheumatoid arthritis patients on methotrexate at the time of reconstructive surgery of the hand. *Orthopedics* 1993;16:1233–1235.

400. Sany J, Anaya JM, et al. Influence of methotrexate on the frequency of postoperative infectious complication in patients with rheumatoid arthritis. *J Rheumatol* 1993;20:1129–1132.

401. Huskisson EC, Hart FS. Severe, unusual and recurrent infections in rheumatoid arthritis. *Ann Rheum Dis* 1972;31:118–121.

402. Volz RG, Lieb M, Benjamin J. Biomechanics of the wrist. *Clin Orthop* 1980;149:112–117.

403. Evans JS, Blair WF, et al. The in vivo kinematics of the rheumatoid wrist. *J Orthop Res* 1986;4:142–151.

404. Backdahl M, Carlsoo S. Distribution of activity in muscles acting on the wrist. *Acta Morphol Neerl Scand* 1961;4:136.

405. Linscheid RL. Dynamic factors affecting carpal stability Paper presented at: the 4th Triennial International Hand and Wrist Biomechanics Symposium; June, 2001; Izmir, Turkey.

406. Yi-Wen C, Strommen J, Fong-Chin SU, et al. Muscle activation during isometric torque generation at wrist joint. Paper presented at: the 4th Triennial International Hand and Wrist Biomechanics Symposium; June, 2001; Izmir, Turkey.

407. McFarland GB Jr, Weathersby HT. Kinesiology of selected muscles acting on the wrist: electromyographic study. *Arch Phys Med Rehab* 1962;April:165–171.

408. Gordon M, Bullouh PG. Synovial and osseous inflammation in failed silicon-rubber prostheses. *J Bone Joint Surg* 1982;64:574–580.

409. Schmalzried TP, Jasty M, Harris WA. Periprosthetic bone loss in total hip arthroplasty, polyethylene wear and the concept of effect joint space. *J Bone Joint Surg* 1992;74:849–863.

410. Archibeck MJ, Jacobs JJ, Roebulk KA, et al. The basic science of periprosthetic osteolysis. *J Bone Joint Surg* 2000;82:1478–1489.

411. Jones LC, Frondoza L, Hungerford DS. Effect of PMMA particles and movement on an implant interface in a canine model. *J Bone Joint Surg* 2001;83:448–458.

412. Harris WH, Davis JP. Modern use of modern cement for total hip replacement. *Orthop Clin North Am* 1988;19:581–589.

413. Dawson WJ. Radius fracture after total wrist arthroplasty. *J Hand Surg* 1989;14:630–634.

414. Ferlic DC, Jolly SN, Clayton ML. Salvage for failed implant arthroplasty of the wrist. *J Hand Surg* 1992;17:917–923.

415. Beer TA, Turner RH. Wrist arthrodesis for failed wrist implant arthroplasty. *J Hand Surg* 1997;22:685–693.

416. Carlson JR, Simmons BP. Wrist arthrodesis after failed wrist implant arthroplasty. *J Hand Surg* 1998;23:893–898.

417. Alnot JY. Rheumatoid arthritis of the wrist with adult onset. *Acta Orthop Belg* 2000;66:329–336.

418. Kraft G, Detels P. Position of function of the wrist. *Arch Phys Med Rehab* 1972;53:272–275.

419. Pryce JC. The wrist position between neutral and ulnar deviation that facilitate the maximum power grip strength. *J Biomechanics* 1980;13:505–511.

420. O'Driscoll SW, Horii E. et al. The relationship between wrist position, grasp size, and grip strength. *J Hand Surg* 1992;17:169–177.

421. Stanley JK, Tolat AR. Long-term results of Swanson silastic arthroplasty in the rheumatoid wrist. *J Hand Surg* 1993;18:381–388.

422. Sorbie C. Arthroplasty in the rheumatoid upper extremity: a plea for earlier referral. *Orthopedics* 2000;23:11–12.

423. Stanley JK. Conservative surgery in the management of rheumatoid disease of the hand and wrist. *J Hand Surg* 1992;17:339–342.

424. Kushner I, Dawson NV. Aggressive therapy does not substantially alter the long-term course of rheumatoid arthritis. *Rheum Dis Clin North Am* 1993;19:163–173.

425. Lehman, Domer, Bodell. Review of the rheumatoid wrist and a new classification algorithm. *J Am Soc Surg Hand* 2003 *(in press)*.

426. Meyerdierks EM, Mosher JF, Werner FW. Limited wrist arthrodesis: a laboratory study. *J Hand Surg* 1987;12:526–529.

427. Garcia-Elias M, Cooney WP, An KN, et al. Wrist kinematics after limited intercarpal arthrodesis. *J Hand Surg* 1989;14:791–799.

428. Viegas SF, Patterson RM, Peterson PD, et al. Evaluation of the biomechanical efficacy of limited intercarpal fusions for the treatment of scapholunate dissociation. *J Hand Surg* 1990;15:120–128.

429. Short WH, Werner FW, Fortino BS, et al. Distribution of pressures and forces on the wrist after simulated intercarpal fusion and Kienböck's disease. *J Hand Surg* 1992;17:443–449.

430. Buchanan TS, Moniz MJ, Dewald JP, et al. Estimation of muscle forces about the wrist joint during isometric tasks using an EMG coefficient method. *J Biomech* 1993;26:547–560.

431. Tolbert JR, Blair WF, Andrews JG, et al. The kinetics of normal and prosthetic wrists. *J Biomech* 1985;18:887–897.

432. Sirkett D, Miles AW, Miilineux G, et al. Three dimensional constraint modelling of the wrist. Paper presented at: the 8th Congress of the IFSSH; June, 2001; Istanbul, Turkey.

80

DENERVATION OF THE WRIST

MICHAEL SAUERBIER

HISTORICAL PERSPECTIVE

Partial or total wrist arthrodeses are considered definitive solutions or salvage procedures for treating the painful arthrotic wrist (1–11). They can be performed at any stage of the patient's history, once osteoarthrosis is confirmed. Limited wrist arthrodesis or a proximal row carpectomy (PRC) may relieve pain and stop progressive wrist degeneration. These procedures frequently allow return to full activity after a substantial postsurgery recovery period (8). Because of the limitation in range of motion, the long convalescences, and low demands, especially in the elderly, many patients are reticent to undergo such a procedure, and other options are desirable (8). Denervation of the wrist joint represents an appealing alternative for pain relief while maintaining wrist motion with a minimal recovery period (12). The purpose of this surgical method is to cut off the afferent pain transmission A-delta and C-delta fibers of the articular wrist capsule (13).

The idea of reducing joint pain by denervation of articular sensory branches was originally described by Camitz (14) in 1933 for the hip joint and refined in 1942 by Tavernièr and Truchet (15). Later, many authors published their results of hip denervation; however, there has been very limited experience using this method in other joints.

It was the German surgeon Albrecht Wilhelm who performed the first denervation of the radiocarpal joint in 1959 at the Department of Surgery of Würzburg University in a patient with a 30-year-old scaphoid nonunion with progressive osteoarthrosis. In 1966, Wilhelm described the technique and surgical anatomy of the denervation of the wrist joint and published the first clinical series of wrist denervation in 21 patients (16). The innervation of the wrist joint was described first by Wilhelm and later, in further publications, by others.

SURGICAL ANATOMY AND BIOMECHANICS

The wrist is the junction between forearm and hand and provides a mechanism allowing wrist extension, flexion, radial deviation, ulnar deviation, and a limited amount of axial rotation. The kinematics and biomechanics of the wrist joint have been studied extensively, and a substantial amount of basic knowledge of the normal and the pathologic wrist has been described since the 1980s. There are many causes of chronic wrist pain, such as posttraumatic, degenerative, or inflammatory arthropathies. Most arthropathies follow predictable patterns of degenerative changes, whereby specific regions of the carpal articular surfaces undergo degenerative changes, whereas others are not included (8). Typical examples for these patterns are the scapholunate advanced collapse (11,17–19) (SLAC) or the scaphoid nonunion advanced collapse (SNAC) (1,2,5).

Anatomic investigations of the nerve supply of the wrist from Wilhelm (20), Buck-Gramcko (21), Dellon et al. (22), and others (13,23–27) have shown that the innervation of the wrist is selectively supported by intraarticular branches from the following nerves: (a) the posterior interosseous nerve (PIN), (b) the superficial radial nerve (SRN), (c) the lateral antebrachial cutaneous nerve, (d) the median nerve, (e) the anterior interosseous nerve (AIN), (f) the ulnar nerve, and (g) the posterior antebrachial cutaneous nerve (Fig. 1).

Posterior Interosseous Nerve

The PIN is purely sensory after innervating the muscle belly of the extensor indicis proprius and runs onto the base of the fourth extensor compartment with the distally directed division of the anterior interosseous artery (Fig. 1A) (13). Before the nerve reaches the dorsal aspect of the radius, a branch passes for the innervation of the distal radioulnar joint (DRUJ) (Fig. 1A). Typically, the PIN is found with the anterior interosseous artery on the radial aspect of the fourth compartment, where the nerve is especially easy to isolate because of a generous coat of epineurium, which doubles or triples the cross-sectional area of the nerve (13). At the radiocarpal joint, the nerve spreads into three to four longer main branches that run divergently against the bases of the metacarpal bones 2 to 5. At the level of the radiocar-

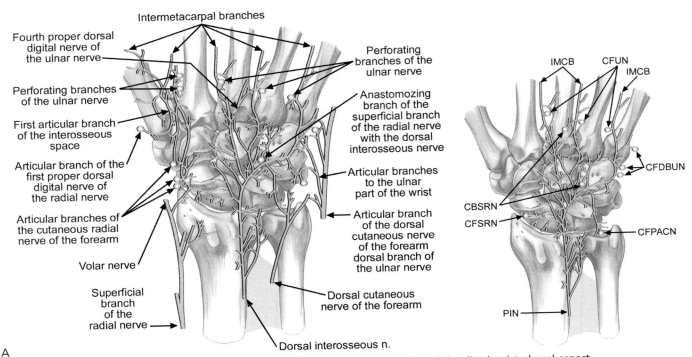

FIGURE 1. A: Innervation of the wrist dorsally. **B:** Innervation of the distal wrist, dorsal aspect. CBSRN, connecting branches of the superficial radial nerve, perforating the superficial fascia; CFDBUN, connecting fibers of the dorsal branch of the ulnar nerve; CFPACN, connecting fibers of the posterior antebrachial cutaneous nerve; CFSRN, connecting fibers of the superficial radial nerve; CFUN, connecting fibers of the ulnar nerve; IMCB, intermetacarpal branches, supplying the metacarpophalangeal joints; n., nerve; PIN, posterior interosseous nerve.

pal joint capsule, the nerve innervates the central two-thirds of the dorsal wrist joint capsule.

Anterior Interosseous Nerve

The AIN is adjacent to the PIN within 2 mm (28). The nerves are separated only by the thin membranous region of the distal interosseous membrane (IOM) of the forearm (13). Some small branches can be found in the pronator quadratus muscle; however, the main branch reaches the wrist capsule. The AIN appears at this level much smaller than the PIN at the base of the fourth extensor compartment. The AIN innervates the palmar capsular side of the DRUJ and the radiocarpal joint (13).

Superficial Radial Nerve

The first articular branch of the SRN arises at the level of the radial styloid and innervates the radiocarpal joint in the proximal part of the radial snuffbox. This branch connects in this area with very tiny branches of the lateral antebrachial cutaneous nerve as well as with a branch of the PIN. More distally, the articular branch of the first interosseous space arises from the first dorsal digital nerve or from its branches in the proximal part of the first interosseous space. At the bases of the first and second metacarpals, it divides

into various branches and has connections with small fibers of the deep branch of the ulnar nerve. Also, there are recurrent fibers that run with the radial artery in a proximal direction innervating the inter- and carpometacarpal joints 1 and 2. There are more small fibers that innervate the metaphalangeal joint of the thumb and other directions of the first metacarpal bone (29–33).

Lateral Antebrachial Cutaneous Nerve

Wilhelm described that the lateral antebrachial cutaneous nerve anastomoses in the distal forearm with the palmar cutaneous branch of the median nerve (31). Two of its branches run distally together with the radial artery and innervate the radiopalmar area of the radiocarpal joint, as well as the radial section of the carpus, including the scaphotrapeziotrapezoid (STT) and the trapeziometacarpal joints.

INDICATIONS

The principal indication for denervation of the wrist is painful restriction of wrist motion (13,31,34,35). In most situations, these symptoms are caused by posttraumatic or idiopathic arthrosis of the carpal bones or the radiocarpal joint. The majority of the patients have from nonunited fractures of the carpus (SNAC wrist), ligamentous injuries of the carpus (scapholunate dissociation followed by SLAC wrist), lunotriquetral tears, or intraarticular fractures and fracture dislocations of the radius, including injuries of adjacent areas such as the DRUJ or the triangular fibrocartilage complex (TFCC). Other indications are Kienböck's and Preiser's disease.

It has to be recognized that denervation of the wrist is not a definite solution for progressive arthrosis of the wrist joint (2,8). The procedure is an alternative to salvage procedures, if the arthrosis is not in a late or severe state. The patients have to be selected carefully and need to be aware preoperatively that the surgery cannot prevent progressive radiocarpal collapse or arthrosis at the whole wrist joint (13). The ideal patient has an early stage of arthrosis and an acceptable range of motion. Another good example might be made, as stated by Berger (13), by the condition of chronic static irreducible scapholunate dissociation. Usually, such a situation would be treated with a salvage operation such as an STT or scaphocapitate fusion or a PRC (2–6,9,18,36). In this scenario, performing the salvage operation might be considered, but the wrist denervation procedure may provide considerable advantages such as immediate pain relief and functional enhancement. If the denervation procedure fails, a salvage procedure is still the treatment of choice as the next step. It can be done at any point during the course of treatment, if necessary (8,13).

Another good indication is a heavy-working patient between the ages of 55 and 60 years who wants to work a few more years before retirement but not undergo extensive wrist surgery and rehabilitation with the risk of more restricted range of motion and the inability to return to work.

CONTRAINDICATIONS

There are only a few contraindications for isolated wrist denervation. One is symptomatic reflex dystrophy in its initial or severe state (31). Another contraindication is failed preoperative testing or blocking of the nerves at the wrist joint with local anesthesia (13).

PREOPERATIVE EVALUATION

A history of trauma or development of symptoms is obtained in the office when the patient visits initially. The patient is asked to determine which maneuvers of the wrist produce pain and in which areas. Several clinical tests, such as the Watson test, the scapholunate ballottement test, the lunotriquetral ballottement test, the pisiform lift test or the fovea sign, and others, have to be performed by the hand surgeon. It is mandatory to get conventional x-rays in the posteroanterior and lateral views to determine the severity

of arthrosis. In selected cases, a computed tomography scan or a wrist arthroscopy is helpful to define the stage of the disease. The severity of an arthrosis in the DRUJ can be determined very reliably with axial computed tomography scans in pronation, supination, and neutral positions. Wrist arthroscopy is mandatory for the evaluation of patients who have TFCC injuries or degenerative tears (Palmer type-2A–2E). Wrist arthroscopy is also a good diagnostic option for early SNAC and SLAC (stage I) problems because it helps to define whether a scaphoid reconstruction with resection of the radial styloid or a dorsal capsulodesis after scapholunate instability in combination with a radial styloidectomy is possible (8). It might also be indicated in Kienböck's stage IIIa/b for decision making whether a revascularization of the lunate or a limited wrist fusion is possible or whether a wrist denervation should be performed (37).

Additionally, grip strength, range of motion for extension/flexion, ulnar/radial deviation, and pronation/supination are recorded with a computerized Jamar (DEXTER, Cedaron, Inc., Davis, CA) (5,6). In the author's department, every patient undergoing wrist surgery has to fill out a DASH (*d*isabilities of the *a*rm, *s*houlder, and *h*and) questionnaire (38,39) preoperatively for prospective outcome evaluation. The DASH questionnaire is a subjective outcome tool that is focused on the patient's activities of daily living (ADL) (4–6,38,39).

PREOPERATIVE INJECTION

The indication for a wrist denervation may become obvious after a preoperative test injection of 1% lidocaine. The author does it with every patient who is a possible candidate for a wrist denervation. On the day before the wrist denervation procedure, the patient is examined by an occupational therapist. The patient has to perform a test series with various types of ADL. Grip strength is checked without local anesthesia. This examination is called a *null series*. The next day, the patients do the same series after injecting the nerves that will be cut during the denervation procedure (*stress series*). If the symptoms improve significantly after the so-called stress series, the patient will undergo the wrist denervation procedure the next day. If the symptoms do not improve, other surgical options have to be discussed.

The preoperative injection is performed by a physician. The distal forearm and wrist are prepared in the manner typically used by the treating hand surgeon. First, the DRUJ is identified by palpating the ulnar head. The point of skin penetration for the injection is determined 1 fingerbreadth proximally to the most proximal level of the ulnar head (Fig. 2). The injection is carried out through the IOM so that the point of the injection must be centered between the radius and ulna. A standard 25-gauge needle with a 10-

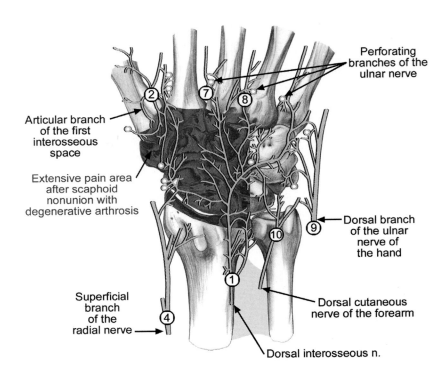

Perforating branches of the ulnar nerve

Articular branch of the first interosseous space

Extensive pain area after scaphoid nonunion with degenerative arthrosis

Dorsal branch of the ulnar nerve of the hand

Superficial branch of the radial nerve

Dorsal cutaneous nerve of the forearm

Dorsal interosseous n.

FIGURE 2. Preoperative injection for blocking the posterior interosseous nerve/anterior interosseous nerve. Dorsal aspect of the wrist with numbers indicating the sequence and points of injection to block the different nerve branches. n., nerve.

cc syringe containing 1% lidocaine is forwarded 5 mm into the injection point, where 2 cc of the lidocaine is injected under low pressure (13). The needle is then advanced another 5 mm through the proximal part of the IOM, where a second shot of 2 cc lidocaine is deposited (13). If a complete wrist denervation is considered for surgery, the next steps for preoperative nerve blocks should be followed according to Wilhelm's suggestions (31).

The articular branch of the SRN in the first interosseous space is injected dorsally and subcutaneously between the bases of the first and second metacarpals with 0.5 cc lidocaine. In the next step, the articular branches of the lateral antebrachial cutaneous nerve are injected 3 cm proximally to the palmar wrist crease and ulnarly from the radial artery with 1 cc lidocaine. It is important to block the articular branch of the SRN because this branch contributes tremendously to radial-sided wrist problems. The injection site of this branch is 4 cm proximal to the radial styloid, with 3 cc lidocaine injected in a transverse direction. The palmar branch of the median nerve can be injected 1 cm proximally to the palmar wrist crease above the tendon of the flexor carpi radialis muscle. One cc of local anesthesia is infiltrated subcutaneously between the radial artery and the palmaris longus tendon. Perforating fibers of the deep branch of the ulnar nerve can be injected with 0.5 cc dorsally, directly above intermetacarpal joints 1 and 2. The dorsal branch of the ulnar nerve and the articular branch of the medial antebrachial cutaneous nerve are infiltrated above the ulnar edge of the ulnar head with a subcutaneous infiltration of 3 cc lidocaine in a palmar direction consecutively up to the level of the extensor carpi ulnaris. Finally, the posterior antebrachial cutaneous nerve can be blocked

with an injection over the posterior aspect of the ulnar head with a subcutaneous infiltration of 1 cc lidocaine in a transverse direction.

Thirty minutes after the injections, the patient undergoes the examination, as described above, with an occupational therapist. The pain is rated under resting and stress conditions with a visual analogue scale from 0 to 100. The patient is also asked about any sensory deficits in the anatomic areas of the median or ulnar nerve. Any severe change in sensory levels in these peripheral nerves invalidates the test (13).

SURGICAL MANAGEMENT

The wrist denervation procedure can be performed under local anesthesia together with sedation, intravenous anesthesia (Bier block), regional anesthesia (brachial plexus anesthesia), or general anesthesia. Regional anesthesia is preferable in the majority of the author's patients. The patient is positioned on the operating table in a supine position, and a pneumatic tourniquet (300 mm Hg) is wrapped around the upper arm in a standard manner. For identification of the small branches of the nerves, the author recommends loupe magnification with 2.5× glasses.

Incisions

The author does not routinely carry out a complete wrist denervation as proposed by Wilhelm (12,16,29–31,35-37), Buck-Gramcko (12,16,29–31), and others (38–53) because no significant differences between partial and complete

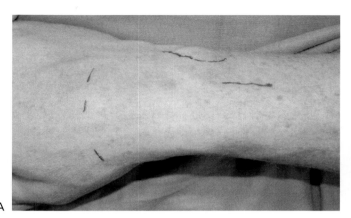

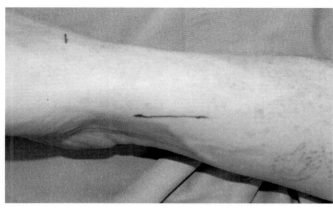

A   B

FIGURE 3. A,B: Outlines for the incision for wrist denervation.

wrist denervation were found in the author's patient group. This is discussed later in this chapter.

Initially, the incision to resect the PIN and the AIN is carried out dorsally on the distal forearm (Figs. 3 and 4). The incision line is drawn on the skin in a longitudinal direction, spanning 3 to 4 cm, extending proximally from the DRUJ (13). After exposing the superficial ante-brachial fascia, it is opened at the radial edge of the extensor pollicis longus muscle, ulnar to the dorsal tuber-cle of the radius. After retraction of the extensor pollicis longus muscle and the digital extensors of the fourth compartment ulnarly, the PIN can be explored over the periosteum of the distal part of the radius and the proxi-mal part of the IOM. It can be easily dissected from the IOM and the perforating anterior interosseous artery. First, the PIN should be resected for at least 1.5 cm very

proximally to eliminate the articular branch of the DRUJ as well. Then the IOM is incised 2 cm in length, and the deep head of the pronator quadratus muscle is exposed. The AIN is found lying immediately anterior to the IOM or within the dorsal 1 mm of the pronator quadratus (13). It may be hidden temporarily from visual exposure, adjacent to the incision line in the IOM. The terminal sensory branch of the AIN is seen more distally, and a 2-cm segment is electrocoagulated and resected. Proxi-mally, there can be several diverging nerve branches that should be left in place. The author always tries to protect the anterior interosseous artery, which lies adjacent to the AIN. The wound is irrigated then with saline solution, and the incised IOM can be left open, as well as the deep antebrachial fascia. The skin is closed with nonresorbable 5-0 sutures.

Dorsal approach   Dorsal approach

AIAp
PIN (area of resection)
Radius

DRUJ
Ulna
IOM

Distal PIN
AIN (area of resection)
Proximal PIN (resected)

AIA
PQ
IOM

FIGURE 4. Resection of the posterior interosseous nerve (PIN)/anterior interosseous nerve (AIN) through a single approach. AIA, anterior interosseous artery; AIAp, perforating anterior interosseous artery; DRUJ, distal radioulnar joint; IOM, interosseous membrane; PQ, pronator quadratus muscle.

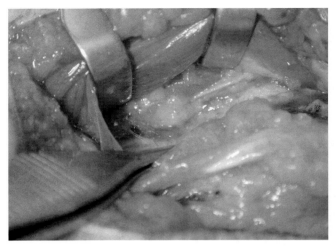

FIGURE 5. Dissection of the articular branches of the lateral cutaneous nerve and the articular branch of the superficial radial nerve.

The next stage of the procedure is the dissection of articular branches of the lateral cutaneous nerve of the forearm and the articular branch of the SRN. A 4 to 6-cm-long curvilinear palmar incision is made from the trapezium to the distal radius region (Fig. 5). The radial artery is explored and denuded over a length of approximately 2 cm. Articular fibers and accompanying venous vessels are electrocoagulated. The SRN and its radiopalmar branches are preserved. Then, the articular branches of the SRN are dissected carefully in a manner of an epifascial mobilization of the soft tissue layers in radial and dorsoradial directions. All branches that descend towards the carpus are coagulated. A branch from the dorsal radial nerve of the thumb to the first carpometacarpal joint, which is arising adjacent to the radial styloid, is coagulated.

Next, the sheath of the flexor carpi radialis is opened, and the palmar cutaneous branch of the median nerve is freed until it passes superficially in the subcutaneous tissue at the distal palmar wrist crease. After irrigation of the wound with saline solution, the skin is closed with nonresorbable 5-0 sutures.

For the resection of the articular fibers of the dorsal branch of the ulnar nerve, a 3-cm curvilinear incision is made, dorsoulnarly encircling the ulnar head. The sensory branch of the ulnar nerve is frequently found deeply embedded in the fascia over the distal joint capsule. The nerve is elevated and all of its deep branches are divided and electrocoagulated, with care not to injure the dorsal transverse cutaneous sensory branch, which remains with the skin. Finally, the skin is undermined blindly with the index finger in the proximal direction to include contributions from the medial or posterior cutaneous nerves or both. The wound is then closed with nonresorbable monofilament 5-0 sutures. Closing of all incisions should be possible without drainage. A light compression dressing

is applied, and splinting is necessary unless another surgical procedure is associated. The sutures are removed between days 12 and 14 postoperatively.

Postoperative Management

The procedure can be carried out on an outpatient basis. The patient should get oral pain medication with nonsteroidal antiinflammatory drugs, such as diclofenac or ibuprofen, for 5 to 7 days if they do not have a history of gastroenterologic diseases. The patient is instructed to protect the wound from moisture and contamination for a week but is otherwise unrestricted. ADL are allowed as tolerated.

RESULTS

One-hundred-forty-five patients were treated with an isolated wrist denervation at the Department of Hand, Plastic, and Reconstructive Surgery/BG Trauma Center Ludwigshafen from 1993 to 2000. Of these, 84 (65%) were reexamined and included in the study. The majority of the patients were men. The mean follow-up time was 46 months. The main indication for wrist denervation was radiocarpal arthrosis in 58 patients (65.5%); other indications included chronic wrist pain after scapholunate or lunotriquetral ligament instability and disorders at the TFCC. Thirty-seven patients underwent a complete wrist denervation according to Wilhelm's technique (31), including the denervation of the bases of the carpometacarpal joints 1 to 4. The other 47 patients were operated on as described in an earlier section.

Pain was evaluated under stress and resting conditions with a visual analogue scale from 0 to 100. Grip strength and range of motion were measured with an electronic computerized Jamar Dynamometer (DEXTER, Cedaron Medical, Inc., Davis, CA). The patient's ADL and general quality of life were estimated with the DASH questionnaire.

Pain was reduced from 69.1 preoperatively to 49.8 postoperatively under stress and remained unchanged under resting conditions. There were no statistical differences between the groups (partial vs. total denervation). Eighteen of the 84 patients had complete pain relief under stress conditions. The average duration of pain relief was 37 months (6 to 91 months). Active range of motion for extension/flexion was 63% and was 57% for ulnar/radial deviation, without any significant differences in the two denervation groups. The average total DASH score was 38 points for all 84 patients, again demonstrating no significant differences between partial (without bases of the metacarpals) and total wrist denervation. Eight patients underwent additional surgery, including total wrist arthrodesis, four-corner arthrodesis, and PRC. Thirty-one patients experienced partial loss of sensation at the dorsal wrist side. Forty-nine patients felt that they were "somewhat satisfied" with the procedure, nine patients were "partially satisfied," and 26 patients were "not satisfied" with the postoperative result at the time of follow-up evaluation.

DISCUSSION

Denervation of the wrist is an established standard procedure for various wrist arthropathies and was developed by the German surgeon Albrecht Wilhelm (12,16,20). After Wilhelm's description of the surgical technique, it was Buck-Gramcko (34), again a German hand surgeon, who published a multicenter study in 1977 with 195 examined patients. The average follow-up time was 4.1 years. The results of this study demonstrated that 68.7% of the patients had complete or at least some pain relief during heavy work. The best results were seen in patients with scaphoid nonunion and Kienböck's disease. Buck-Gramcko confirmed his results in another follow-up study with 242 patients, showing good or excellent results in 66.5% of the patients (35). Other authors could also demonstrate satisfying results after this procedure (40,42,45,49,51). Wilhelm recently reported (31) that in 24 patients, after an average follow-up time of 10.5 (6 to 14) years, 62.5% showed good or excellent results in terms of pain relief. The grip strength decreased over time from 66.7% compared with the contralateral hand after 1.2 years of follow-up to 50.0% after 10.5 years. Wilhelm could demonstrate that a deterioration of results over the years was mostly related to the progress in degenerative changes in the already existing wrist arthropathies (31). An increase of degenerative changes attributable to the denervation procedure was not found in Wilhelm's study. Ishida et al. (45) reported on 13 complete and 4 partial denervations, but only 24% of the patients were satisfied at a mean follow-up of 51 months. Because of the disappointing results, they concluded that denervation surgery alone was not sufficient. Ekerot et al. (41) reported that 70% improved in a series of 46 patients. Röstlund et al. (52) obtained good results with a simplified four-nerve neurotomy. Grechenig et al. (53) confirmed satisfying results in 17 out of 22 patients after a mean follow-up of 50 months.

Unfortunately, all of these studies are retrospective studies, and tools, such as a visual analogue scale for pain control pre- and postoperatively, or outcome measurements, such as the DASH questionnaire (4–6,38,39), are not included in these protocols. The patients' subjective expectations and results were not respected, and little information is available on such outcomes.

Interestingly, the author's data are a little different from previous studies. The author thinks this is related to the existence of more sophisticated outcome tools. The so-called objective data, such as grip strength and range of motion, do not really describe the patient's point of view after such a procedure (39). The author was surprised about the complication rate after questioning the patients very critically about their results. Interestingly, there was no difference in loss of sensation at the dorsal wrist side between the patients with denervation including the carpometacarpal joints and those with denervation excluding these joints. Our data show that there is no difference in pain relief whether a carpometacarpal denervation is performed or not. The author thinks that a partial wrist denervation, with only resection of the PIN and the AIN from a dorsal approach (13), serves the patient well in most situations because these nerve fibers innervate at least two-thirds of the wrist joint. In the author's opinion, total wrist denervation is an extensive procedure, as we know that there is always a risk of loss of sensation at the dorsum of the wrist. Some other surgeons feel that a total wrist denervation is not possible without substantial risk of loss of desired neural function (52).

The technique described by Berger (13) is technically easy because of the neighborhood of the AIN and the PIN to each other in an accessible region of the forearm. This approximation allows the possibility of preoperative assessment with anesthetic nerve blocks reliable, which should allow the prescreening of patients who will likely not benefit from the procedure. The distribution of the AIN and the PIN covers the central two-thirds of the carpus, both anteriorly and posteriorly. However, causes of pain do exist in the radial and ulnar margins of the carpus, and the isolated resection of the AIN and the PIN does not denervate these regions predictably. The author thinks that if a patient has additional substantial pain in either the radial or ulnar area of the wrist, a denervation of these regions should be carried out in the same procedure.

In our series and in the literature, there are no Charcot-like changes in the wrist postdenervation. Even if there were, it is unlikely that they would represent any more serious challenges for treatment than the existing degenerative changes (13).

The author was able to do some outcome studies after various wrist arthropathies. A series of 60 patients after total wrist arthrodesis showed residual pain in a lot of patients and a DASH score of 51 points (4). The DASH results after STT fusions in 26 patients reached 26 points and clearly demonstrate that partial wrist fusions have good results (6). The results after four-corner arthrodesis with complete scaphoid excision (DASH score 28) were better from the patients' subjective point of view, compared with the wrist denervation series (5). This might be due to the fact that the author always resects the PIN during a wrist salvage procedure from a dorsal approach and that the arthrotic changes in the wrist are eliminated with these salvage operations (5–7,54). Surprisingly, the complication rates after partial wrist fusions were less than after selective total wrist denervation. Recently, the author has begun to resect both the PIN and the AIN from this approach during a standard wrist procedure from the dorsal approach (13).

Despite the fact that our results after wrist denervation seem to be a little bit less predictable than in other studies, the satisfaction rate of the patients is acceptable. The advantage of the procedure is that it leaves open the possibility of other, more difficult treatment options. If the procedure fails or if patients realize progressively worsening pain over time, salvage procedures, such as partial (2,3,5,6) or total wrist arthrodesis (4), PRC (55), or wrist arthroplasty, can be considered at any time (56–58).

Denervation of the wrist is an attractive option for the patient who desires pain relief with a short operative recovery time, while maintaining a satisfying range of motion and grip strength. It might be worthwhile in the future to conduct more outcome studies with a randomized study design. It would be very interesting to compare partial versus complete wrist denervation in a prospective, randomized manner and also to compare partial wrist fusion versus wrist denervation. However, the results of our retrospective outcome studies about partial wrist fusions demonstrate overall superior results, compared with the wrist denervation procedure.

REFERENCES

1. Krakauer JD, Bishop AT, Cooney WP. Surgical treatment of scapholunate advanced collapse. *J Hand Surg [Am]* 1994;19(5):751–759.
2. Krimmer H, Krapohl B, Sauerbier, M, et al. Der posttraumatische karpale Kollaps (SLAC- und SNAC-wrist)—Stadieneinteilung und therapeutische Möglichkeiten. *Handchir Mikrochir Plast Chir* 1997;29:228–233.
3. Lanz U, Krimmer H, Sauerbier M. Advanced carpal collapse: treatment by limited wrist fusion. In: Büchler U, ed. *Wrist instability*. London: M. Dunitz, 1996:139–145.
4. Sauerbier M, Kluge S, Bickert B, et al. Subjective and objective outcomes after total wrist fusion in patients with radiocarpal arthrosis or Kienböck's disease. *Chir Main* 2000;19:223–231.
5. Sauerbier M, Linsner G, Tränkle M, et al. Midcarpal arthrodesis with complete scaphoid excision and interposition bone graft in the treatment of advanced carpal collapse (SNAC/SLAC wrist): operative technique and outcome assessment. *J Hand Surg [Br]* 2000;25(4):341–345.
6. Sauerbier M, Tränkle M, Erdmann D, et al. Functional outcome with scapho-trapezio-trapezoid arthrodesis in the treatment of Kienböck's disease. *Ann Plast Surg* 2000;44:618–625.
7. Sauerbier M, Bickert B, Tränkle M, et al. Operative Behandlungsmöglichkeiten bei fortgeschrittenem karpalen Kollaps (SNAC/SLAC wrist). *Unfallchirurg* 2000;103:564–571.
8. Sauerbier M, Berger RA. Limited wrist arthrodesis. In: Hastings H, Weiss APC, eds. *Arthritic surgery of the hand and wrist*. Philadelphia: Lippincott Williams & Wilkins, 2002.
9. Tränkle M, Sauerbier M, Linsner G, et al. Die STT-Arthrodese zur Behandlung der Lunatumnekrose im Stadium III:

funktionelle Ergebnisse. *Handchir Mikrochir Plast Chir* 2000;32:419–423.
10. Tomaino MM, Miller RJ, Cole I, et al. Scapholunate advanced collapse wrist: proximal row carpectomy or limited wrist arthrodesis with scaphoid excision? *J Hand Surg [Am]* 1994;1:134–142.
11. Watson HK, Goodman ML, Johnson TR. Limited wrist arthrodesis. Part II: intercarpal and radiocarpal combinations. *J Hand Surg [Am]* 1981;6(3):223–233.
12. Wilhelm A. Die Denervation der Handwurzel. *Hefte Unfallheilkd* 1965;81:109–114.
13. Berger RA. Partial denervation of the wrist: a new approach. *Tech Hand Upper Extr Surg* 1998;2:25–35.
14. Camitz H. Die deformierende Hüft-Gelenksarthritis und speziell ihre Behandlung. *Acta Orthop Scand* 1933;4:193–213.
15. Tavernièr L. L'denervation de la hanche dans les coxarthries. *Rev Orthop Belg* 1949;15:272–277.
16. Wilhelm A. Die Gelenkdenervation und ihre anatomischen Grundlagen. Ein neues Behandlungsprinzip in der Handchirurgie. *Hefte Unfallheilkd* 1966;86:1–109.
17. Watson HK, Ballet FL. The SLAC wrist: scapholunate advanced collapse pattern of degenerative arthritis. *J Hand Surg [Am]* 1984;9(3):358–365.
18. Krimmer H, Hahn P, Prommersberger KJ, et al. Diagnostik und Therapie der skapholunären Dissoziation. *Aktuelle Traumatol* 1996;26:264–269.
19. Ashmead D, Watson HK, Damon C, et al. Scapholunate advanced collapse wrist salvage. *J Hand Surg [Am]* 1994;19(5):741–750.
20. Wilhelm A. Zur Innervation der Gelenke der oberen Extremität. *Z Anat Entwicklungsgesch* 1958;120:331–371.
21. Buck-Gramcko D. Zur Denervation des Handgelenkes und der Mittelgelenke der Finger. *Handchirurgie* 1969;1:179–181.
22. Dellon AL, MacKinnon SE, Daneshwar A. Terminal branch of the anterior interosseous nerve as a resource of wrist pain. *J Hand Surg [Br]* 1984;9(3):316–322.
23. Dubert T, Oberlin C, Alnot JY. Anatomie des nerfs articulaires du poignet. *Ann Chir Main* 1990;9:15–21.
24. Filogamo G, Robecchi M. Innervazione delle capsule e dei legamenti delle articolazioni superiore. *Arch Ital Anat Embriol* 1950;55:334–355.
25. Fukumoto K, Kojima T, Kinoshita Y, et al. An anatomic study of the innervation of the wrist joint and Wilhelm's technique for denervation. *J Hand Surg [Am]* 1993;18(3):484–489.
26. Gray J, Gardener E. The innervation of the joints of the wrist and hand. *Anat Rec* 1965;151:261–266.
27. Dellon AL. Partial dorsal wrist denervation: resection of the distal posterior interosseous nerve. *J Hand Surg [Am]* 1985;10(4):527–533.
28. Wilhelm A. Die Schmerzausschaltung an der Handwurzel durch Denervation. In: Wachsmuth W, Wilhelm A, eds. *Die Operationen an der Hand*. Bd X, Teil 3 der *Allg u Spez Chir Operationslehre*. Berlin-Heidelberg-New York: Springer, 1972:274.
29. Wilhelm A. Handgelenkdenervation. In: Buck-Gramcko D, Nigst H, eds. *Bibliothek für Handchirurgie: Handgelenksverletzungen*. Stuttgart: Hippokrates, 1988:194.

30. Wilhelm A. Denervation of the wrist. *Tech Hand Upper Extr Surg* 2001;5:14–30.

31. Rüdinger N. *Die Gelenknerven des Menschlichen Körpers.* Erlangen: Enke, 1857.

32. Rüdinger N. *Die Anatomie der Menschlichen Rückenmarksnerven*, 2. Abt. Tafel VII. Stuttgart: Cotta, 1870.

33. Buck-Gramcko D. Denervation of the wrist. *J Hand Surg [Am]* 1977;2(1):54–61.

34. Buck-Gramcko D. Denervation of the wrist joint. In: Tubiana R, ed. *The hand*, vol. 4. Philadelphia: W.B. Saunders, 1993:822.

35. Sauerbier M, Tränkle M, Erdmann D, et al. Therapeutische Möglichkeiten zur Behandlung der Lunatumnekrose. *Trauma Berufskrankh* 2000;2:232–238.

36. Buck-Gramcko D. Wrist denervation procedures in the treatment of Kienböck's disease. *Hand Clin* 1993;9:517–520.

37. Buck-Gramcko D, Lankers J. Ergebnisse in der Therapie der Mondbeinnekrose. Untersuchungen an 91 Patienten. *Handchir Mikrochir Plast Chir* 1990;22:28–38.

38. Cozzi EP, Nemirovski CE. Denervación articular de la muneca y de la mano. *Rev Ortop Traumatol Latinoam* 1971;16.

39. Hudak PL, Amadio PC, Bombardier C, et al. Development of an upper extremity outcome measure: the DASH (disabilities of the arm, shoulder and hand). *Am J Ind Med* 29;602–608.

40. Amadio PC. Outcomes assessment in hand surgery. What's new? *Clin Plast Surg* 1997;24:191–194.

41. Ekerot L, Holmberg J, Eiken O. Denervation of the wrist. *Scand J Plast Reconstr Surg* 1983;17:155–157.

42. Geldmacher J, Legal HR, Brug E. Results of denervation of the wrist and wrist joint by Wilhelm's method. *Hand* 1972;4:57–59.

43. Helbig B. Zusätzliche Indikation zur Denervierungsoperation am Handgelenk nach Wilhelm. *Orthop Prax* 1980;80:393–396.

44. Helmke B, Geldmacher J, Luther R. Indikation, Technik und Ergebnisse der Handgelenksdenervation nach Wilhelm bei knöchernen Veränderungen im Handwurzelbereich. *Orthop Prax* 1977;13:96–98.

45. Ishida O, Tsai TM, Atasoy E. Long-term results of denervation of the wrist joint for chronic wrist pain. *J Hand Surg [Br]* 1993;18(1):76–80.

46. Kojima T. Denervation for wrist joint pain and its results. *J Jpn Soc Surg Hand* 1985;2:636–639.

47. Lanz U, Lehmann L. Denervazione del polso: indicazioni e resultati. *Riv Chir Della Mano* 1976;13:79–84.

48. Marcacci G. I risultati a distanza delle enervazioni articolari. *Minerva Ortop* 1954;5:309–312.

49. Martini AK, Frank G, Küster HH. Klinische Erfahrungen mit der Handgelenksdenervation nach Wilhelm. *Z Orthop* 1983;121:767–679.

50. Meine J, Buck-Gramcko D. Die Denervation des Handgelenkes: eine gültige Alternative? *Handchir* 1974;6:137–139.

51. Partecke BD, Buck-Gramcko D. Die Denervation des Handgelenkes bei sekundär-arthritischen Veränderungen nach distaler intraartikulärer Radiusfraktur. In: Buck-Gramcko D.

52. Röstlund T, Somnier F, Axelsson R. Denervation of the wrist joint—an alternative to conditions of chronic pain. *Acta Orthop Scand* 1980;51:609–616.

53. Grechenig W, Mähring M, Clement HG. Denervation of the radiocarpal joint. *J Bone Joint Surg* 1998;80:504–507.

54. Wulle Ch. Risultati della denervazione nell' arto superiore. *Riv Chir Della Mano* 1976;13:85–87.

55. Ferreres A, Suso S, Foucher G, et al. Wrist denervation: surgical considerations. *J Hand Surg [Br]* 1995;20(6):769–772.

56. Stegmann B, Brug E, Stedtfeld HW. Erfahrungen mit der Handgelenksdenervation nach Wilhelm als Auxiliärmaßnahme in der operativen Therapie der Naviculare-Pseudarthrose und Lunatummalazie. *Hefte Unfallheilkd* 1980;148:156–158.

57. Bickert B, Sauerbier M, Germann G. Scapholunate ligament reconstruction using the MITEK bone anchor: technique and preliminary results. *J Hand Surg [Br]* 2000;25(2):188–192.

58. Wyrick JD, Stern PJ, Kiefhaber TR. Motion-preserving procedures in the treatment of scapholunate advanced collapse wrist: proximal row carpectomy versus four-corner arthrodesis. *J Hand Surg [Am]* 1995;20(6):965–970.

81

CONGENITAL DISORDERS: CLASSIFICATION AND DIAGNOSIS

SCOTT H. KOZIN

Congenital anomalies affect 1% to 2% of newborns, and approximately 10% of these children have upper extremity abnormalities (1,2). These anomalies require an accurate diagnosis and communication of relevant information to the family. A standardized classification system that is user friendly and reliable facilitates accurate diagnosis and consistency between facilities. Development of such a system is an arduous task that requires an extensive understanding of limb anomalies, potential causes, and varying presentations. The clinician who is involved in the care of children with congenital anomalies must also possess a basic understanding of embryogenesis, limb formation, and inheritance patterns. This knowledge affords the physician the ability to diagnosis, to discuss, and to treat these challenging cases. Communication between family and physician is an integral part of the treatment paradigm. Relay of fictitious information is misleading and must be avoided at all costs. Appropriate referral is necessary for children and families who require genetic testing or multidisciplinary management, or both.

This chapter discusses the classification and the diagnosis of congenital anomalies of the upper extremity. The sequencing of the human genome and investigation into the molecular basis of limb development have provided new information regarding the etiology of limb malformation. This knowledge has already altered our dialect with affected families and has enhanced our diagnostic approach to children who are born with limb anomalies. In the future, genetic manipulation may prevent certain limb deformities and may offer hope to families who have these genetic idiosyncrasies.

CLASSIFICATION OF LIMB ANOMALIES

A valuable classification system should provide diagnostic, therapeutic, and prognostic information. A classification scheme should also be practical and applicable to the majority of cases that are encountered. Adequate detail must be included to separate different types of congenital anomalies without making the system overly complex. Increasing the numbers of categories and inclusion criteria often creates a system that is cumbersome and less reliable between observers. A balance between sufficient details without excessive convolution creates a workable system that is practical and readily accepted by numerous disciplines. A uniform system facilitates the development of a registry and monitoring of congenital anomalies.

There are numerous classification systems for upper extremity limb anomalies that are based on embryology, teratologic sequencing, or anatomy, or a combination of these. Each proposal has merit at the time of its inception, although many systems become outdated as our understanding of limb development and genetics expands (1,3). Embryologic classification attempts to define the defect according to malformation during limb development (3). Teratologic sequencing grades congenital anomalies according to the severity of expression (4,5). Anatomic classification schemes provide useful descriptive analyses and often offer therapeutic guidelines for treatment based on pathoanatomy. Currently available classification systems will most likely be archaic in the future, as our understanding of limb malformation advances. This section discusses various classification systems that are divided according to their basis of foundation.

Embryologic Schemes

The most widely accepted classification of congenital limb anomalies was pioneered by Frantz and O'Rahilly (6) and was published by Swanson (7). This work eliminated much of the confusing Greek and Latin terminology and was accepted by the American Society for Surgery of the Hand, the International Federation of Societies for Surgery of the Hand, and the International Society for Prosthetics and Orthotics. This system is based on embryonic failure during development and relies on clinical diagnosis for categorization. Each limb malformation is classified according to the most predominant anomaly and is placed into one of seven categories (Table 1). Different clinical presentations

TABLE 1. EMBRYOLOGIC CLASSIFICATION OF CONGENITAL ANOMALIES

Classification (group)	Subheading	Subgroup	Category
1: Failure of formation	Transverse arrest	Shoulder	—
		Arm	—
		Elbow	—
		Forearm	—
		Wrist	—
		Carpal	—
		Metacarpal	—
		Phalanx	—
	Longitudinal arrest	Radial deficiency	—
		Ulnar deficiency	—
		Central deficiency	—
		Intersegmental	Phocomelia
2: Failure of differentiation	Soft tissue	Disseminated	Arthrogryposis
		Shoulder	—
		Elbow and forearm	—
		Wrist and hand	Cutaneous syndactyly
			Camptodactyly
			Thumb in palm
			Deviated or deformed digits
	Skeletal	Shoulder	—
		Elbow	Synostosis
		Forearm	Proximal
			Distal
		Wrist and hand	Osseous syndactyly
			Carpal bone synostosis
			Symphalangia
			Clinodactyly
	Tumorous conditions	Hemangioma	—
		Lymphatic	—
		Neurogenic	—
		Connective tissue	—
		Skeletal	—
3: Duplication	Whole limb	—	—
	Humeral	—	—
	Radial	—	—
	Ulnar	Mirror hand	—
	Digit	Polydactyly	Radial (preaxial)
			Central
			Ulnar (postaxial)
4: Overgrowth	Whole limb	—	—
	Partial limb	—	—
	Digit	Macrodactyly	—
5: Undergrowth	Whole limb	—	—
	Whole hand	—	—
	Metacarpal	—	—
	Digit	Brachysyndactyly	—
		Brachydactyly	—
6: Constriction band syndrome	—	—	—
7: Generalized skeletal abnormalities	—	—	—

of similar categories of embryonic failures are explained by varying degrees of damage within the organization of the limb mesenchyme (7).

Group 1 is divided into transverse or longitudinal failure of formation. Transverse deficiencies are also called *congenital amputations* and are termed according to the anatomic level of limb termination. The most common site of amputation occurs at the proximal one-third of the forearm and is referred to as a *short below-the-elbow defect* (Fig. 1). Rudi-

mentary digits can be located on the end of the amputation stump (Fig. 2). A vascular insult during limb development is the most prevalent explanation for these deficiencies (8). The recent illegal use of misoprostol (Cytotec) to induce abortion has lent further evidence to a vascular etiology (9). Misoprostol induces uterine contractions and vaginal bleeding with the potential for termination of pregnancy. However, misoprostol ingestion may induce vascular disruption to the developing embryo without abortion. Con-

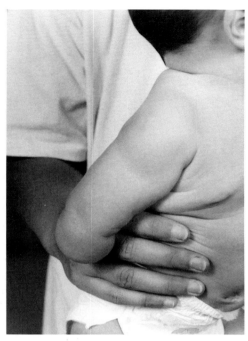

FIGURE 1. A 10-month-old infant with a right, short below-the-elbow congenital amputation.

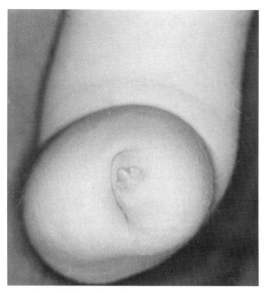

FIGURE 2. Short below-the-elbow congenital amputation with rudimentary digits on the end of the stump.

sequential findings include terminal transverse limb defects and other hemorrhage-related problems. Early chorionic villous sampling and failed attempts at pregnancy termination by dilatation and curettage have also been associated with transverse limb deficiencies and lend further support to vascular disruption as an underlying etiology (10).

Longitudinal deficiencies are named according to bones that are partially or completely absent. All completely or partially absent bones are named. In general, these deficiencies can be divided into radial (preaxial), ulnar (postaxial), or central forms. The central type includes deficiencies of the second, third, and fourth rays (digits and underlying carpus). There is considerable variability in the amount of insufficiency (i.e., phenotype), which is detailed in specific classification schemes that are based on teratologic sequencing and anatomic abnormalities (11,12). Phocomelia is another form of longitudinal deficiency that is characterized by an intercalary or intersegmental deficiency. The absent segment is variable, but includes a portion of the limb between the shoulder and hand (6). In profound cases, the hand appears to emanate from the glenohumeral joint (Fig. 3).

Group 2 infers failure of differentiation or separation of parts. This grouping implies development of all the essential components but failure of arrangement into a proper finalized form. This failure of differentiation can affect skeletal, dermal, fascial, muscular, ligaments, or neurovascular components, or a combination of these, of the limb. This category includes a heterogeneous group of disorders that are further subdivided according to anatomic abnormali-

ties. Syndactyly is the most common presentation of a group 2 anomaly and occurs with an incidence of approximately 2 to 3 per 10,000 live births (Fig. 4) (13–15). Inheritable, spontaneous, and syndromic forms have been identified with various similarities and dissimilarities. Inheritable syndactylism is associated with genetic defects that involve particular candidate regions on the second chromosome (14). The mode of transmission is considered autosomal dominant with variable expressivity and incomplete penetrance. This terminology signifies familial propa-

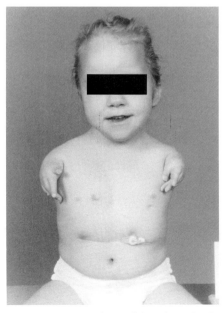

FIGURE 3. Bilateral phocomelia with hands projecting from the shoulder girdles.

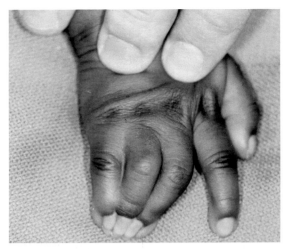

FIGURE 4. A 3-month-old child with complete long-ring–small-finger syndactyly and common fingernail (synonychia).

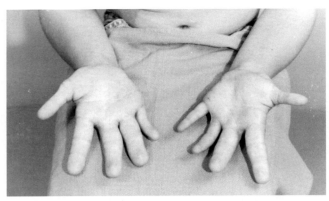

FIGURE 6. Bilateral digital macrodactyly in a child with Klippel-Trénaunay-Weber syndrome (hemangiomas, varicose veins, limb hypertrophy).

gation, although the syndactyly may skip a generation (incomplete penetrance) and may not be present in full form (variable phenotype) (15). Familial syndactyly is associated with syndactyly of the second and third toes. Syndactyly also is more prevalent in male offspring, which may indicate a decreased penetrance in females.

Group 3 anomalies represent duplication of parts and are most commonly observed as polydactyly. Postaxial or ulnar polydactyly often demonstrates familial propagation and racial preference (16). The duplication is transmitted via an autosomal-dominant pattern and occurs more commonly in black individuals. Preaxial duplication or radial polydactyly also demonstrates racial predilection toward white children but is usually unilateral and sporadic (Fig. 5) (17,18). Further subdivision into various categories has been performed according to the extent of duplication (19). Genetic analysis of a particular form of polydactyly (ring-finger duplication) combined with syndactyly (synpolydactyly) has been linked to a gene mutation (*HOXD13* gene), which is located on chromosome 2 (2q31) (20).

Group 4 abnormalities are listed as overgrowth and can present as diffuse hypertrophy of the entire limb or isolated enlargement of various parts. This category is uncommon in occurrence but dramatic in presentation. Underlying etiologies for limb overgrowth (e.g., vascular abnormalities or malformations) must be considered during patient evaluation (21,22). In addition, overgrowth can be a constituent of a variety of syndromes (e.g., neurofibromatosis or Klippel-Trénaunay-Weber syndrome) (Fig. 6).

Group 5 deformities correspond to undergrowth or hypoplasia of the limb or its parts. Hypoplasia is subdivided according to anatomic locale and is prevalent in many disorders (Fig. 7). For example, brachydactyly (shortened digit) is a consistent finding in children with Poland's syndrome (23).

Group 6 anomalies occur with constriction band syndrome (also known as *amniotic disruption sequence*). These deficiencies are not hereditary, and their cause remains controversial, with intrinsic and extrinsic theories (7,15,24). The intrinsic concept postulates that the amniotic bands represent a localized lack of mesodermal development, similar to a normal skin crease. The depth of the mesodermal defect determines the severity of clinical presentation. The extrinsic theory postulates that the amniotic membrane traps the developing hand or an amniotic band encircles the affected part, thus leading to a variable amount of injury (vascular

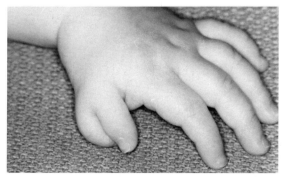

FIGURE 5. Radial polydactyly or thumb duplication shown in an infant.

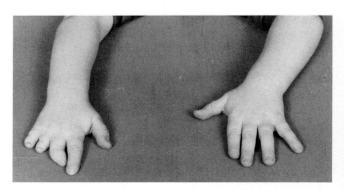

FIGURE 7. Hypoplastic right hand, primarily involving the ulnar digits.

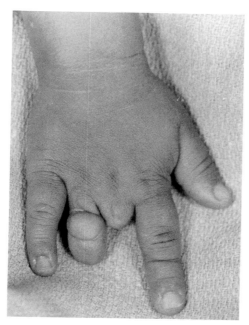

FIGURE 8. Amniotic disruption sequence or constriction band syndrome affecting the right hand with varying severity across the digits.

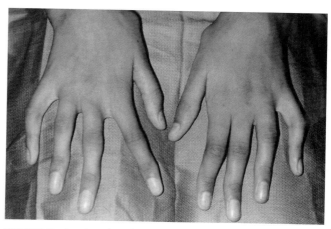

FIGURE 9. Arachnodactyly in a child with Marfan syndrome.

insult). Currently, the extrinsic hypothesis is favored, as amnion has been found in the constriction ring, and the bands tend to occur in a straight line across multiple digits. Amniotic bands can cause mild digital damage, initiate an embryonic repair process, and yield variable amounts of circumferential stricture (Fig. 8). Severe damage can lead to complete vascular ischemia and complete truncation of the affected parts. Amniotic band formation has also been associated with the use of misoprostol as an illegal abortion agent during the first trimester (9). In these cases, uterine contraction or vaginal bleeding, or both, may liberate amniotic bands or cause a vascular injury to the affected part.

Group 7 anomalies occur in conjunction with generalized skeletal abnormalities. Examples include dwarfism, Ollier's disease, and Marfan syndrome (Figs. 9 and 10). The specific clinical findings depend on the underlying syndrome and the phenotypic expression of the deformity. Systemic problems are common, and comprehensive evaluation is warranted.

This classification scheme represents a valiant attempt to comprehensively classify congenital anomalies. The worldwide adoption of a uniform classification does enhance research efforts into incidence, etiology, treatment, and outcome (25). However, valid criticisms of this system have arisen concerning the difficulty with classifying the "predominant" deformity and the inability to categorize peculiar anomalies (26–31). This has resulted in modifications to allow placement of an anomaly into multiple categories and the addition of additional diagnoses to particular categories (26,29). However, a more critical problem with this system concerns the underlying premise for categorization (30). Astute observation and the explosion of genomic and

proteomic research have outdated much of the information regarding embryogenesis and pathogenesis of limb malformations that is used in this system (3,25,32,33). Defects in human limb formation have been linked to mutations in genes that encode signaling proteins, receptor molecules, and transcription factors (Table 2) (3,33). It is essential to incorporate this information into contemporary embryologic classification schemes (3).

Embryology Update

Embryogenesis of the upper extremity commences with formation of the upper limb bud on the lateral wall of the

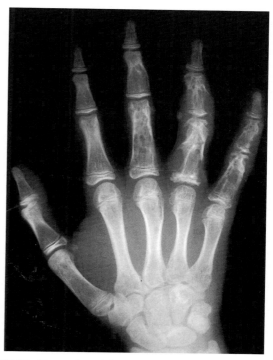

FIGURE 10. X-ray of a right hand that demonstrates multiple enchondromas (Ollier's disease) of the long, ring, and small digits.

TABLE 2. GENETIC CLASSIFICATION OF LIMB DEFECTS

Molecular defect	Syndrome	Limb defect	Gene	Chromosome
Transcription factor	Holt-Oram	Radial deficiency	TBX5	12q24.1
	Synpolydactyly	Syndactyly, polydactyly, brachydactyly	HOXD13	2q31-q32
	Townes', Brock's	Polydactyly	SALL1	16q12
	Waardenburg's, type 1 and 3	Syndactyly	PAX3	2q35
	Hand-foot-genital	Brachydactyly	HOXA13	7p15-p14.2
	Saethre-Chotzen	Brachydactyly, syndactyly	TWIST	7p21
	Ulnar mammary	Deficiency and duplication	TBX3	12q24.1
	Pallister-Hall	Polydactyly	GL13	7p13
	Creig cephalopoly syndactyly	Syndactyly, polydactyly	Gl13	7p13
Signaling protein	Grebe	Severe brachydactyly	CDMP1	20q11.2
	Hunter-Thompson	Brachydactyly	CDMP1	20q11.2
	Aarskog	Brachydactyly	FGD1	Xp11.2
Receptor protein	Apert's	Syndactyly	FGFR2	10q26
	Pfeiffer's	Brachydactyly, syndactyly	FGFR1 FGFR2	8p11.2-p11.1
	Jackson-Weiss	Syndactyly, brachydactyly	FGFR2	10q26
Unknown	Split-hand-foot	Syndactyly, fusion	—	7q21, Xq26, 10q24
	Tarsal-carpal coalition	Brachydactyly, fusions	—	17q
	Nager's	Posterior limb deficiency	—	9q32

embryo 4 weeks after fertilization and is complete 8 weeks after fertilization (2,3,34). The majority of upper extremity congenital anomalies occur during this period of rapid limb development. The limb bud is formed by migration and multiplication of the dorsal somatopleure (ectoderm and underlying undifferentiated somatic mesoderm) from the eighth to tenth somites to the lateral wall. A thickened layer of ectoderm condenses over the limb bud (apical ectodermal ridge), which acts as a signaling center to guide the underlying mesoderm to differentiate into appropriate structures (3,33). The limb develops in a proximal-to-distal direction, and the apical ectodermal ridge is responsible for this process. Within the posterior margin of the limb bud resides an additional signaling center, the zone of polarizing activity, which is responsible for anterior-to-posterior (radioulnar) development (3,33). The hedgehog pathway is located within the zone of polarizing activity, and the signaling molecule that is necessary for limb orientation is the Sonic hedgehog compound (35). The Wnt (Wingless type) signaling pathway resides in the dorsal ectoderm and secretes factors that induce the underlying mesoderm to adopt dorsal characteristics (36,37). This process mediates the development of dorsal-to-ventral axis configuration and dorsalization of the limb. The apical ectodermal ridge, the zone of polarizing activity, and the Wnt pathway all function in a coordinated effort to ensure proper limb patterning and growth during embryogenesis (3). Abnormalities of these crucial areas directly affect limb formation and indirectly prohibit adequate functioning of the remaining signaling centers.

The arm and forearm appear before the hand plate, which appears by 5 weeks' gestation in the form of a paddle that is covered by the apical ectodermal ridge. Condensation of the mesoderm forms the skeletal anlagen, which eventually undergoes initial chondrification and subsequent ossification

(2,34). The ingrowth of vessels and nerves into the developing extremity occurs during the fifth through eighth weeks of gestation. Joint formation begins with the condensation of chondrocyte precursors along dense plates as a precursor to joint articulation. Subsequent joint cavitation ensues with formation of a joint cavity that requires motion for formal remodeling. By the eighth week, embryogenesis is complete, and all limb structures are present. Subsequently, the fetal period commences with differential growth of existing structures, and this process continues until birth.

The fragile period of embryogenesis has been altered in animal models by experimental embryologists. This information has provided insight into limb malformation and has enhanced our appreciation of the factors that are responsible for limb development. The identification of the molecular factors that are involved in intricate cell-to-cell interaction has begun to unravel the mysteries of embryogenesis. In addition, the delineation of responsible genetic mutations or receptor abnormalities, or both, has focused our attention on endogenous causes rather than exogenous teratogens (3). Crucial centers that are responsible for limb axis development have been surgically manipulated in animal models to recreate comparable anomalies that are seen in humans. This information will undoubtedly lead to innovative treatment options and will amend current classification schemes. Currently, the relationship between the experimental embryologist, the clinical geneticist, and the treating physician is immature and evolving. However, advances in medicine happen with cross-fertilization between physicians, specialists, and scientists. Future study and collaboration will offer diagnostic studies and sound answers to parents who struggle to understand the pathogenesis of their child's limb malformation.

Experimental embryologists have noted that genes and developmental programs are strongly preserved among

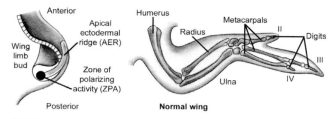

FIGURE 11. Normal wing development in the chicken embryo requires an intact apical ectodermal ridge and zone of polarizing activity.

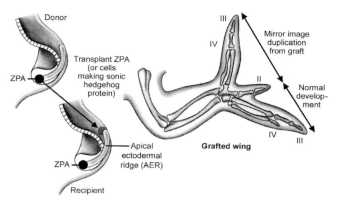

FIGURE 12. Transplantation of a portion of the zone of polarizing activity (ZPA) results in duplication of the digits along the radioulnar axis.

widely disparate species (3,38,39). This conservation allows study of different organisms and provides insight into the development of the hominoid limb. Animal models have been used to dissect and to manipulate the crucial signaling centers that affect limb development and orientation (Fig. 11). Transplantation of the zone of polarizing activity (or the Sonic hedgehog signaling molecule) to the anterior part of the developing chick limb bud results in duplication of the elements along the radioulnar axis (Fig. 12) (33,35). This effect is dose dependent, as high concentrations of transplanted material result in an increased number of duplicated digits. The malpositioning or duplication of this signaling center offers a plausible explanation for the rare mirror hand deformity (Fig. 13). In a mouse model, inactivation of the Wnt pathway prevents dorsalization of the limb and results in ventral pads on both sides of the foot. (37). The apical ectodermal ridge also appears integral to limb formation. This ridge secretes proteins (e.g., fibroblast growth factors) that influence the development of the underlying tissues (40). Removal of the apical ectodermal ridge during embryogenesis yields a truncated limb that is similar to a congenital amputation (Fig. 14) (33). As embryogenesis progresses, the apical ectodermal ridge disperses around the hand paddle. This fragmentation results in longitudinal interdigital necrosis between the digits. Failure of the ridge to separate is the most prevalent explanation for syndactyly and represents a failure of mesenchyme differentiation.

A variety of genes that control limb development have been defined. Many of these genes transcend species, and analogies between primitive species (e.g., the fruit fly) and humans have become apparent. The *HOX* genes are a major group of patterning genes that are expressed sequentially during limb development. In humans, these genes are located on four different chromosomes (*HOXA* through *HOXD*), and mutations have been linked to limb anomalies (3). Syndactyly, combined with ring-finger duplication (synpolydactyly), has been linked to a *HOXD13* gene mutation, which is located on chromosome 2 (2q31) (20). The classic autosomal-dominant syndactyly has also been localized to a specific candidate region of a responsible gene on chromosome 2 (2q34-q36) (14).

Molecular factors may also explain limb defects that occur after normal limb development. For example, amniotic disruption sequence (also known as *amniotic band deformity*) often results in terminal deficiencies. Vascular disruption contributes to the formation of these anomalies, and risk factors include chorionic villus sampling, prostaglandin ingestion, ergotamine, and trauma (9,10). Variable phenotypes are common and are related to the degree of injury and the response to this injury. Infants with a limited capacity to recover from the hypoxia-reperfusion injury may be predisposed to severe deficiencies. The identification of genetic biomarkers for particular reperfusion factors may assist in the identification of vulnerable infants. These infants may war-

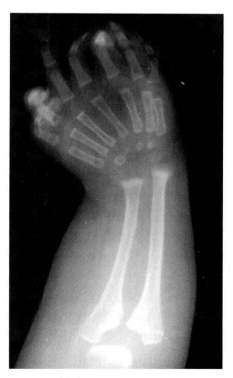

FIGURE 13. X-ray of left upper extremity with duplication of the ulnar and multiple digits that is characteristic of a mirror hand.

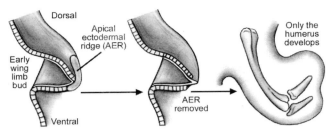

FIGURE 14. Removal of the apical ectodermal ridge during embryogenesis results in truncation of limb formation.

rant frequent ultrasound monitoring for early diagnosis of constriction band formation and even consideration for *in utero* band release before limb truncation (41).

A classification system that is based on the particular genetic or molecular abnormality would organize deformities according to their root of existence. Early classification schemes have emerged, although frequent modifications are necessary, as advances in gene mapping and molecule identification are occurring at an escalating rate (Table 2) (3). In addition, this type of classification may be excessively cumbersome, because multiple gene mutations appear to be necessary for a resultant limb malformation. This inherent redundancy of genetic information provides certain protection to the developing embryo. Ultimately, parallel classification systems may exist with an embryologic scheme that is used for diagnosis and potential genetic treatment options and a teratologic or anatomic scheme that is designed to guide practical management principles for the treating physician.

Embryologic Classification Variants

Several Japanese authors have noted numerous similarities and differences between various congenital anomalies and have proposed a classification scheme that is based on embryologic failure and that differs from Swanson's classification (7,25,42–47). The major difference is the classification of typical and atypical (also known as *severe symbrachydactyly*) cleft hand into similar or disparate categories of embryologic malformation (Table 3). This astute insight and perception warrant discussion, as this scheme highlights the combination of basic embryologic failure and clinical findings.

Clinical Features

Typical cleft hand and syndactyly can occur in the same hand and have many apparent similarities that may indicate a parallel mode of occurrence (25,43). Typical cleft hand and syndactyly are often hereditary, affect both hands, involve the feet, and usually include the long digit (45). These associated findings indicate an interrelated pathogenesis of these distinctly different entities. In contrast, atypical cleft hand is not hereditary and is usually unilateral. The hand is also smaller than the hand on the normal side, and the feet are not involved. Atypical cleft hand is often com-

TABLE 3. CHARACTERISTICS OF CLEFT HAND

	Typical cleft hand	Atypical cleft hand
Clinical features		
Involvement	Bilateral	Unilateral
Inheritance	Familial	Spontaneous
Syndactyly	Common	Rare
Anatomic findings		
Arterial supply	Ring finger may have three digital arteries	Vestigial supply to central digits
Tendon	Dual tendons to ring finger common	Minimal
Skeleton	Hypertrophy adjacent to cleft	Hypoplasia
Classification	Abnormal number of digits	Failure of formation

bined with ipsilateral pectoralis muscle anomalies (e.g., Poland's syndrome), which can also be found in anomalies that are considered failures of formation (e.g., transverse arrest and radial deficiency) (Fig. 15) (23,45,47).

Anatomic Abnormalities

Anatomic differences exist between typical and atypical cleft hands that infer different pathogenesis. X-ray scrutiny of typical cleft hands reveals thickening of the adjacent proximal phalanges, if the cleft metacarpal is present, or thickening of the adjacent metacarpals, if the central metacarpal is absent (Fig. 16) (25,46). In contrast, atypical cleft hands possess hypoplasia of the remaining skeleton without findings that are consistent with enlargement (44).

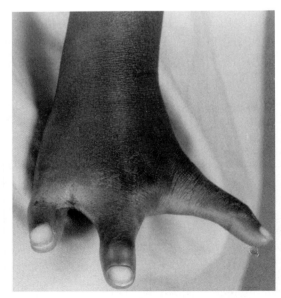

FIGURE 15. Isolated atypical cleft hand or symbrachydactyly in a 10-year-old girl without a familial history or lower extremity involvement.

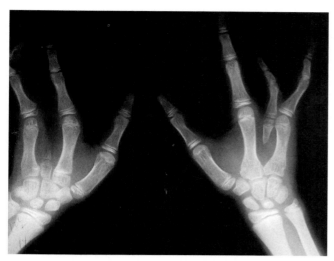

FIGURE 16. X-ray of untreated bilateral typical cleft hands with thickening of the adjacent metacarpals and the phalanges that surround the cleft.

Arteriograms of typical cleft hands have occasionally visualized three digital arteries to the ring finger (25). Surgical exploration has revealed dual tendons that insert into the extensor apparatus of the ring finger. Atypical cleft hands often have residual nubbins without a discrete arterial supply or tendon structure.

These clinical features and anatomic differences support the separation of typical and atypical cleft hand into different etiologies. Typical cleft hand and syndactyly appear interrelated and distinctly embryologically different from atypical cleft hand and radial deficiency (25,45,46). This information supports the merging of typical cleft hand and syndactyly into a single category that is defined as an abnormal number of digits that are attributed to impairment of mesenchymal tissue distribution and abnormality of the apical ectodermal ridge, respectively (25,45). These findings suggest that typical cleft hand may result from fusion of digital rays rather than a lack of constituents. In contrast, atypical cleft hand seems to be caused by necrosis

of mesenchymal tissue (failure of formation) with attempts at regeneration.

The resultant classification delineates six categories of embryologic failure that are modifications of the scheme that was proposed by Swanson (7,25) (Table 4). The first category involves abnormality of formation (i.e., failure of formation), secondary to necrosis of mesenchymal tissue, and can occur with or without regeneration. This includes atypical cleft hand, transverse amputations, radial deficiency, and ulnar deficiency. The regeneration of tissues explains the presence of distal structures, such as a thumb in radial deficiency, nubbins in congenital amputations, or phocomelia (Figs. 2 and 3). The second category encompasses anomalies in the number of digits due to abnormalities in the distribution of mesenchyme or the apical ectodermal ridge. This includes typical cleft hand, syndactyly, and polydactyly (Fig. 5). Additional categories include congenital constriction band syndrome, generalized skeletal abnormalities, failure of differentiation, and abnormal growth (overgrowth or undergrowth).

Teratologic Sequence Classification

Congenital anomalies can be classified or ranked according to their severity of expression, as variable phenotypes are common. This notion was proposed by Müller (4) and forms the basis for many classification schemes. The concept of variable expressivity rationalizes placing malformations that may appear quite different into similar categories (e.g., symbrachydactyly). These classification systems are quite popular, as the extent of pathology often determines function and provides a basis to guide treatment (31). For example, teratologic sequencing of thumb hypoplasia is an established classification scheme that was initiated by Müller (4) and subsequently was modified by Blauth (48) and Manske et al. (49). The five-category system of increasing severity of hypoplasia describes anatomic anomalies and directs treatment (Table 5) (50,51).

A type 1 deficiency represents the least involvement with generalized thumb hypoplasia without discrete absence of

TABLE 4. MODIFIED EMBRYOLOGIC FAILURE CLASSIFICATION

Category	Subcategory	Examples
Failure of formation	With regeneration	Phocomelia, radial and ulnar deficiency, symbrachydactyly
	Without regeneration	Terminal transverse deficiency
Abnormal number of digits	Slight impairment of mesenchymal tissue	Simple syndactyly, polydactyly, typical cleft hand, duplicated thumb
	Moderate or severe impairment	Complicated syndactyly, extensive thumb duplication
Congenital constriction band syndrome	—	—
Generalized skeletal abnormalities	—	Multiple hereditary exostosis, dwarfism
Failure of differentiation	—	Radioulnar synostosis, metacarpal synostosis
Over- or undergrowth	—	Macrodactyly, limb hypertrophy

TABLE 5. THUMB DEFICIENCY CLASSIFICATION

Type	Findings	Treatment
1	Minor generalized hypoplasia	Augmentation
2	Absence of intrinsic thenar muscles	Opponensplasty
	First web space narrowing	First web release
	Ulnar collateral ligament insufficiency	Ulnar collateral ligament reconstruction
3	Similar findings as type 2, plus:	Reconstruction
	Extrinsic muscle and tendon abnormalities	Pollicization
	Skeletal deficiency	—
	Stable carpometacarpal joint	
	Unstable carpometacarpal joint	
4	Pouce flottant or floating thumb	Pollicization
5	Absence	Pollicization

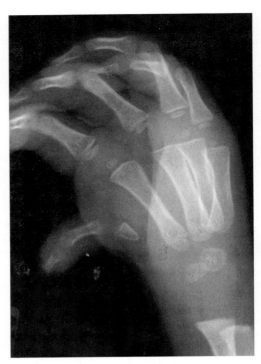

FIGURE 18. X-ray of a type 3B thumb with absence of the proximal metacarpal and carpometacarpal joints.

structures. A type 2 deficiency is more involved and is characterized by thumb–index web space narrowing, thenar muscle absence, and insufficiency of the thumb metacarpophalangeal ulnar collateral ligament. Type 3 hypoplasia possesses the intrinsic anomalies that are associated with a type 2 deformity and adds additional skeletal and extrinsic musculotendinous abnormalities (e.g., flexor pollicis longus). Type 3 anomalies are divided into 3A and 3B, depending on the presence or absence of a stable carpometacarpal joint, respectively (Figs. 17 and 18) (49). The status of the carpometacarpal joint is crucial and directly affects the treatment recommendation (31,49,51,52). Type 4 deficiency represents a severe expression of thumb hypoplasia and denotes a residual digit or *pouce flottant*. Type 5 is the most involved teratologic presentation and is noted by complete absence of the thumb.

A similar methodology has been applied to classify radial deficiencies according to the extent of absence (11,53,54). The severity is classified into four types and is based on x-ray interpretation (Table 6). The user must be aware that ossification of the radius is delayed in radial deficiency, and the differentiation between total and partial absence (types 3 and 4) cannot be established until the patient is approximately 3 years of age (55). A type 1 deficiency is the mildest expression and is characterized by mild radial shortening of the radius without considerable bowing. Minor radial deviation of the hand is apparent, although considerable thumb hypoplasia may be evident (Fig. 19). A miniature radius with distal and proximal physeal abnormalities and moderate deviation of the wrist characterize a type 2 deficiency. A type 3 deficiency is partial absence of the radius, most commonly the distal portion, and severe wrist radial deviation. Complete absence of the radius is a type 4 deformity and is the most common variant (Fig. 20). The hand tends to develop a perpendicular relationship with the forearm (Fig. 21).

A modified classification of radial longitudinal deficiency has been developed to combine thumb and carpal anomalies into a single scheme (Table 7) (12). This strategy recognizes that radial deficiency refers to anomalies along the preaxial corridor, which can affect the radius or thumb, or both. This scheme applies the principles of teratologic sequencing to form an inclusive classification that grades thumb and radius deficiencies based on x-ray findings. An appreciation of the delayed ossification of the radius and carpus in preaxial deficiency must be considered during

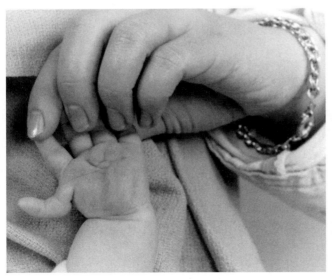

FIGURE 17. A 3-month-old infant with hypoplastic thumb without a palpable proximal metacarpal and devoid of carpometacarpal stability.

TABLE 6. RADIAL DEFICIENCY CLASSIFICATION

Type	X-ray findings	Clinical features
1: Short radius	Distal radial epiphysis that is delayed in appearance Normal proximal radial epiphysis Mild shortening of radius without bowing	Minor radial deviation of the hand Thumb hypoplasia is the prominent clinical feature that requires treatment
2: Hypoplastic	Distal and proximal epiphysis present Abnormal growth in both epiphyses Ulna is thickened, shortened, and bowed	Miniature radius Moderate radial deviation of the hand
3: Partial absence	Partial absence (distal, middle, proximal) of radius Distal one-third or two-thirds absence most common Ulna thickened, shortened, and bowed	Severe radial deviation of the hand
4: Total absence	No radius present Ulna thickened, shortened, and bowed	Most common type Severe radial deviation of the hand

Note: Because ossification of the radius is delayed in radial clubhand, the differentiation between total and partial absence (types 3 and 4) cannot be established until the patient is approximately 3 years of age.
Note: Centralization is required for types 2, 3, and 4.

application of this scheme. Radial-sided carpal bones appear even later than the ulna and begin to ossify at approximately 8 years of age, which delays determination of carpal anomalies until that age (12,56,57). A type N deficiency is the mildest form of radial deficiency and is characterized by a normal radius, normal carpus, and only thumb hypoplasia. A type 0 deficiency includes thumb hypoplasia and carpal anomalies but a normal radius. A type 1 deficiency incorporates thumb hypoplasia, carpal anomalies, and a slightly shortened radius (Fig. 18). Abnormalities of the proximal radius are common in types 0 and 1 (Fig. 22). Progressive hypoplasia of the radius is evident in a type 2 deficiency, whereas a type 3 anomaly is missing a physis altogether. A type 4 deficiency represents the extreme manifestation, with thumb and carpal anomalies combined with complete absence of the radius (Fig. 20).

The method of teratologic sequencing for classification has also been applied to ulnar deficiency by numerous authors (58–64). Bayne (63) combined the schemes of Ogden et al. (59) and Riordan (60) into a single classification (Table 8). A type 1 deficiency has a proximal and distal epiphysis, although the ulna is hypoplastic. Absence of the distal or middle one-third of the ulna is regarded as a type 2 deficiency, and total agenesis of the ulna is a type 3 defi-

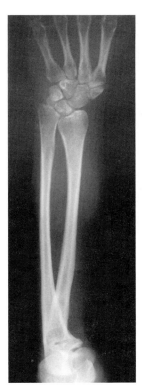

FIGURE 19. Adult with a type 1 radial deficiency and absent thumb.

ciency. A type 4 deficiency indicates fusion of the radius to the ulna or a radiohumeral synostosis (Fig. 23).

Müller (4) applied the concept of teratogenic sequencing to the developing hand plate in an effort to explain the

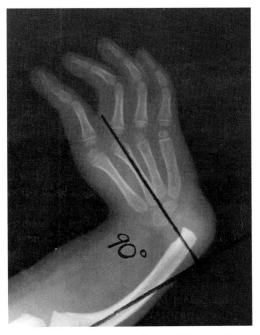

FIGURE 20. X-ray of a type 4 radial deficiency with complete absence of the radius.

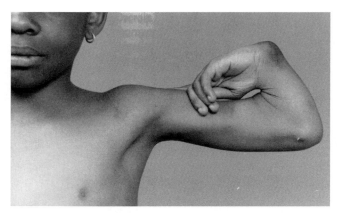

FIGURE 21. A 12-year-old patient with type 4 radial deficiency and a perpendicular relationship between the hand and the forearm.

Anatomic Classification

Classification of congenital anomalies can also be based on anatomic findings or the extent of involvement, or both. This is also a common methodology for classification and has been applied to numerous conditions. The concepts of variable pathoanatomy and teratologic sequencing are frequently combined into these classifications. Many of these schemes use x-ray findings to determine the basis for the degree of deficiency. The user must consider the age of the child and the degree of ossification before definitive categorization (12,56). These methods of classification are popular and practical, and many guide treatment recommendations. The classification of syndactyly and ulnar deficiency is related to first web configuration.

Syndactyly

The extent and intensity of digital union are variable in syndactyly, which guides the classification scheme (13,15). The basic terminology includes *complete*, *incomplete*, *simple*, and *complex*. The term *complicated* is a modifier that provides additional information regarding the pathoanatomy. The extent of syndactyly is incomplete if the skin bridge does not extend the full length of the involved digits or is complete when the connection encompasses the entire length. Complete syndactyly can also produce a shared or common fingernail (synonychia) (Fig. 4). The intensity of syndactyly is soft tissue alone (simple) or in conjunction with bone (complex). Complex implies fusion of adjacent phalanges or interposition of accessory bones. There are also atypical forms of syndactyly that are labeled complicated and that present with convoluted soft tissue abnormalities or a hodgepodge of abnormal bones. Many of these atypical configurations occur in accordance with a variety of syndromes and defy standard terminology and classification. The term *complicated* can be incorporated into the subtypes of simple and complex syndactyly to create a classification scheme that guides treatment (Table 9) (15).

spectrum of deficiencies that is associated with symbrachydactyly. The concept begins with a brachydactylous hand that can progress into a variety of central defects and culminates in a monodactylous or adactylous hand (Fig. 24). The reduction can start at the index finger and proceeds in an ulnar direction or begins at the middle digit and progresses outward. The specific pathway of reduction and the extent of progression determine the ultimate expression. This premise can explain the multitude of clinical manifestations that are associated with symbrachydactyly. A variant of this original hypothesis is the centripetal suppression theory, which suggests that a progressive deficiency is dependent on the insult to the developing limb bud (65). A mild deformity results from minimal inhibition of the hand plate and is expressed as a simple cleft without missing tissue. A more severe form involves bony and tissue reduction that begins in the central digits. Progressive insult yields increasing digital suppression, beginning with the radial side and advancing to the ulnar digits. Successive involvement results in a monodactylous or adactylous hand, similar to the end result that was noted by Müller (4) (Fig. 25).

TABLE 7. GLOBAL CLASSIFICATION OF RADIAL LONGITUDINAL DEFICIENCY

Type	Thumb anomaly	Carpal anomaly[a]	Distal radius	Proximal radius
N	Absent or hypoplasia	Normal	Normal	Normal
0	Absent or hypoplasia	Absence, hypoplasia, or coalition	Normal	Normal, radioulnar synostosis, or radial head dislocation
1	Absent or hypoplasia	Absence, hypoplasia, or coalition	>2 mm shorter than ulna	Normal, radioulnar synostosis, or radial head dislocation
2	Absent or hypoplasia	Absence, hypoplasia, or coalition	Hypoplasia	Hypoplasia
3	Absent or hypoplasia	Absence, hypoplasia, or coalition	Physis absent	Variable hypoplasia
4	Absent or hypoplasia	Absence, hypoplasia, or coalition	Absent	Absent

Note: X-rays must be of children who are older than 8 years of age to allow for ossification of the carpal bones.
[a]Carpal anomaly implies hypoplasia, coalition, absence, or bipartite carpal bones. Hypoplasia and absence are more common on the radial side of the carpus, and coalitions are more frequent on the ulnar side.

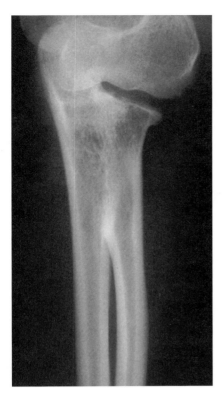

FIGURE 22. X-ray of the proximal radius reveals a proximal radioulnar synostosis in the adult patient who is depicted in Figure 19.

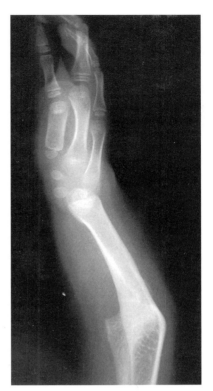

FIGURE 23. X-ray of a type 4 ulnar deficiency with absent ulna and radiohumeral synostosis.

Ulnar deficiency has been classified according to the anatomy of the first web space. This scheme is based on surgical indications, which primarily involve the thumb and first web abnormalities (66–67). A critical analysis of the thumb–index web space and thumb composition in ulnar deficiency has yielded four different anomalies (Table 10). Type A is a normal first web space and thumb, although forearm deformities are still prevalent. Type B is mild first web deficiency and mild thumb hypoplasia. Type C is moderate to severe first web deficiency and thumb hypoplasia that is defined as diminished motion, malrotation, and absent motors (Figs. 26 and 27). Type D is the extreme manifestation with complete absence of the thumb. Interestingly, the progressive deficiency of the first

web space and thumb does not correlate with severity of forearm and elbow anomalies (68). Therefore, a two-tiered classification may be applicable, with separate categories for forearm deficiencies and hand anomalies.

DIAGNOSIS

Patient Evaluation

The diagnosis and treatment of children with upper extremity anomalies require patience, empathy, knowledge, and a support staff. Children with mild differences (e.g., simple syndactyly) can be treated solely from a medical standpoint. However, children with considerable anomalies or with an underlying syndrome require medical, psychological, financial, and social assistance. This type of care is best provided at an institution that is familiar with the care of challenged children, as these facilities offer the services that are necessary for inclusive care. A hand surgeon evaluating children and families in need of such tertiary care should refer the patient without hesitation. After such transfer of care, families often are extremely grateful and feel indebted to the referring physician.

The initial evaluation of a child with a congenital anomaly is a combination of art and science. The concept of treating a child should be thought of as a privilege rather

TABLE 8. CLASSIFICATION OF ULNAR DEFICIENCIES

Type	Grade	Characteristics
1	Hypoplasia	Hypoplasia of the ulna with presence of distal and proximal ulnar epiphysis, minimal shortening
2	Partial aplasia	Partial aplasia with absence of the distal or middle one-third of the ulna
3	Complete aplasia	Total agenesis of the ulna
4	Synostosis	Fusion of the radius to the ulna

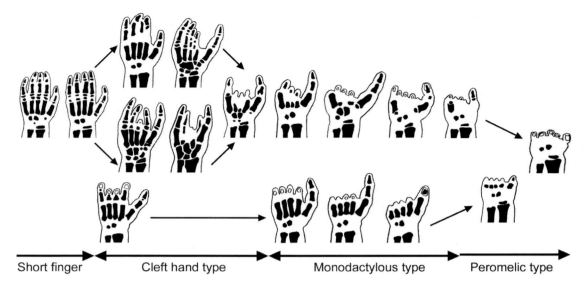

Short finger | Cleft hand type | Monodactylous type | Peromelic type

FIGURE 24. Diagram of Müller's concept (4) of teratogenic sequencing applied to symbrachydactyly. Reduction can start at the index finger and proceeds toward the ulnar side of the hand or begins in the long digit and progresses in a radial and ulnar direction.

than as a patient encounter. For parents to entrust the care of their child to any physician communicates extreme confidence and represents a unique opportunity. The establishment of a trusting relationship requires a conscientious and caring physician. The assessment cannot be hurried, as the family often has numerous questions that must be answered entirely. The conversation portion of the initial assessment usually takes considerably longer than the physical examination portion. The rapport between doctor and family should be in lay terminology with an avoidance of medical jargon, except for important terminology concerning the named diagnosis. Misconceptions concerning the

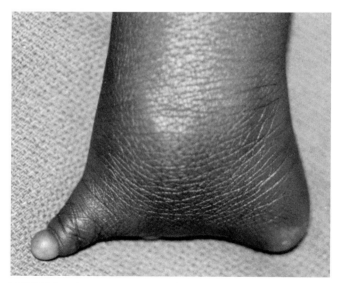

FIGURE 25. Severe expression of symbrachydactyly with adactylous hand.

TABLE 9. SYNDACTYLY CLASSIFICATION

Simple syndactyly (SS)	Standard (SSs)	Straightforward simple syndactyly of nonborder digit. Surgery can be delayed until 18 months of age.
	Complicated (SSc)	Simple syndactyly that is associated with additional soft tissue interconnections, syndromes (e.g., Poland's syndrome, central deficiency), or abnormal bony elements (e.g., hypoplasia). Treatment must be individualized, and the physician should beware of neurovascular anomalies.
	Urgent (SSu)	Soft tissue syndactyly of border digits or digits of unequal length, girth, or joint level. Requires early separation to prevent angular and rotational deformity of the tethered digit.
Complex syndactyly (CS)	Standard (CSs)	Complex syndactyly of adjacent phalanges without additional bony anomalies (e.g., delta phalanx, symphalangism).
	Complicated (CSc)	Complex syndactyly that is associated with additional bony interconnections (e.g., transverse phalanges, symphalangism, polysyndactyly) or syndromes (e.g., constriction band syndrome). Treatment must be individualized, and the digits may function better as a unit.
	Unachievable (CSu)	Complex syndactyly with severe anomalies of the underlying bony structures that often prohibits formation of a five-digit hand without extensive surgical intervention.

TABLE 10. CLASSIFICATION OF ULNAR DEFICIENCY ACCORDING TO FIRST WEB SPACE ABNORMALITY

Type	Grade	Characteristics
A	Normal	Normal first web space and normal thumb
B	Mild	Mild first web deficiency and mild thumb hypoplasia with intact opposition and extrinsic tendon function
C	Moderate to severe	Moderate to severe first web deficiency and similar thumb hypoplasia with malrotation into the plane of the digits, loss of opposition, and dysfunction of the extrinsic tendons
D	Absent	Absence of the thumb

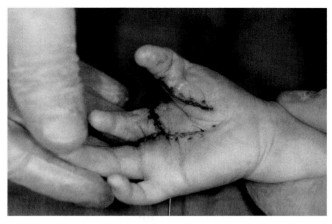

FIGURE 27. Intraoperative photograph after rotation of a flap from the cleft to recreate the first web space and transposition of index digit.

anomaly and its underlying pathogenesis are common and should be dispelled. This dialogue between physician and family should be reciprocal, with input from both parties. A rambling monologue from the physician must be avoided, as this discourse prohibits family participation.

The history should be comprehensive and should include questions concerning familial occurrence of limb anomalies, prenatal problems, birth history, and child development. The family history is particularly pertinent in congenital anomalies with known familial propagation, such as polydactyly and syndactyly. Many of these anomalies are transmitted with variable expressivity and incomplete penetrance. This indicates the possibility of the anomaly skipping a generation (incomplete penetrance) or being present in less than full form (variable phenotype). Therefore, careful questioning about any family members with congenital anomalies is the most efficacious method to generate relevant information. The prenatal history is important with regard to possible causes, although this questioning is usually unproductive. First trimester exposure to viral infections or potential teratogens should be assessed and documented. Inquiry includes questions about

previous pregnancies, stillbirths, or miscarriages. The birth history should include the duration of pregnancy, the time and length of delivery, the position at time of birth (e.g., breech presentation), and the posture of the affected limbs. Details about the achievement of developmental milestones (e.g., sitting, standing, walking, and talking) are important, as the presence of a congenital anomaly does not negate the possibility of additional problems, such as cerebral palsy. Review of any available records is also helpful to provide an accurate baseline and update of previous treatment. Clinical photographs are routinely taken as part of the initial evaluation. These pictures are placed in the medical record and provide documentation of the original presentation. Perusal of the initial photographs is often invaluable during subsequent evaluations and can be used to assess change after surgery. Videotaping is another popular medium for documentation, although it is costly and time consuming. The advent of digital video combined with electronic charting may facilitate its routine application over time.

Additional support team members are consulted when supplementary needs become evident. These services include other physicians (e.g., physiatrists, geneticists, cardiologists, nephrologists, endocrinologists), social services, and nurse specialists. The hand surgeon must be aware of hand anomalies that are associated with other conditions and direct referral patterns. The hand specialist cannot presume that appropriate workup has been performed and should enlist the services of colleagues. For example, a child with radial deficiency must be evaluated for systemic conditions, including heart, kidney, and blood dyscrasias.

Accurate diagnosis of limb anomalies also requires a basic knowledge of potential genetic and chromosomal causes to direct referral for genetic analysis and counseling. The role of the clinical geneticists is expanding, and genetic testing for limb malformations is gradually increasing in its availability and clinical applicability. Genomic and proteomic research is identifying the genetic material that is

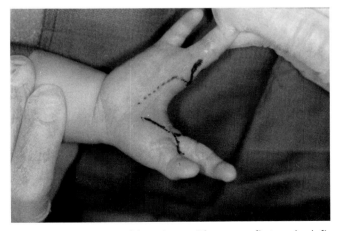

FIGURE 26. A 3-year-old patient with severe first web deficiency or type C ulnar deficiency.

responsible for limb malformation. Currently, only a small number of limb anomalies have been mapped to specific chromosomal segments and even fewer have been identified at the molecular level. Certain recognized etiologies have been defined that necessitate genetic evaluation (Table 2). These mutations may affect a single gene, multiple genes, or entire chromosomes. The clinician who is involved in the evaluation of children with congenital anomalies must keep abreast of the expanding developments in this area to ensure appropriate referral.

Imaging Modalities

X-rays of the affected limbs are usually performed, although many parts remain cartilaginous and invisible. Advanced imaging modalities (e.g., magnetic resonance imaging, computerized tomography, angiography) are reserved for specific indications. The x-ray is a valuable tool to use during discussions with the family, especially when the anomaly is compared to a normal extremity.

Physical Examination

The child needs to be examined gradually and carefully without unnecessary handling. Age-appropriate toys and props are used during the examination and provide valuable information in terms of hand usage and dexterity (Fig. 28). Multiple brief periods of examination are better tolerated than prolonged manipulation. Parents can be asked to participate in the examination, as the child usually responds better to a caregiver than a physician. The examination can occur while a parent is holding the child, and playful activities can be incorporated into the evaluation. A concurrent evaluation by the physician and the therapist is beneficial and allows the development of parallel treatment goals. Therapists are helpful in facilitating the assessment and adding additional expertise with regard to normative developmental skills and potential therapeutic modalities.

The physical examination should include a complete musculoskeletal examination. The affected limbs are examined from hand to hemithorax, and unilateral anomalies warrant careful inspection of the contralateral limb to ensure normality. Bilateral anomalies are often asymmetric, and mild expression can exist unrecognized. The posture of the limb and the use of the extremity during activities provide baseline information that requires documentation. In the newborn child, movement is difficult to elicit, and primitive reflexes are used to assess motion. Moro's reflex, asymmetric tonic neck response, and stimulation of palmar grasp are commonly used. As the child ages, gross movement patterns and integration of the affected hand into functional activities are pertinent observations. Absolute active range-of-motion measurements and manual muscle testing are not practical to assess in an infant or young child. However, limitation of active movement requires

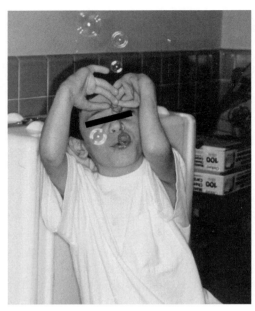

FIGURE 28. Manual dexterity can be evaluated in children by using tasks such as blowing bubbles.

assessment and documentation of passive range of motion. Any other abnormalities, such as facial asymmetry, webbing, hairy patches, birthmarks, dimples, and abnormal genitals, should be noted. Many syndromes are diagnosed by associated findings. For example, a broad-based radially deviated thumb that is combined with abnormal facies and hirsutism is characteristic of Rubinstein-Taybi syndrome, and ulnar polydactyly that is associated with dwarfism and dysplasia of the teeth is consistent with Ellis-van Creveld syndrome (also known as *chondroectodermal dysplasia*).

After the initial evaluation, the physician may have a definitive diagnosis and a sound understanding of the problem. This perpetuates a logical discussion with the family regarding diagnosis and treatment. An overall plan should be provided with realistic goals and expectations. The proposal should include the timing of surgery, the number of procedures, postoperative management, the duration of therapy, and the ultimate goal. Because congenital hand anomalies are not life threatening and do not require urgent intercession, decisions regarding definitive treatment should not be expected during the initial consultation. Parents need time to process the abundance of information that is provided and to weigh the potential treatment options. Most congenital anomalies do not warrant early surgical intervention, except for complex border syndactylies or progressive angular deformities. Therefore, delay and reevaluation are recommended to allow familiarity between the physician and the family along with parental acceptance of the deformity.

In certain cases, the diagnosis or management is not straightforward or easily explainable. The physician should not be hesitant to elicit assistance from colleagues, experts, and published sources. Families are typically responsive to this suggestion, as long as the matter is handled carefully. Additional consultation is better than advising erroneous information, which negatively affects the physician-family relationship and may be detrimental to the care of the child. Advances in technology have facilitated worldwide conferencing and appraisal. Digital photography allows capturing of valuable information that can be attached to electronic mail. The internet has provided a readily accessible network for dissemination of cases to specialists in congenital hand surgery. The American Society for Surgery of the Hand (http://www.hand-surg.org) has established a listserv for solicitation of opinions regarding complicated cases. The internet also provides access to established sites for the retrieval of data concerning congenital anomalies and potential differential diagnosis. The National Institutes of Health web site (http://www.ncbi.nlm.nih.gov) allows internet access to online mendelian inheritance in humans and valuable updated information regarding genes and disease. This source is readily available, frequently updated, and invaluable when evaluating a child with an unfamiliar or rare syndrome.

The worldwide web has also provided a substantial avenue for families to obtain knowledge regarding their child's anomaly. Some of this information is factual and relevant, whereas other material is hypothetical and inappropriate (69). The family is usually unable to decipher the reliability of the information, and this task is left to the evaluating physician. Families with children who have anomalies not only yearn for additional information, but also seek confirmation that other kids have similar anomalies. The internet and virtual chat rooms have created a means for contact between families with similar difficulties. These meetings may be helpful or detrimental, depending on the information that is conveyed.

Facilities that concentrate on congenital ailments are more apt to provide supplemental information regarding various anomalies and support organizations. Support groups may be available to help the family handle the stress and to buffer the disappointment. Literature regarding particular differences is often available, and monthly institutional publications are offered. Referral to other reputable publications that provide germane information is important (e.g., Superkids, Newton, MA, http://www.super-kids.org). In addition, families are encouraged to tour the hospital after the evaluation, which provides immediate exposure to congenitally different children.

Surgical Planning and Preparation

The timing and goals of surgery are discussed well before the details of the procedure. The specific timing should consider underlying medical problems, developmental level, the number of proposed procedures, and postoperative management. In general, hand reconstruction should be completed by school age. However, this represents an oversimplification, as consideration of many issues is necessary during surgical planning. In addition, certain procedures (e.g., distraction osteogenesis) cannot easily be performed on such an immature skeleton.

Before elective surgery, parents often request additional discussion and a preoperative counseling session. This conference is scheduled within 6 weeks of surgery, with ample time allotted for conversation. Because congenital anomalies are relatively uncommon, patients often request the chance to talk to a family who has undergone a similar operation. This request is accomplished via a phone conference, without physician or staff participation, that is arranged with an agreeable family. In addition, photographs of other children with similar anomalies that depict the preoperative condition and the postoperative result are accessible to the family. During their preoperative visit, the family and child tour the hospital, including portions of the operating suite, to acquaint them with the layout (operating and recovery rooms) along with the process of the events surrounding surgery.

Patients often express concerns about anesthesia for their child. These questions are directly referred to the pediatric anesthesiologist to allay any fears, to familiarize the family and physician with each other, and to allow management of any issues. Complicated cases require formal anesthesia consultation well before the planned surgical procedure. This evaluation must allow ample time to obtain any requested preoperative studies without jeopardizing the planned procedure.

Emotional Issues

Parents also feel directly responsible for their child's anomaly and express considerable guilt and confusion (70). The physician must be understanding of this reaction and must not be afraid to address these issues. Many of the perceived reasons for having an anomalous child are erroneous and can be dispelled by using scientific facts. However, responsibility is a natural response and may never dissipate entirely. Periods of remorse are common and often parallel phases of blame. The physician must understand that having a child with a congenital anomaly is a life-altering event, and families manage by a variety of coping mechanisms. These means of adjustment are not consistent among families, and physician participation is important, although primarily supportive. Marital difficulties are common, and financial worries are pervasive, especially in severely affected children with multisystemic involvement.

Parents of children who are born with congenital anomalies are also extremely concerned about peer pressure and chiding. The physician should acknowledge this probability and should promote supplementary support and increased parental affection during these times. Literature is available to help the child and family explain their limb anomalies, although parental discussion is the mainstay to understanding. School-age playmates are acutely aware of congenital limb differences, which are a source of discussion and possible teasing. As a congenitally different child grows, he or she develops inward and outward coping mechanisms to handle his or her anomaly. The physician should act as part of the child's support system with open discussions regarding his or her anomaly and questions about peer discourse. These conversations are often insightful and revealing to the physician and the family.

REFERENCES

1. Flatt AE. Classification and incidence. In: Flatt AE, ed. *The care of congenital hand anomalies,* 2nd ed. St. Louis: Quality Medical Publishers, 1994:47–63.

2. Kozin SH, Thoder J. Congenital anomalies of the upper extremity. In: Baratz ME, Watson AD, Imbriglia JE, eds. *Orthopedic surgery: the essentials.* New York: Thieme Medical Publishers, 1999:657–673.

3. Bamshad M, Watkins WS, Dixon ME, et al. Reconstructing the history of human limb development: lessons from birth defects. *Pediatr Res* 1999;45:291–299.

4. Müller W. *Die angeborenen Fehlbildungen der menschlichen Hand.* Leipzig, Germany: Thieme Verlag, 1937.

5. Buck-Gramcko D. Teratologic sequences. In: Buck-Gramcko D, ed. *Congenital malformations of the hand and forearm.* London: Churchill Livingstone, 1998:17–20.

6. Frantz CH, O'Rahilly R. Congenital skeletal limb deficiencies. *J Bone Joint Surg* 1961;43:1202–1224.

7. Swanson AB. A classification for congenital limb malformations. *J Hand Surg* 1976;1:8–22.

8. Hoyme HE, Jones KL, Van Allen MI, et al. Vascular pathogenesis of transverse limb reduction defects. *J Pediatr* 1982;101:839–843.

9. Gonzalez CH, Marques-Dias J, Kim CA, et al. Congenital abnormalities in Brazilian children associated with misoprostol misuse in first trimester of pregnancy. *Lancet* 1998;351:1624–1627.

10. Burton BK, Schulz CJ, Burd LI. Spectrum of limb disruption defects associated with chorionic villous sampling. *Pediatrics* 1993;91:989–993.

11. Bayne LG, Klug MS. Long-term review of the surgical treatment of radial deficiencies. *J Hand Surg* 1987;12:169–179.

12. James MA, McCarroll HR, Manske PR. The spectrum of radial longitudinal deficiency: a modified classification. *J Hand Surg* 1999;24:1145–1155.

13. Eaton CJ, Lister GD. Syndactyly. *Hand Clin* 1990;6:555–574.

14. Bosse K, Betz RC, Lee YA, et al. Localization of a gene for syndactyly type 1 to chromosome 2q34-q36. *Am J Hum Genet* 2000;67:492–497.

15. Kozin SH. Syndactyly. *J Am Soc Surg Hand* 2001;1:1–13.

16. Watson BT, Hennrikus WL. Postaxial type-B polydactyly. Prevalence and treatment. *J Bone Joint Surg* 1997;79:65–68.

17. Ezaki MB. Radial polydactyly. *Hand Clin* 1990;6:577–588.

18. Cohen MS. Thumb duplication. *Hand Clin* 1998;14:17–27.

19. Wassel HD. The results of surgery for polydactyly of the thumb. A review. *Clin Orthop* 1969;125:175–193.

20. Muragaki Y, Mundlos S, Upton J, et al. Altered growth and branching patterns in synpolydactyly caused by mutations in HOXD13. *Science* 1996;272:548–551.

21. Upton J, Coombs C. Vascular tumors in children. *Hand Clin* 1995;1:307–337.

22. Upton J, Coombs CJ, Mulliken JB, et al. Vascular malformations of the upper limb: a review of 270 patients. *J Hand Surg* 1999;24:1019–1035.

23. Ireland DC, Takoyama N, Flatt A. Poland's syndrome: a review of 43 cases. *J Bone Joint Surg* 1976;58:52–58.

24. Wiedrich TA. Congenital constriction band syndrome. *Hand Clin* 1998;14:29–38.

25. Miura T. New ideas on classification of congenital malformations. In: Buck-Gramcko D, ed. *Congenital malformations of the hand and forearm.* London: Churchill Livingstone, 1998:9–16.

26. Leung PC, Chan KM, Cheng JC. Congenital anomalies of the upper limb among the Chinese population in Hong Kong. *J Hand Surg* 1982;7:563–565.

27. Ogino T, Minami A, Fukuda K, et al. Congenital anomalies of the upper limb among the Japanese in Sapporo. *J Hand Surg* 1986;11:364–371.

28. Cheng JC, Chow SK, Leung PC. Classification of 578 cases of congenital upper limb anomalies with the IFSSH system—a 10 years' experience. *J Hand Surg* 1987;12:1055–1060.

29. De Smet L, Matton G, Monstrey S, et al. Application of the IFSSH (3) classification for congenital anomalies of the hand: results and problems. *Acta Orthop Belg* 1997;63:182–188.

30. Luijsterburg AJ, van Huizum MA, Impelmans BE, et al. Classification of congenital anomalies of the upper limb. *J Hand Surg* 2000;25:3–7.

31. McCarroll HR. Congenital anomalies: a 25-year overview. *J Hand Surg* 2000;25:1007–1037.

32. Nelson K, Holmes LB. Malformations due to presumed spontaneous mutations in newborn infants. *N Engl J Med* 1989;320:19–23.

33. Riddle RD, Tabin CJ. How limbs develop. *Sci Am* 1999;280:74–79.

34. Beatty E. Upper limb tissue differentiation in the human embryo. *Hand Clin* 1985;1:391–403.

35. Riddle RD, Johnson RL, Laufer E, et al. Sonic hedgehog mediates the polarizing activity of the ZPA. *Cell* 1993;75:1401–1416.

36. Riddle RD, Ensini M, Nelson C, et al. Induction of the LIM homeobox gene Lmx 1 by WNT7a establishes dorsoventral pattern in the vertebrate limb. *Cell* 1995;83:631–640.

37. Parr BA, MvMahon AP. Dorsalizing signal Wnt-7a required for normal polarity of D-V and A-P axes of the mouse limb. *Nature* 1995;374:350–353.

38. Serrano N, O'Farrell PH. Limb morphogenesis: connections between patterning and growth. *Curr Biol* 1997;7:186–195.

39. Shubin N, Tabin C, Carroll S. Fossils, genes and the evolution of animal limbs. *Nature* 1997;388:638–648.
40. Cohn MJ, Izpisua-Belmonte JC, Abud H, et al. Fibroblast growth factors induce additional limb development in the flank of chick embryos. *Cell* 1995;80:739–746.
41. Crombleholme TM, Dirkes K, Whitney TM, et al. Amniotic band syndrome in fetal lambs I: fetoscopic release and morphometric outcome. *J Pediatr Surg* 1995;30:974–978.
42. Miura T. A clinical study of congenital anomalies of the hand. *Hand* 1981;13:59–68.
43. Miura T, Suzuki M. Clinical differences between typical and atypical cleft hand. *J Hand Surg* 1984;9:311–315.
44. Ogino T, Minami A, Kato H. Clinical features and roentgenograms of symbrachydactyly. *J Hand Surg* 1989;14:303–306.
45. Miura T, Nakamura R, Horii E. The position of symbrachydactyly in the classification of congenital hand anomalies. *J Hand Surg* 1994;19:350–354.
46. Ogino T. Teratogenic relationship between polydactyly, syndactyly, and cleft hand. *J Hand Surg* 1990;15:201–209.
47. Ogino T. Cleft hand. *Hand Clin* 1990;6:661–671.
48. Blauth W. Der hypoplastische Daumen. *Arch Orthop Unfallchir* 1967;62:225–246.
49. Manske PR, McCarroll HR Jr, James MA. Type III-A hypoplastic thumb. *J Hand Surg* 1995;20;246–253.
50. Lister G. Reconstruction of the hypoplastic thumb. *Clin Orthop* 1985;195:52–65.
51. Kozin SH, Weiss AA, Weber JB, et al. Index finger pollicization for congenital aplasia or hypoplasia of the thumb. *J Hand Surg* 1992;17:880–884.
52. Graham TJ, Louis DS. A comprehensive approach to surgical management of the type IIIA hypoplastic thumb. *J Hand Surg* 1998;23:3–13.
53. Lourie GM, Lins RE. Radial longitudinal deficiency. A review and update. *Hand Clin* 1998;14:85–99.
54. Damore E, Kozin SH, Thoder JJ, et al. The recurrence of deformity after surgical centralization for radial clubhand. *J Hand Surg* 2000;25:745–751.
55. Heikel HV. Aplasia and hypoplasia of the radius. Studies on 64 cases and on epiphyseal transplantation in rabbits with the imitated defect. *Acta Orthop Scand Suppl* 1959;39:1–155.
56. Gruelich WW, Pyle SI. *Radiographic atlas of skeletal development of the hand and wrist,* 2nd ed. Stanford, CA: Stanford University Press, 1959:136–149.
57. Hensinger RN. Hand. In: Hensinger RN, ed. *Standards in pediatric orthopedics: tables, charts, and graphs illustrating growth.* New York: Raven Press, 1986:136–149.
58. Kümmell W. Die missbildungen der extremitaeten durch defect, verwachsung und ueberzahl. *Bibliotheca Med (Cassel)* 1895;3:1–83.
59. Ogden JA, Watson HK, Bohne W. Ulnar dysmelia. *J Bone Joint Surg* 1976;58:467–475.
60. Riordan DC. The upper limb. In: Lovell W, Winter RB, eds. *Pediatric orthopaedics,* vol. 2. Philadelphia: JB Lippincott Co, 1978:685–719.
61. Swanson AB, Tada K, Yonenobu K. Ulnar ray deficiency: its various manifestations. *J Hand Surg* 1984;9:658–664.
62. Miller JK, Wenner SM, Kruger LM. Ulnar deficiency. *J Hand Surg* 1986;11:822–829.
63. Bayne LG. Ulnar club hand (ulnar deficiencies). In: Green DP, ed. *Operative hand surgery,* 3rd ed. New York: Churchill Livingstone, 1993:288–304.
64. Schmidt CC, Neufield SK. Ulnar ray deficiency. *Hand Clin* 1998;14:65–76.
65. Maisels DO. Lobster-claw deformities of the hand. *Br J Plast Surg* 1970;23:269–281.
66. Broudy AS, Smith RJ. Deformities of the hand and wrist with ulnar deficiency. *J Hand Surg* 1979;4:304–315.
67. Johnson J, Omer GE Jr. Congenital ulnar deficiency: natural history and therapeutic implications. *Hand Clin* 1985;1:499–510.
68. Cole RJ, Manske PR. Classification of ulnar deficiency according to the thumb and first web space. *J Hand Surg* 1991;22:479–488.
69. Beredjiklian PK, Bozentka DJ, Steinberg DR, et al. Evaluating the source and content of orthopaedic information on the internet. The case of carpal tunnel syndrome. *J Bone Joint Surg* 2000;82:1540–1543.
70. Bradbury E. Psychological issues for children and their parents. In: Buck-Gramcko D, ed. *Congenital malformations of the hand and forearm.* London: Churchill Livingstone, 1998:48–56.

82

CONGENITAL DISORDERS: SYNDACTYLY

TADAO KOJIMA
YUICHI HIRASE

SURGICAL ANATOMY

Skin

Various types of skin deficiencies are seen with the different forms of syndactyly. Mansfield (1) reported that skin loss was underestimated in many surgical procedures, and, for this reason, estimation of skin deficiency has been practiced in cases of syndactyly release. Kilian and Neimkin (2) reported a 22% deficiency of skin, according to the surgical design. Eaton and Lister (3) reported that skin deficiency was produced by two components, the fused region and the web space of the adjoining finger. In the normal hand, the abduction range is 70 to 90 degrees in the first web space and more than 35 degrees for the fingers (4), owing to the existence of elastic skin in the web space. The normal commissure of the finger has a dorsal slope of 40 to 45 degrees, the texture of dorsal skin, and non–hair-bearing skin.

Fascial Interconnection

The existence of fascial structures that connect the fingers is seen in the separation of syndactyly. This fascial interconnection is often hypertrophic and is identified as Cleland's ligament, the interosseous fascia, the superficial palmar fascia, or the intermetacarpal ligament (3). Lösch and Duncker (5) demonstrated that Cleland's ligament in syndactyly arose from the lateral site of the phalanx and ran to the mid-region of the syndactylic space, fused in the midline, and, finally, attached to the dermis of the palmar skin. In syndactyly between the thumb and index finger, this fascial structure becomes the transverse intermetacarpal ligament, which is not seen in the normal hand (4). In the case of syndactyly with digits of different length, these abnormal bands tether and flex the longer digits and result in secondary deformity of the joint and bone.

Neurovascular Bundle

The most common abnormality is distal bifurcation of the common digital artery and nerve in the web space (3,6).

This is especially common in complex syndactyly and symbrachydactyly. Loop formation of the nerve is sometimes observed around the artery.

Bone

There are various bone abnormalities, ranging from the simple type of osseous fusion of only the distal phalangeal bone to more extensive complicated forms, which are seen in complex syndactyly. In association with growth, the secondary osseous deformity becomes more marked due to fascial interconnection.

PATHOPHYSIOLOGY

In the term *syndactyly*, the Greek root *syn* means *together*. Therefore, *syndactyly* means webbed fingers (7). The type of syndactyly in which the fingers are webbed to the fingertip is classified as *complete syndactyly*, whereas those cases in which web formation does not extend to the fingertip are classified as *incomplete syndactyly*. The type of syndactyly in which the web space is made only of soft tissue is called *simple syndactyly*, whereas those cases that involve bridging skeletal elements are called *complex syndactyly*. A hybrid form of syndactyly, in which skeletal abnormalities exist, such as hidden polydactyly, clinodactyly, symphalangism, or brachydactyly, with side-to-side fusion is defined as *complicated syndactyly* (3). Syndactyly occurs not only in isolation, but also in association with other kinds of abnormalities. It is often observed together with congenital hand anomalies, such as polydactyly, cleft hand, and constriction ring syndrome.

PATHOGENESIS

Swanson (8) reported a practical classification that was based on embryologic failure. This classification was developed by the Committees of the American Society for Surgery of the Hand and the International Federation of

TABLE 1. CLASSIFICATION OF CONGENITAL HAND DEFORMITIES

Failure of formation of parts (arrest of development)
   Transverse deficiencies
      Amputations: arm, forearm, wrist, hand, digits
   Longitudinal deficiencies
      Phocomelia: complete, proximal, distal
      Radial deficiencies (radial club hand)
      Central deficiencies (cleft hand)
      Ulnar deficiencies (ulnar club hand)
      Hypoplastic digits
Failure of differentiation (separation) of parts
   Synostosis: elbow, forearm, wrist, metacarpals, phalanges
   Radial head dislocation
   Symphalangism
   Syndactyly
      Simple
      Complex
      Associated syndrome
   Contracture
      Soft tissue
         Arthrogryposis
         Pterygium cubitale
         Trigger digit
         Absent extensor tendons
         Hypoplastic thumb
         Thumb-clutched hand
         Camptodactyly
         Windblown hand
      Skeletal
         Clinodactyly
         Kirner's deformity
         Delta bone
Duplication
   Thumb (preaxial) polydactyly
   Triphalangism and hyperphalangism
   Finger polydactyly
      Central polydactyly (polysyndactyly)
      Postaxial polydactyly
   Mirror hand
      Ulnar dimelia
Overgrowth: all or portions of upper limb
   Macrodactyly
Undergrowth
Congenital constriction band syndrome
Generalized skeletal abnormalities
   Madelung's deformity

Adapted from Swanson AB. A classification for congenital limb malformations. *J Hand Surg* 1976;1:8–22.

Societies for Surgery of the Hand (Table 1). Swanson and Tada (9) later formed a subclassification in 1983. Since then, this classification has been adopted in many countries. However, there has been some conflict regarding Swanson's classification, which is based on embryology. Several investigators (10,11) point out that polydactyly, syndactyly, and typical cleft hand, which affect the central ray, are caused by a common teratologic mechanism. Ogino (11,12) indicated that these anomalies should be classified in the same category based on clinical and experimental studies. He modified Swanson's classification by adding a category of abnormal induction of digital rays that includes these anomalies (13). The Japanese Society for Surgery of the Hand adopted this modified Swanson's classification in 1996.

INCIDENCE

Maccollum (14) reported that syndactyly occurred in 1 in 2,000 to 2,500 births. This is a similar incidence to that reported by Skoog (15) (approximately 1 in 2,000 births) and Flatt (16) (approximately 1 in 2,000 to 2,500 births).

The reported frequency of syndactyly in congenital hand anomalies varies: 19.1% in Iowa (reported by Flatt) (16), 14.9% in Hong Kong (reported by Leung et al.) (17), and 4.1% in Sapporo (reported by Ogino et al.) (12). As Ogino reported, this difference seems attributable to the particular category that is adopted for associated syndactyly, such as typical cleft hand, radial ray deficiency, polydactyly, and constriction ring syndrome. Oka et al. (18) reported the appearance of congenital hand anomalies during a 14-year period from 1973 to 1986 in Miyagi prefecture of Japan. This investigation was reliable for determining the incidence of congenital hand anomalies in Japan because it was performed by plastic and orthopedic surgeons. In this report, syndactyly comprised 10% of all congenital hand anomalies, with a prevalence of 1.4 in 10,000 births, and 80% of cases of syndactyly occurred between the middle and ring fingers.

CLINICAL SIGNIFICANCE

A commissure with almost normal elasticity is necessary for abduction of the thumb and fingers. A finger pulp with an almost normal nail and good sensation and form is necessary for grasp of the hand. Many cases of syndactyly, including associated syndactyly, require separation of the fingers to improve function. It is important to perform surgery at the appropriate time and age.

EVALUATION

Clinical History and Physical Examination

The design for separation and the method of making a commissure must be adequately considered before surgery is based on the type of syndactyly (complete or incomplete, simple or complex, pure or complicated). The size of skin deficiency should also be evaluated. In cases of complex or complicated syndactyly, it should be considered whether separation of fingers is possible. For this purpose, the condition of the bone is evaluated by x-ray, and the condition of the extensor and flexor tendons and the digital artery is evaluated by echography, magnetic resonance imaging, and angiography (6,19). Digital subtraction angiography has also been useful for this purpose (20).

The level of the normal palmar-digital crease of the adjoining finger is used to determine the web height for plasty of the commissure. However, as the availability of this method is limited to isolated single syndactyly with a normal palmar-digital crease, Richterman et al. (21) indicated that radiographic analysis by x-ray was an accurate and reproducible method that could be applied to postoperative evaluation of web height.

SURGICAL MANAGEMENT

Options and Indications

Operative methods for syndactyly have been reported since the beginning of the nineteenth century and have continued to progress until now. The purpose of surgery for syndactyly is to make an almost normal finger with a normal-shaped commissure, fingertip, and fingernail, without deformity or contracture. It is ideal to create such a result by a single procedure. However, there are some operative problems in creating the commissure and covering the skin defect on the lateral side of the finger during the separation. It is important to consider the final results and the advantages and disadvantages of conventional methods and to select the optimal method.

The treatment of syndactyly is by operation. There are a few cases in which surgery is not recommended, such as those patients with severe anomalies or severe mental retardation. However, surgery is generally performed in most cases at the appropriate time.

Timing of Operation

Since the report of Davis and German (22), most authors, with some exceptions, have recommended surgery before the age of 2 years. The main reason to delay surgery until after 2 years of age is the high rate of reoperation because of skin contracture if the surgery is done before 1.5 years of age (3,23). A report has highlighted the possibility of hypertrophic scarring occurring frequently after surgery in infancy (15). Also, it has been noted that surgery in the infantile hand is too difficult technically, with some problems in postoperative treatment (23). In addition, some opinions recommend delaying surgery until the patient is 4 or 5 years of age because of the large amount of infant fat under the skin, which presents some difficulty in accurately assessing dissection planes and incision placement (1). Since the 1970s, earlier operations have been performed because of the improved safety of general anesthesia, the use of loupe magnification, the improvement of surgical equipment, and the change of thinking regarding infant fat. The recommendation for earlier operation is also supported by the fact that the infantile functional pattern of the hand is established between 6 months and 2 years of age (3,24). The authors recommend earlier operation because postoperative treatment is easier in a 1-year-old baby than it is in a 2-year-old child and does not cause psychological stress to the baby.

HISTORICAL REVIEW OF SPECIFIC SURGICAL METHODS

Plasty of Commissure

The report of Davis and German (22) describes several methods to make a tunnel before separation. Rudtorffer (1801) separated the syndactyly after epithelialization of a tunnel, which was made by means of a leaden thread that was passed from the dorsum to the palmar aspect at the base of the syndactyly. Velpeau (1847) separated the syndactyly and then sutured the margins, which were cut from the epithelialized commissure, which was made by Rudtorffer's method, to the fingertip. This method was advanced by Felizet (1892) and Pieri (1949), who made a tunnel by using a flap.

Simple Division

Didot (1849) separated syndactyly by means of broad rectangular flaps, which were elevated in dorsal and palmar sites from the base of syndactyly to the fingertip, and sutured each flap at the commissure. Nelaton (1932) made similarly shaped, but larger, flaps and sutured them directly to make the commissure.

Free Skin Graft

Lennander (1891) separated the syndactyly in a relatively straight line and first performed free split-thickness skin grafting from the commissure to the lateral sites of the fingers. Kanavel (1932) made a T-shaped incision in the dorsal and palmar sites at the base of the finger and performed free full-thickness skin grafting from the commissure to the lateral sites of the fingers.

Triangular Flap Method

Zeller (1801) first performed triangular flap transfer to make the commissure. Agnew (1883) elevated a long triangular flap from the base of the web to the fingertip in cases with sufficient commissure skin and sutured this flap to the palmar side. Bidwell (1913) combined this triangular flap with a rectangular flap for separation of the fingers. Alternatively, Norton (1881) first elevated two triangular flaps from the dorsal and palmar sides. Subsequently, in 1943 and 1956, Cronin (25,26) combined this method with a zigzag incision for separation of the fingers. Blackfield (1955) made the tip of the triangular flap round. Nylen

(1957), Mansfield (1961) (1), Skoog (1965) (15), Zachariae (1955) (27), Velasco (1967), and Millesi (1970) also used a triangular flap for separation of the fingers. These methods are still being used as of 2003.

Rectangular Flap Method

Although Dieffenbach (1834) first used a dorsal rectangular flap for syndactyly, it had not been used for quite some time. Oldfield (1948) used a horseshoe-shaped flap, in which the tip of the rectangular flap was made round. Since the 1950s, there have been many reports of the use of a rectangular flap by Bauer et al. (1956) (28), Emmett (1963), Marumo et al. (1970) (29), Henz and Littler (1971) (30), and Dobyns (1988) (4). Flatt (1977) (16) made the tip of the rectangular flap oblique and combined it with a zigzag incision to cover the skin defect without the use of a skin graft in one finger. To prevent postoperative web creep, the rectangular flap was inserted a little deeper. Buck-Gramcko (1971) (31) made the tip of the flap into a diamond shape. Katsumata et al. (1984) (32) made an M-shaped rectangular flap to insert into the base of the finger in the palmar site where the reversed Y-shaped incision is initially made. Upton (1990) (24) made a small longitudinal incision in the central tip of the rectangular flap and inserted a small triangular flap into it. Moss and Foucher (1990) (33) made the central portion of the flap narrower to fix the shape of the commissure and made a small triangular flap at the palmar base of the finger to transpose to both sides of the rectangular flap. A procedure to elevate the rectangular flap from the palmar side was first described by Villechaise (1927) and was used by Barsky (1958) and Blauth (1973).

Island Flap Method

Colville (1989) (34) used V-Y advancement of a dorsal diamond-shaped island flap to make the commissure. Sherif (1998) (35) created the commissure by V-Y advancement of a dorsal metacarpal flap, like Colville's technique, and described that branches of the dorsal metacarpal artery nourished this island flap.

Separation Method of Syndactyly

Simple Longitudinal Separation

Simple longitudinal separation was performed by Zeller (1810) and Dieffenbach (1834), followed by Norton (1881). Lennander (1891) covered one finger with a flap and the other finger with a skin graft. Blackfield (1955) performed Z-plasty at the level of the joint to avoid lateral scar formation and separated the skin defect region for free full-thickness skin graft. Nylen (1957) also made a small incision at the level of the joint for a free full-thickness skin

graft. These methods progressed to the small triangular flap method by Skoog (1965) (15). Didot (1849) and Nelaton (1884) performed a technique by using a rectangular flap that was based on the side of finger. Bidwell (1913) combined this technique with a dorsal triangular flap for commissure plasty. Cogswell (1913) and Oldfield (1945) also combined this technique with a dorsal rectangular flap. Colville (1989) (34) elevated rectangular flaps in each phalanx, so as not to cross the finger crease, and covered one finger with this flap and the other finger with a free skin graft. Faniel (1911) elevated four large triangular flaps by making a large Z-shaped incision on the dorsal and palmar sides and covered the donor site area with the flaps.

Zigzag Incision

The first report of use of a zigzag incision for separation of fingers was made by Cronin (1943) (25), following the experience of Faniel who indicated the advantages of a large Z-shaped incision. Cronin initially made a zigzag incision only on the palmar side and a longitudinal incision on the dorsal side, but, subsequently, he also made a zigzag incision on the dorsal side of the web (26). This method greatly influenced Zachariae (1955) (27), Webster (1955) (36), Bauer et al. (1956) (28), Barsky (1958), and Flatt (1977) (16). Buck-Gramcko (1971) (31) modified Cronin's method by extending the tip of the triangular flap to the midline of the finger and indicated the necessity of a skin graft to the lateral sides of the fingers to decrease the tension on the linear scar. Henz and Littler (1977) (30), Kilian and Neimkin (1985) (2), Brown (1997) (23), and Dobyns (1988) (4) used zigzag incisions and performed free full-thickness skin grafting to both fingers. Bunnell (1964) (7) and Kelikian (1974) used a slightly curved incision by making the tip of the zigzag incision round. On the other hand, Zachariae (1955 and 1966) (27,37) initially used a zigzag incision to the midline of the finger but later changed to a larger zigzag incision method to reach the whole area of the dorsal and palmar sides of the finger.

Operative Treatment without Skin Graft

Since a non–skin grafting method, as reported by Zeller and Diot, resulted in scar contracture and web formation, many procedures with skin graft have subsequently been performed. However, there are also some trials of non–skin grafting methods. Raus (1984) (38) performed Zeller's method for separation of the fingers under local anesthesia for newborn babies within 24 to 72 hours after birth, but its long-term results have not been published. Niranjan and De Carpentier (1990) (39) described a method to avoid skin grafting by a combination of a dorsal trilobed flap and a round tip–shaped zigzag incision. Ekerot (1996) (40) performed a similar method to Niranjan, but skin grafting and secondary reconstruction in three cases were necessary. In the conventional dorsal rectangular flap method, a flap for commissure plasty is elevated in the dorsum of the finger. As described before by Colville, Sherif produced the commissure by advancement of an island flap in the dorsum of the hand. However, skin grafting is necessary in some cases, and the resulting scar on the dorsum of the hand is a disadvantage of this method.

Surgical Method for Complete Syndactyly Fingertip Separation

In complete syndactyly in which the distal phalanx is fused, separation of the fingers, along with coverage of the exposed distal phalangeal bone and creation of the lateral nail fold, is a problem. Thomson (1971) (41) used two small abdominal flaps for coverage. Johansson (1982) (42) separated the region from the nail to the fused part of the distal phalanx and covered the exposed bone with a triangular flap that was pedicled in the mid-thenar region. The pedicle of the flap was cut at 10 days after surgery, and the syndactyly was separated 2 to 3 months later. Van der Biezen and Bloem (1992) (43) used double-opposing palmar flaps for coverage after separation of the distal phalangeal bone, and, 2 weeks later, division of flaps and separation of fingers were performed at the same time. Buck-Gramcko (1990) (44) made a well-shaped lateral nail wall by the pulp flap technique to rotate distally two small triangular flaps in the pulp region. Sugihara et al. (1991) (45) made the lateral nail wall by rotating distally two small narrow rectangular flaps from the dorsal and palmar sides. Sommerkamp et al. (1992) (46) performed free composite grafting from the lateral side of the great toe and was successful in obtaining a relatively normal contour and satisfactory pad.

Tissue Expanders for Syndactyly

Morgan and Edgerton (1985) (47) used a tissue expander for a case of postoperative recurrence after syndactyly operation and successfully performed separation without free skin grafting. Van Beek and Adson (1987) (48) reported 11 cases of the upper extremity, including three cases of syndactyly. In their report, they described one case of symbrachydactyly to the proximal interphalangeal joint in which separation of the fingers and commissure plasty were possible at the same time without performing a free skin graft. Ishikura and Tsukada (1992) (49) described approximately five cases, including three cases of primary repair, and reported the exposure of the tissue expander in one case. The authors used this technique for 11 hands of ten patients (including six cases of complete syndactyly and three cases of complex syndactyly) (Fig. 1). Of the 21 expanders inserted, five expanders (24%) became exposed. However, expanders were useful to decrease the amount of grafted skin (50).

AUTHORS' PREFERRED TREATMENT: TECHNIQUE

The authors and Marumo et al. (29) described their preferred method in 1976. To obtain a balance of the size of the finger compared to the adjoining fingers, the authors recommend the use of local flaps and free skin graft for each finger and do not recommend the performance of skin grafting in one finger and flap coverage in the other finger. The authors described the method to locate the dorsal rectangular flap to one side and to perform skin grafting of the proximal and distal phalanges of one finger and of the middle phalanx of the other finger. The authors later modified this technique to make the palmar zigzag incision larger (51).

First, the adjoining commissure level is confirmed, and a mark is made at the mid-point of the interdigital space. In the next step, a dorsal rectangular flap is designed with a trapezoidal shape, more than 7 mm at the tip and broader at the base of the flap. The length of the flap is decided by measuring the dorsal slope of the adjoining commissure (Fig. 2A). By designing the flap to be 2 to 3 mm longer than the length of the dorsal slope of the adjoining commissure, the flap can obtain the surplus skin that is required. The position of the dorsal rectangular flap is decided by which finger's proximal phalanx is covered by the triangular flap. In the case of syndactyly with different-length fingers, as a rule, the triangular flap covers the proximal phalanx whose palmar-digital crease is lower. Then, the design of the triangular flap in one finger is made by the zigzag incision design on the palmar side. The height of the triangular flap is made the same as the length of the rectangular flap. A line is made from the top of the triangular flap to the mid-lateral line of the middle phalanx of the other finger through the mid-point of the proximal finger crease of syndactyly. This line is curved distally and radially at the proximal phalanx of one finger. The line runs distally from the middle phalanx of the other finger to the pulp through the mid-point of the distal finger crease (Fig. 2B). The design of the distal phalanx is decided by the existence of surplus skin between the nails. In cases with surplus skin, the flap covers one side of the fingertip. In cases with insufficient skin, skin grafting is performed on both sides or Buck-Gramcko's method is used (44), especially for cases that involve the distal phalangeal osseous fusion. If the fingertip is tapering, and there is not enough skin, a two-staged operation by the Van der Biezen and Bloem method (43) is selected. In elevating the large triangular flap, care must be taken not to make it too thin. A Kirschner wire with a 0.8- or 1.0-mm diameter is inserted from the fingertip to the metacarpophalangeal joint with the finger fully extended and in slight abduction. By suturing the flaps, a skin defect is produced in the proximal and distal phalanges of one finger and the middle or distal phalanx of the other finger (Fig. 2C). Full-thickness skin is harvested from the medial

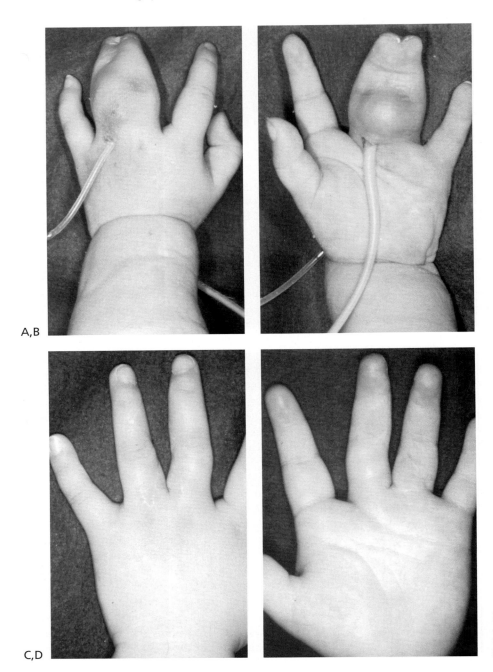

A,B

C,D

FIGURE 1. Case of complete syndactyly applied-tissue expander. **A,B:** Expansion was completed on the dorsal and palmar sides. **C,D:** Postoperative views after 1 year.

inframalleolar region of the foot for grafting, and compression is applied. It is important to perform skin grafting with the finger in slight abduction. If the finger is in strong abduction, a discrepancy is made in the graft. For the grafted skin, the tie-over method or simple compression is performed, but care must be taken not to apply strong compression. The fingertip is kept visible at all times to check the vascularity. The elbow joint is fixed at 90 degrees in a long arm cast. In cases in which the separated bone and joint are exposed because of skin deficiency in complex syndactyly, the tissue expander method is selected (50). Also, in some cases of complete syndactyly, the tissue

expander method is selected to decrease the amount of skin graft (Fig. 3).

POSTOPERATIVE MANAGEMENT

In the postoperative period, the fingertip is checked for circulatory abnormalities. Postoperatively, infants generally do not complain of pain, but if the patient complains of pain, it is necessary to check whether the dressing is too tight and to reapply the compression bandage in the case of congestion of the fingertip. The compression dressing

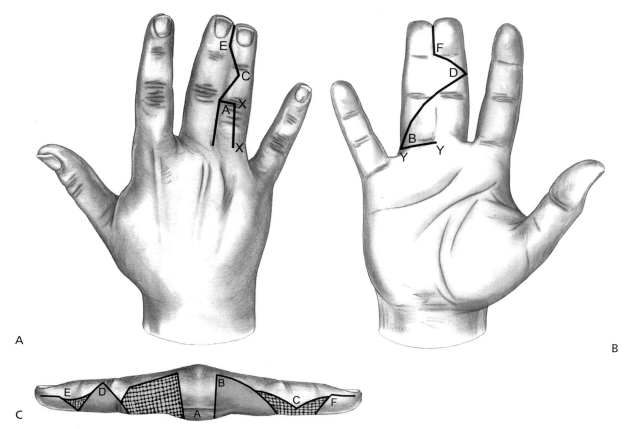

FIGURE 2. Incision design for simple complete syndactyly. **A:** A dorsal rectangular flap (*A*) and small zigzag incision (*A, C, E*) are designed on the dorsal side. **B:** A large zigzag incision is designed on the palmar side (*B, D, F*). The base (*YY*) of triangular flap (*B*) should coincide with the height (*XX*) of the dorsal rectangular flap. **C:** When each flap is elevated and sutured in position, one skin defect in one finger and two skin defects in the other finger result. The shaded areas indicate skin defects, which are covered with full-thickness skin grafts.

is removed at 1 week postoperatively, and a light recompression dressing is applied until 2 weeks postoperatively. On the tenth postoperative day, the sutures are removed, and flexion and extension exercises of the finger are started after removal of the Kirschner wire at 2 weeks postoperatively.

POSTOPERATIVE REHABILITATION

Special rehabilitation is not necessary postoperatively. Massage with ointment by the parents is recommended. If the grafted skin takes with an adequate incision design, and the wound is healed primarily, a postoperative splint is not necessary. However, if wound healing is not obtained primarily, a postoperative splint is necessary. Careful observation for scar contracture and joint or nail deformity is necessary. If there is scar contracture, and the full range of extension and flexion is impossible in the proximal interphalangeal and distal interphalangeal joints, reoperation is performed before the development of bone or joint deformity.

COMPLICATIONS

Postoperative complications consist of web recurrence, flexion contracture of the finger, lateral deviation, rotation deformity, nail deformity, and pigmentation of the skin graft. All of these problems, except pigmentation of the skin graft, result from scar contracture.

Prevention of Scar Contracture

Scar contracture results from inadequate skin incision design, necrosis of the wound margin, poor take of the skin graft, or necrosis of the flap.

1. The first step in prevention of contracture is to make an adequate skin incision design. Incisions are made so as not to cross a skin crease at an angle that is close to 90 degrees. In cases in which such an incision cannot be avoided, Z-plasty or an additional incision is necessary. This problem is one reason why the authors made the palmar zigzag incision larger and the dorsal zigzag incision smaller, so as not to produce contracture. To

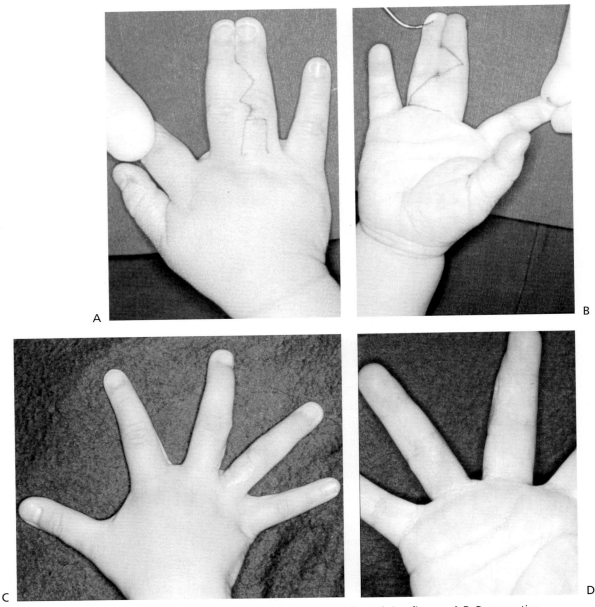

FIGURE 3. Case of complete syndactyly between the middle and ring fingers. **A,B:** Preoperative views and incision designs. **C,D:** Postoperative views after 2 years.

prevent web creep, it is important to use the same textured skin as the dorsal slope, considering the dorsal slope of the normal commissure, and a rectangular flap with sufficient length and width is designed by observing the adjoining commissure. It makes sense to use the methods by Katsumata et al. (32), Upton (24), and Moss and Foucher (33) for prevention of creep.

2. It is important to obtain primary wound healing to prevent scar contracture. Primary wound healing is gained by adequate suture of the surgical margin without tension and complete survival of skin grafts and flaps. For this, adequate design of incisions is necessary. To decrease the tension on the surgical margin, adequate resection of infant fat is necessary (24,25,52).

3. Complete take is important in skin grafting. For this purpose, care must be taken with hemostasis and adequate compression. In skin grafting, split- and full-thickness skin grafts have been used for a long time. However, it has become clear in follow-up studies (53–55) that full-thickness skin grafts produce less contracture, and, therefore, full-thickness skin grafts are now more commonly used.

4. Aside from problems in incision design, the technique for undermining the flap is critical in preventing flap necrosis. When elevating a large triangular flap across

the midline of the finger, care should be taken not to make the flap too thin.

5. The groin region is the most common donor site for skin grafts, but skin grafting from this region may produce postoperative pigmentation, which is a problem in people of Asian descent. Webster (36) reported that skin grafts that were harvested from the area below the internal malleolus of the medial pedal region produced less pigmentation with a normal color and were more functional and aesthetic than skin that was harvested from other hair-bearing areas of the body. The authors have used this area as the donor site since the 1970s and have found that skin that is taken from this area did not produce pigmentation (53). In infants, there is more surplus skin in this area than in adults, and a width of 2 cm can be sutured directly by undermining the skin over the medial malleolus proximally.

CLINICAL RESULTS

There are not a lot of reports that adequately describe evaluation of the postoperative results. Brown (23) reported that further operation was necessary in 45% of cases, and contracture was seen in 44% of cases, especially in split-thickness skin graft cases. Toredo and Ger (54) evaluated 35 patients with 97 treated webs. In these, 52% of cases needed a secondary operation; web recurrence of more than 1 cm was seen in four cases, and web recurrence of less than 1 cm was seen in 30%. Hair growth was seen in 11% of cases, and hyperpigmentation was seen in 5% of cases. Percival and Sykes (55) reported that web creep developed in 22% of 100 patients with 218 webs, significant flexion contracture occurred in 26%, and secondary operation was necessary in 42%.

In general, approximately 50% of cases needed a secondary operation. Thus, web recurrence and contracture occur more frequently than expected. The authors performed a 10-year follow-up for 25 cases with 28 hands out of 208 cases in total (146 syndactyly, 162 symbrachydactyly), which were operated on at the Jikei University School of Medicine over 25 years between 1969 and 1994. Web recurrence, including web formation of less than 3 mm, was seen in 50%; flexion contracture, including cases with a slight degree of contracture, was seen in 46%; deviation was seen in 50%; and rotation was seen in 32%.

RECOMMENDED TREATMENT AND TECHNIQUES

Based on the historical review of the operative techniques for syndactyly and the authors' experience, the authors' recommended treatment and techniques are as follows: To make the commissure, a dorsal rectangular flap is recommended. So as not to produce web creep, small triangular flaps (24,33) are useful. To separate the fingers, a zigzag incision is made that is small on the dorsal side and large on the palmar side. For elevation of a large palmar triangular flap, care is taken not to make the flap too thin. In rotating and suturing flaps, infant fat is often resected to reduce tension on the flap. Grafted skin is harvested from the medial inframalleolar region of the foot for full-thickness skin grafts to the skin defect. In cases of bone fusion of the distal phalanx with one broad nail plate, Buck-Gramcko's method is recommended, and, in cases of tapering fingertip without surplus skin, a two-staged method, such as that described by Van der Biezen, is performed. For simple syndactyly, operation is performed when the patient is approximately 1 year of age. In complex syndactyly, if discrepancy of the finger length exists, early operation is recommended.

REFERENCES

1. Mansfield OT. Syndactyly. *Br J Plast Surg* 1961;13:249–252.
2. Kilian JT, Neimkin RJ. Syndactyly reconstruction by a modified Cronin method. *South Med J* 1985;78:414–418.
3. Eaton CJ, Lister GD. Syndactyly. *Hand Clin* 1990;6:555–575.
4. Dobyns JH. Syndactyly. In: Green DP, ed. *Operative hand surgery,* 3rd ed. New York: Churchill Livingstone, 1933:346–363.
5. Lösch GM, Duncker HR. Anatomy and surgical treatment of syndactylism. *Plast Reconstr Surg* 1972;50:167–173.
6. Mantero R, Grandis C, Auxilla E. Arteriographic findings in congenital malformations of the hand. *Handchir Mikrochir Plast Chir* 1983;15:71–76.
7. Boys JH. *Bunnell's surgery of the hand,* 4th ed. Philadelphia: JB Lippincott Co, 1964.
8. Swanson AB. A classification for congenital limb malformations. *J Hand Surg* 1976;1:8–12.
9. Swanson AB, Tada K. A classification for congenital limb malformations. *J Hand Surg* 1983;8:693–702.
10. Miura T. Syndactyly and split hand. *Hand* 1978;10:99–103.
11. Ogino T. A clinical and experimental study on teratogenic mechanism of cleft hand, polydactyly and syndactyly. *J Jpn Orthop Assoc* 1979;53:535–543.
12. Ogino T, Minami A, Fukuda K, et al. Congenital anomalies of the upper limb among the Japanese in Sapporo. *J Hand Surg* 1986;11:364–371.
13. Ogino T. Current classification of congenital hand deformities based on experimental research. In: Saffer P, Amadio PC, Foucher G, eds. *Current practise in hand surgery.* London: Martin Dunitz, 1997:337–341.
14. Maccollum DW. Webbed fingers. *Surg Gynecol Obstet* 1940;71:782–789.
15. Skoog T. Syndactyly A. clinical report on repair. *Acta Chir Scand* 1965;130:537–549.
16. Flatt AE. *The care of congenital hand anomalies.* Saint Louis: CV Mosby, 1977.

17. Leung PC, Chan KM, Cheng JC. Congenital anomalies of the upper limb among the chinese population in Hong Kong. *J Hand Surg* 1982;7:563–565.
18. Oka I, Watanabe H, Nagumo M, et al. Incidence of congenital anomalies in hand. *J Jpn Soc Surg Hand* 1988;5:771–774.
19. Ueba Y, Nishijima N, Hamanishi T, et al. Angiography in the treatment for congenital anomalies of the hand. *J Jpn Soc Surg Hand* 1984;1:269–272.
20. Mantero R, Rossello MI, Grandis C. Digital subtraction angiography in preoperative examination of congenital malformations. *J Hand Surg* 1989;14:351–352.
21. Richterman IE, DuPree CO, Thoder J, et al. The radiographic analysis of web height. *J Hand Surg* 1998;23:1071–1076.
22. Davis JS, German WJ. Syndactylism (coherence of the fingers and toes). *Arch Surg* 1930;21:32–75.
23. Brown RM. Syndactyly—a review and long term results. *Hand* 1977;9:16–27.
24. Upton J. Congenital anomalies of the hand and forearm. In: McCarthy JG, ed. *Plastic surgery*, 1st ed. Philadelphia: WB Saunders, 1990:5279–5293.
25. Cronin TD. Syndactylism. Experience in its correction. *Tristate Med J* 1943;15:2869–2871.
26. Cronin TD. Syndactylism: results of zigzag incision to prevent postoperative contracture. *Plast Reconstr Surg* 1956;18:460–468.
27. Zachariae L. Syndactylism. *J Bone Joint Surg* 1955;37:356.
28. Bauer TB, Tondra JM, Trusler HM. Technical modification in repair of syndactylism. *Plast Reconstr Surg* 1956;17:385–392.
29. Marumo E, Kojima T, Suzuki S. An operation for syndactyly, and its results. *Plast Reconstr Surg* 1976:561–567.
30. Henz VR, Littler JW. The surgical management of congenital hand anomalies. In: Convers JM, ed. *Reconstructive plastic surgery*, 2nd ed. Philadelphia: WB Saunders, 1977:3306–3349.
31. Buck-Gramcko D. Indikation und Zeitpunkt der oprative Behandlung angeborener Handfehrbildungen. *Zeitschrift Kinderchir Grenzgebiete* 1971;10:220–229.
32. Katsumata H, Fujuta S, Kiryu M. Follow-up study of interdigital cleft plasty with dorsal M-shaped flap. *J Jpn Soc Surg Hand* 1984;1:285–288.
33. Moss AL, Foucher G. Syndactyly: can web creep be avoided? *J Hand Surg* 1990;15:193–200.
34. Colville J. Syndactyly correction. *Br J Plast Surg* 1989;42;12–16.
35. Sherif MM. V-Y dorsal metacarpal flap; a new technique for the correction of syndactyly without skin graft. *Plast Reconstr Surg* 1998;101:1861–1865.
36. Webster JP. Skin grafts for hairless areas of the hands and feet. *Plast Reconstr Surg* 1955;15:83–101.
37. Ebskov B, Zachariae L. Surgical method in syndactylism; evaluation of 208 operations. *Acta Chir Scand* 1966;131:258–268.
38. Raus EE. Repair of simple syndactylism in the healthy newborn. *Orthop Rev* 1984;9:448–502.
39. Niranjan NS, De Carpentier J. A new technique for the division of syndactyly. *Eur J Plast Surg* 1990;13:101–104.
40. Ekerot L. Syndactyly correction without skin grafting. *J Hand Surg* 1996;21:330–337.
41. Thomson HG. Isolated acrosyndactyly: avoiding post-operative contracture. *Br J Plast Surg* 1971;24:357–260.
42. Johansson SH. Nagelwallbildung durch Thenarlappen bei kompletter Syndactylie. *Handchirurgie* 1982;14:199–203.
43. Van der Biezen JJ, Bloem JJ. The double opposing palmar flaps in complex syndactyly. *J Hand Surg* 1992;17:1059–1064.
44. Buck-Gramcko D. Progress in the treatment of congenital malformation of the hand. *World J Surg* 1990;14:715–724.
45. Sugihara T, Ohura T, Umeda T. Surgical method for treatment of syndactyly with osseous fusion of the digital phalanges. *Plast Reconstr Surg* 1991;87:157–164.
46. Sommerkamp TG, Ezaki M, Carter PR, et al. The pulp plasty: a composite graft for complete syndactyly fingertip separations. *J Hand Surg* 1992;17:15–20.
47. Morgan RF, Edgerton MT. Tissue expansion in reconstructive hand surgery. Case report. *J Hand Surg* 1958;10:754–757.
48. Van Beek AL, Adson MH. Tissue expansion in the upper extremity. *Clin Plast Surg* 1987;14:535–542.
49. Ishikura N, Tsukada S. Reconstruction of syndactyly using tissue expander. *J Jpn Soc Surg Hand* 1992;9:155–158.
50. Uchida M, Kojima T, Fukumoto K. Use of tissue expander in the surgical treatment of congenital hand malformations. *J Jpn Soc Surg Hand* 1997;13:900–903.
51. Kojima T. Syndactyly and its operative procedures. *J Jpn Soc Surg Hand* 1993;9:924–930.
52. Chang BW, Shaw Wilgis EF. A systematic approach to repair of syndactylism. *Ann Plast Surg* 1992;28:252–256.
53. Uchida M, Kojima T, Uchida T, et al. Long-term follow-up study of surgical treatment for syndactyly. *J Jpn Soc Surg Hand* 1996;12:743–745.
54. Toredo LC, Ger E. Evaluation of the operative treatment of syndactyly. *J Hand Surg* 1979;4:556–564.
55. Percival NJ, Sykes PJ. Syndactyly: a review of the factors which influence surgical treatment. *J Hand Surg* 1989;14:196–200.

83

CONGENITAL DISORDERS: POLYDACTYLY

EMIKO HORII

Polydactyly is the most common congenital hand malformation. The Congenital Hand Committee of the International Federation of Societies for Surgery of the Hand decided in 1995 to discontinue the terms *preaxial* and *postaxial* (1). The polydactyly that includes the thumb is referred to as *radial polydactyly*, whereas polydactyly that involves the little finger is referred to as *ulnar polydactyly*. *Central polydactyly*, which includes polydactyly that involves the index, middle, and ring rays, is often observed in association with syndactyly. In this chapter, surgical treatment for radial and ulnar polydactyly is discussed.

RADIAL POLYDACTYLY

Classification: Types 1 through 7

The Wassel classification is the most widely used classification of radial polydactyly (2), and several modifications have been reported (1,3,4) (Fig. 1). Delayed ossification of initially entirely cartilaginous phalanges occasionally requires minor reclassification (5). Two initially radiographically distinct areas of ossification may fuse into a single phalangeal component at skeletal maturity. The existence of three phalanges in the excised digit (usually the radial digit) is not an important factor for surgical planning. Relying on the radiographically visible skeleton, thumb polydactyly is classified into four groups by the level of bifurcation. Excluding triphalangism, these are the distal phalangeal type, the proximal phalangeal type, the metacarpal type, and others (6,7). The existence of three phalanges in the preserved digit is important accompanying information.

Preoperative Evaluation

Physical Examination

The size of the fingernail is compared to the unaffected side. When the two digits are evenly developed, or the nail size is less than 60% of the unaffected side, the preserved digit is small, perhaps too small for adequate function (8). The preserved digit is carefully examined for joint mobility and stability. When finger creases are shallow or absent, little or no motion is present. When lateral bending deformity of the interphalangeal (IP) joint or narrowing of the first web space is observed, a preoperative corrective splint may be useful to reduce contracture preoperatively (9). Careful examination is often best confirmed under anesthesia, just before surgery. The skeletal structure may be felt by palpation, even if it is unseen on x-ray. The family should be informed that (a) other body systems must be checked, (b) surgery is not simple ablation but includes reconstruction, (c) the remaining thumb will never be identical to a normal thumb, and (d) a reconstructed thumb requires physical review for several years.

Preoperative X-Ray

A true anteroposterior view on x-ray is essential to identify the branching type and to evaluate the angulation of the digit. Corrective osteotomy is scheduled only when the bony axis is obviously deviated. When the space of the IP joint is too wide for just one epiphysis, an accessory phalanx may exist. When the epiphysis of the distal phalanx is observed in early infancy, it can be an ossification of an accessory phalanx (10).

Timing for Surgery

The author prefers to operate on radial polydactyly when the patient is 6 to 9 months of age, when the child's hand is larger, and anesthesia is safer. When the preserved digit is too small, a need for complicated osteotomy exists, or management of a delta phalanx is necessary, surgery is postponed until the patient is 1 year of age or older.

Treatment

Surgical treatment is based on the level of involvement and the degree of involvement. The essential surgical steps include reduction and reconstruction (11). Usually, the radially situated digit is excised, and the ulnar digit is pre-

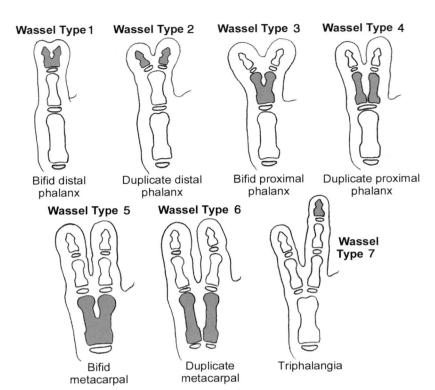

Wassel Type 1 — Bifid distal phalanx

Wassel Type 2 — Duplicate distal phalanx

Wassel Type 3 — Bifid proximal phalanx

Wassel Type 4 — Duplicate proximal phalanx

Wassel Type 5 — Bifid metacarpal

Wassel Type 6 — Duplicate metacarpal

Wassel Type 7 — Triphalangia

FIGURE 1. An illustration of the Wassel classification of thumb polydactyly. Type 4 is the most common.

served and reconstructed, but this is reversed if the radial digit is more robust or functional.

Distal Phalangeal Type

Evenly Developed

The Bilhaut procedure is a well-described technique in which a central wedge is excised, and the two remaining peripheral portions are coapted (Fig. 2A,B). Commonly, this procedure makes a wide thumb with a central split ridge (Fig. 2C,D) (8,12–17). For this reason, the usual preference is to fillet out the smaller bone, retaining only the soft tissue that is needed to augment the preserved digit (Fig. 3A,B) (18). An obliquely situated epiphysis sometimes causes ulnar bending at the IP joint, but this deformity gets less noticeable with growth. A corrective osteotomy may be scheduled after bone maturation, if necessary.

Ulnar Digit Dominant

Removal of the smaller digit (usually the radial digit), partial resection of the head of the proximal phalanx, centralization of the retained distal phalanx, and repair of the radial collateral ligament usually create a good-looking functional thumb (19–27). A corrective osteotomy is rarely needed. Care should be taken to create balanced finger pulp, if augmenting tissue is brought to that distal level.

Proximal Phalangeal Type

Approximately 50% of radial polydactyly is classified into the proximal phalangeal type (6,25,28). Several subdivisions of surgical reconstruction have been reported (5,21,29).

Evenly Developed

In the evenly developed type of radial polydactyly, the ulnar digit is usually small (Fig. 4). Instability or stiffness of the IP joint is often observed. The Bilhaut procedure is still occasionally used; however, it is technically demanding and often creates a stiff thumb with a wide, deformed nail (8,12–17). The author recommends reconstructing the ulnar digit by using soft tissue flaps from the radial digit (Fig. 5) (18). The basic surgical technique is the same as for the unbalanced type. A corrective osteotomy is sometimes required for this type of polydactyly. The tendons are sometimes hypoplastic and may have an eccentric or anomalous insertion; if so, centralization of the insertion of both tendons and deletion of anomalous connections are required, even if this means detaching and reinserting the tendons (19).

Ulnar Digit Dominant

In ulnar digit–dominant radial polydactyly, the skin incision is a racquet incision with a nearly straight dorsal longitudinal incision and a palmar zigzag incision (Fig. 6). Each of the digits has flexor and extensor tendons. Usually, a single proximal flexor or extensor tendon diverges into two separate tendons, with each inserting on a different digit. The extrinsic tendons to the radial digit are excised, unless they are needed. The abductor pollicis brevis tendon inserts into the radial side of the proximal

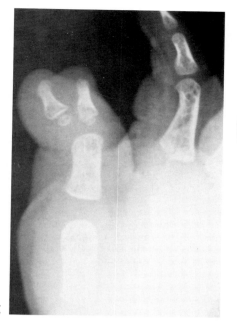
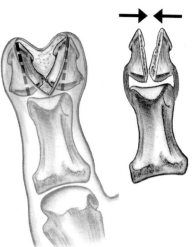
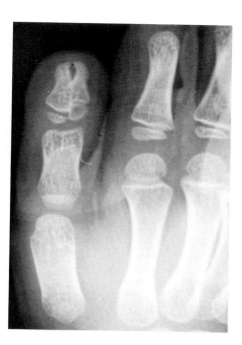

A–C

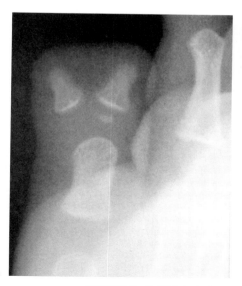

D

FIGURE 2. A: Distal phalangeal–type thumb polydactyly (Wassel type 2); both digits are evenly developed. **B:** Bilhaut procedure. Coaptation of the lateral tissues from each thumb with central part excision. **C,D:** X-ray and photograph 6 years after Bilhaut procedure. The nail in the right thumb is wide with a central ridge. A difference in epiphyseal level causes growth disturbance.

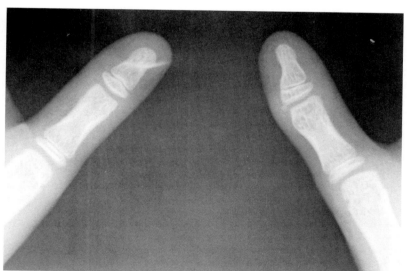

A

B

FIGURE 3. A: Distal phalangeal–type thumb polydactyly. Resection of the radial digit and repair of the radial collateral ligament were performed. **B:** Seven years after surgery. Slight ulnar bending remains owing to the trapezoidal epiphysis.

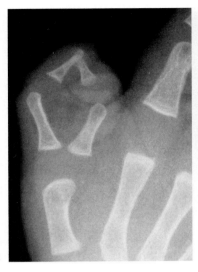
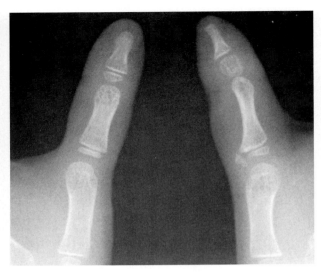

A,B

FIGURE 4. **A:** Proximal phalangeal–type thumb polydactyly. The radial and ulnar digits are small. Preoperative splint is effective to improve ulnar bending at the interphalangeal joint. **B:** Eight years after resection of the radial digit, which is associated with ligament reconstruction and tendon reinsertion. The right thumb is in good alignment, although instability at the interphalangeal joint, which is due to the thick epiphysis, is observed.

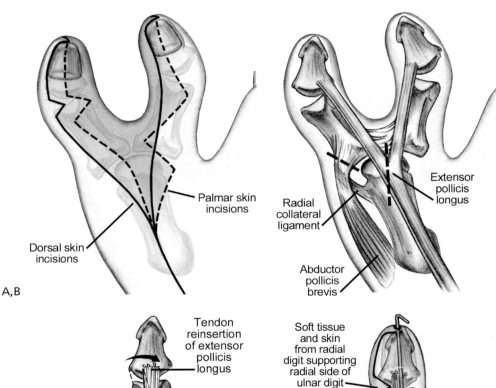

A,B

Palmar skin incisions

Dorsal skin incisions

Extensor pollicis longus

Radial collateral ligament

Abductor pollicis brevis

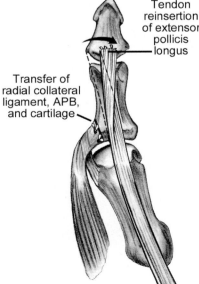
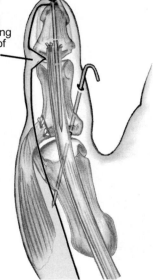

C,D

Tendon reinsertion of extensor pollicis longus

Transfer of radial collateral ligament, APB, and cartilage

Soft tissue and skin from radial digit supporting radial side of ulnar digit

FIGURE 5. **A:** Reconstruction of evenly developed proximal phalangeal–type polydactyly. Soft tissue from the radial digit is used to support the radial side of the ulnar digit. **B:** The metacarpal joint is stabilized by the abductor muscles, the radial collateral ligament, and the cartilage. **C:** Tendon reinsertion is usually essential to rebalance. **D:** The interphalangeal and metacarpophalangeal joints were temporally fixed by Kirschner wire for 3 to 4 weeks. APB, abductor pollicis brevis.

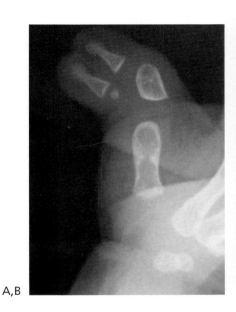
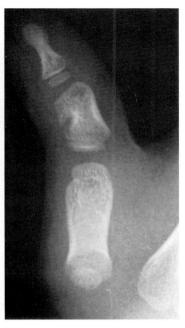

A,B

FIGURE 9. A: The proximal phalanx of the ulnar digit is trapezoidal, and the interphalangeal (IP) joint is bent radially. Open wedge osteotomy of the proximal phalanx and reinsertion of the extensor tendon are necessary at the initial surgery. **B:** Three years after surgery. The thumb is bent radially at the IP joint. The proximal phalanx shows a trapezoidal shape. Recorrection of the bony axis and stabilization of the IP joint are necessary.

joint that they need reconstruction by using osteotomy, ligament augmentation, or other methods (Fig. 11) (29,35).

Stiffness of Joints

Stiffness is sometimes seen at the IP joint, owing to joint hypoplasia, abnormal tendon insertions or interconnections, and hypoplastic tendons. Release of adherent tendons seldom helps. Tendon transfer or graft may be considered. Stiffness is a difficult residual problem to correct; fortunately, it is rarely a functional problem.

In spite of meticulous surgical reconstruction, a reoperation rate as high as 25% has been reported. Parents wish for their child to have a normal thumb after surgery. They have

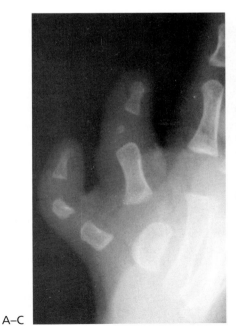
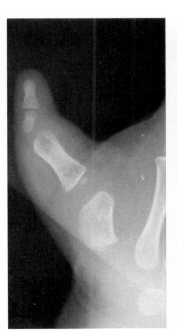
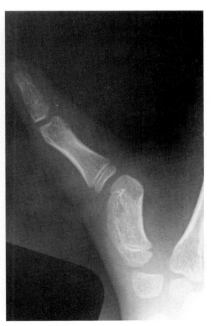

A–C

FIGURE 10. A: Thumb polydactyly with triphalangism. The ulnar digit has an ossicle between phalanges. The first metacarpus is trapezoidal in shape. **B:** X-ray at 2 years of age shows that the retained digit has an accessory phalanx that is adjacent to the distal phalangeal epiphysis. **C:** X-ray 6 years after excision of the accessory phalanx with securing the collateral ligament. The distal phalangeal epiphysis is thick but stable. Abduction deformity is observed at the metacarpophalangeal joint due to the delta metacarpus.

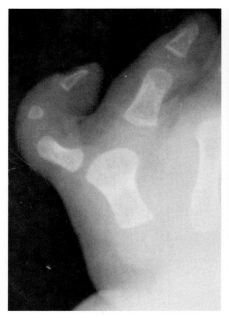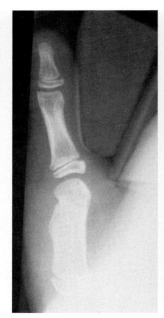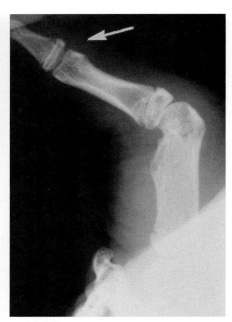

A–C

FIGURE 11. A: Proximal phalangeal–type polydactyly shows ulnarward bending. Closing wedge osteotomy of the first metacarpus is necessary at the initial surgery to rebalance the bony axis. **B,C:** Ten years after surgery, the thumb has severe instability at the metacarpophalangeal joint *(arrow)*. Reconstruction is necessary.

to be informed of the potential need for additional surgical procedures as growth occurs. The frequency of secondary deformity is related to the degree of preoperative deformity and instability, as well as the surgical craftsmanship.

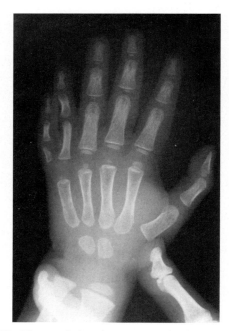

FIGURE 12. Ulnar polydactyly type A. The hypoplastic ulnar digit was excised, and the hypothenar muscles were transferred to the radial digit.

ULNAR POLYDACTYLY

Classification

Ulnar polydactyly is classified into types A and B. When the extra ulnar digit is well formed and articulates with the little-finger metacarpal or with a duplicated little-finger metacarpal, it is classified as type A (Fig. 12). When a small, poorly formed digit is connected to the little finger, it is classified as type B. Type B is often inherited as an autosomal-dominant trait. This is particularly common in black babies (36,37). Type B polydactyly of the little finger is often associated with chromosomal abnormalities or is related to syndromes, such as Ellis-van Creveld syndrome (3).

Treatment

Ulnar polydactyly seldom causes hand dysfunction. Type B polydactyly is simply excised. For type A polydactyly, transfer of the abductor digiti minimi or corrective osteotomy is occasionally necessary (38). Inherent hypoplasticity of the little finger sometimes results in a restricted range of motion, but secondary reconstruction is seldom required.

REFERENCES

1. Light TR. Polydactyly: terminology and classification. In: Buck-Gramcko, ed. *Congenital malformations of the hand*

and forearm. New York: Churchill Livingstone, 1998:217–224.

2. Wassel HD. The results of surgery for polydactyly of the thumb: a review. *Clin Orthop* 1969;64:175–195.

3. Ezaki M. Radial polydactyly. *Hand Clin* 1990;6:577–588.

4. Wood VE. Polydactyly and the triphalangeal thumb. *J Hand Surg* 1981;3:436–444.

5. Islam S, Watanabe H, Fujita S. Contrast arthrography in thumb polydactyly with variable morphological patterns. *J Hand Surg* 1992;17:178–184.

6. Flatt A. Extra thumbs. In: Flatt A, ed. *The care of congenital hand anomalies.* St. Louis: Quality Medical Publishers, 1994:120–136.

7. Blauth W, Olason AT. Classification of polydactyly of the hands and feet. *Arch Orthop Trauma Surg* 1988;107:334–344.

8. Dobyns J, Lipscomb PR, Cooney WP. Management of thumb duplication. *Clin Orthop* 1985;195:26–44.

9. Iwasawa M, Misuo K, Hirose T, et al. Improvement in the surgical results of treatment of duplicated thumb by preoperative splinting. *J Hand Surg* 1989;14:941–945.

10. Makino H, Miura T, Nakamura R, et al. Histological analysis of triphalangism associated with polydactyly of the thumb. *Cong Anom* 1993;33:55–62.

11. Townsend DJ, Lipp EB Jr, Chun K, et al. Thumb duplication, 66 years' experience—a review of surgical complications. *J Hand Surg* 1994;19:973–976.

12. Andrew JG, Sykes PJ. Duplicate thumbs: a survey of results in twenty patients. *J Hand Surg* 1988;13:50–53.

13. Cheng JC, Chan KM, Ma GF, et al. Polydactyly of the thumb: a surgical plan based on ninety-five cases. *J Hand Surg* 1984;9:155–164.

14. Karchinov K. The treatment of polydactyly of the hand. *Br J Plast Surg* 1962;15:362–367.

15. Manske PR. Treatment of duplicated thumb using a ligamentous/periosteal flap. *J Hand Surg* 1989;14:728–733.

16. Naasan A, Page RE. Duplication of the thumb. A 20-year retrospective review. *J Hand Surg* 1994;19:355–360.

17. Tonkin MA, Rumball KM. The Bilhaut-Cloquet procedure revisited. *Hand Surg* 1997;2:67–74.

18. Miura T. Duplicated thumb. *Plast Reconstr Surg* 1982;69:470–479.

19. Dobyns JH. Duplicate thumbs (preaxial polydactyly). In: Green DP, ed. *Operative hand surgery,* 2nd ed. New York: Churchill Livingstone, 1988:435–447.

20. Hartrampf CR, Vasconez LO, Mathes S. Construction of one good thumb from both parts of a congenitally bifid thumb. *Plast Reconstr Surg* 1974;54:148–152.

21. Hung L, Cheng JC, Bundoc R, et al. Thumb duplication at the metacarpophalangeal joint. Management and a new classification. *Clin Orthop* 1996;323:31–41.

22. Light TR. Thumb polydactyly. In: Green DP, ed. *Operative hand surgery,* 5th ed. New York: Churchill Livingstone, 1988:432–440.

23. Light TR. Treatment of preaxial polydactyly. *Hand Clin* 1992;8:161–175.

24. Seidman GD, Wenner SM. Surgical treatment of the duplicated thumb. *J Pediatr Orthop* 1993;13:660–662.

25. Marks TW, Bayne LG. Polydactyly of the thumb: abnormal anatomy and treatment. *J Hand Surg* 1978;3:107–116.

26. Stranc MF, Robertson GA. An intraarticular approach to correction of the bifid thumb. *Ann Plast Surg* 1979;3:35–38.

27. Tada K, Yonenobu K, Tsuyuguchi Y, et al. Duplication of the thumb. A retrospective review of two hundred and thirty-seven cases. *J Bone Joint Surg* 1983;65:584–598.

28. Ogino T, Ishii S, Takahata S, et al. Long-term results of surgical treatment of thumb polydactyly. *J Hand Surg* 1996;21:478–486.

29. Horii E, Nakamura R, Sakuma M, et al. Duplicated thumb bifurcation at the metacarpophalangeal joint level: factors affecting surgical outcome. *J Hand Surg* 1997;22:671–679.

30. Kawabata H, Tada K, Masada K, et al. Revision of residual deformities after operations for duplication of the thumb. *J Bone Joint Surg* 1990;72:988–998.

31. Miura T. An appropriate treatment for postoperative Z-formed deformity of the duplicated thumb. *J Hand Surg* 1977;2:380–386.

32. Ogino T. Radially deviated type of thumb polydactyly. *J Hand Surg* 1988;13:315–319.

33. Islam S, Fujita S. Triphalangism in thumb polydactyly: an anatomic study on surgically resected thumbs. *Plast Reconstr Surg* 1991;88:831–836.

34. Wood VE. Treatment of the triphalangeal thumb. *Clin Orthop* 1976;120:188–200.

35. Kawabata H, Masatomi T, Shimada K, et al. Treatment of residual instability and extensor lag in polydactyly of the thumb. *J Hand Surg* 1993;18:508.

36. Woolf CM, Woolf RM. A genetic study of polydactyly in Utah. *Am J Hum Genet* 1970;22:75–88.

37. Woolf CM, Myrianthopoulos NC. Polydactyly in American negroes and whites. *Am J Hum Genet* 1973;25:397–404.

38. Light TR. Little finger polydactyly. In: Green DP, ed. *Operative hand surgery,* 2nd ed. New York: Churchill Livingstone, 1988:461–464.

84

CONGENITAL DISORDERS: HYPOPLASTIC THUMB

JULIA A. KATARINCIC

ANATOMY, PATHOMECHANICS, AND PATHOPHYSIOLOGY

Hypoplasia of the thumb is included in the group 5 or undergrowth category of upper extremity malformations (1). Included in this category are malformations that range from those in which the hypoplasia is difficult to recognize to a pouce flottant to complete aplasia of the thumb. Thumb hypoplasia has been reported to comprise 3.5% of congenital upper extremity malformations (2). It may occur as an isolated malformation along with a more global radial hypoplasia. Looking at a group of 98 patients with thumb hypoplasia, James et al. (3) found 63% to have bilateral involvement, 59% to have radial dysplasia, and 86% to have other anomalies.

Buck-Gramcko (4,21) has modified the Blauth classification of thumb hypoplasia into five types (Table 1) (Fig. 1). Type 1 is a mildly hypoplastic thumb. The osseous structures may be slightly smaller, and the opponens pollicis and abductor pollicis brevis are mildly hypoplastic, but the ulnar collateral ligament of the metacarpophalangeal (MCP) joint is competent.

Type 2 thumbs are slightly more hypoplastic, with more hypoplasia of the bones and thenar musculature. The phalanges, trapezium, and scaphoid may be small, in addition to a small metacarpal. There have been case reports of all of the median innervated thenar muscles being absent, or, in other cases, only a hypoplasia of the opponens pollicis and adductor pollicis brevis are absent (5). The extrinsic thumb flexor, the flexor pollicis longus (FPL), or extensor, extensor pollicis longus (EPL), may also be absent or hypoplastic. The FPL may also have an aberrant origin, such as from the index flexor digitorum profundus, or an aberrant insertion (6). The ulnar collateral ligament is always hypoplastic and unstable. The first web space may also be narrowed.

Type 3 thumbs were subclassified by Manske et al. (7) into types 3A and 3B. In type 3 thumbs, the osseous structures are small, especially the proximal metacarpal and the opponens hypoplastic. In type 3A thumbs, the carpometa-carpal joint (CMC) is present. In type 3B thumbs, the CMC is unstable, because the proximal metacarpal is so hypoplastic. All type 3 hypoplastic thumbs have an unstable MCP joint with associated first web contracture.

A type 4 hypoplastic thumb is termed a *pouce flottant*. The thumb consists of rudimentary phalanges. There is a small soft tissue attachment of variable size between the thumb and the hand that usually contains a single neurovascular bundle. The thenar muscles are not present. In a type 5 hypoplastic thumb, the thumb is completely absent.

EVALUATION

As with every child who is seen in an orthopedic office, a complete history, including a prenatal history, should be taken. A number of syndromes are associated with thumb hypoplasia or a more global radial hypoplasia, including Fanconi's anemia, thrombocytopenia, VATER association (*v*ertebral anomalies, *a*nal atresia, *t*racheoesophageal fistula, *e*sophageal atresia, *r*enal defects), Holt-Oram syndrome, Cornelia de Lange's syndrome, diastrophic dwarfism, and a 13q deletion (8). Communication with the pediatrician is important in these children to ensure appropriate diagnostic testing is performed, if it is indicated. This may include a complete blood cell count, echocardiogram, and renal ultrasound. It can be interesting to note the size of the parents' thumbs.

The parents and child should be asked, if appropriate, about functional deficit, which, depending on the age of the child, includes whether the child is able to do such things as hold a bottle or toy, hold a pen, ride a bicycle, or climb on the monkey bars. Children with a mildly hypoplastic thumb may have no limitations, and no intervention is needed.

On physical examination, the child should be assessed for any associated syndromes. The spine should be examined for any scoliosis or hairy patches. Looking at the upper extremity, the muscles of the chest wall, specifically the pec-

TABLE 1. CLASSIFICATION OF HYPOPLASTIC THUMBS

Type 1	All structures are minimally shortened and narrowed
Type 2	Mild underdevelopment of all structures; short bones; smaller diameter; mild hypoplasia of thenars; unstable thumb metacarpophalangeal joint; narrow first web space
Type 3A	Stable carpometacarpal joint; significant decrease in the size of the thumb; severe hypoplasia of the intrinsic and extrinsic musculature; unstable metacarpophalangeal joint; narrow first web space.
Type 3B	Type 3A with an unstable carpometacarpal joint
Type 4	Pouce flottant; rudimentary phalanges
Type 5	Complete aplasia of the thumb

toralis major, should be examined. Muscle strength and range of motion of both limbs should be performed. Elbow and wrist stability should be checked. The length of the radius should be evaluated.

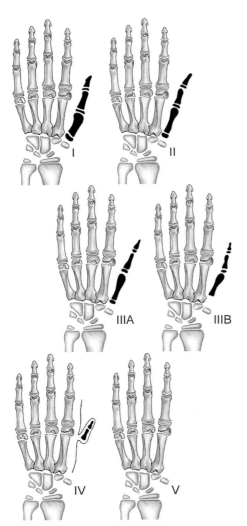

FIGURE 1. Classification of thumb hypoplasia.

The overall size of the thumb should be examined. Is the length adequate for it to be opposable to other fingers? The size of objects that the child is able to pick up should be noted. If the child is doing prehensile activities between the index and long fingers, the second web space may be enlarged, and the index finger may have assumed a slightly pronated posture. Thumb opposability and thenar muscle strength should be measured. Next, the stability of the ulnar collateral ligament of the MCP joint must be assessed. The stability of the CMC should also be evaluated.

If the child has a long, skinny thumb, Holt-Oram syndrome may be the diagnosis. If one is evaluating a child with relatively normal thumbs and radial hypoplasia, the child may have thrombocytopenia and an absent radius. If the hypoplastic thumb is a type 4 or pouce flottant, the size of the rudimentary thumb and the soft tissue attachment between the thumb and hand should be noted. It is also important to assess the quality of the index finger. As the degree of thumb hypoplasia increases, the index finger is more likely to be stiff. This is important to note because this may affect the technical aspects of pollicization, if it is indicated.

Plain radiographs should be taken of all the thumbs. The size of the bony structures and, most importantly, the quality of the CMC should be evaluated. Radiographs of the entire forearm should also be taken to rule out an associated radial dysplasia.

NONOPERATIVE TREATMENT

The role of nonoperative treatment in a child with a hypoplastic thumb is limited. In a child with a type 1 or minimally hypoplastic thumb with good pinch and grasp, surgery is not indicated. There may be a select child in this group who benefits from therapy for thenar strengthening or for activities of daily living, but few require this. In children with more advanced thumb hypoplasia, splinting or therapy, including thenar strengthening, is not helpful in improving the function. Splinting may be helpful for stability in a child who, for medical reasons, is not a surgical candidate. The use of a functional pediatric test, such as the Jebson test, by therapists may help evaluate the function of the children and help determine if surgical intervention is warranted.

SURGICAL TREATMENT

The child's potential for grip and pinch plays a major role in the decision to operate on a child with a hypoplastic thumb. The thumb is an essential component for prehensile grasp. The inability to do prehensile activity because of poor thumb function is an indication for treatment of the hypoplastic thumb. One has to remember that these children are different from those who have had a traumatic injury or amputation of the thumb because of the lack of normal cerebrocortical representation.

Most children develop prehensile patterns of hand use at approximately 6 to 12 months of age (9). It is reasonable to offer reconstructive thumb surgery at 1 to 2 years of age. The children are usually large enough by 1 year of age that there is minimal risk with general anesthesia, and the structures around the thumb are large enough to make the surgery technically easier. If the surgery is delayed until the child is 3 or 4 years of age, the patterns of hand usage may be so well developed that retraining of the child is more difficult postoperatively. Also, the child is closer to school age, and it may take time to become facile with writing. If the child undergoing a pollicization is also undergoing surgery for radial aplasia, the pollicization is usually performed 6 months after the wrist surgery.

The classification of a hypoplastic thumb is important because, in almost all cases, it dictates the treatment plan. Types 1, 2, and 3A thumbs are reconstructible. In types 3B and 4 thumbs, amputation and pollicization are the standard treatments. A cultural bias may factor into treatment decision. In some cultures, loss of a digit is not acceptable, so amputation of a type 3B or type 4 (pouce flottant) thumb and pollicization may not be options. It may be necessary to reconstruct the thumb even if the function may not be as good as a pollicized index finger. In the type 5 or absent thumb, pollicization is the surgery that is recommended.

In a reconstructible thumb, the treatment for a hypoplastic thumb may include skeletal lengthening, web deepening, MCP stabilizations, and an opponensplasty. Types 2 and 3A hypoplastic thumbs are usually considered for reconstruction. Type 1 hypoplastic thumbs usually present with little or no functional deficit, and surgery is rarely required. Most commonly performed are an opponensplasty with or without an MCP stabilization by ulnar collateral ligament reconstruction.

Opponensplasty

Multiple types of opponensplasty have been described (10–13). The Huber transfer has been classically described for an opponensplasty in a child. This muscle is usually always present in these children. The length and cross-sectional area are appropriate. The muscle can be harvested through an incision on the ulnar border of the hand and passed subcutaneously across the palm of the hand to the base of the thumb. The muscle is flipped, as if turning the page of a book, as it crosses the hand. It can be inserted into the extensor mechanism and capsule of the MCP joint with the thumb in a near maximally opposed position. During harvesting, the origin on the pisiform should be protected to prevent damage to the neurovascular bundle (14,15) (Fig. 2).

A second opponensplasty uses the flexor digitorum superficialis (FDS) to the long or ring finger. This is prefera-

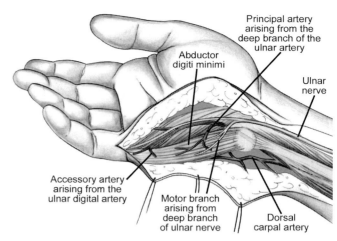

FIGURE 2. Neurovascular pedicle of the abductor quinti muscle and the proximity to the origin on the pisiform.

ble when the MCP joint is unstable and the ulnar collateral ligament requires reconstruction. The superficialis is harvested through a palmar incision over the proximal interphalangeal (PIP) joint. A second incision is made just proximal to the mid-palm, and the tendon is brought out through this incision. Using the transverse carpal ligament as a pulley, the FDS is inserted into the radial side of the thumb MCP joint to provide opposition. The second tail of the tendon can be brought around to the ulnar side of the joint, and the ulnar collateral ligament can be reconstructed.

Postoperatively, children who undergo opponensplasty are casted for 1 month. They are next placed in a removable thumb spica splint for the next 6 months. The splint is worn at night for the entire 6 months and is weaned during the day as opposition strength improves. The therapists can help the children improve the strength and dexterity of the thumb over the first few months after the cast is removed.

Collateral Ligament Reconstruction

An isolated MCP stabilization is rarely indicated. Usually, a child with a type 2 or 3A hypoplastic thumb with an unstable MCP joint also benefits from an opponensplasty, so the procedure that was described previously, using an FDS transfer, is performed. In the rare case that an isolated ulnar collateral ligament is required, local tissue, including periosteum of the metacarpal, can be used, or a slip of palmaris can be used if the local soft tissue is deficient. These children should also be casted for 1 month and then slowly mobilized by using a splint as appropriate.

For completeness, chondrodesis should also be included for an unstable MCP joint. In children in whom no good soft tissue exists to stabilize the joint, or in a child who has a collapsed thumb that is also hypoplastic, this procedure may be a good option. Stability of the MCP joint can be obtained without damage to the physis.

Web Space Release

The first web space may also be tight, especially as the degree of thumb hypoplasia increases. The need to deepen this web is a subjective decision, but it is an easy way to aesthetically and functionally lengthen the thumb. For deepening of the first web, a two- or four-flap Z-plasty and a dorsal butterfly flap have been described. The advantage of the Z-plasty is that it provides a 75% (two-flap) or a 164% (four-flap) increase in the web width, and the web provides an easy place to make the incision. Although using a dorsal butterfly flap does not increase the web width as much, a nice dorsal skin flap is created that is cosmetically better and keeps scarring volarly in the palm rather than in the center of the web. For these two reasons, the author prefers a web deepening with the dorsal butterfly flap. No skin graft is required for either operation, so they are well tolerated with a low complication rate. These children should be casted for 2 weeks, and afterward, intermittent splinting and an elastomer or silicone pad to soften the scar should be used.

Skeletal Lengthening

The decision to perform bony lengthening is subjective as well. Often, after providing opponens strength or deepening the web, the children are able to pinch and grasp things sufficiently. If the length of the thumb is still an issue, lengthening can be considered (15). The length requirements in these children are usually small enough that a one-stage lengthening that uses iliac crest bone graft or a toe phalangeal graft can be considered (16).

Pollicization

In children with a type 3B, 4, or 5 hypoplastic thumb, thumb reconstruction is usually achieved through pollicization of the index finger. In patients with a type 3B hypoplastic thumb who refuse to undergo amputation and pollicization, a free-vascularized metatarsal transfer has been suggested for first CMC stabilization followed by reconstruction of the hypoplastic digit. A recent report of five cases with almost 8 years' follow-up shows limited pinch, which leaves narrow indications for this procedure. It is probably best used in cases in which amputation of a type 3B thumb is refused by the parents, because pollicization, the alternative, gives a superior functional result (17). Results in the Japanese literature have been more positive toward reconstruction, but one has to remember the strong cultural bias of the Japanese toward avoiding amputation (18,19).

Pollicization was first described in the literature by Gosset (20). It remains a popular procedure, because long-term studies show maintenance of good functional and cosmetic results. The basic concept is to pronate the index finger approximately 120 degrees and to translate it proximally to be able to perform

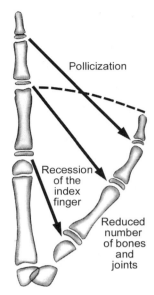

FIGURE 3. Transposition of the osseous structures from the index finger to the new thumb.

prehensile activities. The distal interphalangeal joint of the finger becomes the thumb interphalangeal joint, the finger PIP joint becomes the thumb MCP joint, and the finger MCP joint becomes the thumb CMC (Fig. 3). The extensor digitorum communis and finger flexors are left *in situ* to act as the EPL and FPL, respectively. The dorsal interosseus becomes the abductor brevis, and the volar interosseus becomes the adductor of the pollicized digit.

Multiple incisions have been described for this technique. Buck-Gramcko (21) has described an incision that results in excellent cosmesis and allows all of the structures to be well visualized intraoperatively (Figs. 4 and 5). Once the incisions are made, the neurovascular bundles should be identified. The radial bundle is present 85% to 90% of the time. If it is

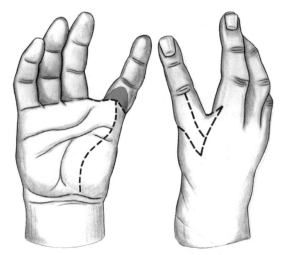

FIGURE 4. Skin incisions for a pollicization for type 5 thumb hypoplasia.

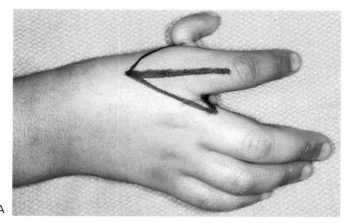

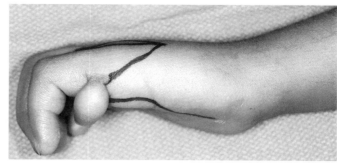

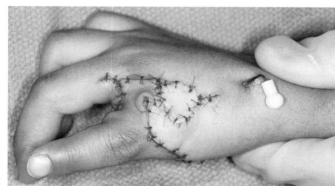

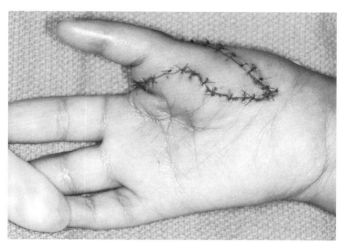

FIGURE 5. A–D: Preoperative planning of incisions and postoperative photos of a pollicization of a type 4 thumb. For cultural reasons, the parents requested that some part of the abated thumb be used in the reconstruction, so a small skin graft was placed dorsally.

difficult to see the bundles, the metacarpal can be transected dorsally and flipped up, so that the bundles can be easily visualized. The fat around the neurovascular pedicles should be left undisturbed to minimize arterial spasm and to protect the venae comitantes, which can provide an additional source of venous drainage. The radial neurovascular bundle to the long finger can be divided to allow the index finger to be rotated. Also, in this dissection, one should try to preserve one or two large dorsal veins to prevent outflow problems.

The level of the index metacarpal resection is through the physis. The remainder of the proximal index metacarpal shaft can be resected, leaving 3 to 5 mm of bone at the base for the skeletal stabilization.

Before the skeletal stabilization is performed, the proper length of the pollicized digit should be decided. The tip of the digit should be at the level of the long-finger PIP joint. It is appropriate, in the case of a stiff index finger, to leave the pollicized digit slightly longer to allow stronger pinch.

The metacarpal head is fully extended and then sutured, with two sutures placed at 90 degrees to the base of the index metacarpal. This prevents hyperextension of the pollicized digit with use (Fig. 2). Before stabilization, the digit should be pronated 120 to 140 degrees to allow for tip pinch. A small Kirschner wire is placed across the metacarpal base for added stability.

The extensor indicis proprius and extensor digitorum communis can be imbricated, if needed, and act as the EPL and abductor pollicis longus, respectively. The first dorsal interosseous is woven into the radial portion intrinsics to act as the abductor pollicis brevis, and the palmar interosseous is woven into the ulnar intrinsic to act as the adductor pollicis (Table 2; Fig. 6). The FPL is left alone to shorten on its own with use. The skin flaps are loosely closed with absorbable sutures. Once the closure is done, it is easier to understand the incision.

Postoperatively, the child is hospitalized overnight, with frequent neurovascular checks. If there is a concern about an inflow problem or venous congestion, the cast should be loosened. If necessary, the child may be taken back to the operat-

TABLE 2. MUSCULAR REROUTING IN THE POLLICIZED DIGIT

Original muscle	Subsequent muscle
Extensor digitorum communis (index finger)	Abductor pollicis longus
Extensor indicis proprius	Extensor pollicis longus
First dorsal interosseous	Abductor pollicis brevis
First volar interosseous	Adductor pollicis

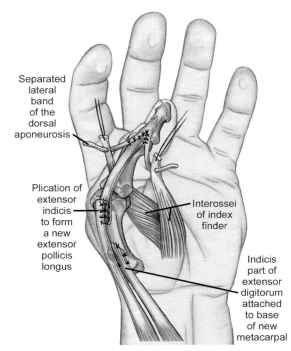

Separated
lateral
band
of the
dorsal
aponeurosis

Plication of
extensor
indicis
to form
a new
extensor
pollicis
longus

Interossei
of index
finder

Indicis
part of
extensor
digitorum
attached
to base
of new
metacarpal

FIGURE 6. Imbrication of the extensor pollicis longus and the extensor digitorum communis and insertion of the interossei into the intrinsics for muscular rebalancing.

ing room, and some of the sutures should be removed. The child is in a long arm thumb spica cast for 4 weeks. At that point, the pin is removed, and the child is placed in a forearm-based thumb spica splint. The child is started on an exercise program that is designed to improve the function of the new thumb. Therapy and improvement in hand usage are a slow process because of the cortical retraining that is required. With patience and encouragement, the child develops a good pattern of usage. The splint is worn full time for 6 weeks and then at night for an additional 4 to 6 months.

Reported complications of pollicization are rare. The infection rate is low. Growth disturbances in the pollicized digit are rarely reported. There are only rare cases of reported vascular compromise.

Secondary procedures have been reported to be necessary in up to 50% of children. Manske and McCarroll (22) reported on 40 patients, with 18 requiring a secondary opponensplasty. Most of these children had an associated radial dysplasia. Sykes et al. (23) also reported on secondary procedures, including opponensplasty, scar revision, and rotational osteotomies, in 36% of his children.

Long-term follow-up of children who undergo pollicization has shown good clinical results (24–26). Manske et al. (24) looked at a group of 28 children, and, compared to the normal thumb, the pollicized digit had 50% total active motion, and tasks took 22% longer. Kozin et al. (25) reported on a group of ten thumbs in 14 patients at an average of 9 years of follow-up. Grip strength was 67% of the normal side, and manual dexterity was 70% of the normal side. Importantly, Clark et al. (26)

presented a group of patients who demonstrated good continued thumb function at a 27-year follow-up.

CONCLUSION

Thumb hypoplasia has been well described and classified in types 1 to 5. In type 1, no intervention is required. In types 2 and 3A, reconstruction is possible. In types 3B, 4, and 5, amputation and pollicization should be performed. Postoperatively, in a child with isolated thumb hypoplasia, good functional results can be expected. In children with associated radial hypoplasia, results are not as good, but hand function is still improved.

REFERENCES

1. Swanson AB, Swanson C, de Groot, et al. A classification for congenital limb formation. *J Hand Surg* 1983;8:693–702.
2. Flatt AE. *The care of congenital hand anomalies,* 2nd ed. St. Louis: Quality Medical Publishing, 1994:741.
3. James M, McCarroll HR Jr, Manske PR. Characteristics of patient with hypoplastic thumbs. *J Hand Surg* 1996;21: 104–113.
4. Blauth W. Der hypoplastische Daumen. *Arch Orthop Unfall Chir* 1967;62:225–246.
5. Su CT, Hoopes JE, Daniel R. Congenital absence or the thenar muscles innervated by the median nerve. *J Bone Joint Surg* 1976;58:115–118.
6. Blair WF, Omer GE. Anomalous insertion of the flexor pollicis longus—an anatomy note. *J Hand Surg* 1983;8:93–94.
7. Manske PR, McCarroll HR Jr, James M. Type IIIA hypoplastic thumb. *J Hand Surg* 1995;20:246–253.
8. Edgerton MT, Snyder GB, Webb WL. Surgical treatment of congenital thumb deformities. *J Bone Joint Surg* 1965;47: 1453–1474.
9. Jones KL. *Smith's recognizable patterns of human malformation,* 4th ed. Philadelphia: WB Saunders, 1988.
10. Manske PR, McCarroll HR Jr. Abductor digiti minimi opponensplasty in congenital radial dysplasia. *J Hand Surg* 1978;3:552–559.
11. Littler JW, Cooley SG. Opposition of the thumb and its restoration by abductor digiti quinti transfer. *J Bone Joint Surg* 1963;45:1386–1396.
12. Ogino T, Minimi A, Fukuda K. Abductor digiti minimi opponensplasty in a hypoplastic thumb. *J Hand Surg* 1986;11:372–377.
13. Cooney WP, Linscheid RL, An KN. Opposition of the thumb: an anatomic and biomechanical study of tendon transfers. *J Hand Surg* 1984;9:777–786.
14. Dunlap J, Manske PR, McCarthy JA. Perfusion of the abductor digiti quinti after transfer on a neurovascular pedicle. *J Hand Surg* 1989;14:992–995.
15. Matev IB. Thumb reconstruction in children through metacarpal lengthening. *Plast Reconstr Surg* 1979;64:665–669.
16. Carroll RE, Green DP. Reconstruction of hypoplastic digits using toe phalanges. *J Bone Joint Surg* 1975;57:727.

17. Foucher G, Medina J, Navarro R. Microsurgical reconstruction of the hypoplastic thumb, type IIIB. *J Reconstr Microsurg* 2001;17:9–15.

18. Shibata M, Yoshizu T, Seki T, et al. Reconstruction of a congenital hypoplastic thumb with use of a free vascularized metatarsal phalangeal joint. *J Bone Joint Surg* 1998;80:1469–1476.

19. Tsujino A, Itoh Y, Hyashi K. Reconstruction of the floating thumb by transplanting the fourth metatarsal. *J Bone Joint Surg* 1994;76:551–554.

20. Gosset J. La pollicisation de l'index. *J Chir* 1949;65:403–411.

21. Buck-Gramcko D. Pollicization of the index finger: methods and results in aplasia and hypoplasia of the thumb. *J Bone Joint Surg* 1971;53:1605–1618.

22. Manske PR, McCarroll HR Jr. Index finger pollicization for the congenitally absent or nonfunctioning thumb. *J Hand Surg* 1985;10:606–612.

23. Sykes PJ, Chandraprakasam T, Percival NJ. Pollicization of the index finger in congenital anomalies. A retrospective analysis. *J Hand Surg* 1991;16:144–147.

24. Manske PR, Rotman MB, Dailey LA. Long-term functional results after pollicization for the congenitally deficient thumb. *J Hand Surg* 1992;17:1064–1072.

25. Kozin SH, Weiss AA, Webber JB, et al. Index finger pollicization for congenital aplasia or hypoplasia of the thumb. *J Hand Surg* 1992;17:880–884.

26. Clark DI, Chell J, Davis TR. Pollicization of the index finger. *J Bone Joint Surg* 1998;80:631–635.

85

CONGENITAL DISORDERS: RADIAL AND ULNAR CLUB HAND

DIETER BUCK-GRAMCKO

In the classification for congenital limb malformations (1), which was adopted by the International Federation of Societies for Surgery of the Hand, one can find three longitudinal deficiencies of the forearm and hand. These are radial, central, and ulnar deficiencies. Synonyms that are still used frequently are radial club hand, cleft hand, ulnar hemimelia, and others. Their incidence is different, although it seems to be impossible to give true or exact numbers of incidence, because the numbers in the reports differ considerably. Flatt (2) has seen, among his 2,758 cases with congenital deformities, 127 patients with radial club hands, 106 patients with central defects, and only 34 patients with ulnar hypoplasia. Birch-Jensen (3) has reported, in his careful analysis, 19 ulnar and 73 radial defects. In my own clinical material of approximately the same number of patients as Flatt, I have counted 223 patients with radial deficiencies, 164 patients with ulnar deficiencies, and 89 patients with central deficiencies, with the numbers of involved arms in each group being 270, 200, and 137, respectively. This shows that many patients have a bilateral involvement and that ulnar deficiencies are not as rare as is often described.

The term *radial* or *ulnar deficiency* is more comprehensive than club hand. Deficiency includes also the distal deformities in which only the thumb or the ulnar fingers and their metacarpals are involved, and the forearm is normal. In club hands, the forearm must be involved, even in a different severity. Therefore, in this chapter, deformities of digits with normal forearm bones are not included.

RADIAL CLUB HAND

Occurrence

As was already mentioned, it is impossible to give correct numbers for the incidence of radial club hand. In the literature, numbers between 1 in 30,000 and 1 in 100,000 live births are reported. Radial club hands occur as isolated deformities without any other malformations or as a part of a syndrome, the most frequent of which are Fanconi's anemia; Holt-Oram syndrome (in combination with congenital heart defects); thrombocytopenia–absent radius syndrome, in which the thumb is always present; and the VATER association (*v*ertebral anomalies, *a*nal atresia, *t*racheoesophageal fistula, *e*sophageal atresia, *r*enal defects). Because many of these patients suffer also from cardiac defects, limb deformities, and a single umbilical artery, this combination is sometimes called the *VACTERLS association* (*v*ertebral anomalies, *a*nal atresia, *c*ardiac defects, *t*racheoesophageal fistula, *e*sophageal atresia, *r*enal defects, *l*imb deformities, *s*ingle umbilical artery). Other non-syndrome-associated anomalies are cardiac, gastrointestinal, genitourinary, craniofacial, musculoskeletal, and chromosomal anomalies or blood dyscrasias.

Most radial club hands occur sporadically. Only approximately 20% are hereditary, mainly those that exist in combination with syndromes. Best known as an external cause of radial club hand is thalidomide; its ingestion between the thirty-fourth and the fiftieth day after the last menstrual period produces limb malformations. In the hands and the forearms, the radial one-half is involved almost exclusively; phocomelia is minimal, if not completely absent. In Germany, orthopedic surgeons had to deal with an overabundance of patients in the years of and after the thalidomide tragedy of 1959 to 1961, so that many patients with radial club hand remained untreated until an age of 8 to 10 years; this was the reason for so many therapeutic problems.

Morphology

The leading symptom of radial club hand, the deformity of the radius, shows a great variety. It starts with simple hypoplasia of the styloid process and ends with the complete absence of the radius (Fig. 1). Synostoses between the radius and the ulna, as is shown in Figure 2, are seen in several cases (4). For didactic, as well as for therapeutic, purposes,

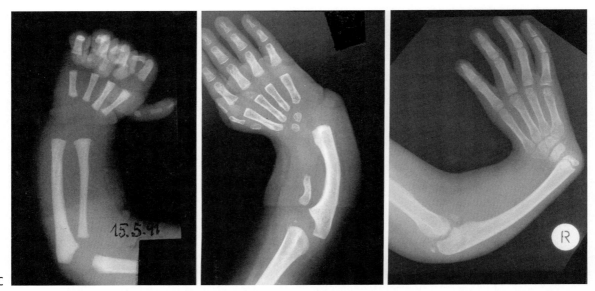

A–C

FIGURE 1. Different types of radial deficiencies. **A:** Hypoplasia of the radius with grade IV thumb hypoplasia (1 day of age). **B:** Partial aplasia of the radius with grade III thumb hypoplasia (9 months of age). **C:** Complete aplasia of the radius and the thumb (10 years of age).

there exists an approved classification. The differentiation in hypoplasia and partial and complete aplasia not only concerns the bone deformity, but also corresponds to abnormalities of muscles, tendons, nerves, and blood vessels. In general, one can say that the more bone that is missing, the more abnormal in number and course are the soft tissues. These anomalies include hypoplasia or aplasia of the radial muscles (mainly the extensors) with abnormal origins or insertions, or both, and abnormal course of the arteries and the nerves. Usually, the superficial branch of the radial nerve is missing and is replaced by a branch of the median nerve that runs radially far beneath the skin

of the concavity of the deviated wrist. It makes any lengthening of the short radial soft tissue more difficult.

The radial deviation at the wrist, which is associated with some palmar subluxation, depends not only on the lack of bony support for the carpal bones and, ultimately, for the whole hand, but also on this muscular imbalance. Although some of the radial extensors may be hypoplastic or even aplastic, the remaining muscles are short (secondary to the deviation), and the finger flexors run radially to the center of rotation, so that any function with finger flexion increases the radial deviation (Fig. 3). This problem also exists postoperatively in cases with incomplete correction of the deviation.

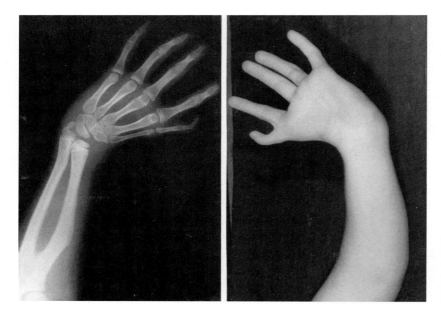

FIGURE 2. Hand and forearm of a thalidomide patient who is 11 years of age. Hypoplastic radius and ulna are fused proximally by a synostosis. The carpal bones show deformation; the triphalangeal thumb is syndactylized partially with the index finger.

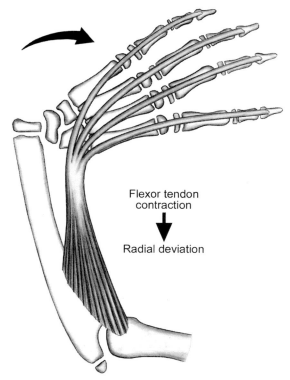

FIGURE 3. Diagram that demonstrates the adverse effect of the flexor muscles that run radial to the center of rotation: any contraction increases the radial deviation.

In contrast to the fact that there is a variety of congenital malformations that are limited to the thumb ray with normal radius, all deformities of the radius variety of club hand are associated with malformations of the thumb ray, including the radial carpal bones (Fig. 4). The scaphoid and tra-

pezium are hypoplastic or absent, as are the bones (metacarpal and phalanges). Intrinsic muscles and the tendons of the forearm muscles that connect to the thumb are missing or are, at least, defective. A hypoplastic thumb can be fixed by partial or complete syndactyly to the index finger, or the thumb may have, particularly in the thalidomide cases, an additional middle phalanx (Fig. 2). With the exception of hands with thumb hypoplasia of grades I and II, these thumbs are unstable and weak, are without motion, and therefore are functionally useless. The resulting necessity for pollicization of the index finger is a valuable additional part of the treatment, although the results are not as good as in cases of thumb hypoplasia without radial club hand, in regard to the involvement of the extrinsic muscles.

The anomalies of the extensor muscles and tendons are also the main reason for the limited mobility of the joints of the radial fingers, especially in the metacarpophalangeal joints. The range of motion in the finger joints decreases from the little finger to the index finger, particularly in the flexion. This influences function, even postoperatively after axial correction and pollicization.

Another problem in radial club hand concerns the ulna. In many cases, this bone is curved (Fig. 1B), so that the surgical correction also has to include an osteotomy of the ulna. Vilkki (5) was able to demonstrate in long-term follow-up examinations (40 years!) of the previous patients of Heikel (6) that the growth of a nonoperated ulna in radial club hand is only approximately 60% to 65% of the growth in normal forearms. He has also shown that, in these early years, a centralization resulted in further damage to ulnar growth, so that this bone was a mean of approximately 5 cm shorter than it was in the nonoperated arms.

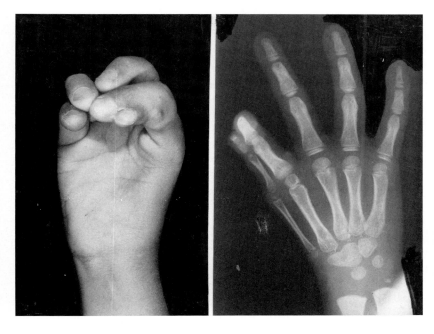

FIGURE 4. Right hand of a patient with hypoplasia of the radius—the typical appearance of a thalidomide patient. The thumb is hypoplastic and triphalangeal and is fixed to the index finger by complete syndactyly. The radial carpal bones and the styloid process of the radius are missing; the capitate and the trapezoid are synostotic (6 years of age).

Surgical Treatment

Conservative management cannot alter the deformity and the muscular imbalance, so that there is no place for it in the management of radial club hand, with the exception of daily stretching of the wrist from birth until the operation.

Historical Perspectives

The high number of recommended procedures is an expression of the fact that surgery in the radial club hand is difficult, and the results are unsatisfactory. One of the reasons for the bad outcome of this surgery is the fact that, in most of the procedures, only the bones are considered, and the muscles are ignored. The principle of the centralization procedure, in which the head of the ulna is placed under and in the central carpal bones, has been applied in different modifications since 1893 (7–10). Many of the results have been disappointing, because the epiphyseal plate of the ulnar head was damaged or an improved muscle balance was not restored. Disappointed by many unsatisfactory results in his series of 63 centralizations between 1969 and 1979, Buck-Gramcko (11) developed a new technique, which was published in 1985 under the term *radialization*. This term is used because the head of the ulna is positioned under the radial carpal bones and not at its center. This leads to better mechanical advantages, because the lever arm to the ulnar side is much longer and more powerful by the radial positioning of the ulnar head and the transposition of the radial wrist muscles. The mobility is better, because no carpal bones have to be excised. A further improvement of the results was gained by preoperative distraction of the soft tissues around the wrist. This facilitates considerably the operation, avoids the excision of carpal bones, and takes any pressure to the distal end of the ulna, which would otherwise damage the growth plate (12,13).

Recently, Vilkki (14) has developed a quite different procedure: a vascularized transplantation of the second metatarsophalangeal joint after some distraction. He has reported good results in a 10-year follow-up period.

Interesting correlations between the initial deformity, the age, the amount of correction, and the recurrence were found in the careful analysis of Damore et al. (15); as a consequence, they have altered their current approach and recommend early radialization.

Indications

Since the introduction of the preoperative distraction, the indications for radialization are more expanded, because a severe fixed contracture in radial deviation at the wrist is no longer a contraindication. The main contraindication that still exists is the lack of radial wrist muscles combined with weakness of the ulnar wrist muscles and the flexors. This means that, even after radialization, these weak muscles cannot prevent a recurrence of the radial deviation. In these cases, an early ulnocarpal fusion with careful preservation of the growth plate is the only possible treatment with a permanent axial correction.

Optimal Age

Although the age for the surgical intervention depends on the age of the referral of the child, it is preferable to perform the axial correction as early as possible, that is, in the first year of life. The reason is that the radial deviation is more contracted and the finger joints are more restricted in their mobility in the elder child. However, an operation in a young patient requires that the surgeon have experience with such a delicate operation and is trained in microsurgery.

Surgical Technique

The preoperative distraction of the wrist has proven so advantageous that it now applies to all patients with radial club hand, not only to those with severe contractures in radial deviation, as was practice in previous years. A distraction device is used that is specifically constructed for use in small children (CFK-Mini-fixator, LITOS GmbH, Hamburg, Germany). It is light weight (60 g), has high stability, is radiolucent, and combines the possibilities of longitudinal distraction and axial correction (Fig. 5). Daily lengthening is of a distance of 0.75 mm on the radial side and stops after 4 to 8 weeks, when both carbon fiber half-rings are approximately parallel. It is important to prevent flexion contractures of the digits by daily exercises or even by an additional splint.

An interruption of 2 to 3 weeks allows the swelling to decrease, so that the fixator can be removed, and the open radialization is performed. A closed reduction of the ulnar head results in an early recurrence, because only the bones are treated, and the establishment of a better muscle balance is ignored.

The operation is performed in a bloodless field and starts with an S-shaped incision (Fig. 6A). After identification and careful preservation of the two important nerve branches (the dorsal branch of the ulnar nerve and the abnormal branch of the median nerve) and the radial artery, the extensor retinaculum is elevated from the radial to the ulnar side. The extensor tendons, which are often tiny, are dissected, and all abnormal insertions to the retinaculum or the periosteum of the carpal or metacarpal bone are released. The necessary mobilization of the hand is gained by the division of all fasciae, especially on the radial side of the wrist and the joint capsule. The insertions of the radial wrist muscles (flexor and extensor, if present) are detached, so that the distal end of the ulna is mobilized enough for its transposition under the radial carpal bones, which may still be cartilaginous. The position is secured by a Kirschner wire with a diameter of 1.2 to 2.0 mm, depending on the width of the medullary canal of the ulna.

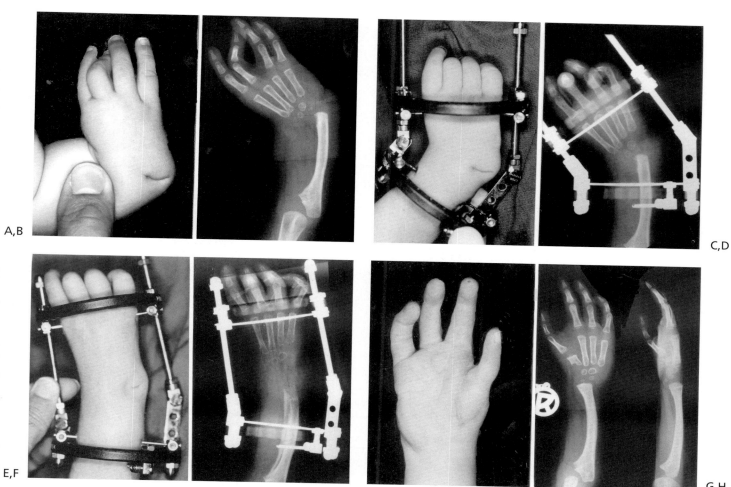

FIGURE 5. Clinical **(A)** and radiologic **(B)** appearance of a hand and forearm of a patient with aplasia of the radius and the thumb. **A,B:** Preoperative condition (2 years of age). **C,D:** Distraction device at the beginning of the preoperative distraction. **E,F:** Condition at the end of the distraction. Note the altered distance and angulation of the two carbon fiber half-rings. **G,H:** The result 1 year later, after pollicization of the index finger, shows good position of the head of the ulna under the radial carpal bones and excellent axial correction, as well as good appearance of the new thumb.

The wire is inserted retrograde in an oblique direction through the scaphoid, into the base of the second metacarpal, and outside through the skin. The hand is reduced in slight overcorrection (i.e., ulnar deviation) over the head of the ulna, and the Kirschner wire is driven in a central direction with its blunt end in the ulna to avoid perforation of the cortical bone. In the case of a curved ulna, an osteotomy is performed. The fixation after straightening is done by the same wire, which is stable enough in these small children. After suture of the capsular remnants, the extensor retinaculum is realigned between the bones and the extensor tendons to prevent copious adhesions.

An important step of the operation is the creation of a good muscle balance by transposition of the radial wrist muscles (flexor and extensor, which often have a common muscle belly). These previously detached muscles are pulled with their tendons between the ulna and the finger extensors to the ulnar side and are sutured end to side to the tendon of the extensor carpi ulnaris, because they are not long enough to find an insertion on the base of the fifth metacarpal (Fig. 6B). The extensor carpi ulnaris tendon is shortened with the same suture, because it is too long in the corrected position. The wound is closed after careful hemostasis and excision of the excess skin and subcutaneous tissue on the preoperative convexity of the wrist region. During the postoperative immobilization in a long arm plaster splint, the fingers need some extension exercises, because they are in a flexed position, as a consequence of the increased distance between origin and insertion after axial correction.

In some cases of severe radius hypoplasia, at radialization, the short radius is ignored, because it does not participate in articulation and has limited further growth (Fig. 7).

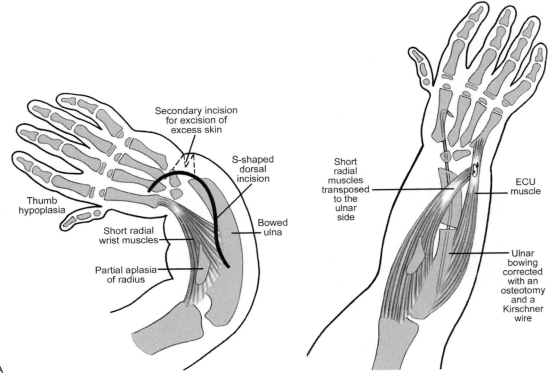

FIGURE 6. Diagrams of the surgical technique, which is demonstrated in a case of partial aplasia of the radius and grade IV thumb hypoplasia. **A:** The S-shaped dorsal incision and the additional incision (*dotted line*) for the excision of the excess skin at the ulnar side of the wrist. **B:** After radialization, the head of the ulna is positioned under the radial carpal bones, the bowing of the ulna is corrected by an osteotomy, and the short radial wrist muscles are transposed to the ulnar side and sutured end to side to the tendon of the extensor carpi ulnaris (ECU). The corrected position is held in ulnar deviation of the wrist by a Kirschner wire.

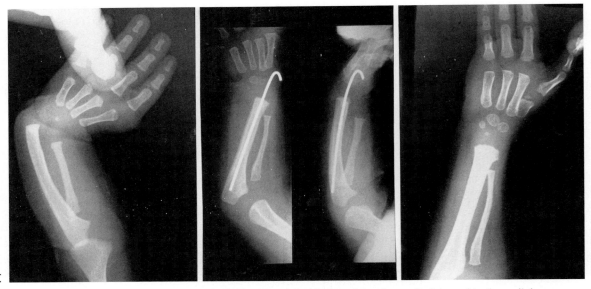

FIGURE 7. In severe hypoplasia of the radius **(A)**, this short bone has to be ignored in the radialization **(B)**. The result 15 months later **(C)** shows not only a limited further growth of the radius, but also an excellent axial correction and the typical broadening of the distal ulna in consequence to the altered force transmission.

Postoperative Management

The immobilization is maintained for 3 weeks, and, in cases of ulnar osteotomy, it is maintained for an additional 3 weeks. The child is allowed to use the hand after this time, but, in patients with a tendency to flexed finger position, a night splint is worn. The Kirschner wire is removed approximately 6 months postoperatively during the next operation, the index finger pollicization, or at an isolated procedure at approximately the same time. Subsequently, a static night splint is worn to control the wrist position, but only for a few months and never for a prolonged period of time.

Complications

The most frequent complications that have been seen are small wound margin necroses, but skin grafting was necessary only in a few instances. In the 194 radializations that have been performed since 1979, I have seen one deep infection and one fracture of the ulna. An unstable wrist occurred four times, and problems with the Kirschner wire (fracture, migration, wrong position with subsequent delayed union of the ulna osteotomy) occurred in 12 patients. These complications have not influenced the final results, as they were the result of partial necrosis of the ulna epiphysis, which results in an unequal growth with increasing obliquity of the articular surface of the distal ulna. I have seen this in 19 patients, but I have never seen it since I have applied the preoperative distraction. Therefore, I see the cause not so much as surgical damage to the epiphyseal plate but more as an increased pressure to the growth plate that is caused by inadequate ulnar shortening (which we have performed in some earlier cases) or inadequate carpal bone excision.

Results

My experiences with the great number of operated radial club hands have led to a learning process that has resulted in modifications of the surgical technique. One of these recognitions was the importance of sufficient muscles in number and in strength. When there are no good radial wrist muscles, which are necessary for the reinforcement of the "antirecurrent" pull of the extensor carpi ulnaris, early recurrence is seen. Only an ulnocarpal fusion can help in this situation, as a primary operation or as a secondary correction in previous patients.

Although the mobility in the new ulnocarpal joint is always sufficient for performing all activities of daily life, the range of motion is restricted particularly in extension and ulnar abduction. Although flexion and radial abduction are usually normal, the extension is, in most patients, possible only to neutral position or an additional 10 to 15 degrees. The same range is seen for the ulnar abduction. Also, the range of motion in the fingers remains incomplete, but the overall function is remarkably improved by the pollicization of the index finger.

Late Treatment

Besides the already mentioned index finger pollicization, which should follow the radialization at an interval of approximately 6 months, a considerable improvement of the function of the arm as a whole and appearance can be gained by distraction lengthening of the forearm. I have done this usually in patients of 8 to 10 years of age who have asked for such a treatment. The lengthening during this time-consuming procedure is approximately 4 to 6 cm. The distraction can be repeated and can also be combined with some axial correction, if necessary.

ULNAR CLUB HAND

The manifestations of ulnar deficiencies appear in such great variety that a classification is impossible. The different combinations of the abnormalities of the fingers, the metacarpal and carpal bones, the ulna, the radius, the elbow, the upper arm, and the shoulder are so diverse that they cannot fit into a classification system. Nevertheless, there exist several classifications that take into consideration mostly only the deformities of one structure or one part of the extremity, the ulna and radius, the elbow, or the radial side of the hand (16–18). Therefore, they are not related to the clinical picture of the whole arm or to therapeutic measures.

Occurrence

Almost all ulnar deficiencies are sporadic. Only in cases in which the ulnar defect is a part of a syndrome is inheritance described, mostly in an autosomal-dominant pattern. These cases include combinations with orofacial malformations, Cornelia de Lange's syndrome, Schinzel syndrome, and FFU (femur-fibula-ulna) syndrome, which was described 1967 by Kühne et al. (19) and is the European synonym for the American Proximal Femoral Focal Deficiency (PFFD), which was described in 1969 by Aitken (20). The ulnar club hand differentiates from congenital pseudarthroses of the ulna with or without neurofibromatosis.

In contrast to radial deficiencies, cardiac, gastrointestinal, genitourinary, and hematopoietic anomalies are uncommon. Most of the associated anomalies concern the musculoskeletal system and belong to the syndromes that were mentioned in the last paragraph. Their incidence is reported to be between 25% and 50%.

Morphology

There is no typical picture of an ulnar club hand (Fig. 8). The deformities are found in all parts of the arm without

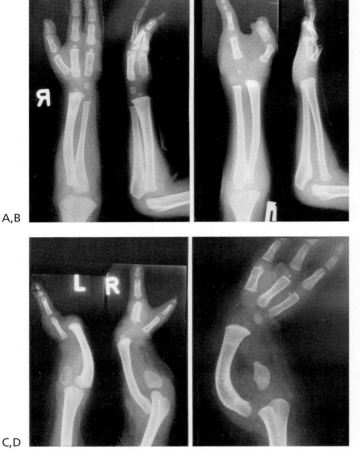

A,B

C,D

FIGURE 8. Different types of ulnar deficiencies. **A:** Hypoplasia of the ulna with oligodactyly (2 years of age); the remaining digits are normal, with the exception of a symphalangia in the index finger. **B:** Hypoplasia of the ulna with congenital dislocation of the radial head and severe finger deformation (2 years of age). **C:** Bilateral ulnar deficiency in a patient who is 2 years of age with partial aplasia of both ulnae, severe digital deformities with reduction in the number of digits, dislocation of the radial head at the right elbow, and beginning radiohumeral synostosis (*left*) (the cartilaginous growth plate is radiologically still visible). **D:** Partial absence of the ulna with dislocation of the head of the bowed radius and absence of the fourth and fifth digital rays (2 years of age).

any regularity and in numerous combinations. Therefore, the description should follow the different localizations of the arm in a direction from distal to proximal.

Hand

A reduced number of digital rays is typical for ulnar deficiencies. In most hands, the missing digits are the little and ring fingers, but, in rare cases, the thumb can be absent. In my own clinical material (21) of 200 involved forearms in 164 patients, only 17 patients (8.5%) showed a full complement of digits; there were 31 hands with four fingers (15.5%), 87 hands with three fingers (43.5%), 48 hands

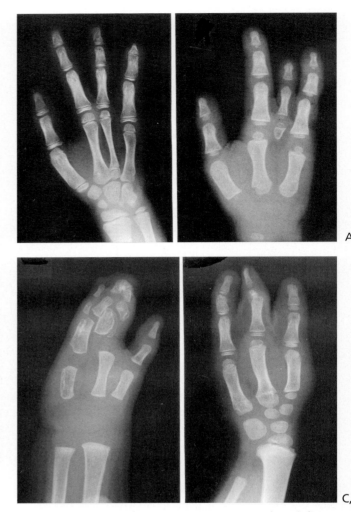

A,B

C,D

FIGURE 9. Skeletal deformities that are seen in ulnar deficiencies. **A:** Hypoplasia of a digital ray, particularly in the metacarpal (8 years of age). **B:** Partial aplasia of a metacarpal (2 years of age). **C:** Severe bone deformities with phalangeal synostoses, longitudinal bracketed epiphyses, and additional rudimentary bones (14 months of age). **D:** Reduced digital number with deformed carpal bones and phalanges (8 years of age).

with two fingers (24%), and 17 hands with only one finger (8.5%). In these numbers, the 33 hands with oligodactyly but with normal ulnae are not included. Many of the present digits are abnormal; some are hypoplastic or are missing a phalanx or a metacarpal, whereas others show an additional rudimentary finger or bones with longitudinal bracketed epiphyses or tendon anomalies (Fig. 9). At the phalangeal or metacarpal level, synostoses are also seen. In 92 hands (46%) of our patients, a syndactyly was present, mostly a complete one. Often this finding is combined with a bone bridge between the terminal phalanges (Figs. 9 and 10), especially if there are only two fingers present.

The reason that Cole and Manske (17) have chosen to base their classification on the radial side of the hand is that, in the primarily ulnar-sided deformity, a surprisingly high number of anomalies of the thumb and first web are

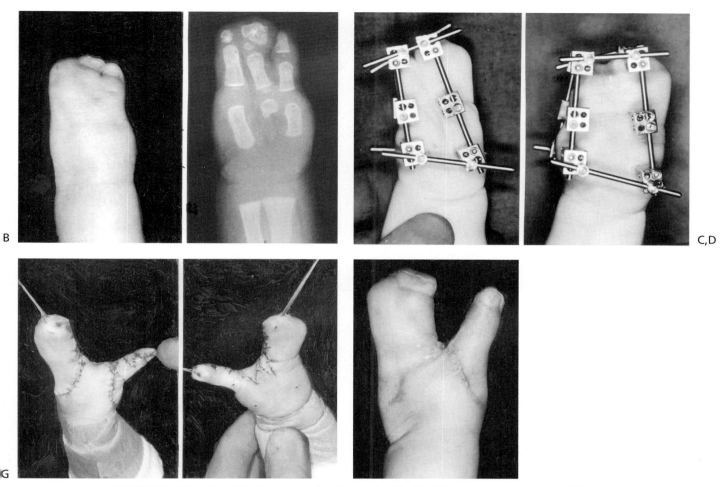

B

C,D

G

FIGURE 10. Oligodactyly in the hand of a 13-month-old girl with complete syndactyly of the deformed three digits and partial absence of the second metacarpal **(A,B)**. To gain more skin for the syndactyly separation, a transverse soft tissue distraction with a special small device was applied. **C:** At the beginning of the distraction. **D:** Six weeks later. **E,F:** At the syndactyly separation, an almost complete skin cover with local skin was possible. **G:** The result shows the new first web space.

found. They consist of hypoplasia or aplasia of the thumb; a rotational deformity, so that the thumb is lying in the plane of the fingers; and narrowing of the first web space or even a complete syndactyly. In my patients, with the exception of the monodactylous hands, in 136 of 183 hands, a radial-sided involvement was noted. This percentage (74%) corresponds exactly with the numbers of Cole and Manske.

Wrist

An ulnar angulation is seen in some patients but is not essential and is never seen in such a high degree as in radial club hands. It is caused by bowing of the radius and a slant of the distal articular surface. The role of a fibrocartilaginous anlage, which is present in forearms with partial absence of the ulna, is discussed controversially. Although Riordan (22,23) believes that the bowing of the radius is increased by the slowly growing anlage with its insertions at

the distal radius and the carpus and recommends its early excision, other observations (24–27) have shown the minor effect of the excision on the ulnar deviation. It seems to be better to control the ulnar angulation and to excise the anlage only in patients with progression of the condition and in whom the angulation exceeds 30 degrees.

O'Rahilly (28) has given exact information on carpal bones that has been confirmed by many reports. Absence is seen in correlation to the missing digital rays; only the pisiform is absent in almost all cases. In approximately 30% to 40%, synostoses of the carpal bones are seen. Many of the carpals show abnormal shapes (Fig. 9).

Forearm

With the exception of some patients with hypoplasia of the ulna, the forearm is shorter than normal (Figs. 11 and 12). The ulna shows hypoplasia and partial or complete absence;

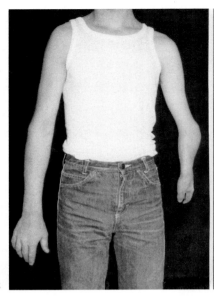
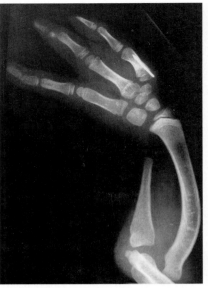

A,B

FIGURE 11. In ulnar deficiencies, the involved extremity is remarkably shorter, as is demonstrated in a patient with partial aplasia of the ulna and dislocation of the radial head [the clinical photograph (A) was taken at 16 years of age, and the radiogram (B) was taken at 8 years of age].

these types can be combined with different anomalies of the hand and elbow, without any correlation in the severity of the deformities. The radius may be normal in many forearms with ulnar hypoplasia, but, in combination with partial or complete aplasia, there are bowings with a slanted distal and dislocated ulnar head or fusion to the distal humerus (Fig. 8).

In my own series of 200 involved arms in 164 patients, hypoplasia of the ulna was seen in 59.5%, partial aplasia was seen in 22.5%, and complete absence was seen in 18%. There were 61 congenital dislocations of the radial head (30.5%) and 35 radiohumeral synostoses (17.5%) in different combinations; the exact numbers were recently reported (21). The anomalies of the muscles, tendons, nerves, and

blood vessels are mentioned only in a few publications, at best in the fundamental report by Stoffel and Stempel (29). In general, there are not as many abnormalities of these structures as there are in the radial club hand.

Elbow

The configuration of the articular surfaces of the elbow joint is almost normal only in patients with ulna hypoplasia, but, in many of these cases, the coronoid process is also lower. In all other ulnar deficiencies, there is at least hypoplasia of all articular parts. In cases of congenital dislocation of the head of the radius, the opposite part, the capitulum humeri, is also

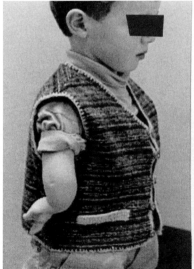
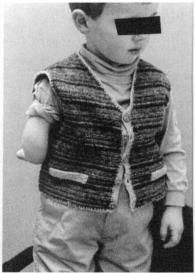
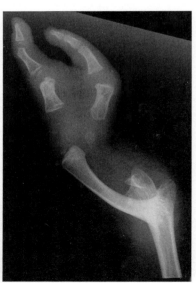

FIGURE 12. In patients with radiohumeral synostoses, the involved extremity is short and shows a dorsal angulation in extreme pronation at the elbow—a position without any functional use (3 years of age).

deformed. The most severe deformity, ankylosis of the elbow or radiohumeral synostosis, is combined with a rotational deformity of the short arm in extreme pronation and with a dorsal angulation at the elbow level (Fig. 12). Any function of the hand, which always has a reduced number of digits, is possible only with compensatory rotation in the shoulder joint. The frequency of these deformities in my patients was already mentioned in the last paragraph.

Upper Arm and Shoulder

The deformities of the upper arm and shoulder are not mentioned in most reports. Even in my series, only shoulder mobility, which was almost unrestricted in all cases, was described. Reported anomalies are hypoplasia of the muscles and hypoplasia of the humerus and the glenoid.

Surgical Treatment

Conservative treatment, which is the often-recommended splinting to prevent any progression of the ulnar angulation of the wrist, is useless and bothers the mother and the child.

Surgical treatment primarily consists of operations of the hand, as has been reported from many authors. In my patients, 242 (92.3%) of all 262 operations were performed at the hand. Depending on the type of deformity, several different procedures have to be applied. In my patients, the most frequent operation was a syndactyly separation, which was performed in 63 hands, followed by a widening of the first web space in 52 hands. For the skin closure at the first web space, the rotational advancement flap (Fig. 13) has proven successful (30). Other procedures were rotational

osteotomies of the first metacarpal (in 28 hands) or, in cases of hands with only two fingers, of both metacarpals (in 21 hands) and the removal of rudimentary digital parts or additional fingers (in 36 hands). Many of these procedures were combined in the same stage.

In hands with only two digits with complete syndactyly, skin closure after syndactyly separation and widening of the web space is difficult. It can be facilitated by the application of a modern technique, the transverse soft tissue distraction. A specially developed distraction device extends, after division of a distal bone bridge, the narrow skin bridge so far in the course of 5 to 6 weeks that, in the final stage, a direct skin closure is possible (Fig. 10). The period of approximately 2 weeks after the distraction is important, as it allows the extended skin and the edema to settle.

The rotational osteotomy of the first metacarpal in hands with adducted nonrotated thumbs, which are lying in the same plane as the other metacarpals, provides, in combination with a widening of the first web space, excellent results (25). More problematic may be the late outcome in hands with only two digital rays. Osteotomies of both metacarpals lead to sufficient pinch, but the pull of the interossei acts in a derotational sense on the growing bone, so that, finally, the fingers lie again in approximately the same plane. This can be prevented, except for a sufficient rotation of approximately 90 degrees of the distal bone parts, by a transposition of the insertions of the interossei to the opposite side of the base of the proximal phalanx; after this procedure, the pull of the muscles acts in a correct rotational sense and influences the bone growth in this direction.

In our patients, some further operations were performed in the hand: six pollicizations of the index finger in cases of

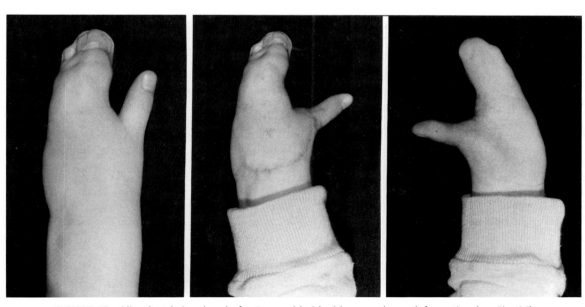

A–C

FIGURE 13. Oligodactyly in a hand of a 4-year-old girl with severe bone deformation (see Fig. 9C) and narrow first web space **(A)**. After widening of the first web space and skin cover with a dorsal rotation-advancement flap **(B)**, a wide abduction of the thumb is possible **(C)**.

absence of the thumb, 14 separations of metacarpal synostoses, and eight metacarpal stabilizations in hands with absence of the proximal three-fourths of one metacarpal.

The only procedure at the wrist level is the excision of the cartilaginous anlage, which is still discussed controversially. In our patients, it was done only in seven cases: three times in combination with the construction of a one-bone forearm, the other time in response to an increasing ulnar deviation. In these patients, the tendons of the flexor and extensor carpi ulnaris were transposed to the radial side to increase the forces for radial deviation. Special attention is necessary not to damage the ulnar nerve, which lies close to the tendinous insertions.

In the forearm, the indication for the construction of a one-bone forearm was formerly limited to an instability between the radius and the existing part of the ulna. Since the introduction of distraction lengthening as a therapeutic measure, both procedures can be combined successfully. In a first stage, the fibrous connections between the two bones are divided, the anlage is resected, and the radius is distracted against the ulna. In most cases, it is possible to bring the dislocated radial head into a better position; sometimes, part of it has to be resected. In a second stage, the proximal parts of the radius and the ulna are fused in the distracted position by osteosynthesis. Such a one-bone forearm can be lengthened again by distraction some years later.

At the level of the elbow, a surgical correction is indicated in only a few instances. A trial of reduction of the dislocated head of the radius with permanent retention in the correct position is impossible in cases of a deformed articular surface of the distal humerus. In contrast, another procedure is more successful in special cases: the rotational angulatory osteotomy in elbows with radiohumeral synostosis (Fig. 12). By rotation and anterior angulation of the forearm, the hand can be brought into a better functional position. Special care is necessary to protect the brachial artery and the major nerves, which are located close to the bones at the osteotomy site. Here again, several years later, distraction lengthening of the proximal radius can improve the function and appearance of the arm. The possible complications and results of these procedures were already mentioned in the previous paragraphs.

REFERENCES

1. Swanson AB, deGroot Swanson G, Tada K. A classification for congenital limb malformation. *J Hand Surg* 1983;8:693–702.
2. Flatt AE. *The care of congenital hand anomalies,* 2nd ed. St. Louis: Quality Medical Publishers, 1994.
3. Birch-Jensen A. *Congenital deformities of the upper extremities.* Odense, Denmark: Andelsbogtrykkeriet, 1949.
4. Blauth W. Zur Morphologie und Therapie der radialen Klump-hand. *Arch Orthop Unfallchir* 1969;65:97–123.
5. Vilkki S. Radiusaplasia ja Henrik Heikelin aineisto. Myöhäissenvantatutokset 35 vuoden kuluttua (in Finnish). *Suomen Orthop Traumatol* 1997;20:205–208.
6. Heikel HV. Aplasia and hypoplasia of the radius. *Acta Orthop Scand* 1959;[Suppl 39]:1–155.
7. Bayne LG, Klug MS. Long-term review of the surgical treatment of radial deficiencies. *J Hand Surg* 1987;1:169–179.
8. Lamb DW. Radial club hand. A continuing study of sixty-eight patients with one hundred and seventeen club hands. *J Bone Joint Surg* 1977;59:1–13.
9. Lamb DW, Scott H, Lam WL, et al. Operative correction of radial club hand. A long-term follow-up of centralization of the hand on the ulna. *J Hand Surg* 1997;22:533–536.
10. Sayre RH. A contribution to the study of club-hand. *N Y Med J* 1893;58:529–532.
11. Buck-Gramcko D. Radialization as a new treatment for radial club hand. *J Hand Surg* 1985;1:964–968.
12. Buck-Gramcko D. Radialization for radial club hand. *Tech Hand Upper Extrem Surg* 1999;3:2–12.
13. Tonkin MA. Radial longitudinal deficiency (Radial dysplasia radial clubhand). In: Green DP, Hotchkiss RN, Pederson WC, eds. *Green's operative hand surgery,* 4th ed. New York: Churchill Livingstone, 1990:344–358.
14. Vilkki SK. Vascularized joint transfer for radial club hand. *Tech Hand Upper Extrem Surg* 1998;2:126–137.
15. Damore E, Kozin SH, Thoder JJ, et al. The recurrence of deformity after surgical centralization for radial clubhand. *J Hand Surg* 2000;25:745–751.
16. Bayne LG. Ulnar club hand (Ulnar deficiencies). In: Green DP, ed. *Operative hand surgery,* 1st ed. New York: Churchill Livingstone, 1982:245–257.
17. Cole RJ, Manske PR. Classification of ulnar deficiency according to the thumb and first web. *J Hand Surg* 1997;22:479–488.
18. Lausecker H. Der angeborene Defekt der Ulna. *Virchows Arch Pathol Anat Physiol Klin Med* 1954;325:211–226.
19. Kühne D, Lenz W, Petersen D, et al. Defekt von Femur und Fibula mit Amelie, Peromelie oder ulnaren Strahldefekten der Arme. Ein Syndrom. *Humangenetik* 1967;3:244–263.
20. Aitken GT. *Proximal femoral focal deficiency. a congenital anomaly.* Washington: National Academy of Science, 1969.
21. Buck-Gramcko D. Ulnar deficiency. In: Tubiana R, Gilbert A, eds. *Surgery of the tendons and nerves and other disorders of the hand.* London: Martin Dunitz, 2001.
22. Riordan DC. Congenital absence of the ulna. In: Lovell WW, Winter RB, eds. *Pediatric orthopaedics.* Philadelphia: JB Lippincott Co, 1978:714–7109.
23. Riordan DC, Mills EH, Alldredge RH. Congenital absence of the ulna. *J Bone Joint Surg* 1961;43:614.
24. Broudy AS, Smith RJ. Deformities of the hand and wrist with ulnar deficiency. *J Hand Surg* 1979;4:304–315.
25. Buck-Gramcko D. Ulnar deficiency. In: Saffar P, Amadio PC, Foucher G, eds. *Current practice in hand surgery.* London: Martin Dunitz, 1997:371–390.
26. Johnson J, Omer GE. Congenital ulnar deficiency. Natural history and therapeutic implications. *Hand Clin* 1985;1:499–510.
27. Marcus NA, Omer GE. Carpal deviation in congenital ulnar deficiency. *J Bone Joint Surg* 1984;66:1003–1007.
28. O'Rahilly R. Morphological patterns in limb deficiencies and duplications. *Am J Anat* 1951;89:135–194.
29. Stoffel A, Stempel E. *Anatomische Studien Ober die Klump hand.* Stuttgart, Germany: Enke, 1909.
30. Buck-Gramcko D. Syndactyly between the thumb and index finger. In: Buck-Gramcko D, ed. *Congenital malformations of the hand and forearm.* London: Churchill Livingstone, 1998:141–147.

86

CONGENITAL DISORDERS: CLEFT HAND

SIMON P. J. KAY
ALASTAIR J. PLATT

To most people, a cleft suggests a wedge-shaped defect in a structure, but, in developmental terms, a cleft is an abnormality of a structure that may be represented by a tissue deficit or by an abnormality in the remaining tissue. Cleft hand is an uncommon condition that may occur unilaterally or bilaterally. The cleft of variable extent usually occurs in the central ray and is commonly associated with syndactyly and other abnormalities in adjacent digits and sometimes with abnormalities in the feet (Fig. 1). It is a striking condition not only for the appearance of the more severe forms but also for the remarkable function that can occur even in the untreated hand. Swanson (1–4) classifies the deformity as a longitudinal failure of formation of parts. In common with other longitudinal deficiencies (e.g., radial and ulnar), this carries the implication that the proximal longitudinal supporting structures (e.g., nerves, vessels, tendons, and intrinsic muscles) of the absent part are themselves deficient.

DEFINITION AND CLASSIFICATION

Central defects of the hand have in the past been divided into *typical* and *atypical*, which broadly correspond to the type 1 and type 2 classification that was devised by Sandzén (5) (Table 1) in 1985. In 1992, at the International Federation of Societies for Surgery of the Hand meeting in Paris (6), it was agreed to use the term *cleft hand* to refer to the *typical* forms, and it was recognized that *atypical* cleft hand formed part of the sequence of symbrachydactyly.

Typical or true cleft hand (Sandzén type 1) (5), with which this chapter is concerned, is manifested by unilateral or bilateral central defects of the hands, usually with one or more digital rays reduced or absent. The resultant defect is truly cleft-shaped (V-shaped), and associated abnormalities may be found in the hand, including syndactyly, triphalangeal thumb, polydactyly, and transverse bones. The condition has a genetic basis and may be hereditary. The feet may also be affected (Fig. 2).

By contrast, the condition of symbrachydactyly (7) (*atypical cleft hand*, Sandzén type 2) is sporadic in occurrence, has no hereditary basis, only ever affects one limb, and shows a teratologic sequence with typically U-shaped central defects. The digital absences resemble intercalary or isolated transverse absences of the fingers, often with small nubbins of finger and nail tissue remaining. This condition is not considered further in this chapter.

The classification of cleft hand has often resulted in unhelpful categories and subdivisions. Blauth and Falliner (8) examined 35 true cleft hands and divided them into three groups, type 1 being cleft hand with aplasia alone, type 2 being cleft hand with synostosis, and type 3 being cleft hand with aplasia and synostosis. They believed that our knowledge of etiology was still too rudimentary to allow classification on the basis of a mechanism of causation. The variations in the subclassifications that were proposed for this rare condition are confusing, and it is easier to use the term *cleft hand* to describe all types of central longitudinal failures of development. Manske and Halikis (9) have provided a morphologic classification (Table 2) that is based on the quality of the first web space, which may be involved in adjacent syndactyly or in the cleft itself. This web space is an important determinant not only of function but also of indications for surgery, and this is now the classification that the authors prefer. This classification acknowledges that, in the more extensive clefts, the cleft may merge with the first web space (producing a wide but competent web) or may even involve a thumb, thus being manifested by the absence of the radial structures.

PATHOGENESIS

Genetics

Although cleft hand occurs sporadically, cases of cleft hand occur in conjunction with cleft foot as a result of abnormal genes that are known as *split-hand and split-foot* (*SHSF*) (10–12). Inheritance of SHSF shows an autosomal-dominant pattern with variable penetrance. Transmission of the abnormal gene from an affected individual results in structural abnormalities in 70% of cases that inherit the gene

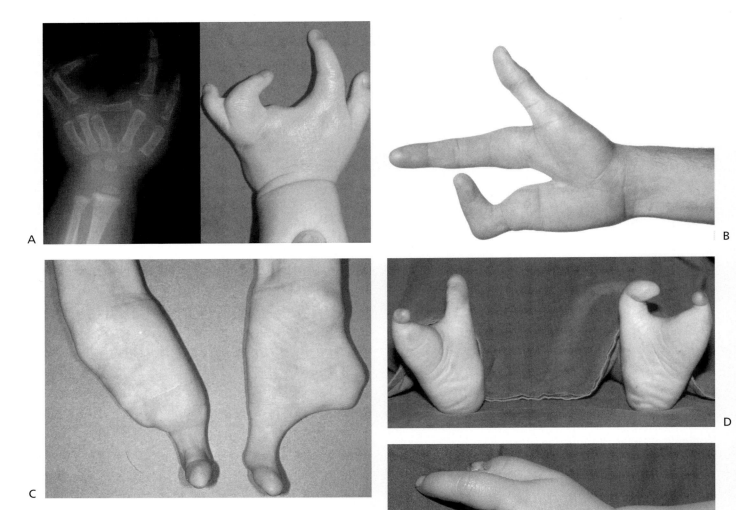

FIGURE 1. A: A typical cleft hand in which the central ray is suppressed, and there is a transverse bone that lies between the cleft borders and articulates with the metacarpophalangeal joints on either side. **B:** Typical cleft hand. Note the deep V-shaped cleft and the adjacent clinodactyly. **C:** Extreme example of typical cleft hand in which only the ulnar border ray is not suppressed. **D:** Typical foot deformity in severe cleft hand and cleft foot. The child usually walks with only the fibular ray being weight bearing. **E:** This child shows a minor cleft with adjacent syndactyly—a common feature of true cleft hand.

TABLE 1. SANDZÉN'S CLASSIFICATION OF CLEFT HAND

Type 1	Frequently bilateral. Often involves the foot. Usually familial. One or more central rays are absent, with a cone-shaped defect extending into the metacarpal region.
Type 2	*Atypical.* Usually unilateral. Does not involve the feet. Sporadic. Uninherited. U-shaped cleft. Partial or complete absence of the metacarpals. Hypoplastic thumb. Hypoplastic little finger.
Type 3	One, two, or three rays are missing. Syndactyly and polydactyly.

Note: Types 1 and 3 now known as *cleft hand*. Type 2 is now known as *symbrachydactyly*.

mutation. In the other 30%, the presence of the mutant gene cannot be determined by examination alone, because no physical abnormalities are present. Cleft hand is phenotypically analogous to the dactyl aplasia mutant in mice (13), in which the central segment of the apical ectodermal ridge degenerates, leaving the radial and ulnar segments intact. A gene in the region of chromosome 3q27 plays a critical role in the formation and maintenance of the apical ectodermal ridge, and missense mutations in this gene have been identified in families who are affected by the SHSF malformation and also in families who are affected by electrodactyly-ectodermal dysplasia-clefting (EEC) syndrome (see the following section, Associated Anomalies). Syndromic associations with the phenotype of true cleft hand are

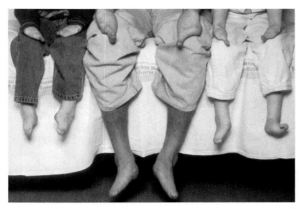

FIGURE 2. This family illustrates the hereditary nature (autosomal dominant) of cleft hand and cleft foot.

summarized in Table 3, and, even in the absence of syndromic associations, a large number of other congenital anomalies have been reported to coexist with the phenotype of cleft hand (Table 4).

Associated Anomalies

Many associated anomalies have been identified in cleft hand. Syndrome complexes that are associated with cleft hand are shown in Table 3. The most common association is with other limb clefts, bilaterally in the upper limbs or associated with foot clefts in the autosomal-dominant condition. *EEC syndrome* (14–16) (Fig. 3) refers to ectrodactyly-ectodermal dysplasia-clefting, and, in this syndrome, cleft hands are associated with oral clefts, anodontia, and cutaneous manifestations of ectodermal dysplasia, including hair, nail, and skin abnormalities. This is an important condition to recognize because the oral cleft may be occult and submucous, and it should be actively sought. More recently, three different forms of EEC syndrome (17) have been identified with phenotypic overlap and differing gene mapping, one of which appears to be allelic for limb mammary syndrome. Thus, the genetic explanation for the dis-

TABLE 3. SYNDROMES THAT ARE ASSOCIATED WITH CLEFT HAND

Cornelia de Lange's syndrome
Oculodigital complex
Orodigital complex
Otodigital complex (Wildervank syndrome)
Silver-Russell syndrome
Electrodactyly-ectodermal dysplasia-clefting syndrome

order of cleft hand is shown to be complex, and it is likely that more than one genetic defect and varying degrees of penetrance can result in the cleft hand phenotype, thus explaining its occurrence in a number of syndromes.

Etiology

A wedge-shaped defect of the apical ectoderm of the limb bud is thought to lead to cleft hand. Maisels' centripetal theory (18) proposed a progression of clefting, from a simple, central, soft tissue defect to complete absence of all digits, in an attempt to explain the progressive spectrum of deformity and the so-called teratologic sequence. Suppression progresses in a radial direction, so that, in the monodactylous form, the little finger is preserved in contrast to severe *atypical* clefts (symbrachydactyly) in which the thumb is the best or last remaining digit. Regardless of whether this theory has a basis in embryogenesis, it does represent the clinical findings.

More recently, Ogino (19–21) has emphasized the association between polydactyly, syndactyly, and cleft hand and has been able to reproduce cleft hand in rats using teratogens, particularly busulphan. It is an important observation in clinical series that central polydactyly is often associated with adjacent-cleft osseous syndactyly, and the same phenomenon has been observed in Ogino's rat model. It is suggested by some that central polydactyly leads to cleft formation by the progressive syndactyly of adjacent rays. Miura (22–24) and Watari and Tsuge (25,26) have also emphasized the importance of central polydactyly in the

TABLE 2. SURGICAL CLASSIFICATION OF CENTRAL DEFICIENCY

Type	Description	Characteristics
1	Normal web	Thumb web space is not narrowed.
2A	Mildly narrowed web	Thumb web space is mildly narrowed.
2B	Severely narrowed web	Thumb web space is severely narrowed.
3	Syndactylized web	Thumb and index rays are syndactylized; web space is obliterated.
4	Merged web	Index ray is suppressed; thumb web space is merged with the cleft.
5	Absent web	Thumb elements are suppressed; ulnar rays remain; thumb web space is no longer present.

TABLE 4. ANOMALIES THAT ARE ASSOCIATED WITH CLEFT HAND

Limb	General
Club feet	Cleft lip and palate
Tibial defects	Congenital heart disease
Hypoplastic patella	Imperforate anus
Pseudarthrosis of the clavicle	Nystagmus
Synostosis of the elbow	Cataract
Radioulnar synostosis	Deafness
Short humerus	Ptosis
Short forearm	Undescended testes
Absent ulna	
Short femur	
Cleft feet	

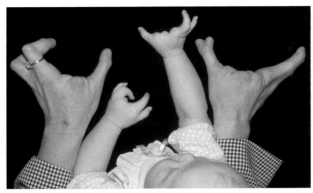

FIGURE 3. A mother and child with ectrodactyly-ectodermal dysplasia-clefting syndrome; note the cleft hands of the mother and child.

etiology of cleft hand. It appears that central synpolydactyly is a condition that is capable of mimicking many of the features of cleft hand but that brings some features of its own, including the findings of common metacarpals.

INCIDENCE

Reports of the incidence of cleft hand vary from as high as 4 per 100,000 live births to as low as 1.4 per 100,000 live births in Denmark. Nutt and Flatt (27,28) found a prevalence of 3.9% in 2,758 anomalous hands. Giele et al. (29),

in a more recent Australian total population study, found that failure of formation represented 15% of all upper limb abnormalities but does not indicate the proportion of central defects.

EVALUATION

Morphology and Appearance

There are many variations in the appearance of cleft hand. The major differences are in the adjacent digital deformities and in the extent of the cleft, which may be minimal or profound and may involve one digital ray or several. Typically, there is absence of the central portion of the hand in the position of the third ray. The cleft may be deep and may extend down to the carpus with complete absence of the central metacarpal (Fig. 4A). There may be loss of all three central rays, leading to the uncommon two-fingered form in which the border digits may be found (Fig. 4B). In the most extreme form of cleft hand, only the ulnar ray is preserved (Fig. 1C).

Several metacarpal variations are seen. The bone may be totally missing in the cleft, or two metacarpals may support one finger, which then resembles a severe compound syndactyly on radiographs. This is especially true in phenotypes of central synpolydactyly. Alternatively, and less commonly, a bifid metacarpal may support two digits. Transverse bones at the metacarpal level are common. These "cross-bones" form

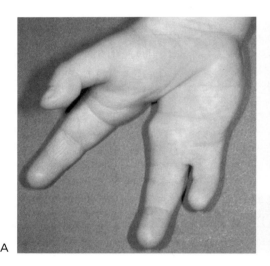

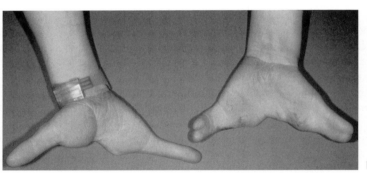

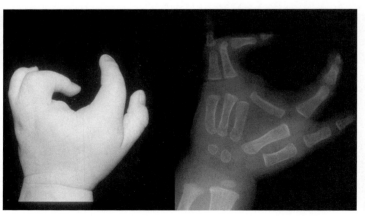

FIGURE 4. A: Typical cleft with absent central ray and with the cleft extending to the carpus. **B:** Bilateral cleft hands with only the border digits present. **C:** Typical cleft hand. Note the transverse bone that articulates with the metacarpophalangeal joints at either border of the cleft and the double metacarpal that supports a single finger. Note also the adjacent clinodactyly, rotation, and syndactyly of the border digits.

a triangle that is attached at either end by a joint or a synostosis to the border rays (Fig. 4C).

The digits that border the cleft are affected in a variety of ways. Syndactyly is frequent, as are angulation and rotation of the digits with delta-shaped phalanges and longitudinally bracketed epiphyses (Fig. 4C).

Flexion contractures of the proximal interphalangeal joints with associated stiffness are seen, and there may be thickening of the fingers due to broad bones or double phalanges. The intrinsic mechanism of the thumb may be severely abnormal, and the thumb, in extreme cases, may be conjoined with the index finger and held in the same plane as the other digit.

Blauth and Falliner (8) found frequent synostosis between the capitate and the hamate, and, later, Imamura and Miura (30) drew attention to the frequent anomalies within the carpus, which have received little documentation or discussion to date, in this condition. In general, the forearm is normal, as is the size of the remaining hand.

The anomaly is often bilateral, and, in the SHSF phenotype, it is associated with comparable defects in the feet. Because of the dominant inheritance of the condition, presentation may be late, despite the dramatic appearance of the hands, because the family may have many members through the generations with such hands and may take a relatively phlegmatic view of the condition.

MANAGEMENT

Nonoperative Treatment

Flatt (28) memorably summed up the severely deformed hand as a "functional triumph, but a social disaster." Although the hands of these children are deformed, the function is often excellent, and little or no disability is apparent. There may be reluctance from a parent with a similar deformity to avoid surgery in the light of their own experiences, because, untreated, they may develop remarkable function. Surgery can, however, improve the stigmatizing deformity while maintaining or improving function.

As with all congenital anomalies of the hand, immediate attention should be paid to the behavioral aspects of the condition. The parental reaction to the birth (31) should be understood and addressed, in particular the grieving reaction that is so frequently seen. Information exchange, explanation, and counseling are all appropriate (32), as is some introduction to the surgical protocol and care pathways. Genetic counseling in this condition is desirable, and full assessment and identification of any associated syndrome are essential.

Surgery for the older patient who has successfully adapted to his or her malformation functionally and who seeks surgery for aesthetic reasons should be approached with caution. These patients may have unrealistic expectations, and their aims should be carefully evaluated before undertaking treatment. In this group of patients, the authors find the use of plaster casts of the hands on which the surgical outcomes can be rehearsed to be helpful for the patient.

Surgical Management

The timing of surgery depends on the anatomic findings. In general, it is sensible to distinguish preventative measures from corrective measures. In the former, one might include the separation of syndactyly between digits of unequal length (especially the thumb and index rays) to prevent rapidly progressive deformity and the removal of transverse bones whose unfettered growth results in widening of the cleft. Most of the other surgical procedures are not time critical and may be left until the child is between 1 and 2 years of age.

During the surgical correction of cleft hand, function should never be compromised for the sake of appearance. The goals of surgery may be summarized as follows:

Release of syndactylies between digits of unequal length
Removal of transverse bone
Closure of the cleft hand and release of thumb adduction contracture, including syndactyly
Correction of deviation of digits

Release of Syndactyly between Digits of Unequal Length

Release of syndactyly between digits of unequal length is most commonly needed in the first cleft between the thumb and the index finger. If left untreated for any length of time, this may result in tethering and deviation of the index finger (Fig. 5) and certainly impedes the development of the thumb prehension patterns. By definition, the first cleft in these cases (Manske and Halikis type 3) is absent, and considerable skin is needed to correct the first web space. It is not essential to correct the tight first web space at the same time as release of the syndactyly, although there are obvious advantages to combining these stages for some patients. If they are combined, the skin required may be provided by the Snow-Littler procedure (33–35) (see the section Closure of the Cleft and Release of the First Web Space) or by transposition of the index finger [Miura and Komada (36)]. However, in some cases of tight syndactyly, this is not sufficient, and the first web space correction may require the transplantation of skin as a vascularized flap.

At the time of correction, the attitude of the thumb ray may also be corrected. In such syndactyly, the thumb often lies in the plane of the palm, and rotation at the metacarpal level can be undertaken to correct this. In such rotation osteotomy, the soft tissues need extensive release circumferentially and over most of the length of the metacarpal, together with attention to the direction of pull of the long

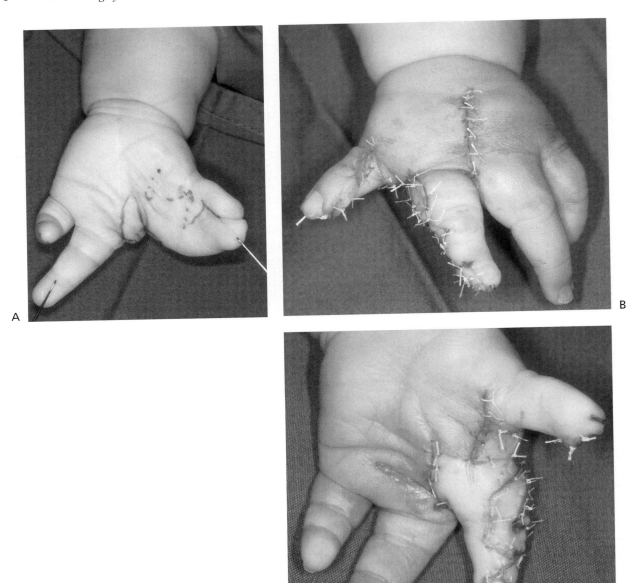

FIGURE 5. A: Syndactyly between the thumb and index fingers, as part of true cleft hand. **B,C:** This is separated at the same time as transposition of the index ray and closure of the cleft.

tendons. Without these precautions, recurrence of the rotatory deformity is likely.

Removal of Transverse Bone

Whatever other reconstructions are planned, it is almost always sensible to remove transverse bones in the hand, because the presence of growing epiphyses within these malaligned tubular bones forces the cleft ever wider, and there is therefore a preventative element to their removal. In cases in which the bone forms a common joint at the metacarpophalangeal level of an adjacent ray, reconstruc-

tion of the collateral ligament and capsular structures is required (Fig. 6).

Closure of the Cleft and Release of the First Web Space

Direct closure of the cleft by excision of soft tissue is used to treat minor deformities. Local flap reconstruction of a web commissure is essential to create a pleasing appearance and is achieved by placing a U-shaped flap across the new commissure in such a way that the apex of the new commissure does not contain a scar. This is important to create a natural-look-

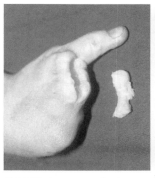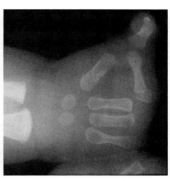

FIGURE 6. Removal of transverse bone that is restricting the mobility of the digital ray and forcing the cleft wider with growth.

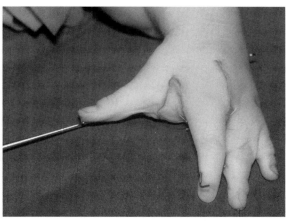

FIGURE 7. This cleft has been closed with the use of the cleft skin as a palmarly based flap to transpose to the first web space for widening of that structure in the method of Snow and Littler. Such closure is often not possible without supplementary skin grafts.

ing commissure and to avoid the deep, V-shaped commissure that is often associated with cracking and instability of the scar at its apex. This is accompanied by excision of an unsatisfied metacarpal, if this is present, and, in more extensive clefts, may also involve translocation of a normal adjacent ray onto the base of the resected metacarpal. Recurrent drifting apart of the metacarpals should be prevented by construction of the transverse metacarpal ligament. Such construction may be achieved with a free tendon graft and may be protected by temporary trans-metacarpal wiring. In the presence of a residual metacarpal, the extensor and the flexor to the suppressed finger are often present and may be used for this purpose. Tsuge and Watari (26) have also described an ingenious method of reconstruction of the transverse metacarpal ligament by using parts of the first annular pulleys from the adjacent clefts.

More severe clefts require more substantial treatment. Often, these clefts are associated with adduction contractures of the thumbs, and several methods have been devised to make use of the skin that is excised from the cleft to resurface the first web release with appropriate and well-matched material. Release of the first web space may require release of the first dorsal interosseous and the adductor (which may also be absent). These should be released at their origins, and, often, partial section or subperiosteal elevation suffice.

The best known and most beautifully illustrated of the techniques that transfer skin from the cleft at closure to the released first web space is that of Snow and Littler. The preshaped commissural skin from the cleft is used as a palmarly based transposition flap to resurface the new thumb web, although, often, some supplementation with full-thickness skin grafts is required (Fig. 7). The operation also involves an osteotomy and ulnar translocation of the index-finger metacarpal onto the base of the middle-finger metacarpal. This translocation is difficult, and the osteosynthesis is performed in close proximity to the deep motor branch of the ulnar nerve. Care must be taken to control rotation during this transfer, as in all metacarpal osteotomies, and careful flexion of the transposed ray and comparison with adjacent rays are advised before finally securing the osteosynthesis.

Translocation of the index metacarpal may require extensive release of the thumb web contracture and subperiosteal dissection of the origin of the first dorsal interosseous muscle to allow translocation to occur. An interosseous Kirschner wire between the transposed digit and its ulnar neighbor not only facilitates the ligament repair but also controls rotation. In some cases, the authors have found that simple closure of the cleft by approximation of the metacarpals without osteotomy is possible if the cleft space metacarpal has been excised, including its base. This should only be performed in cases in which closure is simple and without tension, and, again, care should be taken to check that the approximation of the two metacarpals has not caused rotation. Some have recommended the creation of intertendinous junctions between the flexor tendons or the extensor tendons to prevent excessive spreading of the reconstruction, although the authors have not found that necessary.

Although the Snow-Littler procedure has the attraction of elegance and the appeal of transferring a complete commissure, in practice, the planning and execution can be difficult, and the transposed flap may not lie exactly as required and may need to be supplemented with skin grafts. In addition, the flap can experience partial necrosis, as its length substantially exceeds its breadth. Rider et al. (35) have shown a low rate of flap necrosis, but one-third of their cases required secondary revision, and, in the tightest first web spaces, supplementary skin grafting was required. The lack of reconstruction of a transverse metacarpal ligament was not associated with radiologically or clinically increased divergence of the digits.

Because of these difficulties, other solutions have been proposed. The best known of these is the solution of Miura and Komada (36) in which, after the transposition, the thumb web is simply recreated by interdigitation of the dorsal and palmar flaps. This procedure is undoubtedly simpler and produces pleasing results. Principles from either or both of these

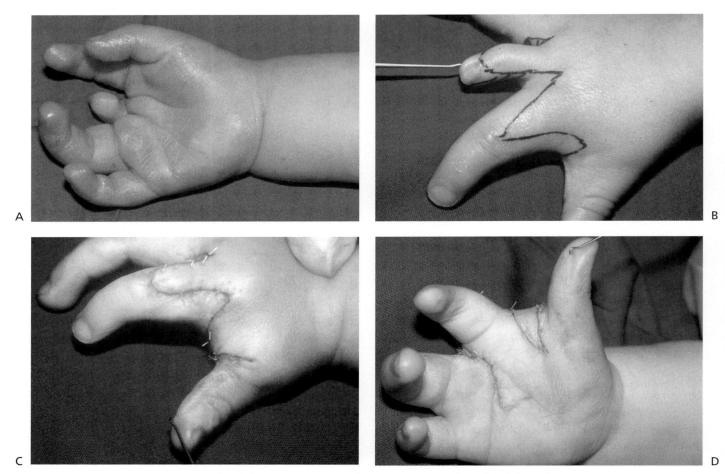

FIGURE 8. **A–D:** This cleft requires excision of the rudimentary ray in the cleft, with transposition of the radial finger and widening of the first web space. This is accomplished by a large flap from the dorsum of the index, which, in turn, is closed with a smaller step-down or bilobed flap design from the cleft ray.

techniques may be used in the great variety of architectures that are seen in cleft hand. Modifications of this principle can be designed as required and may include the use of bilobed flaps (37) from the dorsum in cases with digital remnants that are to be excised in the cleft (Figs. 8 and 9).

Release of Syndactyly and Correction of Digital Deviation

Release of syndactyly and correction of digital deviation follow the principles that have been described elsewhere. However, some caution should be exercised in extreme cases [described by Flatt (28) as "profound cleft hand"] in which only border digits may be present, because little benefit may accrue from surgery to correct angulation. In such cases, and especially in those cases that present late, care should be exercised in planning surgery, because the enthusiastic straightening of digits, the separation of clefts, or the closure of clefts may deny the patient an already established and essential prehension pattern. It is all too easy in these cases to end up with a hand that looks better and functions worse. In some cases, the ulnar digit may

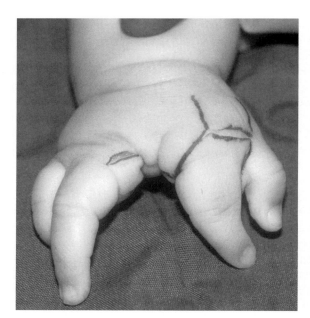

FIGURE 9. The same hand as in Figure 5. Note the design of a small U-shaped flap to resurface the new commissure.

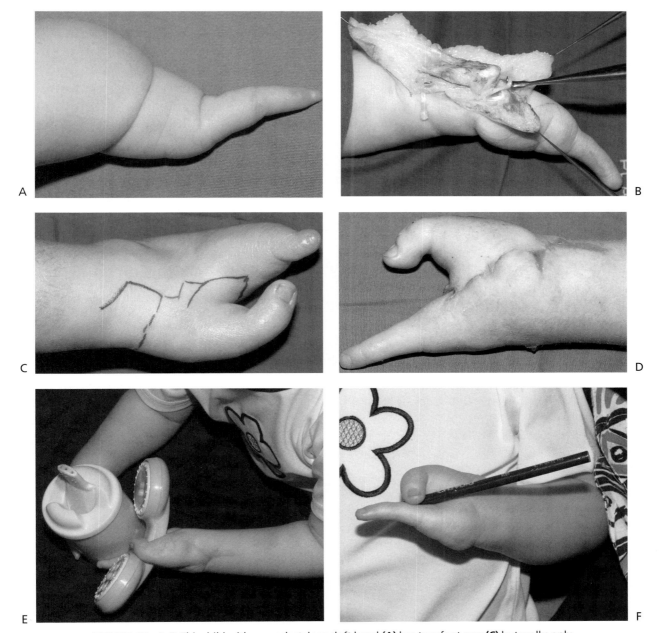

FIGURE 10. A–F: This child with monodactylous cleft hand **(A)** has two foot rays **(C)** but walks only on the fibular ray, leaving the tibial ray available as a transfer. Exploration of the hand **(B)** yielded the surprising finding of confluent flexor and extensor tendons that had excursion similar to a pulley system over the distal end of the cleft. Transfer was microsurgically simple, with vessels found on exploration, as expected (no angiogram was required), and useful prehension established.

be the best and most competent digit, and, on rare occasions, it may be appropriate to perform a form of ulnar pollicization by stabilization, rotation, and reanimation.

When many digits are absent, some authors have suggested microvascular toe transfer (38–40). It is now recognized that this may be effective in longitudinal deficiencies within the hand, but the indications in severe cleft hand remain controversial. Similarly, case reports of microsurgical transfer of supernumerary digits in cleft hand are controversial in terms of indications. The authors, however, have found toe

transfer useful in the case of monodactyly cleft hand. In this condition, the ulnar digit is the only remaining digit and is often stiff and inflexible, offering the child no opportunity for prehension with the hand. This is almost always associated with a significant abnormality in the foot, and the authors' experience has been that the feet in these patients are often highly abnormal, with only the border digits remaining. The child always walks on the fibular ray of the foot, and the tibial ray may be abnormal, with clinodactyly, and often makes no contact with the ground. Figure 10 shows a child in whom the tibial rays were microvascularly transplanted to the hand to create radial digits. The procedure was approached with some concern because of the lack of information about such cases in the literature, but a number of interesting observations were made. First, the authors were surprised to find useful longitudinal enabling structures for the absent rays in the hands. These included the flexor and extensor tendons that were confluent around the distal part of the limb, as a rope around a pulley, and thus had good excursion and gliding structure. Second, vessels and cutaneous nerves were easily found on exploration (angiography was not performed in the foot or the hand). The location of the vessels was aided preoperatively with a 10-MHz Doppler probe.

Despite the preoperative abnormality of the tibial ray in the foot and its clearly uncosmetic appearance in the hand, useful function was achieved, and, although the power and range of grip were limited, this child went from having no prehension in either hand to having useful holding and manipulative abilities in each hand.

CONCLUSION

Surgical treatment for children with central longitudinal deficiency is challenging and can give excellent functional and aesthetic results. In more severe forms, the ingenuity of the surgeon is taxed, and, sometimes, surgery has little to offer. In these cases, the surgeon may agree with the parents whose experience over generations tells them that, despite the adverse appearance, children adapt and learn to use their hands in a way that might have been considered impossible by many when they were born. Surgery should not impair function, but improved appearance is a valid goal, as is improved function. Surgical correction should be planned according to a schedule that recognizes the urgency of some aspects of treatment and the discretionary or optional nature of others. The overriding determinant of function is the first web space, and this structure is at the center of the most useful classification. Microvascular transfers from the foot can be useful in highly selected cases.

REFERENCES

1. Swanson AB. A classification for congenital limb malformations. *J Hand Surg* 1976;1:8–22.
2. Swanson AB, Barsky AJ, Entin MA. Classification of limb malformations on the basis of embryological failures. *Surg Clin North Am* 1968;48:1169–1179.
3. Swanson AB, Swanson GD, Tada K. A classification for congenital limb malformation. *J Hand Surg* 1983;8:693–702.
4. Swanson AB, Entin MA. Classification of limb malformations on the basis of embryological failures. *Surg Clin North Am* 1968;48:1169–1179.
5. Sandzén SC Jr. Classification and functional management of congenital central defect of the hand. *Hand Clin* 1985;1:483–498.
6. Manske PR. Symbrachydactyly instead of atypical cleft hand. *Plast Reconstr Surg* 1993;91:196.
7. Buchler U. Symbrachydactyly. In: Gupta A, Kay S, Scheker L, eds. *The growing hand.* London: Mosby, 2000.
8. Blauth W, Falliner A. Morphology and classification of cleft hands. *Handchir Mikrochir Plast Chir* 1986;18:161–195.
9. Manske PR, Halikis MN. Surgical classification of central deficiency according to the thumb web. *J Hand Surg* 1995;20:687–697.
10. Zlotogora J. On the inheritance of the split hand/split foot malformation. *Am J Med Genet* 1994;53:29–32.
11. Zguricas J, Bakker WF, Heus H, et al. Genetics of limb development and congenital hand malformations. *Plast Reconstr Surg* 1998;101:1126–1135.
12. Caldwell BD. Genetics of split hand and split foot. A case study. *J Am Podiatr Med Assoc* 1996;86:244–248.
13. Ianakiev P, Kilpatrick MW, Toudjarska I, et al. Split-hand/split-foot malformation is caused by mutations in the p63 gene on 3q27. *Am J Hum Genet* 2000;67:59–66.
14. Rodini ES, Richieri–Costa A. EEC syndrome: report on 20 new patients, clinical and genetic considerations. *Am J Med Genet* 1990;37:42–53.
15. Miller CI, Hashimoto K, Shwayder T, et al. What syndrome is this? Ectrodactyly, ectodermal dysplasia, and cleft palate (EEC) syndrome. *Pediatr Dermatol* 1997;14:239–240.
16. Tekin M, Ohle C, Johnson DE, et al. Counseling dilemmas in EEC syndrome. *Genet Couns* 2000;11:19–24.
17. van Bokhoven H, Hamel BC, Bamshad M, et al. p63 Gene mutations in EEC syndrome, limb-mammary syndrome, and isolated split hand-split foot malformation suggest a genotype-phenotype correlation. *Am J Hum Genet* 2001;69:481–492.
18. Maisels DO. Lobster-claw deformities of the hand. *Hand* 1970;2:79–82.
19. Ogino T. Teratogenic relationship between polydactyly, syndactyly and cleft hand. *J Hand Surg* 1990;15:201–209.
20. Ogino T. Cleft hand. *Hand Clin* 1990;6:661–671.
21. Ogino T. Congenital anomalies of the hand. The Asian perspective. *Clin Orthop* 1996;323:12–21.
22. Miura T, Nakamura R, Horii E. Congenital hand anomalies in Japan: a family study. *J Hand Surg* 1990;15:439–444.
23. Miura T. Clinical features of embryological failures. *Nagoya J Med Sci* 1993;56:19–26.
24. Miura T, Nakamura R, Horii E. The position of symbrachydactyly in the classification of congenital hand anomalies. *J Hand Surg* 1994;19:350–354.
25. Watari S, Hagiyama Y, Tsuge K. Recent knowledge on the cleft hand: its pathologic pattern and scope. *Hiroshima J Med Sci* 1984;33:81–100.
26. Tsuge K, Watari S. Surgical treatment of cleft hand and its associated deformities. *Bull Hosp Jt Dis Orthop Inst* 1984;44:532–541.
27. Nutt JN III, Flatt AE. Congenital central hand deficit. *J Hand Surg* 1981;6:48–60.
28. Flatt AE. *The care of congenital hand anomalies.* St. Louis: CV Mosby, 1977.

29. Giele H, Giele C, Bower C, et al. The incidence and epidemiology of congenital upper limb anomalies: a total population study. *J Hand Surg* 2001;26:628–634.

30. Imamura T, Miura T. The carpal bones in congenital hand anomalies: a radiographic study in patients older than ten years. *J Hand Surg* 1988;13:650–656.

31. Bradbury ET, Hewison J. Early parental adjustment to visible congenital disfigurement. *Child Care Health Dev* 1994;20:251–266.

32. Kay S, Bradbury E. Talking with parents and children. In: Gupta A, Kay S, Schecker L, eds. *The growing hand.* London: CV Mosby, 2000:83–87.

33. Buck-Gramcko D. Cleft hands: classification and treatment. *Hand Clin* 1985;1:467–473.

34. Glicenstein J, Guero S, Haddad R. Median clefts of the hand. Classification and therapeutic indications apropos of 29 cases. *Ann Chir Main Memb Super* 1995;14:253.

35. Rider MA, Grindel SI, Tonkin MA, et al. An experience of the Snow-Littler procedure. *J Hand Surg* 2000;25:376–381.

36. Miura T, Komada T. Simple method for reconstruction of the cleft hand with an adducted thumb. *Plast Reconstr Surg* 1979;64:65–67.

37. Sykes P, Kay S. The cleft hand. In: Gupta A, Kay S, Schecker L, eds. *The growing hand.* London: CV Mosby, 2000.

38. Berger A, Reichert B. Heterotopic finger transfer in ulnar ray deficiency associated with contralateral postaxial polydactyly: a case report. *J Reconstr Microsurg* 1993;9:27–32.

39. Upton J. Heterotopic finger transfer in ulnar ray deficiency associated with contralateral postaxial polydactyly: a case report. *J Reconstr Microsurg* 1993;9:109–110.

40. Vilkki SK. Advances in microsurgical reconstruction of the congenitally adactylous hand. *Clin Orthop* 1995;314:45–58.

87

CAMPTODACTYLY AND CLINODACTYLY

SCOTT H. KOZIN

Camptodactyly and clinodactyly are abnormal deviations of the fingers in the sagittal and coronal planes, respectively (1,2). Camptodactyly is a painless flexion contracture of the proximal interphalangeal (PIP) joint that is usually gradually progressive (3). There is no intraarticular or periarticular swelling. The metacarpophalangeal and distal interphalangeal joints are not affected, although they may develop compensatory deformities. The definition of camptodactyly has been expanded to include reducible (also known as *flexible*) and irreducible (also known as *fixed*) forms, which create disparity among reports (4,5). The physician must differentiate between flexible and fixed deformities, as different treatment algorithms apply.

CAMPTODACTYLY

Incidence

Camptodactyly is believed to occur in less than 1% of the population, although most patients are asymptomatic and may not seek medical attention (1,6). Camptodactyly is bilateral in approximately two-thirds of the cases, although the degree of contracture is usually not symmetric (Figs. 1 through 3). The fifth finger is most commonly involved (2,7). Other digits can be affected, although the incidence decreases toward the radial side of the hand (Figs. 4 and 5).

Demographics

Camptodactyly has been divided into three categories (2,8,9). A type 1 deformity is the most common form and becomes apparent during infancy. The deformity is usually an isolated finding and is limited to the fifth finger. This *congenital* form affects men and women equally. A type 2 deformity has similar clinical features, although they are not apparent until preadolescence (Figs. 1 through 3). This *acquired* form of camptodactyly develops between 7 and 11 years of age and affects women more than men (6). This type of camptodactyly usually does not improve spontaneously and may progress to a severe flexion deformity (1,10).

A type 3 deformity is often a severe deformity that usually involves multiple digits of both extremities and is associated with a variety of syndromes. The extent of involvement between hands is often asymmetric. This syndromic camptodactyly can occur in conjunction with craniofacial disorders, short stature, and chromosomal abnormalities (Figs. 6 and 7) (Table 1) (1,2,4).

Hereditary Factors

Most cases of camptodactyly are sporadic in occurrence. However, camptodactyly can be inherited and is considered an autosomal-dominant trait with variable expressivity and incomplete penetrance (3,11,12). This terminology signifies familial propagation, although the camptodactyly may skip a generation (incomplete penetrance) and may not be present in full form (variable phenotype).

Pathophysiology

The forces around the PIP joint create a balance between flexion and extension. Any slight alteration in this equilibrium generates an imbalance and leads to a deformity. In camptodactyly, this inequity can result from an increase in the flexion force or a decrease in the extension force around the PIP joint. The resultant deformity is initially passively correctable (i.e., flexible or reducible camptodactyly) but often develops into a fixed or irreducible contracture over time. This concept of imbalance of the flexion-extension forces is the basis to understanding and treating camptodactyly (10,13–15).

The exact etiology that underlies camptodactyly remains unknown, and there is no consensus about the pathogenesis of the condition. Almost every structure around the PIP joint has been implicated as the principal cause or a contributing factor in the formation of camptodactyly (3,5). Proposed skin and subcutaneous tissue changes include a deficiency or contracture within the dermis and fibrotic changes within the subcutaneous tissue or fascia, or both (16,17). Conceivable periarticular alterations consist of contractures of the collateral ligaments or the volar plate, or

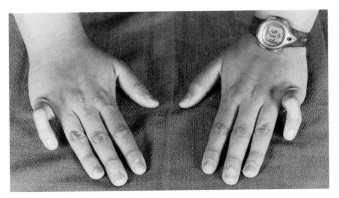

FIGURE 1. A 15-year-old girl with acquired camptodactyly that affects both small fingers.

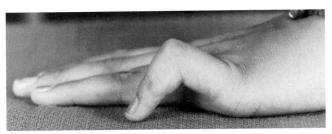

FIGURE 2. Left small finger with proximal interphalangeal flexion deformity and compensatory metacarpophalangeal hyperextension.

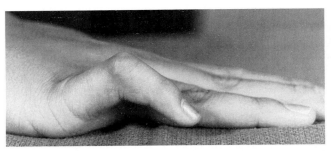

FIGURE 3. Right small finger with a lesser degree of proximal interphalangeal flexion deformity.

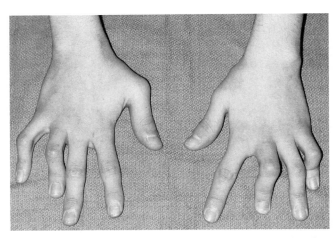

FIGURE 4. A 14-year-old patient with camptodactyly that affects both hands and multiple digits.

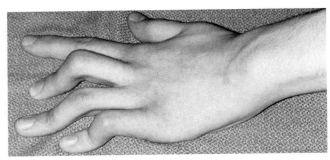

FIGURE 5. Left hand with involvement of the long, ring, and small fingers.

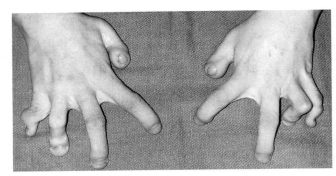

FIGURE 6. A 16-year-old patient with orofaciodigital syndrome and type 3 camptodactyly that affects both hands.

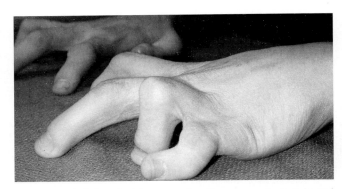

FIGURE 7. Left hand with severe ring finger camptodactyly and small finger clinodactyly.

TABLE 1. GENERALIZED CONDITIONS THAT ARE ASSOCIATED WITH CAMPTODACTYLY

Craniofacial disorders
   Orofaciodigital syndrome
   Craniocarpotarsal dystrophy (Freeman-Sheldon syndrome)
   Oculodentodigital dysplasia
Chromosomal disorders
   Trisomy 13 through 15
Short stature
   Camptomelic dysplasia type 1
   Mucopolysaccharidosis
   Facial-digital-genital (Aarskog-Scott syndrome)
Others
   Osteoonychodysostosis (Turner-Kieser syndrome)
   Cerebrohepatorenal (Zellweger syndrome)
   Jacob-Downey syndrome

both (18). Possible musculotendinous anomalies involve abnormalities of the flexor tendons, intrinsic muscles (lumbricals or interossei, or both), and extensor apparatus (3,7,13,15,16,19–25). Potential abnormalities in the restraining ligaments around the finger include anomalies of the transverse or oblique retinacular ligaments (15). Plausible bone and joint deformities include atypical configurations of the PIP joint, specifically the head of the proximal phalanx and the base of the middle phalanx (17,26). Even an abnormality within the spinal cord at the eighth cervical and first thoracic nerve segments has been implicated as a potential cause of camptodactyly (3).

The most prevalent anomalies that are associated with camptodactyly affect the flexor digitorum superficialis and intrinsic musculature (lumbricals and interossei) (3,10, 16,17,21,25). The normal flexor digitorum superficialis of the small finger has considerable structural variability (17,27,28). The flexor digitorum superficialis muscle can originate from the tendon of the ring finger flexor digitorum superficialis or as a separate muscle belly. Generally, the tendon runs parallel with the index finger flexor digitorum superficialis, although it may course adjacent to the ring flexor digitorum superficialis. Less commonly, the superficialis to the small finger may be completely absent (27). In camptodactyly, the flexor digitorum superficialis tendon has been described as contracted, underdeveloped, or devoid of a functional muscle (3,11,15,16). The tendon may originate from the palmar fascia or the transverse carpal ligament instead of a muscle belly (3,10,24,25). This abnormal musculotendinous architecture cannot elongate during periods of rapid growth (i.e., infancy and adolescence), which creates a tenodesis effect and a subsequent PIP joint flexion deformity (Fig. 8).

An aberrant lumbrical muscle has also been implicated as the principal cause of camptodactyly (4,16,21). Similar to the flexor digitorum superficialis, the normal lumbrical

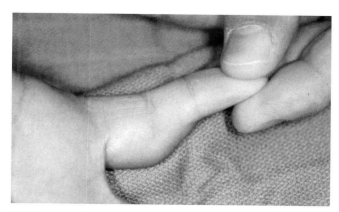

FIGURE 9. Palmar skin pterygium across camptodactyly of the small finger.

to the small finger has considerable variability (29–31). The typical insertion into the extensor apparatus was found in 60% to 72% of anatomic specimens, with an abnormal insertion recognized in 17% to 35%. Furthermore, as much as 5% of specimens lacked the lumbrical muscle altogether. In camptodactyly, the lumbrical may have an abnormal origin or insertion, although a consistent anomaly has not been reported (4,16,21,23). An abnormal origin has been reported from the transverse carpal ligament or from the ring flexor tendons (23). Aberrant insertions are more common and include an attachment directly into the metacarpophalangeal joint capsule, onto the flexor digitorum superficialis tendon, into the ring finger extensor apparatus, or within the lumbrical canal (6,7,16,21). The deficiency of the lumbrical muscles leads to an intrinsicminus deformity, which may lead to camptodactyly. This concept is supported by examination of the active PIP joint extension, with the metacarpophalangeal joint positioned in extension and flexion. In flexible camptodactyly, enhanced PIP joint extension during metacarpophalangeal joint flexion is often evident. This finding implies abnormal function of the intrinsic tendons and normal performance of the extrinsic tendons (6).

Persistent PIP joint contracture leads to secondary changes in the surrounding structures. The palmar skin may appear to bowstring across the PIP joint, similar to a pterygium (Fig. 9). Abnormal fascial bands can form beneath the skin, mimicking Dupuytren's contracture. Consequential changes in the bone and joint configuration of the PIP joint can ensue as a response to continual joint flexion (3,4,17,25).

Diagnosis

History

The type 1 or congenital form of camptodactyly presents with a flexion deformity that is noted at birth or during infancy (8,10,13). The type 2 or acquired form begins with a subtle deformity that is gradually progressive (Figs. 1

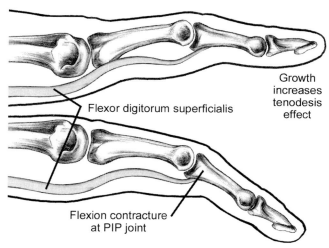

Flexor digitorum superficialis

Growth increases tenodesis effect

Flexion contracture at PIP joint

FIGURE 8. Diagram of tenodesis effect of abnormal flexor digitorum superficialis, which causes proximal interphalangeal (PIP) joint contracture during growth.

TABLE 2. DIFFERENTIAL DIAGNOSIS OF FLEXION DEFORMITIES OF THE FINGERS

Diagnosis	Distinguishing feature
Pterygium syndrome	Multiple pterygiums; usually includes the knee and elbow
Arthrogryposis	Multiple joint involvement, waxy skin and underdeveloped musculature, ulnar deviation of the digits
Symphalangism	No active or passive joint motion, absence of skin creases
Boutonnière deformity	History of trauma and pain, joint swelling, reciprocal distal interphalangeal joint hyperextension
Beals' syndrome (39,40)	Congenital contractural arachnodactyly; kyphoscoliosis; external ear deformities; flexion contractures of the proximal interphalangeal joint, elbows, knees
Marfan syndrome	Arachnodactyly without flexion contractures, loose ligaments, eye problems, dissecting aortic aneurysms
Juvenile palmar fibromatosis (mimics Dupuytren's contracture)	Metacarpophalangeal joint involvement, characteristic skin changes with nodules adherent to dermis
Trigger fingers	Metacarpophalangeal joint involvement, palpable click on finger extension
Inflammatory arthritis	Widespread joint involvement, swelling around joints or tendons

through 3). The contracture remains mild up to the age of 10 years and is rarely disabling. This small amount of flexion may go unnoticed by the patient and family, and a delay in seeking evaluation and treatment is common. Often, the specific onset of the PIP joint flexion is unknown. During the growth spurt of adolescence, the PIP flexion deformity progresses and can advance to 90 degrees (3,17,32). A gradual worsening of the PIP joint position can continue until 20 years of age (3). The main complaint of the patient and family is the angulation of the finger and the appearance of the hand. Pain is not a common complaint and may indicate an alternative diagnosis (Table 2).

The history should search for other potential causes of a PIP joint flexion deformity, such as trauma, inflammatory arthropathies, and arthrogryposis (Fig. 10). The differential diagnoses are often excluded by an astute history and thorough physical examination (Figs. 11 and 12). There is an uncommon deformity in infancy that is termed *late extenders* that can be confused with camptodactyly (33). The child cannot fully extend the PIP joint of the involved fingers, but passive motion is complete. Splint application and therapy for passive motion result in a gradual restoration of extension. These children most likely have a hypoplasia of the extensor mechanism, similar to a congenital clasped thumb.

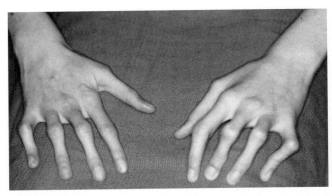

FIGURE 10. A 15-year-old girl with congenital contractural arachnodactyly that affects both hands.

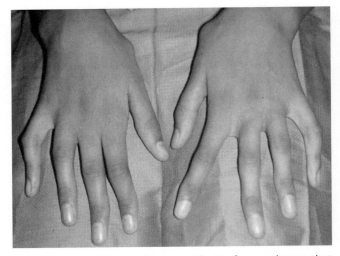

FIGURE 11. An 11-year-old girl with Marfan syndrome that appears to be similar to camptodactyly.

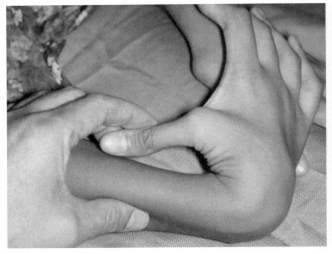

FIGURE 12. Further examination of the hand reveals excessive laxity of the soft tissues.

Examination

The preoperative status of the digit dictates the recommended treatment. The active and passive motion of the PIP joint is recorded with a goniometer. A flexible deformity must be differentiated from a fixed flexion contracture. The end feel of a contracted PIP joint that is placed in extension is fundamental information that is pertinent to the proposed treatment. A rubbery or soft end point implies probable improvement with therapeutic modalities, such as stretching and splinting. Active PIP joint flexion is preserved in camptodactyly, and the patient should be able to make a full fist.

The examination requires individual inspection and careful inventory of the potential causes for the flexion deformity. The examination begins with an inspection of the skin, including its integrity, tenseness, and presence or absence of a pterygium. Occasionally, a fascial band can be palpated beneath the skin along the palmar aspect of the proximal phalanx (16). A fixed PIP joint flexion contracture implies shortening and thickening of the flexor tendon sheath, checkrein ligaments, or volar plate, or a combination of these (34). The amount of passive PIP joint extension is assessed while varying the positions of the wrist and the metacarpophalangeal joint. Flexion of the wrist and the metacarpophalangeal joint can often increase the amount of passive PIP joint extension (Fig. 13). This finding implies tightness of the extrinsic flexors, primarily the flexor digitorum superficialis.

A flexible deformity with an extension lag indicates the possibility of attenuation of the central slip. The central slip tenodesis test is useful to determine its integrity (35). In a normal hand, simultaneous flexion of the wrist and the

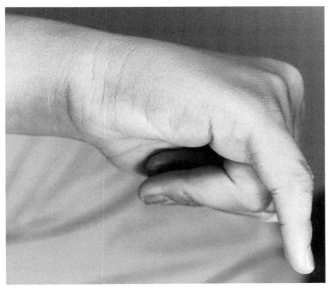

FIGURE 13. The 15-year-old patient who was depicted in Figure 1 with a decrease in proximal interphalangeal joint flexion posture during concomitant metacarpophalangeal joint flexion.

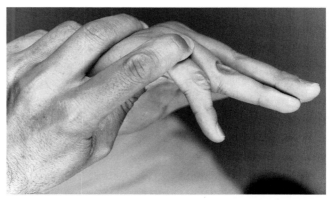

FIGURE 14. Almost full, active proximal interphalangeal joint extension is achieved when the metacarpophalangeal joint is held in flexion.

metacarpophalangeal joints results in complete PIP joint extension. An extension lag during this maneuver infers central slip attenuation that may require augmentation at the time of surgery.

The degrees of active PIP joint extension should also be assessed with the metacarpophalangeal joint positioned in extension and flexion. Compensatory metacarpophalangeal hyperextension frequently develops in response to a PIP joint that is postured in flexion (Fig. 2). Holding the joint in flexion prohibits this abnormal posture. Full active extension during metacarpophalangeal positioning implies that hyperextension of the joint is a considerable part of the problem (Fig. 14). This assessment is similar to the Bouvier's test for ulnar nerve palsy, which assesses the ability of the extrinsic extensors to achieve active PIP joint extension (36).

Isolated function of the flexor digitorum superficialis and flexor digitorum profundus to the involved digits must be assessed. The flexor digitorum superficialis of the small and ring digit can be interconnected. This anomaly prohibits independent PIP joint flexion of the small finger and is present in one-third of individuals (17). Therefore, inability to flex the PIP joint of the small finger while holding the remaining digits in full extension may not imply absence of the flexor digitorum superficialis (Fig. 15). The test should be repeated with liberation of the ring finger and a similar assessment of active PIP joint flexion (Fig. 16). This two-part evaluation prevents an erroneous conclusion regarding the absence of the flexor digitorum superficialis to the small finger. An independent flexor digitorum superficialis to the small finger is a potential donor for tendon transfer. A dependent flexor digitorum superficialis must be separated from the ring finger at the time of surgery to be a suitable donor for transfer.

X-Rays

Anteroposterior and lateral x-rays are routinely performed to assess the joint space configuration and the status of the

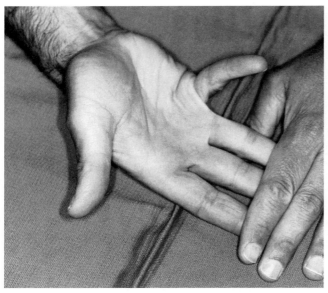

FIGURE 15. Apparent absence of the flexor digitorum superficialis function in the small finger.

surrounding bones. The lateral x-ray is the most informative view to assess abnormalities around the PIP joint (Fig. 17). In long-standing cases, the x-rays are invariably abnormal, with changes on both sides of the joint secondary to the prolonged flexion deformity (2,10,17,37). The proximal phalanx head often loses its normal convexity and appears misshapen. The flexed middle phalanx base creates an indentation along the palmar neck of the proximal pha-

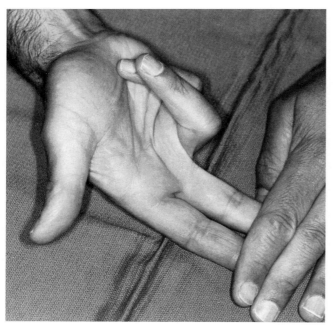

FIGURE 16. Repeat testing with liberation of the ring finger reveals the interconnection of the flexor digitorum superficialis between the ring and small fingers.

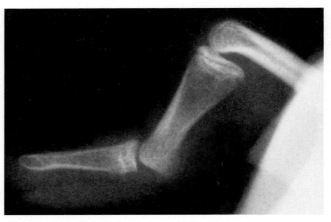

FIGURE 17. Lateral x-ray of a small finger with camptodactyly with palmar subluxation and flattening of the middle phalanx base.

lanx. The base of the middle phalanx can be subluxed in a palmar direction and may appear flat.

Differential Diagnosis

Multiple ailments present with a flexion deformity of fingers, and these diagnoses require consideration during the evaluation of a patient with suspected camptodactyly (Figs. 10 and 11) (Table 2) (1,2,4,38–40). The majority of these etiologies can be excluded by a thorough history and astute physical examination. Finger contractures that are associated with syndactyly, central deficiencies, or brachydactyly are not regarded as camptodactyly.

Treatment

Indications

Conservatism is the tenet for treatment of mild camptodactyly. A contracture of less than 30 to 40 degrees does not create a functional handicap or interfere with activity of daily living (2,3,5,25). The patient should be instructed to accept his or her deformity and to avoid surgical intervention. Static splinting at night is recommended to prevent progression of the deformity and subsequent surgical intervention. The static splint is fabricated from a thermoplastic material and is affixed to the finger with Velcro straps.

The natural history of camptodactyly is no improvement or progression of the deformity in 80% of individuals (10). Severe involvement hinders various occupational and sporting endeavors, such as using a computer keyboard, playing a musical instrument, or wearing a baseball glove (Fig. 18) (1,3). This extreme flexion warrants treatment, although restoration of full motion is not a realistic expectation or a reasonable goal. Bony changes are not a contraindication to surgery, although the expected outcome is downgraded (4).

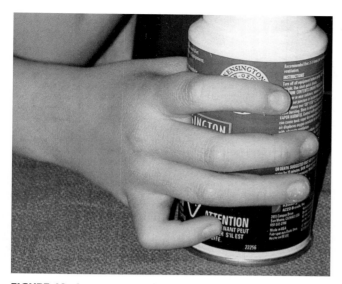

FIGURE 18. Severe camptodactyly creates difficulty in grasping large objects.

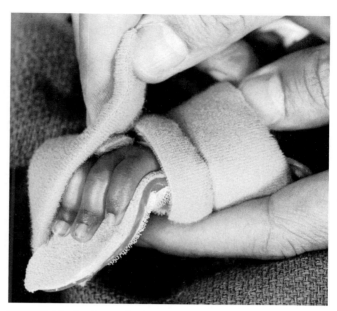

FIGURE 19. An 8-month-old patient with camptodactyly of the long, ring, and small fingers who was treated with a forearm-based splint and dorsal strap to position the proximal interphalangeal joints in less flexion.

Nonoperative

A preliminary period of nonoperative treatment is almost always attempted to resolve any fixed flexion deformity (8,15,25,41). Formal therapy is usually required to provide adequate stretching, splinting (static and dynamic), and even serial casting. A mild prolonged stretch is necessary to elongate the tight palmar structures and is followed by static splinting (8). Serial splinting or casting in incremental amounts of extension can lead to improvement of a PIP joint contracture. Dynamic splinting can be added to the treatment regimen, although static progressive splinting is often more efficacious in rigid deformities (1). In infants, the splints must be forearm based for adequate fit and to decrease the chances of removal (Fig. 19) (4). The amount of splint wear per day varies among reports concerning conservative management (15,25,41). Hori et al. (41) used dynamic splinting 24 hours per day for "a few months," followed by 8 hours per day after correction was achieved. Miura et al. (15) requested the splint to be worn "day and night" but accepted 12 hours per day in young children. Benson et al. (8) recommended 15 to 18 hours of splint wear per day in the young infant and 10 to 12 hours per day as the child grew older. Irrespective of the initial splinting regimen, part-time splinting needs to be continued for a long period of time. Complete discontinuation of the splint should be delayed until the late teens or closure of the growth plate, which indicates cessation of longitudinal growth of the finger (1,15,41).

Operative

Operative treatment is reserved for a severe deformity that has not responded to conservative management. The operative treatment of camptodactyly reflects the perceived pathol-

ogy, and multiple procedures have been recommended. Proposed surgical treatment includes division of some or all offending agents, including fascia, skin, tendons, tendon sheath, capsule, collateral ligaments (3,17,21,42); reconstruction or augmentation of the extensor mechanism (3,6,17); and bony procedures around the PIP joint (18,26).

There are numerous problems that must be addressed at the time of surgery. The first concerns are the amount of PIP joint contracture and the status of the periarticular structures. Preoperative stretching and splinting may have diminished the initial deformity, but residual contracture is common. The second issue is the altered balance around the PIP joint and the possibility of anomalous anatomy. These problems are not mutually exclusive, and both may be addressed by manipulation of similar anatomic structures. For example, a flexor digitorum superficialis transfer may relieve a PIP joint contracture and may restore balance between the flexion and extension forces.

Approach

The PIP joint can be approached by using a palmar or midlateral incision, depending on the magnitude of the contracture and the status of the skin (6). The surgeon must decide whether a local skin rearrangement (e.g., Z-plasty) is adequate to accommodate a complete extension of the PIP joint or whether a supplemental skin graft is required (Fig. 20). A palmar longitudinal approach with Z-plasty lengthening is used for a mild to moderate flexion contracture (4,16,17). A full-thicknesss skin graft is selected for a severe PIP joint contracture. The incision is extended into the palm in a zigzag fashion for complete exploration of the

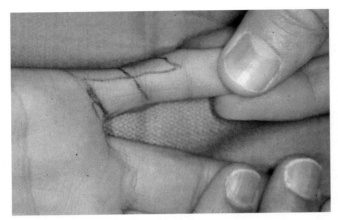

FIGURE 20. Palmar longitudinal incision that is segregated into Z-plasties for moderate camptodactyly.

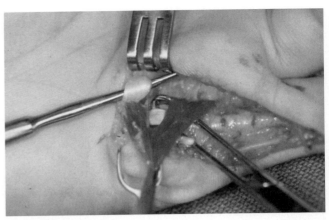

FIGURE 22. Resection of an abnormal lumbrical that is inserted into the metacarpophalangeal joint capsule.

digit. The proximal extent of the dissection ends at the transverse carpal ligament. Skin shortage within the palm is not an issue, and Z-plasty lengthening is not required. Flexible camptodactyly without a fixed flexion can be approached with a mid-lateral incision over the digit combined with a zigzag incision in the palm.

Deeper Dissection

The degree of the PIP joint contracture and the involvement of the periarticular structures dictate the extent of the release that is required. A graduated release of the offending agents is performed until adequate PIP joint extension is obtained. After the skin incision, any abnormal fascia and linear fibrous bands are released during exposure of the deeper structures (4,17). Additional release of the flexor tendon sheath, the flexor digitorum superficialis tendon, the checkrein ligaments, the collateral ligaments, and the palmar plate may be necessary to obtain sufficient extension (16,34).

The digit is explored for anomalous structures, with specific examination of the intrinsic muscles and flexor digi-

torum superficialis. Any anomalous origin or insertion of the lumbrical or interosseous muscles is resected (4,16,17). The lumbrical should be explored along its entire length to assess for any abnormality (Fig. 21). The lumbrical can insert directly into the metacarpophalangeal joint capsule, onto the flexor digitorum superficialis tendon, or into the ring finger extensor apparatus (Fig. 22). Traction to an anomalous lumbrical muscle does not result in PIP joint extension. An anomalous palmar interosseous muscle can pass into the ring finger, although partial division of the intermetacarpal ligament may be required to completely assess its course. The palmar interosseous is assessed, but diligent exploration is not always performed.

The flexor digitorum superficialis tendon is identified proximal to the first annular pulley (Fig. 23). Traction is applied to the tendon in a proximal and distal direction to assess its excursion and insertion. Deficient proximal excursion with concomitant inability to flex the PIP joint indicates abnormalities of insertion. This requires release of the flexor digitorum superficialis tendon through a third annu-

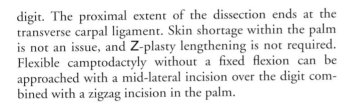

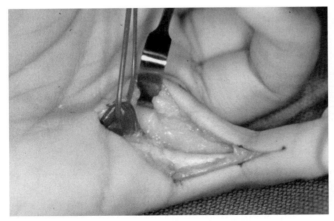

FIGURE 21. Isolation and exploration of the lumbrical to the small finger.

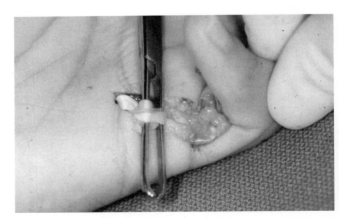

FIGURE 23. Isolation of the flexor digitorum superficialis tendon proximal to the first annular pulley and assessment of available excursion.

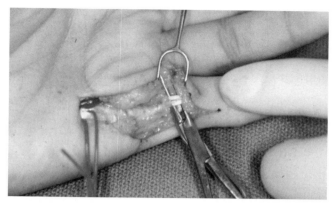

FIGURE 24. Division of the flexor digitorum superficialis through a third annular pulley window.

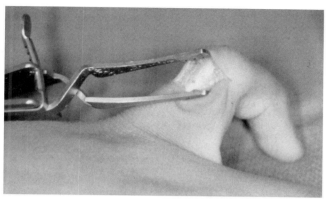

FIGURE 26. Isolation of the lateral band and the extensor mechanism.

lar pulley window. Lack of distal excursion implies proximal pathology or aplasia of the muscle and necessitates excision of the flexor digitorum superficialis. In these instances, the tendon is traced into the palm and is released from its abnormal site of origin.

Tendon Transfer

The presence of distal excursion in the flexor digitorum superficialis makes the tendon suitable for transfer. The preoperative status of the flexor digitorum superficialis is an important consideration. An independent flexor digitorum superficialis to the small finger can be transferred without further dissection. However, a dependent flexor digitorum superficialis must be separated from the ring finger to become a suitable donor for transfer. Failure to achieve independent function is a relative contraindication to transfer of the small-finger flexor digitorum superficialis tendon.

Transfer of the flexor digitorum superficialis tendon to the extensor apparatus lessens the PIP joint flexion force and augments PIP joint extension (3,4,16). The flexor digitorum superficialis tendon is transected just distal to the PIP joint through a third annular pulley window (Fig. 24).

The tendon is withdrawn into the palm proximal to the first annular pulley (Fig. 25). The lateral band and central slip are isolated over the dorsum of the digit (Fig. 26). A tendon passer is placed from dorsum of the finger into the lumbrical canal, beneath the intermetacarpal ligament, and into the palm (Figs. 27 and 28). The tendon passer is used to grasp the flexor digitorum superficialis tendon and to guide the tendon through the lumbrical canal (Figs. 29 and 30). The flexor digitorum superficialis tendon is attached to the lateral band and central slip via a weave technique. The tendon is tensioned with the metacarpophalangeal joint positioned in 30 degrees of flexion and the PIP joint held in full extension. A tendon braider facilitates the passage of the flexor digitorum superficialis tendon through the extensor mechanism. The coaptation sites are sutured with a nonabsorbable braided polyester stitch.

When the flexor digitorum superficialis tendon of the small finger is anomalous, an alternative donor for transfer is necessary. The flexor digitorum superficialis tendon from the adjacent ring finger can also be harvested and passed into the small finger extensor apparatus. In instances of multidigit camptodactyly, numerous flexor digitorum

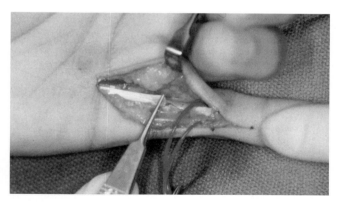

FIGURE 25. The divided flexor digitorum superficialis tendon is pulled into palm. A vessel loop is placed around the flexor digitorum profundus tendon.

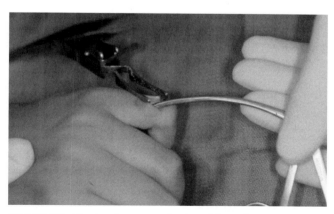

FIGURE 27. The tendon passer is placed from the extensor surface through the lumbrical canal.

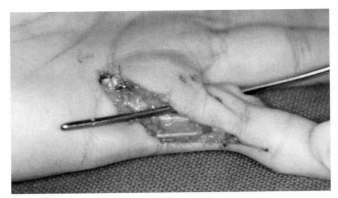

FIGURE 28. The tendon passer is positioned in the palmar incision.

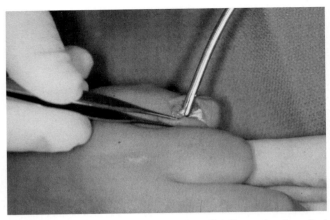

FIGURE 30. The flexor digitorum superficialis tendon is pulled through the lumbrical canal toward the extensor mechanism.

superficialis tendons can be used as donors. The flexor digitorum superficialis tendon can also be split and transferred into two adjacent digits, similar to a modified Stiles-Bunnell transfer (43).

After tendon transfer, the skin is closed using a Z-plasty or an application of a full-thickness skin graft (Fig. 31). The extremity is immobilized with the wrist in neutral, the metacarpophalangeal joints in 70 degrees of flexion, and the interphalangeal joints straight. Kirschner wire fixation of the PIP joint is controversial. Prolonged wire fixation can lead to loss of finger flexion and restricted grasp. In contrast, no internal fixation can foster early recurrence of the flexion deformity. The choice is usually made at the time of surgery and depends on the degree of preoperative PIP joint contracture, the ease of obtaining extension, and the end feel of the joint in extension (Fig. 32). If Kirschner wire fixation is chosen, the duration is limited to 3 weeks.

Alternative transfers have been described to restore PIP joint extension. The extensor indicis proprius tendon is accessible and expendable and can be rerouted through the lumbrical canal (44). The tendon is braided into the radial intrinsic or central slip, and tension is adjusted with the central slip tenodesis test.

Postoperative Care

Three weeks after surgery, the cast is removed, and the sutures are removed. A thermoplastic splint is fabricated with the wrist in neutral, the metacarpophalangeal joints in 70 degrees of flexion, and the interphalangeal joints straight. Another option is to use an ulnar wristlet sling that maintains the metacarpophalangeal joint in flexion and encourages PIP joint extension (Fig. 33) (45). The splint and the wristlet attempt to position the metacarpophalangeal joint in flexion to enable the extrinsic extensors to extend the PIP joint until the intrinsic tendon transfer is capable (Fig. 34). In addition, metacarpophalangeal joint flexion slackens the transferred flexor digitorum superficialis and protects the tendon transfer.

At this time, therapy is initiated with the focus on scar management and teaching the patient to activate the transferred tendon consistently. Scar massage should be with lotion to decrease the friction over the surgical site. The superficial (incision) and the deeper scar around the tendon transfer should be addressed. If the patient appears to have

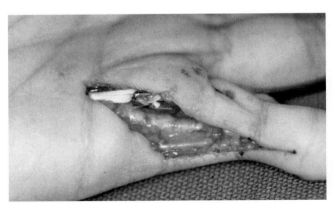

FIGURE 29. The tendon passer grasps the flexor digitorum superficialis tendon.

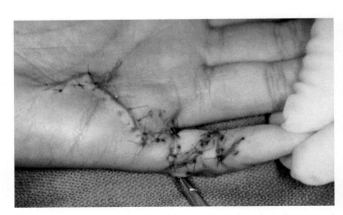

FIGURE 31. Z-plasty closure after camptodactyly release and reconstruction.

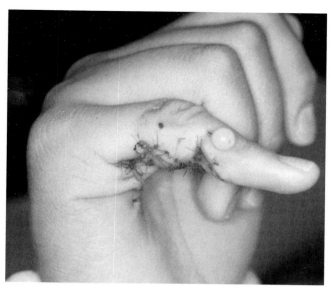

FIGURE 32. Kirschner wire fixation after proximal interphalangeal joint release and flexor digitorum superficialis tendon transfer.

signs of hypertrophy of the incision, the therapist may consider the use of supplemental products, such as a silicone gel or elastomer pad. This treatment provides prolonged pressure and may facilitate better organization of collagen (46,47). Ultrasound is another modality that can encourage tissue mobilization, although this technique is usually reserved for recalcitrant scar formation after the tendon transfer has healed (6 to 7 weeks after surgery).

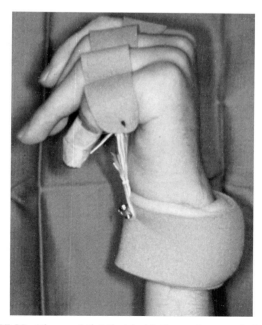

FIGURE 33. Ulnar wristlet that holds the metacarpophalangeal joint in flexion. The distal interphalangeal joint is splinted to concentrate the flexor digitorum profundus action on proximal interphalangeal joint flexion.

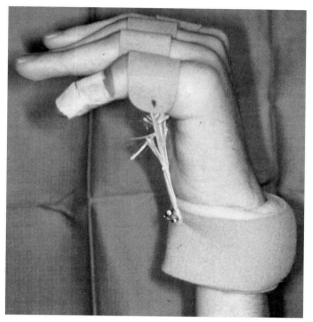

FIGURE 34. The ulnar wristlet positions the metacarpophalangeal joint in flexion to protect the intrinsic transfer and to allow extrinsic proximal interphalangeal joint extension.

Early tendon gliding is the most efficacious method to prevent deep scar formation that can limit motion. The patient must learn to consistently fire the transferred muscle without compensatory motion from adjacent musculature. During the first several days, the therapist attempts to palpate an isolated contraction of the transfer in an antigravity plane. The connection is often taught by having the patient complete the original function of the transferred muscle in an isometric manner. For example, the patient may be cued to attempt isolated PIP joint flexion of the donor digit, which should activate the flexor digitorum superficialis tendon and should yield PIP joint extension. If the patient is unable to isolate the transfer, biofeedback may be helpful in the reeducation process. As the patient achieves a consistent contraction, therapy may progress to functional activities that use PIP joint extension.

During week 6, the patient may engage in some light resistive strengthening. If the patient is firing the transfer, the splint may be removed during the day except during strenuous activity that places the tendon transfer at risk for rupture. During weeks 7 and 8, more resistance may be added to the strengthening program. The intrinsic transfer should be protected for at least 12 weeks after surgery (6,45). Subsequently, the splint is discontinued for all activity, and unrestricted use is allowed. Prolonged nighttime splinting until the late teens is required to prevent recurrence (15).

Salvage Procedures

Severe flexion deformity of the PIP joint with secondary bony changes is often not amenable to contracture release and tendon transfer. In these instances, bony realignment is the only method to correct the excessive flexion. This adjustment can be made by a dorsal closing wedge osteotomy of the proximal phalanx or a PIP joint fusion (chondrodesis or arthrodesis). The osteotomy corrects the posture of the finger and shifts the arc of motion. The overall amount of PIP joint motion remains unchanged, which results in loss of full flexion and impaired grasp (2,26).

A PIP joint chondrodesis or arthrodesis can also be used to reposition the finger into a better alignment, although any remaining motion is sacrificed. A chondrodesis requires removal of the cartilage from the proximal phalanx head and the base of the middle phalanx. The physis of the middle phalanx is preserved to allow continued longitudinal growth. The PIP joint is placed in approximately 40 degrees of flexion, and percutaneous Kirschner wires are placed for internal fixation. An arthrodesis is performed in a similar fashion without preservation of the growth plate. Additional options for internal fixation are available, including tension band, interosseous wire, or screw (48–52).

Outcome

Camptodactyly is difficult to treat and even more difficult to consistently achieve successful results. McCarroll (5) noted different preoperative findings among outcome reports after surgical reconstruction of camptodactyly. The most noteworthy differences concerned the presence or absence of a fixed PIP joint flexion deformity and the amount of active extension of the PIP joint when the metacarpophalangeal joint is positioned in flexion. In addition, many reports combine different types of camptodactyly into a single cohort, which confounds the outcome after treatment. These considerable differences obscure the surgical results, as fundamental differences in pathoanatomy may be present before the procedure.

Conservative treatment with splinting and passive stretching has resulted in an improvement in the amount of PIP joint contracture (8,15,25,41). Supervised therapy and a compliant patient are prerequisites to implementation of conservative management. The best results are obtained in a well-motivated patient with a mild deformity (25). Prolonged diligent splinting is necessary to achieve a satisfactory outcome. Hori et al. (41) reported on 24 patients (34 fingers) with small finger camptodactyly who were treated with a splinting regimen. The splints were worn 24 hours per day until adequate correction was obtained, followed by 8 hours per day until maturity. The average follow-up time was almost 4 years. Twenty fingers had almost full extension, nine had improved extension, three were unchanged, and two fingers were worse. The average flexion contracture improved from 40 to 10 degrees after treatment.

Benson et al. (8) treated 22 patients (59 digits) with a therapy program and reported their results at a mean follow-up of 33 months. Type 1 or infantile camptodactyly (13

patients or 24 PIP joints) improved from a 23-degree flexion contracture to 4 degrees shy of full extension. Type 2 or adolescent camptodactyly (four patients or five PIP joints) were relatively noncompliant with therapy and achieved minimal correction. Two patients underwent an attempt at surgical correction, and both digressed after the procedure, with a worsening of the PIP joint contracture. Type 3 camptodactyly (five patients or 30 PIP joints) possessed a diverse amount of deformity. Twelve PIP joints lacked at least 15 degrees of extension and improved to an average of 1 degree shy of full extension after the splinting protocol.

Multiple surgical procedures have been reported for camptodactyly. The technique is variable, and the results are scattered with respect to outcome. Smith and Kaplan (3) performed an isolated tenotomy of the flexor digitorum superficialis at the wrist or the hand in 12 fingers with camptodactyly. The site of transection had no effect on the amount of correction that was achieved. The flexion deformity decreased by at least 33% in all fingers without a loss in finger flexion strength. Unfortunately, the exact amount of PIP joint flexion is not discussed.

Jones et al. (6) reported on a small cohort of six patients who underwent severance of the flexor digitorum superficialis combined with transfer of the tendon to the extensor apparatus. The residual PIP joint contracture averaged 15 degrees (with a range from 0 to 25 degrees) without mention of any sacrifice in flexion.

Engber and Flatt (10) analyzed the treatment of camptodactyly in 66 patients. Thirty-four patients were evaluated only once and were excluded from the follow-up data. Fourteen patients were treated without surgery by various forms of stretching and splinting. Six patients improved, and eight progressed despite conservative treatment. Corrective and salvage types of surgery were performed on 24 hands to lessen the contracture. Twenty hands underwent release of the palmar structures with or without transfer of the flexor digitorum superficialis. Seven hands improved, six remained the same, and seven worsened after surgery. Slightly better results were noted when the flexor digitorum superficialis was transferred. Four hands underwent osteotomy or arthrodesis to better align the finger. The authors concluded that surgical intervention is not uniformly satisfying.

Siegart et al. (25) reviewed 57 patients with "simple" camptodactyly, although multiple digital involvement was common. Thirty-eight fingers were treated with surgery, and 41 digits were treated by therapy. Seven patients were unavailable for follow-up evaluation. The remaining patients had a mean follow-up of more than 6 years. Surgery consisted of release of the contracted structures with or without transfer of the flexor digitorum superficialis. Abnormalities of the lumbrical muscle were found in two patients, whereas eight patients had anomalies of the flexor digitorum superficialis. In ten patients, the PIP joint was pinned in extension. The results were classified according to the ultimate improvement in PIP joint extension without a

TABLE 3. CLASSIFICATION OF OUTCOME AFTER TREATMENT FOR CAMPTODACTYLY

Classification	Criteria
Excellent	Correction to full extension with less than 15 degrees of loss of PIP joint flexion
Good	Correction to within 20 degrees of full PIP joint extension or a more than 40-degree increase in PIP joint extension, with less than 30 degrees of loss of flexion
Fair	Correction to within 40 degrees of full PIP joint extension or a more than 20-degree increase in PIP joint extension, with less than 45 degrees of loss of flexion
Poor	Less than 20 degrees of improvement in PIP joint extension or less than 40 degrees of total PIP joint motion

PIP, proximal interphalangeal.
Adapted from Siegert JJ, Cooney WP, Dobyns JH. Management of simple camptodactyly. *J Hand Surg* 1990;15:181–189.

simultaneous loss of flexion (Table 3). In the operative group, there were 25 poor, six fair, seven good, and no excellent results. The overall improvement in extension was only 10 degrees, and ten patients lost a significant amount of flexion. An additional six patients developed ankylosis of the PIP joint. In the conservative group, there were six poor, eight fair, 27 good, and no excellent results. Seigart et al. (25) concluded that camptodactyly appears superficially to be a simple problem. In reality, however, it is a "long-term and frustrating problem to both patient and doctor."

Ogino and Kato (24) encountered 35 cases of camptodactyly over a 14-year period. Surgical treatment was performed on six patients after failure of conservative treatment and a strong patient desire. The flexor digitorum superficialis was hypoplastic in five patients, without proximal continuity to its muscle belly. Preoperative active extension deficit averaged 71 degrees, and active flexion averaged 93 degrees. At a mean follow-up of 27.5 months, the active extension deficit improved to 23 degrees, and flexion diminished to an average of 80 degrees. The amount of PIP joint flexion contracture reduced from a mean of 57.5 degrees to 16 degrees.

McFarlane et al. (16,21) are fervent supporters of abnormalities within the intrinsic system as the principal defect that underlies camptodactyly. A series of 53 surgical patients were assessed for preoperative, operative, and postoperative data to ascertain the cause of deformity and the results of treatment. An abnormal lumbrical muscle was found in all cases, and flexor digitorum superficialis anomalies were also noted in nearly one-half of the patients. These abnormalities were found to be interdependent, and each had an adverse effect on outcome. Overall, the PIP joint contracture improved from 49 degrees to 25 degrees. The return of finger flexion was prolonged, and only 33% of the patients regained full flexion at 1 year. Positive predictors of outcome

were a PIP joint contracture of less than 45 degrees and independent flexor digitorum superficialis function.

Smith et al. (17) assessed the surgical management of camptodactyly in a cohort of 16 patients (18 fingers) who were followed for a mean of 2.8 years (with a range from 8 months to 9 years). A unified surgical approach was applied to the majority of patients with a graduated release of contracted structures and a thorough assessment for anomalous elements. The results were classified according to Siegart et al. (25) with inclusion of parameters for extension and flexion (Table 3). Excellent or good results were reported in 15 fingers or 83% (six excellent and nine good). Two fingers were rated as fair, one was poor, and all had preoperative bony deformities. These satisfactory results are in direct contrast to the series that was reported by Seigart et al. (25). The dissimilar outcome between these series is difficult to explain but may be related to different durations of follow-up, patient compliance, underlying pathoanatomy, and surgical technique.

Koman et al. (13) reported on eight patients who were seen at birth with severe flexion deformities of multiple digits (27 fingers) without a predilection for the small finger. This cohort is distinctly different from other reports of camptodactyly. Many of these children had associated anomalies, including two children with arthrogryposis and one with Marfan syndrome. All patients underwent initial hand therapy and splinting. Surgery was performed on six children (20 digits) between 13 months and 8.5 years of age. Follow-up on all patients was longer than 2 years. Eight digits had surgery that was limited to the palmar aspect, with release of the contracted structures and lengthening of the flexor digitorum superficialis. Twelve digits had surgery on the palmar side, combined with reconstruction of the extensor mechanism on the dorsal surface. Reconstruction was performed by lateral band realignment and transfer of the flexor digitorum superficialis. No improvement was noted in the eight digits that underwent an isolated palmar approach. Ten of the 12 fingers that had a combined approach demonstrated less than 20 degrees of residual flexion deformity and a "functional" grasp and release. This group of children represents a subset of camptodactyly that appears to benefit from extensor mechanism reconstruction by lateral band realignment and transfer of the flexor digitorum superficialis to augment intrinsic power.

Complications

Surgery for camptodactyly is fraught with early and late complications. A higher incidence of surgical complications occurs in severe camptodactyly with a fixed deformity. Release of these contracted fingers can result in injury to the neurovascular structures from laceration, tension during extension of the digit, or subsequent scarring (25). Skin slough is also more common in digits with considerable contracture. After skin loss, exposure of the tendon may require valiant techniques for coverage, such as a cross-finger flap. These complications often have a deleterious effect on outcome.

Loss of motion after surgery is a serious concern and can be limited by diligent postoperative care. Release of the flexor digitorum superficialis tendon violates the tendon sheath and leads to scar formation. Immediate distal interphalangeal motion prevents adhesion formation around the flexor digitorum profundus tendon (4). A confounding factor occurs when a concomitant PIP joint release is required, which is notorious for loss of motion. To lessen the chances of losing flexion, the duration of PIP joint immobilization should be limited to 3 weeks. Lack of full extension is better tolerated than deficient flexion, and early mobilization fosters restoration of flexion (17). Despite early motion of the flexor digitorum profundus and the PIP joint, return of flexion is slow and may take 6 to 12 months (16). A small residual flexion deficit is common, but this amount must be minimized to prevent impairment in grasp. Complete ankylosis of the PIP joint has been reported after camptodactyly reconstruction (10,25). This complication is associated with attempts at remodeling the joint surface, which should be avoided (10).

CLINODACTYLY

Clinodactyly is more common than camptodactyly but is less problematic. The abnormal deviation is in the coronal or radioulnar plane (1,53). Clinodactyly typically affects the small-finger distal interphalangeal joint, and the deviation is usually in a radial direction (Fig. 35). A deviation of less than 10 degrees is so common that it may be considered normal (1,53). On occasion, clinodactyly can involve

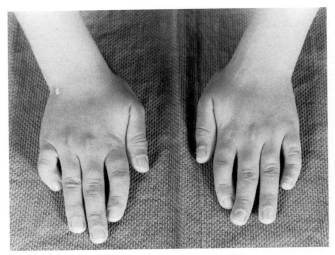

FIGURE 36. Clinodactyly that affects both hands and multiple digits.

several digits (Fig. 36). The deformity is usually fixed, and there is no intraarticular or periarticular swelling.

Incidence and Demographics

Clinodactyly is reported to occur between 1.0% and 19.5% of normal children, and most are bilateral (1,54). The exact incidence is probably higher, as most patients are asymptomatic and do not seek medical attention. Clinodactyly can be inherited and is considered an autosomal-dominant trait with variable expressivity and incomplete penetrance (53,54). Clinodactyly is also associated with many syndromes and chromosomal abnormalities, most notably Down syndrome, with an incidence between 35% and 79% (1,55–58). Thumb clinodactyly is also a prominent feature of Apert's syndrome (59), Rubinstein-Taybi syndrome (60), diastrophic dwarfism (61), and triphalangeal thumbs (Fig. 37) (62).

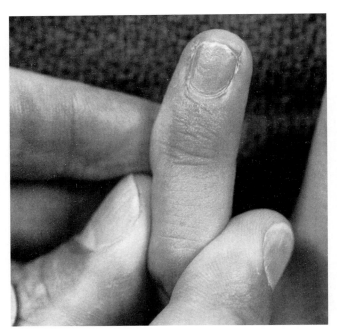

FIGURE 35. Clinodactyly of the small finger with radial deviation of the distal interphalangeal joint.

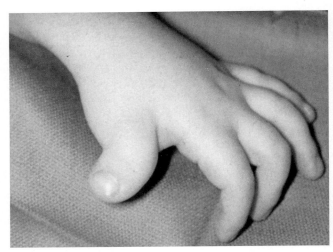

FIGURE 37. A 5-year-old patient with Rubinstein-Taybi syndrome and associated thumb clinodactyly.

Pathophysiology

The normal alignment of the interphalangeal joints is perpendicular to the long axis of the bone. Clinodactyly is a deviation from this normal orientation. Typical clinodactyly is caused by malalignment of the distal interphalangeal joint that is attributed to inclination of the middle phalanx articular surface (1,53). The fact that the middle phalanx is the last phalanx to ossify may be a factor in its involvement in clinodactyly.

Abnormal deviation of a digit can be caused by other pathology. An anomalous orientation of the growth plate can alter the configuration of the phalanx and can cause coronal deviation of the finger (1,63). This condition is known as a *delta phalanx*, a *longitudinal bracketed diaphysis*, or a *longitudinal epiphyseal bracket*. This entity must be considered during the evaluation of a child with clinodactyly.

Classification

Clinodactyly has been classified according to the extent of the deformity and the presence or absence of associated findings (Table 4) (64). The complicated cases often have a concomitant rotational deformity (Fig. 38).

Diagnosis

History

Typical clinodactyly presents with radial deviation of the small finger, which is noted at birth or during infancy (Fig. 35). The primary complaint of the patient and family is often related to the appearance of the finger rather than a functional problem. A thorough history is necessary to ensure that this represents an isolated anomaly and is not part of a syndrome.

Examination

The angulation of the distal interphalangeal joint is measured with a goniometer. The active and passive motion of

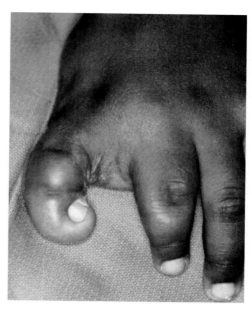

FIGURE 38. An 8-year-old patient with complicated clinodactyly that is attributed to underlying macrodactyly.

the distal interphalangeal joint is assessed and recorded. The deformity is usually fixed, and only slight passive correction is achievable via opening of the joint space. The other fingers and thumb are assessed for coronal deviation or additional anomalies.

X-Rays

X-rays of the affected part are a routine component of the evaluation. The alignment of the digits and the configuration of the bony constituents are assessed. An inclination of the middle phalanx articular surface is characteristic of typical or simple clinodactyly. However, the surrounding bones are scrutinized for anomalies that may contribute to the malalignment. A longitudinal epiphyseal bracket (also known as a *delta phalanx* or a *longitudinal bracketed diaphysis*) tends to occur in the phalanges (Fig. 39) (1,64,65). The longitudinal epiphyseal bracket represents a functioning physis and epiphysis along the side of the phalanx that courses in a proximal-to-distal direction. The surface that overlies the longitudinal physis is covered by articular cartilage, and active enchondral ossification occurs along the involved side of the phalanx (63). The abnormal growth plate may bracket part of or the entire phalanx. This orientation prevents appropriate longitudinal growth of the finger and may promote progressive angulation.

The longitudinal epiphyseal bracket is highly variable in morphology, and, before ossification of the epiphysis, the ultimate shape of the phalanx and the extent of the abnormal epiphysis and physis cannot be determined (53,63). Successive x-ray films reveal the specific configuration of the bone and growth plate. The longitudinal epiphyseal bracket tends to be C-shaped and is situated along the

TABLE 4. CLASSIFICATION OF CLINODACTYLY

Classification	Criteria
Simple	Bony deformity of middle phalanx with less than 45 degrees of angulation (with a range from 15 to 45 degrees)
Simple complicated	Bony deformity of middle phalanx with greater than 45 degrees of angulation (with a range from 45 to 60 degrees)
Complex	Bony and soft tissue deformity with less than 45 degrees of angulation (with a range from 15 to 45 degrees, with syndactyly)
Complex complicated	Bony and soft tissue deformity with 45 to 60 degrees of angulation with polydactyly or gigantism

Adapted from Cooney WP. Camptodactyly and clinodactyly. In: Carter P, ed. *Reconstruction of the child's hand*. Philadelphia: Lea & Febiger, 1991.

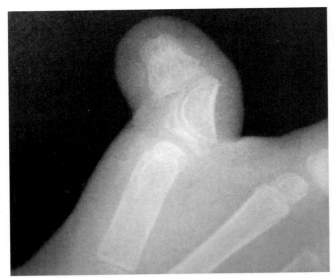

FIGURE 39. Thumb clinodactyly that is secondary to a longitudinal epiphyseal bracket.

shorter side of the bone (63). Magnetic resonance imaging can be used for early delineation of the longitudinal epiphyseal bracket (Fig. 40).

Treatment

Indications

Conservatism and observation are the mainstays of treatment for simple camptodactyly. Mild and moderate forms of clinodactyly do not require surgery. Corrective procedures are reserved for severe angulation with digital overlap during fist formation. Clinodactyly that is secondary to a delta phalanx requires treatment that is directed toward the abnormal growth plate (63,66,67). Clinodactyly that is associated with syndactyly, polydactyly, or macrodactyly necessitates treatment of the primary malformation (Fig. 38).

Nonoperative

In contrast to camptodactyly, splinting is not recommended for clinodactyly (1,53,63). The underlying deformity is a bony malformation, and it is unlikely that splinting would impart any benefit. In complex clinodactyly that is attributed to a longitudinal epiphyseal bracket, progressive angulation can occur over time. However, the rate of development and the magnitude of the deformity are unpredictable. This variation is related to the growth potential within the cells and the morphology of the bracket (63). Therefore, observation of the digit is preferred until progressive angulation is demonstrated or until skeletal maturity is reached.

Operative

Operative treatment is reserved for a severe deformity that interferes with function. The basic treatment is an osteotomy of the middle phalanx to realign the digit. A variety of surgical techniques have been described to complete this task. The exact procedure depends on the underlying etiology, the amount of deformity, the status of the soft tissues, and the surgeon's preference.

In simple uncomplicated clinodactyly, a closing wedge osteotomy provides ample correction of the deformity (Fig. 41). The wedge is removed from the middle phalanx along the convex side of the deformity. A mid-lateral approach

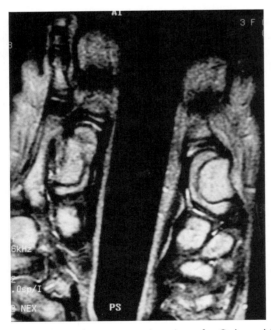

FIGURE 40. Magnetic resonance imaging of a C-shaped longitudinal epiphyseal bracket that involves both metatarsals.

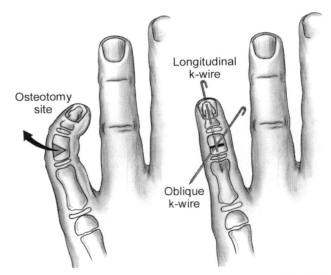

FIGURE 41. Diagram of osteotomy along the convex side of the middle phalanx to realign the digit. k-wire, Kirschner wire.

with elevation of the extensor apparatus allows adequate exposure of the middle phalanx. The wedge is configured with the base along the ulnar border of the finger and the apex along the radial edge. The amount of wedge resection can be planned before surgery or can be determined at the time of surgery. During surgery, a 0.035-in. Kirschner wire is drilled perpendicular to the shaft at the proposed osteotomy site in the diaphysis. A 25-gauge needle is placed into the distal interphalangeal joint in the coronal plane. The angle between the Kirschner wire and the needle subtends the configuration of the wedge. A second Kirschner wire is placed retrograde from the fingertip into the distal phalanx and across the distal interphalangeal joint. This wire serves as a joystick in the distal fragment and provides fixation after wedge osteotomy. The positions of the Kirschner wires and needle are confirmed by mini fluoroscopy.

The osteotomy is performed with a bone biter or small oscillating saw. The saw must have a fine kerf to prevent excessive bone removal. The first cut is performed along the Kirschner wire and is advanced two-thirds through the middle phalanx. The transverse Kirschner wire is removed. A second cut is carried out parallel to the needle, such that the wedge meets along the radial border of the digit. The periosteum and a portion of the cortex along the radial side are not disrupted to preserve some stability. The wedge of bone is removed, and the finger is angulated into ulnar deviation. This maneuver cracks the remaining radial cortex and aligns the finger. The longitudinal Kirschner wire is advanced across the osteotomy site to provide provisional stability. The position of the longitudinal Kirschner wire, the alignment of the digit, and the status of the osteotomy site are verified by mini fluoroscopy. Additional stability can be obtained by placement of a second Kirschner wire in an oblique direction.

In simple complicated clinodactyly, the amount of wedge resection can result in an excessive amount of shortening. An opening wedge osteotomy can be performed along the concave side to lengthen the digit (Fig. 42). The skin may require Z-plasty lengthening to accommodate the increase in length. This type of osteotomy is considerably more difficult than a closing wedge.

In complicated clinodactyly, the underlying malformation must be addressed. Syndactyly, polydactyly, and macrodactyly have their individual treatment regimens that manage the bone and soft tissue anomalies. Clinodactyly that is secondary to a longitudinal epiphyseal bracket is the most common cause of complicated syndactyly. Multiple procedures have been proposed to correct the underlying physeal abnormality (Fig. 43). In general, the longitudinal epiphysis is cut, and the growth plate along the convex side of the bone is ablated. The horizontal portion of the epiphysis must be preserved to allow for longitudinal growth. In mild deformities, a closing wedge osteotomy of the phalanx can be performed to realign the digit. An opening wedge provides simultaneous lengthen-

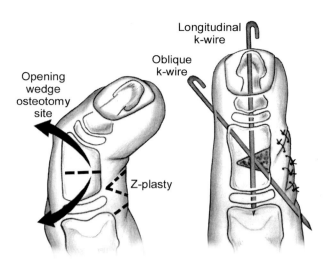

FIGURE 42. Diagram of opening wedge osteotomy and Z-plasty of the skin to correct clinodactyly and to preserve length. k-wire, Kirschner wire.

ing of the digit, and an autograft or allograft can be placed into the defect. A reversed wedge graft has also been described, which resects a wedge from the convex side and inserts the segment into the concave side (66). An opening or reverse wedge can lead to fusion of the graft across the horizontal portion of the epiphysis. This results in a physeal bar with partial or complete growth arrest and a recurrent angular deformity or a shortened digit. Irrespec-

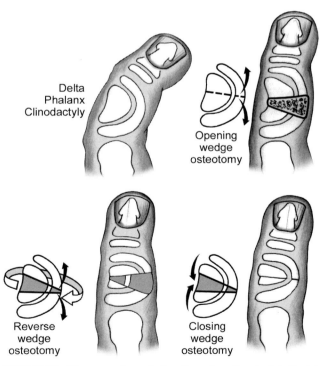

FIGURE 43. Diagram of surgical options for clinodactyly that is secondary to a longitudinal epiphyseal bracket.

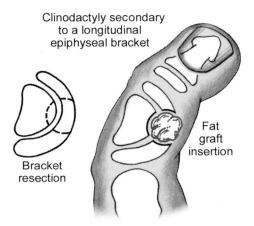

Clinodactyly secondary
to a longitudinal
epiphyseal bracket

Fat
graft
insertion

Bracket
resection

FIGURE 44. Diagram of a resection of the longitudinal growth plate and fat graft insertion for clinodactyly that results from a longitudinal epiphyseal bracket.

tive of the type of osteotomy, Kirschner wires are used for internal fixation until union.

A prophylactic procedure has been described for young children with progressive deformity (63, 67). The operation is performed when the child is approximately 3 years of age. A mid-lateral approach along the digit provides exposure to the apex of the longitudinal epiphyseal bracket. The longitudinal portion of the bracket is excised, and a fat graft is inserted to cover the ends of the split physis (Fig. 44). Over time, the digit gradually straightens as growth of the digit occurs through the horizontal portions of the growth plate.

Complications

Simple clinodactyly that is treated by wedge resection is a relatively straightforward operation. A closing wedge osteotomy can disturb the surrounding tendons and can cause adhesions around the tendons. The resultant limitation of motion can hinder hand function. In addition, the extensor tendons do not tolerate substantial shortening, and an extension lag can develop at the distal interphalangeal joint.

Surgery for complicated clinodactyly is more prone to problems. The longitudinal epiphyseal bracket is a difficult condition to treat. A misplaced osteotomy can inadvertently injure the horizontal portion of the growth plate, which leads to a growth disturbance and a shortened digit.

REFERENCES

1. Flatt AE. Crooked fingers. In: Flatt AE, ed. *The care of congenital hand anomalies*, 2nd ed. St. Louis: Quality Medical Publishers, 1994:47–63.
2. Senrui H. Congenital contractures. In: Buck-Gramcko D, ed. *Congenital malformations of the hand and forearm.* London: Churchill Livingstone, 1998:295–309.
3. Smith RJ, Kaplan EB. Camptodactyly and similar atraumatic flexion deformities of the proximal interphalangeal joints of the fingers. *J Bone Joint Surg* 1968;50:1187–1203.
4. Kay SP. Camptodactyly. In: Green DP, Hotchkiss RN, Pederson WC, eds. *Green's operative hand surgery,* 4th ed. Philadelphia: Churchill Livingstone, 1999:510–517.
5. McCarroll HR. Congenital anomalies: a 25-year overview. *J Hand Surg* 2000;25:1007–1037.
6. Jones KG, Marmor L, Lankford LL. An overview on new procedures in surgery of the hand. *Clin Orthop* 1974;99:154–167.
7. Courtemanche AD. Campylodactyly: etiology and management. *Plast Reconstr Surg* 1969;44:451–454.
8. Benson LS, Waters PM, Kamil NI, et al. Camptodactyly: classification and results of nonoperative treatment. *J Pediatr Orthop* 1994;14:814–819.
9. Weber FP. A note on camptodactylia (Landouzy) and Dupuytren's condition. *Med Press Circ* 1947;217:453–454.
10. Engber WD, Flatt AE. Camptodactyly: an analysis of sixty-six patients and twenty-four operations. *J Hand Surg* 1977;2:216–224.
11. Scott J. Hammer-finger with notes of seven cases occurring in one family. *Glasgow Med J* 1903;60:335–344.
12. Welch JP, Temtamy SA. Hereditary contractures of the fingers (camptodactyly). *J Med Genet* 1966;3:104–113.
13. Koman LA, Toby EB, Poehling GG. Congenital flexion deformities of the proximal interphalangeal joint in children: a subgroup of camptodactyly. *J Hand Surg* 1990;15:582–586.
14. Millesi H. Camptodactyly. In: Littler JW, Cramer LM, Smith JW, eds. *Symposium on reconstructive hand surgery.* St. Louis: CV Mosby, 1974:175–177.
15. Miura T, Nakamura R, Tamura Y. Long-standing extended dynamic splintage and release of an abnormal restraining structure in camptodactyly. *J Hand Surg* 1992;17:665–672.
16. McFarlane RM, Classen DA, Porte AM, et al. The anatomy and treatment of camptodactyly of the small finger. *J Hand Surg* 1992;17:35–44.
17. Smith PJ, Grobbelaar AO. Camptodactyly: a unifying theory and approach to surgical treatment. *J Hand Surg* 1998;23:14–19.
18. Fèvre M. Les locages tendineux digitaux. (Doigts à resort et flexions des doigts par blocages tendineux dans les gaines digitales.) *Rev Orthop* 1936;23:137–142.
19. Inoue G, Tamura Y. Camptodactyly resulting from paradoxical action of an anomalous lumbrical muscle. *Scand J Plast Reconstr Hand Surg* 1994;28:309–312.
20. Magnusson R. La camptodactylie. *Acta Chir Scand* 1942;87:236–242.
21. McFarlane RM, Curry GI, Evans HB. Anomalies of the intrinsic muscles in camptodactyly. *J Hand Surg* 1983;8:531–544.
22. Millesi H. Zur Behandlung der Kamptodaktylie. *Klin Med* 1966;21:329–335.
23. Minami A, Sakai T. Camptodactyly caused by abnormal insertion and origin of lumbrical muscle. *J Hand Surg* 1993;18:310–311.
24. Ogino T, Kato H. Operative findings in camptodactyly of the little finger. *J Hand Surg* 1992;17:661–664.

25. Siegert JJ, Cooney WP, Dobyns JH. Management of simple camptodactyly. *J Hand Surg* 1990;15:181–189.

26. Oldfield MC. Campylodactyly: flexor contracture of the fingers in young girls. *Br J Plast Surg* 1956;8:312–317.

27. Furnas DW. Muscle-tendon variations in the flexor compartment of the wrist. *Plast Reconstruct Surg* 1965;36:320–324.

28. Shrewsbury MM, Kuczynski K. Flexor digitorum superficialis in the fingers of the human hand. *Hand* 1974;6:121–133.

29. Basu SS, Hazary S. Variations of the lumbrical muscles of the hand. *Anat Rec* 1960;136:501–504.

30. Eyler DL, Markee JE. The anatomy and function of the intrinsic musculature of the fingers. *J Bone Joint Surg* 1954;36:1–9.

31. Mehta HJ, Gardner WU. A study of lumbrical muscles in the human hand. *Am J Anat* 1961;109:227–238.

32. Adams W. On congenital contraction of the fingers and its association with "hammer-toe"; its pathology and treatment. *Lancet* 1891;2:111–114,165–168.

33. Barton NE. Late extenders. In: *Hand correspondence newsletter.* Rosemont, IL: American Society for Surgery of the Hand, 1999:43.

34. Curtis RM. Capsulectomy of the interphalangeal joints of the fingers. *J Bone Joint Surg* 1954;36:1219–1232.

35. Smith PJ, Ross DA. The central slip tenodesis test for early diagnosis of potential boutonnière deformities. *J Hand Surg* 1994;19:88–90.

36. Omer GE Jr. Ulnar nerve palsy. In: Green DP, Hotchkiss RN, eds. *Green's operative hand surgery,* 3rd ed. Philadelphia: Churchill Livingstone, 1993:1449–1466.

37. Currarino G, Waldman I. Camptodactyly. *Am J Roentgenol* 1964;92:1312–1321.

38. Beals RK, Hecht F. Congenital contractural arachnodactyly. A heritable disorder of connective tissue. *J Bone Joint Surg* 1971;53:987–993.

39. Ogino T, Kato H, Ohshio I, et al. Clinical features of congenital contractural arachnodactyly. *Congen Anom* 1993;33:85–94.

40. Zancolli E, Zancolli E Jr. Congenital ulnar drift of the fingers. Pathogenesis, classification, and surgical management. *Hand Clin* 1985;1:443–456.

41. Hori M, Nakura R, Inoue G, et al. Nonoperative treatment of camptodactyly. *J Hand Surg* 1987;12:1061–1065.

42. Hefner RA. Inheritance of crooked little finger (streblomicrodactyly). *J Hered* 1929;20:395–398.

43. Smith RJ. *Tendon transfers of the hand and forearm.* Boston: Little, Brown and Company, 1987:253–254.

44. Gupta A, Burke FD. Correction of camptodactyly. *J Hand Surg* 1990;15:168–170.

45. Smith RJ. *Tendon transfers of the hand and forearm.* Boston: Little, Brown and Company, 1987:119–120.

46. Gold MH. Topical silicone gel sheeting in the treatment of hypertrophic scars and keloids. A dermatologic experience. *J Dermatol Surg Oncol* 1993;19:912–916.

47. Widgerow AD, Chait LA, Stals R, et al. New innovations in scar management. *Aesthetic Plast Surg* 2000;24:227–234.

48. Carroll RE. Small joint arthrodesis in hand reconstruction. *J Bone Joint Surg* 1969;51:1219–1221.

49. Faithfull DK, Herbert TJ. Small joint fusions of the hand using the Herbert bone screw. *J Hand Surg* 1984;9:167–168.

50. Lister G. Intraosseous wiring of the digital skeleton. *J Hand Surg* 1978;3:427–435.

51. McGlynn JT, Smith RA, Bogumill GP. Arthrodesis of small joint of the hand: a rapid and effective technique. *J Hand Surg* 1988;13:595–599.

52. Teoh LC, Yeo SJ, Singh I. Interphalangeal joint arthrodesis with oblique placement of an AO lag screw. *J Hand Surg* 1994;19:208–211.

53. Ezaki, M. Angled digits. In: Green DP, Hotchkiss RN, Pederson WC, eds. *Green's operative hand surgery,* 4th ed. Philadelphia: Churchill Livingstone, 1999:517–521.

54. Hersh AH, DeMarinis F, Stecher RM. On the inheritance and development of clinodactyly. *Am J Hum Genet* 1953;5:257–268.

55. Gerald B, Umansky R. Cornelia de Lange syndrome: radiographic findings. *Radiology* 1967;88:96–100.

56. Hefke HW. Roentgenologic study of anomalies of hands in 100 cases of mongolism. *Am J Dis Child* 1940;60:1319–1323.

57. Houston CS. Roentgen findings in the XXXXY chromosome anomaly. *J Can Assoc Radiol* 1967;18:258–267.

58. Snyder CC. Bilateral facial agenesis (Treacher-Collins syndrome). *Am J Surg* 1956;92:81–87.

59. Poznanski AK, Garn SM, Holt JF. The thumb in the congenital malformation syndromes. *Radiology* 1971;100:115–129.

60. Rubenstein JH. The broad thumbs syndrome- progress report 1968. *Birth Defects* 1969;5:25–41.

61. Stover CN, Hayes JT, Holt JF. Diastrophic dwarfism. *Am J Roentgenol* 1963;89:914.

62. Wood VE. Treatment of the triphalangeal thumb. *Clin Orthop* 1976;120:179–193.

63. Light TR, Ogden JA. The longitudinal epiphyseal bracket: implications for surgical correction. *J Pediatr Orthop* 1981;1:299–305.

64. Cooney WP. Camptodactyly and clinodactyly. In: Carter P, ed. *Reconstruction of the child's hand.* Philadelphia: Lea & Febiger, 1991.

65. Poznanski AK, Pratt GB, Manson G, et al. Clinodactyly, camptodactyly, Kirner's deformity, and other crooked fingers. *Radiology* 1969;93:573–582.

66. Carstam N, Theander G. Surgical treatment of clinodactyly caused by longitudinally bracketed diaphysis. *Scand J Plast Reconstr Surg* 1975;9:199–202.

67. Vickers D. Clinodactyly of the little finger: a simple operative technique for reversal of the growth abnormality. *J Hand Surg* 1987;12:335–345.

88

DELTA PHALANX AND MADELUNG'S DEFORMITY

DAVID WHITMAN VICKERS

DELTA PHALANX

The term *delta phalanx* was suggested by Blundell Jones (1) in 1964 to describe a congenital triangular-shaped anomaly of the middle phalanx of a finger with a continuous epiphysis along one side (Fig. 1). Since then, *delta phalanx* has become a term of convenience that is loosely applied to other crudely triangular bones of the hands and feet of similar derivation. The involved bones are not always phalanges and are not necessarily delta shaped. Light and Ogden (2) prefer the term *longitudinal epiphyseal bracket*, and Light and Blevins (3) have classified bones with a longitudinal epiphyseal bracket into five groups. Carstam and Theander (4) have suggested the term *longitudinally bracketed diaphysis*. A delta phalanx is a three-dimensional pyramid, and the more common trapezoidal variety is like a cone that is obliquely truncated at each end. Each delta phalanx produces a curvature of the digit, which is termed *clinodactyly* if it is more than 10 degrees off the longitudinal axis. The mid-zone or isthmus of the continuous epiphysis may be substantial or thin bone or may be represented only by articular cartilage that blends with an underlying continuous physis. There is inclination of the joint surfaces at one or both ends because the bone is incapable of unrestrained growth on this side. Asymmetric bipolar migration of the growth plates or incomplete separation of adjacent phalanges in a polydactylous relationship could be responsible. Genetic factors are important, and there is a dominant familial association in quite a number of multiple deformities that include a delta phalanx. In some societies, there is a close relationship to polydactyly.

The bony component of a delta phalanx appears abnormal on x-rays, even in infancy. It does not grow in an orderly fashion but rather becomes an enlargement of itself by a form of frustrated physeal and appositional growth. Although a delta phalanx grows in early childhood, the clinarthrosis remains, and, further into childhood, the clinodactyly may increase, possibly related to growth spurts or to continuing ossification of the continuous epiphysis.

Clinical Manifestations

The most common example of a delta phalanx is found in the middle phalanx of both little fingers, producing a clinodactyly toward the ring finger (Fig. 2). Somewhat less common is a clinodactyly of the thumb that is secondary to a delta proximal phalanx, usually with radial deviation, but occasionally with ulnar deviation (Fig. 3). A triphalangeal thumb that has a delta mid-phalanx and produces clinodactyly toward the index finger is fairly uncommon. Delta bones elsewhere are quite rare and do not follow any particular pattern. In multiple delta phalanges, the tendency to clinodactyly may cancel out (Fig. 1D).

In clinodactyly of the little finger, there is a variable degree of inclination or clinarthrosis of both interphalangeal joints. Pain is not a feature in children, and they exhibit an adequate range of motion and function. It is frequently familial as an autosomal-dominant trait but is not commonly associated with a syndrome or other pathology other than polydactyly and Down syndrome. A thumb clinodactyly that is secondary to a delta anomaly of the proximal phalanx is generally more extreme and part of a syndrome, especially Rubinstein-Taybi syndrome, for which Wood and Rubinstein (5) have reported a 34% incidence of severe radial angulation. Thumb clinodactyly may also be associated with multiple epiphyseal dysplasia, polydactyly, syndactyly, Apert's and Poland's syndromes, and diastrophic dwarfism. A triphalangeal thumb that contains a delta phalanx produces a clinodactyly toward the index finger, appears long, is unstable, and is usually bilateral. If the extra phalanx is longer, the thumb tends to be less curved and more fingerlike. Some triphalangeal thumbs are actually supernumerary fingers with three normal phalanges. Many varieties of triphalangeal thumb are familial, behaving as an autosomal-dominant trait with a high degree of penetrance. Associated anomalies include polydactyly, cleft hand, and a variety of cardiac defects that should be identified before surgery.

Management

Many cases need no surgery or any other treatment, as they are minor, and other cases are too complex for surgery to be

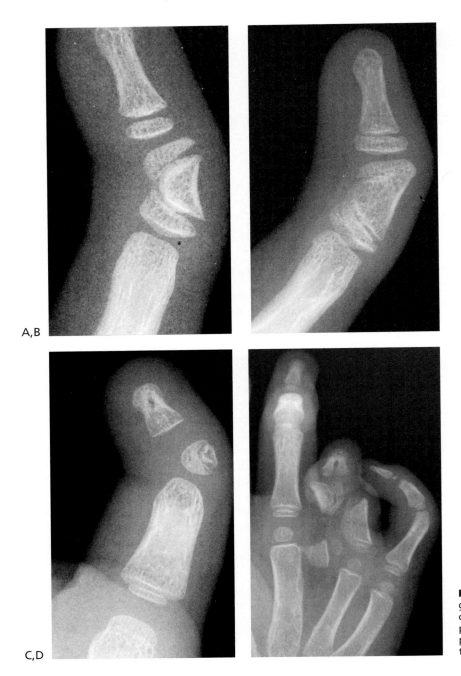

A,B

C,D

FIGURE 1. A: Classic delta phalanx, which would grow and correct nicely after physiolysis. **B:** A distal clinarthrosis with closed physis cannot remodel. The proximal physis responds well to physiolysis. **C:** Delta phalanx in a triphalangeal thumb. Physiolysis is contraindicated. **D:** Complex delta phalanges.

helpful. The surgical possibilities for the treatable group with significant deforming potential involve growth restoration (physiolysis) or osteotomy, or both. During the growth period, the author favors growth restoration, wherever possible, as this is simple, may avoid the need for osteotomy, increases length, and, most importantly, improves joint surfaces. Since Langenskiöld's original report (6) of bone bridge excision in 1975, it is now well accepted that a progressive deformity after partial fusion of a growth plate after trauma is reversible if the fusion is excised and if its recurrence is prevented with interposition of fat. The author, having some experience with this proce-

dure, believed that some congenital growth plate anomalies might also grow more normally if a developmental tether was removed, but this assumed that the remaining growth plate could respond. This theory was confirmed after a physiolysis for Madelung's deformity in 1979 and for delta phalanx in 1980. The author now has experience with 231 Langenskiöld procedures since 1973, including 86 procedures for delta phalanx (7–11).

Blundell Jones (1) made some observations of growth after osteotomy through the continuous epiphysis of a delta phalanx but did not manipulate the conditions for this to be maintained. Carstam and Theander (4) reported a lim-

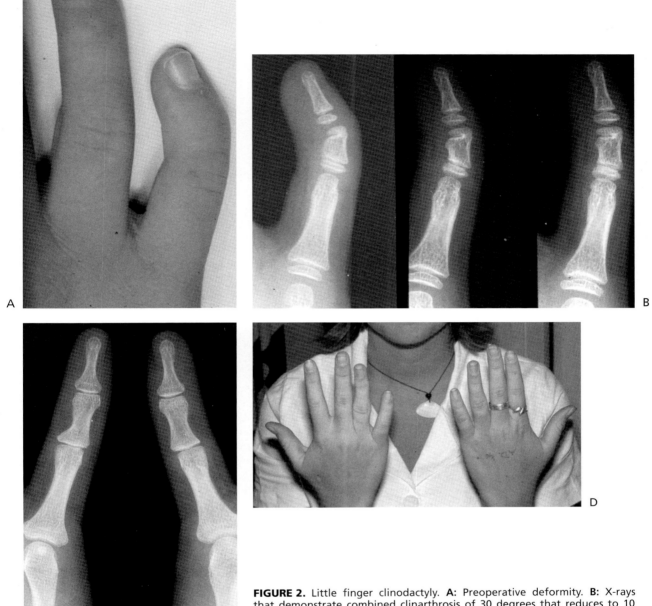

FIGURE 2. Little finger clinodactyly. **A:** Preoperative deformity. **B:** X-rays that demonstrate combined clinarthrosis of 30 degrees that reduces to 10 degrees in 2 years of growth restoration. **C:** X-ray that was taken 11 years after physiolysis without osteotomy. **D:** Clinical appearance at maturity.

ited experience with attempted growth restoration, and Light and Ogden (2) went a step further in proposing a careful osteotomy to leave the physis clear of any bony contact and in using a fat graft according to Langenskiöld's recommendation. The author shares this view.

A clinodactyly that is secondary to a delta or trapezoidal phalanx can be reversed over a period of time by performing a 15-minute physiolysis procedure—nature finishes the job during the remainder of the growth period. Evidence of regrowth in slow-growing phalanges is subtle but progressive. The main benefits are at the joints at which the clinarthrosis decreases, producing an apparent lengthening of the

digit, and there is remodeling of the joint surfaces themselves, which minimizes the development of arthritis later on.

In the little finger, the traditional approach by most surgeons has been to do nothing or to perform an osteotomy—the latter being reserved for significant deformity. There is a considerable middle ground here in which many of the untreated group could be improved quite simply during childhood with a physiolysis procedure, which has the further advantage that, being so simple, both hands can be treated under one anesthetic. The ideal age for this surgery is 4 years of age, as there is plenty of time for growth to

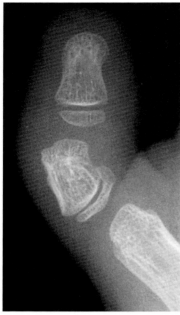
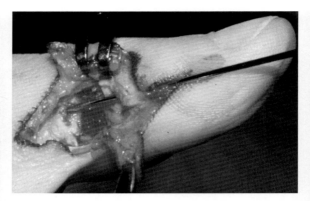
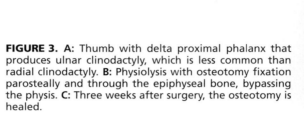
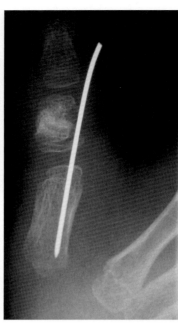

A,B

FIGURE 3. A: Thumb with delta proximal phalanx that produces ulnar clinodactyly, which is less common than radial clinodactyly. **B:** Physiolysis with osteotomy fixation parosteally and through the epiphyseal bone, bypassing the physis. **C:** Three weeks after surgery, the osteotomy is healed.

C

remodel the bone, and any earlier attempted surgery is difficult, because the bone is so small. Despite this, the average age at surgery in the author's series was 8 years because of late presentation. At an older age, a moderate clinodactyly of the little finger is still improved with a physiolysis procedure, even if only 1 or 2 years of growth remain. The only advantage of osteotomy is a more immediate correction, but overcorrection is possible and unacceptable. This never occurs with physiolysis. Clinodactyly of the thumb is generally more significant—beyond the capacity of growth restoration alone. A concomitant osteotomy is usually required. Apart from the angular deformity, these thumbs are usually broad and stubby, so every attempt should be made to preserve length and to produce conditions that are conducive to growth to minimize this appearance. Complex or multiple delta phalanges are so variable in their presentation that it is not possible to discuss a general plan of management. Often, the multiple deformities tend to cancel out in any case. The triphalangeal thumb that contains a delta phalanx is the exception regarding growth restoration, as it is already too long. The morphology of the interposed delta phalanx varies significantly, but, in any particular case, it is usually obvious what should be done to most effectively shorten, straighten, and stabilize the digit. When the delta phalanx is a small mosaic or composite portion of the joint surface, it should be retained or fused *in situ*. When there is a small, additional pyramidal bone that is interposed between two otherwise normal joint surfaces, there is some argument about the management. Excision with ligament reconstruction and Kirschner wire stabilization

for 4 to 6 weeks is possible if the child is less than 5 years of age (12). However, others prefer a fusion of the more appropriate joint in these cases. If the interposed delta or trapezoidal phalanx is longer, dual osteotomies to allow shortening and realignment, along with a fusion of the less satisfactory joint, are required. In the cases in which the triphalangeal thumb is more like an extra finger without a specific delta anomaly, shortening, rotation, and web creation may all be required, possibly a complete pollicization procedure.

Operative Technique: Growth Restoration

Growth restoration (physiolysis) in the little finger is performed under general anesthesia, and a bloodless field is provided by an upper arm pneumatic tourniquet. A midlateral incision is made overlying the apex of the delta phalanx, just long enough to visualize its mid-portion. The subcutaneous tissues are mobilized by blunt dissection, exposing whitish fibrous tissue. Passive movement of the finger reasonably locates the proximal interphalangeal joint, and, with the assistance of magnifying loupes, the initial excision is now made just distal to this joint with a no. 15 scalpel blade. An ellipse of fibrous tissue and cartilage is scalloped out until the scalpel contacts bone in the mid-portion of the phalanx. All soft tissue tethers that are bow strung across the concavity are excised, namely the dorsal and palmar periosteum and other palmar tissues, which may include some of the fibrous flexor sheath. In young children in whom the continuous epiphysis has not ossified, it is not necessary

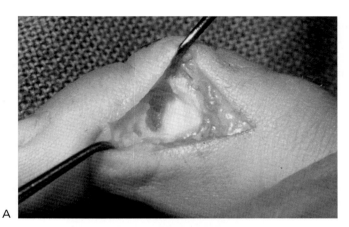

A

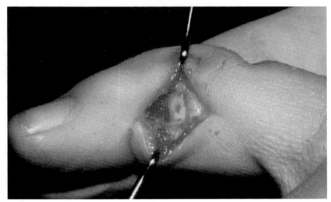

B

FIGURE 4. **A:** In young children without a continuous bony epiphysis, it is not necessary to visualize the epiphyseal bony nucleus, as long as the metaphyseal border of the physis is clearly defined from the dorsal to palmar periosteum. **B:** If the bony epiphysis is visualized, this is still acceptable.

to expose the bony nucleus of the proximal epiphysis, but there must be a clear excision just distal to the vertical cartilaginous component that is the physis (Fig. 4). Sometimes, the physis displays a grey-blue vertical plane that contrasts with the whiter articular or epiphyseal cartilage, but this difference is not always visible. In cases in which there is ossification of the continuous epiphysis, one progressively encounters serial layers of tissue, namely fibrous, cartilaginous, bony isthmus, and physeal, and then the bone of the mid-portion of the phalanx. In these cases, the proximal bony epiphyseal nucleus is visualized as an integral part of the procedure when the bony isthmus is excised. A 1-mm rongeur is now used to nibble a little bone away from the metaphyseal interface, so that the physeal cartilage is prominent to ensure a good contact with the fat graft. All loose flaps of periosteum should be cleanly excised, as they are liable to produce bone that may cross the physis. If there is an open growth plate distally in the phalanx, it is profiled in similar fashion to promote growth. If the distal physis has closed, there is no need for any significant dissection here. A separate incision is made in the ulnar border of the mid-

forearm, avoiding visible veins, to excise a piece of fat to fill the surgical void in the fingers of both hands. Plain bupivacaine 0.25% is now injected subcutaneously in the wounds, and the forearm wound is closed with 5-0 plain catgut suture. Now, the tourniquet is deflated for approximately 5 minutes and then is reinflated, and the cavity in the finger is washed out and gently cleansed of blood clot. The appropriate amount of fat is now inserted into the cavity, so that, when the skin is closed, it completely fills the space but does not protrude through the sutured wound to any extent. Before the dressings are applied, an aerosol adhesive is freely sprayed on the limb to assist in retention of the dressings. A nonstick dressing is now applied to the wound, which is further covered with some cotton wool and a 2.5-cm crepe bandage. The dressings remain undisturbed for 10 days. The opposite little finger is treated in a similar fashion under the same anesthetic, using the other one-half of the piece of fat that was harvested previously. The entire procedure for both hands should take approximately 40 minutes.

Clinodactyly of the thumb that is secondary to a delta anomaly of the proximal phalanx is an important indication for surgery. An osteotomy and fixation are always required, so each thumb is treated in a separate session. A generous, straight, mid-lateral incision is performed on the concave side, and the oblique extensions for the Z-plasty are performed now to enhance exposure. In some cases, the collateral ligament appears to bypass the delta phalanx, linking the metacarpal to the distal phalanx. In one rare case of clinodactyly in ulnar deviation, the insertion of the adductor tendon reached the distal phalanx. These anomalous tissues are released. Using a simple bone cutter, an osteotomy is now carefully advanced across the bone at the mid-point of the concavity, sufficiently distal to the metacarpophalangeal joint to avoid the basal physis. The objective now is to incompletely perform the osteotomy, preserving the opposite cortex, so that a greenstick fracture can be produced by straightening the thumb but preserving some stability. The open wedge thus created is not bone grafted because one cortex and intact periosteum are enough for rapid union. The exposed physis is now defined on the metaphyseal side from dorsal to palmar periosteum. If the osteotomy is inadvertently completed, it is best stabilized by placing the opposite cortex of the proximal fragment more centrally in the distal fragment before fixation. A single parosteal 1-mm Kirschner wire is passed distally in the mid-lateral plane, where there is abundant soft tissue, then in retrograde fashion through the bony epiphysis of the proximal fragment, which is large and looks like the bull's eye of a target (Fig. 3). The wire is now carefully advanced across the joint and up to the basal physis of the metacarpal. In this way, the Kirschner wire does not cross the physis of either bone. Its parosteal location on the open side of the osteotomy is a barrier to redeformity. If this preferred method of fixation is not possible or not stable enough,

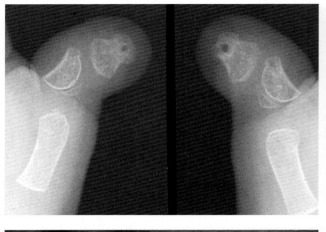

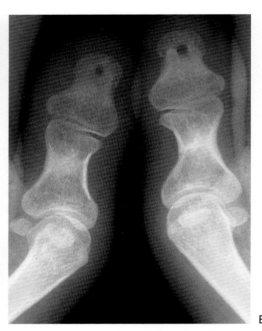

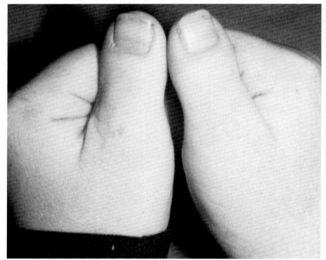

FIGURE 5. A: Thumb in Rubinstein-Taybi syndrome. **B,C:** The result, 14 years after surgery.

then an alternative method, crossing the physis, is acceptable. The exposed physis and the surgical space are now covered with a small, free fat graft that is harvested from the ulnar border of the forearm. Subcutaneous bupivacaine (0.25% plain) is injected into the wounds, which are closed with 5-0 plain catgut suture. After spraying an adhesive aerosol onto the limb generally, cotton wool padding is applied, and the thumb is immobilized in a long arm plaster slab for 3 weeks. The sticky dressing helps stabilize and retain the slab in a busy little child.

Clinical Examples and Results of Surgery

The author has experience with 86 physiolysis procedures for the delta phalanx anomaly since 1980 (little finger, 67; thumb, 14; other, 5). No significant complications developed early or late, and the range of motion was preserved in all cases.

In clinodactyly of the little finger, the general observation is a noticeable decrease in the deformity in the first 3 months after surgery, slowing down for the remainder of the growth period (Fig. 2). Correction of the clinarthrosis at one or both

ends is responsible for axial correction. Growth and correction at the growing end tend to be maintained, and, although the distal physis tends to close as it should, some correction of a distal clinarthrosis is possible if 50% or more of the physis is open at the time of surgery. There was only one case in the entire series (Fig. 1B) in which an osteotomy was still required at maturity because there was deformity at the distal joint that was incapable of natural correction as the distal physis was closed at the time of surgery (10). It is usual for part or all of an injured or deformed physis to close 6 to 12 months before maturity after a physiolysis, but growth by then has slowed to such an extent that deformity does not increase. This has been observed quite early in four cases, without ill effect.

Thumb deformity is more extensive and difficult to treat with physiolysis because the delta phalanx is small, and supplementary osteotomy with fixation is always required (Fig. 3). Despite its complexity, there have been no major complications, and all outcomes were satisfactory. Growth response has not been apparent in approximately 20% of the cases, but this is difficult to assess radiologically, as growth is so slow, and the physis is difficult to visualize. In these cases, the result was no better but no worse than with osteotomy alone. The case with the longest follow-up is illustrated in Figure 5. Further clinical material is available in the other publications by the author that are referenced in this chapter.

Conclusion

A growth restoration operation (physiolysis) is a relatively simple and quick surgical procedure that can optimize the outcome of surgery for deformity that is secondary to delta phalanx. No follow-up procedures are required, and complications are rare. Changing the circumstances for growth early in childhood allows nature to finish the job. The absolute benefit is improvement of the joint surfaces, which cannot be artificially produced. In many cases, this overcomes the need for an osteotomy, which is a more complex procedure. Even in cases of significant deformity in which an osteotomy is still required, paying attention to detail in the region of the physis can quite easily afford the extra benefit of renewed growth in the majority of cases. In 20 years of experience with these procedures, there have been no bad outcomes, and the patients and parents have been universally satisfied.

MADELUNG'S DEFORMITY

The clinical entity of Madelung's deformity is the result of a bony and ligamentous dysplasia at the wrist that produces a palmar displacement of the hand on a short, bowed forearm, which is associated with a dorsal subluxation and prominence of the ulnar head (Fig. 6). The original description by Madelung (13) in 1878 outlined the clinical appearance in fine detail from all perspectives. It may be sporadic or familial. Leri and Weill (14) and Langer (15) further clarified the familial variety of the condition. The lesions in Madelung's deformity are genetically determined, involving the *SHOX* gene pathway to produce a bony dysplasia that centers around the lunate fossa of the radius and a ligament tether of the carpus that prevents its proper advancement with growth. A reverse form of Madelung's deformity has also been known for some time, but intermediate varieties, including chevron carpus, have only recently been recognized as spatially different forms of the same pathologic processes (16). Although, for convenience, three clinical entities are described, there is a continuous spectrum of intermediate forms that depend on the spatial location of the dyschondrosteosis lesions in the anteroposterior axis of the ulnar zone of the distal radius. The deformity is usually bilateral and is much more common in women. It is a feature of Leri-Weill syndrome and is also seen in Turner's syndrome. In Leri-Weill syndrome, the distal radial and ligamentous lesions are more extreme, and lower limb bones are also involved, producing mesomelic (middle segment) dwarfism.

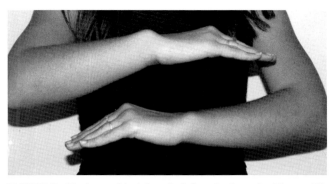

FIGURE 6. Moderate Madelung's deformity (see also Figure 10). A deformity that is similar to Madelung's deformity can be associated with osteochondroma and enchondroma after a fracture and partial fusion of the physis or repetitive stresses in gymnastics. In these cases, the terms *Madelung-like* or *pseudo–Madelung's deformity* are more appropriate.

Genetic Basis

A gene that is termed the *short stature homeobox gene* or *SHOX* has been isolated from the distal short arm of the X chromosome at band Xp22.3 (17,18) and its involvement in Leri-Weill syndrome was confirmed after the identification of mutations, including deletions and, less commonly, point mutations in *SHOX* in sporadic and familial patients (19,20).

The mode of inheritance is effectively dominant because the gene is located on the pseudoautosomal region of the X and Y chromosomes that is inherited in an autosomal manner. However, not all Leri-Weill syndrome patients or primary Madelung's deformity patients have mutations in *SHOX* (21). This suggests that other genes that are potentially regulated by *SHOX* may also be causative of Madelung's deformity.

Thus far, the practical applications in Leri-Weill syndrome of *SHOX* gene testing by fluorescence *in situ* hybridization are in genetic counseling and risk assessment of Madelung's deformity before other signs, or with ambiguous signs, on radiographs.

Histology

Histologic examination of operative material revealed confusion of the orientation and cellular structure of the cartilaginous columns and primary spongiosa and hyperplasia of the anomalous ligament. Cells in the proliferative area demonstrated side-by-side grouping, whereas, elsewhere, nests of chondrocytes were seen containing cells at various stages of disorderly maturation. The size of the proliferative zone was decreased, and the hypertrophic zone was increased. Large islands of hypertrophic osteoid-containing microscopic enchondromata were seen in ectopic locations. The histologic features of dyschondrosteosis are similar to those of achondroplasia. The anomalous radiolunotriquetral ligament had the appearance of normal ligamentous tissue, so its thickness is believed to be due to hyperplasia

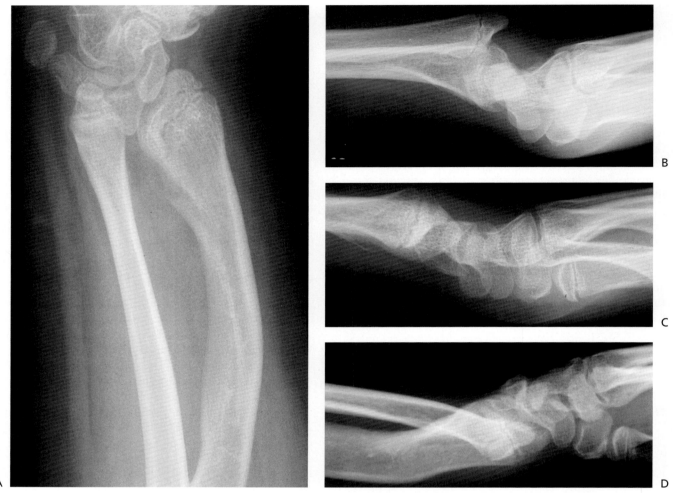

FIGURE 7. A: Dyschondrosteosis. The deep trough and spike that are characteristic of the radio-lunotriquetral ligament are anchored proximal to the growth plate, which does not appear fused. **B:** Madelung's deformity. **C:** Chevron carpus. **D:** Reverse Madelung's deformity.

rather than hypertrophy. It was observed at the microscopic level to blend intimately with the fibrocartilage of the triangular fibrocartilage complex (TFC).

Pathogenesis and Natural History

In 1899, Ranvier (22) proposed that the increase in cartilaginous columns of the growth plate and the bone-forming cells of the periosteum all came from the ossification groove. In over 50 years of research to confirm this, Langenskiöld et al. (23) also demonstrated that the stem cells of the reserve layer of the germinal zone in the growth plate migrate centrifugally to the ossification groove, where some of them add cartilage columns for longitudinal growth, and others move into the cambium layer of the periosteum to produce growth in width. They went further and proposed that a disorder of this process might be the cause of enchondroma, osteochondroma, dyschondrosteosis, and, possibly, achondroplasia. Not only the streaming of the stem cells, but also their maturation from chondrocytes to osteoblasts could be defective.

Madelung's deformity and the spectrum of related conditions, including reverse Madelung's deformity and chevron carpus, are all a result of a bony dysplasia and a pathologic ligament tethering (Figs. 7 and 8). It is likely that both of these conditions occur as a result of a genetic defect in relation to the *SHOX* gene, but it is not clear whether they develop independently or whether one is primary and the other reactive. Trauma is no longer regarded as causative. The author's opinion regarding the pathologic sequence in Madelung's deformity is based on clinical observation and the surgical findings during liberation of the growth plate in 51 cases of Madelung's deformity over a 21-year period (7,9,16,24–26). This is further reinforced by the experience of 94 bone bridge resections for traumatic fusions in various bones since 1973. The dyschondrosteosis lesion is always in the ulnar zone of the distal radius that is destined to support the lunate. This lesion is focused on the palmar aspect in Madelung's deformity, midway in chevron carpus, and the dorsal aspect in reverse Madelung's deformity.

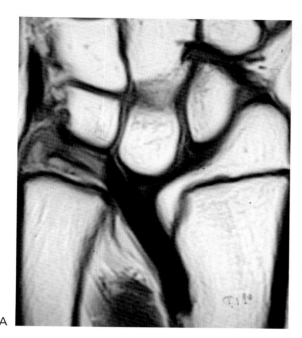

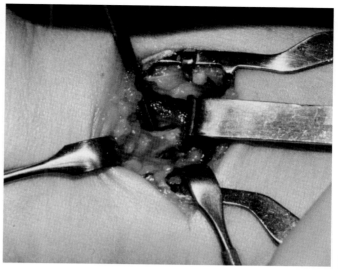

FIGURE 8. A: Magnetic resonance image of the radiolunotrique-tral ligament. **B:** The thick ligament is attached to the lunate.

The pathologic radiolunotriquetral ligament is as large as 1 cm diameter in Leri-Weill syndrome but may only be rudimentary in tall children with sporadic disease. It anchors the carpus to the immovable area of the radius in such a way that the intercalated growth plate is unable to progress. The proximal attachment is believed to be initially epiphyseal, as it should be, but it ceases to advance with growth, is left far behind, and is submerged in metaphyseal bone. The distal attachment is principally to the lunate, as is seen during surgery, with an extension to the triquetral that is only visible on magnetic resonance imaging (MRI). The mid-section lies in a deep metaphyseal trough in the radius.

Because the dyschondrosteosis lesion occurs elsewhere in the skeleton, it seems unlikely that the radial lesion is the result of ligamentotaxis, which causes a compressive lesion according to the Heuter-Volkmann law of cartilage growth. Further evidence that the bony dysplasia is independent is the observation that the anomalous ligament is always palmar, even in reverse Madelung's deformity in which the bony lesion is dorsal. Growth in the ulnar zone initially becomes confused and ineffective, trailing behind the advancing radial epiphysis and turning to face the ulna. The change in orientation in relation to the longitudinal axis further impairs any contribution to growth in length. The author believes that fusion is a late consequence of this process rather than a primary event. A partial fusion would cause tilting of the entire epiphysis, as is seen after trauma, and not a trailing off at one corner. The origin of the anomalous ligament is not thought to be a stress response to frustrated bony growth. It is not known whether the ligament is a new structure, a vestige of an anomalous muscle, or a giant, short, radiolunate ligament. It is more likely to be novel, as its attachment deep into the radial shaft is bizarre. The absence of anomalous ligament development in Madelung-like deformities after fracture, osteochondroma, or enchondroma does not support a hyperplasia or hypertrophy of an existing structure. It is conceivable, however, that the short radiolunate ligament attachment to the radial epiphysis ceased to advance by confusion, fusion, or reorientation early in childhood. It would then be left well behind and submerged by the growth in width of the bone. This theory is supported by the fact that the proximal attachment of the TFC is fused in the usual relationship with the anomalous ligament at its proximal bizarre insertion into the radius. Distally, the TFC moves dorsally and ulnarly. It appears to be more extensile, as it only causes a minor tilting of the distal ulnar epiphysis. There may be some developmental significance in the fact that the fibers of the anomalous ligament, the TFC, and the interosseous membrane are parallel. Linscheid has reported one case of an anomalous pronator quadratus muscle (25,27), and Hutchinson (*personal communication*) has made a similar observation bilaterally. The author currently believes that the bony dysplasia and the anomalous ligament develop independently as a result of a genetic anomaly in the *SHOX* gene pathway.

There are no signs of Madelung's deformity in infancy. The effect of the bony dysplasia and the pathologic ligament is subtle in early childhood, causing a progressive bowing of the radius because of the asymmetric tethers. The ulna, meanwhile, grows straight ahead. Localized evidence of the dysplasia only becomes apparent at approximately 4 years of age when truncation of the ulnar metaphysis of the radius may be detectable on the anteroposterior radiograph (Fig. 9).

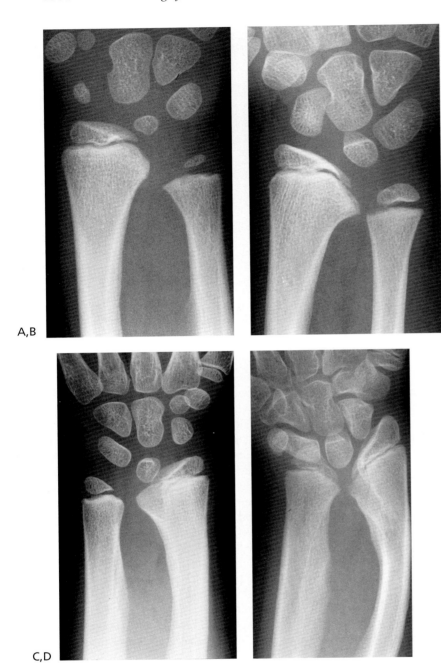

A,B

C,D

FIGURE 9. A: The patient at 6 years of age. Truncation of ulnar metaphysis has changed little since 4 years of age. **B:** The patient at 7.5 years of age. The deformity is now progressive. **C:** Leri-Weill syndrome at 6 years of age. **D:** The patient at 9 years of age. Earlier ligament resection would have modified the deterioration.

During mid-childhood, the dyschondrosteosis lesion becomes more apparent in the zone of the radius that is adjacent to the lunate. The thin tail of the radial epiphysis is slow to ossify and "turns the corner" into the lesion. At approximately 7 years of age and thereafter, there is a likelihood of more rapid deterioration. This could be the climax of physical developments and a hormonal effect.

Clinical Features

The deformity at the wrist that was described by Madelung involves a palmar inclination of the distal radius and causes a subluxation of the hand on a short, dorsally bowed forearm with resultant prominence of the head of the ulna. The hand is effectively suspended beneath the ulna and is frequently in a mildly supinated position. It is much more common in women. Although the condition is bilateral, usually one wrist is more deformed than the other. The tilt of the distal radial articular surface shifts the arc of motion, but there is a real decrease in range as well, especially in supination and dorsiflexion. Rotatory motion is impeded by the dorsal subluxation of the ulna, the bowing of the radius, and the diastasis between the distal ends of the forearm bones. Forced supination of the forearm is painful, especially in sporting activities, such as tennis. Pain otherwise is variable and tolerable. Because the carpus is suspended beneath the distal radius and ulna, instability and soft tissue fatigue are more of a problem than impaction of joint surfaces. A reverse Madelung's deformity is less common and may be seen bilaterally or in the opposite wrist of a patient with Madelung's deformity. The appearance resembles the dinner fork deformity of a Colles' fracture. The distal radial articular surface faces dorsal, so the carpus and hand are displaced dorsally, with the ulnar head being visible and palpable in the palmar aspect of the wrist. The intermediate variety in the spectrum of these dysplastic deformities presents with a short forearm with little deformity. Pain is the notable feature of this "chevron carpus," which the author refers to as the *chevron paradox*, as the minimal apparent deformity produces the maximum pain. The proximal row of the carpus forms a wedge with a pyramid-shaped lunate at the apex, which is fixed to the radius by the strong radiolunotriquetral ligament that severely limits radial and ulnar deviation. Any motion of the wrist causes impaction of the joint surfaces.

Investigations

Plain radiographs are the single most useful investigation in the established case. In the anteroposterior radiograph, the radius clearly exhibits a defect at the location at which the lunate facet normally resides. The tail of the radial epiphysis on the ulnar side turns proximally and narrows down to a point that is adjacent to a broad trough that is produced by the anomalous ligament and the bony dysplasia. A prominent spike of cortical bone forms at the proximal extent of this trough, well proximal to the normal level of the metaphysis and well proximal to any growth activity (Fig. 7A). Signs of actual fusion or bony bar formation are absent but may occur late in the process. The presence of a radiolunotriquetral ligament is detected by examining the trough and spike in the metaphysis, the width of the space between the radius and ulna, and the shape and location of the lunate in this space. The ulna appears relatively straight and longer than the radius. It may overlap the triquetrum. Because the carpus is subluxed in Madelung's deformity, it appears to be too proximal, but the shape of the lunate is normally rounded, as it is not compressed, and the proximal row is not especially wedge shaped. In chevron carpus, however, the lunate is pyramidal and is wedged firmly between the forearm bones at the apex of a wedge-shaped carpus. The scaphoid, being under compression, rotates to demonstrate a ring sign. In chevron carpus, stress radiographs in radial and ulnar deviation reveal no significant motion at the radiocarpal joint, with some compensatory motion at the mid-carpal level. The lateral radiograph demonstrates the abnormal slope of the distal radius, with the notch streaming back into the metaphysis like a translucent cone. This cone is palmar in Madelung's deformity, central in chevron carpus, and dorsal in reverse Madelung's deformity. Likewise, the orientation of the lunate varies from palmar flexed to neutral to dorsiflexed in these three scenarios (Fig. 7).

Although bone age measurements have not been used, it is fortuitous that Greulich and Pyle (28) have provided sequential radiographs of the wrist, which is a useful standard for comparison in doubtful Madelung's deformity cases or for monitoring development in a child who is at risk of Madelung's deformity. In one child who was 5 years of age in a family with Leri-Weill syndrome, the comparative radiographs demonstrated that the distal radial epiphysis was 2 years behind the standard for the child's age, the carpus was 1 year behind, and the remainder of the hand was equal to the standard. This demonstrated a progressive fall off in the dysplasia, centrifugally from the distal radius.

MRI has now replaced tomography and computed tomography when further investigation is indicated. The greatest value of MRI is the imaging of the anomalous radiolunotriquetral ligament in the young child. It may also affect management in a mature patient with a chevron carpus, if proven, in whom division of the ligament alone should relieve pain.

Management

The treatment of Madelung's, reverse Madelung's, and chevron carpus deformities depends on a number of factors, the most important of which is age at presentation. Growth restoration surgery during childhood can be achieved by excision of the bony and ligamentous tethers with a physiolysis procedure that controls progress of the deformity (Figs. 10 and 11). The place of associated hemistapling of the radial styloid is unclear, but this procedure would only be considered when the deformity is close to maturity and is associated with ulnar physiodesis. After maturity, some form of salvage procedure is the only possibility, but this is quite complex and is not generally recommended except in the extreme case. The exception is the painful chevron carpus with a thick anomalous ligament in which a surgical release of the ligament from its distal attachment is indicated. A timely physiolysis procedure can reliably arrest further deformation, can relieve pain, and can improve range of motion. Unfortunately, the usual random presentation is later—in the 10- to 12-year-old age group—after the deformity becomes obvious, and pain develops. The degree of deformity then may not remodel adequately with physiolysis; however, restoration of even a year or two of growth is still helpful for pain relief and improved range of motion. When left unchecked, the dysplastic lesions exert their greatest deformation in the final 1 or 2 years of growth.

Education of the medical community has led to earlier referrals of patients who were previously told that nothing could be done. The majority of cases are of a familial nature, which should allow identification of the problem child in a family with Leri-Weill syndrome. Close observation is also warranted in the offspring of any patient who was treated earlier for Madelung's deformity or in Turner's syndrome, espe-

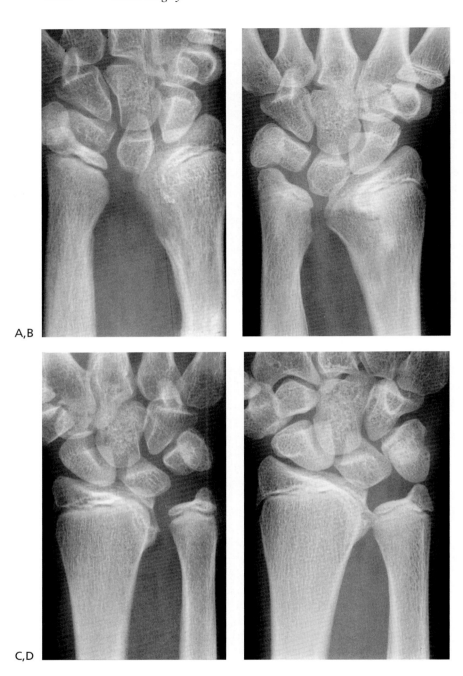

A,B

C,D

FIGURE 10. The same case of moderate Madelung's deformity that was shown in Figure 6. **A:** Right wrist with a major lesion, at 12 years of age. **B:** Right wrist, 17 months after physiolysis. The carpus is decompressed, better supported, and less deformed, with no pain. **C:** Left wrist with a minor lesion, at 12 years of age. **D:** Left wrist, 17 months later, without surgery. The carpus is more compressed and more proximal, with scaphoid ring sign. Subsequent ligament detachment relieved pain and increased mobility.

cially if growth hormone therapy is a consideration. Radiologic monitoring in early childhood has been used in these cases with success (Fig. 9), but more enlightened genetic methods are now available from birth. It is not yet known how early the anomalous ligament can be detected with MRI, nor is it known whether an early detachment of the ligament alone from the lunate may have a useful prophylactic effect.

Surgical Technique

Physiolysis is performed by using general anesthesia and a pneumatic tourniquet. Some experience with growth plate surgery is necessary. A transverse incision that is approximately 4 cm long is made 1 to 2 cm proximal to the most proximal wrist crease. A longitudinal incision would provide easier access but may heal with a poor scar. Palpation of the radial styloid is also a guide, as the bony lesion is 2 to 3 cm proximal to this level. The approach passes either side of the flexor carpi radialis tendon to the radial margin of the digital flexor tendon group. The path is sought to achieve maximum protection of the radial artery and the median nerve, and care is also required that retractors do not kink the nerve. The pronator quadratus is visualized by using blunt dissection, and exposure of the distal radius is improved by releasing

,B

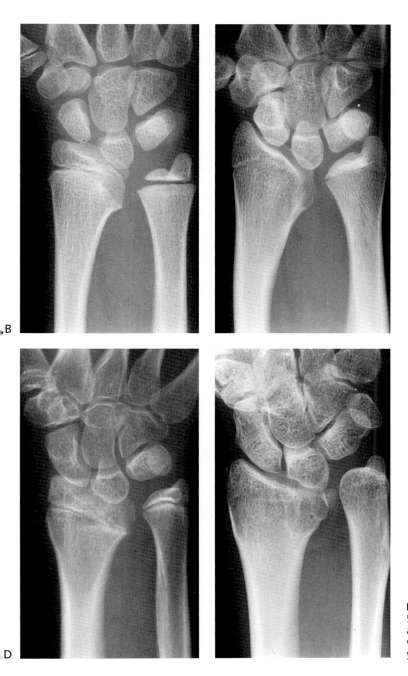

D

FIGURE 11. A,B: Progressive deformity that occurred for 5 years. The scaphoid is vertical, the carpus is compressed, and there is ulnar overgrowth. **C,D:** A similar case that was treated with physiolysis exhibits improvement after 5 years of unrestrained growth.

some of the radial attachment of the distal margin of this muscle. A mass of white tissue is encountered and is composed of joint capsule and a composite of the anomalous ligament and the TFC. It is not easy initially to locate the wrist joint, as the lunate may be fixed when the hand is moved, with motion occurring instead at the midcarpal joint. The lunate is usually palpable in the midline, but, in case of doubt, an exploratory longitudinal incision is made adjacent to this prominence, or radiography is used. At this stage, the anomalous ligament may be detached from the proximal pole of the lunate (Fig. 8B), or, alternatively, the first step may be a longitudinal osteotomy from well proximal to distal several milli-

meters into the ulnar metaphysis of the radius. The osteotome is supinated a little to coincide with the oblique plane of the radial deformity. A magnifying loupe is now used to inspect the bony surface that is thus produced for evidence of growth plate cartilage. The initial osteotomy is usually too shallow, exposing only longitudinal fibrous tissue in the floor of the trough. In this case, a deeper longitudinal osteotomy is made to expose bone, but care is taken distally to preserve as much epiphysis as possible, with minimal intrusion into the wrist joint. The appearance of the physis improves distally just before it changes direction to its normal plane across the radius. The thick ligament that lies in its trough may be further excised, with care being taken to preserve the TFC, which blends with it but is of a different consistency and is more dorsally located. When the ligament is adequately released, the lunate can be distracted away from the radius, which was not possible before. The white line of the physis is now defined from its palmar to its dorsal extent. This should not be too radical, as support for the lunate is always deficient in this condition, so conservation of as much of the epiphyseal bone as possible is advantageous. In this regard, the author has become more conservative in the later cases in his series. It is important to clear the metaphyseal side of the physeal cartilage to make it prominent at the location at which it achieves good contact with the fat graft. This is achieved with a small gouge or ball bur, or the oblique tip of a fine sucker. The epiphyseal bone on the germinal side is not excavated. Now, some fat is harvested from the medial border of the forearm, avoiding the cutaneous veins and nerves. The volume of fat should be sufficient to more than completely fill the surgical cavity. The skin of the donor site is closed and subcutaneous bupivacaine 0.5% plain is injected in all wounds. The tourniquet is now deflated, and sponges are used under manual pressure to minimize bleeding. After most of the ooze has ceased, the tourniquet is reinflated, and blood clots are carefully removed and washed out of the cavity. The fat graft is now pressed into the cavity, and the flexor tendons are released to trap it in place. After skin closure, a short arm plaster slab is applied for comfort until suture removal at 2 weeks. The limb is then left free, and no special therapy is required. When physiolysis is performed close to maturity, the associated procedure of excision physiodesis of the ulna may be considered. This is quite a simple technique, as one is able to excise the physis with a scalpel and then turn the epiphysis back to remove the physeal cartilage and some bone with a rongeur. It is only necessary to use one or two strong sutures to stabilize the osteotomy. This procedure should be restricted to late cases, as subsequent overcorrection is a possibility.

In reverse Madelung's deformity, the procedure is the same. The author has previously used a dorsal approach but, more recently, has found that the standard palmar approach is more suitable, as the abnormal ligament is always palmar, and access to the physis is just as easy when using this approach, despite the fact that the dyschondrosteosis lesion is in its dorsal component. In the case of a chevron carpus, the approach is a little more proximal, but, otherwise, it is similar. Those cases of chevron carpus that seek pain relief after maturity only require a distal release of the anomalous ligament to decompress the lunate. It is not necessary to completely excise the ligament, as there is a risk of injury to the TFC with radical surgery. No bony surgery is indicated.

Osteotomy procedures should be reserved for mature patients with extreme deformities or pain. Various techniques have been described to reorient the distal radius to make the wrist joint more stable and are supplemented by a shortening of the ulna. Some involve a closing wedge

osteotomy, whereas others favor open wedge osteotomies to gain length (24,25,27,29). In open wedge osteotomy, distal to the radial attachment of the anomalous ligament, a release of the ligament is necessary to decompress the carpus, as is emphasized by Carter et al. (30). In cases of marked bowing of the radius, a double osteotomy has been described by the author and Linscheid (25) first to elevate the lunate fossa and to reorient the distal radius and, second, to correct the diaphyseal bowing. In some cases, an ulnar recession is also necessary. Ulnar recession involves a shortening that is proximal to the metaphysis or cuff resection. Because the hand is suspended beneath the distal ulna, a Darrach-type excision alone simply to remove the prominence is not recommended, as it further decreases stability. Recently, there have been attempts at progressive correction of Madelung's deformity by using the Ilizarov frames and principles. Once again, the presence of the radiolunotriquetral ligament must be considered, especially if the hand is distracted, which otherwise could avulse the lunate from the proximal carpal row. A novel approach by Foucher (*personal communication*) and others (31) involves fusion of the lunate into the radial trough defect and further incorporation into a fusion with the distal ulna. A false joint is produced in the distal ulna to mimic a Sauve-Kapandji procedure. The scaphoid and triquetrum are excised from the proximal row of the carpus.

Clinical Experience

Since 1979, the author has performed a physiolysis procedure on 47 wrists with Madelung's deformity, reverse Madelung's deformity, or chevron carpus during growth. Four wrists with chevron carpus were treated after maturity with ligament release alone. Leri-Weill syndrome was present in more than one-half of the group, and the only two men had genetic evidence of this condition. Bilateral surgery, usually in two stages, was performed on 22 wrists. The age range for physiolysis was from a girl who was 10 years of age to a boy who was 14.5 years of age. Nine patients exhibited a chevron carpus or a hybrid form of this condition with a minor Madelung's deformity. Three patients (four wrists) were treated for reverse Madelung's deformity. Only three osteotomies were performed—one at the time of physiolysis in a patient with total radial dysplasia and two after maturity in one patient with extreme deformity at presentation that was unable to be controlled with growth restoration. Improvement in the deformity occurred in two-thirds of the cases, with no change in the remainder, and no patient with mild deformity who was treated at a younger age required an osteotomy at maturity. No patients were made worse by the procedure. Range of motion improved in all except one patient, who had total radial dysplasia. The average gain in supination was 23 degrees, with the maximum gain being 70 degrees. Twenty patients reported no pain, 26 had less pain, and one patient, who developed some instability of the head of the ulna, reported pain of a different nature. Partial denervation could play a part in the degree of pain, but this is unintentional.

Complications were few but included one unintentional lunate osteotomy that healed without consequence, one temporary median nerve palsy, and one distal radioulnar joint instability that was due to partial excision of the TFC. Space does not allow the illustration of many clinical cases; however, the reader is directed to the other publications by the author for more examples.

CONCLUSION

Madelung's deformity is the result of a genetically determined dysplasia of bone and soft tissues at the wrist. A different focus of the same dysplastic process results in other deformities, such as reverse Madelung's deformity and a spectrum of transitional forms between these two extremes, including chevron carpus. The extent of the deformity can be controlled by surgical intervention in mid-childhood by excision of the failed growth plate and anomalous ligament tethers. Physiolysis should be reserved for the child who is beginning to show signs of increasing deformity—usually prominence of the ulnar head—and who is developing pain. Osteotomy is generally reserved for postmature patients with significant pain and deformity. Unfortunately, the usual presentation is late in childhood with a deformity beyond the capacity to recover, although growth restoration surgery is still beneficial, as the final 2 years of growth are the most destructive. Earlier identification of children at risk of significant deformity is achievable in family groups and in Leri-Weill and Turner's syndromes by using genetic and imaging studies and through education of the medical community to refer cases sooner. The place of a simple release of the ligament alone early in childhood has not yet been determined, but increased availability of MRI will assist this research. There is an occasional indication in the mature patient with a painful chevron carpus to detach the anomalous ligament from the lunate to decompress the carpus.

REFERENCES

1. Blundell Jones G. Delta phalanx. *J Bone Joint Surg* 1964;46:226–228.
2. Light TR, Ogden JA. The longitudinal epiphyseal bracket: implications for surgical correction. *J Pediatr Orthop* 1981;1:299–305.
3. Light TR, Blevens A. Congenital angulation of tubular bones in the hand. In: Flatt AE, ed. *The care of congenital hand anomalies,* 2nd ed. St. Louis: Quality Medical Publishers,1994:212–213.
4. Carstam N, Theander G. Surgical treatment of clinodactyly caused by longitudinally bracketed diaphysis ("delta phalanx"). *Scand J Plast Reconstr Surg* 1975;9:199–202.
5. Wood VE, Rubinstein JH. Surgical treatment of the thumb in the Rubinstein-Taybi syndrome. *J Hand Surg* 1987;12:166–172.
6. Langenskiöld A. An operation for partial closure of an epiphyseal plate in children, and its experimental basis. *J Bone Joint Surg* 1975;3:325–330.
7. Vickers D. Premature incomplete fusion of the growth plate: causes and treatment by resection (physiolysis) in fifteen cases. *Aust N Z J Surg* 1980;50:393–401.
8. Vickers D. Clinodactyly: a simple operative technique for reversal of growth abnormality. *J Hand Surg* 1987;12:335–342.
9. Vickers D. *Epiphyseolysis. Current orthopaedics.* Longman Group, 1989:41–47.
10. Vickers D. Delta phalanx. In: Saffar P, Amadio P, Foucher G, eds. *Current practice in hand surgery.* London: Martin Dunitz, 1997:355–365.
11. Vickers D. Delta phalanx. In: Gupta A, Kay S, Scheker L, eds. *The growing hand.* St. Louis: Mosby, 2000:303–308.
12. Buck-Gramcko D. Triphalangeal thumb. In: Buck-Gramcko D, ed. *Congenital malformations of the hand and forearm.* London: Churchill Livingstone, 1998:403–424.
13. Madelung O. Die spontane Subluxation der Hand nach vorne, Verhandl d deutsch. *Gesellsch Chir Berlin* 1878;7:259–276.
14. Leri A, Weill J. Une affection congénitale et symétrique du développement osseux: la dyschondrostéose. *Bull Mem Soc Med Hôp Paris* 1929;53:1491–1494.
15. Langer LO. Dyschondrosteosis: a hereditable bone dysplasia with characteristic roentgenographic features. *Am J Roentgenol* 1965:178–188.
16. Vickers D, Nielsen G. Madelung deformity: surgical prophylaxis (physiolysis) during the late growth period by resection of the dyschondrosteosis lesion. *J Hand Surg* 1992;27:401–407.
17. Rao E, Weiss B, Fukami M, et al. Pseudoautosomal deletions encompassing a novel homeobox gene cause growth failure in idiopathic short stature and Turner syndrome. *Nat Genet* 1997;16:54–63.
18. Ellison JW, Zabihullah W, Young MF, et al. PHOG, a candidate gene for involvement in the short stature of Turner syndrome. *Hum Mol Genet* 1997;6:1341–1347.
19. Belin V, Cusin V, Viot G, et al. SHOX mutations in dyschondrosteosis (Leri Weill syndrome). *Nat Genet* 1998;19:67–69.
20. Shears DO, Vassal HJ, Goodman FR, et al. Mutation and deletion of the pseudoautosomal gene SHOX cause Leri Weill dyschondrosteosis. *Nat Genet* 1998;19:70–73.
21. Schiller S, Spranger S, Schechinger B, et al. Phenotypic variation and genetic heterogeneity in Leri-Weill syndrome. *Eur J Hum Genet* 2000;8:54–62.
22. Ranvier L. *Traité Technique d'Histologie,* 2nd ed. Paris: Savy, 1889.
23. Langenskiöld A, Elima K, Vuorio E. Specific collagen mRNAs elucidate the histogenetic relationship between the growth plate, the tissue in the ossification groove of Ranvier, and the cambium layer of the adjacent periosteum. *Clin Orthop* 1993;297:51–54.
24. Tachdjian M, ed. *Pediatric orthopedics,* 2nd ed, vol. 1. Philadelphia: WB Saunders, 1990:210–222.

25. Vickers D, Linscheid RL. Madelung's deformity. In: Cooney WP, Linscheid RL, Dobyns JH, eds. *The wrist: diagnosis and operative treatment.* St. Louis: Mosby, 1998:966–981.

26. Vickers DW. Madelung deformity. In: Gupta A, Kay S, Scheker L, eds. *The growing hand.* St. Louis: Mosby, 2000:791–798.

27. Dobyns JH. Madelung's deformity. In: Green DP, ed. *Operative hand surgery,* 3rd ed, vol. 1. New York: Churchill Livingstone, 1993:515–520.

28. Greulich WW, Pyle SI. *Radiographic atlas of skeletal development of the hand and wrist,* 2nd ed. Stanford, CA: Stanford University Press, 1959.

29. dos-Reis FB, Katchburian MV, Faloppa F, et al. Osteotomy of the radius and ulna for the Madelung deformity. *J Bone Joint Surg* 1998;80:817–824.

30. Carter P, Ezaki M, Cummings K. Anterior approach for correction of Madelung's deformity: dome osteotomy and Vickers ligament release. *J Hand Surg* 25[Suppl]:21–22(abst).

31. Soler-Minoves JM, Jove-Talavera R, Vila-Ferrer R, et al. Madelung's deformity. A new therapeutic approach. *Ann Chir Main Memb Super* 1993;12:335–341.

89

MACRODACTYLY, CONSTRICTION BAND SYNDROME, SYNOSTOSIS

PAUL C. DELL

Hamartomas of soft tissue frequently occur in the digit and may individually involve the skin or the fat or the lymphatic, vascular, or nerve elements. When enlargement involves more than one soft tissue element and the bony architecture, the term *digital gigantism* (1) should be used to properly describe this condition, irrespective of etiology. Commonly, digital gigantism is associated with hyperplasia or neoplasia of the median or ulnar nerve and follows the sensory distribution of either nerve. In rare instances, the distribution of both nerves is followed. The histology of the involved nerve may demonstrate interfascicular infiltration of fat and fibrous tissue or, in other instances, well-delineated or plexiform neurofibromata. Occasionally, however, digital gigantism may be present without nerve enlargement, and, conversely, hamartomas of the median nerve may be present without digital gigantism. Frequently, the stigmata of cutaneous and skeletal neurofibromatosis may accompany digital gigantism, but, in other instances, they are absent.

Although there is a spectrum of overlapping clinical presentations, there are three relatively distinct varieties of digital gigantism, two of which are associated with accompanying nerve enlargement and one in which the nerve is normal. Classic digital gigantism with lipofibromatous hamartoma (type 1) of the involved nerve is not heritable, is usually unilateral, is not associated with the cutaneous manifestations of neurofibromatosis, and is infrequently accompanied by other congenital anomalies. Digital gigantism as a manifestation of neurofibromatosis (type 2) is heritable, is usually bilateral, and is associated with cutaneous stigmata and other anomalies that are characteristic of von Recklinghausen's disease. The rarer hyperostotic digital gigantism (type 3) is not heritable, is usually unilateral, is associated with other skeletal anomalies in the affected limb, and presents without accompanying nerve pathology. Common to all three variants is overgrowth of multiple cell types within the digit, which is present at birth or noted during early infancy, and involvement of a digit or digits that follows the sensory distribution of the median or ulnar nerve.

TYPES OF GIGANTISM

Type 1: Digital Gigantism with Lipofibromatous Hamartoma

Digital gigantism with lipofibromatous hamartoma of the median or ulnar nerve has been variously described as *macrodactyly* (2,3), *nerve territory–oriented macrodactyly* (4), *megadactyly* (5–7), *macrodystrophia lipomatosa* (8), or *macrodactylia fibrolipomatosis* (9). It is one of the least common congenital anomalies, with an incidence of 0.5% (10), of all anomalies of the hand. The phalanges and soft tissue types are invariably affected (2,5,11), but the metacarpals appear to be inconsistently involved (7,12,13). Metacarpal involvement may be a manifestation of the severity of the disorder or increased patient age. Digital overgrowth may be symmetric, involving equally the radial or ulnar sides of the same digit, or asymmetric. If overgrowth is asymmetric, curvature of the digit results, which is more frequently ulnarly convex. There is fibrotic thickening of the dorsal skin and predominantly palmar soft tissue overgrowth, which may cause the digit to be hyperextended at the distal interphalangeal joint. In milder forms, a symmetrically involved digit may have the appearance of an enlarged normal digit, with preserved active joint motion. Frequently, however, the digit is grotesquely enlarged, and the interphalangeal joints are stiff. Involvement of multiple digits always involves adjacent digits, and abnormal fingers are never separated by a normal finger. Digital gigantism with lipofibromatous nerve hamartoma is unilateral 90% of the time (10). Associated congenital anomalies are limited to syndactyly, which is present in approximately 8% of cases. Café au lait spots, which are characteristic of neurofibromatosis, are not associated with this variant of digital gigantism. There is no heritable factor (2,5,6) that is known, and no chromosomal abnormalities have been identified (2).

DeLaurenzi delineated two types of digital gigantism that were dependent on growth characteristics (2). Enlargement that is present at birth with further growth proportionate to the remaining uninvolved digits was believed to be static. More frequently, disproportionate growth occurs, so that the involved digit (or digits) increases in size at a faster rate than could be attributed to normal growth pattern. This second type, progressive gigantism, was more frequently complicated by palmar overgrowth of soft tissue and metacarpal involvement.

Characteristically, type 1 gigantism is associated with hyperplasia of the ulnar nerve or, more frequently, the median nerve. Digital involvement follows the sensory distribution of the enlarged nerve. Grossly, the median nerve is normal to the level of the distal forearm, where it gradually begins to increase in size. Within and distal to the carpal canal, the median nerve and its branches, including the digital nerves, become strikingly enlarged (14). Patients with type 1 gigantism with hamartoma of the median nerve may present with symptoms of median nerve compression owing to the tremendous size of the nerve within the carpal tunnel.

Type 2: Neurofibromatosis

Neurofibromatosis (von Recklinghausen's disease) is a systemic disorder of considerable complexity that is characterized by hyperplasia and neoplasia in the connective tissues throughout the nervous system. The well-known clinical hallmarks of the disorder include multiple tumors of the peripheral nerves, areas of cutaneous pigmentation (café au lait spots), and pedunculated cutaneous tumors (molluscum fibrosum). Neurofibromatosis is inherited as an autosomal-dominant trait but may also be the result of a spontaneous mutation; it occurs with an approximate rate of 1 in 3,000 live births.

Similar to type 1 gigantism, type 2 gigantism follows the distribution of a major peripheral nerve, most frequently the median nerve, but is unlike other variants of overgrowth. Although the overgrowth of bone as well as soft tissues occurs in types 1 and 2 gigantism, involved digits in neurofibromatosis may demonstrate large osteochondral masses that arise from the physes of the phalanges and metacarpals and are confluent with the epiphyses (15,16). In the young child, these masses are predominantly cartilaginous and, with age, undergo enchondral ossification. As these osteochondromata enlarge, they displace the flexor tendons palmarly and erode the distal aspect of the adjacent phalanx or metacarpal. Although the remaining joint surface may be normal, joint motion is severely limited mechanically.

The peripheral nerve tumors are usually multiple and may be discrete or diffuse (plexiform) neurofibromas. They may occur along the course and at the terminations of peripheral and autonomic nerves and in sympathetic ganglia. Neurofibromas probably arise from the fibrous connective tissue elements of the nerve sheath as well as from Schwann cells, because these tumors contain collagen and reticulin. Similar to what occurs in hamartoma nerve involvement, the affected nerve is enlarged and tortuous

distal from the level of the wrist but, additionally, may include multiple nodular tumor masses along its course.

Type 3: Hyperostotic Digital Gigantism

Occasionally, digital gigantism involves the skeleton and soft tissues of the digit but is not associated with nerve enlargement (type 3). Similar to other types of gigantism, overgrowth in the affected digits involves the phalanges and metacarpals and follows the sensory distribution of the median nerve. Although there are no cutaneous manifestations of neurofibromatosis, osteochondral masses that are identical to those that are formed in neurofibromatosis arise from the physes of the phalanges and metacarpals. As these mature and enlarge, adjacent joint motion is hindered (4). Other associated anomalies include dysplasia of the radiocapitellar joint with subluxation of the radial head, osteocartilaginous loose bodies of the elbow, and, infrequently, hemihypertrophy. There is no apparent heritable factor. Although hyperostotic gigantism may have radiologic findings that are similar to those of neurofibromatosis, the lack of nerve neurofibromas and cutaneous stigmata and the apparent absence of heritability suggest that this is a third variant of digital gigantism.

Treatment

Treatment of the patient with digital gigantism is difficult and often discouraging. Factors that affect treatment include the type of gigantism, the rapidity of progression, the digits involved, and the age of the patient. The major objectives of a treatment plan are to lessen the disparity in the length and circumference between the affected and unaffected digits, to maintain useful sensibility at the fingertip, and to maintain flexion and extension at the metacarpophalangeal joint. To attempt to satisfy these objectives, surgical intervention should begin early. Nonoperative care is not indicated.

Digital gigantism has historically been treated by multiple defatting procedures in combination with partial or complete ray ablation. Bunnell suggested that, in the young child, epiphysiodesis would be effective in controlling length (17). He recommended defatting procedures to additionally lessen the circumference. Subsequently, numerous reports have advocated epiphyseal arrest (6,18) or physeal excision (5) to terminate longitudinal growth. Ablation of the epiphyseal plate does not affect appositional bony growth. Consequently, longitudinal phalangeal osteotomies may be used to narrow the finger. Approximately one-third of the lateral bone may be removed; this procedure is often combined with soft tissue debulking. After longitudinal osteotomies, however, interphalangeal joint motion is probably diminished.

McCarroll (19) reported that excessive finger growth ceased when the distal nerves were totally excised. To maintain sensibility, Tsuge (13) excised only the nerve branches but preserved the digital nerve trunk. All branches were separated from the nerve trunk and were excised along with adipose tissue through lateral incisions. If surgery was necessary bilaterally, within the same finger, the procedures were staged at 3-month intervals. Edgerton and Tuerk (12) recommended reducing the size of the hypertrophic digital nerve by longitudinally excising a portion of nerve as soon after birth as possible. Both authors also advised that further surgery might be necessary to improve the appearance of the digits.

Curvature of a digit can be corrected by a closed wedge osteotomy that removes a generous portion of the bone to achieve some shortening, as well as longitudinal correction. Although this may be done through the middle phalanx, the osteotomy may also be done through an epiphyseal plate, with excision of the physis, or through the proximal interphalangeal joint, with fusion of the proximal and middle phalanges. The resulting soft tissue redundancy from the shortening requires revision at a second stage. Correction of the angular deformity through excision of the distal interphalangeal joint does not permit the same degree of shortening without potential nail growth disturbances.

In the adult, after opportunities for arrest of growth have passed, the involved digits may reach grotesque proportions. Partial amputation may be performed through the middle phalanx or at the terminal phalanx (20). Tsuge (13) modified this technique somewhat by making mid-lateral incisions and raising the nailbed with a thin layer of the dorsal terminal phalanx on a proximally based dorsal flap (Fig. 1). The remaining terminal phalanx and a portion of the middle phalanx are removed, and the nail is inset into the remaining middle phalanx. Skin redundancy occurs dorsally and is resected at a second stage.

The thumb may be adequately shortened by arthrodesis of the metacarpophalangeal joint with resection of generous amounts of proximal and distal phalanges. Redundancy of soft tissue after shortening can be excised secondarily. Millesi (21) has described a unique method of simultaneously shortening and narrowing an enlarged thumb (Fig. 2). This technique entails three features, namely central wedge resection of the thumbnail and distal phalanx, amputation of the terminal portion of the distal phalanx, and a shortening oblique osteotomy of the proximal phalanx.

For the treatment of an adult patient with only one finger affected, particularly if the finger is stiff and grotesquely enlarged, or in those patients in whom previous surgical procedures have failed, ray resection is the procedure of choice (10,22,23). Central ray resection may be combined with ray transfer. After amputation, there may be progressive fatty overgrowth in the palm and at the site of amputation that might require repeated excision.

Author's Preferred Treatment

In the young child with multiple digit involvement, physeal arrest of all involved phalanges and metacarpals prevents fur-

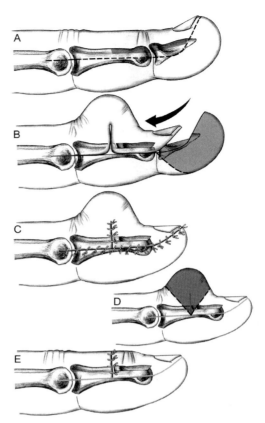

FIGURE 1. Tsuge's method of shortening an enlarged digit. **A:** The nailbed is elevated on a proximally based dorsal flap. **B:** After resection of the distal phalanx, the nail, with an underlying sliver of bone, is inset into the middle phalanx. **C–E:** The dorsal redundancy is resected 3 months later.

ther longitudinal growth but does not stop appositional bony growth. Dorsal cutaneous branches of the digital nerves that are encountered can be transected. Epiphysiodesis is difficult due to the orientation of the physeal plate. Exposure is through a mid-lateral incision by using a small power bur to

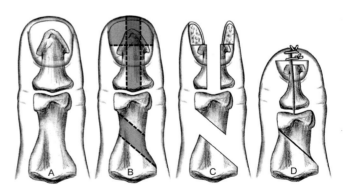

FIGURE 2. **A–D:** Shortening and narrowing of the thumb according to the technique that was described by Millesi. This method involves a central wedge resection of the thumbnail and distal phalanx, amputation of the terminal portion of the distal phalanx, and oblique shortening osteotomy of the proximal phalanx.

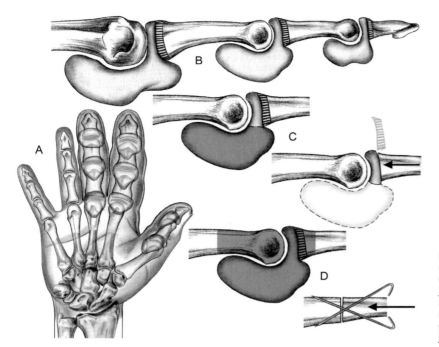

FIGURE 3. A,B: Diagrammatically, the osteochondral masses arise from the epiphyses and, as they enlarge, erode the adjacent bone and restrict joint motion. **C:** Resection of these masses has been disappointing as a method of restoring joint motion. **D:** The mass should be removed with generous amounts of bone on either side of a joint, and the joint should be fused.

ablate the physis. When present, osteochondral masses can be removed at the same time. An alternative to epiphysiodesis is physeal excision with the mass, and shortening of the digit occurs through the fusion mass. Later, redundant skin has to be excised (Fig. 3). Subsequently, longitudinal wedge osteotomies can be performed to narrow the girth of the finger. Parents should be aware that, despite surgical intervention, the finger remains grotesquely enlarged and stiff. Amputation of one digit in the young child is certainly an option to lessen the visual impact. Amputation through the metacarpal physis results in diaphyseal atrophy over time, and ray transfer is not necessary. In the older child, epiphysiodesis is not effective. The surgical objective is to shorten and narrow the finger. Treatment should include phalangeal shortening, often fusing the proximal interphalangeal joint with wedge resection of redundant skin. The middle phalangeal osteotomy should include excision of the physis. At 3-month intervals, longitudinal wedge osteotomies combined with further soft tissue excision can be planned. Amputation of a single finger is still an excellent option.

The principal surgical complication is skin flap necrosis. Whether the problem is due to an underlying inadequacy of blood supply or an inefficiency of cutaneous circulation, the incidence of skin flap problems is substantially higher than would be anticipated. After defatting procedures, the skin may be removed from the excised portion and replaced as a full-thickness skin graft. Mid-lateral incisions and proper staging of procedures are important to avoid this problem.

Surgical restoration of lost interphalangeal joint motion is impossible to achieve. Removal of the large osteochondral masses that are frequently encountered in types 2 and 3 gigantism permits improved passive and active ranges of motion. With time, however, the gain that has been achieved may gradually be lost.

CONSTRICTION BAND SYNDROME

Constriction band syndrome is a random condition that occurs in approximately 1 in 15,000 live births. There is no evidence of an inherited defect. The lesions are usually asymmetric and tend to occur toward the distal end of the limb. The most likely cause is oligohydramnios (24). The smaller uterine volume creates premature rupture of the amniotic sac, which allows the fetal lining to engulf the fingers and produces a vascular compromise. Finger development up to this point has been normal. The extent of constriction bands varies from a mild eccentric band on one aspect of the finger to ischemia and an intrauterine amputation of the distal portion of the finger. Patterson (25) devised a classification system that was based on severity of the defect:

1. Simple constriction ring (Fig. 4)
2. Constriction ring that is associated with deformity of the distal part, with or without lymphedema
3. Constriction ring that is associated with distal soft tissue coalescence (acrosyndactyly)
4. Intrauterine amputation

Type 3, acrosyndactyly, may be further classified into three types (26):

Type 1: Conjoined fingertips with well-formed commissure at the proper depth.

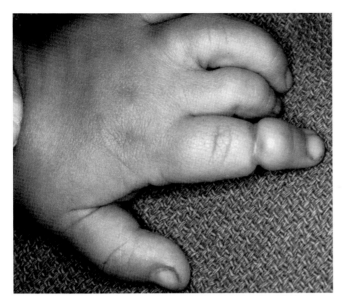

FIGURE 4. Mild constriction bands that can be treated by staged Z-plasties.

Type 2: Distal syndactyly with incomplete commissure formation.

Type 3: Distal syndactyly; absent commissural formation with sinus tract between the involved digits (Fig. 5).

The syndactyly of constriction band syndrome differs from the typical presentation of congenital syndactyly. In constriction band syndrome, normal digital separation has occurred. There is a vascular insult to the distal aspect of the finger that results in raw surfaces that fuse distally. Typically, osseous structures are not involved in the distal syndactyly, and there is a sinus tract that is the remnant of the original

web space. This acrosyndactyly may involve adjacent fingers but, dissimilar to congenital syndactyly, may involve nonadjacent fingers, with the uninvolved finger being forced dorsally or volarly by the fusion mass. Sensibility in constriction band syndrome may be variably affected, depending on the depth of band formation (27,28), whereas sensibility in congenital syndactyly is normal. Sensibility changes and temperature gradients across the constricting band are more likely to occur with proximally located bands.

Treatment

In its mildest presentation, simple constriction rings that are shallow or incomplete may not require any treatment. Bands that are deep and completely circumferential with a viable tip should be treated with Z-plasties. The Z-plasty flap should be as large as possible and should have an angle of approximately 60 degrees. Only one-half of the digital circumference should be done at one operation. The constriction band should be excised, rather than incised, to avoid repositioning of the abnormal tissue into the Z-plasty (29). The procedures should be staged by an interval of 2 or 3 months.

In constriction bands with lymphedema, the same principles apply, that is, excision of the band tissue and Z-plasties. Parents should be made aware that, postoperatively, complete resolution of the lymphedema is unlikely, and any improvement would be seen slowly over the ensuing months. Alternately, amputation of the distal part may be considered.

Author's Preferred Treatment

When the constriction ring is so deep that distal edema is present, progressive distal ischemia may occur. Early Z-plasty

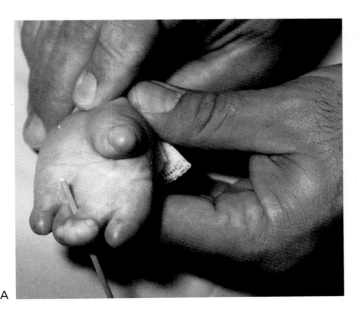

A

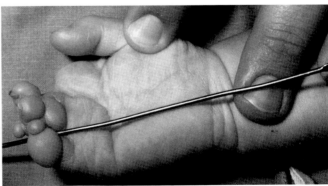

B

FIGURE 5. A,B: Type 3 acrosyndactyly typically has a sinus tract that is more distally located than the ideal level of the commissure.

should be considered. In less severe presentations, release can be done electively. Owing to the differences in skin mobility, larger Z-plasties can be used dorsally, whereas small, more numerous Z-plasties are used volarly. The constriction ring is excised and is not repositioned as part of the flap to decrease residual deformity. The neurovascular bundle should be identified proximal to the ring, and great care should be taken when excising the ring owing to the superficial location of the bundle.

Acrosyndactyly of multiple fingers that is secondary to extensive constriction band syndrome should be released early to allow parallel longitudinal growth of the involved fingers. Distal separation should begin at 6 months of age and is followed by deepening of the commissure to at least the level of the metacarpal head (Fig. 6). The epithelial-lined sinus, at the base of the involved digits, is invariably

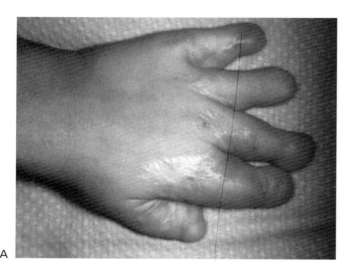

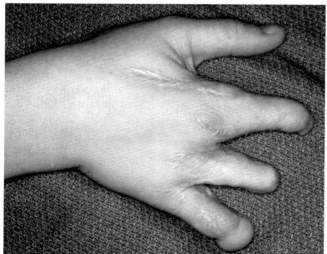

FIGURE 6. A: Early surgical intervention is recommended to allow longitudinal growth of separate digits. This child was originally operated on at 6 months of age. **B:** After multiple staged procedures, the appearance of her hand at 18 years of age is quite acceptable.

more distal than the optimal site for commissural reconstruction and should be excised. Deepening of the web space follows the same principles as congenital syndactyly. Flaps should be defatted and interdigitated, and a dorsal-proximal–based dorsal flap should be used for web reconstruction. Full-thickness skin grafts may be necessary at the base of the proximal phalanx after separation. The epithelial-lined sinus tract can be used as a flap or can be excised. Alternately, an oblique incision through the web produces two flaps to resurface the contiguous phalangeal surfaces. Full-thickness skin grafts are frequently necessary. Poorly covered, pencil-tipped phalanges may be cold sensitive. Preferably, the bone should be shortened somewhat to cover the tips with local full-thickness skin, as opposed to skin grafts. The author has not found it necessary to lengthen the skeleton of involved fingers and would rather ensure that the web space is adequately deepened and the tips well padded. Range of motion is usually lost at the interphalangeal joints but is preserved at the metacarpophalangeal joint. Children should be followed through skeletal maturity to ensure that potential secondary contractures are properly addressed.

ELBOW SYNOSTOSIS

Synostosis of the elbow results primarily from an intrinsic defect in joint formation or secondarily from inadequate muscle formation and limited intrauterine limb motion. Elbow synostosis is rare and frequently presents with other upper extremity malformations, most commonly, ulnar aplasia (30). The elbow is fixed in flexion from 60 to 90 degrees, and, frequently, there is little forearm rotation. The lack of elbow motion significantly interferes with placement of the hand in space and, consequently, hand function. Compensatory trunk, head, and shoulder motion are necessary to accomplish the tasks of toiletry and hygiene (31).

Other than repositioning the elbow in a more optimal degree of flexion, there are no operative indications. All described surgical procedures that were directed at restoring elbow motion have been failures. Failed arthroplasty techniques have included interposition of various biologic and nonbiologic materials with and without continuous passive motion devices (30). If the child cannot compensate through alternate joint motion, or if an associated forearm aplasia places the hand dysfunctionally, a corrective osteotomy is indicated.

RADIOULNAR SYNOSTOSIS

During fetal development, the upper limb begins as a common cartilaginous anlage. At 6 to 7 weeks of embryonic fetal development, segmentation of the humerus, radius, and ulna occurs. As longitudinal segmentation continues

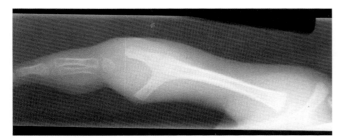

FIGURE 7. Radioulnar synostosis is typically proximal and is a failure of separation within the common cartilaginous anlage.

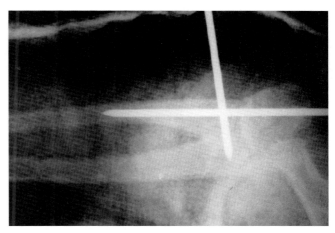

FIGURE 8. When performing a derotational osteotomy through the fusion mass, a longitudinal Kirschner wire is inserted before the osteotomy is performed. After correction, a second, oblique Kirschner wire is inserted to maintain correction.

distally, a separate radius and ulna are formed. During this period of longitudinal segmentation, the proximal ends of the radius and ulna share a common perichondrium and hence are united for a period. Intrinsic genetic or extrinsic teratogenic factors in operation during the period interrupt the normal sequencing and leave the radius and ulna as a common bony mass (Fig. 7). Concurrently, during this period of intrauterine development, the forearm is anatomically positioned in varying degrees of pronation (32,33). Failure of separation of the proximal radius and ulna then leaves the forearm in pronation (34). Although positive family histories have been reported (35,36), radioulnar synostosis is mostly a sporadic event. It is bilateral 80% of the time, which suggests an internally flawed genetic mistake. Associated anomalies include the cardiovascular, thoracic, gastrointestinal, renal, and central nervous systems. Other associated syndromes include acrocephalosyndactyly, arthropyosis, acropolysyndactyly, and Klinefelter's syndrome (34).

The degree of deformity of pronation, the age of the patient, and bilateralism often influence the age at which children present for evaluation. Younger children with unilateral involvement or mild pronation deformities, or both, rarely present until school age. At presentation, the elbow is flexed, the forearm is shortened, and there is hypermobility of the wrist as a compensatory mechanism (37). Shortening is most obvious when involvement is unilateral. Parents should be questioned at length in regard to functional deficits, if any. Many times, the forearm is so pronated that there is backhanded positioning when holding objects. Thirty percent of children present with fixed pronation deformities, less than 60 degrees (34), that are unilateral and are compensated for with increased wrist rotation; these children rarely have functional deficits. These children do not need surgery and should be counseled that operative repositioning of the forearm would be unlikely to improve their function. X-rays demonstrate the fusion mass and variable hypoplasia of the radial head to aplasia in children with no rotation (38). When surgery is indicated, there should be no attempt to provide forearm rotation. Biologic and nonbiologic interposition arthroplasties have been attempted but have been uniformly disappointing in restoring motion. Abnormal muscle development may be

an underlying factor in failures to maintain active forearm rotation, which intraoperatively is attained.

Author's Preferred Treatment

In the child with severe pronation deformity, a derotational osteotomy of the proximal forearm fusion mass is recommended (34). The proximal forearm is exposed through a skin excision along the subcutaneous border of the ulna. Before osteotomy, a longitudinal, smooth Kirschner wire is passed from the olecranon apophysis, down the intramedullary canal of the ulna, and under the fluoroscopic control to control position after the osteotomy (Fig. 8). An osteotomy is performed through the synostosis subperiosteal with an oscillating saw. The forearm is then rotated into approximately 0 to 20 degrees of pronation. A second, percutaneous Kirschner wire is directed obliquely from the ulna to the radius, transfixing the osteotomy. Compensatory wrist hypermobility should be considered when selecting the final position of the forearm (37). Anterior and posterior splints are applied, and the child is carefully monitored postoperatively for compartment syndrome, which has been reported to occur in as much as 36% of patients (34). If compartment syndrome is impending, the child should be immediately returned to the operating room, and the oblique percutaneous Kirschner wire should be removed. This allows the forearm to rotate back into a safer position. After resolution of compartment pressures, the forearm can be rotated once again into the corrected position.

REFERENCES

1. El-Shami IN. Congenital partial gigantism: case report and review of literature. *Surgery* 1969;65:683–688.
2. Barsky AJ. Macrodactyly. *J Bone Joint Surg* 1967;49:1255–1266.

3. Moore BH. Macrodactyly and associated peripheral nerve changes. *J Bone Joint Surg* 1942;24:617–631.
4. Kelikian H. Macrodactyly. In: Kelikian H, ed. *Congenital deformities of the hand and forearm.* Philadelphia: WB Saunders, 1974.
5. Jones KG. Megadactylism: case report of a child treated by epiphyseal resection. *J Bone Joint Surg* 1963;45:1704–1708.
6. Rechnagel K. Megadactylism: report of 7 cases. *Acta Orthop Scand* 1967;38:57–66.
7. Thorne FL, Posch JL, Mladick RA. Megalodactyly. *Plast Reconstr Surg* 1968;41:232–239.
8. Ranawat CS, Arora MM, Singh RG. Macrodystrophia lipomatosa with carpal tunnel syndrome. *J Bone Joint Surg* 1968;50:1242–1244.
9. Yaghmai I, McKowne F, Alizadeh A. Macrodactylia fibrolipomatosis. *South Med J* 1976;69:1565–1568.
10. Wood VE. Macrodactyly. *J Iowa Med Soc* 1969;59:922–928.
11. Tuli SM, Khanna NN, Sinha GP. Congenital macrodactyly. *Br J Plast Surg* 1969;22:237–243.
12. Edgerton MT, Tuerk DB. Macrodactyly (digital gigantism): its nature and treatment. In: Littler JW, Cramer LM, Smith JW, eds. *Symposium on reconstructive hand surgery,* vol. 9. St. Louis: CV Mosby, 1974.
13. Tsuge K. Treatment of macrodactyly. *Plast Reconstr Surg* 1967;39:590–599.
14. Frykman GK, Wood VE. Peripheral nerve hamartoma with macrodactyly in the hand: report of three cases and review of the literature. *J Hand Surg* 1978;3:307–312.
15. Heiple KG, Elmer RM. Chondromatous hamartomas arising from the volar digital plates. *J Bone Joint Surg* 1972;54:393–398.
16. Hensinger RN, Rhyne DA. Multiple chondromatous hamartomas. Report of a case. *J Bone Joint Surg* 1974;56:1068–1070.
17. Boyes JH. *Bunnell's surgery of the hand,* 5th ed. Philadelphia: JB Lippincott Co, 1970.
18. Clifford RH. The treatment of macrodactylism: a case report. *Plast Reconstr Surg* 1959;23:245–248.
19. McCarroll HR. Clinical manifestations of congenital neurofibromatosis. *J Bone Joint Surg* 1950;32:601–617.
20. Dennyson WG, Bear JN, Bhoola KD. Macrodactyly in the foot. *J Bone Joint Surg* 1977;59:355–359.
21. Millesi H. Macrodactyly: a case study. In: Littler JW, Cramer LM, Smith JW, eds. *Symposium on reconstructive hand surgery,* vol. 9. St. Louis: CV Mosby, 1974.
22. Boyes JG Jr, Hamilton JP. Macrodactylism. *N C Med J* 1977;38:151–153.
23. Timoney FX. Macrodactyly. Case report. *Ann Surg* 1944;119:144–147.
24. Torpin R. Amniochorionic mesoblastic fibrous strings and amniotic bands: associated constricting fetal malformations or fetal death. *Am J Obstet Gynecol* 1965;91:65.
25. Patterson TJ. Congenital ring constriction. *Br J Plast Surg* 1961;14:1.
26. Light TR. Growth and development of the hand. In: Carter PR, ed. *Reconstruction of the child's hand.* Philadelphia: Lea & Febiger, 1991:122.
27. Flatt AE. Constriction ring syndrome. In: Flatt AE, ed. *The care of congenital hand anomalies.* St. Louis: CV Mosby, 1977:214.
28. Weeks DM. Radial, median and ulnar nerve dysfunction associated with a congenital constricting band of the arm. *Plast Reconstr Surg* 1982;69:333.
29. Dobyns JH. Congenital ring syndrome. In: Green DP, ed. *Operative hand surgery,* 2nd ed. New York: Churchill Livingstone, 1988:505.
30. Dobyns J, Wood V, Bayne L. Congenital hand deformities. In: Green DP, Ed. *Operative hand surgery,* 3rd ed. New York: Churchill Livingstone, 1993:251.
31. Waters PM, Simmons BP. Congenital abnormalities: elbow region. In: Peimer CA, ed. *Surgery of the hand and upper extremity.* New York: McGraw-Hill, 1995:2049.
32. Morrison J. Congenital radio-ulnar synostosis. *Br J Med* 1892;2:1337.
33. Wilkie DP. Congenital radioulnar synostosis. *Br J Surg* 1914;1:366.
34. Simmons BP, Southmayd WW, Riseborough EJ. Congenital radioulnar synostosis. *J Hand Surg* 1983;8:829.
35. Fahlstrom S. Radio-ulnar synostosis. *J Bone Joint Surg* 1932;14:395.
36. Henson HO, Anderson ON. Congenital radio-ulnar synostosis. *Acta Orthop Scand* 1970;41:255.
37. Oqino T, Hikinok. Congenital radio-ulnar synostosis: Compensatory rotation around the wrist and rotation osteotomy. *J Hand Surg* 1987;12:173.
38. Mital MA. Congenital radio-ulnar synostosis and congenital dislocation of the radial head. *Orthop Clin North Am* 1976;7:375.

90

REPLANTATION

RANDY SHERMAN
WILLIAM C. PEDERSON
A. CHARLOTTA LA VIA

Microsurgical reattachment of a body part that has been amputated represents one of the modern pinnacles of reconstructive hand surgery. Replantation of such parts usually offers a result that is functionally and cosmetically superior to other types of reconstruction, all of which are, by their nature, delayed, multistaged, and dependent on a donor site that carries its own morbidity once it is used. Replantation of extremities involves more than microsurgery, however, as repair of bone, tendon, nerve, and muscle injuries must be undertaken as well. It is these latter components that usually determine the ultimate functional outcome. Functional results that are measured by standard protocols, such as total active motion, two-point discrimination, and grip strength, set the final parameters of success or failure as opposed to viability rates, which were used in much earlier stages of the discipline. This chapter focuses on the indications, technique, and results of replantation of amputated body parts.

EXTREMITY REPLANTATION

Definitions

This section provides a word about commonly used terminology and how it may lead to confusion in practice guidelines. Often mistakenly termed *reimplantation*, the act of reattaching digits or other body parts is termed *replantation*. The term *reimplantation* should be reserved for total joint surgeons who perform revision total hips and knees. When replantation is performed, whether successful or not, it should be assumed that the part was completely severed from the body. The term *revascularization*, no matter how imprecise, denotes repair of all structures, always including, but not limited to, arteries and veins, in an incompletely amputated part, which is essentially dead because of no nutrient blood flow. Oftentimes, its outcome may be worse than that of the more spectacular complete amputation that arrives in a bag because of underappreciation of the terminal nature of the injury by triage personnel (Fig. 1).

History

The first successful replantation of a severed limb was carried out nearly 40 years ago by Malt (1) in Boston when he replanted the completely amputated arm of a 12-year-old boy. Revascularization of incompletely severed digits was proven feasible in the clinical setting by Kleinert and Kasdan (2) in 1963. The first successful digital replantation was performed by Tamai in Japan, as reported in 1965 (3). Since these early reports, replantation of severed extremities has become an accepted procedure (4–8), and the indications, technique, and expected results are discussed in the following sections.

Indications

Although the indications for replantation have not changed significantly over the years, experience with the techniques and results have refined the indications (Table 1). All indications for replantation must take into account the status of the amputated part (sharp amputation vs. crush) and the patient (healthy vs. systemic illnesses.) The degree of tissue injury may mitigate against replantation, even in the case of a clear indication, such as thumb amputation. The indications are not based solely on potential viability but are predicated on the potential for long-term function. Overall, thumb replantation probably offers the best functional return. Even with poor motion and sensation, the thumb is useful to the patient as a post for opposition (9–12) (Fig. 2). A replanted thumb offers the best reconstruction available, toe transfers not withstanding. Although single-finger replantations are generally not performed (13,14) (see the section Contraindications), replantation beyond the level of the sublimis tendon insertion (zone 1) usually results in good function (15,16) (Fig. 3). Multiple finger amputations present reconstructive difficulties that may be challenging to correct without replantation of one or all of the amputated digits (13,17). Oftentimes, in the case of multiple digit amputations, the hand surgeon can use favorably amputated parts (clean cut through diaphyseal segments of

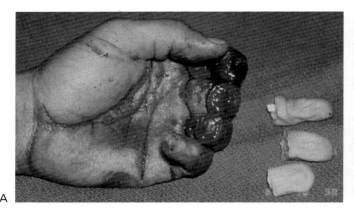

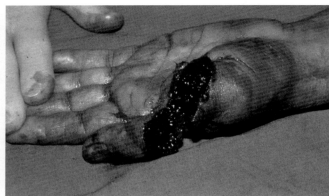

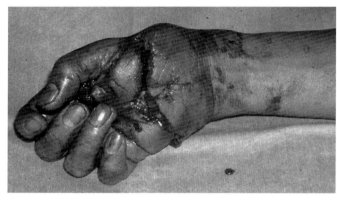

FIGURE 1. A: Multiple digital amputations, cleanly severed; excellent indication for replantation. **B:** Thumb devascularization, still attached with no nutrient blood flow. **C:** Midpalmar devascularization. Note the distal cyanosis. Pulse oximetry would immediately make the diagnosis of a limb-threatening condition.

bone) on nonnative bases; that is, when all four fingers are amputated at the mid-proximal phalanges, there may be a situation that precludes the use of the amputated long finger, as well as some crush to the metacarpophalangeal joint of the index. In this circumstance, the index finger may be replanted onto the long-finger stump. The astute replantation surgeon constantly assesses each amputated part for its best possible use as opposed to just its anatomically correct place. Any hand amputation from zone e (distally) to zone 5 (proximally) offers the chance of reasonable function after replantation (Fig. 4), which is usually superior to available prostheses. Several centers believe that cleanly amputated carpal hands may, when promptly replanted, offer excellent functional recovery potential (18–20). Although usually indicated, the replantation of any hand or arm proximal to the level of the mid-forearm must be carefully considered. The risk of complications goes up and the chance of functional return goes down with amputations

above the elbow. It is generally felt that replantation should be attempted with almost any part in a child. In children, success rates (in terms of viability) are lower, but the functional results are better (21–23). Although there have been a number of reports of successful lower limb replantation (24–29), this area remains controversial. The available lower extremity prostheses make amputation less of a functional problem in the leg than in the upper extremity. The leg contains larger masses of muscle (which tolerate ischemia poorly), and without adequate sensory recovery, the foot is at risk for soft tissue breakdown. Replantation and revascularization of the foot or lower leg, or both, in children may, however, give gratifying results (30–32).

Contraindications

The contraindications to replantation are more relative than the indications, but they must be kept in mind (Table 2). Single-finger replantations at the level of zone 2 (from the first annular pulley to the distal sublimis tendon insertion) are rarely indicated, with the notable exception of the thumb. Amputated parts that are severely crushed and those with multiple-level injuries have poor function even if they survive replantation (33,34) (Fig. 5). Those parts that carry avulsed tendons from the musculotendinous junctions (Fig. 6) are never successfully replanted, no matter how seemingly intact the distal element

TABLE 1. INDICATIONS FOR REPLANTATION

Thumb
Multiple digits
Hand amputation through palm
Hand amputation (distal wrist)
Any part in a child
More proximal arm (sharp only)
Finger distal to sublimis insertion (zone 1)

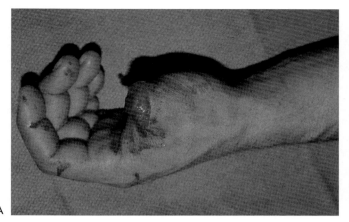

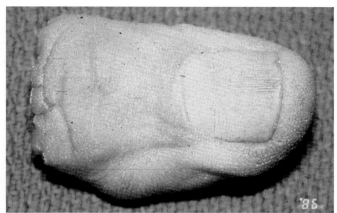

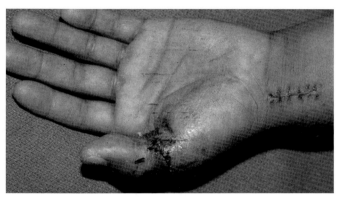

FIGURE 2. A: Clean thumb amputation at middle proximal phalangeal level. This is an excellent candidate for replantation. **B:** Amputated part. Notice how there is no crush component. **C:** Successfully replanted thumb.

appears. Patients with parts of fingers that have been completely degloved (ring avulsions) are generally considered poor candidates for attempted replantation (35) (Fig. 7). Distal amputations at the level of the nailbed are marginally indicated, as there needs to be approximately 4 mm of intact skin proximal to the nail fold for adequate veins to be present. Patients who have severe systemic injury or disease may not tolerate the anesthesia and surgery well, and the consideration of replantation in these patients must weigh the systemic risks versus the potential functional loss of the amputated part (36). Successful replantation has been reported in an octogenarian, but the functional results were poor (37). Experience in patients who have severe mental disease or who experience substance abuse may also be poor. Although the technical aspects of replantation in these individuals may not present a problem, postoperative compliance is usually poor, and rehabilitation is difficult. With appropriate postoperative support, however, reasonable functional results are possible.

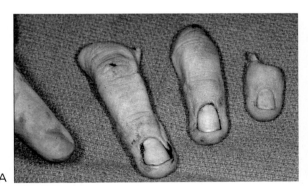

FIGURE 3. A: Multiple digital amputations at the proximal phalangeal level. Clean, with no crush or avulsion component. **B:** Postoperative photograph, immediately after replantation.

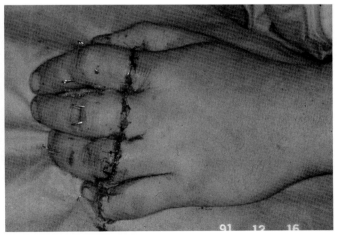

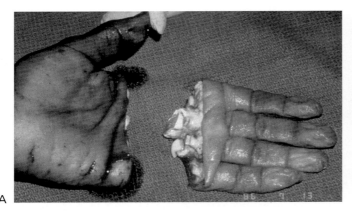

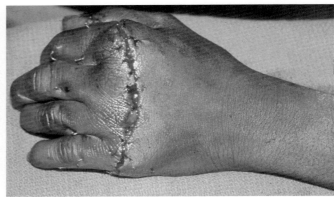

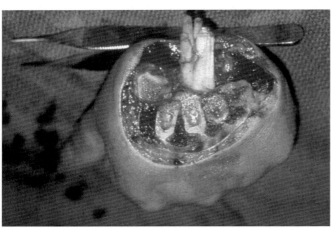

FIGURE 4. A: Distal palmar amputation, which can expect fair functional return. **B:** After replantation. **C:** Proximal palmar amputation, which can expect reasonable functional return.

Patient Management

Although replantation can be successfully performed in a community hospital (38), patients experiencing extremity amputation are often transferred to a center that performs these operations routinely. A clearly written and illustrated protocol, preferably laminated, should be disseminated and posted in all facilities, fixed (e.g., emergency rooms, schools, fire stations) and mobile (e.g., ambulances, helicopters), that may interface with this type of injury (Fig. 8). Before transfer, the patient should be stabilized cardiovascularly, and the amputated part should be cooled to maximize its ischemic tolerance (34,39). The part should be gently cleansed, but attempts at débridement in the emergency room should be avoided. The part should be wrapped in a moist gauze sponge, placed in a container (a

TABLE 2. CONTRAINDICATIONS FOR REPLANTATION

Single digits proximal to flexor digitorum superficialis insertion (zone 2)
Severely crushed or mangled parts
Multiple-level amputations
Replantation in patients with multiple trauma or severe medical problems[a]

[a]Relative contraindication.

sterile bag or a specimen cup), and then placed in ice. Floating the part in cold saline is probably not detrimental (34), but this tends to macerate the tissue if it is in this solution for many hours. Dry ice is to be avoided, as it can freeze the part (Fig. 9). The ischemic tolerance of amputated digits is fairly high, owing to the lack of significant muscle mass (40). The warm ischemic tolerance of digits is generally felt to be in the range of 8 hours, but successful replantation has been reported after cold ischemia times of up to 30 to 40 hours (41–43) and longer (44). With more

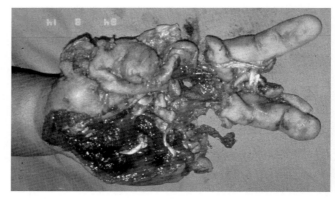

FIGURE 5. A massive crush avulsion that is not a candidate for replantation.

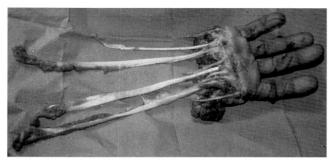

FIGURE 6. Avulsion of tendons at the musculotendinous junctions, as well as multiple-level distal injuries. This is not a candidate for replantation.

proximal amputations, the ischemic tolerance is significantly shorter. The absolute maximum warm ischemic tolerance or major amputations is in the range of 4 to 6 hours, and this may be prolonged by cooling to the 10- to 12-hour

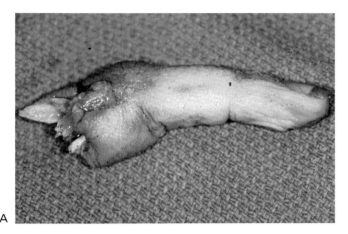

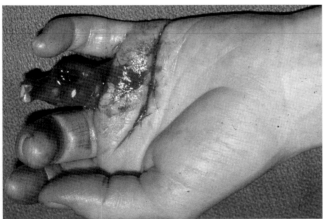

FIGURE 7. A: Urbaniak et al. type 3 ring avulsion amputation. Notice the ribbon sign or faint red midaxial line that denotes probable avulsion of the neurovascular bundle, thus making successful replantation unlikely. **B:** Amputation stump of ring avulsion injury that demonstrates level of separation. No good answer exists for coverage except possible partial free toe transfer. Most of these injuries are treated with completion amputation with possible ray resection.

range (34). Amputated parts with a significant amount of muscle (arms and legs) have poor ischemic tolerance, and delay in replantation can lead to significant metabolic problems after revascularization.

Once the patient arrives, preparation for surgery should proceed rapidly. Repeated examinations of the injured limb should be avoided, as this is painful and may increase the risk of vascular spasm. The patient should be warmed, and intravenous solutions should be administered to keep the blood volume and pressure up. X-rays are taken of the amputated part and the limb that has experienced the amputation. X-rays of both are important because there may be missing bony fragments, and management of this should be planned for and discussed with the patient. The patient is given broad-spectrum antibiotics and tetanus prophylaxis, when appropriate. The operative permit should include permission for *at least* the following: revision amputation, vein grafts, nerve grafts, skin grafts, bone grafts, and, possibly, free flaps for coverage. Brad Edgarton often points out, no matter how hopeless the situation appears, or how contraindicated the replantation attempt seems, after a full, open, and frank discussion with the patient and family, the patient should be assured that everything possible will be done in the operating theater to salvage and restore function. The acute loss of part or all of an extremity is profoundly shocking and extremely difficult to comprehend. Coupled with sometimes unrealistic expectations from

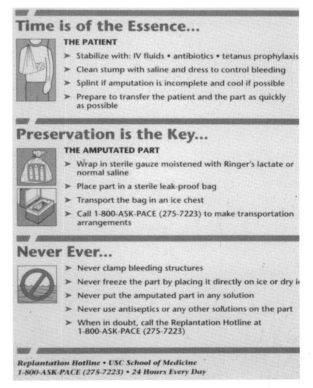

FIGURE 8. Example of a replantation algorithm, simply written with easy-to-follow illustrations.

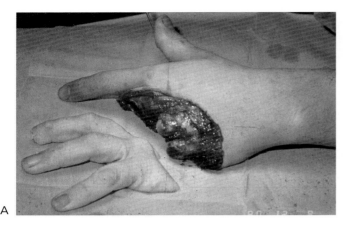

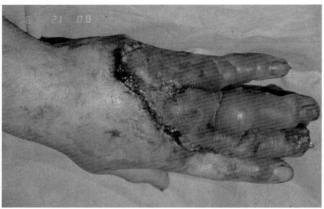

FIGURE 9. A: Cleanly amputated partial hand that was transported on dry ice, a practice that should be avoided. **B:** Severe frostbite injury that manifested itself several hours after successful replantation.

patient and family, a quick dismissal of one's chances to undergo attempted replantation in a major trauma center based solely on written contraindications may frequently lead to unnecessary legal action.

Once the patient has been worked up in the emergency room, the part is taken to the operating room for examination and preparation. When possible, a two-team approach is optimal, one group examining and preparing the amputated part, the other preparing the stump (Fig. 10). Careful examination of the part in the operating room, before the patient is under anesthetic, allows time for appropriate

TABLE 3. OPERATIVE SEQUENCE

Bone shortening and fixation
Tendon repair
Arterial repair
Neurorrhaphies
Venous repairs
Skin coverage or closure

decision making (Table 3). After careful débridement, the digital vessels are dissected out and examined under strong loupe magnification or microscope. A standard microsurgical instrument tray is required, including, but not limited to, jewelers forceps, dissecting scissors, suture scissors, needle holders, dilators, microsuture (9-0 through 11-0), bipolar electrocautery forceps, microvascular occluding and approximating clips (Acland type), background material, and irrigating solutions, including heparinized saline, 2% lidocaine (Xylocaine), papaverine, and streptokinase (Fig. 11). Anastomotic venous couplers have been used successfully to cut down on ischemia time but can be noticed as an annoying foreign body postoperatively (Fig. 12). The vessels must be examined carefully, as their status can give an idea of the severity of injury and whether vein grafts are needed (or in fact whether replantation can be attempted). A corkscrew appearance of the arteries [the "ribbon" sign (45)] implies that an avulsion force has been applied to them, and this segment of vessel should be excised and vein grafted (46). If bruising is noted along the course of the digit at the point at which the neurovascular bundle runs, this implies a severe avulsion injury with disruption of branches of the digital artery at the sites of the bruises. This particular sign should alert the surgeon that revascularization of the amputated part may be unsuccessful.

Once identified, the arteries and nerves are marked—it can be surprisingly difficult to find them later. A 6-0 polypropylene suture that is cut long serves this purpose well. If veins on the dorsal surface are obvious, these are marked as well, but they are often easier to find after completion of the arterial anastomosis. Attention is next turned to the bones and tendons. The bone should be minimally débrided with a curette and managed as an open fracture

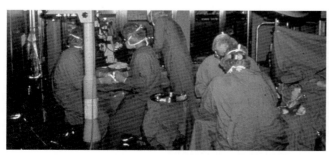

FIGURE 10. Two-team approach to replantation.

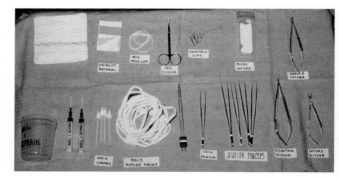

FIGURE 11. Typical replantation microsurgical instrument tray.

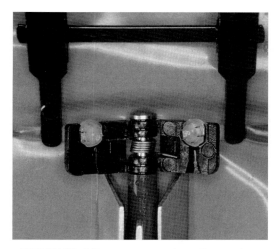

FIGURE 12. Microvenous anastomotic coupler.

(47). Once the bone is cleaned, distal fixation can be placed in the amputated part. The type of fixation used depends on a number of factors, but in fingers, the simplest is usually the best. For this reason, crossed Kirschner wires are usually used and are placed retrograde in the amputated finger first. Interosseous wires can be used to supplement the Kirschner wires (48) but are usually not necessary. Although plates can be used in digital replantation, these are more time intensive and require extensive soft tissue dissection for bony exposure. Plate fixation in replantation at the proximal phalanx level may, however, be indicated to allow early motion (49). Plates offer excellent fixation in amputations through the midmetacarpal level (50), and the distal portion of the plate can be placed on the amputated part in the preparation stage if attention is paid to alignment (relative to the site of amputation and the amount of proximal bone that is available) (Table 4). Periosteal repair should be performed after bony fixation, particularly on the dorsal surface, to decrease adhesions of the tendons to the bone.

After placing the distal bony fixation, attention is turned to the tendons. These may need to be trimmed to give a clean end, but excessive trimming should be avoided. In zone 2, it may be best to repair the profundus only, especially if the tendons are not cleanly cut. A double-core suture technique is usually chosen for the flexor tendons,

TABLE 4. OSTEOSYNTHESIS

Parallel longitudinal Kirschner wires
Crossed Kirschner wires
Intramedullary pins
Interosseous wires
Plate fixation
Screw fixation
External fixation
Bone pegs

and one-half of this suture can be placed in the distal tendon before final bony fixation.

Surgical Technique

At this point, the amputated part is ready for replantation (Fig. 13). The amputated part is kept on ice if the amputation stump is not yet ready. The stump is irrigated with antibiotic-containing saline solution, and nonviable tissue and debris are removed. The proximal bone is minimally débrided, and small, loose, bony fragments are removed. Larger fragments should be cleaned and saved for use, if necessary. The tendons, vessels, and nerves are exposed and made ready for repair. They can be exposed through a Bruner-type zigzag incision in the finger or palm. Once these structures are identified, the amputated part is brought into the field, and bony fixation is completed. This step should proceed rapidly if the distal fixation was properly done. After bony fixation, the tendons are repaired in standard fashion, using the previously placed core suture for the flexor tendons (Fig. 14).

All patients who undergo replantation and who have experienced avulsion of the digit with attached tendon should have release and exploration of the carpal tunnel. As the finger is pulled out, portions of the muscle belly may be avulsed within the carpal tunnel, leading to acute median nerve compression. As this is difficult to diagnose in a patient after replantation surgery, release of the transverse carpal ligament and removal of nonviable muscle fragments should prevent compression of the median nerve. In these individuals, consideration should be given to performing a forearm fasciotomy as well, as swelling can ensue postoperatively owing to the trauma of avulsion of the tendon from muscle, especially if the patient is heparinized.

If the total ischemic time has been short, nerve repair can be done next (Fig. 15). If the surgeon is concerned about ischemia, which is usually the case, then arterial repair takes precedence over nerves. The function of replanted digits is much better if return of sensibility is reasonable (51,52), and special attention should be paid to nerve repairs. The edges must be trimmed back to undamaged nerve, and doing this adequately may not allow primary anastomosis. Nerve gaps should be grafted in most digital replants, unless the likelihood of survival is believed to be low. In the case of a multiple-digit amputation, the most damaged finger may prove useful as a source of parts to repair the other digits—especially nerve and skin grafts (53). Other sources of nerve graft include the medial antebrachial cutaneous nerve from the forearm and the sural nerve. In any case, the finger should not be flexed to allow primary nerve anastomosis, as later movement likely disrupts this repair.

The vascular repairs are done next. Nowhere is precision more linearly correlated with viability (Fig. 16). Although primary repair of the arteries is occasionally possible, vein

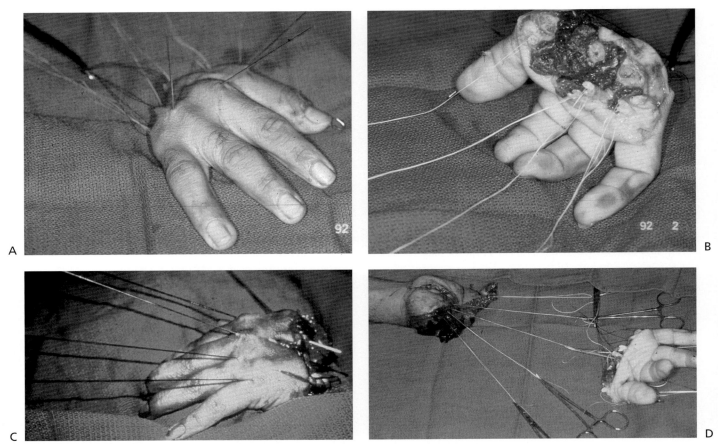

FIGURE 13. A: Preparing the amputated part with Kirschner wire placement, tendon suturing, and nerve identification. **B:** All tendons receive a modified Kessler suture, so that sewing is minimized once the parts are coapted. **C:** The amputated part is now ready to be replaced. **D:** Immediately before replantation.

grafts should be used if any question about the status of the artery exists (54,55). The vessel should be trimmed back until there is no thrombus or intimal separation. Vein grafts of appropriate size for digital arteries can be harvested from the distal volar forearm or dorsal foot. If there is volar skin loss, and coverage of the neurovascular repairs will be a problem, some skin that overlies the vein graft may be taken with the vein graft, and this is used as a small flow-through venous flap (56–58). This obviates the need for skin grafts or another type of flap later. After arterial repair, the finger should rapidly turn pink in color, but this may take a period of 10 to 15 minutes if the digit is cold or if there has been a long ischemia time. Four percent lidocaine or papaverine, or both, placed on the vessels minimizes vasospasm, and the finger should be wrapped with warm sponges after arterial repair is complete. One should wait 10 to 15 minutes and should watch the status of perfusion before repairing veins. If the finger does not show signs of good perfusion after this period, revision of the anastomosis is in order, or a second arterial repair should be performed. Many studies have shown that survival rates are improved with the anastomosis of two arteries per finger

(59–62); however, a single anastomosis with good flow may be adequate (21,63).

Thumb amputations present certain technical difficulties in terms of vascular anastomosis (64). With amputations between the metacarpophalangeal and interphalangeal joints, access to the arteries can be difficult after bony fixation. For this reason, most authors suggest the use of a vein graft from radial artery in the anatomic snuffbox to the amputated segment (9,65), particularly in avulsion injuries (66,67). Anastomosis of the vein graft is performed first to the distal vessel on the amputated part (usually on the back table), followed by proximal anastomosis after bony fixation (68).

There should be brisk bleeding from the veins after the digit is warmed up, and one should select the two veins that are bleeding the most for venous anastomosis (59). Due to the anatomy of the dorsal venous system, it is less common to need vein grafts for venous outflow. The veins are exposed by carefully elevating the dorsal skin off of the venous plexus, and division of one or more branches usually provides a gain in length to allow primary anastomosis. If primary anastomosis is not possible, vein grafts should be used. This is often the case in patients with dorsal skin loss,

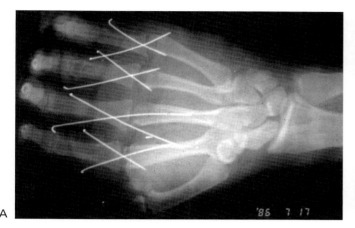

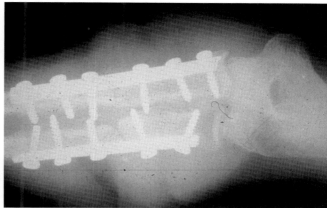

A

B

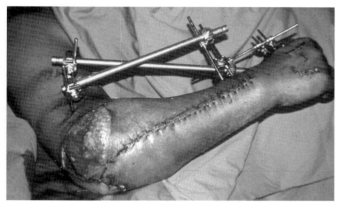

C

FIGURE 14. **A:** Crossed Kirschner wire osteosynthesis. **B:** Plate and screw internal fixation for both-bone proximal forearm reduction. **C:** External fixation for an elbow dislocation-amputation.

in which case, a venous free flap (56,58) or a long venous pedicle flap from an adjacent finger may be necessary (58,69). Once adequate length for primary anastomosis has been gained, the two veins with the most brisk bleeding should be connected. All other bleeding veins should be identified and closed with small vascular clips or with bipolar electrocautery, which maximizes flow via the anastomosed veins. In some instances, there may not be adequate veins for anastomosis (especially in distal replantation). If

brisk retrograde flow is noted in the contralateral digital artery after repair of one artery, the second artery can be anastomosed to a proximal vein to provide outflow for blood (70–72).

If arterial and venous flow is adequate at this point, the skin should be carefully closed. Care must be taken to avoid compression of the veins by skin closure, and a minimal number of sutures should be used. If any question exists as to whether the skin closure may be too tight, small nonmeshed

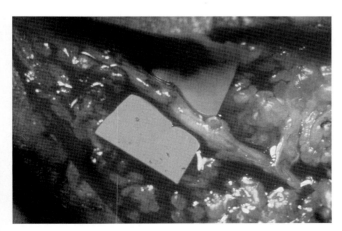

FIGURE 15. Precision neurorrhaphy using 10-0 or 11-0 microsutures.

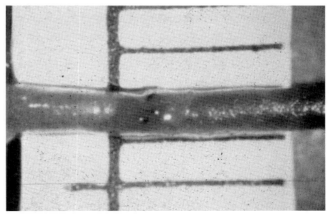

FIGURE 16. Arterial and venous anastomoses must be done as perfectly as possible to maximize success rates.

TABLE 5. DRESSINGS

No compression
Immobilization
Comfort
Aesthetics
Monitoring

TABLE 6. RING AVULSION CLASSIFICATION BY URBANIAK ET AL.

Type 1	Soft tissue injury only; no vascular compromise
Type 2	Soft tissue injury with arterial or venous compromise, or both
Type 3	Total degloving of soft tissues

split-thickness skin grafts should be placed. It is far better to place a small skin graft over the draining veins than to occlude outflow by a too-tight skin closure. The extremity should be placed in a well-padded splint with no circumferential dressings around the digits. An excellent dressing can be made by wrapping the entire extremity in 1-in. foam, which is then wrapped with plaster rolls. This type of dressing cannot become too tight in the postoperative period (Table 5).

Postoperative Management

The patient should be placed in a warm room in the postoperative period. Arterial spasm can be a significant problem in replanted digits, and keeping the environment warm may lessen this problem. An indwelling axillary sheath catheter, through which a constant infusion of bupivacaine hydrochloride (Marcaine) is given to provide pain relief and a chemical sympathectomy, should be placed in the operating room (73,74). This is left in place for approximately 5 days. Although systemic heparinization is widely used in replantation, it is difficult to prove its efficacy (75). Its use is certainly indicated if vascular thrombosis occurs in the operating room or the vessels appear severely damaged (76). Chlorpromazine is a potent peripheral vasodilator and is given orally in the dose of 25 mg three times a day, for this effect and its sedative action on the patient, for 3 to 5 days postoperatively (34). Aspirin is also given at a dose of 325 mg daily for its antiplatelet effect. This aspirin dose is generally given for a total of 3 weeks postoperatively.

Unless there is a circulatory problem, the replanted part should not be manipulated in any way in the immediate postoperative period. Except in the case of major limb replantation, all wounds should be closed at the time of initial replantation. Experience has shown that an early return to the operating room with blood pressure shifts from anesthesia and temperature change can lead to irreversible vascular spasm. Problems can also be encountered after dressing changes, which should be avoided in the first few days postoperatively. When the patient is ready to be discharged, the outer splint and dressing can be removed, but any adherent dressing next to the wound should be left in place.

Ring Avulsion

A special case of digital amputation involves ring avulsions. In this injury, the soft tissue is partially or totally avulsed from the underlying bone and tendon. Urbaniak et al. (35) have classified these into three types (Table 6). Management of type 1 is fairly straightforward, as neurovascular injuries are dealt with in standard fashion. There may be significant damage to the soft tissues in type 2, however, and coverage of the vascular repairs may be necessary. As noted previously, a small venous flow-through flap or some type of local flap from the hand can be used for arterial or venous repair, or both, in these instances (77). The management of type 3 ring avulsions remains somewhat controversial (35,78–84). Most authors agree that replantation of the completely avulsed skin envelope is often unsuccessful, and, even with a successful revascularization of the skin, function is usually poor. Thumb avulsions, on the other hand, should be considered for replantation. If successful, this type of replant usually gives better function than an amputation (66). Experienced authors feel that the best management of patients with type 3 ring avulsions and those with amputation proximal to the sublimis insertion may be primary ray amputation of the finger (35). This gives a functional and cosmetic result, whereas a poorly functioning replantation of a completely avulsed digit may interfere with global hand function.

Monitoring

The primary problem with any technique for monitoring vascular flow is that it must be interpreted and understood by the nursing staff. There are a number of excellent techniques for monitoring the status of tissue perfusion today, but many of them experience technical difficulties and problems with interpretation. For this reason, many surgeons prefer to monitor the vascular status of replanted digits with temperature measurement (85–88) (Fig. 17). In general, the temperature of a well-vascularized digit should be at or above 31°C (89). Although temperatures somewhat below this may be compatible with adequate inflow, a decrease in arterial inflow results in a rapid loss of temperature in the digit. The baseline after surgery should be noted, and any marked decreases in this temperature indicate problems with the artery. Another monitoring technique is the use of a pulse oximeter (90,91). This probe can be placed on the distal digit, and changes in inflow give a rapid change in oxygenation (Fig. 18). Doppler laser flowmetry has also found some advocates, and, if the equipment is available, this technique is sensitive to changes in arterial flow (86,92,93). Photoplethysmography monitoring has been advocated in the past (94), but the interpretation of these data may be difficult for nursing personnel and has largely been supplanted by the previously mentioned techniques.

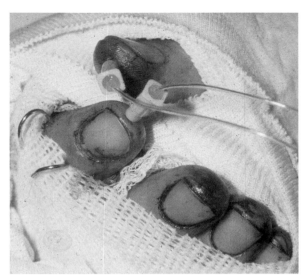

FIGURE 17. Temperature probes that are placed in replanted fingertips.

Management of the Failing Replant

There has been much discussion on the approach to the best management of a replanted extremity that is having vascular difficulties. The only sure way to remedy a vascular problem with a replanted part is to revise the anastomosis. The decision to take a patient back to surgery for salvage depends on the circumstances that are involved in the injury and the findings at surgery. Reported success rates of reoperation for vascular salvage of compromised replants range from 9% to 89% (21,61,63). Some experienced surgeons feel that the initial sur-

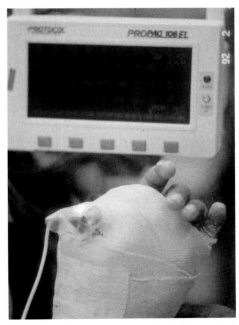

FIGURE 18. Pulse oximetry, although it obscures visual monitoring, probably gives the most useful real-time data.

gery should be the best that can be done and rarely return to surgery to attempt secondary repair of thrombosed vessels. (Urbaniak, *personal communication*). This attitude is certainly applicable to digits, and experience shows that fingers that struggle to survive (with or without vascular revision) are usually functionally the worst. They are often atrophic, have poor sensation, and move poorly. Although a thumb with these attributes may be useful to the patient, digits like this are rarely useful. Replanted hand parts certainly deserve reexploration if they show signs of vascular compromise, and replantations in children should usually be reexplored if problems arise. In the case of severe avulsion or crush injuries, more proximal amputations, and patients who have experienced perioperative systemic complications, a return to surgery for attempted salvage may not be appropriate.

Nonoperative treatment may improve the situation and, in fact, lead to salvage of some compromised replants. If arterial inflow decreases, the dressing should be loosened, and the patient should be heparinized (if not already on heparin). Likewise, an axillary block may improve the situation if vascular spasm is present. If a decrease in arterial flow occurs, however, the primary decision is whether to return the patient to surgery, knowing that reoperation is the option of choice if the digit is to be salvaged.

Venous outflow problems present a somewhat different set of considerations. Distal digital replantation (at or beyond the distal interphalangeal level) may not have adequate veins for reanastomosis (95–97). This type of replant may be appropriate in some patients, and venous outflow may present difficulties. An arteriovenous anastomosis can be performed to the other digital artery in some patients, but, failing this, there must be some provision for venous outflow. Some authors have proposed heparinizing the patient and removing the fingernail (34,98). A heparinized pledget is placed on the nail, and this is removed at intervals to promote bleeding. Our experience with this technique has been less than satisfying. A second, and usually more reasonable option, is the use of leeches.

The medicinal leech, *Hirudo medicinalis* (Fig. 19), secretes a complex protein anticoagulant that is called *hirudin*. Its action is largely local, and systemic side effects are minimal. In the replant with venous outflow obstruction, leeches can provide adequate outflow to allow survival of the part (97,99). It is common to see the statement that leech therapy is only necessary for 2 or 3 days, but this is certainly not the case in the authors' experience. If there is total obstruction of venous outflow, nearly continuous leeching is necessary for at least 5 to 6 days, and the patient may experience significant blood loss (in the 2- to 6-U range). This blood loss represents the primary potential complication of leech therapy, but leeches also have the potential to cause infection. *Aeromonas hydrophila* is a saprophytic organism in the leech's gut that, although not a primary pathogen in humans, can cause significant infection (100–102). One review article found that infection occurred in 7% to 20% of cases of leech application for

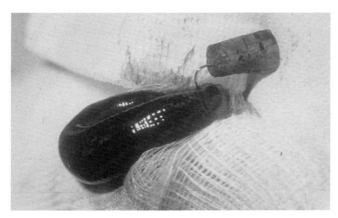

FIGURE 19. A typical example of leech therapy. Bleeding continues at the site for several hours.

venous outflow problems and was associated with a decrease in salvage of the involved tissue (101). Infection is uncommon in tissue with adequate arterial supply, however, and their use should be avoided if the viability of the tissue is questionable (102). To minimize the risk of infection, the patient should be covered with appropriate antibiotic therapy during the period of leech application (103). Studies of leech flora suggest that a third-generation cephalosporin is appropriate prophylaxis in most cases (104).

Complications

Serious complications are unusual in digital replantation and are usually related to the patient's underlying health rather than the surgery itself. The primary operative complications include bleeding (usually from anticoagulation) (105), infection (106), and loss of the replanted digit. If serious bleeding is encountered, the value of the replanted part versus the potential side effects of transfusion should be weighed and discussed with the patient. Infection after digital or hand replantation is unusual and is usually related to the amount of contamination and the adequacy of débridement. The presence of infection can, however, lead directly to vascular thrombosis and loss of the digit or digits. This fact emphasizes the necessity for good initial débridement and coverage with vascularized tissue.

If the initial replantation is successful, late problems are usually reflected in poor motion and function of the replanted part. Nonunion is uncommon but has been reported (107,108). The joints may undergo Charcot's change due to denervation, but this is surprisingly uncommon (109). Late necrosis of the replanted part may occur, particularly if there is poor soft tissue coverage or infection occurs.

Secondary Surgery

The need for secondary surgery after digital replantation is common and is usually related to poor sensation or motion (Table 7).

TABLE 7. SECONDARY PROCEDURES

Corrective osteotomies
Tenolyses
Tendon grafts
Tendon transfers
Neurolyses
Nerve grafts
Arthroplasties
Soft tissue releases

Neurolysis or nerve grafting may be required, particularly if the nerves were not repaired at the initial setting. Tenolysis is frequently necessary, as early motion is not possible in most patients undergoing replantation. This has been shown to be a valuable procedure in postreplant patients (110). Tenolysis may be necessary on the flexor and extensor sides of the digit, as the extensor tendons often become adherent at the site of bone injury. In some cases, staged reconstruction of the tendon by placement of a silastic rod followed by tendon grafting may be necessary. Web space release and flap coverage may be needed in patients with thumb replantation if first web space contracture is not prevented. Request for amputation of a replanted digit by the patient is unusual, even if function is poor.

Major Limb Replantation

As noted previously, replantation of more proximal amputations is indicated in certain situations (Fig. 20). The function of hands that are replanted from the midmetacarpal level to distal wrist (zone 3 to zone 5) is usually quite good, although intrinsic muscle function is usually poor. More proximal amputations through the muscle bellies of the flexors and extensors can function well but are often avulsion injuries that may severely compromise later function. Amputations above the elbow should be considered for replantation in certain instances, but the main goal is often preservation of a functioning elbow for later prosthesis fitting (111). Ischemia time is important in proximal amputations, as the large amount of muscle mass in these amputations tolerates ischemia poorly. Attempting to replant a forearm or arm with a prolonged warm ischemic period can lead to severe metabolic problems and, potentially, death of the patient (112–114). Débridement of nonviable tissue is paramount, and this leads to the problem of soft tissue coverage in many of these patients. Although uncommon in digital replantation, infection, and even systemic sepsis, is the number one complication in major limb replants (106,115). For this reason, major limb replantation is not to be undertaken without a serious commitment to the endeavor.

Technically, there are a few points about major limb replantation that should be noted. Stable bony fixation is important to maximize healing and to avoid motion that could disrupt vascular repairs. The usual sequence of surgery should be modified, however, as revascularization of the

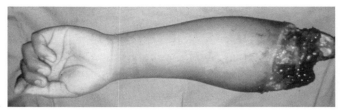

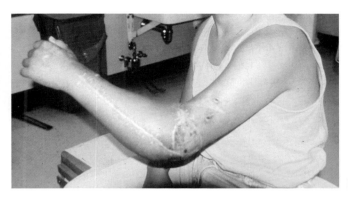

FIGURE 20. A: Major limb dislocation-amputation in which ischemia time must be minimized at all costs, oftentimes requiring temporary revascularization through the use of shunts before bony stabilization. **B:** Several months after successful replantation. Note the scars from compartmental releases on the forearm and hand intrinsics. Volar surfaces are released as well.

ischemic muscle is paramount. Some allow arterial perfusion via a shunt, which is used to perfuse the amputated part while bony fixation is performed (34). A vein graft can also be used, if it is made long enough to allow manipulation of the bone. While the part is receiving arterial blood, the venous effluent is simply allowed to bleed out. For this reason, every patient who is to undergo an attempt at major limb replantation should be typed and cross-matched for multiple units of blood and informed that blood transfusions are *required*.

For forearm and transhumeral amputation, most prefer bony fixation with a plate. If there is significant bony comminution or loss, an external fixator can be used, particularly in the forearm (116). This allows stabilization of the bone fragments while vascular and soft tissue repair is undertaken, with bony reconstruction planned for a later date if the initial procedure is successful. Once the bone is fixed, vascular repair can be done. If an arterial shunt has been used during this period, the artery is repaired first. Vein grafts are often required, unless there is significant bony shortening, and should be used if any question as to damage to the vessel ends exists. The approach to nerves should be individualized. Without return of sensation, the part that is replanted is virtually useless, but unless there is good soft tissue coverage and a high likelihood of success, primary nerve grafting of long gaps is probably not indicated. If the replant is successful, nerves can be prioritized and grafted in a good bed when the wounds are healed.

The final (and often most important) issue in these cases is management of the soft tissue loss. Local tissue is rarely available for coverage of bone and neurovascular repairs, and, thus, regional flaps or free flaps may be needed. The latissimus dorsi can be useful as a pedicled flap for coverage of the upper arm, and the pectoralis major may be useful in smaller, more proximal defects. For most forearm injuries, however, a free flap is required for significant soft tissue loss. Many feel that wound coverage should be obtained at the time of replantation, as exposed bone and neurovascular structures fare poorly if they are not covered with well-vascularized tissue. When the vascular repairs are performed, vein grafts can be taken longer than needed and placed in an extraanatomic position if necessary to avoid exposure.

For coverage of these wounds, muscle is probably the best choice in terms of vascularity and resistance to infection. The surgeon can choose whatever muscle he or she is most comfortable with, but adequate tissue should be transferred to fill dead space and to afford coverage of deep structures. Although thorough initial débridement is vital to success, all patients who undergo major limb replantation should be considered for return to the operating room at 24 to 48 hours to evaluate the wound and further débride nonviable tissue if necessary. For this reason, initial muscle coverage should allow extra tissue if this becomes necessary at the second look; this extra tissue can be removed, if necessary. All patients with proximal replantation should have fasciotomies of the hand and forearm, as the usual clinical parameters of compartment syndrome (pain and sensory changes) are not present in a replanted limb, and an untreated compartment syndrome in the replanted limb renders it useless. Secondary surgery is almost always necessary in major limb replantations and can range from muscle–tendon transfers to nerve grafting (111).

Results

Successful revascularization of the amputated part should be expected in as much as 80% of cases. Success is not measured today by survival, however. Function is the only real measure of success, and, based on this, success can often be predicted by the level of amputation. Single fingers distal to the sublimis insertion usually function well, even without motion at the distal interphalangeal joint. Hands proximal to the mid-palm also usually function well. A replanted thumb is almost always useful, even if it functions as a post for opposition, and is certainly the best reconstruction available. A study compared hand function after thumb amputation and replantation; however, it found little significant difference between the two groups (117). Patients with more proximal amputations and those with crush or avulsion injuries often have poor functional return. Function is usually predicated on the quality of sensory return, and, thus, return of sensation is important. The average sensation of replanted thumbs is approximately 11 mm, with clean amputations having better sensation, and avulsion injuries having poorer sensation. The average two-point discrimination of sharply amputated fingers averages 8 mm, with only 15 mm in patients who experience crush-avulsion–type injuries. Sensation is always better in children than adults (21,23). Motion is usually rather poor, with only approximately 35 degrees of motion in proximal interphalangeal joints that are replanted proximal to the flexor digitorum superficialis insertion. This motion improves to 82 degrees when the amputation is distal to the flexor digitorum superficialis insertion (34).

Cold intolerance is a problem in all patients after replantation, and, although most feel that this improves after approximately 2 years (118), some studies have shown that this persists for many years (119,120). The improvement in cold sensitivity is usually related to the quality of sensory reinnervation, and patients with better sensation usually have less cold intolerance (121–123).

Cost versus Benefit of Upper Extremity Replantation

Questions have been raised about the cost-effectiveness of replantation. In a study from Israel, Engel et al. (124) found that any amputation that would result in greater than a 15% impairment of the hand would benefit from replantation. Based on the American Medical Association *Guides to the Evaluation of Permanent Impairment*, loss of the thumb at the interphalangeal joint results in a 20% impairment of the hand, and loss of the index or middle finger at the proximal interphalangeal joint leads to a 16% impairment (125). These statistics would certainly imply that digital replantation is cost-effective, if one applies the values from Engel's paper. Another study from Sweden found that replantation was twice as costly as amputation and that one-half of these costs were due to nonsurgical factors—primarily, rehabilitation and the costs of time off work (126). A study from Austria, on the other hand, found that 82% of patients who underwent replantation had compensation benefits that were lower than those that would have accrued with amputation of the part (127). Although it is difficult to say exactly how these data compare to that of the United States, one would have to assume that replantation is valuable not only to the patient but also to society in terms of cost.

Lower Extremity

Amputation of the lower extremity is usually secondary to severe trauma, and, owing to the crushing nature of the injury, replantation may not be a viable option. Even without total amputation, foot salvage in the face of severe crushing injuries to the lower leg remains a controversial issue (128–130). The conditions that favor consideration of replantation of the lower extremity are amputations in young healthy patients, sharp amputations, and amputations in the distal one-third of the leg (131). The contraindications for lower extremity replantation mirror those of the upper extremity and include life-threatening associated injuries, crushing or avulsion injuries, and age or chronic illness that

would preclude a prolonged operation (131). The time period of ischemia is also a critical consideration, as prolonged ischemia predicates against success of replantation (132). A significant ischemic period in this group of patients may lead to myonecrosis and renal failure if attention is not paid to this issue (133). These patients require transfusion, with an average of 15 U in one series (134). With sharp amputations in young patients, however, results can be quite good (26,32,134,135). Many patients require further surgery after successful lower extremity replantation, particularly in the face of major limb length discrepancies (136–139).

Although replantation of the great toe has been reported in children (140), this is probably rarely indicated in adults. Replantation of the heel pad has been reported with good results, however (141–144). Larger portions of the foot can be replanted with acceptable function if the amputation is sharp (31,134,145).

With a crushing amputation of the lower leg, problems may arise in terms of coverage of the stump to maintain a functional length for prosthesis fitting. In cases such as this, portions of the foot may be replanted to cover exposed bone in the stump. The plantar surface of the foot has been used for this purpose and is nicknamed the "fillet of sole" (146–148). The dorsal surface can also be transferred based on the posterior tibial-dorsalis pedis system (149). Use of this otherwise discarded tissue provides excellent coverage and obviates the need for distant flap transfer.

NONEXTREMITY REPLANTATION

Microsurgery has been used for replantation of a number of tissues that have been amputated or avulsed. Among those reported have been the ear (150–152), the nose (153–155), the lip (156–158), the scalp (159–161), and even the entire face (162). There have also been a number of reports that concern replantation of the penis (163–165), the amputation of which is often the result of self-mutilation. Although patients presenting with the need for replantation of facial or other body parts are unusual, these types of replantation are discussed in the following sections, with particular emphasis on the problems that are encountered.

Ear Replantation

Loss of the ear from trauma presents a significant reconstructive challenge, and the replantation of an ear obviates the problems that are associated with its loss. Ear replantation presents some formidable difficulties, primarily due to the size and number of vessels. The primary arterial supply (relative to vascular repair) is from the temporal artery. There is a small branch from the temporal artery at approximately the level of the tragus that supplies the anterior surface of the ear. This vessel is quite small, but primary anastomosis is possible by skilled microsurgeons. If the ear has been sharply amputated, this may be possible. Unfortunately, many ear amputations are secon-

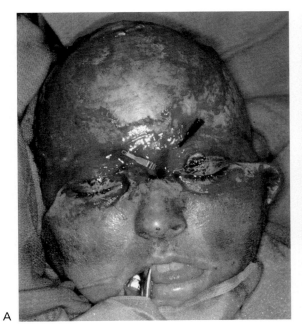

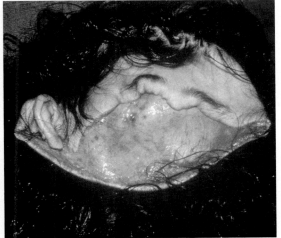

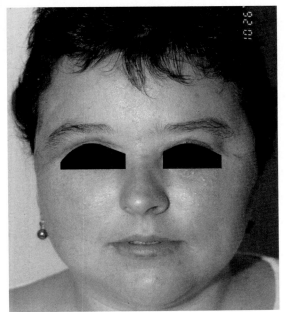

FIGURE 21. A: Total scalp avulsion; the usual pattern. **B:** The avulsed scalp; the subgaleal plane. **C:** Several months after successful replantation.

dary to avulsion and may render primary repair impossible. In these cases, vein grafts may have to be used, or, alternatively, the temporal artery can be freed up and brought posteriorly as a vascular leash for anastomosis to the ear (152). The real problem with ear replantation, however, is the venous drainage. The veins on the posterior surface are extremely small and few in number. Ear replantation can be successful without venous anastomosis, however, and many authors suggest using leeches in lieu of vascular repair for venous drainage (166–169). Others suggest making stab wounds in the posterior ear to allow for drainage (151,170,171). All reports of successful ear replantation have used heparin. If vascular repair is deemed impossible, or if thrombosis occurs, the ear cartilage can be salvaged by wrapping it in the temporoparietal fascia (172). Owing to the relatively few reports of ear replantation, success rates are difficult to estimate. With a successful arterial anastomosis and with the use of heparin and leeches, however, success should be

expected. Even with partial survival of the replanted ear, the cosmetic results are usually superior to reconstruction.

Scalp Replantation

Many cases of replantation of the scalp have been documented since the first case was reported in 1978 (159,173). As in the case of ear replantation, scalp replantation offers a result that is far superior to other types of reconstruction of this defect (Fig. 21). The availability of vessels for anastomosis is related generally to the size of the avulsed portion of scalp. If the entire scalp has been torn off, there are usually vessels of reasonable size available (primarily the temporal artery) (174,175), although vein grafts may be needed to bridge damaged segments (161,176,177). The entire scalp can survive on a single artery and vein if there is adequate flow through these vessels (178,179). The problems reported with

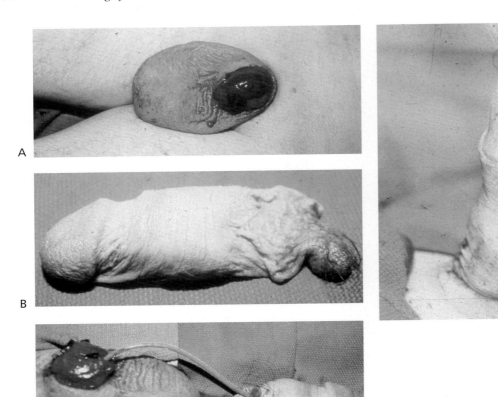

FIGURE 22. A: Penile amputation. **B:** The amputated part. There is no distal injury. **C:** The Foley catheter is analogous to an internal fixator. **D:** Immediately after replantation. Long-term erectile function was restored.

scalp replantation include poor venous outflow, which may necessitate the use of leeches (180) or incisions in the skin to allow venous bleeding (181). The use of a second artery in the scalp for anastomosis to a recipient vein to allow egress of blood has also been reported (161). Hematoma formation under the replanted scalp is one of the more commonly reported complications and can lead to compromise of the tissue (182,183). The results in reported series have generally been good, with only approximately a 5% to 10% total failure rate. Partial loss of the tissue is fairly common, however, with approximately 30% of patients sustaining partial necrosis of the replanted tissue (161,177,183,184). The need for secondary procedures to deal with partial loss and cosmetic concerns is common (185,186), but all reports note good return of hair growth in the surviving segments of scalp.

Lip and Nose Replantation

Traumatic amputation of the lips or nose, or both, remains an unusual occurrence. The largest reported series (from 12 institutions) contains only 13 patients who required lip replantation (158). Nasal amputation that is amenable to replantation has been reported only a few times (one patient had the lip and nose amputated) (153–156,181,187). These injuries occur most commonly due to animal bites (primarily dogs), with a lesser number from human bites. Arterial anastomosis in the amputated lip is reasonably straightforward via the labial artery (158,188,189). As with ear replantation, the primary problem with lip replantation is venous drainage, which is usually addressed with anticoagulation and leeching. Most patients require transfusion with this approach, which averages approximately 6 U (158). Most reported cases have been successful, with loss usually due to inadequate venous drainage.

Penis Replantation

Amputation of the penis is an uncommon injury and is frequently the result of self-mutilation in patients with psychiatric disorders (164,165,190–192). The external genitalia can also be avulsed in machinery (193). Replantation is fairly straightforward, via anastomosis of the dorsal or deep arteries, or both, and dorsal veins (Fig. 22). Venous outflow problems have not been reported, as they have been in tissues of the head and neck. The reported cases have been universally successful, but failures undoubtedly occur. The authors are aware of one case of failure that was due to the patient manipulating the replanted penis in the early postoperative period (after a self-inflicted amputation). With appropriate nerve anastomosis, there can be return of erectile and sexual function in the replanted part (192,194). Complications are primarily related to the urethral injury, and fistula and stricture have been reported (191,193). As with small parts of the head and neck, penile replantation offers a result that is far superior to any available reconstruction.

REFERENCES

1. Malt RA. Clinical aspects of restoring limbs. *Adv Surg* 1966;2:19–33.
2. Kleinert HE, Kasdan ML. Anastomosis of digital vessels *J Kentucky Med Assoc* 1963;63:106.
3. Komatsu S, Tamai S. Successful replantation of a completely cut-off thumb. *Plast Reconstr Surg* 1968;42:374.
4. Berger A, Millesi H. Functional results from replantation surgery: a five year report from the Viennese replantation team. *Aust N Z J Surg* 1980;50:244–247.
5. Kleinert HE, Jablon M, Tsai TM. An overview of replantation and results of 347 replants in 245 patients. *J Trauma* 1980;20:390–398.
6. Buncke HJ, Alpert BS, Johnson-Giebink R. Digital replantation. *Surg Clin North Am* 1981;61:383–394.
7. Zhong-Wei C, Meyer VE, Kleinert HE, et al. Present indications and contraindications for replantation as reflected by long-term functional results. *Orthop Clin North Am* 1981;12:849–870.
8. Tamai S. Twenty years' experience of limb replantation—review of 293 upper extremity replants. *J Hand Surg* 1982;7:549–556.
9. Schlenker JD, Kleinert HE, Tsai TM. Methods and results of replantation following traumatic amputation of the thumb in sixty-four patients. *J Hand Surg* 1980;5:63–70.
10. Ekerot L, Holmberg J, Niechajev I. Thumb replantation or not? *Scand J Plast Reconstr Surg* 1986;20:293–295.
11. Janezic TF, Arnez ZM, Solinc M, et al. Functional results of 46 thumb replantations and revascularisations. *Microsurgery* 1996;17:264–267.
12. Ward WA, Tsai TM, Breidenbach W. Per primam thumb replantation for all patients with traumatic amputations. *Clin Orthop* 1991:90–95.
13. Jones JM, Schenck RR, Chesney RB. Digital replantation and amputation—comparison of function. *J Hand Surg* 1982;7:183–189.
14. Scott FA, Howar JW, Boswick JA Jr. Recovery of function following replantation and revascularization of amputated hand parts. *J Trauma* 1981;21:204–214.
15. Soucacos PN, Beris AE, Touliatos AS, et al. Current indications for single digit replantation. *Acta Orthop Scand Suppl* 1995;264:12–15.
16. Urbaniak JR, Roth JH, Nunley JA, et al. The results of replantation after amputation of a single finger. *J Bone Joint Surg* 1985;67:611–619.
17. Steinau HU, Biemer E. Status of replantation—indications and limits in hand surgery. *Langenbecks Arch Chir* 1990;[Suppl 2]:751–755.
18. Blomgren I, Blomqvist G, Ejeskar A, et al. Hand function after replantation or revascularization of upper extremity injuries. A follow-up study of 21 cases operated on 1979–1985 in Goteborg. *Scand J Plast Reconstr Surg* 1988;22:93–101.
19. Goldner RD, Urbaniak JR. Indications for replantation in the adult upper extremity. *Occup Med* 1989;4:525–538.
20. Meyer VE. Hand amputations proximal but close to the wrist joint: prime candidates for reattachment (long-term functional results). *J Hand Surg* 1985;10:989–991.
21. Saies AD, Urbaniak JR, Nunley JA, et al. Results after replantation and revascularization in the upper extremity in children. *J Bone Joint Surg* 1994;76:1766–1776.
22. O'Brien B, Franklin JD, Morrison WA, et al. Replantation and revascularisation surgery in children. *Hand* 1980;12:12–24.
23. Ikeda K, Yamauchi S, Hashimoto F, et al. Digital replantation in children: a long-term follow-up study. *Microsurgery* 1990;11:261–264.
24. Mamakos MS. Lower extremity replantation—two and a half–year follow-up. *Ann Plast Surg* 1982;8:305–309.
25. Kutz JE, Jupiter JB, Tsai TM. Lower limb replantation. A report of nine cases. *Foot Ankle* 1983;3:197–202.
26. Vilkki SK. Replantation of a leg in an adult with 6-years' follow-up. *Acta Orthop Scand* 1986;57:447–449.
27. Fukui A, Inada Y, Sempuku T, et al. Successful replantation of a foot with satisfactory recovery: a case report. *J Reconstr Microsurg* 1988;4:387–390.
28. Yuksel F, Karacaoglu E, Ulkur E, et al. Replantation of an avulsive amputation of a foot after recovering the foot from the sea. *Plast Reconstr Surg* 2000;105:1435–1437.
29. Betz AM, Stock W, Hierner R, et al. Cross-over replantation after bilateral traumatic lower-leg amputation: a case report with a six-year follow-up. *J. Reconstr Microsurg* 1996;12:247–255.
30. Simonich MP, Schenck RC Jr, McGanity PL, et al. Successful revascularization of a partially avulsed foot in a 6-year-old child. *Texas Med* 1996;92:72–74.
31. Park EH, Mackay DR, Manders EK, et al. Replantation of the midfoot in a child—six-year follow-up with pedobarographic analysis. *J Reconstr Microsurg* 1999;15:337–341.
32. Masuda K, Usui M, Ishii S. A 17-year follow-up of replantation of a completely amputated leg in a child: case report. *J Reconstr Microsurg* 1995;11:89–92.
33. Manktelow RT. What are the indications for digital replantation? *Ann Plast Surg* 1978;1:336–337.
34. Goldner RD, Urbaniak JR. Replantation. In: Green DP, Hotchkiss RN, Pederson WC, eds. *Green's operative hand surgery*, 4th ed. New York: Churchill Livingstone, 1999.
35. Urbaniak JR, Evans JP, Bright DS. Microvascular management of ring avulsion injuries. *J Hand Surg* 1981;6:25–30.
36. Sood R, Bentz ML, Shestak KC, et al. Extremity replantation. *Surg Clin North Am* 1991;71:317–329.
37. Leung PC. Hand replantation in an 83-year-old woman—the oldest replantation? *Plast Reconstr Surg* 1979;64:416–418.
38. Pomerance J, Truppa K, Bilos ZJ, et al. Replantation and revascularization of the digits in a community microsurgical practice. *J Reconstr Microsurg* 1997;13:163–170.
39. Bajec J, Grossman JA, Gilbert D, et al. Upper extremity preservation before replantation. *J Hand Surg* 1987;12:321–322.
40. Morgan RF, Reisman NR, Curtis RM. Preservation of upper extremity devascularizations and amputations for replantation. *Am Surg* 1982;48:481–483.
41. Chiu HY, Chen MT. Revascularization of digits after thirty-three hours of warm ischemia time: a case report. *J Hand Surg* 1984;9:63–67.

42. May JW Jr, Hergrueter CA, Hansen RH. Seven-digit replantation: digit survival after 39 hours of cold ischemia. *Plast Reconstr Surg* 1986;78:522–525.

43. Baek SM, Kim SS. Successful digital replantation after 42 hours of warm ischemia. *J Reconstr Microsurg* 1992;8:455–458; discussion, 459.

44. Wei FC, Chang YL, Chen HC, et al. Three successful digital replantations in a patient after 84, 86, and 94 hours of cold ischemia time. *Plast Reconstr Surg* 1988;82:346–350.

45. Van Beek AL, Kutz JE, Zook EG. Importance of the ribbon sign, indicating unsuitability of the vessel, in replanting a finger. *Plast Reconstr Surg* 1978;61:32–35.

46. Alpert BS, Buncke HJ, Brownstein M. Replacement of damaged arteries and veins with vein grafts when replanting crushed, amputated fingers. *Plast Reconstr Surg* 1978;61:17–22.

47. Tupper JW. Techniques of bone fixation and clinical experience in replanted extremities. *Clin Orthop* 1978:165–168.

48. Gordon L, Monsanto EH. Skeletal stabilization for digital replantation surgery. Use of intraosseous wiring. *Clin Orthop* 1987:72–77.

49. Nunley JA, Goldner RD, Urbaniak JR. Skeletal fixation in digital replantation. Use of the "H" plate. *Clin Orthop* 1987:66–71.

50. Berger A, Meissl G, Walzer L. Problems of fracture fixation in replantation surgery. *Handchirurgie* 1980;12:247–248.

51. Yamauchi S, Nomura S, Yoshimura M, et al. Recovery of sensation in replanted digits—time of recovery and degree of two-point discrimination. *J Microsurg* 1982;3:206–213.

52. Glickman LT, Mackinnon SE. Sensory recovery following digital replantation. *Microsurgery* 1990;11:236–242.

53. Schoofs M, Raoult S, Fevrier P, et al. The strategy of the finger bank. *Ann Chir Main Memb Super* 1994;13:240–246.

54. Hamilton RB, O'Brien BM, Morrison A, et al. Survival factors in replantation and revascularization of the amputated thumb—10 years' experience. *Scand J Plast Reconstr Surg* 1984;18:163–173.

55. Cooney WP. Revascularization and replantation after upper extremity trauma: experience with interposition artery and vein grafts. *Clin Orthop* 1978:227–234.

56. Tsai TM, Matiko JD, Breidenbach W, et al. Venous flaps in digital revascularization and replantation. *J Reconstr Microsurg* 1987;3:113–119.

57. Inoue G, Maeda N. Arterialized venous flap coverage for skin defect of the hand and foot. *J Reconstr Microsurg* 1988;4:255–264.

58. Merle M, Dautel G. Advances in digital replantation. *Clin Plast Surg* 1997;24:87–105.

59. Matsuda M, Chikamatsu E, Shimizu Y. Correlation between number of anastomosed vessels and survival rate in finger replantation. *J Reconstr Microsurg* 1993;9:1–4.

60. Tark KC, Kim YW, Lee YH, et al. Replantation and revascularization of hands: clinical analysis and functional results of 261 cases. *J Hand Surg* 1989;14:17–27.

61. Holmberg J, Arner M. Sixty five thumb replantations. A retrospective analysis of factors influencing survival. *Scand J Plast Reconstr* 1994;28:45–48.

62. Zumiotti A, Ferreira MC. Replantation of digits: factors influencing survival and functional results. *Microsurgery* 1994;15:18–21.

63. Arakaki A, Tsai TM. Thumb replantation: survival factors and re-exploration in 122 cases. *J Hand Surg* 1993;18:152–156.

64. Nystrom A, Backman C. Replantation of the completely avulsed thumb using long arterial and venous grafts. *J Hand Surg* 1991;16:389–391.

65. Shafiroff BB, Palmer AK. Simplified technique for replantation of the thumb. *J Hand Surg* 1981;6:623–624.

66. Stevanovic MV, Vucetic C, Bumbasirevic M, et al. Avulsion injuries of the thumb. *Plast Reconstr Surg* 1991;87:1099–1104.

67. Hetland KR, Reigstad A, Rugtveit A, et al. Thumb replantation. *Nord Med* 1986;101:238–242.

68. Ikeda K, Morikawa S, Hashimoto F, et al. Fingertip replantation: pre-osteosynthesis vein graft technique. *Microsurgery* 1994;15:430–432.

69. Foucher G, Norris RW. The venous dorsal digital island flap or the neutral flap. *Br J Plast Surg* 1988;41:337–343.

70. Koshima I, Soeda S, Moriguchi T, et al. The use of arteriovenous anastomosis for replantation of the distal phalanx of the fingers. *Plast Reconstr Surg* 1992;89:710–714.

71. Smith AR, Sonneveld GJ, van der Meulen JC. AV anastomosis as a solution for absent venous drainage in replantation surgery. *Plast Reconstr Surg* 1983;71:525–532.

72. Suzuki Y, Ishikawa K, Isshiki N, et al. Fingertip replantation with an efferent A-V anastomosis for venous drainage: clinical reports. *Br J Plast Surg* 1993;46:187–191.

73. Berger A, Tizian C, Zenz M. Continuous plexus blockade for improved circulation in microvascular surgery. *Ann Plast Surg* 1985;14:16–19.

74. Matsuda M, Kato N, Hosoi M. Continuous brachial plexus block for replantation in the upper extremity. *Hand* 1982;14:129–134.

75. Davies DM. A world survey of anticoagulation practice in clinical microvascular surgery. *Br J Plast Surg* 1982;35:96–99.

76. Kutz JE, Hanel D, Scheker L, et al. Upper extremity replantation. *Orthop Clin North Am* 1983;14:873–891.

77. Alonso-Artieda M. Reimplantation of an avulsed ring finger using a sensory cross-finger flap. *Br J Plast Surg* 1971;24:293–295.

78. Bieber EJ, Wood MB, Cooney WP, et al. Thumb avulsion: results of replantation/revascularization. *J Hand Surg* 1987;12:786–790.

79. Cao X, Cai J, Liu W. Avulsive amputations of the thumb: comparison of replantation techniques. *Microsurgery* 1996;17:17–20.

80. Chen L, Gu J. Replantation of a completely detached degloved thumb. *Microsurgery* 1996;17:48–50.

81. Cheng GL, Pan DD, Qu ZY, et al. Replantation of avulsively amputated thumb: a report of 15 cases. *Ann Plast Surg* 1985;15:474–480.

82. Hung LK, Leung PC. Salvage of the ring avulsed finger in heavy manual workers. *Br J Plast Surg* 1989;42:43–45.

83. Tsai TM, Manstein C, DuBou R, et al. Primary microsurgical repair of ring avulsion amputation injuries. *J Hand Surg* 1984;9:68–72.

84. Tseng OF, Tsai YC, Wei FC, et al. Replantation of ring avulsion of index, long, and ring fingers. *Ann Plast Surg* 1996;36:625–628.

85. Aihara M, Tane N, Matsuzaki K, et al. The sticker-type temperature indicator in digital replantation: simplified application. *J Reconstr Microsurg* 1993;9:191–195.

86. Hovius SE, van Adrichem LN, Mulder HD, et al. Comparison of laser Doppler flowmetry and thermometry in the postoperative monitoring of replantations. *J Hand Surg* 1995;20:88–93.

87. Vilkki SK. Postoperative skin temperature dynamics and the nature of vascular complications after replantation. *Scand J Plast Reconstr Surg* 1982;16:151–155.

88. Reagan DS, Grundberg AB, George MJ. Clinical evaluation and temperature monitoring in predicting viability in replantations. *J Reconstr Microsurg* 1994;10:1–6.

89. Stirrat CR, Seaber AV, Urbaniak JR, et al. Temperature monitoring in digital replantation. *J Hand Surg* 1978;3:342–347.

90. Keller H, Lubbers DW. Reflection photometry of oxygen supply of skin flaps and replanted fingers. *J Reconstr Microsurg* 1986;2:241–245.

91. Matsen FA 3rd, Bach AW, Wyss CR, et al. Transcutaneous PO2: a potential monitor the status of replanted limb parts. *Plast Reconstr Surg* 1980;65:732–737.

92. Heden PG, Hamilton R, Arnander C, et al. Laser Doppler surveillance of the circulation of free flaps and replanted digits. *Microsurgery* 1985;6:11–19.

93. Lowdon IM, Toby EB, Ecker J, et al. Laser Doppler monitoring of replants using a small prism probe. *Microsurgery* 1989;10:175–177.

94. Doyle DJ, Eng P. A microminiature photoplethysmograph probe for microvascular surgery. *Microsurgery* 1984;5:105–106.

95. Barnett GR, Taylor GI, Mutimer KL. The "chemical leech": intra-replant subcutaneous heparin as an alternative to venous anastomosis. Report of three cases. *Br J Plast Surg* 1989;42:556–558.

96. Earley MJ. Microsurgical revascularisation of the thumb pulp with a discussion of the venous drainage of the thumb. *J Hand Surg* 1985;10:347–350.

97. Foucher G, Norris RW. Distal and very distal digital replantations. *Br J Plast Surg* 1992;45:199–203.

98. Tsai TM, McCabe SJ, Maki Y. A technique for replantation of the finger tip. *Microsurgery* 1989;10:1–4.

99. Lineaweaver WC, O'Hara M, Stridde B, et al. Clinical leech use in a microsurgical unit: the San Francisco experience. *Blood Coagul Fibrinolysis* 1991;2:189–192.

100. Lowen RM, Rodgers CM, Ketch LL, et al. *Aeromonas hydrophila* infection complicating digital replantation and revascularization [See comments]. *J Hand Surg* 1989;14:714–718.

101. de Chalain TM. Exploring the use of the medicinal leech: a clinical risk-benefit analysis. *J Reconstr Microsurg* 1996;12:165–172.

102. Lineaweaver WC, Hill MK, Buncke GM, et al. *Aeromonas hydrophila* infections following use of medicinal leeches in replantation and flap surgery. *Ann Plast Surg* 1992;29:238–244.

103. Lineaweaver WC, Furnas H, Follansbee S, et al. Postprandial *Aeromonas hydrophila* cultures and antibiotic levels of enteric aspirates from medicinal leeches applied to patients receiving antibiotics. *Ann Plast Surg* 1992;29:245–249.

104. Hermansdorfer J, Lineaweaver W, Follansbee S, et al. Antibiotic sensitivities of *Aeromonas hydrophila* cultured from medicinal leeches. *Br J Plast Surg* 1988;41:649–651.

105. Poole MD, Bowen JE. Two unusual bleedings during anticoagulation following digital replantation. *Br J Plast Surg* 1977;30:267–268.

106. Wang SH, Young KF, Wei JN. Replantation of severed limbs—clinical analysis of 91 cases. *J Hand Surg* 1981;6:311–318.

107. Kuwata N, Kawai S, Doi K. Clinical and experimental studies of bone union in reimplantation of digits: a preliminary report on ischemic interval. *Microsurgery* 1984;5:31–35.

108. Strauch B, Greenstein B, Goldstein R, et al. Problems and complications encountered in replantation surgery. *Hand Clin* 1986;2:389–399.

109. Vanderhooft E, Sack J. Charcot arthropathy following digital replantation. *J Hand Surg* 1995;20:683–686.

110. Jupiter JB, Pess GM, Bour CJ. Results of flexor tendon tenolysis after replantation in the hand. *J Hand Surg* 1989;14:35–44.

111. Wood MB, Cooney WP III. Above elbow limb replantation: functional results. *J Hand Surg* 1986;11:682–687.

112. Hales P, Pullen D. Hypotension and bleeding diathesis following attempted arm replantation. *Anaesth Intensive Care* 1982;10:359–361.

113. Makris G, Papasoglou O, Kalakonas P, et al. Proceedings: metabolic changes and late results in two cases of reimplantation of the upper limb. *J Cardiovasc Surg (Torino)* 1973;14:615–618.

114. Doi K, Kawai S, Kotani H, et al. Multiple organ failure after revascularisation of lower limb. Paper presented at: 7th Symposium of the International Society of Reconstructive Microsurgery; 1983; New York.

115. Russell RC, O'Donoghue J, Morrison WA, et al. The late functional results of upper-limb revascularisation and replantation. *J Hand Surg* 1984;9:623–633.

116. Weiland A, Robinson H, Futrell JW. External stabilization of a replanted upper extremity: case report *J Trauma* 1976;16:239–241.

117. Goldner RD, Howson MP, Nunley JA, et al. One hundred eleven thumb amputations: replantation vs. revision. *Microsurgery* 1990;11:243–250.

118. Backman C, Nystrom A, Bjerle P. Arterial spasticity and cold intolerance in relation to time after digital replantation. *J Hand Surg* 1993;18:551–555.

119. Povlsen B, Nylander G, Nylander E. Cold-induced vasospasm after digital replantation does not improve with time. A 12-year prospective study. *J Hand Surg* 1995;20:237–239.

120. Povlsen B, Nylander G, Nylander E. Natural history of digital replantation: a 12-year prospective study. *Microsurgery* 1995;16:138–140.

121. Povlsen B. Cold-induced vasospasm after finger replantation; abnormal sensory regeneration and sensitisation of cold nociceptors. *Scand J Plast Reconstr Surg* 1996;30:63–66.

122. Isogai N, Fukunishi K, Kamiishi H. Patterns of thermoregulation associated with cold intolerance after digital replantation. *Microsurgery* 1995;16:556–565.

123. Nunley JA, Penny WH III, Woodbury MA, et al. Quantita-

tive analysis of cold stress performance after digital replantation. *J Orthop Res* 1990;8:94–100.

124. Engel J, Luboshitz S, Jaffe B, et al. To trim or replant: a matter of cost. *World J Surg* 1991;15:486–492.

125. American Medical Association. *Guides to the evaluation of permanent impairment,* 4th ed. Chicago, IL: American Medical Association, 1993.

126. Holmberg J, Lindgren B, Jutemark R. Replantation-revascularization and primary amputation in major hand injuries. Resources spent on treatment and the indirect costs of sick leave in Sweden. *J Hand Surg* 1996;21:576–580.

127. Gasperschitz F, Genelin F, Karlbauer A, et al. Decrease in disability pension following replantation. *Handchir Mikrochir Plast Chir* 1990;22:78–81.

128. Pederson WC, Sanders WE. Bone and soft-tissue reconstruction. In: Rockwood CA, Green DP, Bucholz RW, et al., eds. *Rockwood and Green's fractures in adults,* 4th ed. Philadelphia: Lippincott–Raven Publishers, 1996.

129. Lange RH, Bach AW, Hansen SR, et al. Open tibial fractures with associated vascular injuries: prognosis for limb salvage. *J Trauma* 1985;25:203–208.

130. Yakuboff KP, Stern PJ, Neale HW. Technical successes and functional failures after free tissue transfer to the tibia. *Microsurgery* 1990;11:59–62.

131. Walton RL, Rothkopf DM. Judgment and approach for management of severe lower extremity injuries. *Clin Plast Surg* 1991;18:525–543.

132. Chen ZW, Zeng BF. Replantation of the lower extremity. *Clin Plast Surg* 1983;10:103.

133. Hierner R, Betz AM, Comtet JJ, et al. C. Decision making and results in subtotal and total lower leg amputations: reconstruction versus amputation. *Microsurgery* 1995;16:830–839.

134. Gayle LB, Lineaweaver WC, Buncke GM, et al. Lower extremity replantation. *Clin Plast Surg* 1991;18:437–447.

135. Yaffe B, Borenstein A, Seidman D, et al. Successful replantation of both legs in a child—5-year followup: case report. *J Trauma* 1991;31:264–267.

136. Datiashvili RO, Chichkin VG. Successful replantation of the lower leg after 42-hour ischemia: case report. *J Reconstr Microsurg* 1992;8:447–453.

137. Datiashvili RO. Simultaneous replantation of both lower legs in a child: a long-term result. *Plast Reconstr Surg* 1993;91:541–547.

138. Datiashvili RO, Oganesian OV, Chichkin VG, et al. Rehabilitation of patients after lower limb replantations by the bone distraction method. *J Trauma* 1993;35:368–374.

139. Mirzoyan AE. Reimplantation and lengthening with use of the Ilizarov apparatus after a traumatic amputation of the leg. A case report. *J Bone Joint Surg* 1996;78:437–438.

140. Sakamoto K, Kozuki K, Maki H. Replantation of the great toe: two case reports. *Foot Ankle Int* 1998;19:638–640.

141. Chiang YC, Wei FC, Chen LM. Heel replantation and subsequent analysis of gait. *Plast Reconstr Surg* 1993;91:729–733.

142. Libermanis O. Replantation of the heel pad. *Plast Reconstr Surg* 1993;92:537–539.

143. Macionis V. Heel replantation. *Br J Plast Surg* 1998;51:473–475.

144. Sanger JR, Matloub HS. Successful replantation of the heel pad: a seven-year follow-up. *Ann Plast Surg* 1989;22:350–353.

145. Hsiao CW, Lin CH, Wei FC. Midfoot replantation: case report. *J Trauma* 1994;36:280–281.

146. Russell RC, Vitale V, Zook EC. Extremity reconstruction using the "fillet of sole" flap. *Ann Plast Surg* 1986;17:65–72.

147. Pribaz JJ, Morris DJ, Barrall D, et al. Double fillet of foot free flaps for emergency leg and hand coverage with ultimate great toe to thumb transfer. *Plast Reconstr Surg* 1993;91:1151–1153.

148. van der Wey LP, Polder TW. Salvage of a through-knee amputation level using a free fillet of sole flap. *Microsurgery* 1993;14:605–607.

149. Dubert T, Oberlin C, Alnot JY. Partial replantation after traumatic proximal lower limb amputation: a one-stage reconstruction with free osteocutaneous transfer from the amputated limb. *Plast Reconstr Surg* 1993;91:537–540.

150. Lewis EC, Fowler JR. Two replantations of severed ear parts. *Plast Reconstr Surg* 1979;64:703–705.

151. Katsaros J, Tan E, Sheen R. Microvascular ear replantation. *Br J Plast Surg* 1988;41:496–499.

152. Kind GM, Buncke GM, Placik OJ, et al. Total ear replantation. *Plast Reconstr Surg* 1997;99:1858–1867.

153. Tajima S, Ueda K, Tanaka Y. Successful replantation of a bitten-off nose by microvascular anastomosis. *Microsurgery* 1989;10:5–7.

154. Niazi Z, Lee TC, Eadie P, et al. Successful replantation of nose by microsurgical technique, and review of literature. *Br J Plast Surg* 1990;43:617–620.

155. Hammond DC, Bouwense CL, Hankins WT, et al. Microsurgical replantation of the amputated nose. *Plast Reconstr Surg* 2000;105:2133–2136.

156. James NJ. Survival of large replanted segment of upper lip and nose. Case report. *Plast Reconstr Surg* 1976;58:623–625.

157. Holtje WJ. Successful replantation of an amputated upper lip. *Plast Reconstr Surg* 1984;73:664–670.

158. Walton RL, Beahm EK, Brown RE, et al. Microsurgical replantation of the lip: a multi-institutional experience. *Plast Reconstr Surg* 1998;102:358–368.

159. Buncke HJ, Rose EH, Brownstein MJ, et al. Successful replantation of two avulsed scalps by microvascular anastomoses. *Plast Reconstr Surg* 1978;61:666–672.

160. Fogdestam I, Lilja J. Microsurgical replantation of a total scalp avulsion. Case report. *Scand J Plast Reconstr Surg* 1986;20:319–322.

161. Cheng K, Zhou S, Jiang K, et al. Microsurgical replantation of the avulsed scalp: report of 20 cases. *Plast Reconstr Surg* 1996;97:1099–1106.

162. Thomas A, Obed V, Murarka A, et al. Total face and scalp replantation. *Plast Reconstr Surg* 1998;102:2085–2087.

163. Cohen BE, May JW Jr, Daly JS, et al. Successful clinical replantation of an amputated penis by microneurovascular repair. Case report. *Plast Reconstr Surg* 1977;59:276–280.

164. Wei FC, McKee NH, Huerta FJ, et al. Microsurgical replantation of a completely amputated penis. *Ann Plast Surg* 1983;10:317–321.

165. Zenn MR, Carson CC III, Patel MP. Replantation of the penis: a patient report. *Ann Plast Surg* 2000;44:214–220.

166. de Chalain T, Jones G. Replantation of the avulsed pinna: 100 percent survival with a single arterial anastomosis and substitution of leeches for a venous anastomosis. *Plast Reconstr Surg* 1995;95:1275–1279.

167. Concannon MJ, Puckett CL. Microsurgical replantation of an ear in a child without venous repair. *Plast Reconstr Surg* 1998;102:2088–2093.

168. Nath RK, Kraemer BA, Azizzadeh A. Complete ear replantation without venous anastomosis. *Microsurgery* 1998;18:282–285.

169. Cho BH, Ahn HB. Microsurgical replantation of a partial ear, with leech therapy. *Ann Plast Surg* 1999;43:427–429.

170. Juri J, Irigaray A, Juri C, et al. Ear replantation. *Plast Reconstr Surg* 1987;80:431–435.

171. Turpin IM. Microsurgical replantation of the external ear. *Clin Plast Surg* 1990;17:397–404.

172. Chun JK, Sterry TP, Margoles SL, et al. Salvage of ear replantation using the temporoparietal fascia flap. *Ann Plast Surg* 2000;44:435–439.

173. Van Beek AL, Zook EG. Scalp replantation by microsurgical revascularization: case report. *Plast Reconstr Surg* 1978;61:774–777.

174. Gatti JE, LaRossa D. Scalp avulsions and review of successful replantation. *Ann Plast Surg* 1981;6:127–131.

175. Nahai F, Hester TR, Jurkiewicz MJ. Microsurgical replantation of the scalp. *J Trauma* 1985;25:897–902.

176. McCann J, O'Donoghue J, Kaf-al Ghazal S, et al. Microvascular replantation of a completely avulsed scalp. *Microsurgery* 1994;15:639–642.

177. Arashiro K, Ohtsuka, H, Ohtani, K. et al. Entire scalp replantation: case report and review of the literature. *J Reconstr Microsurg* 1995;11:245–250.

178. Nahai F, Hurteau J, Vasconez LO. Replantation of an entire scalp and ear by microvascular anastomoses of only one artery and one vein. *Br J Plast Surg* 1978;31:339–342.

179. Eren S, Hess J, Larkin GC. Total scalp replantation based on one artery and one vein. *Microsurgery* 1993;14:266–271.

180. Henderson HP, Matti B, Laing AG, et al. Avulsion of the scalp treated by microvascular repair: the use of leeches for postoperative decongestion. *Br J Plast Surg* 1983;36:235–239.

181. Jeng SF, Wei FC, Noordhoff MS. Replantation of amputated facial tissues with microvascular anastomosis. *Microsurgery* 1994;15:327–333.

182. Biemer E, Stock W, Wolfensberger C, et al. Successful replantation of a totally avulsed scalp. *Br J Plast Surg* 1979;32:19–21.

183. Zhou S, Chang TS, Guan WX, et al. Microsurgical replantation of the avulsed scalp: report of six cases. *J Reconstr Microsurg* 1993;9:121–125.

184. Chen IC, Wan HL. Microsurgical replantation of avulsed scalps. *J Reconstr Microsurg* 1996;12:105–112.

185. Cho BC, Lee DH, Park JW, et al. Replantation of avulsed scalps and secondary aesthetic correction. *Ann Plast Surg* 2000;44:361–366.

186. Sadove AM, Moore TS, Eppley BL. Total scalp, ear, and eyebrow avulsion: aesthetic adjustment of the replanted tissue. *J Reconstr Microsurg* 1990;6:223–227.

187. Sanchez-Olaso A. Replantation of an amputated nasal tip with open venous drainage. *Microsurgery* 1993;14:380–383.

188. Schubert W, Kimberley B, Guzman-Stein G, et al. Use of the labial artery for replantation of the lip and chin. *Ann Plast Surg* 1988;20:256–260.

189. Crawford CR, Hagerty RC. Survival of an upper lip aesthetic complex using arterial reanastomosis only. *Ann Plast Surg* 1991;27:77–79.

190. Yamano Y, Tanaka H. Replantation of a completely amputated penis by the microsurgical technique: a case report. *Microsurgery* 1984;5:40–43.

191. Sanger JR, Matloub HS, Yousif NJ, et al. Penile replantation after self-inflicted amputation. *Ann Plast Surg* 1992;29:579–584.

192. Lidman D, Danielsson P, Abdiu A, et al. The functional result two years after a microsurgical penile replantation. Case report. *Scand J Plast Reconstr Surg* 1999;33:325–328.

193. Matloub HS, Yousif NJ, Sanger JR. Temporary ectopic implantation of an amputated penis. *Plast Reconstr Surg* 1994;93:408–412.

194. Szasz G, McLoughlin MG, Warren RJ. Return of sexual functioning following penile replant surgery. *Arch Sex Behav* 1990;19:343–348.

91

VASCULAR INJURIES: ACUTE OCCLUSIVE CONDITIONS

JOEL S. SOLOMON

In most hand surgery practices, the treatment of acute hand ischemia is relatively rare. Because of abundant collateral circulation, most upper extremity injuries, even those with known damage to a major vessel, do not result in hand ischemia (Fig. 1). Vascular compromise secondary to obvious trauma proximal to the elbow is usually referred to a vascular surgeon. In contrast, devascularizing trauma to the forearm, wrist, hand, or digits is typically referred to a hand surgeon, as therapeutic intervention often requires a thorough knowledge of regional anatomy and microsurgical skills. The hand surgeon may also be called upon to evaluate the rare patient with spontaneous acute hand or digit ischemia in the absence of trauma. Accurate diagnosis and timely intervention can be both limb sparing and lifesaving. Upper extremity vascular anatomy is reviewed in Chapter 4, Basic Vascular Pathophysiology of the Hand, Wrist, and Forearm. Other related chapters include Raynaud's Syndrome (Chapter 94), Replantation (Chapter 90), Thoracic Outlet Syndrome (Chapter 51), and Compartment Syndromes and Ischemic Contracture (Chapter 92).

PRESENTATION

The classic presentation of acute limb ischemia is summarized by the "six Ps": *pain, pallor, pulselessness, poikilothermia (coolness), paresthesias,* and *paralysis.* The presentation of an individual patient, however, may vary considerably. At one extreme, the surgeon may be consulted to see a young, otherwise healthy patient with a stab wound to the arm, a local pulsatile hematoma, a pulseless distal extremity, and sluggish capillary refill in the digits. In this patient, the diagnosis and site of injury are clear. Such a patient can be adequately evaluated with a thorough history and physical examination and treated via emergent arterial repair and possible fasciotomies. At the other extreme is the patient who presents with chronic pain and cold intolerance in the extremity and the recent onset of fingertip discoloration. Such patients may or may not have a history of trauma and

require a more extensive evaluation to determine the etiology of their symptoms. Often, there are primary and secondary causes of upper extremity ischemia. What appears to the patient as an acute presentation may represent an acute exacerbation of a chronic vascular disease process. Because of abundant collateral vessels, injury or disease of a major upper extremity vessel is less likely to cause limb-threatening ischemia than it would in the lower extremity. Nevertheless, upper extremity vascular injury may result in distal ischemia and tissue loss. The clinical presentation of a particular injury may be influenced by peripheral vascular disease diffusely affecting collateral pathways. Similarly, injury of a major upper extremity vessel may lead to profound, sympathetically mediated vasoconstriction that renders an intact collateral pathway incapable of providing sufficient blood flow to prevent distal ischemia and tissue loss.

HISTORY

The common causes of acute upper extremity ischemia are listed in Table 1. The majority of conditions can be diagnosed purely by history and physical examination.

Penetrating Trauma

Gunshot, Stab, and Projectile Injuries

The most common cause of acute upper extremity arterial insufficiency is penetrating trauma (1). Stab and gunshot injuries can divide major vessels. Alternatively, the blast effect from a projectile can cause vessel contusion and thrombosis. Angiography may be necessary when the site of vascular injury cannot be easily defined. Acute ischemia of the hand secondary to a gunshot or stab wound mandates rapid operative intervention. Untreated vascular injuries with adequate collateral flow may eventually become symptomatic. During the hours immediately after injury, the extremity may develop compartment syndrome. Undetec-

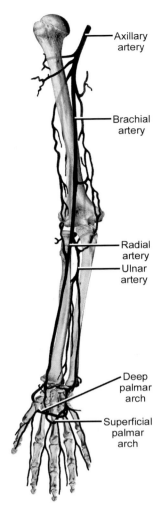

FIGURE 1. Note the parallel sources of circulation to the digits via the superficial and deep palmar arterial systems. In most patients, the entire hand is adequately perfused with maintained flow in either the ulnar artery (and the superficial palmar arch) or the radial artery (and the deep palmar arch).

ted intimal injury may lead to delayed thrombosis or distal embolization. Over the course of weeks to months, injured vessels may become symptomatic because of aneurysm formation with distal embolization or formation of an arteriovenous fistula.

Arterial Cannulation

Radial artery cannulation for continuous blood pressure monitoring typically causes temporary thrombosis in 20% to 40% of patients (2). For patients with "radial dominant" circulation, such injuries can have devastating consequences, such as ischemic necrosis of the thumb (3). A decreased complication rate has been demonstrated with the use of smaller (20-gauge) catheters, cannulation for less than 20 hours, and aspirin therapy (2,4). Thrombosis may lag decannulation by several days (2). Symptomatic radial artery thrombosis after

TABLE 1. CAUSES OF ACUTE UPPER EXTREMITY ISCHEMIA

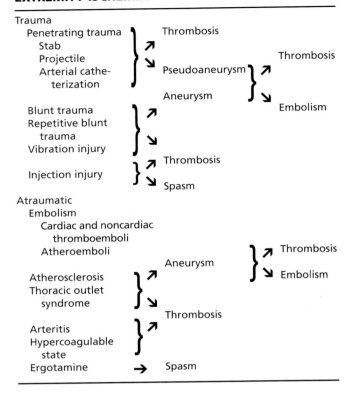

decannulation has been effectively treated by either thrombolytic infusion or surgical reconstruction with vein graft (5,6). Brachial artery access for cardiac catheterization and related procedures has a reported incidence of thrombotic complications in 1% to 4% of patients (1). Preferred treatment is surgical reconstruction with direct repair, interposition graft, or patch angioplasty.

Injection Injuries

The introduction of substances into an artery may be caused by industrial accident or iatrogenic injury but is usually the result of intravenous drug abuse. Such injuries can cause vessel damage over a great distance. Intraarterial injection may lead to decreased flow and thrombosis through a variety of mechanisms, including chemical endarteritis, vasospasm, and embolic occlusion by insoluble substances. These injuries are difficult to treat and require an aggressive approach. Initial treatment consists of anticoagulation and treatment of vasospasm. Thrombolytic infusion is a reasonable first-line therapy but is often ineffective (6,7). Success has been reported with prostacyclin infusion (7,8).

Blunt Trauma

Blunt trauma to an extremity can cause vessel contusion, intimal injury, and subsequent thrombosis. Symptoms may not present immediately, as there may be multiple converging influences that, over time, lead to vessel thrombosis. A crush injury, for example, may cause intimal damage that remains subclinical until local soft tissue swelling and systemic hypotension decrease arterial flow and allow for vessel thrombosis. Alternatively, damage to the vessel wall may lead to aneurysm formation weeks after the injury and may present as acute ischemia from thrombosis or distal thromboembolization. Circulation must be evaluated before and after reduction of fractures and dislocations. Anterior dislocation of the shoulder or subsequent closed reduction rarely causes disruption of the axillary artery (9). Posterior dislocation of the elbow or humerus fracture may cause brachial artery injury via contusion, compression, or laceration (1). Undetected vascular injury from supracondylar humerus fractures remains a common cause of Volkmann's contracture in children (10). Any persistent blood flow abnormality after reduction of a fracture or dislocation must be investigated, usually with angiography.

Distant History of Trauma: Aneurysm

The appearance of symptoms from an aneurysm can follow the inciting traumatic event by a period of hours to several years (11). Injury to the internal elastic lamina of an artery can cause a localized area of vessel expansion, or a *true aneurysm*. Turbulent flow in this area of vessel deformity predisposes to thrombosis. Acute ischemia can result from vascular thrombosis itself or from recanalization with distal embolization of the thrombus. True aneurysms in other parts of the body are usually the result of atherosclerosis. In the upper extremity, however, true aneurysms are almost exclusively the result of blunt trauma (11). They are most commonly seen at the level of the wrist (e.g., hypothenar hammer syndrome) but may occur anywhere in the upper extremity (11). Axillary artery aneurysm as a result of compression by crutches has been reported (12).

Alternatively, penetrating trauma to an artery can cause a false aneurysm, or *pseudoaneurysm* (11,13). After a penetrating arterial injury, a hematoma develops that eventually fibroses. Recanalization of this organized hematoma, which forms a saclike protrusion from the parent vessel, is a pseudoaneurysm (Fig. 2). Mycotic aneurysms, a consequence of vessel wall infection, may result from septic emboli or any type of penetrating trauma. Such aneurysms are most commonly seen in the setting of intravenous drug abuse (14). Upper extremity aneurysms of any type may present as distal ischemia or a pulsatile mass. The mass effect of an aneurysm can also cause symptoms of nerve compression. Aneurysms are treated with resection and then ligation or reconstruction. Reconstruction can often be performed via primary repair (14). The decision to reconstruct is usually based on an intraoperative assessment of distal perfusion after resection.

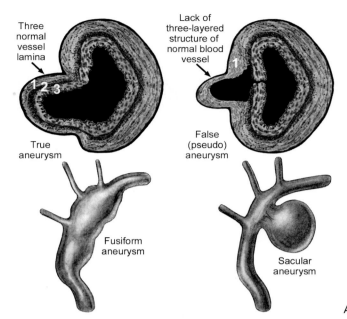

FIGURE 2. A: True aneurysms most often result from blunt trauma with damage to the internal elastic lamina. The aneurysm wall, although abnormal, contains elements of the three normal vessel lamina. **B:** False aneurysms result from penetrating trauma. They project from the side of a vessel and lack the three-layered structure of a normal blood vessel wall.

Repetitive Blunt Trauma or Vibration

Vibration and repetitive blunt trauma may cause vascular injury and thrombosis or aneurysm formation. Hand ischemia and Raynaud's phenomenon have been reported in workers using vibrating pneumatic tools (5). In hand surgery, the most common presentation of vascular injury from repetitive blunt trauma is the hypothenar hammer syndrome. Manual laborers who frequently use the hypothenar palm as a hammer can develop thrombosis of the ulnar artery as it exits Guyon's canal and passes over the hook of the hamate. Thrombosis may result from periadventitial thickening and vascular compression or from injury to the internal elastic lamina and subsequent aneurysm formation (Fig. 3) (15). The syndrome is most common in male laborers in the fifth decade of life who smoke (16). Patients usually complain of chronic ulnar-sided hand pain and cold intolerance but may present with acute ischemia due to vessel thrombosis or distal embolization. Local compression of the neighboring ulnar nerve may lead to complaints of numbness in the ring and small fingers. On examination, these patients have a positive Allen's test (see Physical Examination) and indications of hand ischemia. Some may have a palpable thrombosis of the ulnar artery (15). Ischemia or embolization may lead to gangrene in the digits, particularly the ring and small fingers. Hypothenar hammer syndrome is treated by aneurysm resection and ulnar artery reconstruction if necessary (17). Often, aneurysm resection alone provides excellent relief of symptoms by removing a source for embolization and eliminating a

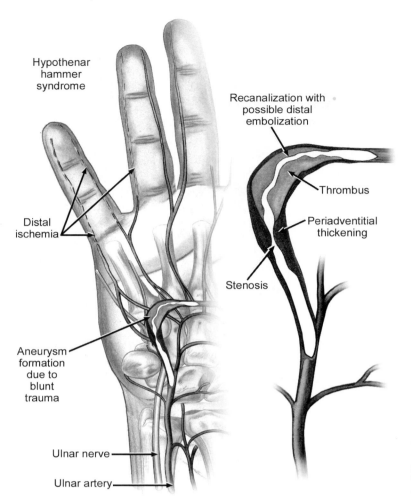

FIGURE 3. Blunt trauma may cause distal ischemia because of aneurysm formation, periadventitial fibrosis, or vessel thrombosis. Aneurysms themselves may thrombose. Recanalization may cause ischemia from distal embolization of the thrombus.

source of increased sympathetic tone (15). Some authors perform intraoperative digital plethysmography to determine whether further reconstruction is needed after aneurysm resection (15,17). Although the role of adjunctive thrombolytic infusion has not been defined, catheter-directed thrombolysis alone is usually not sufficient therapy (18).

Atraumatic Presentation

Embolism

In the absence of trauma, unilateral symptoms suggest embolism, one of the most common causes of acute hand ischemia. Embolism comes from the Greek *embolus,* which means "plug" (19). The term describes the pathologic situation in which a solid particle, composed of platelet–fibrin thrombus, cholesterol debris, or foreign material, obstructs a vessel lumen. Emboli tend to lodge at vessel bifurcations, obstructing flow in both the parent vessel and collaterals (20). Their presentation is, therefore, often dramatic with the acute onset of profound ischemia. The majority of upper extremity emboli lodge in the distal brachial artery at its bifurcation into

the radial and ulnar arteries (19). More than 70% of upper extremity emboli come from the heart (16), and two-thirds to three-fourths of these are associated with atrial fibrillation (19). Dysfunctional contraction of the atria leads to stasis and clot formation, particularly within the left atrial appendage. Transmural myocardial infarction can also cause intracardiac thrombus formation and distal embolization. Acute ischemia in the extremities from distal embolization can be the presenting sign of a recent myocardial infarction. Rare sources of cardiac emboli include tumor emboli from an atrial myxoma, septic emboli in patients with bacterial or fungal endocarditis, and emboli from thrombus or vegetations associated with prosthetic heart valves. Thorough imaging of the heart must be performed on all patients with suspected embolic disease.

Noncardiac emboli are largely the result of atherosclerosis of more proximal vessels. In addition, subclavian artery emboli may occur at a site of poststenotic dilatation in the setting of thoracic outlet syndrome. Microemboli from more distal arteries obstruct smaller vessels in the forearm, hand, and digits (16). Such emboli can cause acute ischemia to the hand; however, other more subtle presentations, such as fingertip ulceration or Raynaud's phenomenon, are also common. An appropriate workup usually involves vascular imaging from the heart to the fingertips with arteriography through a femoral artery access and echocardiography. Despite extensive investigation, 10% to 15% of embolic sources remain undetermined (21,22). Treatment usually involves embolectomy and definitive treatment of the embolic source. Catheter-directed thrombolysis may be the therapy of choice in some patients.

Native Arterial Thrombosis

Advanced atherosclerosis, often in association with diabetes and renal failure, can cause arterial occlusion (23). Deposition of lipids in the intimal layer of an artery leads to vessel stenosis and the development of a thrombogenic atherosclerotic core that is separated from the arterial lumen by a fibrous cap. Disruption of the fibrous cap with exposure of the core can lead to acute thrombosis. Patients with renal failure and hypercalcemia can exhibit extensive vessel wall calcification and occlusion.

Hypercoagulable State

The presentation of patients with thrombosis due to a hypercoagulable state is often dramatic (19). The most frequently implicated hypercoagulable states result from malignancy, antiphospholipid syndrome, antithrombin III deficiency, and vasculitis (19). A full hematologic workup for a hypercoagulable state should proceed in patients who have no history of trauma, no documented embolic source, and no arteriographic evidence of atherosclerosis. *Purpura fulminans* is acute ischemia and necrosis of the distal extremities associated with meningococcemia and some other types of sepsis (24). The condition appears to result from a combination of vasculitis, vasoconstriction, and disseminated intravascular coagulation. There are no proven treatments, but prostacyclin appears to be of benefit (24,25). Patients who survive their sepsis typically require amputations.

Intoxication

Ergotamine compounds, used in the treatment of migraine, are profound vasoconstrictors. Even when taken at prescribed dosages, patients may have unusual responses to the drug with severe vasospasm and upper extremity ischemia. Some antibiotics and other drugs are known to potentiate the effects of ergotamine (26). Treatment involves anticoagulation and vasodilators.

PHYSICAL EXAMINATION

After a detailed history, thorough physical examination with the aid of a handheld Doppler flowmeter is often sufficient to establish a diagnosis and formulate a treatment plan. The extremity must be inspected for color and capillary refill. Fingertips should be examined for evidence of chronic ischemic ulceration. Nailbeds should be inspected for splinter hemorrhages suggestive of microembolism. Palpation of upper extremity pulses should be performed from the axilla to the wrist. An irregular pulse may raise suspicion of a primary cardiac abnormality leading to distal embolization. Palpation may also reveal masses consistent with aneurysm or hematoma. Auscultation down the extremity may reveal a systolic bruit suggestive of aneurysm or a sustained bruit suggestive of arteriovenous fistula. A brachial pressure should be documented; however, more information can be gained by making segmental pressure measurements down the extremity (see below). All findings should be compared to the opposite, uninvolved upper extremity.

The presence of a distal pulse may be misleading in that palpable distal pulses may represent reconstitution of flow through collateral pathways, such as retrograde filling of the radial or ulnar arteries by the palmar arch vessels. An Allen's test can be performed to isolate the contributions of the radial and ulnar arteries to distal flow. The hand is exsanguinated, usually by having the patient make a tight fist. The examiner then manually compresses the radial and ulnar arteries along the volar wrist. The patient relaxes the fingers, and the return of color to the hand is monitored after the release of compression of one of the two arteries. The test is then repeated, with compression of the other artery released. In this manner, the contribution of antegrade blood flow to the hand through the radial and ulnar arteries can be evaluated independently. Similarly, a digital Allen's test can assess the contribution of radial and ulnar proper digital vessels to the perfusion of a digit.

LABORATORY EVALUATION

Electrocardiogram

More than half of all patients presenting with acute extremity ischemia have abnormal electrocardiograms (ECGs) (27). The cardiac comorbidities of such patients are, in large part, responsible for the 10% to 25% mortality rate associated with acute peripheral artery occlusion (19). In patients with suspected peripheral vascular disease, an ECG may identify those with cardiac ischemia due to associated coronary artery disease. ECG can also diagnose atrial fibrillation and recent myocardial infarction, conditions that may point to a source of thromboembolism. If indicated, a more thorough cardiac evaluation should be performed and can influence the mode of therapy, patient monitoring, and overall prognosis.

Pulse Oximetry

The pulse oximeter is an easy and rapid way to assess pulsatile blood flow to the digits (28). A pulsatile waveform, the frequency of which corresponds to the heart rate, assures some degree of distal perfusion. Unfortunately, a normal oximeter reading may persist in the face of drastically reduced digital pressure, making oximetry an insensitive test of digital ischemia (29).

Doppler

The Doppler ultrasonic flowmeter measures blood flow velocity by detecting the shift in the frequency of sound waves that are reflected off of moving red blood cells. The output is transmitted as an audible signal, the pitch of which varies with red blood cell velocity. The handheld probe can be used to trace arteries across the wrist and out to the digital tips. In conjunction with digital compression of the radial or ulnar arteries at the wrist, the Doppler can be used to locate areas of obstruction and to distinguish between anterograde and retrograde flow through the palmar arch and dorsal radial artery (Fig. 4).

In combination with occlusive blood pressure cuffs, the Doppler probe can be used to document segmental systolic pressures. Segmental pressure measurements are among the most valuable measures for assessing vascular injury. The measurement of the systolic pressure can be compared at different levels of the arterial tree within one extremity or to corresponding levels of the arterial tree in the opposite upper extremity. A pressure difference of greater than 15 mm Hg, either between neighboring levels in an extremity

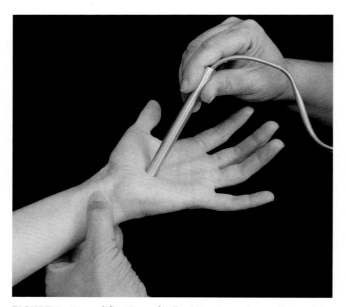

FIGURE 4. A modification of Allen's test can be performed by using the Doppler to measure palmar arch flow while alternately compressing the radial and ulnar arteries. Obliteration of the radial Doppler pulse at the wrist, with compression of the ulnar artery, indicates retrograde flow in the radial artery at this level via the palmar arch vessels and suggests a more proximal radial artery injury. Doppler flow in the ulnar artery can be similarly assessed with compression of the radial artery at the wrist.

or between corresponding levels in the two upper extremities, is unusual (20). A normalized "index" can be calculated by taking the ratio of a segmental pressure measurement to that of the brachial artery pressure in the same extremity. Digital brachial indices can be calculated using small pneumatic cuffs designed for the digits. The normal range for the digital brachial index is 0.78 to 1.27 (30). An index of less than or equal to 0.7 or an absolute digital pressure of less than 70 mm Hg indicates severely compromised distal flow (20). Nevertheless, digital pressures may be normal in the face of complete occlusion of one of the paired proper digital arteries (20). Because of technical limitations, distal pressures can be greatly overestimated when examining calcified, noncompressible vessels that are often seen in diabetes and end-stage renal disease.

Duplex Ultrasound

Doppler flow velocity information can be combined with traditional ultrasound imaging techniques (B-mode). These duplex scans can give both anatomic and flow information. They can identify and gradate stenotic lesions, as well as identify areas of occlusion and collateral flow. Although the resolution of ultrasound imaging is far inferior to contrast angiography, it has the advantages of no ionizing radiation, lower cost, and noninvasiveness. Moreover, its resolution is sufficient to differentiate patent and occluded digital arteries with an accuracy of greater than 85% (31). Duplex imaging can be useful for detecting aneurysms, but arteriography is more effective in defining the extent of vascular injury and planning operative intervention.

Echocardiography

On occasion, patients may present with acute upper extremity ischemia that appears to result from embolism, although no proximal embolic source can be detected by arteriography. In such patients, transesophageal echocardiography may be more sensitive than arteriography in demonstrating ulcerated atherosclerotic plaques of the aortic arch. Transesophageal echocardiography allows better visualization of embolic sources in the heart and thoracic aorta than conventional transthoracic echocardiography (22,32).

Pulse-Volume Recordings

Pulse-volume recordings quantitate flow by detecting minute changes in the volume of a limb or digit that occur with the pulsatile perfusion of blood. Volume changes are usually detected by an air-filled cuff or by detecting changes in the reflectance of light, as with a pulse oximeter (Fig. 5). The output waveform in normal vessels demonstrates the normal triphasic pattern of expansion-contraction-expansion that occurs with each heartbeat. Alterations of this normal pattern can reveal hemodynamically signifi-

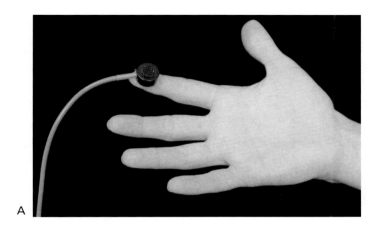

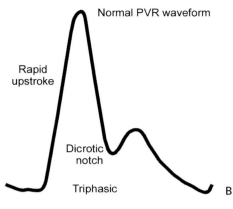

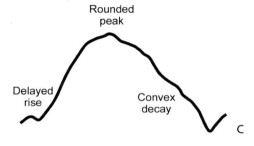

FIGURE 5. A: A small photoplethysmograph applied to the pad of the index finger can measure a pulse-volume recording (PVR). **B:** The normal PVR waveform is triphasic, with a rapid upstroke and a dicrotic notch. **C:** Decreased flow to the digit can give rise to an obstructive PVR waveform with a delayed rise, a rounded peak, and a convex decay.

cant stenosis that might not be detected by segmental pressure measurements (33).

Contrast Angiography

Contrast angiography remains the gold standard for evaluating the anatomy of the upper extremity vasculature. Radiopaque contrast material is injected into the arterial circulation via a femoral artery access site in the groin. Fluoroscopy is then used to visualize the passage of contrast material down the arterial tree from the aortic arch to the terminations of the digital vessels. In addition to demonstrating the anatomy of the dominant circulation and collaterals, the technique can also identify stenoses, occlusions, vascular malformations, and, with the injection of vasodilators, vasospasm. Current digital subtraction methods allow for improved vascular imaging with smaller amounts of contrast material. In the absence of trauma, it is usually appropriate to image both upper extremities, whether symptoms are unilateral or bilateral. The comparison of the two extremities may help to pinpoint the cause of ischemia or to identify the presence of subclinical vascular disease on the unaffected side.

Although an excellent test for imaging the vascular system, contrast angiography should not be used as a screen for extremities suspected to have compromised blood flow. The test is expensive, time-consuming, and carries potential risks

of arterial puncture, radiation exposure, and dye load to the patient. On the other hand, contrast angiography can be very helpful when the site of vascular injury is unknown, or when multiple levels of arterial injury are suspected (e.g., shotgun wounds, multiple stab wounds). Embolus may appear as a convex filling defect in an otherwise normal vessel and often occurs at a vessel branch point. Lack of collateral vessels proximal to the defect suggests an acute event. A tapered, irregular filling defect with multiple collateral vessels is more consistent with spontaneous arterial thrombosis in the context of chronic atherosclerosis.

Magnetic resonance angiography (MRA) is an emerging technology that may hold great promise for investigations of upper extremity vasculature (34). Unlike traditional contrast angiography, there is no ionizing radiation. In addition, there is no risk of allergic reaction to iodine contrast or potential toxicity to the kidney. MRA requires high-resolution equipment and specialized computer processing. Under the best of circumstances, however, MRA remains inferior to modern contrast angiography.

TREATMENT

Treatment of acute upper extremity ischemia has two objectives: (a) to restore adequate perfusion and (b) to address the inciting pathology (Fig. 6). For a patient with a

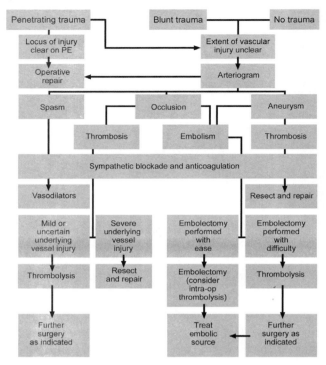

FIGURE 6. Treatment of acute upper extremity ischemia with salvageable limb. PE, physical examination.

stab wound to the arm and laceration of the brachial artery, these two objectives are one and the same. For a patient with embolic occlusion, restoration of perfusion and treatment of the embolic source are totally separate. Because of the relatively high risk of heart disease in patients presenting with upper extremity ischemia, it is frequently worthwhile to see whether adequate perfusion can be restored with temporizing measures while the patient is stabilized and prepared for surgery. For patients presenting with acute ischemia, sympathetic blockade or intraarterial vasodilator administration may restore sufficient collateral blood flow to allow for continued observation. Surgical reconstruction can be performed on an elective basis if indicated (15). Observation of a compromised but viable extremity must be differentiated from delay in the treatment of critical ischemia. In the absence of adequate perfusion, delay in treatment may be the most influential determinant of outcome. When treatment is delayed more than 8 hours after the onset of symptoms, mortality and limb loss increase (21).

Preoperative Measures

The natural history of untreated ischemia is often tissue necrosis. The extent of tissue necrosis and the prognosis for limb salvage, however, depend on a variety of factors that influence the metabolic supply and demand of the affected tissues. Primary determinants of perfusion include the degree of vascular obstruction, the extent of collateral chan-

nels, systemic blood pressure, and sympathetic tone. Exacerbating influences may include peripheral vascular disease, compartment syndrome, arterial thrombosis, thrombus propagation, venous thrombosis, and distal embolization.

Preoperative measures directed at maximizing distal perfusion are directed toward (a) maintaining systemic arterial pressure, (b) relieving arterial spasm, and (c) preventing thrombosis of collateral pathways. For patients with penetrating trauma to the extremity, division of a major limb artery, and distal ischemia, the treatment program is direct. The patient must be stabilized and transported to the operating room for vascular repair. In these cases, therapies directed at relieving arterial spasm and preventing thrombosis are misguided and possibly harmful. For most other patients, treatment of vessel spasm and thrombosis should be considered.

In the acutely ischemic limb, sympathetic blockade and vasodilator administration may restore sufficient collateral blood flow to allow for continued observation and surgical reconstruction on an elective basis (15). A long-lasting sympathetic blockade can be achieved via the administration of brachial plexus block or axillary block anesthesia. These methods have the added benefit of excellent pain relief. If systemic anticoagulation is planned, applying the anesthetic block first may decrease the likelihood of iatrogenic hematoma. If preoperative plans include angiography, thought should be given to the intraarterial infusion of vasodilator.

Thrombus formation is a predictable consequence of significant arterial injuries, whether by trauma or peripheral vascular disease. Propagation of the thrombus can further exacerbate an injury by occluding collateral flow. For this reason, aggressive anticoagulation is a major component of the treatment of acute ischemia not involving penetrating trauma. If there is no history of penetrating trauma and physical examination does not reveal a palpable hematoma, systemic anticoagulation with heparin may be indicated. If a hypercoagulable state or disseminated intravascular coagulation is suspected, anticoagulation should proceed in consultation with a hematologist. Anticoagulation is the first-line therapy in the treatment of embolism (21). Often, anticoagulation is continued indefinitely as treatment for the embolic source (e.g., refractory atrial fibrillation) (21). Heparin should also be used as a first-line therapy in the treatment of arterial injection injuries. In patients with disease localized to digital end arteries who may have few therapeutic alternatives, chronic anticoagulation with aspirin and dipyridamole can reduce pain and tissue loss (35).

Arterial Repair or Bypass

Arterial reconstruction should be embarked on only with proper deference to the patient's overall condition and the ability to undergo what could be a lengthy procedure. Perioperative mortality after limb revascularization remains around 12% (36). For patients with a lengthy period of ischemia, reperfusion can cause systemic toxicity with the efflux of acid, potassium, and inflammatory mediators from the limb. The entry of these compounds into the systemic circulation immediately after the restoration of blood flow to the limb can cause cardiac dysrhythmia. The triad of peripheral muscle infarction, myoglobinemia, and myoglobinuric renal failure has been termed *reperfusion syndrome* (19). Furthermore, prolonged ischemia can lead to compromised vessel wall integrity and consequent edema. Such edema may be of a sufficient degree to increase the pressure within fascial compartments above end capillary pressure and, thereby, obstruct flow (see Chapter 92, Compartment Syndromes and Ischemic Contracture). At the microvascular level, edema of the capillary endothelium from ischemic injury and reperfusion can cause capillary obstruction. This chain of events is termed the *no-reflow phenomenon*. Obstruction of microvascular pathways leads to progressive thrombosis and abnormal shunting of blood flow through low-resistance pathways. Tissue death then proceeds despite what, at first, appears to be the successful restoration of flow.

Arterial repair can successfully restore flow and prevent tissue loss. Brachial artery laceration or acute thrombosis at a brachial artery access site is best treated by direct repair (37). If both the radial and ulnar arteries are injured and repaired, the long-term patency of at least one of these repairs is approximately 90% (38). The use of interposition vein grafts does not lower patency rates (39). Patency rates are lowered by factors that make for a hostile, local soft tissue bed, including tissue necrosis and infection. The long-term patency of radial or ulnar artery repair in the face of maintained flow in the other vessel is reported to vary between 47% and 68% (38,40,41). Flow in the uninjured vessel is seen to increase over time. This relatively low patency rate, compared to that seen in most microvascular reconstructions, is thought to be the result of turbulent blood flow due to back pressure from the remaining patent forearm vessel. If there is no distal ischemia, the decision to reconstruct an isolated radial or ulnar artery injury is usually based on the patient's overall health and the morbidity associated with such a repair. Microsurgical revascularization procedures extending out into the palm can be very effective. Preliminary data suggest a patency rate greater than 50% (6). Resection and reconstruction is the treatment of choice for aneurysms causing distal ischemia or embolization (16,42).

Thrombolytic Therapy

Pharmacologic activation of the body's thrombolytic enzymes is a powerful mode of therapy that is still finding its place in the treatment of upper extremity ischemia. Methods for catheter-directed infusion of fibrinolytic agents directly into an arterial thrombus were popularized in the 1970s (43). Application of the technique continues to grow. Agents used for thrombolysis include tissue plasminogen activator, urokinase, and streptokinase. When infused, these enzymes lead to the local generation of the enzyme plasmin, which dissolves clots by virtue of its fibrinolytic activity. Patients require intensive care unit monitoring during thrombolysis because of the risk of spontaneous hemorrhage. Progress is monitored with arteriographic imaging every 6 to 12 hours. After successful thrombolysis, patients are anticoagulated with heparin for 7 to 10 days (5).

Most information on the efficacy of thrombolytic therapy for the treatment of acute upper extremity ischemia is extrapolated from data on its use in the lower extremity. Recent multicenter trials comparing the results of surgery to thrombolysis in patients presenting with acute (<14 days) lower extremity ischemia have demonstrated comparable or superior results of thrombolysis with respect to limb salvage and survival (36,44–46). Whether for treatment of spontaneous thrombosis, bypass graft thrombosis, or thromboembolism, thrombus dissolution occurs in approximately 70% of cases over a period of approximately 36 hours (44). Long-term patency 1 year after successful thrombolysis and angioplasty in the treatment of lower extremity native vessel occlusion approaches 90% (47). Preliminary data suggest that long-term patency may be higher in patients treated for thromboembolism (19). In the presence of arterial injury or disease, thrombolysis may restore perfusion only temporarily. Maintained flow usually requires therapy directed at the site of vessel damage. Initial treatment with a thrombolytic can clarify the lesion underlying a local thrombosis and allow for an endovascular or lesser open surgical procedure for definitive treatment (36,46). "Pretreatment" with a thrombolytic also allows definitive treatment to be performed electively on a well-prepared patient. Very few studies have explored the role of thrombolytic therapy in the upper extremity. The technique has shown benefit in patients with ischemia from thromboembolism as well as atherosclerosis and anatomic abnormalities (18,48,49). Catheter-directed thrombolysis may be particularly effective in the digital end arteries, where therapeutic alternatives are limited (49). Thrombolytic infusion has also been used intraoperatively as an adjunct to thrombectomy. Preliminary results suggest improvement in distal perfusion (50). Of course, embolization of atherosclerotic plaque would not be expected to improve with fibrinolysis. The role for thrombolysis in the treatment of ischemia from upper extremity aneurysms is uncertain (18).

Patients not responding to thrombolysis require embolectomy and possible arterial reconstruction. Although restoration of flow in the digital end arteries of the hand has been reported after infusion of a thrombolytic from a catheter situated in the proximal forearm, the inability to pass a guidewire across an occlusion or place the thrombolysis

TABLE 2. CONTRAINDICATIONS TO THROMBOLYTIC THERAPY

Absolute
  Established cerebrovascular event (including transient ischemic attacks) within the last 2 mos
  Active bleeding diathesis
  Recent gastrointestinal bleeding (<10 d)
  Neurosurgery (intracranial, spinal) within last 3 mos
  Intracranial trauma within last 3 mos
Relative major
  Cardiopulmonary resuscitation within last 10 d
  Major nonvascular surgery or trauma within last 10 d
  Uncontrolled hypertension: >180 mm Hg systolic or >110 mm Hg diastolic
  Puncture of noncompressible vessel
  Intracranial tumor
  Recent eye surgery
Minor
  Hepatic failure, particularly those with coagulopathy
  Bacterial endocarditis
  Pregnancy
  Diabetic hemorrhagic retinopathy

From The Working Party on Thrombolysis in the Management of Limb Ischemia. Thrombolysis in the management of lower limb peripheral arterial occlusion—a consensus document. *Am J Cardiol* 1998;81:207–218, with permission.

catheter within the substance of the thrombus is associated with a high failure rate in the lower extremity (51) (18,48,49). Contraindications to thrombolytic therapy are listed in Table 2 (52). As would be expected, bleeding complications are more common with thrombolytic therapy than with surgery alone and can be expected in approximately 10% of patients (44,46). Although such complications are most often the result of bleeding at the arterial access site, the most serious of these complications is intracranial hemorrhage. With present methods, intracranial hemorrhage is seen in 1% to 2% of patients (45,46).

Embolectomy or Thrombectomy

Surgical embolectomy was first performed in the early 1900s and continues to be performed today using a balloon catheter developed by Fogarty in the 1960s. For the larger emboli of cardiac origin, many favor transbrachial embolectomy under local anesthesia because of its simplicity and excellent results (16,37). Embolectomy of forearm vessels can be performed with a 3-mm Fogarty catheter (23). Embolus at or distal to the wrist can be performed with a 2-mm Fogarty catheter; however, there is a significant risk of causing further damage to these small vessels (23). Embolectomy in the palm and digits is rarely indicated. If performed, the involved vessels should be treated under direct vision (16). Systemic anticoagulation is instituted for 5 to 7 days after embolectomy and may be continued indefinitely (16). In cases of nonembolic arterial thrombosis, vessel wall damage often exists. In such cases, thrombectomy is not recommended, as it may further damage the vessel wall, causing thrombus extension and an exacerbation of ischemia (19,53).

REFERENCES

1. Hammond DC, Gould JS, Hanel DP. Management of acute and chronic vascular injuries to the arm and forearm. *Hand Clin* 1992;8:453–463.
2. Bedford RF, Wollman H. Complications of percutaneous radial-artery cannulation: an objective prospective study in man. *Anesthesiology* 1973;38:228–236.
3. Samaan HA. The hazards of radial artery pressure monitoring. *J Cardiovasc Surg (Torino)* 1971;12:342–347.
4. Bedford RF, Ashford TP. Aspirin pretreatment prevents post-cannulation radial-artery thrombosis. *Anesthesiology* 1979;51:176–178.
5. Newmeyer WL. Vascular disorders. In: Green DP, ed. *Operative hand surgery*, 3rd ed. New York: Churchill Livingstone, 1993:2251–2308.
6. Jones NF. Acute and chronic ischemia of the hand: pathophysiology, treatment, and prognosis. *J Hand Surg [Am]* 1991;16:1074–1083.
7. Gouny P, Gaitz JP, Vayssairat M. Acute hand ischemia secondary to intraarterial buprenorphine injection: treatment with iloprost and dextran-40. *Angiology* 1999;50:605–606.
8. Andreev A, Kavrakov T, Petkov D, et al. Severe acute hand ischemia following an accidental intraarterial drug injection, successfully treated with thrombolysis and intraarterial iloprost infusion. *Angiology* 1995;46:963–967.
9. Raskin KB. Acute vascular injuries of the upper extremity. *Hand Clin* 1993;9:115–130.
10. Ashbell TS, Kleinert HE, Kutz JE. Vascular injuries about the elbow. *Clin Orthop* 1967;50:107–127.
11. Ho PK, Weiland AJ, McClinton MA, et al. Aneurysms of the upper extremity. *J Hand Surg [Am]* 1987;12:39–46.
12. Abbott WM, Darling RC. Axillary artery aneurysms secondary to crutch trauma. *Am J Surg* 1973;125:515–520.
13. Spittel JA. Aneurysms of the hand and wrist. *Med Clin North Am* 1958;42:1007–1010.
14. Ho PK, Yaremchuk MJ, Dellon AL. Mycotic aneurysms of the upper extremity, report of two cases. *J Hand Surg [Br]* 1986;11:271–273.
15. Koman LA, Urbaniak JR. Ulnar artery thrombosis. *Hand Clin* 1985;1:311–325.
16. Koman LA, Ruch DS, Smith BP, et al. Vascular disorders. In: Green DP, Hotchkiss RN, Pederson WC, eds. *Green's operative hand surgery*, 4th ed. New York: Churchill Livingstone, 1999:2254–2302.
17. Rothkopf DM, Bryan DJ, Cuadros CL, et al. Surgical management of ulnar artery aneurysms. *J Hand Surg [Am]* 1990;15:891–897.
18. Wheatley MJ, Marx MV. The use of intra-arterial urokinase in the management of hand ischemia secondary to palmar and digital arterial occlusion. *Ann Plast Surg* 1996;37:356–363.
19. Greenberg RK, Ouriel K. Arterial thromboembolism. In: Rutherford RB, ed. *Vascular surgery*, 5th ed. Philadelphia: Saunders, 2000:822–835.

20. Sumner DS. Evaluation of acute and chronic ischemia of the upper extremity. In: Rutherford RB, ed. *Vascular surgery*, 5th ed. Philadelphia: Saunders, 2000:1122–1139.

21. Elliott JP, Hageman JH, Szilagyi DE, et al. Arterial embolization: problems of source, multiplicity, recurrence, and delayed treatment. *Surgery* 1980;88:833–845.

22. Rubin BG, Barzilai B, Allen BT, et al. Detection of the source of arterial emboli by transesophageal echocardiography: a case report. *J Vasc Surg* 1992;15:573–577.

23. Pederson WC. Management of severe ischemia of the upper extremity. *Clin Plast Surg* 1997;24:107–120.

24. Willis TMS, Hopp RJ, Romero JR, et al. The protective effect of brachial plexus palsy in purpura fulminans. *Pediatr Neurol* 2001;24:379–381.

25. Norman P, House AK. Surgical complications of fulminating meningococcaemia. *Br J Clin Pract* 1990;44:36–37.

26. Fukui S, Coggia M, Goeau-Brissonniere O. Acute upper extremity ischemia during concomitant use of ergotamine tartrate and ampicillin. *Ann Vasc Surg* 1997;11:420–424.

27. Kuukasjarvi P, Riekkinen H, Salenius JP, et al. Prevalence and predictive value of ECG findings in acute extremity ischemia. *J Cardiovasc Surg* 1995;36:469–473.

28. Rozenberg B, Rosenberg M, Birkhan J. Allen's test performed by pulse oximeter. *Anaesthesia* 1988;43:515–516.

29. Levinsohn DG, Gordon L, Sessler DI. The Allen's test: analysis of four methods. *J Hand Surg [Am]* 1991;16:279–282.

30. Sumner DS. Noninvasive assessment of upper extremity and hand ischemia. *J Vasc Surg* 1986;3:560–568.

31. Langholz J, Ladleif M, Blank B, et al. Colour coded duplex sonography in ischemic finger artery disease—a comparison with hand arteriography. *Vasa* 1997;26:85–90.

32. Mariano MC, Gutierrez CJ, Alexander J, et al. The utility of transesophageal echocardiography in determining the source of arterial embolization. *Am Surg* 2000;66:901–904.

33. Kleinert JM, Gupta A. Pulse volume recording. *Hand Clin* 1993;9:13–46.

34. Holder LE, Merine DS, Yang A. Nuclear medicine, contrast angiography, and magnetic resonance imaging for evaluating vascular problems in the hand. *Hand Clin* 1993;9:85–113.

35. Morris-Jones W, Preston FE, Greaney M, et al. *Ann Surg* 1981;193:462–466.

36. Ouriel K, Veith FJ, Sasahara AA. A comparison of recombinant urokinase with vascular surgery as initial treatment for acute arterial occlusion of the legs. *N Engl J Med* 1998;338:1105–1111.

37. Katz SG, Kohl RD. Direct revascularization for the treatment of forearm and hand ischemia. *Am J Surg* 1993;165:312–316.

38. Gelberman RH, Nunley JA, Koman LA, et al. The results of radial and ulnar arterial repair in the forearm. *J Bone Joint Surg* 1982;64A:383–387.

39. Keen RR, Meyer JP, Durham JR, et al. Autogenous vein graft repair of injured extremity arteries: early and late results with 134 consecutive patients. *J Vasc Surg* 1991;13:664–668.

40. Stricker SJ, Burkhalater WE, Ouellette AE. Single-vessel forearm arterial repairs: patency rates using nuclear angiography. *Orthopedics* 1989;12:963–965.

41. Nunley JA, Goldner RD, Koman LA, et al. Arterial stump pressure: a determinant of arterial patency? *J Hand Surg [Am]* 1987;12:245–249.

42. Kaufman JL. Atheroembolism and microthromboembolic syndromes (blue toe syndrome and disseminated atheroembolism). In: Rutherford RB, ed. *Vascular surgery*, 5th ed. Philadelphia: Saunders, 2000:836–845.

43. Dotter CT, Rosch J, Seaman AJ. Selective clot lysis with low-dose streptokinase. *Radiology* 1974;111:31–37.

44. Ouriel K, Shortell CK, DeWeese JA, et al. A comparison of thrombolytic therapy with operative revascularization in the initial treatment of acute peripheral arterial ischemia. *J Vasc Surg* 1994;19:1021–1030.

45. Ouriel K, Veith FJ, Sasahara AA. Thrombolysis or peripheral arterial surgery: phase I results. *J Vasc Surg* 1996;23:64–75.

46. The STILE Investigators. Results of a prospective randomized trial evaluating surgery versus thrombolysis for ischemia of the lower extremity: the STILE trial. *Ann Surg* 1994;220:251–268.

47. Suggs WD, Cynamon J, Martin B, et al. When is urokinase treatment an effective sole or adjunctive treatment for acute limb ischemia secondary to native artery occlusion? *Am J Surg* 1999;178:103–106.

48. Widlus DM, Venbrux AC, Benenati JF, et al. Fibrinolytic therapy for upper-extremity arterial occlusions. *Radiology* 1990;175:393–399.

49. Coulon M, Goffette P, Dondelinger RF. Local thrombolytic infusion in arterial ischemia of the upper limb: mid-term results. *Cardiovasc Intervent Radiol* 1994;17:81–86.

50. Beard JD, Nyamekye I, Earnshaw JJ, et al. Intraoperative streptokinase: a useful adjunct to balloon-catheter embolectomy. *Br J Surg* 1993;80:21–24.

51. Ouriel K, Shortell CK, Azodo MVU, et al. Acute peripheral arterial occlusion: predictors of success in catheter-directed thrombolytic therapy. *Radiology* 1994;193:561–566.

52. Working Party on Thrombolysis in the Management of Limb Ischemia. Thrombolysis in the management of lower limb peripheral arterial occlusion—a consensus document. *Am J Cardiol* 1998;81:207–218.

53. Hill SL, Donato AT. The simple Fogarty embolectomy: an operation of the past? *Am Surg* 1994;60:907–911.

92

COMPARTMENT SYNDROMES AND ISCHEMIC CONTRACTURE

MICHAEL J. BOTTE

Acute compartment syndrome is a condition of increased tissue fluid pressure within a fascial muscle compartment that reduces muscle capillary blood perfusion below a level necessary for tissue viability (1–38). Muscle and nerve are particularly vulnerable to injury from these sustained pressures and the accompanying ischemia. If untreated, sustained elevated pressures cause irreversible damage. Muscle undergoes necrosis, fibrosis, and contracture. Coexisting nerve injury causes further muscle dysfunction, sensibility deficits, or chronic pain, or a combination of these. The result is a dysfunctional, deformed limb that is known as *Volkmann's ischemic contracture* (39–70).

A separate entity of reversible compartment syndrome that is precipitated by exercise or repetitive motion also exists. The signs and symptoms are transient, and there are no neurologic sequelae. This form is known as *exertional compartment syndrome* (28,71–94). In the following review, three main aspects of compartment syndrome are discussed. These are acute compartment syndrome, Volkmann's ischemic contracture, and exertional compartment syndrome. Because of its relationship to compartment syndrome and clinical importance, a severe form of compartment syndrome, *crush syndrome*, is also discussed (20,95).

ACUTE COMPARTMENT SYNDROME

Historical Aspects

Case reports of extremity contracture after injury have been cited as early as 1840 (96). Most acquired contractures were believed to be a result of direct neurologic injury. Richard von Volkmann (97) was among the first to discuss these acquired contractures, providing in-depth reports as early as 1869. He originally described the condition as an "inflammatory myositis." In 1881, von Volkmann (98) further expounded on the process, describing in greater detail the course and progression of muscle ischemia, paralysis, and subsequent contracture. He concluded that the contractures were a consequence of decreased arterial blood flow and attributed the pathology to application of tight, constricting bandages to an injured limb that resulted in muscle necrosis and contracture. A distinguishing feature of Volkmann's early analysis was the connection of ischemia and muscle necrosis to the cause of contracture:

> The paralysis is caused by the death of primitive muscle fibers which have been deprived of oxygen. The contractile substance coagulates, falls into pieces, and is afterwards absorbed. The following contracture may be considered simply as a condition closely akin to rigor mortis, and indeed the limbs, if, as is usually the case, all muscles of a part are equally affected by the ischemia, assume the well known position as after death (97).

In 1884, Leser (99) further described the clinical features of these acquired contractures and attempted to design animal models to evaluate the disease process. His pathologic evaluations were among the first to confirm that muscle necrosis was a part of the condition. His contributions were so important that the syndrome had subsequently been referred to as *Volkmann-Leser contracture* by some authors (96,100).

In 1890, Hildebrand (101) provided additional animal studies based on Leser's results and noted that, in addition to muscle injury, nerve involvement was also a factor in the pathologic process. Hildebrand was among the first to refer to the contracture as *Volkmann's contracture*.

In 1900, Bernays (41) reviewed the work of Volkmann, Leser, and others and provided his own detailed description of the pathology of ischemic muscle and associated contracture, noting that the muscle injury and contractures could range from mild to severe. He also made an early reference to the potential physician liability and litigation in these cases.

In the following decades, several authors contributed theories of etiology. Thomas (100) provided an extensive review of cases and available literature on Volkmann's contracture in 1908. In 1922, Brooks (102–104) attributed venous obstruction as a factor in contracture formation. The concept of increased pressure initially described by Volkmann remained as the early consistent feature, and Jones (105) further noted, in 1928, that the reigning opinion was that contracture was "due to pressure from within or without, or both." Arterial spasm and injury were noted as related factors by Leriche in 1928 (106), Griffiths in 1940 (57), and Foisie in 1942 (108). A version of the so-called *four Ps* for diagnosis of compartment syndrome was a contribution by Griffiths (57) in 1940, noting "*p*ain with passive extension, *p*ainful or painless onset, *p*allor, or *p*uffiness."

Methods of treatment were also evolving, with most advances reported after the turn of the century. Before 1911, treatments had placed emphasis on managing the sequelae of ischemic contracture. Nonoperative methods consisted mainly of limb mobilization and muscle stretching. Operative management included tendon lengthening, contracture release, and bone-shortening techniques (to relax the tension on the contracted muscles) (96,109). In 1911, Bardenheuer (110) provided the first account of fasciotomy in the forearm of patients with impending Volkmann's contracture. He described an *aponeurectomy*, which consisted of incision of the deep antecubital and forearm fascia. In 1914, Murphy (111) suggested early fasciotomy as a means of preventing paralysis and contracture when pressure was increased within a fascial-enclosed muscle space after hemorrhage and edema. Although the pathogenesis remained relatively poorly understood, Jepson (112,113) demonstrated the effects of early fascial decompression on injured muscle in 1926. Other authors included Jorge in 1925 (114), Moulonquet and Seneque in 1928 (63), and Massart in 1935 (115), all of whom stressed the need for fasciotomy in selected patients. The operative techniques were not discussed in detail. In 1939, Garber (116) recommended exploration of the median and ulnar nerves and the brachial artery along with decompression of forearm compartments. The operative technique for fasciotomy was described by Benjamin in 1959. In his series of several cases of impending Volkmann's ischemic contracture, Benjamin (39) recommended a transverse division of the fascia of the antecubital fossa followed by a longitudinal division of the deep forearm fascia.

As the pathogenesis became more clearly understood, Eechler and Lipscomb described a stepwise technique that included division of forearm skin, subcutaneous tissue, and fascia (51). In the mid-1970s, the concept of increased tissue pressure was accepted as the common basis of the disease process (11–14,20–25,117–124). Matsen and Clawson (11) provided a "unified concept of compartment syndrome" in 1975. Matsen indicated that the increased tissue pressure could be caused by a decrease in the size of the compartment or an increase in the volume of its contents. This resultant increased tissue pressure leads to decreased tissue perfusion and results in necrosis of muscle and nerve. The appreciation of increased tissue fluid pressure leads to the development of more accurate methods of measurement, including the methods by Whitesides et al. (infusion technique) (35–38), Hargens and Mubarak (wick and slit

catheter techniques) (7,25,118,123,125), and Matsen et al. (continuous monitoring technique) (13). More recently, pressure measurement and monitoring have been performed with portable, commercially made transducers (27). These contributions, which related to tissue pressure measurements, helped establish the urgency that was required for operative decompression. In addition, these techniques have allowed further assessment of compartment syndrome when physical exam is difficult or limited, such as in the obtunded or unconscious patient or those with a coexisting proximal peripheral or spinal nerve injury.

The surgical anatomy was more clearly delineated by Eaton and Green (49), who emphasized surgical decompression from the proximal forearm to the wrist and proposed secondary wound closure with split-thickness skin grafts and relaxing incisions. Whitesides et al. (37) included carpal tunnel release in their descriptions of forearm decompression from the distal arm to the mid-palm. Newmeyer and Kilgore (126) recommended wide exposure of all three possible areas of involvement, including the forearm flexor and extensor compartments and the intrinsic muscles of the hand. Gelberman (4,5,54) discussed and popularized a volar approach that used a single longitudinal curvilinear incision for forearm decompression that allowed incision of the palmar antebrachial fascia and transverse carpal ligament, as well as exposure of the forearm neurovascular structures and mobile wad. This extensile exposure was similar to the combined exposure of the median and ulnar nerves, as described by Henry (127). More recently, additional reports and studies have led to descriptions of fasciotomy of compartments in the shoulder region, the arm, and the intrinsic muscles of the hand (128–131).

Multiple studies and reports on the pathogenesis, sequelae, and treatment of compartment syndrome have since been performed (7,8,11–29,118–125,132–157). Microcirculatory impairment that is secondary to sustained increase in intracompartmental interstitial pressure is now accepted as the critical factor that causes compartment syndrome and, ultimately, Volkmann's ischemic contracture. The use of fasciotomy to relieve the pressure and to prevent ischemic contracture is historically well established (4,15,22,23,37, 54,158). In addition, the concept of the less severe recurrent or chronic form of compartment syndrome (exertional compartment syndrome) has also been appreciated, along with the treatment of elective fasciotomy (28,71–80,83–94). For established deformity from ischemic contracture, methods of surgical reconstruction were outlined by Seddon (66,67), Goldner (56,159–161), Gelberman (54), Tsuge (69,70), and Smith et al. (162,163). Techniques used to correct or improve deformity include infarct excision, muscle and tendon lengthening or recession, contracture release, tendon transfer, and, in selective joints, arthrodesis (54,56,66,67,69, 70,159–162). Advances in microvascular and microneural surgery have allowed the development of free tissue transfer to augment function (164–170).

Despite the advances in diagnosis, prevention, and management, acute compartment syndrome remains a relatively common clinical problem, especially in trauma centers and acute care facilities. Subsequent ischemic contractures continue to occur and can result in severe, challenging clinical presentations.

Muscle Compartments and Associated Anatomy

Skeletal Muscle Compartment

Skeletal muscles are individually surrounded by their own thin fibrous epimysial sheath. Groups of muscles are additionally enclosed by deep fascia, forming discrete compartments. Compartment boundaries also include interosseous membranes and bone (128,129,171).

The contents of an anatomic compartment include muscles, arteries, veins, and nerves. The upper extremity is divided into several compartments with single or multiple muscle, nerve, and vascular components. The muscle and nerve components of the various compartments are the primary and secondary tissues of injury, respectively, in the pathologic process of compartment syndrome (128,172,173).

Fascial Components and Related Structures

The fascia has been divided into superficial and deep components. The superficial fascia is a less distinct layer of connective tissue that forms the thin superficial layer that contains the membrane for the fatty tissues beneath the skin.

The deep fascia is the thicker, more distinct layer that surrounds the muscles and extends between muscles. The term *fascia* is usually used to denote the deep fascia. It can be adherent to the epimysium but, in most instances, is structurally separate (128,129). The deep fascia is more involved in the mechanics of compartment syndrome than the superficial fascia. The deep fascia may form a substantial and relatively unyielding envelope around individual muscle and septae between muscles and compartments.

The two fascial layers are usually joined by loose areolar tissue that provides a plane of dissection between the two fascial layers. As noted by Doyle (128), a notable exception to the thin superficial fascia that is seen in most areas of the upper extremity is the thick and substantial palmar aponeurosis in the hand. In thermal or electrical burns, the superficial fascia and skin may form an unyielding and constricting eschar and may play a role in the production of compartment syndrome (along with the deeper fascia and intramuscular edema) (174).

Histologically, fascia is composed of sheets of collagenous bundles and fibroblasts with parallel, wavelike rows of collagen (128,129,175). Fibers from one sheet interweave with adjoining layers and contribute to the overall strength of the fascial layer.

Garfin et al. (176) have shown that removal of fascia reduces the force of muscle contraction by nearly 15%. This apparently occurs because of the reduction of the volume-containing ability of the fascia, thus allowing the muscle to balloon out and thereby lose contractile efficiency.

The subfascial connective tissue components of muscle consist of the *epimysium,* the *perimysium,* and the *endomysium.* The epimysium is usually separate from and deep to the muscle fascia. It is a connective tissue sheath that directly contacts and encloses the muscles. The epimysium is composed of type I collagen and contributes to the outer fascial envelope that surrounds muscles and muscle groups. Deep to the epimysium is the perimysium, a thin connective tissue layer that surrounds groups (fasciculi) of muscle fibers. The perimysium contains vascular structures, nerves, and neuromuscular spindles. This layer contains type I and III collagen. The perimysial fibers are inward extensions of the epimysium. Individual muscle fibers are surrounded by a delicate network of connective tissue, the *endomysium.* This layer is the site of metabolic exchange between muscle and blood. Capillaries and small nerves are also found in this layer (177). The endomysium contains types III, IV, and V collagen. The endomysium is continuous with the more substantial connective tissue, the *perimysium* (128).

Anatomic Compartments of the Upper Extremity

Upper extremity muscle compartments have been described by Henry, Garfin, Doyle, Bojsen-Miller, Sotereanos, and others (127–129) and are listed in Table 1. The major compartments consist of those of the deltoid, anterior arm, posterior arm, forearm mobile wad, volar forearm, pronator quadratus compartment, dorsal forearm, central palmar compartment of the hand, adductor compartment, and the thenar, hypothenar, interosseous compartments (128). Although the carpal tunnel is not a true muscle compartment, it can have the physiologic properties of a closed compartment and is anatomically relevant in acute carpal tunnel syndrome (178–180). It is therefore included in the description of the anatomic compartments. The appreciation of these separate compartments and the specifics of their anatomy and boundaries assist in the assessment and operative management.

Deltoid Compartment

The deltoid compartment contains only the deltoid muscle (Fig. 1). The compartment is bounded by the deep fascia of the deltoid muscle on the anterior, lateral, and posterior aspects and by the humerus medially (128,129). The fascia sends multiple septae between its fasciculi and is continuous with the fascia of the pectoralis major anteriorly and the fascia of the infraspinous posteriorly (128,177). On the superior aspect, the fascia is attached to the clavicle, the acromion, and

TABLE 1. MUSCLE COMPARTMENTS AND FASCIAL SPACES OF THE UPPER EXTREMITY

Compartment	Principal muscles
Deltoid compartment	Deltoids
Anterior compartment of the arm	Biceps brachii
	Brachialis
	Coracobrachialis
Posterior compartment of the arm	Triceps muscle (three heads)
Mobile wad compartment of the forearm	Brachioradialis
	Extensor carpi radialis longus
	Extensor carpi radialis brevis
Volar compartment of the forearm	Pronator teres
	Flexor carpi radialis
	Flexor digitorum superficialis
	Flexor carpi radialis
	Flexor carpi ulnaris
	Flexor digitorum profundus
	Flexor pollicis longus
	Palmaris longus
Dorsal compartment of the forearm	Extensor digitorum communis
	Extensor carpi ulnaris
	Extensor digiti quinti
	Extensor pollicis longus
	Abductor pollicis longus
	Extensor pollicis brevis
Carpal tunnel[a]	Extrinsic digital flexor tendons
Central palmar compartment of the hand	Extrinsic flexor tendons
	Lumbricals
Thenar compartment	Abductor pollicis brevis
	Flexor pollicis brevis
	Opponens pollicis
Hypothenar compartment	Abductor digiti minimi
	Flexor digiti minimi
	Opponens digiti minimi
Adductor compartment of the hand	Adductor pollicis
Interosseous compartments of hand	Dorsal interosseous (four)
	Palmar interosseous (three)

[a]Although not a true muscle compartment, the carpal tunnel is listed here because it can have the physiologic properties of a closed compartment in the presence of compartment syndrome.

the crest of the spine of the scapula. On the inferior aspect, the fascia is continuous with the brachial fascia.

The deltoid arises from the clavicle, the acromion, and the spine of the scapula, forming a thick, curved, triangular-shaped muscle. The central part of muscle is multipenniform, usually with four intramuscular septae that extend from the acromion to join three ascending septae from the deltoid tuberosity. The septae are connected by short muscle fibers. The deltoid muscle fasciculi are large and present as coarse longitudinal striations. The fibers converge distally in a short tendon of insertion on the lateral aspect of the humerus (128,129).

The deltoid is innervated by the axillary nerve. The nerve enters the compartment on its deep surface and is accompanied by the posterior humeral circumflex artery. These two structures pass through the quadrangular space

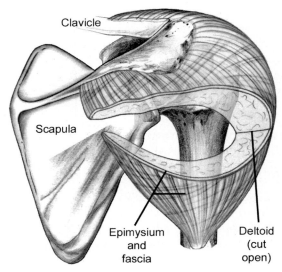

FIGURE 1. Deltoid compartment (posterior view). The epimysium and fascia form one layer that encloses this muscle.

to reach the deltoid compartment. The axillary nerve then divides into anterior and posterior branches. The anterior branch, with the posterior circumflex humeral artery, curves around the humeral neck to traverse the curved deep surface of the muscle to reach its anterior border. The anterior branch of the axillary nerve gives off a few small branches that pierce the muscle, some of which continue on to ramify within the skin over the lower part of the muscle. The posterior branch of the axillary also extends along the deep surface of the deltoid to reach the posterior border of the muscle. The posterior branch pierces the deep fascia at the inferior and posterior aspects of the muscle and continues distally as the upper lateral cutaneous nerve of the arm. The deltoid muscle receives its vascular supply from the acromial and deltoid branches from the thoracoacromial artery, posterior and anterior circumflex humeral subscapular artery, and the deltoid branch of the profunda brachii artery (128).

Anterior Compartment of the Arm

The anterior compartment of the arm is composed of the biceps, brachialis, and coracobrachialis muscles (Fig. 2) (128,129). The compartment is enveloped by fascia anteriorly, medially, and laterally. The posterior margins are enclosed by the medial and lateral intermuscular septa and the humerus.

The musculocutaneous nerve innervates the coracobrachialis and the biceps with separate branches to each head of the biceps. The brachialis receives dual innervation from the musculocutaneous and radial nerves, with the radial nerve supplying a small lateral portion of the muscle. Nerves that traverse the compartment include the median, radial, ulnar nerves, the musculocutaneous nerve and its sensory terminal branch, and the lateral antebrachial cuta-

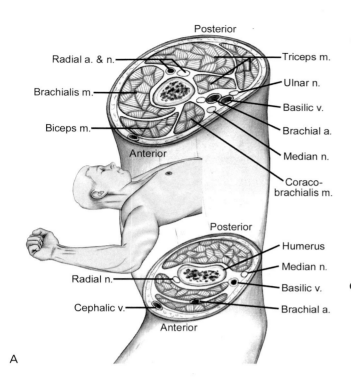

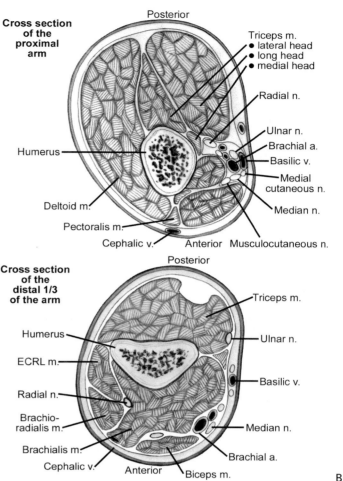

FIGURE 2. Muscle (m.) compartments of the arm. **A:** The biceps and brachialis (and coracobrachialis) comprise the major muscles of the anterior compartment of the arm. The triceps comprises the posterior compartment of the arm. **B:** Cross sections of the compartments of the arm through the proximal **(above)** and distal **(below)** two-thirds of the arm. a., artery; ECRL, extensor carpi radialis longus; n., nerve; v., vein.

neous nerve. The radial nerve enters the anterior arm compartment in the region of the middle and distal two-thirds of the arm by piercing the lateral intermuscular septum and continues distally under the deep surface of the brachioradialis to enter the forearm in the longitudinal interval between the brachioradialis and the brachialis (128).

The vascular supply to the anterior compartment of the arm is largely from the brachial artery and the anterior circumflex, which supply all three muscles. The brachialis also receives branches from the superior and inferior ulnar collateral arteries, the anterior ulnar recurrent artery, the radial collateral branch of the profunda brachii, and the radial recurrent artery. The basilic vein penetrates the brachial fascia medially in the mid-portion of the arm (128).

Posterior Compartment of the Arm

The posterior compartment of the arm consists of the three heads of the triceps muscle (Fig. 2) (128,129). The fascia that envelops the triceps is relatively thick, covering the posterior aspect of the compartment. The anterior margins of the compartment are enclosed by the medial and lateral intermuscular septa and the humerus.

The radial nerve supplies the three heads of the triceps, with separate branches to each head. The radial nerve passes through the major portion of the posterior compartment. The ulnar nerve also passes through the distal portion of the posterior compartment. The nerve enters the compartment at the medial intermuscular septum at the mid-arm and continues anterior to the medial head of the triceps, accompanied by the superior ulnar collateral artery, to enter the cubital tunnel at the elbow (128).

The vascular supply to the posterior compartment of the arm is from the circumflex humeral artery; the branches of the profunda brachii, including the deltoid, middle collateral, and direct branches; the superior and inferior ulnar collateral arteries; and the interosseous recurrent artery (128).

Mobile Wad Compartment of the Forearm

The *mobile wad*, noted by Henry (127), is a distinct muscle compartment that contains the brachioradialis, the extensor carpi radialis longus, and the extensor carpi radialis brevis (Fig. 3). These muscles functionally form a separate fascial compartment, due to fascial extensions from the antebrachial fascia (that is continuous with the brachial fascia). The ante-

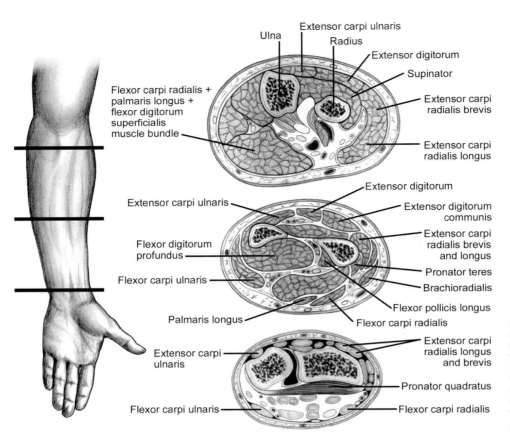

FIGURE 3. Muscle compartments of the forearm. The forearm consists of three major compartments: the volar, dorsal, and mobile wads. Illustrated here are transverse sections through the left forearm at various levels. In the lower illustration, the pronator teres is depicted. This muscle forms a separate compartment.

brachial fascia forms extensions that pass from superficial to deep to reach the underlying bone, creating septae between muscles that anatomically sequester the mobile wad as a separate group. Recognition of this compartment as separate from the neighboring forearm and arm compartments is an important consideration during fasciotomy to ensure complete forearm decompression (128).

The brachioradialis and the extensor carpi radialis longus are usually innervated by branches from the radial nerve trunk. The extensor carpi radialis brevis is usually innervated by the posterior interosseous nerve (57%) or by branches from the superficial sensory branch of the radial nerve (32%) (128).

The vascular supply to the mobile wad includes several sources. The brachioradialis receives vascularity from the radial collateral branch of the profunda brachii, the inferior ulnar recurrent artery, the radial artery directly, and the radial recurrent artery. The extensor carpi radialis longus and brevis receive vascularity from the radial collateral continuation of the profunda brachii, the radial recurrent, the interosseous recurrent, and the posterior interosseous arteries (128).

Volar Compartment of the Forearm

The volar compartment of the forearm contains the extrinsic digital and wrist flexor muscles and the pronator teres (Fig. 3) (128). The antebrachial fascia surrounds the muscles on the volar surface, and, along with the radius, ulna,

and interosseous ligament, forms an anatomic compartment. The compartment can be subdivided into a superficial group and a deep group. The superficial group contains the pronator teres, the flexor carpi radialis, the palmaris longus, and the flexor carpi ulnaris. The deep group consists of the flexor digitorum superficialis, the flexor digitorum profundus, and the flexor pollicis longus. The deep group is likely to be more involved and more severely afflicted in acute compartment syndrome and associated ischemic contractures, especially the flexor digitorum profundus and the flexor pollicis longus (which are deeply situated and bounded, in part, by bone and the rigid interosseous ligament).

The pronator quadratus, although situated in the volar forearm, is considered as a separate compartment, because decompression of the volar compartment of the forearm without specifically addressing the pronator quadratus does not usually adequately decompress the muscle (see the following discussion) (128).

The median nerve innervates most of the volar forearm compartment muscles, with the exception of the flexor carpi ulnaris and flexor digitorum profundus to the small and ring fingers (which are innervated by the ulnar nerve). The anterior interosseous nerve, a branch from the median nerve trunk, usually supplies the flexor pollicis longus and the flexor digitorum profundus to the index and long fingers (as well as the pronator quadratus).

The vascular supply to the volar forearm compartment is from the radial and ulnar arteries (in the form of the primary, recurrent, interosseous, and collateral branches) and the anterior interosseous artery, which arises from the common interosseous artery from the proximal portion of the ulnar artery (128).

Pronator Quadratus Compartment

The pronator quadratus, which is located in the distal palmar forearm, has recently been shown to occupy a functionally separate fascial compartment (Fig. 3) (181). The muscle is enclosed anteriorly by a well-defined fascial sheath that measures 0.4 to 0.5 mm in thickness. This sheath, along with the relatively rigid posterior boundaries of the interosseous ligament and distal radius and ulna, forms a distinct fascial space. Dye that is experimentally injected into this compartment does not communicate with the other forearm compartments (181). Clinical correlations of compartment syndrome that involve the pronator quadratus support the concept that the muscle occupies its own compartment (128,182,183). The pronator quadratus is innervated by the anterior interosseous nerve and receives its blood supply from the anterior interosseous artery (128).

Dorsal Compartment of the Forearm

The dorsal compartment of the forearm contains the extrinsic digital extensors (extensor digitorum communis, extensor digiti minimi, extensor indicis proprius), the thumb extrinsic extensors and abductors (extensor pollicis longus and brevis, abductor pollicis longus), the extensor carpi ulnaris, and the supinator (Fig. 3). The antebrachial fascia surrounds the extensor muscles and, along with the radius, ulna, and interosseous ligament, forms a distinct anatomic compartment (128,129). The dorsal compartment of the forearm has been subdivided into a superficial layer and a deep layer. The superficial layer contains the extensor digitorum communis, extensor digiti minimi, and extensor carpi ulnaris. The deep layer contains the supinator, the abductor pollicis longus, the extensor pollicis longus and brevis, and the extensor indicis (128).

The dorsal compartment of the forearm is innervated by the posterior interosseous nerve. The extensor digitorum communis and extensor digiti minimi receive vascularity from the posterior interosseous artery, the interosseous recurrent artery, and associated anastomosing vessels (including a continuation of the anterior interosseous artery, the dorsal carpal arch, and the dorsal metacarpal, digital, and perforating arteries). The extensor carpi ulnaris is supplied by the posterior interosseous and interosseous recurrent arteries (128).

Carpal Tunnel

The carpal tunnel is not a true muscle compartment. It does not usually contain muscle bellies and is not a true enclosed space because it is open at both ends. However, it has the physiologic properties of a closed compartment (180). Cobb et al. (184,185) studied the pressure dynamics of the carpal tunnel and flexor compartment of the forearm. The authors found that, despite the carpal tunnel being an open anatomic compartment, it functions as a relatively closed compartment with respect to transfer of pressure from the flexor compartment of the forearm under conditions that mimic elevated tissue pressure. The carpal tunnel should therefore be considered a compartment in the presence of compartment syndrome, because the median nerve is vulnerable from the increases in pressure. These considerations are important from an assessment standpoint and from aspects of operative management (acute carpal tunnel syndrome is discussed in Acute Compartment Syndrome of the Wrist).

Central Palmar Compartment of the Hand

The central palmar compartment of the hand is a triangular-shaped space (apex proximal) that begins at the distal margin of the carpal tunnel and ends near the interdigital web spaces. The compartment consists of single space in the proximal palm and a series of eight smaller compartments in the distal part, and the anatomic space can be considered a separate compartment (128,186). It is located between the thenar and hypothenar compartments. Septae from the palmar aponeurosis at the radial and ulnar margins separate the central compartment from the thenar and hypothenar compartments. The septa on the radial margin begins as an extension of the wall of the carpal canal and extends distally over the fascia, covering the adductor pollicis and first dorsal interosseous muscles. It ends at the proximal phalanx, forming the radial and volar margins of the lumbrical canal to the index finger (128). The septa on the ulnar margin begins on the ulnar side of the carpal canal and is attached to the shaft of the little finger metacarpal. The septa separates the central and hypothenar compartments. The roof of the central palmar compartment is formed by the longitudinal and transverse fibers of the palmar fascia. The floor is formed by the fascia of the palmar interosseous muscles, the deep transverse metacarpal ligament, and the adductor fascia. Between the two septae at the margins, there are seven intermediate septae that, along with the marginal septa, divide the distal aspect of the central space into four canals to accommodate the flexor tendons and four canals to accommodate the lumbricals and the neurovascular bundles (128). Thus, the central palmar compartment is a single space in the proximal palm and a series of eight smaller compartments in the distal part (128,186). In addition to the flexor tendons and lumbrical muscles, this compartment also includes the superficial and deep palmar arches, the common digital arteries, and the common and proper digital nerves from the median and ulnar nerves. This central palmar compartment is not consistently considered a separate compartment by all authors (178).

The first and second lumbricals are innervated by the branches from the median nerve-derived common digital nerves. The third and fourth lumbricals are innervated by the deep terminal branch of the ulnar nerve. The third lumbrical frequently receives a branch from the median nerve-derived common digital nerve. The vascular supply to the first and second lumbricals is from the first and second dorsal metacarpal and dorsal digital arteries, the arteria radialis indicis, and the first common palmar digital artery. The third and fourth lumbricals are supplied by the second and third common palmar digital arteries, the third and fourth dorsal digital arteries, and their anastomoses with the palmar digital arteries (128).

Thenar Compartment of the Hand

The thenar compartment of the hand includes the abductor pollicis brevis, the flexor pollicis brevis, and the opponens pollicis (Fig. 4). The compartment is covered palmarly by the thenar fascia, which attaches to the palmar surface of the thumb metacarpal and wraps around the thenar muscles to enclose the deep surface as well. The thenar fascia then attaches to the deep ulnar side of the metacarpal, thus enveloping the thenar muscles by a U-shaped sheet of fascia. The thumb metacarpal comprises the radial margin of the compartment (128,178).

The thenar muscles are usually innervated by the recurrent (motor) branch of the median nerve. The flexor pollicis brevis has two heads, the superficial and deep heads. The superficial head is frequently innervated by the recurrent motor branch of the median nerve, whereas the deep head is supplied by the deep branch of the ulnar nerve. The opponens pollicis may also receive a branch from the deep branch of the ulnar nerve. The vascular supply to the the-nar muscles is from the primary branches from the radial artery, from branches from the first palmar metacarpal artery, and from the radialis indicis, the princeps pollicis, and the deep palmar arch (128).

Hypothenar Compartment of the Hand

The hypothenar compartment of the hand includes the abductor digiti minimi, the flexor digiti minimi, and the opponens digiti minimi (Fig. 4). The compartment is covered radially by the ulnar septum of the central palmar compartment. The ulnar septum attaches to and blends with the hypothenar fascia (which is itself a thinner continuation of the palmar fascia). The hypothenar fascia wraps around the ulnar border of the hypothenar muscles to reach the ulnopalmar aspect of the small finger metacarpal. The small finger metacarpal comprises the deep surface of the hypothenar compartment (128,129,178).

The hypothenar muscles are innervated by the deep branch of the ulnar nerve. The vascular supply is from the deep palmar branch of the ulnar artery, the branches from the superficial palmar arch, and the branches from the digital artery to the little finger (128).

Adductor Compartment of the Hand

The adductor compartment contains only the adductor pollicis muscle (Fig. 4). The compartment is covered palmarly by the adductor fascia. This fascia extends radially from the long finger metacarpal and attaches on the ulnar aspect of the thumb metacarpal. The distal border is bound by the convergence of the adductor fascia into the fascia over the first dorsal interosseous muscle. The compartment is covered dorsally by the fascia that covers the first and second interosseous spaces (128,186).

The adductor pollicis muscle is innervated by the deep branch of the ulnar nerve. The vascular supply is from the princeps pollicis and the radialis indicis, which may be combined as the first metacarpal artery. Branches from the deep palmar arch also supply the adductor pollicis.

Interosseous Compartments of the Hand

The hand has four dorsal interosseous compartments and three palmar interosseous compartments (Fig. 4). The second, third, and fourth dorsal interosseous compartments and the associated first, second, and third palmar interosseous compartments are each bound by a metacarpal on the radial and ulnar margins. Although several discussions combine the dorsal and palmar interosseous compartments into one *interosseous* compartment, in the strictest sense, each represents a separate compartment for the dorsal and palmar interosseous muscle (128,178). The dorsal aspect of each interosseous compartment is enclosed by the dorsal interosseous fascia. The volar aspect

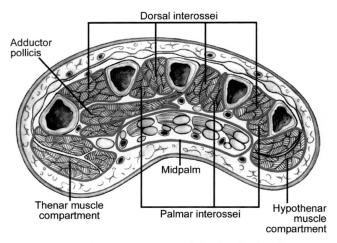

FIGURE 4. Muscle compartments of the hand. The illustration shows a cross section of the mid-palm that depicts the major fascial compartment of the hand.

of the interosseous compartments is enclosed by the volar interosseous fascia.

The first interosseous compartment is unique in that it contains only the first dorsal interosseous muscle. It usually has no palmar interosseous muscle, although controversy exists as to the possible presence of a palmar interosseous muscle in this first web space (177). The first interosseous compartment is bound by the thumb metacarpal radially and the index-finger metacarpal ulnarly (Fig. 4). The dorsal aspect of the first interosseous compartment is covered by the dorsal interosseous fascia. The palmar aspect of the first interosseous compartment is comprised of a fascia that separates the first dorsal interosseous muscle from the adductor pollicis.

The dorsal and palmar interosseous muscles are innervated by the deep branch of the ulnar nerve. The vascular supply to the dorsal interossei is from the dorsal metacarpal, the second to fourth palmar metacarpal arteries, the princeps pollicis and radialis indicis arteries, and perforating branches from the deep radial arch. The vascular supply to the palmar interossei is from the deep palmar arch, princeps pollicis, radialis indicis, palmar metacarpal arteries, and common and proper digital arteries (128).

Compartment of the Digits

The digits do not contain true muscle compartments, because there are no skeletal muscle bellies present. However, as in the carpal tunnel, the digits do have nerves that pass through unyielding "fascial" compartments that are bounded by Cleland's and Grayson's ligaments, along with digital skin (which is anchored by these ligaments and is restrictive when edematous) (Fig. 5) (158,178). The ligaments and skin can result in a type of physiologic compartment that places the palmar digital nerves at risk or susceptible to pressure increases. These pseudocompartments have implications for operative decompression, as discussed in the section Operative Management.

Pathogenesis of Compartment Syndrome

For compartment syndrome to occur, a prerequisite usually includes an intact fascia or constricting skin and subcutaneous tissue. These constricting envelopes are needed to precipitate and maintain the increased intracompartmental tissue fluid pressure. Normal resting intramuscular pressure is usually less than 6 mm Hg. An inciting event usually causes an initial increase in tissue fluid pressure from edema or hemorrhage (1,2,8,11,25,116,187–197). This initial increase in pressure decreases capillary flow and causes localized muscle ischemia. Ischemia promotes vasodilation and increased capillary permeability, which result in additional intracompartmental edema and continued increase in tissue fluid pressure. The intramuscular pressure can increase to more than 100 mm Hg because of the low com-

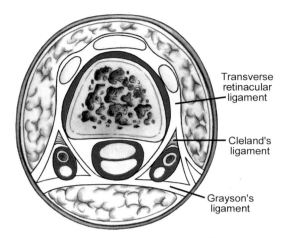

FIGURE 5. Compartments of the digit. The digit has no skeletal muscle; therefore, there are no true muscle compartments. However, the fascial spaces do form potential physiologic compartments, which are bounded by the fascial bands that contain the neurovascular bundles.

pliance of intracompartmental tissues, which are confined by the inelastic fascia and bone (8,23). Rising compartment pressure ultimately leads to compartmental tamponade, microcirculatory impairment, and sustained ischemia (8). This self-perpetuating cycle of increasing ischemia was originally outlined by Matsen and Clawson (11) and further expanded by Hargens and Akeson (Figs. 6 and 7) (7,27,188).

Muscle and nerve tissue are especially vulnerable to ischemia and incur irreversible damage if sufficient pressures are maintained (7,14,34,120–124,138,184,198–206). Normal muscle tissue fluid pressure is usually less than 8 mm Hg. Animal studies have shown that pressures that are maintained at greater than 30 mm Hg for 8 hours are able to cause irreversible damage to muscle and significant nerve conduction impairment (7,15–17,120–122, 124,144). The amount of damage that is sustained is dependent on the extent and duration of the pressure. In other studies, functional impairment of skeletal muscle could be noted after 2 to 4 hours of ischemia, becoming irreversible after 4 to 12 hours. Abnormal function of peripheral nerves starts after 30 minutes of ischemia, with irreversible functional loss after 12 to 24 hours (120). The time between injury and onset of compartment syndrome may vary from hours to days (Fig. 8).

The deepest forearm compartments, especially those adjacent to bone, develop high interstitial pressures during compartment syndrome (39,69,70,189). In the forearm, the flexor digitorum profundus and flexor pollicis longus muscles, with their deep locations that are bound in part by bone and the relatively stiff interosseous ligament, are usually the most severely affected (69,70). Interstitial pressures and associated muscle ischemic injury are often marked in these muscles, especially in the central one-third of the

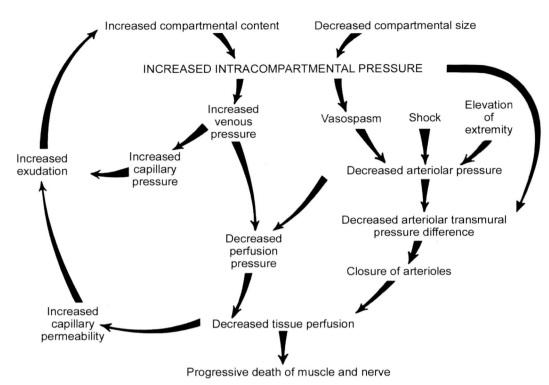

FIGURE 6. Physiologic aspects of the formation of compartment syndrome. Matsen's unified concept of compartment syndrome.

muscle belly in which collateral circulation may be the poorest. The flexor digitorum superficialis and pronator teres are usually affected to a lesser degree than the deeper flexors. The wrist flexors, forearm extensors, and brachioradialis are usually the least affected (69,70).

Causes of Compartment Syndromes

There are numerous events that lead to acute upper extremity compartment syndrome (and the related acute carpal tunnel syndrome). Most of the described causes pertain to compartment syndrome that involves the forearm. The causes or inciting events have been categorized by Matsen, further classified by Hargens and Mubarak (25), and more recently reviewed by Yamaguchi and Viegas (207) (Table 2). These causes can be divided into two large groups: (a) those events that reduce or restrict the dimensions of the closed compartment and (b) those events that increase the volume of the compartment. The former group includes placement of constrictive casts, splints, or dressings (176,187,208,209); tight fascial closures (25); prolonged external limb pressure during unconsciousness after drug overdose; external pressure caused by pneumatic tourniquets (48,124,210–218); and unprotected limb placement that leads to compression during extended surgery (25,144,207,219). The latter group includes edema or hemorrhage from trauma (including fractures, muscle tears, soft tissue crush inju-

ries, gunshot wounds) (2,9,189,220–250); high-pressure injection injuries (251–254); extravasations of fluids from vascular lines or from invasive procedures (191, 255–271); spontaneous hematoma from coagulation abnormalities, such as hemophilia (195,196,257,262,265, 266,272–285); edema from infection (286–290); thermal or electrical burns; frostbite; snake bites (188,291–299); edema after revascularization of arterial injury (39,300–303) or from venous obstruction (300); edema induced by ischemia from prolonged use of surgical tourniquets (48,124,210,211,214,215); edema from strenuous exercise (78,304,305); and anatomically related abnormalities (19,248,306–310).

Trauma (Fractures and Soft Tissue Injury)

Compartment syndrome from fractures occurs more often in closed fractures in which the fascial sheath is maintained. In children, supracondylar humerus fractures are common, well-documented causes, especially when compounded with the application of tight-fitting casts or brachial artery injury or occlusion (227,235,246,311,312). In adults, both-bone forearm fractures (2,313) or distal radius fractures (220,228,241,250,314,315) are more common injuries that result in compartment syndrome. Open fractures with large disruption of the deep forearm fascia usually do not result in compartment syndrome, because the fascial disruption decompresses the compartment. However, open

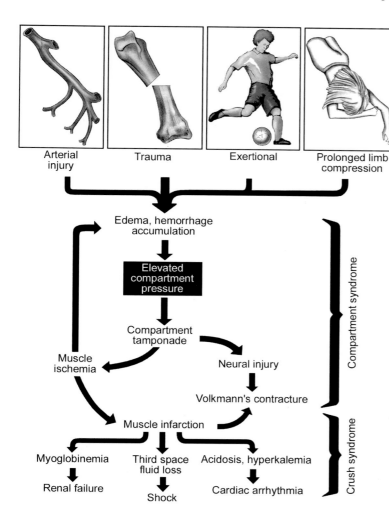

FIGURE 7. Pathophysiology of a compartment syndrome, as originally depicted by Hargens and Akeson, to include the crush syndrome. A variety of conditions may initiate a sequence of events that produces a compartment syndrome. These conditions include arterial injury, trauma, exercise, or prolonged limb compression that is associated with alcohol or drug overdose. Common to all compartment syndromes are elevated intramuscular pressure and subsequent ischemia. Without decompression, a self-perpetuating ischemia-edema process occurs, and irreversible damage, including Volkmann's contracture, may result. If many compartments are involved, a crush syndrome may occur with subsequent renal failure, shock, and possible death.

fractures may still result in compartment syndrome if a sufficient portion of the deep fascia or skin remains intact (222,316) (especially evident in gunshot wounds that are associated with open fractures). Tight, constricting casts or occlusive dressings that are placed on an edematous extremity postreduction of an acute supracondylar or forearm fracture or distal radius fracture or that are placed at the time of an operative procedure do not allow further swelling and risk compartment syndrome.

Supracondylar Fractures

In children, the extension type of supracondylar fracture is the well-recognized injury that is associated with compart-

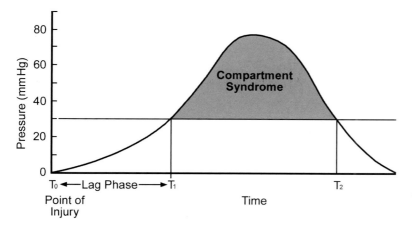

FIGURE 8. The time between injury and the onset of a compartment syndrome may vary from hours to days (with a lag phase from T_0 to T_1). The ischemia of the muscle and nerves of the compartment does not take place until the pressure rises to greater than 30 mm Hg (*horizontal line*). Thus, the time from injury to diagnosis and treatment is only a relative indicator of the ischemia period unless one has monitored the tissue pressure from the point of injury.

TABLE 2. CLASSIFICATION OF ACUTE COMPARTMENTAL SYNDROMES

Decreased compartment size
    Constrictive dressings and casts
    Closure of fascial defects
    Thermal injuries and frostbite
    Localized external pressure
    Pneumatic tourniquet
Increased compartment contents
    Primary edema accumulation
        Postischemic swelling
            Arterial injuries
            Arterial thrombosis or embolism
            Reconstructive vascular and bypass surgery
            Replantation
            Prolonged tourniquet time
            Arterial spasm
            Cardiac catheterization and angiography
            Ergotamine ingestion
        Prolonged immobilization with limb compression
            Drug overdose with limb compression
            General anesthesia with limb compression
        Increased capillary pressure or permeability
            Exercise
            Venous obstruction
            Thermal injuries and frostbite
            Exertion, seizures, and eclampsia
            Venous disease
            Intraarterial injection
            Venomous snake bite
            Infection
    Primarily hemorrhage accumulation
        Hereditary bleeding disorders (e.g., hemophilia)
        Anticoagulant therapy
        Vessel laceration
    Combination of edema and hemorrhage accumulation
        Fractures
            Supracondylar elbow
            Both-bone forearm
            Distal radius
        Soft tissue injury
            Crush
            Severe muscle tear, contusion
            Gunshot wounds
            Iatrogenic (i.e., postoperative bleeding, inflammation)
    Miscellaneous
        Intravenous infiltration (e.g., blood, saline)
        High-pressure injection

Adapted from Mubarak SJ, Hargens AR, eds. *Compartment syndromes and Volkmann's ischemic contracture.* Philadelphia: WB Saunders, 1981:75; and Matsen FA III, Clawson DK. Compartmental syndrome: a unified concept. *Clin Orthop* 1975;113:8–14.

ment syndrome. Constricting casts, splints, or occlusive dressings that are placed on an acute fracture or immediately postsurgery have been associated with development of compartment syndrome (227,235,246,311,312). In addition, immobilization of the elbow that is flexed more than 90 degrees increases the risk of compartment syndrome. Mubarak and Carroll (24) reported 55 children with various injuries in 58 limbs who subsequently developed ischemic contractures. Fractures of the humerus were the most common initiating cause of upper extremity compartment syndrome (of ten cases, nine involved extension-type supracondylar fractures, and one involved fracture of the humeral shaft). Supracondylar fractures that underwent closed reduction and immobilization with the elbow flexed to more than 90 degrees were prone to produce compartment syndrome of the forearm.

Pirone et al. (246) have noted poorer outcomes and higher complications, including ischemic contracture and cubitus varus, when the supracondylar fractures were treated with closed reduction and the application of a cast, as compared to those that were treated operatively with internal fixation or traction.

Eaton and Green (50) reported 19 patients with Volkmann's ischemia of the forearm. Of twelve patients (63%) who developed ischemia after skeletal trauma, supracondylar fractures were responsible for 83%. Seven patients (37%) developed ischemia after soft tissue or vascular trauma.

Bajpai et al. (317) reviewed 138 cases of Volkmann's contracture and noted supracondylar fractures to be the initiating injury in 32 cases (23%). This was second only to both-bone forearm fractures, which accounted for 44 cases (32%). Fractures of the ulna accounted for eight cases (6%).

Fracture of the Distal Radius

Fractures of the distal radius are also common inciting injuries that can lead to compartment syndrome of the forearm or acute carpal tunnel syndrome, or both (220,228,241, 250,314,315). Stockley et al. (250) reported five cases of acute compartment syndrome of the volar forearm that developed after fractures of the distal radius. Four of those cases involved intraarticular fracture of the radius, and three of the four cases had comminuted displaced extraarticular fracture components. One case involved displaced transverse fractures of the distal radius and ulna metaphyses (207,250). Cooney et al. (228) reported four patients who developed a Volkmann's ischemic contracture after a distal radius fracture. Three patients had a constricting cast that was retained despite the patient's complaints of persisting pain. Shall et al. (249) described two cases of compartment syndrome in the forearm that were associated with distal radius fractures.

Gunshot Wounds and Both-Bone Forearm Fractures

Gunshot wounds to the forearm can lead to compartment syndrome, especially when they are associated with fracture of the radius and ulna (232,243). Most injuries involve low-velocity gunshot injuries. Compartment syndrome was noted to develop in 10% of 131 cases of low-velocity gunshots to the forearm. Moed and Yamaguchi (207,243) stress that patients are potentially at increased risk for compartment syndrome when the gunshot injury is associated with a fracture of the proximal one-third of the forearm; close monitoring is required. Elstrom et al. (232) studied 29 patients who sustained gunshot wounds to the forearm with associated fractures of the radius or ulna. Three patients (10%) developed "impending Volkmann's ischemia."

Soft Tissue Injury

Soft tissue trauma without fracture can also frequently lead to compartment syndrome. These injuries usually result from crush injuries, severe contusions, sustained external pressure, or from muscle tears or avulsions. Crush injuries include those from cement blocks, iron gates, logs, steel shelves, large rocks, and car bodies (318). Severe muscle contusions in sports injuries have been noted to result in compartment syndrome (194,207). Compartment syndrome can also occur from muscle ruptures in weight lifters, or avulsions from muscle origins or insertions, and has been described as occurring in the triceps, pectoralis, and flexor digitorum superficialis (207,223,319,320).

High-Pressure Injection Injuries

Industrial and commercial injection devices can inject water, steam, grease, paint, cleaning solvents, or other organic and inorganic solvents at high pressure. The injected material can penetrate the skin and track down tendon sheaths or directly penetrate into a muscle compartment. Compartment syndrome occurs from the volume of fluid injected or from an intense inflammatory response that is caused by the organic or caustic fluids, or both (251–254).

Needle Injection Injuries, Intravenous Fluids, and Peripheral Nerve Blocks

Injections from hypodermic needles, extravasation of intravenous fluids, and the use of arterial lines have initiated several cases of compartment syndrome (207). Ouellette and Kelly (131) described compartment syndrome of the hand that was precipitated by intravenous injection of a drug in 14 patients. In addition, two cases were noted to have been precipitated by use of an arterial line. Several case reports describe compartment syndrome developing after intravenous infusion of hypertonic saline solution (258,261,321). Forearm compartment syndrome that was caused by automated injection of computed tomography contrast material has been described by Bentson et al. (191). The use of thrombolytic therapy has also been associated with compartment syndrome (284,322,323).

Pneumatic Tourniquet Use

Although rare, compartment syndrome of the upper extremity has been attributed to the use of pneumatic tourniquets (214). Cases of compartment syndrome from the use of pneumatic tourniquets have involved the arm (210) and the forearm (211). The development of compartment syndrome may be related to the drop of tissue pH that can occur after 2 hours of tourniquet ischemia. With the fall in tissue pH, there is an increase in capillary permeability and a prolongation of clotting time (324).

Sustained Pressure, Drug Overdose, and the Obtunded Patient

Sustained external pressure on an extremity precipitates compartment syndrome. This can occur in the drug-overdosed patient and often involves the forearm. The unconscious patient may lie for hours with the limb compressed against the floor by the body or with the weight of the head, thus causing ischemia that leads to forearm compartment syndrome (213,267,325,326). Severe crush syndromes that involve the upper limb also precipitate forearm compartment syndrome (see the previous discussion) (20,95,170,197,213,217,221,224,226,240,325,327–339). Sustained external pressure can also occur on an extremity during operative procedures if the limb is not well padded or is improperly positioned during extended surgery.

Vascular Injuries

Vascular injuries can produce compartment syndrome locally or more distally (207). Holden (59) divided Volkmann's contracture into two types based on etiologic factors. In type 1, a proximal arterial injury gives rise to ischemia distally; in type 2, a direct injury gives rise to ischemia at the site of the injury. In types 1 and 2, compartment syndrome develops. The extent and the degree of the ischemic zone are usually more severe in type 1 than in type 2 (69,70,207).

Revascularization and Replantation

After major limb revascularization or replantation, postischemic increased capillary permeability produces edema and swelling and can result in compartment syndrome (207,301). Prophylactic extremity fasciotomy is usually recommended after revascularization of a limb that has been avascular for several hours (340,341).

Coagulopathies and Hematoma

Compartment syndrome of the upper limb has been incited by bleeding in patients with hemophilia (196,266,277,279). Although patients with coagulopathies may recall minor trauma that is associated with the bleeding, spontaneous bleeding without trauma is more frequent. Compartment syndrome has also been noted to occur in patients with hemophilia or leukemia after venipuncture and associated bleeding (266,342). Fractures in the patient with hemophilia may also precipitate bleeding that leads to compartment syndrome.

Infection

Infection is a rare, but recognized, potential inciting event that can lead to compartment syndrome. Schnall et al. (289) reviewed 236 patients and noted four cases of compartment syndrome that were associated with infection. All four had positive cultures for β-hemolytic streptococci. Two separate cases of compartment syndrome have been described that were associated with infection of the hand with *Vibrio vulnificus* (288,290). Goldie et al. (287) have described an unusual case of a recurrent compartment syndrome and ischemic contracture that was associated with chronic osteomyelitis of the ulna. The patient had a closed fracture of the forearm, which developed hematogenous osteomyelitis. The patient subsequently developed compartment syndrome and ischemic muscle contracture. Although not true compartment syndrome, carpal tunnel syndrome is known to have been precipitated by infection, especially granulomatous infections or those that resulted in severe tenosynovitis.

Burns

Thermal and electrical burns cause compartment syndrome by producing intramuscular edema from severe inflammation (293,297,343). Burned, constricted skin loses elasticity, especially if an eschar forms. The burned skin acts similarly to an occlusive dressing by not allowing the extremity to expand in response to the edema. Pressure in the muscle deep to the eschar thus can increase.

Snake Bites

Snake bites from pit vipers (i.e., rattlesnakes, water moccasins, copperheads) cause intense inflammation and edema (188,291,292,295,296,298,344). Approximately 98% of venomous snake bites are inflicted by pit vipers. The venom contains enzymes, nonenzymatic proteins, and peptides that include hemotoxin, neurotoxin, venotoxin, cardiotoxin, and necrotizing factors. Compartment syndrome is more likely to develop if venom is injected deep to the muscle fascia. In most cases, however, snake fangs do not reach deep enough to enter the muscle fascia, and the venom is injected subcutaneously (188,291,292,295,296,298,344). It is also possible to sustain a pit viper snake bite without envenomation, in which the snake does not or cannot inject venom. An inflammatory response and compartment syndrome should not occur.

Exercised-Induced Acute Compartment Syndrome

Exercise has been noted to precipitate the two types of compartment syndrome, acute and exertional (chronic, recurrent) (see the following section for chronic compartment syndrome). Two cases of exercise-induced *acute* compartment syndrome in the forearm extensor muscle have been reported (78,94,207). One developed after strenuous use of a manual boring tool that was used for making holes in thick ice (78). The other occurred from paddling a canoe (94).

Exercise-Induced Chronic Exertional Compartment Syndrome

Exertional compartment syndrome is a condition of transient symptoms that are precipitated by exercise and does not result in the sequelae of Volkmann's contracture (71–73,75,78,79,83–90,93,345–349). Case reports have described chronic exercise-induced compartment syndrome that is related to repetitive motion, strenuous work, or sustained muscle contraction (71,80,83,91,345) (see the section Exertional Compartment Syndrome).

Diagnosis of Compartment Syndrome

Clinical Examination

The diagnosis of acute compartment syndrome is made clinically and is confirmed by measurement of intracompartmental tissue fluid pressure (3,5,8,14,23,75,193,313,320, 350–353). Clinical findings include (a) a swollen, tense, tender compartment, (b) pain (usually out of proportion to that expected from the existing injury), (c) sensibility deficits, and (d) motor weakness or paralysis. Pain is usually accentuated with passive stretch of the afflicted muscles by passive manipulation of the neighboring joints. Passive stretch is not always reliable, because any injury to the limb (such as fracture or blunt trauma) may result in pain with passive stretch of the overlying muscles. Paresthesia, hypesthesia, or anesthesia that is produced by compartment syndrome is located in the area that is distal to the compartment, in the sensory distribution of the nerves that traverse the compartment. Sensibility deficits usually precede motor dysfunction (7,8,144,146). Sensibility is evaluated and monitored by using light touch, sharp-dull discrimination, two-point discrimination, monofilament testing, and vibrometry. Motor strength is subjectively graded using the 0 to 5 scale, with 5 being normal strength, 4 being subjective weakness (good function), 3 being the ability to move the associated joint through a full range against gravity (fair function), 2 being the ability to move the associated joint through a full range with gravity eliminated (poor function), 1 being minimal palpable muscle contraction with little or no limb movement (trace function), and 0 being no palpable muscle contraction (no function). Evaluation of grip strength by using a grip dynamometer and lateral and chuck pinch strength by using a pinch dynamometer provides additional quantitative data. Total active and passive motion of all joints is recorded (44). Serial sensibility and motor evaluation by using these quantitative methods aid in assessing the course (improvement or deterioration) in impending compartment syndrome.

The pulses usually remain intact with acute compartment syndrome. Circulatory impairment in compartment syndrome involves the small vessels, in which intracompartmental pressures cause collapse of the thin-walled capillaries. The larger arteries, however, are not affected, because their higher pressure (a usual systolic arterial pressure of approximately 120 mm Hg) is usually far greater than the pressure of the muscle that is afflicted with compartment syndrome (usually 30 to 60 mm Hg). Because the blood flow of these larger arteries is not usually impeded, distal arterial pulses should remain intact (23,25). It may still be difficult to clinically palpate these intact pulses, because there may be soft tissue swelling or edema that often accompanies injuries that are associated with compartment syndrome. Doppler examination is helpful in these situations and can demonstrate intact pulses in the presence of severe soft tissue swelling. Color, temperature, capillary refill, and turgor of the digits may appear normal, because major arterial flow to the limb is preserved. If there is true loss of pulses in a cool, blanched extremity without capillary refill, arterial injury or occlusion should be expected.

As an aid to diagnosis of compartment syndrome, Hargens and Mubarak (8,25) have emphasized the six Ps that are characteristic of acute compartment syndrome: high *p*ressure, *p*ain (especially with passive stretch), *p*aresthesias, *p*aresis, *p*ink skin color, and *p*ulse (distal pulse present).

Intracompartmental Tissue Fluid Pressure Measurement

Although the diagnosis of compartment syndrome is made clinically, confirmation is aided with measurement of intracompartmental tissue fluid pressure. Intracompartmental pressure can be measured by using the infusion technique, which was developed by Whitesides et al. (35–38); the wick or slit catheter technique, which was developed by Mubarak and Hargens (7,21,23,25,118,123,125); or the continuous monitoring infusion technique, which was developed by Matsen et al. (11,13,15–19) (Fig. 9). More recently, easy-to-use hand-held transducers have become available. These have a needlelike probe that is inserted into the muscle. The unit digitally displays the intramuscular pressure (Stryker Intracompartment Pressure System, Stryker Corporation, Kalamazoo, MI) (8). In addition, electronic catheter systems have become available with transducer-tipped catheters that provide accurate dynamic response to changes in intramuscular pressure without artifacts from saline columns (8,354). Although the more recent devices are becoming easier to use and are potentially more reliable, it should be emphasized that these devices are not infallible and have potential measurement error. The clinical findings and impressions should outweigh specific measured compartment pressure values in making the diagnosis and proceeding with treatment.

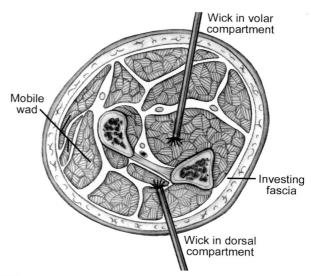

FIGURE 9. Cross section of the proximal forearm that demonstrates placement of wick catheters.

From these different methods of pressure measurement, the threshold pressure that is considered indicative of a diagnosis of compartment syndrome (and further supporting treatment indications) has varied from 45 mm Hg, as proposed by Matsen, to 20 mm Hg below diastolic, as proposed by Whitesides (11,13,15–19,35–38). Based on the animal studies (showing sustained pressures of 30 mm Hg and causing irreversible muscle and nerve damage), Mubarak and Hargens believe that clinical findings, along with compartment pressures of 30 mm Hg or greater, are indicative of compartment syndrome (7,21,23,25,118,123,125). This pressure value has since become an accepted pressure threshold for the diagnosis and the indicated fasciotomy in the presence of clinical findings. These authors, as well as Heppenstall, Whitesides, Matsen, Gelberman, and Szabo, have also emphasized the importance of the difference between systemic mean arterial pressure and compartment pressure. Systemic blood pressure has an effect on extremity perfusion; therefore, a lower threshold for fasciotomy should be considered in the hypotensive patient (8,15,37,178,214,355).

Roentgenographs

Standard roentgenographs are indicated in the edematous injured extremity to assess possible fractures, dislocations, or foreign bodies.

Magnetic Resonance Imaging, Computed Tomography, and Ultrasound

Magnetic resonance imaging, computed polytomography, and ultrasound have been shown to be able to help delineate areas of edema or muscle necrosis and have been investigated as methods to evaluate compartment syndrome

(202,356–359). However, their routine use for the diagnosis of acute compartment syndrome is not indicated, and treatment should not be delayed to obtain these studies.

Arteriography and Doppler Flowmetry

Arteriography and Doppler flowmetry have value in demonstrating the patentcy of associated arteries. However, these studies are not of value in the evaluation of increased muscular pressures. Matsen and Rorabeck (18) and Rowland (158) have emphasized that, in the presence of arterial damage with prolonged periods of ischemia, fasciotomy should be performed immediately, and arteriography should be performed while the patient is on the operating table to allow vascular repair to be carried out, if needed. Arteriography that is performed before the patient is taken to the operating room may excessively delay surgical decompression (18,158).

Pulse Oximetry

Pulse oximetry has been investigated as a potential method of evaluating increased tissue fluid pressure in compartment syndrome. However, findings show it currently not to be of use as an aid in compartment syndrome evaluation (158,360,361).

Delay in Diagnosis

Delay in diagnosis is more likely to occur in the patient with multiple trauma, burns, or concomitant central or peripheral nerve dysfunction or in those with communication problems (Table 3). Patients with cognitive deficits from traumatic brain injury or drug and alcohol intoxication are difficult to assess, especially when they are unresponsive and uncooperative or show no appreciable pain. The diagnosis is based on the clinical findings of a palpable

TABLE 3. PATIENTS IN WHOM DIAGNOSIS OF COMPARTMENT SYNDROME IS OBSCURE

Central nervous system injury patients
  Traumatic brain injury
  Cerebrovascular accident
  Spinal cord injury
Multiple trauma patient
Severe burn patient
Patients who are under general or regional anesthesia for operative procedures
Patients who are under sedation
Critically ill patients
Drug-overdosed patient
Alcohol intoxication
Mentally ill or disabled patients
Infants and young children

Adapted from Ouellette EA. Compartment syndromes in obtunded patients. *Hand Clin* 1998;14:431–450.

tense compartment, which is verified with direct measurement of the compartment pressure. Even in an obtunded patient, there may be signs of pain with passive stretch if the patient is carefully evaluated. These signs include a transient increase in heart rate or blood pressure or the patient's facial wincing or withdrawing of the extremity during passive stretch test (178).

The diagnosis can also be delayed and more difficult to establish when spinal cord or peripheral nerve injuries coexist. Motor and sensory deficits may incorrectly be attributed solely to these more proximal injuries, or, conversely, the compartment syndrome diagnosis may be overlooked if the patient shows little or no pain because of these more proximal nerve injuries. A high index of suspicion is necessary in these groups of patients to make a timely diagnosis of acute compartment syndrome. As noted previously, the diagnosis is made based on the clinical findings of a palpable tense compartment and is verified with direct measurement of the compartment pressure.

Differential Diagnosis

Differential diagnosis of forearm compartment syndrome includes arterial injuries and peripheral or central nervous system injury (25,26) (Table 4). Clinically, all of these conditions may have pain and motor or sensory deficits, and they often coexist in the multiple trauma patient. With arterial occlusion or injury, pulses are diminished or absent but should be intact in compartment syndrome or nerve injuries. Passive muscle stretch induces pain in compartment syndrome and arterial occlusion but should not cause discomfort in isolated nerve injuries. With nerve injuries, relatively little pain and minimal edema exist, and the diagnosis may be assisted by exclusion of the other conditions. Doppler evaluation, arteriography, and compartment tissue fluid pressure measurements are helpful when several of these conditions exist concomitantly.

In the presence of obvious arterial damage with prolonged periods of ischemia, arterial exploration and repair

TABLE 4. DIFFERENTIAL DIAGNOSIS OF COMPARTMENT SYNDROME, ARTERIAL INJURY, AND NERVE INJURY, BASED ON THE FIVE PS

	Compartment syndrome	Arterial injury	Nerve injury
Pressure in compartment	+	−	−
Pain with stretch	+	+	−
Paresthesia or anesthesia	+	+	+
Paresis or paralysis	+	+	+
Pulses intact	+	−	+

Adapted from Hargens AR, Mubarak SJ. Current concepts in the pathophysiology, evaluation, and diagnosis of compartment syndrome. *Hand Clin* 1998;14:371–383; and Mubarak SJ. Treatment of acute compartment syndromes. In: Willy C, Sterk J, Gerngrofs H, eds. *Das Kompartment-Syndrom.* Berlin: Springer-Verlag, 1998:128.

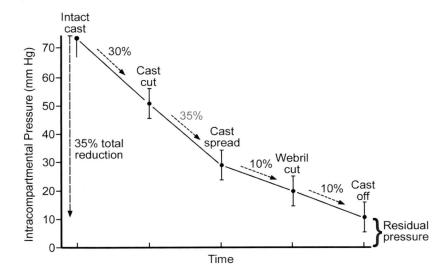

FIGURE 10. Graph that demonstrates reduction of intracompartmental pressure of a casted canine limb with sequential cast cutting, cast spreading, Webril cutting, and complete cast removal.

and prophylactic fasciotomy should be performed emergently. If needed, an arteriogram is obtained while the patient is on the operating table, and vascular repair is carried out as indicated. As emphasized previously, arteriography that is performed in a radiology suite before the patient is taken to the operating room may excessively delay operative management.

Treatment of Acute Compartment Syndrome: General Principles

The management goals of acute compartment syndrome are to restore microcirculation to muscle and nerve and therefore to minimize permanent injury to avoid the sequelae of ischemic contracture. Initial treatment of *impending* compartment syndrome may be nonoperative. Management of *established* compartment syndrome is operative decompression of muscle compartments by fasciotomy. The following discussion addresses principles of nonoperative and operative management. Management, including operative technique, of specific compartment syndromes is then discussed.

Nonoperative Management

In the patient who presents with a tight-fitting cast or occlusive dressing with increased pain or neuritic and vascular symptoms, the patient should initially undergo loosening or removal of the dressing. Splitting of a cast or removal of any occlusive splints is the initial treatment of impending compartment syndrome. If symptoms remain after cast splitting, then cutting or complete removal of cast padding and dressing material is undertaken. Dressings and cast padding can contribute to volume containment and increased intracompartmental pressure (Fig. 10) (176). If symptoms persist, fasciotomy is indicated.

Acute median neuropathy that develops after closed reduction of distal radius fractures can occur, especially if the wrist is immobilized in marked flexion (180,314, 362,363). Intracarpal interstitial fluid pressures have been shown to increase by a mean of 9 mm Hg and 29 mm Hg when the wrist has been placed in 20 degrees and 40 degrees of flexion, respectively, from a neutral position. In addition, intracarpal pressure has increased by 17 mm Hg when the wrist was positioned from neutral to 20 degrees of extension (147). Therefore, a symptomatic patient who wears a cast with the wrist placed in a position of marked flexion or extension should undergo cast splitting followed by repositioning, as necessary. If accentuated wrist flexion is required to maintain fracture reduction, alternative methods of immobilization or operative stabilization should be considered (314).

Repositioning of the elbow, especially with a supracondylar fracture, may also influence the course of impending compartment syndrome. If an elbow was immobilized in flexion greater than 90 degrees, gentle extension of the forearm may help relieve pain and reverse early symptoms (24–26).

In the patient who presents with borderline clinical findings of compartment syndrome or in whom increasing pressures appear likely to develop, the patient may be monitored closely with serial examinations and continuous intracompartmental pressure evaluation by using an indwelling catheter. If the diagnosis remains borderline or unclear, it is usually preferable to proceed with operative decompression rather than to delay treatment. The sequela of untreated or delayed compartment syndrome is so debilitating that fasciotomy in these borderline situations is usually indicated.

There is no indication for the use of elevation or ice in established compartment syndrome. Sympathetic blocks are not effective to increase perfusion, because maximal local vasodilation is already present (50,158).

Hyperbaric oxygen has been used experimentally to treat impending compartment syndrome (251,364–366). Findings suggest that muscle necrosis and edema are reduced after

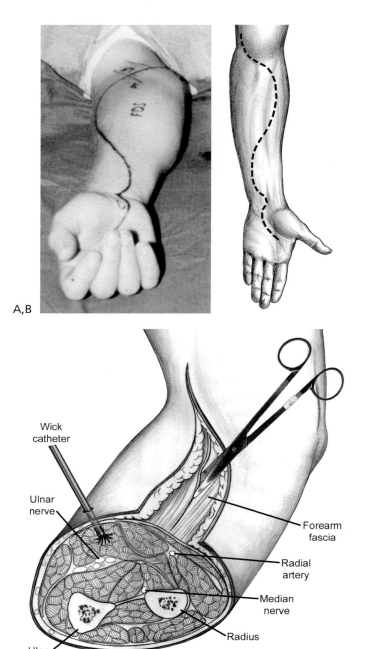

A,B

C

FIGURE 11. A: Photograph of an upper extremity with compartment syndrome. Note the swelling and the tense appearance of the flexor compartments of the forearm. The incision is marked in preparation for fasciotomy. Additional clinical findings in this patient included severe forearm pain; sensibility deficits in the thumb, index, and long fingers; and weakness of digital and thumb flexion. Forearm pain was accentuated with passive extension of the digits. **B:** Illustration, as described by Gelberman, that depicts the incision that is used for flexor compartment release and median nerve decompression. The incision is extended distally for carpal tunnel release. **C:** Cross section of left forearm, with the wick catheter placed and the fasciotomy incision illustrated.

immediate treatments. However, these studies are experimental and preliminary. Further studies are necessary to establish the indications or role of hyperbaric oxygen in the management of acute compartment syndrome (365,366). Fasciotomy should not be delayed to administer a trial of hyperbaric oxygen.

Operative Management

If symptoms do not resolve quickly with nonoperative treatment, fasciotomy is indicated (Fig. 11) (3,5,22,23,29,35,37, 49,51,52,158,331,343,367–371). Operative procedures are performed on an urgent basis without delay. If a patient has recently eaten, regional anesthesia, such as axillary block, should be performed to avoid the time delay that is usually required for general anesthesia. It has been shown that, in more than 90% of patients with compartment syndrome, a treatment delay of more than 12 hours led to irreversible soft tissue and nerve damage (371,372).

Fasciotomy is also indicated at the time of limb revascularization if ischemia time has been 4 to 6 hours. The postrevascularization edema may precipitate compartment syndrome; thus, fasciotomy is indicated as prophylaxis (4,107,300,301,373).

Compartment pressure is decompressed by incision of the enclosed fascial sheath. Intracompartmental microcirculation is hopefully restored. Release of constricting skin may also be indicated to fully decompress the compartment. Coexisting fractures, such as supracondylar elbow fractures, both-bone forearm fractures, and distal radius fractures, are usually stabilized operatively as indicated at the time of fasciotomy. Skin incisions are left open in anticipation of further swelling. In open fractures, fasciotomy is performed, wounds are débrided, and fractures are stabilized. In contaminated wounds, external fixation or limited internal fixation may be preferable to standard internal fixation methods. Secondary closure or skin grafting is performed when wounds permit, usually in 5 to 10 days.

Pre- and postoperative urine myoglobin should be monitored in patients with severe long-standing compartment syndrome or when multiple compartments are involved. Muscle ischemia of 4 hours can give rise to myoglobinuria, which can reach its maximum 3 hours after circulation is restored (25,197,224,226,326,328,329,331,336,374–377). Significant myoglobinuria produces renal failure. If myoglobinuria is suspected, medical consultation is obtained, adequate hydration is maintained for a high urinary output, and attempts are made to keep the urine alkalinized. Myoglobinuria renal failure most commonly occurs after the prolonged compartment syndrome in a drug-overdosed patient or from multiple compartment involvement in crush victims. Serum creatine phosphokinase (CPK) and lactate dehydrogenase can also be elevated.

Patients with compartment syndrome due to snake bites also require medical therapy in addition to compartment decompression. Medical therapy includes intravenous fluid replacement, antivenin administration (after skin test for sensitivity to horse serum), antibiotics, and tetanus prophylaxis (188,291,292,295,296,298,344).

SPECIFIC COMPARTMENT SYNDROMES: DIAGNOSIS AND OPERATIVE MANAGEMENT

Acute Compartment Syndrome of the Shoulder

Compartment syndrome that involves the shoulder is relatively rare, especially when compared to the frequency of compartment syndrome of the forearm (5,130,378). Drug-overdose limb compression or patients who have crush syndrome, or both, are often the causes (5). Intramuscular pressures of the deltoid have been noted to be as high as 80 mm Hg (197).

The shoulder compartment consists of the three heads of the deltoid muscle. Symptoms of shoulder compartment syndrome include deltoid pain, local tenderness, and a tense swollen muscle compartment. There is usually pain with active shoulder abduction or passive adduction. Hypoesthesia over the lateral aspect of the shoulder is consistent with associated compression of the upper lateral brachial cutaneous nerve (cutaneous branch of the axillary nerve), which travels within the compartment (129). Differential diagnosis includes trauma (proximal humerus fracture or dislocation) and infection, especially those conditions that are associated with induration that is secondary to a necrotizing process or abscess in a drug-abuse patient.

Decompression of the deltoid compartment can usually be performed with a single incision that starts over the anterior deltoid, curves superiorly and laterally, lateral to the acromion, and continues posteriorly to reach the posterior deltoid. All three heads of the deltoid can be decompressed with this approach.

Operative Technique: Fasciotomy of the Shoulder (Deltoid) Compartment

In fasciotomy of the shoulder compartment, an incision is placed on the anterior aspect of the deltoid muscle to decompress the anterior deltoid (5,129,197). The incision then curves superiorly and laterally, lateral to the acromion, to course over the lateral deltoid. The incision continues posteriorly to reach the posterior deltoid. Care is taken to avoid injury to the upper lateral brachial cutaneous nerve (the cutaneous branch of the axillary nerve), which becomes subcutaneous from the posterolateral aspect of the deltoid and courses anteriorly with multiple small branches to reach the skin over the lateral shoulder. Overlying the deltoid muscle, the epimysium and fascia may not be separable. Therefore, once the deltoid fascia is exposed,

multiple epimysial-fascial incisions are placed to fully decompress the muscle (197). In addition, because the deltoid is a multipennate muscle that is divided by multiple septae, adequate exposure is necessary to incise the septae as needed. Tissue pressure measurement after fasciotomy is especially valuable to verify adequate decompression of the deltoid (5). The anterior and posterior portions of the incision can be extended distally for additional exposure to decompress coexisting compartment syndrome of the anterior or posterior arm, respectively. The skin is left open to prevent further compression by tight skin closure. A bulky, well-padded shoulder dressing is applied. (However, motion is started in a therapy program as soon as the patient's comfort permits, usually within the first 7 to 10 days or when skin coverage and closure are accomplished.)

Postoperative Care

After fasciotomy, the shoulder is protected in a bulky dressing to protect the open incision. Elevation of the shoulder by raising the head of the bed helps decrease edema. The shoulder is protected initially in a sling or immobilizer while the muscle recovers. Therapy is initiated as soon as the patient's comfort permits. Active and passive mobilization of the shoulder can be started while the bulky dressing is still in place. The elbow, wrist, and digits are also actively mobilized early, because dependent edema with secondary stiffness of these areas may occur if neglected. Wounds are checked in the operating room after approximately 5 days, and the wound is closed if edema resolution and skin relaxation permit. Application of gentle skin traction techniques by using Steri-Strips (3M, St. Paul, MN), vessel loops, or skin traction devices can assist skin relaxation. If the skin cannot be closed secondarily over several days, the open areas can be covered with split-thickness skin grafts. Therapy to maximize motion and strength is continued in the postoperative period until functional level has maximized.

Acute Compartment Syndrome of the Arm

Compartment syndrome that involves the arm above the elbow is relatively rare, especially when compared to the frequency of compartment syndrome of the forearm (5,130,378).

A common cause or initiating event that leads to compartment syndrome of the arm is prolonged exposure of the upper limb to body weight against a solid object or floor (in obtunded patients) (328,329,378). Additionally, patients with compartment syndrome of the arm have been victims of the crush syndrome (5). Other reported causes of compartment syndrome that is specific to the arm have included isolated case reports that are associated with blunt trauma (194,238,379), fracture of the humerus shaft and of the distal humerus (234), rupture of the triceps (223), rupture of the long head of the biceps (242), transfer of the latissimus dorsi for brachial plexus palsy (380), compression by pneumatic tourniquet (147,210), bleeding disorders (266,277,284), vascular injury after transaxillary arteriography (310), and accidental intramural injection of local anesthetic during axillary block anesthesia (which leads to occlusion of the axillary artery) (267).

There are two muscle compartments of the arm: the anterior compartment, which contains the brachialis, the biceps, and the coracobrachialis, and the posterior compartment, which contains the triceps (see the section Anatomic Compartments of the Upper Extremity). It has been postulated that, because the fascia of the arm is thinner, it cannot by itself limit swelling and is therefore more accommodating to increased intracompartmental volume that is caused by hemorrhage or tissue edema (130,381). Because of the thin fascia, the skin may be the only limiting boundary to swelling in the arm. This is seen relatively commonly in patients with circumferential burns, in whom pressure from the rigid skin can lead to a compartment syndrome in the entire extremity (293). In addition to the fascia being relatively thin, the fascia is pierced obliquely by several subcutaneous veins that drain the upper limb. Once the compartmental pressure rises to a level that occludes these subcutaneous veins, a further increase in compartmental pressure is felt to be unlikely (242). The muscle compartments of the arm communicate with those of the shoulder girdle, making it less likely for swelling or bleeding in this area to develop into a compartment syndrome (223).

The clinical signs of compartment syndrome of the arm are usually not as obvious, or as quick to appear, as in compartment syndrome of the forearm (130). Besides the usual findings of swollen, tense compartments, pain out of proportion to the associated injury, and sensibility changes and weakness, a specific finding that is unique to the arm includes severe pain in the arm with passive flexion or extension of the elbow or shoulder in a patient without fracture. Because several nerves pass through the arm compartments, acute compartment syndrome of the arm can present with clinical signs that are related to dysfunction of the musculocutaneous, radial, ulnar, or median nerves (128–130).

Operative decompression of the two compartments of the arm is usually performed through two separate incisions (5,130). When two incisions are used, the anterior compartment is decompressed through a single medial incision, and the posterior compartment is decompressed through a single posterolateral incision. The posterior compartment can also be decompressed through a straight posterior incision (5,130,284).

Alternatively, a single medial incision along the medial intermuscular septum can be used to decompress both compartments (130,210). An advantage of the single-incision technique is that secondary closure can usually be accomplished without the need for skin grafts.

The two-incision technique allows a more extensive decompression and provides more flexibility for individual muscle and nerve inspection or exploration. It may also be more adaptable for fixation of concomitant fractures. Tourniquets are not used, to avoid pressure on the ischemic muscle, and, because of the proximal exposure that is needed, a tourniquet is not feasible.

Operative Technique: Fasciotomy of the Anterior Compartment of the Arm through a Medial Incision (Author's Preferred Technique, as Part of a Two-Incision Technique)

In fasciotomy of the anterior compartment, an incision is placed on the medial aspect of the arm. It starts just medial to the lateral bicipital sulcus (to avoid the cephalic vein) (5,130,284). The incision extends proximally toward the acromion. The subcutaneous tissue is incised to expose the deep brachial fascia. Care is taken to avoid injury to several neurovascular structures with this medial approach, including the medial antebrachial cutaneous nerve and the basilic vein, both of which are superficial to the fascia. The fascia of the anterior compartment of the arm is then incised. The brachial artery and median nerve lie deep to the fascia in this vicinity, and care is taken to avoid injury. In the more proximal aspect of the incision, the musculocutaneous nerve lies anterolateral to the median nerve before the nerve enters the deep surface of the biceps muscle. Also in this area, the medial brachial cutaneous nerve lies in the subcutaneous tissue, superficial to the fascia. The ulnar nerve is also protected in the proximal portion of the incision, where it lies posterior to the brachial artery. In the distal one-half of the arm, the ulnar nerve crosses the intermuscular septum to lie in the subcutaneous tissue of the posterior compartment before it enters the cubital tunnel. This approach allows exploration of these neurovascular structures as needed but also places them at risk for injury during fasciotomy. The incision is extended to the vicinity of the acromion, and the deltoid fascia is incised if indicated (378).

Operative Technique: Fasciotomy of the Posterior Compartment of the Arm through a Posterolateral Incision (Author's Preferred Technique, as Part of a Two-Incision Technique)

In fasciotomy of the posterior compartment, an incision is placed on the posterolateral aspect of the arm (130,378). It starts distally near the tip of the olecranon and extends along the lateral side of the triceps compartment. The subcutaneous tissue is incised to expose the deep brachial fascia. The fascia of the posterior compartment of the arm is then incised. In general, this is a relatively safe operative approach. There may be small branches of the posterior brachial cutaneous nerve that are present in the subcutaneous tissue that provide sensibility to the posterior arm. There may also be, in the most distal aspect of the incision, branches of the medial antebrachial cutaneous nerve. These small branches, if visualized, should be protected.

Operative Technique: Fasciotomy of the Posterior Compartment of the Arm through a Posterior Approach (Author's Preferred Technique when Only the Posterior Compartment Is Involved)

In the posterior approach to fasciotomy of the posterior compartment, an incision is placed on the posterior aspect of the arm (130,284). The incision commences distally near the tip of the olecranon and extends proximally to the proximal arm. With the arm internally rotated, the incision can be extended proximally to reach the posterior fascia of the deltoid. The subcutaneous tissue is incised to expose the deep brachial fascia. The fascia of the posterior compartment is then incised. As with the posterolateral incision approach that was described previously, there may be small branches of the posterior brachial cutaneous nerve present in the subcutaneous tissue that provide sensibility to the posterior arm. There may also be, in the most distal aspect of the incision, branches of the medial antebrachial cutaneous nerve. These small branches, if visualized, should be protected.

If internal fixation of the humerus is desired, the humerus can be exposed through a triceps splitting approach. The radial nerve is identified and protected. This approach allows access to the middle two-thirds of the humeral shaft (127).

Operative Technique: Fasciotomy of the Anterior and Posterior Compartments of the Arm through a Single Incision

In fasciotomy of the anterior and posterior compartments through a single incision, the incision is placed along the medial intermuscular septum, commencing near the elbow and extending to the axilla (130). The subcutaneous tissues are incised to expose the deep brachial fascia. The medial intermuscular septum is then identified, and the fascia is exposed anteriorly and posteriorly to the septum. The fascia of the anterior and posterior compartments of the arm is then incised. As noted previously in the description of the fasciotomy of the anterior compartment through a medial approach, there are multiple neurovascular structures that are at risk in this area. These include the basilic vein (superficial to the fascia) and the brachial artery (deep to the fascial), the median and ulnar nerves (both subfascial), the musculocutaneous nerve (proximally), and the medial antebrachial and medial brachial cutaneous nerves (both within the subcutaneous tissue).

In all methods of fasciotomy of the arm, a bulky, well-padded long arm dressing is applied. Plaster splints are incorporated to immobilize the elbow initially while the muscle recovers. (However, motion is started in a therapy program as soon as the patient's comfort permits, usually within the first 7 to 10 days or when skin coverage and closure are accomplished.)

Postoperative Care: Fasciotomy of the Arm

After fasciotomy, the extremity is elevated in the bulky dressing to promote edema reduction. Wounds are checked in 3 to 5 days in the operating room, and the proximal and distal few centimeters of the wound are closed as skin relaxation permits. Application of gentle skin traction techniques using Steri-Strips, vessel loops, or skin traction devices can assist skin relaxation. When edema resolves, the skin is eventually closed secondarily or is covered with split-thickness skin grafts. Complete coverage is usually accomplished within 10 days. If initial wounds are contaminated, repeat débridements are carried out in the operating room as indicated and eventually are closed secondarily, skin grafted, or allowed to heal by secondary intention.

Therapy is initiated as soon as the patient's comfort permits. Active and passive mobilization of the digits can be started while the bulky dressing is still in place. The elbow and shoulder are also mobilized as soon as patient comfort permits or immediately after skin coverage and closure. Therapy to maximize motion and strength is continued in the postoperative period until functional level has maximized.

A special note is mentioned regarding the digits. With operative procedures that are located more proximally on the shoulder, arm, or forearm, the dependent position and lack of use of the digits may result in edema and secondary stiffness of the hand. The digits should not be neglected, and therapy for mobilization and edema control of the hand should be initiated early in the postoperative period.

Acute Compartment Syndrome of the Forearm

The forearm is the most common upper extremity location that is involved in compartment syndrome (1,4,5,8,69,70, 368,382). The volar compartment is more commonly involved than the dorsal compartment, but involvement of both is common. The mobile wad is usually involved when the volar and dorsal compartments are afflicted. The causes of compartment syndrome of the forearm are numerous and were outlined previously (207).

Compartment syndrome of the forearm presents with swollen tense compartments, pain that is out of proportion to the associated injury, and, eventually, sensibility changes (paresthesias followed by numbness) and weakness (mild paresis to paralysis).

In volar forearm compartment syndrome, weakness is manifested by the loss of digital, thumb, and wrist flexion. There is usually pain with passive extension of the digits. Pulses should be preserved, but they are often difficult to detect (without Doppler) because of associated edema. The digits are held in a position of flexion, especially when passive digital extension is found to cause pain. Compromise of the median nerve is usually seen before ulnar nerve involvement, possibly due to its relatively deeper course in the forearm or its proximity to the deep muscles, which are most likely to be ischemic. The deeply situated flexor muscles are usually the most severely afflicted. Due to their deep location (which increases their vulnerability to high interstitial pressures and ischemia) and their proximity to the rigid bone structures and the firm interosseous ligament, the flexor digitorum profundus (especially to the ring and long fingers) and the flexor pollicis longus are usually the most severely affected, followed by the flexor digitorum superficialis and pronator teres, and, lastly, the wrist flexors (1,5,44,69,70,128).

In dorsal forearm compartment syndrome, weakness is manifested by the loss of digital, thumb, and wrist extension. Passive digital and wrist flexion may increase the pain. The hand may assume a posture of digital and wrist extension to avoid stretch of these involved muscles. Sensory deficits of the hand may be minimal, because the ulnar nerve and the proximal radial nerve pass through the volar compartment. In addition, the superficial branch of the radial nerve has a relatively superficial course, which may help minimize its compression (128).

In compartment syndrome of the mobile wad, clinical manifestations unique to this compartment include weakness and pain on resisted flexion of the elbow with the forearm in mid-rotation, which are caused by involvement of the brachioradialis. There are also weakness of the radial wrist extensors and pain with passive stretch by flexion of the wrist (128).

The technique of forearm fasciotomy was described and popularized by Gelberman et al. (4,5). Operative decompression of the volar compartment of the forearm and of the mobile wad compartment is released through a single volar incision that extends from the distal arm to the distal end of the carpal tunnel (Fig. 11) (1,4,5,44). Compartment syndromes that involve the forearm extensor (posterior) compartment are released through a dorsal incision. When the volar and dorsal compartments are involved, it is preferable to release the volar compartment first, as the relaxation that is afforded by the skin and fascia possibly decompresses the dorsal compartment as well. Clinical evaluation and intraoperative compartmental pressure measurements can be used to determine whether the dorsal compartment requires decompression as well. Tourniquets are not routinely used during fasciotomy because of preexisting muscle and nerve ischemia. Tissue pressure measurement capability should be available intraoperatively.

The intrinsic muscles of the hand and the carpal tunnel are also evaluated and released separately as indicated, by using several separate incisions for complete release (see the following discussion for more detail). Compartment syndromes above the elbow are released, as indicated, by using one incision for the anterior brachium, one for the posterior brachium, and one for the deltoid compartment (see the previous discussion) (4,5,130).

Operative Technique: Fasciotomy of the Volar Forearm and Mobile Wad

In fasciotomy of the volar forearm and mobile wad, the volar incision originates on the medial aspect of the arm 2 cm proximal to the medial epicondyle (Fig. 11) (1,4,5,44). The incision is extended obliquely across the antecubital fossa to reach the volar aspect of the mobile wad. The incision is continued distally, curving slightly ulnarly, and reaching the midline at the junction of the middle and distal two-thirds of the forearm. Continuing distally in the volar forearm, the incision is extended just ulnar to the palmaris longus tendon to avoid injury to the palmar cutaneous branch of the median nerve. The incision crosses the wrist crease at an angle and extends into the mid-palm for carpal tunnel release. It is carried no further radially than the mid-axis of the ring finger. The subcutaneous tissues are incised to expose the deep fascia. The fascia is incised, and the muscles mobilized to ensure decompression. Clinical examination and intraoperative pressure measurements are repeated to verify adequate decompression.

The median nerve is at risk for compression in four anatomic regions and requires sequential decompression at each of these sites. These include, from proximal to distal, the lacertus fibrosus, the pronator teres, the proximal arch and deep fascial surface of the flexor digitorum superficialis, and the carpal tunnel (135,222,383). The nerve is identified in the proximal portion of the incision and is traced distally to the lacertus fibrosus. The lacertus fibrosus, a fascial extension of the biceps tendon, lies anterior to the median nerve at the elbow. The lacertus fibrosus is incised longitudinally along the course of the median nerve to allow complete decompression and exposure of the nerve. The nerve is then explored to the proximal edge of the pronator teres to ensure that there are no areas of constriction between the humeral and ulnar heads of the muscle. The pronator teres is myotomized, as needed, to ensure nerve decompression. The median nerve continues distally deep to the proximal edge of the flexor digitorum superficialis and extends within the fascia of its deep surface. The muscle is mobilized to allow visualization of the nerve, and the fascia is released as needed. Division of the transverse carpal ligament is then carried out. Median nerve decompression is therefore ensured from the distal arm to the mid-palm.

If preoperative findings indicate ulnar nerve compression in the arm or forearm, the nerve is explored as well. Nerve compression often occurs at the elbow within the cubital tunnel or in the interval between the humeral and ulnar heads of the flexor carpi ulnaris or proximal to the elbow, where it continues deep to the arcade of Struthers and pierces the medial intermuscular septum of the arm. The subcutaneous tissues are mobilized to permit exploration and decompression of the ulnar nerve along its course through the cubital tunnel. The arcade of Struthers and the edge of the medial intermuscular septum (between the flexor and extensor compartments of the arm) are released in the proximal portion of the wound. The nerve is explored distally as it passes between the ulnar and humeral heads of the flexor carpi ulnaris, and the muscle or epimysial edges are myotomized as needed. All tight fibrous bands are released, preserving the vincula leashes that contain segmental blood supply to the nerve. Addition procedures, such as anterior nerve transposition or epicondylectomy, are performed if the nerve appears edematous or is under tension along its bed in the cubital tunnel. If severe hand edema or intrinsic compartment syndrome of the hand, or both, exist, decompression of the ulnar nerve in the wrist through Guyon's canal or in the palm may be indicated.

If radial nerve dysfunction exists preoperatively, decompression of the radial nerve within the radial tunnel may be indicated. Potential sites of compression of the radial nerve in the forearm include the fibrous bands that lie anterior to the radial head at the entrance to the radial tunnel, the fan-shaped leash of vessels (the leash of Henry, or the radial recurrent vessels that cross the radial nerve to supply the brachioradialis and extensor carpi radialis longus muscles), the tendinous margin of the extensor carpi radialis brevis, the arcade of Frohse (which forms the oval ligamentous band over the deep branch of the radial nerve as it enters the supinator muscle), and the superficial head of the supinator muscle and associated facial bands. The volar incision may be used to expose the proximal portion of the radial tunnel, curving the proximal portion of the incision more laterally over the mobile wad to expose the radial nerve. The dorsal incision can be used to reach the more distal portion of the radial nerve (i.e., within the supinator) for complete exposure and decompression.

The skin is loosely approximated to cover exposed areas of the median nerve (and ulnar and radial nerves). This includes closure of the skin over the carpal tunnel. The remaining portions of the wounds are packed open, and a bulky, compressive, long arm hand dressing with plaster splints is applied. Secondary wound closure or skin grafts are performed when edema has subsided, usually in 5 to 10 days.

Operative Technique: Fasciotomy of the Dorsal Forearm

If extensor and flexor compartment syndromes coexist, the dorsal compartment is reexamined, and pressures are remeasured after volar forearm decompression (1,4,5,44). If the dorsal compartment remains clinically edematous or

firm, or if pressures exceed 30 mm Hg, dorsal fasciotomy is carried out. A straight longitudinal incision is used. It begins 2 cm lateral to and 2 cm distal to the lateral epicondyle and is extended distally toward the midline of the wrist for 7 to 10 cm. Skin edges are mobilized, and the dorsal fascia is incised directly in line with the skin incision. Clinical examination and intraoperative pressure measurements are repeated to verify adequate decompression.

Wounds are packed open, and a bulky, compressive, long arm hand dressing with plaster splints is applied. Secondarily, wound closure or skin grafts are performed when edema has subsided, usually in 5 to 10 days.

Postoperative Care: Forearm Fasciotomy

After fasciotomy, the extremity is elevated in the bulky dressing to promote edema reduction. Wounds are checked in 3 to 5 days in the operating room, and the proximal and distal few centimeters of the wound are closed as skin relaxation permits. Application of gentle skin traction techniques using Steri-Strips, vessel loops, or skin traction devices can assist skin relaxation. When edema resolves, the skin is eventually closed secondarily or is covered with split-thickness skin grafts. Complete coverage is usually accomplished within 10 days. If initial wounds are contaminated, repeat débridements are carried out in the operating room, as indicated, and, eventually, the wounds are closed secondarily, skin grafted, or allowed to heal by secondary intention. Commercial skin closure devices are available that may aid in closure (367,384).

Hand therapy is initiated as soon as the patient's comfort permits, usually within the first few days after the fasciotomy. Active and passive mobilization of the digits can be started while the bulky dressing is still in place. Therapy to maximize motion and strength is continued in the postoperative period until functional level has maximized. The shoulder and elbow are mobilized in a comprehensive therapy program to prevent potential secondary stiffness in these areas as well.

Acute Compartment Syndrome of the Wrist

The occurrence of compartment syndrome in the wrist (acute carpal tunnel syndrome), along with that in the hand, is second in frequency only to compartment syndromes of the forearm. As in those of the hand, arm, and shoulder, a compartment syndrome of the wrist is a condition that can more easily go unrecognized and thus requires a higher degree of clinical suspicion and awareness to secure the diagnosis in a timely fashion.

The wrist has essentially one significant compartment, the carpal tunnel. As in the fascial compartments of the digits, the carpal tunnel is not a true muscle compartment. It contains no muscle (normally) and is open at both ends. Physiologically, however, it behaves similarly to a closed

TABLE 5. CAUSES OF ACUTE CARPAL TUNNEL SYNDROME

Trauma
    Fracture of the distal radius (180,220,385,386,388,389)
    Fracture dislocation of metacarpal bases (390)
    Fracture of the scaphoid (244)
    Crush injury (131,180)
    Palmar subluxation of the distal ulna (153)
    Intravenous injections (131)
    Intraarterial injections (178)
    Complications of arterial line use (131)
    Burns (158,178)
    Snake bites (158,178)
    Tendon rupture (153)
    Gunshot wound (131,180)
    Prolonged compression after drug overdose (131)
Coagulopathies and hemorrhagic and vascular disorders
    Hemophilia (275,281)
    Oral anticoagulant therapy (272–274,276)
    Thrombosis (19,308,309)
    Leukemia (280)
    Bleeding from giant cell tumor (394)
    Hemarthrosis from pigmented villonodular synovitis (387)
    Rupture or calcification of persistent median artery (19, 306–309)
    Calcification and enlargement of persistent median artery (306)
Inflammatory disorders
    Acute gout (395)
    Pseudogout (393)
    Hemorrhagic tenosynovitis (284)
Infection
    Granulomatous infections
    Acute abscess
    Pyogenic tenosynovitis
Iatrogenic
    Constrictive dressings and casts (158,178)
    Wrist immobilization in acute flexion (180,220,315)
    Postoperative complications (wrist fracture fixation, arthrodesis) (131,180)

compartment, as it is bounded by synovium proximally and distally (178,180,184,206,385–387). Acute carpal tunnel syndrome can arise from trauma (fractures of the distal radius or carpal fracture dislocations) (228,241,250,314, 315,388–390) or, less commonly, from a variety of infectious (usually granulomatous) (286,391,392) or rheumatologic, hematologic, or anatomic abnormalities (179,180, 306–309,363,393–400) (Table 5).

The carpal tunnel behaves similarly to a closed fascial compartment, and it is well recognized that the median nerve is vulnerable to increases in pressure from chronic or acute causes. In chronic carpal tunnel syndrome, pressures average less than 32 mm Hg. Symptoms are often transitory or vary in a degree that is related to activity, type of day, or effect of management. The symptoms are usually reversible (to some degree) after carpal tunnel release (179,180,386). Gelberman and Szabo (179,180,200, 205,314,362,363,401) have investigated and discussed the threshold tissue fluid pressure for nerve dysfunction in the carpal canal. Although

some functional loss occurred at 40 mm Hg, motor and sensory responses were completely blocked at a threshold tissue fluid pressure of 50 mm Hg. It was suggested that between 40 and 50 mm Hg, there exists a critical pressure threshold at which the peripheral nerve is acutely jeopardized (200,402). It appears that systemic blood pressure also affects the threshold tissue fluid pressure (403). Patients with hypertension (i.e., higher perfusion pressures) may tolerate greater magnitudes of compression pressure, and, more importantly, patients with lower perfusion pressures (i.e., hypotension, shock) may have lower limits of pressure tolerance (403,404).

Compartment syndromes of the forearm and hand can result in increased pressure in the carpal tunnel. Therefore, as noted previously, decompression of the forearm also includes carpal tunnel decompression, as well as critical evaluation and appropriate treatment of the hand compartments. Similarly, it is possible that compartment syndromes that affect the hand compartments may indirectly increase the pressure in the carpal tunnel through the lumbrical canals and the flexor tendon sheaths (178). It is therefore important to assess the status of the carpal tunnel when assessing the compartments of the hand (5,179,362). The urgency of *acute* carpal tunnel syndrome is similar to that of acute compartment syndrome (314,362,402,405,406).

Clinical findings of acute carpal tunnel syndrome are similar to those of carpal tunnel syndrome; however, the signs and symptoms are more usually pronounced, especially pain, and are usually progressive. Usually, as in most compartment syndromes, there is an inciting event. In acute carpal tunnel syndrome, the event is usually trauma (or infection) that involves the distal radius or the carpus or injuries that involve injections, vascular extravasation, or bleeding from coagulopathies. The symptoms may be mild at first and progress into severe pain, loss of sensibility, and weakness of the thenar muscle (and radial lumbricals). Provocative tests, such as Phalen's test or Tinel's sign, are also positive and may be quite painful or difficult to perform (positive Tinel's sign and Phalen's test). The signs and symptoms can progress rapidly to complete median nerve dysfunction.

Acute carpal tunnel syndrome must be distinguished from acute median neuropathy and contusion or acute stretch (which result in a neurapraxia or axonotmesis). The diagnosis can usually be made largely from patient history. If the patient notes immediate nerve dysfunction after blunt trauma, fracture, or other injury to the carpal region, and there is no progression of symptoms, the lesion is likely to be a neurapraxia or axonotmesis. Neurapraxia is especially likely if the patient notes some spontaneous improvement after the initial insult. The neurapraxia (or axonotmesis) should spontaneously recover in time, with the neurapraxia recovering over hours or days, and the axonotmesis recovering over weeks or months. Operative management is usually not indicated in these situations. If the patient notes that sensibility and strength of the hand were initially intact after the injury, and the patient progressively developed numbness or painful paresthesias in the thumb, index, long, and radial ring fingers (as well as thenar weakness), acute carpal tunnel syndrome has likely developed. The gradual increase in pressure of the carpal tunnel after the initial insult has resulted in progressive loss of median nerve dysfunction. If the diagnosis remains in question, or if symptoms and signs are mild or borderline, carpal tunnel measurements can be considered as an adjunct to the clinical diagnosis of acute carpal tunnel syndrome.

The carpal tunnel pressure measurements can be performed by advancement of the needle at a point that is 0.5 cm proximal to the proximal wrist crease, entering at a point that is midway between the tendons of the palmaris longus (if present) and the flexor carpi ulnaris. The needle is advanced distally at a 45-degree angle until it reaches the osseous floor. It is then withdrawn approximately 0.5 cm. Confirmation of the needle tip placement within the flexor compartment can be accomplished by actively or passively flexing and extending the digits and by feeling or observing deflection of the needle tip by action of the passing flexor tendons. This measurement is ideally made with the wrist in neutral flexion and extension to prevent false pressure recordings that are induced by wrist position (178).

A history of progressive nerve dysfunction, with signs and symptoms of carpal tunnel, especially those with increasing pain that is out of proportion to the associated injury, should provide a reliable diagnosis. These clinical findings and the appropriate history should outweigh findings of pressure measurements, because pressure measurement tests are not infallible. If symptoms are minimal, and pressure measurements are not consistent with those of compartment syndrome, the patient can be closely monitored with serial examinations (using quantitative methods, such as monofilament testing for sensibility), and the pressure can be monitored with an indwelling catheter into the carpal canal.

It must be emphasized that, if acute carpal tunnel syndrome is suspected, operative decompression is emergently indicated and should not be delayed. It is the author's opinion that more management errors are made in the undesirable delay of decompression, as compared to those errors of perhaps unwarranted decompression in borderline situations. The morbidity of carpal tunnel release is minimal compared to that of the permanent nerve dysfunction that can result from delay in decompression of acute compartment syndrome.

After the diagnosis of acute carpal tunnel syndrome, initial treatment is removal of any constricting bandages or splitting or removal of tight-fitting casts. If the wrist was placed in acute flexion or extension for positioning after fracture or dislocation reduction, the wrist should be gently placed in a neutral position. If symptoms do not quickly resolve, carpal tunnel release is indicated.

Operative Technique: Decompression of the Carpal Tunnel for Acute Carpal Tunnel Syndrome

Decompression of the carpal tunnel is performed for isolated acute carpal tunnel syndrome or as part of a comprehensive decompression of compartment syndrome of the hand or of the forearm (178). The technique of decompression is performed in a similar manner as it is for carpal tunnel syndrome. However, the incision that is used for acute carpal tunnel syndrome can be extended proximally 4 to 5 cm proximal to the wrist crease in a similar manner to that originally described by Telesnik. This more extensive exposure allows release of the distal portion of the deep antebrachial fascia. The incision is placed somewhat ulnarly in the palm and in the distal forearm to avoid injury to the palmar cutaneous branch of the median nerve, which lies along the ulnar aspect of the flexor carpi radialis tendon (178,180,363,407). With coexisting compartment syndrome of the hand, the incision can be extended a few centimeters distally to ensure decompression of the midpalmar space of the hand (see the section Muscle Compartments and Associated Anatomy). The skin is closed, and a bulky hand dressing is applied, with plaster splints holding the wrist in slight extension.

Postoperative Care: Acute Carpal Tunnel Release

After acute carpal tunnel release, the extremity is elevated in the bulky dressing to promote edema reduction. The wrist is placed in slight extension to position the median nerve away from the healing incision. Marked extension is avoided because it may place additional tension on the median nerve. Splinting is continued for 3 to 4 weeks; however, therapy for gentle wrist and digital mobilization is initiated early in the postoperative period, as soon as the patient's comfort permits. Active and passive mobilization of the digits can be started while the bulky dressing or splint is in place. Therapy to maximize motion and strength is continued in the postoperative period until functional level has maximized.

Acute Compartment Syndrome of the Hand

The occurrence of compartment syndrome in the hand, along with that of the wrist, is second in frequency only to compartment syndromes of the forearm. As in those of the arm and shoulder, compartment syndrome of the hand is a condition that can easily go unrecognized and thus requires a higher degree of clinical suspicion and awareness to secure the diagnosis in a timely fashion. The compartments of the hand are complex (see the section Muscle Compartments and Associated Anatomy), and, in the most detailed descriptions, as many as 10 to 11 separate compartments are described. These include the mid-palm, thenar, hypothenar, adductor, four dorsal interosseous, and three palmar interosseous compartments (178,131,408). The digits, which do not contain true muscle compartments, do have unyielding connective tissue compartments that are bounded by Cleland's and Grayson's ligaments. The digits thus have physiologic compartments that are susceptible to pressure increases. Ortiz and Berger (178) emphasize that it is important that all compartments be appropriately addressed during examination, and, if necessary, a comprehensive fasciotomy of the hand should be performed. Unlike the forearm, the muscle compartments of the hand are isolated and must be released individually to achieve an adequate decompression (158,178,409).

The causes of compartment syndrome are described in detail in the section Causes of Compartment Syndromes. More specific to the compartment syndrome of the hand are crush injuries, multiple fractures, arterial injuries with ischemia, burns, limb compression syndromes, and snake bites (178,207). Compartment syndrome of the hand has also been noted to develop from several iatrogenic causes, including constrictive bandages and casts, intravenous extravasation, and multiple attempts at intravenous or intraarterial injections (especially in those with coagulopathies). Compartment syndrome of the hand can also occur after limb revascularization, due to compartment pressure increases from increased capillary permeability and edema that follows reperfusion of ischemia.

The clinical findings of compartment syndrome of the hand are similar to those of the forearm and arm, with the presence of swollen tense compartments, pain out of proportion to the associated injury, and sensory and motor deficits. In addition, there are clinical manifestations that are more specific to the hand, and the examination is more complex. The diagnosis may not be as obvious and may go unrecognized if the examiner does not have awareness and a high index of suspicion.

As a result of swelling, the hand may rest in a position of intrinsic minus (with extension at the metacarpophalangeal joints and flexion at the proximal interphalangeal joints) (178). Passive stretch of the intrinsic muscles of the hand must be tested, although this may be difficult to discern or examine in the presence of pain from contusion or fractures. Ortiz and Berger (178) have emphasized several prudent aspects of the physical examination of the hand, including the need for assessment of each individual compartment for an impending, early, or limited syndrome. Each of intrinsic muscles can be evaluated by passively abducting and adducting the digits while maintaining the metacarpophalangeal joints in extension and the proximal interphalangeal joints in flexion. The thenar compartment muscles are evaluated separately by passive stretch by maneuvering the thumb into radial abduction. The hypothenar compartment muscles are similarly evaluated by using passive stretch by maneuvering the small finger into extension and adduction. The adductor compartment of the thumb is evaluated by passively maneuvering the thumb into palmar abduction, thereby stretching the adductor pollicis. The carpal tunnel can be specifically evaluated by passive dorsiflexion or palmar flexion of the wrist (similar to Phalen's test

for carpal tunnel syndrome). The passive dorsiflexion and palmar flexion increase the carpal tunnel pressure and possibly aggravate the symptoms or neurologic deficits (178).

As with evaluation of each individual muscle, each potentially involved nerve should also be examined systematically (178). It is imperative to rule out excessive pressures in any compartment through which a nerve passes. At the level of the wrist, the median and ulnar nerves are of concern. Motor and sensory components of these nerves should be evaluated. For the median nerve at the wrist, the evaluation is similar to that of carpal tunnel syndrome. An assessment of thumb palmar abduction strength determines function of the recurrent motor branch of the median nerve (and indirectly evaluates the median nerve). The cutaneous sensibility of the palmar aspects of the thumb, index, and long fingers is evaluated with quantitative methods, such as two-point discrimination or monofilament testing. The ulnar nerve at the wrist is evaluated in a similar manner to assessment of ulnar tunnel syndrome. This includes assessment of the strength of the intrinsic muscles of the digits, the hypothenar muscles, and thumb adduction. Intrinsic function of the fingers is assessed by having the patient actively extend the proximal interphalangeal joints of each finger against resistance while holding the metacarpophalangeal joints in flexion. Individual digital abduction and adduction are also tested. Sensibility evaluation includes cutaneous testing of the palmar and dorsal aspects of the small finger and the ulnar aspect of the ring finger. Because the dorsal branch of the ulnar nerve exits the ulnar nerve trunk proximal to the wrist, the preservation of dorsal sensibility to the small and ulnar ring fingers in the presence of palmar sensibility loss indicates the probable location of compression or dysfunction in Guyon's canal (178).

As noted earlier, arterial pulses should remain intact in the presence of compartment syndrome, because systolic arterial pressure usually far exceeds the intramuscular pressures that are seen in compartment syndrome. However, in injuries of the hand, significant edema and soft tissue swelling may make pulses difficult to palpate. Doppler examination should verify the presence of pulses.

In unconscious or obtunded patients, or in those with spinal or proximal peripheral nerve injury, physical findings (i.e., pain that is exacerbated by passive stretch) are not easy to evaluate. The diagnosis is based on the likelihood of a compartment syndrome, given the clinical findings of a palpable tense compartment, which is verified with direct measurement of the compartment pressure. As noted by Ortiz and Berger (178), even in an obtunded patient, there may be signs of pain with passive stretch if the patient is carefully evaluated. These signs include a transient increase in heart rate or blood pressure or the patient's wince or withdrawal of the extremity during test.

Evaluation of intramuscular tissue fluid pressures is performed as an adjuvant to the clinical examination in the diagnosis of compartment syndrome. To completely evaluate compartment syndrome of the hand, it would be necessary to assess each of the 11 compartments of the hand (178). Clinical judgment is usually sufficient to identify the compartments that are at the most risk or those that are suspected of compartment syndrome, and measurements are directed accordingly. Measurements in the hand are usually made by placement of the measurement needle directly into the suspected compartment. A direct dorsal approach is used to evaluate any of the four dorsal interosseous compartments. To reach the palmar interosseous compartments, the needle is advanced deeper through the dorsal interosseous compartment along the radial aspect of the ring and small metacarpals, and along the ulnar aspect of the index metacarpal compartments. The thenar and hypothenar measurements are performed with direct needle insertion into the compartment with a direct palmar approach. In measurement of the thenar compartment, appreciation of Kaplan's cardinal point helps avoid injury to the motor recurrent branch of the median nerve.

Although the measurement of tissue fluid pressures of the intrinsic compartments of the hand is well described, the difficult nature and questionable reliability of these studies have been noted (158,371). The clinical findings are of more significance than those of the tissue fluid measurements. The pressure measurements are used as an adjunct to the clinical exam and are perhaps most useful in the obtunded patient or in those with a more proximal nerve injury in which clinical exam may be less reliable.

After the diagnosis of compartment syndrome of the hand, initial treatment is removal of any constricting bandages or casts. If symptoms do not quickly resolve, fasciotomy of the involved compartments is indicated. In most cases, all of the compartments of the hand are involved and warrant decompression.

The use of prophylactic fasciotomy after revascularization of an ischemic hand has been discussed by several authors (39,107,207,300–303,341,373). Prophylactic fasciotomy of the hand should be considered and carried out in most cases when revascularization is performed after 4 to 6 hours of ischemia (178).

Operative decompression of the hand is accomplished by the use of as many as four incisions (131,178). The carpal tunnel is decompressed through an additional incision, as described previously (Fig. 12). The carpal tunnel decompression also allows decompression of the midpalmar space.

The skin incisions are left open. A bulky hand dressing is applied, with plaster splints holding the digits in an intrinsic-plus position (80 to 90 degrees of flexion of the metacarpophalangeal joints and 0 to 10 degrees of extension at the proximal interphalangeal joints).

Operative Technique: Fasciotomy of the Dorsal and Palmar Interosseous Compartments and the Adductor Compartment of the Hand

In fasciotomy of the dorsal and palmar interosseous compartments and the adductor compartment of the hand, the dorsal

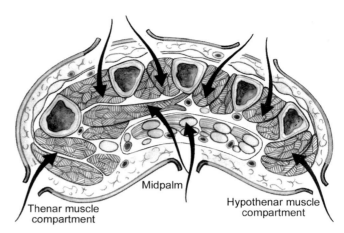

FIGURE 12. Fasciotomy of the hand. Cross section through the mid-palm that demonstrates the pathways (*arrows*) that are used to release the dorsal interosseous, palmar interosseous, the adductor pollicis, thenar, carpal tunnel, and hypothenar compartments. The dorsal incisions, which are 3 to 4 cm in length, are centered over the mid-portion of the metacarpals.

and palmar interosseous muscles and the adductor pollicis are decompressed through a dorsal incision. The first and second interosseous space muscles are released through a single incision that is placed over the index metacarpal. The incision is extended along each side of the metacarpal to incise the fasciae of the first and second dorsal interosseous compartments. Blunt dissection is continued deeper along the radial and ulnar sides of the index metacarpal to reach and incise the fasciae of the adductor compartment and the first palmar interosseous compartment, respectively. The adductor compartment can also be reached by deeper blunt dissection along the ulnar aspect of the index metacarpal. The third and forth interosseous compartments are released through a single incision that is placed over the ring metacarpal. The incision is extended along each side of the ring metacarpal to incise the fasciae of the third and fourth dorsal interosseous compartments. Blunt dissection is continued deeper along the radial and ulnar sides of the ring metacarpal to reach and incise the fasciae of the second and third palmar interosseous compartments (178) (Fig. 12).

Operative Technique: Fasciotomy of the Thenar Compartment

In fasciotomy of the thenar compartment, the thenar compartment is approached directly through a longitudinal incision that is placed along the radiopalmar aspect of the thumb metacarpal. Direct dissection allows incision of the thenar muscle fascia (178) (Fig. 12).

Operative Technique: Fasciotomy of the Hypothenar Compartment

In fasciotomy of the hypothenar compartment, the hypothenar compartment is approached directly through a longitudinal incision that is placed along the ulnar aspect of the small finger. Direct dissection allows incision of the hypothenar fascia (178) (Fig. 12).

Postoperative Care: Hand Compartment Syndrome Decompression

After fasciotomy, the extremity is elevated in the bulky dressing to promote edema reduction. Wounds are checked in approximately 5 days in the operating room and are closed as skin relaxation permits. Application of gentle skin traction techniques by using Steri-Strips, vessel loops, or skin traction devices can assist skin relaxation. The incisions are closed secondarily in 5 to 10 days or when swelling permits. Split-thickness skin grafts are rarely needed but are used if they are necessary. On the thenar and hypothenar eminences, full-thickness skin grafts allow replacement of similar thick skin (as opposed to split-thickness skin grafts). If initial wounds are contaminated, repeat débridements are carried out in the operating room, as indicated, and wounds are eventually closed secondarily, skin grafted, or allowed to heal by secondary intention.

Hand therapy is initiated as soon as the patient's comfort permits. Active and passive mobilization of the digits can be started while the bulky dressing is still in place. Therapy to maximize motion and strength is continued in the postoperative period until functional level has maximized.

Decompression of the Digits

When severe swelling of the digits is present, consideration is made for operative decompression. As noted previously, the digits do not contain true muscle compartments but do have unyielding connective tissue compartments that are bounded by Cleland's and Grayson's ligaments. The digits thus have physiologic compartments that are susceptible to pressure increases. Although theoretically possible, measurement of the interstitial fluid pressure has not been popularized, and the indications for fascial decompression are based on clinical impression, that is, from the amount of edema or soft tissue swelling and from sensibility function. Digital fasciotomy incisions are carried out through midaxial lateral incisions. Incisions that are placed along the ulnar sides of the index, long, and ring fingers and along the radial aspects of the small finger and thumb avoid incision scars in the areas of pinch and along the outside border of the small finger.

Operative Technique: Decompression of the Digits

Each of the digits is decompressed through a single midaxial longitudinal incision (Fig. 13). The incisions are placed along the ulnar sides of the index, long, and ring fingers and along the radial aspects of the small finger and thumb.

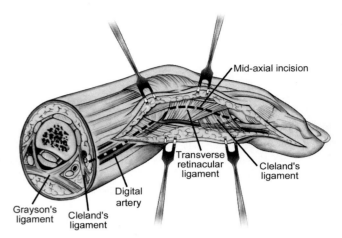

FIGURE 13. Decompression of a digit through a midaxial incision.

The associated neurovascular bundle is identified and explored to release associated constriction fascial bands from Grayson's or Cleland's ligaments. Dissection is extended deeper into the digit along the palmar aspect of the flexor tendon sheath. Vertical bands of connective tissue are released (178). If severe swelling is present with dysfunction of neurovascular bundles on the ulnar and radial aspects of the digit, a second longitudinal incision can be placed to decompress the neurovascular bundle. Alternatively, a single palmar Bruner incision can be placed to decompress both bundles.

The incisions are left open, but the skin is loosely approximated (if possible) to cover the neurovascular bundles. A bulky hand dressing is applied with the digits in an intrinsic plus position (80 to 90 degrees of flexion of the metacarpophalangeal joints and 0 to 10 degrees of extension at the proximal interphalangeal joints). The incisions are closed secondarily in 5 to 10 days or when swelling permits.

Postoperative Care

After fasciotomy, the extremity is elevated in the bulky dressing to promote edema reduction. Wounds are checked in approximately 5 days in the operating room, and the wounds are closed as skin relaxation permits. Hand therapy is initiated as soon as the patient's comfort permits. Active and passive mobilization of the digits can be started while the bulky dressing is still in place. Therapy to maximize motion and strength is continued in the postoperative period until functional level has maximized.

Role of Prophylactic Fasciotomy for Impending Compartment Syndrome in Limb Replantation

Compartment syndrome can occur after revascularization or replantation of a limb that contains muscle compartments. Prolonged ischemia, followed by reperfusion, leads to significant ultracellular changes with resultant increased capillary permeability, increased tissue edema, and venous collapse, thus resulting in loss of local perfusion (301,410). Therefore, the limb is subjected to a type of compartment syndrome and has continued ischemia, despite restoration of perfusion from revascularization.

With ischemia times of less than 3 hours, muscle fibers can recover with few residual changes. After 5 to 7 hours, irreversible damage ensues (215,411). Unfortunately, the average reported ischemia times of replanted or revascularized upper extremities usually range between 5 and 10 hours. Therefore, even with rapid emergency replantation or revascularization, most limbs are at risk for these cellular changes and compartment syndrome (301–303,383,412).

To prevent the continued limb ischemia and development of compartment syndrome after revascularization, the use of prophylactic fasciotomy has been discussed by several authors (39,107,207,300–303,341,370,373). Fasciotomy has been advocated for an amputated part that contains a muscle compartment and in all major replantation procedures of the upper extremity. The fascial incisions are similar to those that were discussed in the section Acute Compartment Syndrome. In replantation of a limb above the elbow, decompression of the volar and dorsal forearm compartments, as well as the several intrinsic compartments of the hand, is indicated. In revascularization of the proximal arm, the brachial fascia may also require incision.

Based on the biochemistry, animal models, and clinical experience with ischemia and perfusion, prophylactic fasciotomy of all compartments that are involved is indicated at the time of replantation of any upper extremity amputation (301). The reader is referred to the excellent further discussion by Hofmeister and Shin (301), who have reviewed several studies regarding the complex biochemistry of ischemia and perfusion and the role of prophylactic fasciotomy (413–421).

CRUSH SYNDROME

Crush syndrome represents one of the most severe presentations of acute compartment syndrome. It is a potentially fatal condition, and, therefore, special discussion is included here (20,95,170,197,213,217,221,224,226,240,325,327–334,337–339). This entity should be kept in mind in any patient who presents with compartment syndrome, especially when multiple compartments are involved, or in patients with a history of prolonged limb compression (i.e., in drug overdose victims or in those with a delay in diagnosis). Crush syndrome is the systemic result of extensive soft tissue injury and compartment syndrome. It is characterized by myoglobinemia, myoglobinuria, acidosis, hyperkalemia, cardiac arrhythmia, renal failure, and hypovolemic shock. Crush syndrome is well recognized as a potentially fatal condition, and the early literature that relates to the syndrome stems from war-time experi-

ences. von Schroeder (95) reviewed the historic aspects and noted that the syndrome was perhaps first described in 1812 by Larey (422). Larey examined soldiers with skin and muscle necrosis in pressure regions after succumbing to carbon monoxide poisoning (240). Historically relevant and war-related descriptions appeared in the German literature in the first quarter of the twentieth century (423–425). In 1923, it was recognized that renal failure and myoglobin were involved in the syndrome after laboratory developments that allowed for the differentiation of myoglobin and hemoglobin (426). During World War II, crush injuries in association with renal failure were discussed in the English literature, and myoglobin was isolated from the urine (95,224,328,329).

The relationship between the amount of myonecrosis and the magnitude of renal failure was subsequently established, and the related factors of acidosis and renal hypoperfusion due to hypotension were considered. The term *crush syndrome* has been in common use since the 1950s (224). Mubarak and Owen (20,197) emphasized the nature of the disorder in their discussions on acute compartment syndrome. von Schroeder (95) has discussed the etiology, pathophysiology, and treatment of this serious disorder in a recent excellent review.

Etiology of Crush Syndrome

Descriptions of crush syndrome have included patients who were crushed or buried during war as the result of explosions or those who were trapped in coal mine accidents. Accounts have also occurred from collapsing masonry during construction or from earthquakes. Common peace-time descriptions have resulted from extremity compression in unconscious victims of drug overdose (217,325,326,337,422) or carbon monoxide poisoning (422,427,428). Crush syndrome has also occurred while the patient is under anesthesia in the knee-chest position (429,430) or on a fracture table (146). It has occurred as a result of blunt muscle trauma from child abuse (431) and has been noted in torture victims (327). Crush syndrome has also been noted to result from pneumatic antishock garments (military antishock trousers) (332). Other variations or related etiologies of crush syndrome and myoglobinemia include hereditary muscle diseases, prolonged exercise, convulsions, malignant hyperthermia, influenza, and snake venom (95,375,425).

Pathophysiology of Crush Syndrome

Damage to muscle results in myoglobinemia from prolonged compression, compartment syndrome ischemia, or direct trauma. Myoglobin is a protein that is synthesized by muscle for oxygen transport and storage. It is present in high concentrations in type I oxidative muscle fibers (95). At least 200 mg of muscle must be damaged before myoglobin appears in the urine (374). Other injury factors, such as the direct effect of mycotoxic drugs, complete immobility, hypoxemia, acidosis, and decreased blood flow, may contribute to the rapid progression of myonecrosis (95).

Muscle compression is perhaps the most common cause of crush syndrome that is presently encountered in trauma units and emergency rooms. Forearm compartment pressures have been shown to reach an average of 178 mm Hg with the forearm underneath the rib cage when lying on a hard floor, 102 mm Hg with the forearm under the leg, and 55 mm Hg with the forearm under the head (213). These pressures are significant and capable of inducing the vicious cycle of compartment syndrome that can lead to crush syndrome (197).

Compression of a muscle causes ischemia, compartment syndrome, pressure-stretch myopathy (432), and reperfusion injury. This results in the release of oxygen free radicals and massive accumulation of calcium in damaged muscles (334). A unique form of compartment syndrome develops that contains necrotic muscle. Microscopically, there is a loss of functional integrity of the muscle sarcolemma and damage to the microcirculation and vessel endothelium with infiltration of neutrophils into reperfused vessels. Compartment edema occurs that results in third space fluid loss, which causes hypovolemia and contributes to shock. Although a small degree of myoglobin and the accompanying potassium and phosphorus from damaged muscles can be handled by normal functioning kidneys, renal failure occurs, with increasing amounts of muscle involved (376). There is a correlation between the severity of the crush syndrome and renal failure. Myoglobin precipitates in the distal convoluted tubules of the nephrons, particularly under acidotic conditions, and causes occlusion of the tubules that results in an obstructive nephropathy (95). Myoglobin contains iron, which may be nephrotoxic (376); however, iron-stimulated hydroxyl formation is not nephrotoxic (337). Oxygen free radicals, nephron hypoxia, and renal hypoperfusion contribute to nephrotoxicity and prerenal renal failure (95).

Hyperkalemia from damaged muscle can cause cardiac arrhythmia and associated electrocardiogram changes, such as peaked T waves, wide QRS complexes, and depressed ST segments. With increasing potassium levels, T waves disappear, and heart block and cardiac arrest can occur. Abnormal cardiac function can contribute to underperfusion of vital organs and shock (95).

Drugs and poisons may also contribute to cardiac arrhythmias and muscle damage. Acidosis results from inadequate tissue perfusion, muscle damage, respiratory depression, uremia, renal failure, hyperkalemia, and lactic acid. Drugs or toxins such as aspirin, methanol, and ethylene glycol can also produce acidosis. Acidosis contributes to cardiac instability, and a vicious cycle ensues (95).

Clinical Presentation of Crush Syndrome

As noted by von Schroeder, the mental status, vital signs, and appearance of a patient with crush syndrome are usually obvious and require resuscitative measures; however, the diagnosis of crush syndrome itself is often delayed (95). For this reason, a high index of suspicion is important, especially in patients with a history of prolonged or severe limb compression. Unfortunately, a clear history is often not available from a comatose or obtunded patient. The possible causes that explain the state of an obtunded hypotensive patient, such as brain injury, other trauma, drugs, and poisons, should be considered. An estimation of the duration of immobility should be sought (95). In a study of 11 patients, the duration of immobility that leads to a crush syndrome was 4 to 48 hours, with a mean of 12 hours (20).

Patients typically have neurologic, respiratory, and cardiac depression. These can be caused by drugs, toxins, trauma, or by the crush syndrome itself. Hypovolemia can be caused by dehydration and third space fluid loss. Shock and cardiac arrhythmia can follow. Oliguria or anuria can be the first clue of a crush syndrome but may also represent the hypovolemic or hypotensive state of a patient (95).

The injured extremity may be overlooked, as resuscitative measures are the main focus. Examination of the extremities may be unremarkable, because findings can be subtle. Conversely, obvious signs, such as profoundly swollen and tight compartments, may be present, and the skin may be tense and shiny, erythematous, or blistered (20,95,197,213,335,339,428).

Pulses are unreliable in diagnosing compartment syndrome. Pulses can be present, weak, or absent (213) and should not be used as an indicator of compartment status. Theoretically, as noted in the discussion of acute compartment syndrome, pulses should be intact, because arterial diastolic and systolic pressures (120 mm Hg and 75 mm Hg) are usually far greater than the tissue fluid pressures of compartment syndrome (i.e., 30 to 60 mm Hg) (1,8,25). However, severe edema or soft tissue swelling often prevents identification of pulses by palpation. Doppler evaluation is often helpful and can frequently demonstrate the presence of peripheral pulses, even with moderate or severe surrounding edema that prevents palpable identification of pulses (95).

Compartments may be painful, and pain may be heightened by muscle stretch. In the severely obtunded patient, subtle signs of pain with passive muscle stretch may be seen by a transient increase in pulse or blood pressure or by facial grimacing or limb withdrawal. Typically, however, with a severe crush, there is no voluntary movement. Paresthesias and pallor can also be important clues when they are present. Compartment pressures should be measured to help in decision making, particularly in the comatose or obtunded patient. Potential differential diagnoses, such as fracture, venous thrombosis, arterial injury, or cellulitis, should not distract from or delay the correct identification of a compartment syndrome.

Laboratory Findings in Crush Syndrome

Muscle injury results in muscle enzymes, myoglobin, potassium, creatinine, and phosphorus being released into the circulation. The enzymes include serum glutamic oxaloacetic acid, lactic dehydrogenase, and CPK. CPK levels are often high (greater than 10,000 IU), and isoenzyme determination may be necessary to rule out underlying myocardial damage. CPK levels merely indicate muscle damage; the levels do not necessarily indicate a compartment or crush syndrome and are therefore nonspecific. For example, large increases in CPK may be seen in fracture patients who do not develop compartment syndromes. The CPK elevation does, however, draw attention to the potential of such syndromes and the possibility of impending renal failure (95,433).

Urine analysis is helpful, provided that the patient is not completely anuric. In crush syndrome, the urine is usually dark in color from myoglobin and may present as reddish brown to brown in color. Protein is present, but glucose and ketones are not. Importantly, urine dipstick analysis suggests or reveals large amounts of blood, because myoglobin is not differentiated from hemoglobin by the benzidine test. The differentiation is made on microscopic examination of the urine, which shows no red blood cells, and myoglobin can be quantitated by spectrophotographic methods. Other cells and debris are also usually absent. Serum creatinine and urea nitrogen can be used as indicators of renal function. Creatinine clearance calculations are the most reliable method for clinical assessment of glomerular filtration rate. Hyperkalemia is also an indicator of muscle damage and impaired renal function and must be treated (see the following discussion) to prevent its arrhythmic effect on the myocardium. Blood gases, including pH, must be monitored frequently and corrected as indicated (95).

Classification of Crush Syndrome

Mubarak and Owen (20,197,213) presented a classification of crush syndrome that was based on 11 cases. These were divided into three stages based on CPK (Table 6). In their series, Mubarak and Owen (20) found 23 compartments that were involved in three patients with stage III crush syndrome. The classification system is based on the severity of the crush syndrome. It does have some prognostic value, but differentiation between the groups may be difficult. The spectrum of crush syndrome spans from mild to severe. Nevertheless, even mild crush syndrome from a single compartment can result in serious symptoms, including renal dysfunction (95).

Management of Crush Syndrome

Zager (377), Mubarak and Owen (20), and von Schroeder and Botte (95) have outlined the medical management aspects of crush syndrome. Management consists of urgent medical consultation with resuscitative and supportive measures for the patient as a whole and the correct and timely diagnosis and treatment of the accompanying compartment syndrome (95). Hypotension is managed with

TABLE 6. CLASSIFICATION OF CRUSH SYNDROME

Stage I
One or two compartments are involved.
Creatine phosphokinase is elevated to greater than 10,000 IU.
Myoglobinuria is present.
Stage II
Several compartments are involved.
Creatine phosphokinase is greater than 20,000 IU.
Myoglobinuria is present.
Serum creatinine and urea nitrogen are elevated.
Patients are not oliguric.
Patients are hypotensive.
Stage III
Multiple compartments are involved.
Shock, oliguria, metabolic acidosis, hyperkalemia, and possible cardiac arrhythmias are present.
Patients develop renal failure.
Considered "full blown" crush syndrome.

Adapted from Mubarak SJ, Owen CA. Compartmental syndrome and its relation to the crush syndrome: a spectrum of disease. *Clin Orthop* 1975;113–181; and von Schroeder HP, Botte MJ. Crush syndrome of the upper extremity. *Hand Clin* 1998;14:451–456.

intravenous crystalloid. In the presence of renal failure, fluid balance is carefully monitored and controlled. Invasive volume and pressure monitoring aid in determining and adjusting volume status. Unless there is a history of blood loss, blood and plasma transfusions are usually not necessary, because hypovolemia is typically due to third space fluid loss and dehydration. Furthermore, blood products can contribute to the already present hyperkalemia. Hyperkalemia should be treated by intravenous administration of calcium gluconate to suppress the myocardial effects of high potassium levels. Internal cation exchange resins reduce potassium levels. Bicarbonate and insulin together with glucose promote cellular potassium uptake. Diuretics also promote potassium loss in the urine, but dialysis may be required to treat severe cases of hyperkalemia. Furosemide and mannitol diuresis can be instituted to achieve 500 mL of urine per hour; urine alkalization should be achieved with intravenous bicarbonate (217,289,335,377). Dialysis may be necessary (434).

Predictors of renal failure include the presence of dehydration, elevated serum CPK, potassium and phosphorus levels, and the degree of depression of serum albumin levels. A venous bicarbonate concentration of less than 17 mmol/L may also predict the development of renal failure (435). Alkalization of the urine to a pH of greater than 6.5 prevents further precipitation of myoglobin. Alkalization also promotes dissolution of some of the accumulated myoglobin and facilitates its excretion (377). Mannitol protects the kidneys by its osmotic diuretic action, by scavenging oxygen free radicals, and by inhibiting tubular sodium resorption (221,432). Dialysis is necessary if renal failure is severe and if potassium levels are high. Respiratory support and monitoring for cardiac arrhythmias are necessary. Antibiotics must be initiated immediately at the first signs of infection or sepsis. Pharmacologic treatment that is directed toward the prevention of reperfusion injury is under investigation (334).

The treatment of an acute compartment syndrome is fasciotomy, as was described previously. However, the role of fasciotomy in crush syndrome is somewhat controversial. If the muscle is necrotic, fasciotomy does not reverse the status of the muscle but exposes the dead tissue to the potential for infection. Such infection can advance rapidly and can develop severe sequelae, such as hemorrhage, systemic sepsis, and necrotizing or deep space infection, and possibly results in amputation or death (377).

Compartment pressure measurements (with clinical correlation) can assist the decision making with respect to fasciotomy. If the pressures are high, further muscle damage may ensue, and the compartment syndrome and crush syndrome can worsen (330). Under such circumstances, the fasciotomy is indicated and is intended to prevent further local effects of increased pressure (20,240,377). This also benefits the patient by decreasing the systemic effects of a crushed extremity. Fasciotomy also allows débridement of the necrotic muscle (422) and thus lessens the metabolic load that is the impetus for the crush syndrome. In Mubarak and Owen's series (20), fasciotomy was a part of the protocol for treatment. There were no amputations or deaths in their series, but fasciotomy did not necessarily change the outcome of the limb; in fact, most patients have residual limb contractures. Frequent operations are usually necessary to débride necrotic muscle. Closure of the skin or skin grafting should be done as soon as there is a clean bed of tissue within the compartment. A meshed split-thickness skin graft is used if the wound edges cannot be approximated for closure (377).

Several authors have indicated that fasciotomy may be contraindicated unless there is clear evidence of significant limb ischemia or if an open injury is present (221,333,335,432). Débridement of muscle may cause bleeding that is difficult to control. Because necrotic muscle can still bleed from traversing vessels, bleeding should not be used as a criterion to determine viability of muscle. Distinguishing between viable and nonviable muscle is often difficult, but they may be distinguished by eliciting a contraction with thermocautery or a nerve stimulator in viable muscle. Fasciotomy and débridement do create the potential problem of infection (377). Despite the controversy, if ongoing compartment syndrome is suspected, the treatment is fasciotomy.

In the crush syndrome, amputation as a possible outcome must be discussed early in the course of treatment with the patient and family (338). Severe infection, such as gas gangrene, necrotizing fasciitis, or profound diffuse hemorrhage, may require an amputation as a life-saving procedure.

Theoretically, hyperbaric oxygen may be of benefit to injured tissues that are still viable (364–366). However, the clinical role of hyperbaric oxygen remains controversial (335), and administration is often not possible from the practical point of view. Furthermore, necrotic muscle does not respond to any form of oxygen. Indicated operative procedures, such as fasciotomy or débridement, should not be delayed to provide a trial of hyperbaric oxygen (377).

The systemic treatment of crush syndrome can potentially have a good outcome, particularly if it is instituted within 6 hours (330). Death from crush syndrome can be avoided if diagnosis is not delayed and if appropriate medical and surgical treatment are initiated. Delays occur from prolonged time before hospitalization, distraction by medical problems, inability to make a diagnosis, the absence of typical signs and symptoms, and the delay in treatment due to a reluctance to anesthetize seriously ill patients (197). Measurement of compartment pressures may decrease delays of diagnosis, may promote more rapid operative management, and may improve outcome. Although the outcome of a crushed limb is difficult to predict (335), the prognosis of the extremity is often poor. Volkmann's contracture subsequently develops in many extremities. In a series of patients with crush syndrome and associated compartment syndrome, Mubarak and Owen reported 80% poor results (20).

VOLKMANN'S ISCHEMIC CONTRACTURE

Pathogenesis of Volkmann's Ischemic Contracture

Muscle and nerve are highly vulnerable to changes in oxygen tension. Muscle undergoes necrosis after 4 hours of experimentally produced ischemia by tourniquet application (120–122). With prolonged ischemia, substantial myonecrosis is followed by fibroblastic proliferation within the muscle infarct (66,67). A variable amount of longitudinal and horizontal contraction takes place as the muscle cicatrix matures and may progress over a 6- to 12-month period after original acute ischemic insult. Necrotic muscle often adheres to surrounding structures, thus fixing the muscle position, and further reduces excursion and mobility. Secondary compression of surrounding structures occurs, with peripheral nerves being particularly vulnerable (7,55,122,144,146,200,402). Limitation of muscle excursion from fibrotic proliferation leads to loss of joint motion and subsequent joint ligament and capsule contracture (Fig. 14). Peripheral nerve injury, which occurs from the original ischemic insult as well as from secondary compression from muscle fibrosis and limb contracture, further contributes to limb dysfunction. Besides motor loss, neuropathy after ischemic contracture can lead to chronic pain, paresthesias, and loss of limb sensibility.

Upper Limb Deformity in Volkmann's Contracture

The deepest compartments, especially those that are adjacent to bone, usually have high interstitial pressures during compartment syndrome (5,66,67,69,70). The flexor digi-

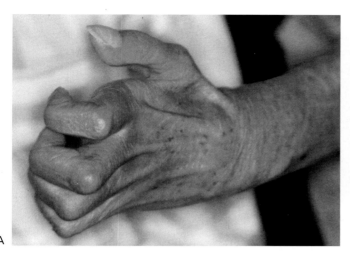

A

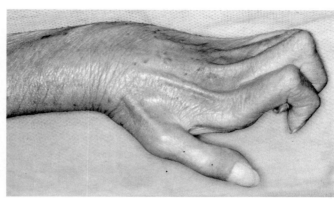

B

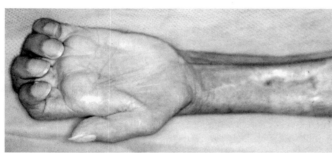

C

FIGURE 14. A–C: Photographs of the upper extremity of a patient with established Volkmann's contracture. Unrecognized compartment syndrome originally occurred after revascularization of the extremity with brachial artery injury. Note the hyperextension at the metacarpophalangeal joints and the flexion at the interphalangeal joints. The deformed extremity is dysfunctional, with sensory and motor deficits in the median and ulnar nerve distributions. Fixed contractures are present at the elbow, the wrist, and the digits. The forearm muscle mass is fibrotic with a firm "woody" consistency that is due to muscle fibrosis. The flexor digitorum profundus, flexor pollicis longus, and flexor digitorum superficialis are all severely involved.

torum profundus and flexor pollicis longus muscles are affected most often (Figs. 15 and 16). In the mildest contractures, only a portion of the flexor digitorum profundus undergoes necrosis, which usually involves the ring and long fingers. In severe contractures, all four digits are involved (Fig. 14). The flexor digitorum superficialis and pronator teres are usually less severely affected. In the most severe cases, however, the digital and wrist flexors and extensors, as well as the compartments above the elbow, may be involved (5,66,67,69,70).

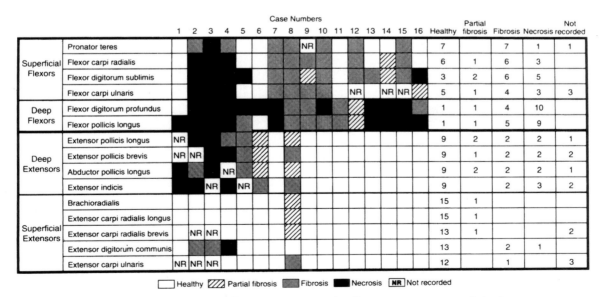

FIGURE 15. Muscles that were affected in 16 cases of Volkmann's contracture of the forearm. Note the frequent involvement of the deep forearm flexor muscles. (From Seddon HJ. Volkmann's contracture: treatment by incision of the infarct. *J Bone Joint Surg* 1956;38:152, with permission.)

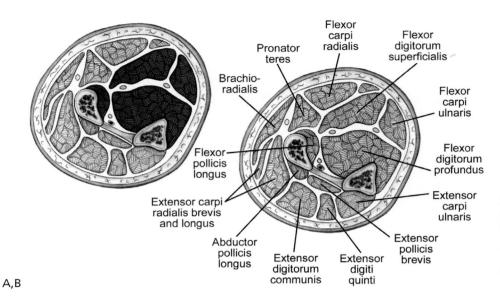

Flexor
carpi
radialis

Pronator
teres

Flexor
digitorum
superficialis

Brachio-
radialis

Flexor
carpi
ulnaris

Flexor
digitorum
profundus

Flexor
pollicis
longus

Extensor
carpi
radialis brevis
and longus

Extensor
carpi
ulnaris

Extensor
pollicis
brevis

Abductor
pollicis
longus

Extensor
digitorum
communis

Extensor
digiti
quinti

A,B

FIGURE 16. Cross section of Volkmann's contracture of the forearm. **A:** The shaded areas represent the degree of involvement of the various muscles. The diagram is based on the data that were provided in Figure 2. **B:** Key to the muscles. The plane of section is through the upper one-third of the forearm.

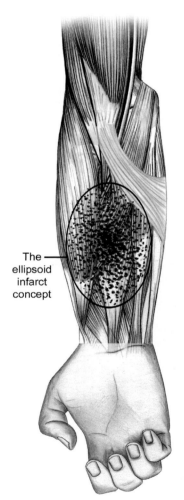

The
ellipsoid
infarct
concept

FIGURE 17. The ellipsoid infarct concept, as proposed by Seddon and Tsuge. Circulation is most severely impaired in the center of the muscle belly. The muscles that are most severely affected are the flexor digitorum profundus and the flexor pollicis longus.

The common involvement of the deep flexors of the forearm is attributed to their deep compartment location, which increases their vulnerability to high interstitial pressures and ischemia (66,67). With compression from within, the circulation to the deep portions of muscle is compromised, whereas collateral circulation to more superficial portions of the muscle may be retained. In the forearm, muscle degeneration commonly occurs in the middle one-third of the muscle belly, being most severe closer to bone, with less involvement toward the proximal and distal surfaces. If compartment syndrome is not treated, swelling may ultimately resolve, but necrotic muscle undergoes fibrosis. An ellipsoid section or cord of cicatrix can develop within the muscle or group of muscles (Fig. 17). The characteristic deformity of ischemic contracture may take weeks or months to develop. When the arm, forearm, and hand are severely involved, deformity in the upper limb usually consists of elbow flexion, forearm pronation, wrist flexion, thumb flexion and adduction, digital metacarpophalangeal joint extension, and interphalangeal joint flexion (44,69,70,73,436). The metacarpophalangeal joint extension and proximal interphalangeal joint flexion give rise to a claw hand type of deformity (Fig. 14). Although extremity deformity may initially be manually flexible (especially in milder cases), chronic muscle imbalance and lack of joint motion may ultimately lead to fixed deformity from secondary joint capsule, ligament, and skin contracture.

Volkmann's contracture may lead to an intrinsic-minus–appearing deformity of the hand, which is characterized by hyperextension at the metacarpophalangeal joints and flexion at the interphalangeal joints. The deformity is usually a result of compartment syndrome that involves the forearm extrinsic muscles (flexors and extensors), which undergo necrosis, fibrosis, and contracture. This extrinsic overpull of the more powerful extrinsic finger flexors and extensors overpowers the weaker intrinsic muscles, thus producing the intrinsic-minus deformity (5,46,223,437,438).

An additional factor in the pathomechanics of all upper extremity deformities is the amount of peripheral nerve injury that is superimposed on the muscle injury. Muscle injury usually causes contracture; nerve injury causes muscle paralysis. Concomitant median and ulnar neuropathy in the forearm or wrist contributes to intrinsic muscle weakness, thereby contributing to intrinsic-minus or claw hand deformity.

If an untreated compartment syndrome is limited to the intrinsic muscles of the hand (as in an isolated hand crush injury), different clinical outcomes may develop, depending on the degree of muscle necrosis (with fibrosis and contracture) and the amount of local nerve damage. Muscle necrosis and fibrosis contribute to an intrinsic-plus hand if the interossei and lumbricals undergo contracture that flexes the metacarpophalangeal joints and extends the proximal interphalangeal joints. The thenar muscles, adductor pollicis, and first dorsal interosseous can contribute to thumb flexion or adduction (439,440). Conversely, local motor nerve injury results in paretic intrinsic muscles and contributes to an intrinsic-minus deformity. The final clinical outcome is dependent on the relative amount of intrinsic muscle and nerve involvement.

Compartment syndrome of the arm flexors may lead to elbow flexion contraction. If the anterior (flexor) compartment and posterior (extensor) compartments of the arm are involved, and muscle contracture develops, there is often still a flexion deformity that is secondary to the larger, stronger elbow flexors, as compared to the elbow extensors. Compartment syndrome of the shoulder that leads to contracture often causes generalized shoulder stiffness. Isolated tightness of the anterior, lateral, or posterior portions of the deltoid can give rise to more specific tightness or contracture. Relatively few data exist regarding reconstruction of shoulder and elbow deformities in ischemic contractures.

Several additional factors can contribute to the deformity of ischemic contracture. Although the more classic deformity has already been described, variability in the presentation of deformity can exist. This can be due to additional factors, such as adhesions or deformity from associated fractures, overpull or adhesions from crushed fibrotic muscle, or additional or unrecognized nerve injury from crush or penetrating injuries.

Diagnosis and Classification of Ischemic Contractures

The diagnosis is based on the clinical findings that were described previously, which follow a suspected or confirmed acute compartment syndrome. Once the diagnosis is made, ischemic contractures of the upper extremity can be classified according to the severity of involvement (40,46,66,67,441–443). The simplest classification system, which was popularized by Seddon (66,67), Tsuge (69,70), and Gelberman, describes mild, moderate, and severe involvement and is useful for determining treatment

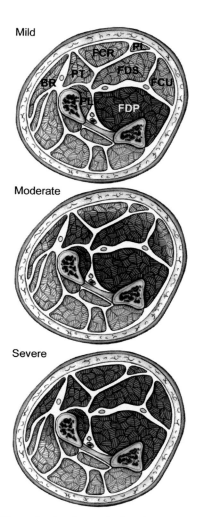

FIGURE 18. The extent of muscle involvement in the three types of Volkmann's contractures. BR, brachioradialis; FCR, flexor carpi radialis; FCU, flexor carpi ulnaris; FDP, flexor digitorum profundus; FDS, flexor digitorum superficialis; FPL, flexor pollicis longus; PL, palmaris longus; PT, pronator teres.

options (Fig. 18). The classification is based on contractures of the forearm.

Mild Contractures

Mild or localized ischemic contracture is limited to a portion of the deep extrinsic finger flexors and usually involves only two or three fingers. The long and ring fingers are most frequently involved. A deep cordlike area of indurated cicatrix may be palpable within the flexor forearm, and the tenodesis effect of involved digits may be present. Hand sensibility is normal, and strength is normal or minimally impaired. Intrinsic muscles are not involved, and fixed joint contractures do not develop. Most mild types of Volkmann's contracture are caused by fractures or crush injuries to the forearm or elbow and usually occur in young adults (24,42,44,46,50,51,54–57,197,444).

Moderate Contractures

Moderate ischemic contractures are considered the classical type and primarily involve the flexor digitorum profundus and flexor pollicis longus muscles. Less frequently, the flexor digitorum superficialis, flexor carpi radialis, and flexor carpi ulnaris are involved. The wrist and thumb become flexed, and the hand assumes an intrinsic-minus hand deformity from extrinsic muscle contracture (5,24,25,44,46,69,342,445).

In moderate contractures, secondary compression neuropathies may develop, especially at specific anatomic sites at which nerves pass beneath ligaments and fibrous arcades or through contracted muscles. The median nerve is frequently involved and is compressed at the lacertus fibrosus, pronator teres, or flexor digitorum superficialis or within the carpal tunnel. The ulnar nerve may be compressed at the elbow between the humeral and ulnar heads of the flexor carpi ulnaris, at the arcade of Struthers, or at the medial intermuscular septum of the arm. The radial nerve and the posterior interosseous nerve, which are rarely involved, may be compressed within the radial tunnel, at the arcade of Frohse, or within the supinator muscle (5,24,25,44,46,69,342).

Moderate contractures of the upper extremity are often caused by supracondylar fractures of the humerus. They usually occur in children who are 5 to 10 years of age (5,44,46,312).

Severe Contractures

Severe contractures involve most or all of the forearm flexors and variable degrees of forearm extensors. Secondary complications of joint contracture, neuropathy, malunion or nonunion of fractures, and cutaneous scar contracture are common. Causes of severe contracture include devascularizing crush injuries, prolonged ischemia after brachial artery injury, or continuous external compression during unconsciousness from drug overdose. Young adults and children most often sustain severe contractures (5,24,25,44,46,69,342).

Management of Volkmann's Ischemic Contracture

The main goals of management of Volkmann's ischemic contracture are to maximize limb function, to decrease any associated pain, and, if possible, to restore limb sensibility.

Nonoperative Management

Treatment of mild contractures depends on the severity of deformity and the time interval between injury and initiation of treatment. Contractures of the deep forearm flexors, with normal hand sensibility and preservation of remaining extrinsic muscle strength, can often be managed nonoperatively with a comprehensive hand rehabilitation program that uses a team approach (5,24,25,44,46,69,159,160,342). Hand therapy, which uses active and passive mobilization, strengthening, and static and dynamic extension splinting, is used to maintain or improve thumb web space width, to strengthen weak thumb intrinsic muscles, and to correct or to improve digital flexion contractures. Splinting techniques for Volkmann's contracture have been described in detail by Goldner (56,159,160). Bivalved pancake plaster casts or custom splints can be alternated with low-profile, lightweight synthetic digital extension and thumb opposition splints. Serial digital casting can be considered as well but is rarely required for mild contractures. A C-bar may be incorporated into the splint to maintain thumb position. Early in the rehabilitation program, static and dynamic splinting is alternated at 2-hour intervals during the day. At night, plaster or custom synthetic extension splints are worn. Recently, commercial dynamic splints have become available and are effective if fitting is satisfactory. These can be used on the digital contractures or on the wrist and elbow. Strengthening with progressive active mobilization against resistance is instituted. A satisfactory outcome can usually be expected when mild contractures are treated soon after their development by using these techniques (56,159,160).

Operative Management of Ischemic Contractures

When mild contractures are encountered late or do not respond to a nonoperative rehabilitation program, operative treatment is considered (24,42,44,46,50,51,54–57,197,444, 446). If the contracture is limited to one or two digits, and a cordlike indurated mass is palpable, simple excision of the infarcted muscle or lengthening of the involved flexor tendon is recommended (5,44,46,55,66,67,69,70). The flexor digitorum profundus to the ring and long fingers most often requires infarct excision.

Reconstruction of Mild Contractures
Operative Technique: Infarct Excision of Mild Contractures. Excision of infarcted muscle is performed through a curved, longitudinal incision on the palmar forearm. Dissection is carried out through the subcutaneous tissues. The deep fascia is incised to identify and protect the radial artery, the median nerve, and the ulnar artery and nerve. The flexor digitorum superficialis and flexor carpi radialis are retracted radially, and the flexor carpi ulnaris is retracted ulnarly to expose the flexor digitorum profundus. Cordlike areas of indurated muscle are isolated and excised (5,44, 46,55,66,67,69,70).

If the contracture is isolated to the pronator teres, myotomy or excision is performed. If contracture and induration involve three or four digits, flexor tendon lengthening may be required (5,44,46,55,66,67,69,70,447) (see the following discussion).

Postoperative Care. When the infarct is excised, mobilization and progressive strengthening in a hand therapy program are initiated as soon as the patient's comfort permits.

Operative Technique: Flexor Tendon Lengthening. Flexor tendon lengthening may be used to reconstruct mild contractures; for a discussion of this operative technique, see the section Reconstruction of Moderate to Severe Contractures.

Reconstruction of Moderate to Severe Contractures

Treatment of moderate to severe contractures may be divided into four phases: phase 1, release of secondary nerve compression; phase 2, treatment of contractures; phase 3, tendon transfers for restoration of lost function; and phase 4, salvage procedures for the severely contracted or neglected extremity (44,46,55,69,70).

Phase 1: Release of Secondary Nerve Compression. After muscle infarct, peripheral nerves can become compressed within a constricting cicatrix or at specific anatomic locations at which space is minimal. Because improvement of nerve function is related to the severity and duration of compression, early nerve decompression is required to minimize further dysfunction. Nerves may sustain compression for longer periods than muscle and still show some reversibility, particularly in regaining sensibility function (5,44,46,55,66,67,69,70). When continuity is maintained, nerves may show signs of gradual recovery over a 12-month period (66,67). In severe contractures with extensive fibrosis, all three major forearm nerves may become compressed. Forearm nerve decompression is optimally undertaken early, as soon as the patient's condition permits (448). A nerve stimulator may be helpful for verification of conductivity and nerve isolation, especially in heavily scarred areas.

Median Nerve. The median nerve, which often lies in the central area of the forearm constricting cicatrix, is at risk for compression at the lacertus fibrosus, the two heads of the pronator teres, and the proximal arch of the flexor digitorum superficialis and within the carpal tunnel. Return of median nerve function is essential for restoration of useful extremity function. Sensory and motor loss, which is consistent with median neuropathy, warrants aggressive management for decompression.

An incision that is similar to that used for forearm decompression in acute compartment syndrome is used for median nerve decompression (see the section Acute Compartment Syndrome of the Forearm).

OPERATIVE TECHNIQUE: MEDIAN NERVE DECOMPRESSION IN THE FOREARM AND CARPAL TUNNEL. In median nerve decompression in the forearm and carpal tunnel, the volar incision originates on the medial aspect of the arm 2 cm proximal to the medial epicondyle (5,178,180,363, 407,448). The incision is extended obliquely across the antecubital fossa to reach the volar aspect of the mobile wad. The incision is continued distally, curving slightly ulnarly and reaching the midline at the junction of the middle and distal two-thirds of the forearm. Continuing distally in the volar forearm, the incision is extended just ulnarly to the palmaris longus tendon to avoid injury to the palmar cutaneous branch of the median nerve. The incision crosses the wrist crease at an angle and is extended into the mid-palm for carpal tunnel release. It is carried no further radially than the mid-axis of the ring finger. The subcutaneous tissues are incised to expose the deep fascia. The fascia is incised, and the muscles are mobilized.

The median nerve is isolated along its course and is sequentially exposed at each of the four anatomic sites of compression (5,44,46,69,70). The nerve is first identified in the proximal portion of the incision and is traced distally to the lacertus fibrosus. The lacertus fibrosus, a fascial extension of the biceps tendon, lies anterior to the median nerve at the elbow. The lacertus fibrosus is incised longitudinally along the course of the median nerve to allow complete decompression and exposure of the nerve. The nerve is then explored to the proximal edge of the pronator teres to ensure that there are no areas of constriction between the humeral and ulnar heads of the muscle. The pronator teres is myotomized as needed to ensure nerve decompression. If the pronator teres is fibrotic, portions of cicatrix are excised. The median nerve continues distally deep to the proximal edge of the flexor digitorum superficialis and extends within the fascia of its deep surface. This muscle is mobilized to allow visualization of the nerve, and the fascia is released as needed. The nerve is freed of adhesions. Portions of fibrotic muscle are excised, as needed, to mobilize the nerve. Division of the transverse carpal ligament is then carried out. Median nerve decompression is therefore ensured from the distal arm to the mid-palm.

POSTOPERATIVE CARE. As in standard carpal tunnel release, the wrist is splinted for 3 to 4 weeks in slight extension to prevent the nerve from adhering to the healing incisional scar. Digital and elbow motion should be initiated as soon as patient comfort permits. Because of patient discomfort, reluctance to move the digits is common, and assistance with a formal hand therapy program is helpful. After the course of wrist immobilization, wrist mobilization and progressive strengthening (along with the digits, elbow, and shoulder) are undertaken. The elbow and shoulder should not be neglected, as secondary stiffness can occur.

Ulnar Nerve. The incidence of ulnar nerve compression in ischemic contractures is lower than that of the median nerve. The ulnar nerve is often compressed at the elbow as it passes between the humeral and ulnar heads of the flexor carpi ulnaris or proximal to the elbow, where it continues deep to the arcade of Struthers and pierces the medial intermuscular septum of the arm. Decompression in the arm, elbow, and forearm is indicated if there are signs and symptoms of ulnar neuropathy (5,44,46,69,70,448).

OPERATIVE TECHNIQUE: ULNAR NERVE DECOMPRESSION IN THE FOREARM.   In ulnar nerve decompression in the forearm, a longitudinal incision is placed in the medial arm near the arcade of Struthers and along the edge of the medial intermuscular septum. The incision then continues along the course of the ulnar nerve, through the cubital tunnel, and into the proximal forearm. The subcutaneous tissues are mobilized in the proximal portion of the incision; the ulnar nerve is identified and traced distally. The arcade of Struthers and the edge of the medial intermuscular septum (between the flexor and extensor compartments of the arm) are released in the proximal portion of the wound. The nerve is then explored more distally as it passes posteriorly to the medial humeral epicondyle and then extends between the ulnar and humeral heads of the flexor carpi ulnaris. The muscle or epimysial edges are myotomized as needed. Fibrotic muscle and tight fibrous bands are excised or released, preserving vincula leashes that contain segmental blood supply to the nerve. Additional procedures, such as anterior nerve transposition or epicondylectomy, are performed if the nerve appears to be edematous or under tension along its bed in the cubital tunnel. If cicatrix or myofibrosis is extensive throughout the forearm to the wrist, decompression of the ulnar nerve may also be indicated through Guyon's canal or into the palm.

POSTOPERATIVE CARE.   After nerve decompression, wounds are closed primarily, the hand is placed in a bulky hand dressing, and hand therapy for mobilization and strengthening is initiated in 3 weeks.

Radial Nerve in the Arm and Forearm.   Although the radial nerve is rarely involved in compression neuropathies after ischemic contracture, decompression of the radial nerve in the radial tunnel or of the posterior interosseous nerve may be required, as they pass through the tendinous origin of the supinator muscle (the arcade of Frohse), within the muscle itself, or are compressed by tendinous bands or vascular leases. Nerve compression at this level is manifested by motor loss of digital and thumb extensors and ulnar wrist extensors. Radial wrist extensor strength and radial nerve sensibility remain intact, as these nerve branches arise proximally to the usual areas of compression.

OPERATIVE TECHNIQUE: DECOMPRESSION OF THE RADIAL NERVE IN THE FOREARM.   In decompression of the radial nerve in the forearm, the radial nerve and the posterior interosseous nerve are explored through a longitudinal incision that is placed on the proximal one-half of the posterior forearm along an imaginary line that extends between the lateral epicondyle and the radial styloid. The interval between the extensor carpi radialis brevis and the extensor digitorum communis is developed. This interval is more easily defined and developed in the distal portion of the incision and is traced proximally. The extensor carpi radialis brevis is retracted radially, and the extensor digitorum communis is retracted ulnarly. The supinator is identified, along with the posterior interosseous nerve proximally, where it enters the muscle. Nerve compression may be encountered from tight tendinous bands of the arcade of Frohse, by a vascular leash that crosses the nerve transversely in this vicinity, or by the supinator muscle itself. The appropriate structures are divided to decompress the nerve.

If a more proximal compression of the radial nerve is suspected, the incision is extended proximally to develop the interval between the brachialis and the brachioradialis. The brachialis and biceps are retracted ulnarly, and the brachioradialis is retracted radially to expose the radial nerve in the intramuscular interval. The nerve is explored, and constricting fascial bands or small vascular leashes are transected or cauterized, respectively.

POSTOPERATIVE CARE.   After nerve decompression, wounds are closed primarily, the hand is placed in a bulky hand dressing, and hand therapy for mobilization and strengthening is initiated in 3 weeks.

Phase 2: Release of Contracture.   Although variable, fixed contractures that develop over time usually produce characteristic deformities of elbow flexion, forearm pronation, wrist flexion, digital clawing (intrinsic minus), and thumb adduction and flexion (5,44,46,55,66,67,69,70). Operative correction is indicated for deformities that are refractory to passive mobilization, splinting, or serial casting. Seddon (66,67) has recommended at least 6 months of preliminary splinting before contracture release. Common procedures that are used to correct established forearm contractures include infarct excision, flexor tendon lengthening or excision, or flexor pronator recession (5, 44,46,55,66,67,69,70). For the severely clenched fist deformity, the superficialis-to-profundus transfer can be considered. Operative procedures are often performed at the time of, or subsequent to, nerve decompression. Intrinsic contractures of the hand often coexist and are addressed at the time of extrinsic release (see the section Reconstruction of Intrinsic Hand Deformities in Ischemic Contracture).

A chief disadvantage of tendon lengthening is the additional weakening that is produced in these previously impaired muscles. However, release of severe contractures is usually functionally advantageous to achieve maximal strength. Tendon transfers are performed at a later time, if they are needed to augment strength (5,44,46,55,66, 67,69,70). In the nonfunctional, severely deformed extremity, contracture release is useful to facilitate extremity hygiene in the palm, wrist crease, or antecubital fossa or to facilitate dressing and positioning (44,46).

Operative Technique: Infarct Excision. If an indurated mass of muscle infarct is palpable, it can be separated and excised. Infarct excision can often be performed within 1 to 6 months after initial injury. A longitudinal palmar incision is placed on the forearm. Dissection is carried out through the fascia to the palpable cord in the muscle. The infarct cord is usually ellipsoid. A longitudinal incision is placed into the muscle, and the muscle fibers are split to reach the cord. The functionless muscle and the contracted cicatrix are isolated and removed (66,67). The deep digital flexors and the thumb flexor are usually the most extensively involved. The pronator teres and pronator quadratus may be released or, if fibrotic, are excised. The forearm and wrist are gently manipulated into supination and extension, respectively, and are immobilized in the corrected position.

POSTOPERATIVE CARE. The hand and wrist are initially splinted in a corrected position. The digits and wrist are mobilized as soon as the patient's comfort permits. A formal therapy program for active and passive motion and strengthening is then initiated.

Operative Technique: Digital Flexor Tendon Lengthening. Goldner notes that infarct excision may not be necessary and advocates Z-lengthening of the flexor tendons proximal to the wrist (56,160). A slightly curved or longitudinal incision is made on the distal one-half of the palmar forearm. The median nerve, the ulnar nerve and artery, and the radial artery are identified and protected. The median nerve, which lies between the flexor digitorum profundus and the flexor digitorum superficialis (on the deep surface of the flexor digitorum superficialis and within its fascia), may be within the cicatrix. The flexor digitorum profundus, flexor digitorum superficialis, flexor pollicis longus, and pronator teres are identified and lengthened by using Z-lengthening incisions to accomplish digital and thumb extension and forearm supination. When forearm fibrosis is extensive, and digital contractures are severe, the infarcted muscle cords are excised. In the severely fibrotic forearm, the flexor digitorum superficialis can be excised.

If minimal fibrosis is present, the tendons may be lengthened by fractional lengthening. Fractional lengthening is performed by placing multiple incisions in the tendinous portions that are proximal to the distal end of the junction, leaving the muscle fibers intact to preserve continuity. The tendon is passively lengthened, opening gaps in the tendinous portion to achieve lengthening (Fig. 19).

If there is severe, fixed digital flexion in a nonfunctional hand, the superficialis-to-profundus transfer is fea-

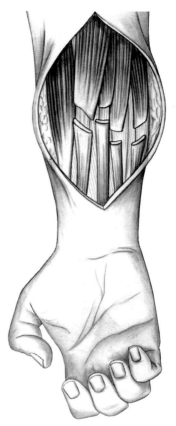

FIGURE 19. Fractional lengthening or release for established contracture.

sible to assist with hygiene and dressing. This transfer provides a large amount of extrinsic digital flexor lengthening while restricting finger hyperextension and preventing possible overcorrection. The procedure usually achieves more correction than Z-lengthening or fractional lengthening (Fig. 20).

Operative Technique: Superficialis-to-Profundus Transfer to Lengthen Flexor Tendons. In the superficialis-to-profundus transfer, a longitudinal, curved incision is made on the palmar aspect of the distal two-thirds of the forearm (449). The median nerve, the ulnar nerve and artery, and the radial artery are protected. The flexor digitorum superficialis and the flexor digitorum profundus are exposed. The tendons of the flexor digitorum superficialis are sutured together at an equal length in an en masse fashion 1 to 2 cm proximal to the wrist. A straight needle and a 3-0 nonabsorbable suture are used. The tendons are transected distal to the level of the suture. The tendons of the flexor digitorum superficialis are then reflected, providing access to the flexor digitorum profundus. The tendons of the flexor digitorum profundus are sutured together at an equal length in an en masse fashion proximally in the forearm at or near the level of the musculotendinous junction. A 3-0

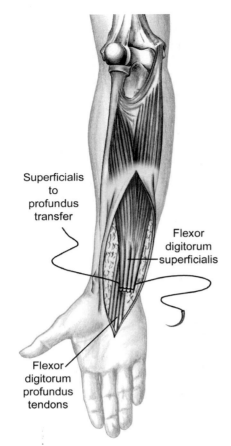

Superficialis
to
profundus
transfer

Flexor
digitorum
superficialis

Flexor
digitorum
profundus
tendons

FIGURE 20. Superficialis-to-profundus transfer.

nonabsorbable suture is used. These tendons are transected just proximal to the level of the suture. The digits are then extended to the desired corrected position. Slight digital flexion should be retained to prevent possible overcorrection. The proximal portion of the flexor digitorum superficialis is sutured to the distal portion of the flexor digitorum profundus. The wrist flexors and flexor pollicis longus tendons are lengthened at the same time, if desired (Fig. 20) (449).

POSTOPERATIVE CARE. After flexor tendon lengthening, a bulky dressing is applied. The digits are immobilized for 4 weeks. Mobilization and strengthening are initiated in a comprehensive therapy program.

Operative Technique: Flexor Pollicis Longus Lengthening. A gentle, curved longitudinal incision is placed on the distal one-third of the radiopalmar forearm (439). The flexor carpi radialis tendon, the median nerve with its palmar cutaneous branch, and the radial artery are identified and protected. The flexor pollicis longus tendon is located deep to the flexor carpi radialis tendon. The tendon is lengthened by fractional lengthening in the musculotendinous portion or by Z-lengthening through the tendinous portion

(depending on the length of coexisting tendon and muscle in the musculotendinous junction that are encountered at the time of dissection). Fractional lengthening is performed by placement of two to three incisions into the tendinous portion that is proximal to the musculotendinous junction, leaving the connecting muscle fibers intact to preserve continuity of the muscle. The thumb is extended to the desired corrected position, creating gaps at the incisions of the tendinous portion and thereby lengthening the muscle–tendon unit. With Z-lengthening or fractional lengthening, care is taken to avoid overcorrection. Residual flexion of 10 to 20 degrees is desirable. A bulky dressing is applied, and the thumb is immobilized in the corrected position for 3 to 4 weeks (Fig. 21) (439).

POSTOPERATIVE CARE. The hand and wrist are immobilized for 4 weeks after tendon lengthening. The digits and the wrist are then mobilized and strengthened in a comprehensive hand therapy program.

Flexor Pronator Slide. The flexor pronator slide, which was described by Page in 1923 (450), has since gained acceptance and has been shown to be more effective than infarct excision alone in obtaining a lasting correction (66,67,69,70).

The flexor pronator slide has been criticized for the occasional unpredictability of the correction that is achieved, the risk of recurrence of deformity with growth, the possibility of overcorrection, and the resultant decrease in grip strength, particularly at the distal interphalangeal joint (132,135,186,208,405,413,451). Overcorrection can result in the extremity developing a position of forearm pronation and wrist extension. Despite these potential problems, the procedure has gained popularity and has proven effective in achieving satisfactory results in a large group of patients with moderate to severe contractures (69,70).

OPERATIVE TECHNIQUE: FLEXOR PRONATOR SLIDE. In the flexor pronator slide, an incision is placed on the medial aspect of the elbow, originating approximately 6 cm proximal to the medial humeral condyle (Fig. 22). The incision is extended to the junction of the middle and distal two-thirds of the forearm. Subcutaneous tissue is separated from the deep fascia on the ulnar and radial sides of the incision. The ulnar nerve is isolated at the level of the elbow and is transposed anteriorly. The origins of the pronator teres, flexor carpi radialis, palmaris longus, and humeral head of the flexor carpi ulnaris are systematically released, followed by detachment of the flexor digitorum superficialis. The muscles are sharply dissected subperiosteally and are mobilized. The ulnar head of the flexor carpi ulnaris and the broad origin of the flexor digitorum profundus are released from the anterior aspect of the ulna. The dissection is extended across the interosseous membrane, and the flexor

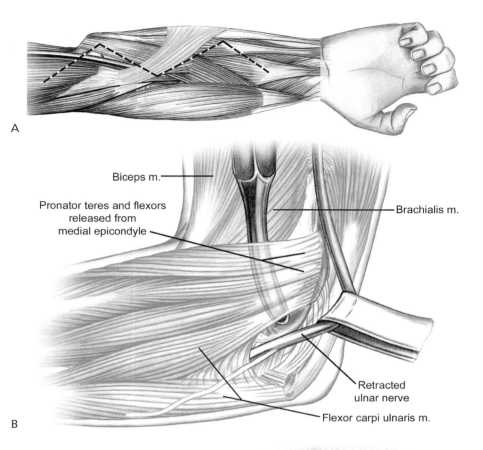

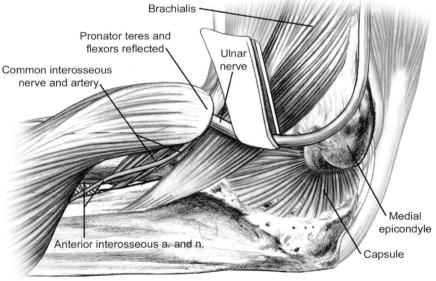

FIGURE 21. Methods to correct the contracted thumb. **A:** Thenar origin and adductor pollicis recession. The origins of the abductor pollicis brevis, flexor pollicis brevis, and the opponens pollicis are gently freed from their attachments on the transverse carpal ligament. If needed, the adductor pollicis is released. The distal portion of the transverse carpal ligament often requires release to allow adequate access to the most proximal origin of the adductor pollicis. After thumb position correction, the muscles are allowed to reattach in a more radial and distal position. **B:** Release of the first dorsal interosseous is performed through a dorsal incision along the ulnar margin of the thumb metacarpal. The muscle (m.) is released from its origin from the metacarpal. The insertion of the adductor pollicis can be released at the distal margin of the incision. **C:** Lengthening of the flexor pollicis longus is performed through its tendinous portion by Z-lengthening **(A)** or fractional lengthening **(B)** if there is an adequate myotendinous junction. a., artery; n., nerve.

pollicis longus is released from the anterior radius. The interosseous artery, vein, and nerves require protection during release of the flexors from the interosseous membrane. The muscles are allowed to slide distally 2 to 3 cm as the digits and wrist are passively extended to a corrected position. If needed, the incision is extended distally to the palmar wrist capsule, and the pronator quadratus is released. Excision of the infarcted muscle and nerve decompression

may also be performed at this time. Tendon transfers, if warranted, are performed secondarily.

POSTOPERATIVE CARE. After flexor pronator slide, the extremity is immobilized for 3 weeks with the elbow at 90 degrees, the forearm supinated, and the wrist and digits extended. A hand therapy program is then initiated for mobilization and strengthening.

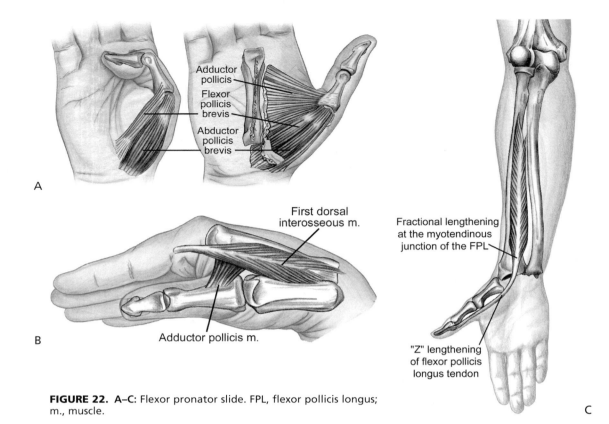

FIGURE 22. A–C: Flexor pronator slide. FPL, flexor pollicis longus; m., muscle.

Phase 3: Tendon Transfers to Restore or Reinforce Function. Among the most desirable functions to restore in the patient with ischemic contractures are finger and thumb flexion and thumb opposition (5,44,46,69,70,439). Tendon transfers are usually delayed until decompressed nerves have recovered maximally and until contractures have been corrected with mobilization and splinting or with operative release or lengthening. A series of tendon transfers has been developed to provide digital flexion and thumb opposition (56,69,70,159–161,442,452). Because forearm extensors are usually the least involved muscles in ischemic contractures, these muscles are often suitable donors. In 1947, Phalen and Miller (452) described transfer of the extensor carpi radialis longus to the flexor digitorum profundus and transfer of the extensor carpi ulnaris, lengthened by tendon graft, to the thumb for opposition. The flexor digitorum superficialis tendons are excised if they are nonfunctional. The extensor pollicis brevis can be used to reinforce the extensor carpi ulnaris–opponens transfer. Alternative transfers to augment thumb opposition include the well-described extensor indicis proprius opponensplasty [popularized by Zancolli (442) and Burkhalter et al. (453)] and the abductor digiti quinti opponensplasty [described by Huber (454)].

When flexor tendons have been severely weakened by previous lengthening, reinforcement by transfer of the extensor carpi radialis longus to the flexor digitorum pro-fundus and transfer of the extensor carpi ulnaris to the flexor pollicis longus can be performed. Techniques are described by Goldner (56,159–161).

Operative Technique: Transfer of the Extensor Carpi Radialis Longus to the Flexor Digitorum Profundus. In transfer of the extensor carpi radialis longus to the flexor digitorum profundus, a volar forearm incision is placed, and the flexor digitorum tendons are isolated from the remaining fibrous muscle mass. Full passive extension of the digits and free gliding of the flexor tendons are required. Through a dorsal incision, the extensor carpi radialis longus tendon is detached from its insertion into the second metacarpal, and the muscle and tendon are mobilized freely on the dorsum of the forearm. The muscle is rerouted deep to the brachioradialis and inserted into the flexor digitorum profundus tendons by using a tendon weave to obtain appropriate tension. Tension is adjusted so that the digits are held in 45 degrees of flexion at the metacarpophalangeal joints and 45 degrees at the interphalangeal joints. Nonabsorbable suture is used for tenorrhaphy.

POSTOPERATIVE CARE. The wrist and digits are immobilized in 20 degrees of flexion, using a bulky long arm hand dressing and plaster splints. Active mobilization is initiated in 3 weeks, and gentle extension is obtained by the use of night splints and mild, manual, intermittent stretching. At the end of 6 weeks, dynamic splinting with outriggers is used as necessary. Full active extension may not be possible because of limited extrinsic tendon excursion and persistent fibrosis of the digit (56,159–161).

Operative Technique: Transfer of the Extensor Carpi Ulnaris That Is Lengthened by a Tendon Graft to Augment Opposition. If the flexor pollicis longus tendon has been excised because of extensive fibrosis, the extensor carpi radialis longus may be transferred to this tendon as well as the digital flexors.

If thumb weakness remains, especially when it involves the intrinsics, the extensor carpi ulnaris, which is lengthened by a tendon graft, is used to augment opposition (137).

A dorsal incision is used to detach the extensor carpi ulnaris tendon approximately 5 cm proximal to its insertion into the small-finger metacarpal. The tendon is elongated by a free tendon graft that is taken from the second or third extrinsic toe extensor or from the plantaris (or palmaris longus if present and not affected by scarring or severe adhesive contracture). The tendon graft is used to lengthen the extensor carpi ulnaris. The graft is attached to the distal, mobilized end of the extensor carpi ulnaris by using a Pulvertaft tendon weave technique. The lengthened extensor carpi ulnaris tendon is transferred around the ulnar aspect of the forearm and is inserted into the tendon of the abductor pollicis brevis. A Pulvertaft tendon weave is used to secure the graft into the abductor pollicis brevis.

POSTOPERATIVE CARE. The hand is immobilized with the thumb in palmar abduction for 3 weeks. A hand therapy program is then initiated for mobilization and strengthening.

Operative Technique: Brachioradialis Tendon Transfer to the Flexor Pollicis Longus to Augment Thumb Flexion. To augment thumb flexion, the brachioradialis may be transferred to the flexor pollicis longus (54,56,159–161,442).

Through a radiovolar incision, the brachioradialis is mobilized along its course from its tendinous insertion to the muscle in the proximal forearm. Care is taken to protect the superficial branch of the radial nerve. The muscle is detached distally, transferred volarly, and attached to the distal segment of the flexor pollicis longus tendon under slight tension.

POSTOPERATIVE CARE. The extremity is immobilized for 4 weeks with the thumb in flexion. A hand therapy program is then initiated for mobilization and strengthening.

Operative Technique: Transfer of the Biceps to the Thumb and Digital Flexors to Augment Thumb and Digital Flexion. If the radial nerve has been damaged, and its innervated muscles are not available for transfer, the biceps may be used to augment digital flexion.

The biceps insertion is detached from the radius through an incision in the proximal forearm. The muscle is lengthened by a tendon graft, obtained from a toe extensor or plantaris, and passed subcutaneously from the elbow to the junction of the middle and distal two-thirds of the forearm. The distal forearm tendon segments of the thumb and finger flexors are isolated and sutured with firm tension into the elongated biceps tendon. Flexion of the elbow helps maintain a tight transfer of the biceps. Segments of the flexor digitorum superficialis are excised from the distal forearm and hand and are used to reinforce tenorrhaphy sites at the elbow and the distal forearm.

POSTOPERATIVE CARE. The extremity is immobilized with the elbow in flexion and with the digits slightly flexed for 4 weeks. A hand therapy program is then initiated for mobilization and strengthening.

After this procedure, patients may obtain the ability to flex the digits when the elbow is extended and the wrist is dorsiflexed. The hand may function as a hook with a weak pinch, and patients are able to use the hand for carrying light objects (56,160,161).

Phase 4: Salvage of the Severely Contracted or Neglected Forearm. The procedures of phases 2 and 3 usually provide satisfactory results, and additional operative procedures are rarely indicated (5,44,46,56,69,70,159–161, 442,452). However, additional measures are occasionally required for reconstruction of severe contractures, especially in the neglected forearm. Described procedures for these involved extremities include proximal or distal row carpectomy (which provides limb shortening to allow wrist extension while maintaining flexibility), radial and ulnar shortening, wrist arthrodesis, and digital joint arthrodesis. Proximal or distal row carpectomy may be performed before tendon transfer in severe deformities. Interphalangeal joint arthrodesis in a more functional position can correct severe fixed contractures, especially when adequate donor muscles are not available for transfer. Arthrodesis that is combined with phalangeal shortening relieves tension on the digital neurovascular structures, as the digit is extended to a more functional position. After interphalangeal joint arthrodesis, the limb can function as a hook, which is generally superior to a prosthesis, especially if sensibility is retained (101,160). Radial and ulnar shortening and wrist arthrodesis are rarely indicated for treatment for salvage of Volkmann's contracture.

Reconstruction of Intrinsic Hand Deformities in Ischemic Contracture

The hand deformity that is associated with Volkmann's contracture is complex and requires a systematic therapeutic approach (62,100,160,162,163,178,317,451,455–471). Intrinsic contractures are usually addressed only after extrinsic finger flexors have been released. Fixed extrinsic contractures create a claw hand (intrinsic minus) deformity, which is characterized by hyperextension at the metacarpophalangeal joints and flexion at the proximal and distal interphalangeal joints. After extrinsic muscle release, as the proximal and distal interphalangeal joints are pulled out of flexion, intrinsic tightness may be revealed. If a tight clenched-fist deformity was originally present and then released, an intrinsic-plus deformity of the hand may develop.

Fixed myostatic contracture of the intrinsic muscles is treated with intrinsic lengthening, recession, or release. Lengthening is performed on the lateral bands of the extensor hood mechanism at the level of the proximal phalanx. Recession is performed at the origin of the interosseous muscles at the metacarpal level. Release of the intrinsic muscles is performed through the tendinous portion at the level of the metacarpophalangeal joints. Complete release of intrinsic contractures may not be desirable, because retaining some metacarpophalangeal joint flexion prevents recurrence of the claw hand deformity. If intrinsic contracture is severe, the oblique fibers of the extensor hood may be released to permit flexion of the interphalangeal joints (162,163,468,472). Alternatively, an interosseous muscle slide procedure can be considered for intrinsic contracture. The intrinsic muscle slide procedure effectively loosens tight but functional interossei, while preserving function. The procedure has been criticized as being extensive, traumatic, and the cause of moderate bleeding. Therefore, the distal intrinsic release is usually optimal.

The more significant hand impairments are not always caused by intrinsic contractures but rather by secondary problems from sequelae of extrinsic muscle contractures in the forearm. Loss of median and ulnar nerve sensibility, intrinsic paralysis that is secondary to median and ulnar motor nerve paralysis, and interphalangeal joint flexion deformities that are secondary to contracture of the extrinsic flexors cause severe functional deficits. Proper management of these problems, as described in phases 1 and 2, should significantly improve hand function.

Author's Preferred Operative Technique: Distal Intrinsic Contracture Release

In distal intrinsic contracture release, a 4-cm incision is placed over the dorsum of the proximal phalanx (468,472). Dissection is carried out ulnarly and radially to expose the palmar edge of the lateral bands. Each lateral band and its oblique fibers are transected. Care is taken to preserve the transverse fibers of the intrinsic apparatus, as well as the central and lateral slips of the extensor tendon.

Postoperative Care

Flexion exercises are begun 2 to 3 days postoperatively, provided that extrinsic lengthening was not performed (468,472).

Operative Technique: Interosseous Muscle Slide

In interosseous muscle slide, a dorsal transverse incision is placed at the level of the mid-shafts of the metacarpals. The digital extensors are isolated and retracted radially, then ulnarly. Subperiosteal dissection is performed to free the interossei from their origins on the metacarpals. Capsulectomy of the metacarpophalangeal joints may be required.

Thumb flexion or adduction deformity can accompany the claw hand in Volkmann's contractures. The deformity may result from intrinsic and extrinsic contractures (5,46,55,439,440). Flexion contracture of the interphalangeal joint, which is attributable to the flexor pollicis longus, may be corrected with tendon lengthening or release (as noted previously). Residual flexion or adduction deformities can be due to thenar muscle or adductor pollicis contracture, contracture of the first dorsal interosseous, joint capsule contracture, or skin contracture of the first web, or a combination of these. The abductor pollicis brevis and the flexor pollicis brevis contribute to flexion deformity at the metacarpophalangeal joint. The adductor pollicis, opponens pollicis, and first dorsal interosseous contribute palmar adduction of the thumb metacarpal (440). Procedures that are recommended for correction of these thumb deformities are directed at the specific contributing muscles. These procedures include thenar origin release, adductor pollicis release (at its origin or insertion), first dorsal interosseous release, deepening of the thumb web space, fusion of the metacarpophalangeal joint or interphalangeal joint, or excision of the trapezium (439,440).

When the flexor pollicis brevis, abductor pollicis brevis, and opponens pollicis are involved, recession of their origin is performed. If needed, the adductor pollicis is released at this time through the same incision (Fig. 21). This procedure allows the muscles to reattach with the thumb in a corrected position. Function is preserved, and overcorrection is avoided (439).

Postoperative Care
The digits are splinted in the intrinsic-minus position, and the interosseous muscles are permitted to reattach more distally. Early active interphalangeal flexion exercises are encouraged.

Technique: Thenar Origin and Adductor Pollicis Recession

In thenar origin and adductor pollicis recession, a curved incision is placed in the palm along the thenar crease (Fig. 21) (439). Dissection is extended to the base of the thenar muscles. The flexor pollicis brevis and abductor pollicis brevis are identified at their origin from the transverse carpal ligament. These muscles are elevated from their attachments on the transverse carpal ligament, taking care to protect the recurrent motor branch of the median nerve. The proximal phalanx of the thumb is extended, allowing the released thenar muscles to slide radially. Exposure of the opponens pollicis is provided, and its origin is released in a similar fashion. The thumb is held in a corrected position for 3 to 4 weeks.

If the adductor pollicis is involved, it is released at the time of thenar origin release. The muscle is identified in the distal aspect of the incision, deep and distal to the flexor pollicis brevis. The adductor pollicis is released from its origin on the third metacarpal or near its insertion. To release the muscle from its origin, the digital neurovascular bundles and flexor tendons to the index and long fingers are identified and retracted. The adductor pollicis is traced to its origin on the third metacarpal. The deep palmar vascular arch and the deep branch of the ulnar nerve pierce the muscle between its transverse and oblique heads. The neurovascular structures are protected, and the muscle is freed from the third metacarpal. Partial release of the distal portion of the transverse carpal ligament assists exposure of the proximal portion of the muscle. If the adductor pollicis is to be released from its tendinous insertion, the muscle is traced radially and released (439). The thumb is held in a corrected position for 3 to 4 weeks.

Postoperative Care

Mobilization and strengthening are initiated after the period of immobilization.

Technique: Release of the First Dorsal Interosseous

Release of the origin of the adductor pollicis has the advantage of preserving function. Release at the insertion, although technically easier, obliterates the muscle's function.

A longitudinal incision is placed on the dorsum of the hand along the palpable ulnar margin of the thumb metacarpal (Fig. 21). Branches of the radial sensory nerve are protected. The tendon of the extensor pollicis longus is identified along the radial margin of the incision. The dissection is continued ulnarly to the extensor pollicis longus tendon to expose the broad origin of the first dorsal interosseous from the ulnar margin of the thumb metacarpal. The muscle is freed from its origin, and the thumb metacarpal is abducted in the plane of the palm to a corrected position. The insertion of the adductor pollicis can be released at this time if the incision is extended distally to the metacarpophalangeal joint. The tendinous insertion is visible at the ulnar margin of the base of the proximal phalanx, distal to the first dorsal interosseous muscle. The tendon is released through this tendinous portion, including release of the attachments to the ulnar sesamoid. The thumb is immobilized for 4 weeks (439).

Postoperative Care

Mobilization and strengthening are initiated after the period of immobilization.

Technique: Arthrodesis of the Thumb Interphalangeal Joint

When fixed flexion deformity exists at the interphalangeal joint of the thumb, arthrodesis provides a satisfactory means of correction.

A curved dorsal incision is placed over the flexed interphalangeal joint (439). The articular surfaces of the interphalangeal joint are denuded of cartilage, the joint is positioned in 10 to 15 degrees of flexion and 10 degrees of pronation. Internal fixation is accomplished by using crossed 0.045-in. wires, screws, or a wire loop. The joint is immobilized for 4 to 6 weeks or until fusion is evident.

Postoperative Care

Mobilization and strengthening are initiated after the period of immobilization.

Free Tissue Transfers for Ischemic Contracture

The severely contracted upper extremity after ischemic insult remains a challenging problem, despite the procedures that were previously described. Free transfer of vascularized muscle, nerve, and skin offers potential additional methods of reconstruction. Several isolated case reports or small studies have been reported (69,70,164–170,473–475). Transfer of the lateral head of the pectoralis major to the flexor forearm in a patient with Volkmann's contracture was reported by Chien et al. in 1977 (164). Satisfactory results have been achieved by using a free vascularized superficial radial nerve graft that is transferred to an irreparably damaged median nerve (69,70,167). Chuang et al. (165,166) have achieved an 80% success rate in free muscle transfer in nine patients who underwent ten transfers for Volkmann's contracture. Free tissue transfer has become increasingly popular, and reconstruction of forearm muscles by using gracilis, rectus femoris, latissimus dorsi, or pectoralis muscles has been described by Manktelow et al. (168,169), McLaren (170), and Chuang (165–167). The early results of these procedures are promising, especially in their role in the reconstruction of severe, neglected Volkmann's contracture in which few adequate donor muscles are available for tendon transfers.

EXERTIONAL COMPARTMENT SYNDROME

Exertional compartment syndrome is characterized by intracompartmental pressures that transiently rise after repetitive motion or exercise, thereby producing temporary, reversible ischemia, pain, weakness, and, occasionally, neurologic deficits (10,28,71,73–77,83–88,115,190,343,356,357,476–480).

It has been specifically defined by Mubarak and Hargens (8) as a condition in which exercise induces high pressure within a closed space that is bounded by bone, fascia, or both, thus resulting in decreased tissue perfusion and ischemic pain. *Exertional* compartment syndrome is a separate, relatively benign affliction that should not be confused with *acute* compartment syndrome. This form of compartment syndrome is usually not associated with the permanent sequelae of ischemic contractures (73).

Exertional compartment syndrome is also referred to as *chronic* or *recurrent* compartment syndrome. Symptoms eventually resolve over minutes or hours but reoccur when activity or exercise is resumed. Although noted to occur in the forearm (71,80,83,94) or hand (73,91), exertional compartment syndrome is more commonly reported in the lower extremity (28,31,10,76,77,84,88,90,348,357,476–479) and, occasionally, in the trunk (480,481). Because the symptoms are transient and induced by activity, the terms *exercised-induced* or *intermittent compartment syndrome* have also been used to describe chronic, recurrent, or exertional compartment syndrome (73).

Pathophysiology of Exertional Compartment Syndrome

In acute compartment syndrome, there is usually an obvious inciting event or injury that precipitates the syndrome (7,8,11,25,118–125,144–146,190,208). In exertional compartment syndrome, however, the exact cause is often not as clear, and the pathogenesis remains less well understood. With normal exercise, there is usually a transient increase in intracompartmental pressure from edema. In most patients, this short-lived increase rapidly resolves. In the patient with exertional compartment syndrome, the increased pressure remains elevated for an extended period of time. Sustained pressure, although temporary, leads to intracompartmental ischemia, which produces symptoms (Fig. 23) (28). With rest, the symptoms of exertional compartment syndrome do resolve over several minutes or hours, and there is no residual neurologic or muscular sequela.

In the upper extremity, exertional compartment syndrome has been linked to the repetitive motion in sports (such as tennis), in musicians who use stringed instruments, and in assembly line workers who are involved with repetitive tasks. Case reports have described exertional compartment syndrome that involves the first dorsal interosseous muscle of the hand (91,345) and of the compartments of the forearm (71,80,83). The activities that precipitated the compartment syndrome include routine strenuous work activity and repetitive motion. One patient developed recurrent symptoms while motorcycle racing (71).

Most information on exertional compartment syndrome has been obtained from patients in whom the syndrome involves the lower extremities (10,28,31,76,77,84,88,90, 348,357,476–479). Several related theories exist as to the

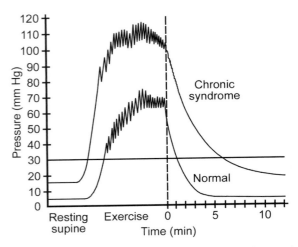

FIGURE 23. Comparison of muscle pressure activity in a patient with chronic compartment syndrome and a healthy patient. In this case, the anterior leg compartment was involved and was used as an example. The anterior compartment pressures were recorded with the wick catheter in place during exercise in a patient who had a chronic anterior compartment syndrome and in a healthy patient. The resting pressure of the chronic syndrome patient is elevated compared to that of the healthy patient. During exercise, the pressure rises to greater than 100 mm Hg and remains greater than 30 mm Hg for more than 5 minutes in the patient with the chronic compartment syndrome.

pathogenesis. In general, lower extremity exertional compartment syndrome is more easily linked to exercise or activity. The specific activity is felt to cause a disturbance of microvascular flow owing to elevated intramuscular pressure, which leads to tissue ischemia, depletion of high-energy phosphate stores, and extreme cellular acidosis (25,26,335). The result is a condition of intermittent and reversible elevation of intracompartmental pressures (25,26,71,356,478). Anatomic factors are believed to contribute to the development of chronic compartment syndrome. These include a limited compartment size, increased intracompartmental volume, constricted fascia, loss of compartment elasticity, poor venous return, or increased muscle bulk (25,26,80,89,94). Styf et al. (91, 480,481) suggested that exertional compartment syndrome may be related to occlusion of larger vessels by local muscle herniation as they traverse the interosseous membrane. Martens and Moeyersoons (263) attributed the exertional compartment syndrome to noncompliance of the deep fascia that does not accommodate the increase in muscle volume that normally occurs during exercise. Detmer et al. (75) noted an increased thickness of the fascia in 25 of 36 biopsies from leg compartments of patients with exertional compartment syndrome. Exercise-induced muscle hypertrophy and abnormal swelling of pathologic muscle within a normal fascial envelope have also been suggested as etiologic factors (25,26,85). Soffer et al. (90) described a patient with aberrant, constricting fascial bands of the anterior leg that were believed to be responsible for bilateral exertional compartment syndrome. Martens and Moeyersoons (263) described an anomalous plantaris muscle that contained an aberrant distal muscular extension that appeared to be the cause of exertional compartment syndrome of the superficial posterior compartment. Trauma has also been suggested as a causative factor in exertional compartment syndrome. A specific injury or event is occasionally associated with the development of the syndrome (80,83,348). Fascial scarring, adhesions, or interstitial fibrosis may result in loss of compartment compliance, thus predisposing the compartment to increased pressure with exercise (73).

Diagnosis of Exertional Compartment Syndrome

The diagnosis of exertional compartment syndrome is suspected by history and confirmed with examination and pressure monitoring before and after exercise. At rest, a patient may have few symptoms or signs, and intracompartmental pressures are normal or slightly elevated (83,347). Some patients may present with mild forearm atrophy or slight increased turgor (81). After a period of activity, the patient notes onset of pain, muscle tenseness or tenderness, and, occasionally, extremity numbness, tingling, and weakness (including loss of grip strength and digital extension) (80,347). Symptoms last for minutes or hours and severely limit further activity.

To confirm the diagnosis, a careful baseline physical exam is carried out, including compartment palpation, sensibility evaluation (with two-point discrimination, monofilament testing), motor evaluation (for muscle grading), joint range of motion, and vascular assessment (including color, temperature, capillary refill, and turgor) (73). Radiographs or a bone scan is obtained if a stress fracture is suspected. Vascular and cardiac consultations are obtained if claudication, peripheral vascular disease, or angina is believed to be a contributing factor (73).

Special Studies for Exertional Compartment Syndrome

A stress test is performed to provoke signs and symptoms of chronic compartment syndrome (25,26,83–87,347,348,478, 480). The patient performs the repetitive activity or exercise until symptoms are produced. Reexamination, including sensibility and strength testing, is carried out. Compartmental pressures (as well as any signs or symptoms) are monitored before, during, and after exercise. In a recently reported case, forearm compartment pressure increased from 6 to 32 mm Hg during exercise on the affected side and from 4 to 8 mm Hg on the unaffected side. A resting intramuscular pressure of greater than 15 mm Hg or a 5-minute postexercise pressure of greater than 25 mm Hg, or both, has been believed to be highly suggestive for chronic exertional compartment syndrome.

Adjunct studies include forearm volume analysis and nerve conduction velocities before and after exercise (80,83). Postexercise increased compartment volume has been demonstrated with volumetric analysis, with an increase of 30 cc detected on the abnormal side compared to 10 cc increase on the unaffected side (85). Nerve conduction velocities postexercise may be normal or abnormal (80,83).

Differential Diagnosis for Exertional Compartment Syndrome

Differential diagnosis includes claudication or other vascular abnormalities, myositis, tendinitis, periostitis, chronic strains or sprains, stress fracture, or other compression or systemic neuropathies (73). Cardiac abnormalities with angina or referred extremity pain should also be considered.

Prognosis of Exertional Compartment Syndrome

The prognosis of exertional compartment syndrome is based on the severity of symptoms and the patient's willingness to adjust activities. Elective fasciotomy can be performed if it is needed (80,83). Prognosis after fasciotomy is favorable, with resolution of symptoms usually expected. Postoperative compartment pressure measurements, taken before and after exercises, have shown complete resolution of previously sustained pressure increases that had preoperatively followed exercises (71,80,83,478).

Nonoperative Management of Exertional Compartment Syndrome

Nonoperative management of chronic compartment syndrome can initially be managed with regulation of the patient's activity. Many patients become aware of the activity threshold that induces symptoms and adjust activity level accordingly. A trial of protective splinting to minimize extremity motion during repetitive tasks may be beneficial. In the lower extremity, the use of diuretics has been promising (74). The role of anti-inflammatory medication has not been established. In refractory cases, or when activity adjustment is not practical, elective fasciotomy is indicated (73,75,80,83).

Operative Management of Exertional Compartment Syndrome

Operative Technique: Elective Fasciotomy for Exertional Compartment Syndrome

Fasciotomy for forearm decompression is performed as described previously in the operative techniques for acute compartment syndrome (1,4,5,44). The skin can usually be closed primarily because marked intracompartmental edema is usually not present. Reported operative findings have included moderately tense muscle compartments, thickened fascia, and aponeurotic bands that constrict the median or ulnar nerves in the forearm.

Postoperative Care

The extremity is placed in a bulky hand dressing. The dressing is changed at approximately 5 to 7 days, and a hand therapy program is initiated to regain motion and strength. The patient gradually increases activities, as tolerated, and resumes the repetitive or strenuous activities as comfort permits.

Complications of Exertional Compartment Syndrome

Complications of chronic compartment syndrome are much less severe than those in acute compartment syndrome. Permanent sequelae of ischemic contractures and chronic neuropathy do not usually occur. Surgical wound complications are similar to those that were described for fasciotomy of the volar compartment but are also less severe, because the wounds can often be closed primarily, and the need for skin grafting and the occurrence of scar contracture and cheloid formation are uncommon (73).

REFERENCES

1. Botte MJ, Gelberman RH. Acute compartment syndrome of the forearm. *Hand Clin* 1998;14:391–403.
2. Brostrom LA, Stark A, Svartengren G. Acute compartment syndrome in forearm fractures. *Acta Orthop Scand* 1990;61:50–53.
3. Dellaero DT, Levin LS. Compartment syndrome of the hand: etiology, diagnosis, and treatment. *Am J Orthop* 1996;25:404.
4. Gelberman RH, Garfin SR, Hergenroeder PT, et al. Compartment syndrome of the forearm: diagnosis and treatment. *Clin Orthop* 1981;161:252–261.
5. Gelberman RH. Upper extremity compartment syndromes: treatment. In: Mubarak SJ, Hargens AR, eds. *Compartment syndrome and Volkmann's contracture.* Philadelphia: WB Saunders, 1981:133–146.
6. Halpern AA, Nagel DA. Compartment syndromes of the forearm: early recognition using tissue pressure measurements. *J Hand Surg* 1979;4:258–263.
7. Hargens AR, Akeson WH, Mubarak SJ, et al. Kappa Delta Award paper. Tissue fluid pressures: from basic research tools to clinical applications. *J Orthop Res* 1989;7:902–909.
8. Hargens AR, Mubarak SJ. Current concepts in the pathophysiology, evaluation, and diagnosis of compartment syndrome. *Hand Clin* 1998;14:371–383.
9. Heckman MM, Whitesides TE Jr, Grewe SR, et al. Compartment pressure in association with closed tibial fractures. *J Bone Joint Surg* 1994;76:1285–1292.
10. Leach RE, Hammond G, Stryker WS. Anterior tibial compartment syndrome: acute and chronic. *J Bone Joint Surg* 1967;49:451–462.
11. Matsen FA III, Clawson DK. The deep posterior compartmental syndrome of the leg. *J Bone Joint Surg* 1975;57:34–39.
12. Matsen FA III, Mayo KA, Sheridan GW, et al. The continuous monitoring of intramuscular pressure and its application to clinical compartment syndromes. *Orthop Trans* 1977;1:81.
13. Matsen FA III, Mayo KA, Krugmire RB Jr, et al. A model compartmental syndrome in man with particular reference to the quantification of nerve function. *J Bone Joint Surg* 1977;59:648–653.
14. Matsen FA III, Winquist RA, Krugmire RB Jr. Diagnosis and management of compartment syndromes. *J Bone Joint Surg* 1980;62:286–291.
15. Matsen FA III, Wyss CR, Krugmire RB Jr, et al. The effects of limb elevation and dependency on local arteriovenous gradients in normal human limbs with particular reference to limbs with increased tissue pressure. *Clin Orthop* 1980;150:187.
16. Matsen FA III. *Compartmental syndromes.* New York: Grune & Stratton, 1980:1–162.
17. Matsen FA III, Veith RG. Compartmental syndromes in children. *J Pediatr Orthop* 1981;1:33.
18. Matsen FA III, Rorabeck CH. Compartment syndromes. *AAOS Instr Course Lect* 1989;38:463–472.
19. Maxwell JA, Kepes JJ, Ketchum LD. Acute carpal tunnel syndrome secondary to thrombosis of a persistent median artery. Case report. *J Neurosurg* 1973;38:774–777.
20. Mubarak SJ, Owen CA. Compartmental syndrome and its relation to the crush syndrome: a spectrum of disease. *Clin Orthop* 1975:113–181.
21. Mubarak SJ, Hargens AR, Owen CA, et al. The wick catheter technique for measurement of intramuscular pressure: a new research and clinical tool. *J Bone Joint Surg* 1976;58:1016.
22. Mubarak SJ, Owen CA. Double-incision fasciotomy of the leg for decompression in compartment syndromes. *J Bone Joint Surg* 1977;59:184–187.
23. Mubarak SJ, Owen CA, Hargens AR, et al. Acute compartment syndromes: diagnosis and treatment with the aid of the wick catheter. *J Bone Joint Surg* 1978;60:1091–1095.
24. Mubarak SJ, Carroll NC. Volkmann's contracture in children: etiology and prevention. *J Bone Joint Surg* 1979;61:285.
25. Mubarak SJ, Hargens AR, eds. *Compartment syndromes and Volkmann's ischemic contracture.* Philadelphia: WB Saunders, 1981.
26. Mubarak SJ, Hargens AR. Acute compartment syndromes. *Surg Clin North Am* 1983;63:539–565.
27. Mubarak SJ. Compartment syndromes. In: Chapman MW, ed. *Operative orthopaedics,* 2nd ed. Philadelphia: JB Lippincott Co, 1993:379–396.
28. Mubarak SJ. Surgical management of chronic compartment syndrome of the leg. *Oper Tech Sports Med* 1995;3:259–266.
29. Mubarak SJ. Treatment of acute compartment syndromes. In: Willy C, Sterk J, Gerngrofs H, eds. *Das Kompartment-Syndrom.* Berlin: Springer-Verlag, 1998:127–140.
30. Patman RD. Compartmental syndromes in peripheral vascular surgery. *Clin Orthop* 1975;113:103–110.
31. Rorabeck CH, Macnab I. The pathophysiology of the anterior tibial compartmental syndrome. *Clin Orthop* 1975;113:52–57.
32. Rorabeck CH, Macnab I. Anterior tibial compartment syn-

drome complication fractures of the shaft of the tibia. *J Bone Joint Surg* 1976;58:549–550.

33. Rorabeck CH, Castle GS, Hardie R, et al. Compartmental pressure measurements: an experimental investigation using the slit catheter. *J Trauma* 1981;21:446–449.

34. Whitesides TE Jr, Hirada H, Morimoto K. The response of skeletal muscle to temporary ischemia: an experimental study. *J Bone Joint Surg* 1971;53:1027–1028.

35. Whitesides TE Jr, Haney TC, Morimoto K, et al. Tissue pressure measurements as a determinant for the need of fasciotomy. *Clin Orthop* 1975;113:43–51.

36. Whitesides TE Jr, Haney TC, Hirada H, et al. A simple method for tissue pressure determination. *Arch Surg* 1975;110:1311–1313.

37. Whitesides TE Jr, Hirada H, Morimoto K. Compartment syndromes and the role of fasciotomy, its parameters and techniques. *AAOS Instr Course Lect* 1977;26:179.

38. Whitesides TE Jr. Methods of measurement of tissue pressure. In: Willy C, Sterk J, Gerngrofs H, eds. *Das Kompartment-Syndrom*. Berlin: Springer-Verlag, 1998:85–89.

39. Benjamin A. The relief of traumatic arterial spasm in threatened Volkmann's contracture. *J Bone Joint Surg* 1959;39:711.

40. Benkeddache Y, Bottesman H, Hamdani M. Proposal of a new classification for established Volkmann's contracture. *Ann Chir* 1985;4:134.

41. Bernays AC. On ischemic paralysis and contracture of muscles. *Boston Med Surg J* 1900;542:539–542.

42. Blount WP. Volkmann's ischemic contracture. *Surg Gynecol Obstet* 1950;90:244.

43. Botte MJ, Gelberman RH. Compartment syndrome and ischemic contracture. In: Nickel VL, Botte MJ, eds. *Orthopaedic rehabilitation*, 2nd ed. New York: Churchill Livingstone, 1992.

44. Botte MJ, Gelberman RH. Compartment syndrome and Volkmann's contracture. In: Peimer C, ed. *Surgery of the hand and upper extremity*. New York: McGraw-Hill, 1995:1539–1555.

45. Botte MJ. Compartment syndrome and Volkmann's ischemic contracture: preface. *Hand Clin* 1998;14:xiii–xiv.

46. Botte MJ, Keenan MA, Gelberman RH. Volkmann's ischemic contracture of the upper extremity. *Hand Clin* 1998;14:483–497.

47. Caouette-Laberge L, Bortoluzzi P, Egerszegi EP, et al. Neonatal Volkmann's ischemic contracture of the forearm: a report of five cases. *Plast Reconstr Surg* 1992;90:621.

48. Conner AN. Prolonged external pressure as a cause of ischemic contracture. *J Bone Joint Surg* 1971;53:118–122.

49. Eaton RG, Green WT. Epimysiotomy and fasciotomy in treatment of Volkmann's ischemic contracture. *Orthop Clin North Am* 1972;3:175–185.

50. Eaton RG, Green WT. Volkmann's ischemia: a volar compartment syndrome of the forearm. *Clin Orthop* 1975;113:58–64.

51. Eichler GR, Lipscomb PR. The changing treatment of Volkmann's ischemic contractures from 1955 to 1965 at the Mayo Clinic. *Clin Orthop* 1967;50:215.

52. Ernst CB, Kaufer H. Fibulectomy-fasciotomy: an important adjunct in the management of the lower extremity arterial trauma. *J Trauma* 1971;11:365–380.

53. Finochietto R. Volkmann's contracture of the intrinsic muscles of the hand. *Bol Trab Soc Cir (Buenos Aires)* 1920;4:31.

54. Gelberman RH. Volkmann's contracture of the upper extremity: pathology and reconstruction. In: Mubarak SJ, Hargens AR, eds. *Compartment syndrome and Volkmann's contracture*. Philadelphia: WB Saunders, 1981:183–193.

55. Gelberman RH, Botte MJ. Management of Volkmann's contracture. In: Chapman MW, ed. *Operative orthopaedics*, 2nd ed, vol. 2. Philadelphia: JB Lippincott Co, 1993:1169–1175.

56. Goldner JL. Volkmann's ischemic contracture. In: Flynn JE, ed. *Hand surgery*. Baltimore: Williams & Wilkins, 1975.

57. Griffiths DV. Volkmann's ischemic contracture. *Br J Surg* 1940;28:239.

59. Holden CE. The pathology and prevention of Volkmann's ischemic contracture. *J Bone Joint Surg* 1979;61:296.

60. Lipscomb PR. The etiology and prevention of Volkmann's ischemic contracture. *Surg Gynecol Obstet* 1956;103:353.

61. Matev I. Surgical treatment of spastic "thumb-in-palm" deformity. *J Bone Joint Surg* 1963;45:703.

62. Meyerding HW. Volkmann's ischemic contracture. *JAMA* 1930;94:394–400.

63. Moulonquet P, Seneque J. Syndrome de Volkmann. *Bull Mem Soc Nat Chir* 1928;54:1094.

64. Sarokhan AJ, Eaton RG. Volkmann's ischemia. *J Hand Surg* 1983;8:806–809.

65. Scaglietti O. Sindromi cliniche immediate e tardive da lesioni vascolari nelle fratture degli arti. *Fiforma Med* 1957;71:749–755.

66. Seddon HJ. Volkmann's contracture: treatment by incision of the infarct. *J Bone Joint Surg* 1956;38:152.

67. Seddon HJ. Volkmann's ischemia. *Br Med J* 1964;1:1587–1592.

68. Sorokhan AJ, Eaton RG. Volkmann's ischemia. *J Hand Surg* 1983;8:806.

69. Tsuge K. Treatment of established Volkmann's contracture. *J Bone Joint Surg* 1975;57:925.

70. Tsuge K. Management of established Volkmann's contracture. In: Green DP, Hotchkiss RN, eds. *Operative hand surgery*, 4th ed. New York: Churchill Livingstone, 1999:592–603.

71. Allen MJ, Barnes MR. Chronic compartment syndrome of the flexor muscles in the forearm: a case report. *J Hand Surg* 1989;14:47–48.

72. Balduini FC, Shenton DW, O'Connor KH, et al. Chronic exertional compartment syndrome: correlation of compartment pressure and muscle ischemia utilizing 31P-NMR spectroscopy. *Clin Sports Med* 1993;12:151–165.

73. Botte MJ, Fronek J, Pedowitz RA, et al. Exertional compartment syndrome of the upper extremity. *Hand Clin* 1998;14:477–482.

74. Christensen JT, Eklof B, Wulff K. The chronic compartment syndrome and response to diuretic treatment. *Acta Chir Scand* 1983;149:249–252.

75. Detmer DE, Sharpe K, Sufit RL, et al. Chronic compartment syndrome: diagnosis, management, and outcomes. *Am J Sports Med* 1985;13:162–170.

76. Garfin SR, Mubarak SJ, Owen CA. Exertional anterolateral compartment syndrome. *J Bone Joint Surg* 1977;59:404–405.

77. Goldfarb SJ, Kaeding CC. Bilateral acute-on-chronic exertional lateral compartment syndrome of the leg: a case report and review of the literature. *Clin J Sports Med* 1997;7:59–62.

78. Imbriglia JE, Boland DM. An exercise-induced compart-

ment syndrome of the dorsal forearm: a case report. *J Hand Surg* 1984;9:142–143.

79. Kirby NG. Exercise ischemia in the fascial compartment of the soleus: report of a case. *J Bone Joint Surg* 1970;52:738.

80. Kutz JE, Singer R, Lindsay M. Chronic exertional compartment syndrome of the forearm: a case report. *J Hand Surg* 1985;10:302–304.

81. Kwiatkowski TC, Detmer DE. Anatomical dissection of the deep posterior compartment and its correlation with clinical reports of chronic compartment syndrome involving the deep posterior compartment. *Clin Anat* 1997;10:104–111.

82. Lokiec F, Sievner I, Pritsch M. Chronic compartment syndrome of both feet. *J Bone Joint Surg* 1991;73:178.

83. Pedowitz RA, Toutounghi FM. Chronic exertional compartment syndrome of the forearm flexor muscles. *J Hand Surg* 1988;13:694–696.

84. Pedowitz RA, Hargens AR, Mubarak SJ, et al. Modified criteria for the objective diagnosis of chronic compartment syndrome of the leg. *Am J Sports Med* 1990;18:35–40.

85. Pedowitz RA, Gershuni DH. Diagnosis and treatment of chronic compartment syndrome. *Crit Rev Phys Rehabil Med* 1993;5:301–313.

86. Pedowitz RA, Garrett WE. Chronic compartment syndrome: case reports and literature review. *South Orthop J* 1994;3:244–250.

87. Pedowitz RA, Gershuni DH. Pathophysiology and diagnosis of chronic compartment syndrome. *Oper Tech Sports Med* 1995;3:230–236.

88. Raether PM, Lutter LD. Recurrent compartment syndrome in the posterior thigh. *Am J Sports Med* 1982;10:40–43.

89. Reneman RS. The anterior and the lateral compartmental syndrome of the leg due to intensive use of muscles. *Clin Orthop* 1975;113:69–80.

90. Soffer SR, Martin DF, Stanish WD, et al. Chronic compartment syndrome caused by aberrant fascia in an aerobic walker. *Med Sci Sports Exer* 1991;23:304.

91. Styf J, Forssblad P, Lundborg G. Chronic compartment syndrome in the first dorsal interosseous muscle. *J Hand Surg* 1987;12:757–762.

92. Styf JR. Intramuscular pressure measurements during exercise. *Oper Tech Sports Med* 1995;3:243–249.

93. Takebayashi S, Takazawa H, Sasaki R, et al. Chronic exertional compartment syndrome in lower legs: localization and follow-up with thallium-201 SPECT imaging. *J Nucl Med* 1997;38:972–976.

94. Tompkins DG. Exercise myopathy of the extensor carpi ulnaris muscle. *J Bone Joint Surg* 1977;59:407–408.

95. von Schroeder HP, Botte MJ. Crush syndrome of the upper extremity. *Hand Clin* 1998;14:451–456.

96. Trice M, Colwell CW. A historical review of compartment syndrome and Volkmann's ischemic contracture. *Hand Clin* 1998;14:335–341.

97. von Volkmann R. Krankenheiten der Bewegungsorgane. In: *Handbuch der Chirugie*, 2nd ed. Erlangen: Pitha-Billroth, 1869:846.

98. von Volkmann R. Die Ischaemischen Muskellahmungen und Kontrakturen. *Zentralbl Chir* 1881;8:801–803.

99. Leser E. Untersuchungen uber ischamische Muskellahumungen und Muskelcontracturen. *Samml Klin Vortrage* 1884;3:2087.

100. Thomas JJ. Nerve involvement in the ischemic paralysis and contracture of Volkmann. *Ann Surg* 1908;49:330.

101. Hildebrand O. Die Lehre von den ischamische Muskellahmungen un Kontrakuren. *Samml Klin Vortrage* 1906;122:437.

102. Brooks B. Pathological changes in muscle as a result of disturbances of circulation. An experimental study of Volkmann's ischemic paralysis. *Arch Surg* 1922;5:188.

103. Brooks B. New methods for study of diseases of the circulation of the extremities. *J Bone Joint Surg* 1925;7:316–318.

104. Brooks B, Johnson GS, Kirtley J Jr. Simultaneous vein ligation. An experimental study of the effect of ligation of the concomitant vein on the incidence of gangrene following arterial obstruction. *Surg Gynecol Obstet* 1934;59:496–500.

105. Jones, Sir R. Volkmann's ischaemic contracture with special reference to treatment. *Br Med J* 1928;2:639.

106. Leriche R. Surgery of the sympathetic system. Indications and results. *Ann Surg* 1928;88:449–469.

107. Goldner RD, Howson MP, Nunley JA, et al. One hundred eleven thumb amputations: replantation vs. revision. *Microsurgery* 1990;11:243–250.

108. Foisie PS. Volkmann's ischemic contracture. An analysis of its proximate mechanism. *N Engl J Med* 1942;226:671–679.

109. Rowlands RP, Lond MS. A case of Volkmann's contracture treated by shortening the radius and ulna. *Lancet* 1905;2:1168–1171.

110. Bardenheuer L. Die entstehung und behandlung der ischamischen muskelkontractur und gangran. *Dtsch Z Chir* 1911;108:44.

111. Murphy JB. Myositis. *JAMA* 1914;63:1249.

112. Jepson PN. Ischemic contracture. Experimental study. *Am Surg* 1926;84:785–795.

113. Jepson PN. The classic. Ischemic contracture experimental study. *Clin Orthop* 1975;113:3–7.

114. Jorge J. Retraction ischemique de Volkmann. Rapport d'Albert monchet. *Bull Mem Soc Nat Chir* 1925;51:884.

115. Massart R. La maladie de Volkmann. *Rev Orthop* 1935;22:385.

116. Garber JN. Volkmann's contracture as a complication of fractures of the forearm and elbow. *J Bone Joint Surg* 1939;21:154–168.

117. Ashton H. Critical closure in human limbs. *Br Med Bull* 1963;19:149.

118. Hargens AR, Mubarak SJ, Owen CA, et al. Interstitial fluid pressure in muscle and compartment syndromes in man. *Microvasc Res* 1977;14:1–10.

119. Hargens AR, Akeson WH, Mubarak SJ, et al. Fluid balance within the canine anterolateral compartment and its relationship to compartment syndromes. *J Bone Joint Surg* 1978;60:499–505.

120. Hargens AR, Evans KL, Hagen PL, et al. Quantitation of skeletal muscle necrosis in a model compartment syndrome. Paper presented at: Orthopedic Research Society; February, 1978; Dallas, TX.

121. Hargens AR, Schmidt DA, Goncalves MR, et al. Quantitation of skeletal-muscle necrosis in a model compartment syndrome. *J Bone Joint Surg* 1981;63:631–636.

122. Hargens AR, Romine JS, Sipe JC, et al. Peripheral nerve conduction block by high muscle compartment pressure. *J Bone Joint Surg* 1979;61:192.

123. Hargens AR. *Tissue fluid pressure and composition.* Baltimore: Williams & Wilkins, 1981.

124. Hargens AR, Gershuni DH, Gould RN, et al. Tissue necrosis associated with tourniquet ischemia. XI European Conference for Microcirculation, Garmisch-Partenkirchen, Germany. *Bibliotheca Anatomica* 1981;20:599–601.

125. Hargens AR, Ballard RE. Basic principles for measurement of intramuscular pressure. *Oper Tech Sports Med* 1995;3:237–242.

126. Newmeyer WL, Kilgore ES Jr. Volkmann's ischemic contracture due to soft tissue injury alone. *J Hand Surg* 1976;1:221.

127. Henry AK. *Extensile exposure*, 2nd ed. London: Churchill Livingstone, 1973.

128. Doyle JR. Anatomy of the upper extremity muscle compartments. *Hand Clin* 1998;14:343–364.

129. Garfin SR. Anatomy of the extremity compartments. In: Mubarak SJ, Hargens AR, eds. *Compartment syndromes and Volkmann's ischemic contracture*. Philadelphia: WB Saunders, 1981.

130. Gellman H, Buch K. Acute compartment syndrome of the arm. *Hand Clin* 1998;14:385–389.

131. Ouellette EA, Kelly R. Compartment syndrome of the hand. *J Bone Joint Surg* 1996;78:1515–1522.

132. Aukland K, Reed RK. Interstitial-lymphatic mechanisms in the control of extracellular fluid volume. *Physiol Rev* 1993;73:1–78.

133. Barlow TE, Haigh AL, Walder DN. Evidence for two vascular pathways in skeletal muscle. *Clin Sci* 1961;20:367.

134. Birnstinge M. Vascular injuries. In: Wilson JN, ed. *Watson-Jones fractures and dislocations*, 6th ed, vol. 1. New York: Churchill Livingstone, 1982:215.

135. Blomfield LB. Intramuscular vascular patterns in man. *Proc R Soc Med* 1945;38:617.

136. Brown PW. Aetiology and investigation: introduction. In: Lamb DW, ed. *The paralysed hand*. Edinburgh, Scotland: Churchill Livingstone, 1987.

137. Clark WE, Blomfield LB. The efficiency of intramuscular anastomoses, with observations on the regeneration of devascularized muscle. *J Anat* 1945;79:15.

138. Dahn I, Lassen NA, Westling H. Blood flow in human muscles during external pressure or venous stasis. *Clin Sci* 1967;32:467–473.

139. Davies MG, Hagen PO. The vascular endothelium. A new horizon. *Ann Surg* 1993;218:593–609.

140. Eaton R, Sarokhan. Subacute compartment syndrome of the forearm. Paper presented at: AOA Annual Meeting; May, 1984; Palm Beach, FL.

141. Fronek K, Zweifach BW. Microvascular pressure distribution in skeletal muscle and the effect of vasodilation. *Am J Physiol* 1975;228:791–796.

142. Gershuni DH, Yaru NC, Hargens AR, et al. Ankle and knee position as a factor modifying intracompartmental pressure in the human leg. *J Bone Joint Surg* 1984;66:1415–1420.

143. Guyton AC. A concept of negative interstitial pressure based on pressures in implanted perforated capsules. *Circ Res* 1963;12:399–414.

144. Hargens AR, Botte MJ, Swenson MR, et al. Effects of local compression on peroneal nerve function in humans. *J Orthop Res* 1993;11:818–827.

145. Hargens AR, Villavicencio JL. Mechanics of tissue/lymphatic transport. In: Bronzino JD, ed. *Biomedical engineering handbook*. Boca Raton, FL: CRC Press, 1995:493–504.

146. Hargens AR. Pressure and time thresholds for acute compartment syndromes. In: Willy C, Sterk J, Gerngrofs H, eds. *Das Kompartment-Syndorm*. Berlin: Springer-Verlag, 1998:154–163.

147. Harman JW. The significance of local vascular phenomena in the production of ischemic necrosis in skeletal muscle. *Am J Pathol* 1948;24:625–642.

148. Henke TJ, Becker HP, Gernroof H. Entwicklung der intrakompartimentellen Mefstechnik. In: Willy C, Sterk J, Gerngrofs H, eds. *Das Kompartment-Syndrom*. Berlin: Springer-Verlag, 1998:112–118.

149. Littler JW. The hand and upper extremity. In: Converse JM, ed. *Reconstructive plastic surgery*. Philadelphia: WB Saunders, 1977.

150. Lundborg G, Gleberman RH, Minteer-Convery M, et al. Median nerve compression in the carpal tunnel: functional response to experimentally induced controlled pressure. *J Hand Surg* 1982;7:252–259.

151. Parkes A. Ischemic effects of external and internal pressure on the upper limb. *Hand* 1973;5:105–112.

152. Reneman RS, Slaff DW, Lindbom L, et al. Muscle blood flow disturbances produced by simultaneous elevated venous and total muscle tissue pressure. *Microvasc Res* 1980;20:307–318.

153. Seiler JG III, Havig M, Carpenter W. Acute carpal tunnel syndrome complicating chronic palmar subluxation of the distal ulna. *J South Orthop Assoc* 1996;5:108–110.

154. Sheridan GW, Matsen FA III, Krugmire RB Jr. Further investigations on the pathophysiology of the compartmental syndrome. *Clin Orthop* 1977;123:266–270.

155. Thomas EL, Grisham MB, Jefferson MM. Myeloperoxidase-dependent effect of amines on functions of isolated neutrophils. *J Clin Invest* 1983;72:441–454.

156. von Schroeder HP, Botte MJ. Definitions and terminology of compartment syndrome and Volkmann's ischemic contracture of the upper extremity. *Hand Clin* 1998;14:331–334.

157. Wertheimer P, Dechaume J. Infarctus musculaire d'origine veineuse. Documents experimentaux. *Lyon Chir* 1937;34:224–228.

158. Rowland SA. Fasciotomy: the treatment of compartment syndrome. In: Green DP, Hotchkiss RN, eds. *Operative hand surgery*, 4th ed. New York: Churchill Livingstone, 1999:689–710.

159. Goldner JL. Deformities of the hand incidental to pathological changes of the extensor and intrinsic muscle mechanisms. *J Bone Joint Surg* 1953;35:115–131.

160. Goldner JL. Intrinsic and extensor contractures of the hand due to ischemic and nonischemic causes. In: Flynn JE, ed. *Hand surgery*, 3rd ed. Baltimore: Williams & Wilkins, 1982;849–869.

161. Goldner J. Surgical reconstruction of the upper extremity in cerebral palsy. *Hand Clin* 1988;4:223–265.

162. Smith DC, Mitchell DA, Peterson GW, et al. Medial brachial fascial compartment syndrome: anatomic basis of neuropathy after transaxillary arteriography. *Radiology* 1989;173:149–154.

163. Smith PJ, Mott G. Sensory threshold and conductance testing in nerve injuries. *J Hand Surg* 1986;11:157–162.

164. Chien CW, Daniel RK, Terzis JK. *Reconstructive microsurgery*. Boston: Little, Brown and Company, 1977.

165. Chuang DCC, Chen HC, Wei FC, et al. Compound functioning free muscle flap transplantation (lateral half of soleus, fibula and skin flap). *Plast Reconstr Surg* 1992;89:335.

166. Chuang DCC, Strauch RJ, Wei FC. Technical considerations in two-stage functioning free muscle transplantation (FFMT) reconstruction of both flexor and extensor function of the forearm. *Microsurgery* 1994;15:338.

167. Chuang DCC. Functioning free muscle transplantation. In: Peimer CA, ed. *Surgery of the hand and upper extremity.* New York: McGraw-Hill, 1996:1901–1910.

168. Manktelow RT, Mckee NH. Free muscle transplantation to provide active finger flexion. *J Hand Surg* 1978;3:416.

169. Manktelow RT, Zuker RM. The principles of functioning muscle transplantation: applications to the upper arm. *Ann Plast Surg* 1989;22:1275.

170. McLaren AC, Ferguson JH, Miniaci AP. Crush syndrome associated with use of the fracture-table. *J Bone Joint Surg* 1987;69:1447–1449.

171. Colborn GL, Goodrich JA, Levine M, et al. The variable anatomy of the nerve to the extensor carpi radialis brevis. *Clin Anat* 1993;6:48.

172. Edwards DA. The blood supply and lymphatic drainage of tendons. *J Anat* 1946;80:147.

173. Grant RT, Wright HP. Further observations on the blood vessels of skeletal muscle (rat cremaster). *J Anat* 1968;103:553.

174. Maor P, Levy M, Lotem M, et al. Iatrogenic Volkmann's ischemia—a result of pressure-transfusion. *Int Surg* 1972; 57:415.

175. Saunders RL, Lawrence J, Maciver DA. Microradiographic studies of the vascular patterns in muscle and skin. In: *X-ray microscopy and microradiography.* New York: Academic Press, 1957.

176. Garfin SR, Mubarak SJ, Evans KL. Quantification of intracompartmental pressure and volume under plaster casts. *J Bone Joint Surg* 1981;63:449.

177. Williams PL. *Gray's anatomy,* 38th ed. New York: Churchill Livingstone, 1995.

178. Ortiz JA Jr, Berger RA. Compartment syndrome of the hand and wrist. *Hand Clin* 1998;14:405–418.

179. Szabo RM. Carpal tunnel syndrome—general. In: Gelberman RH, ed. *Operative nerve repair and reconstruction.* Philadelphia: JB Lippincott Co, 1991:869–888.

180. Szabo RM. Acute carpal tunnel syndrome. *Hand Clin* 1998;41:419–429.

181. Sotereanos DG, McCarthy DM, Towers JD, et al. The pronator quadratus: a distinct forearm space? *J Hand Surg* 1995;20:496.

182. Stuart PR. Pronator quadratus revisited. *J Hand Surg* 1996;21:714.

183. Summerfield SL, Folberg CR, Weiss A-P. Compartment syndrome of the pronator quadratus: a case report. *J Hand Surg* 1997;22:266.

184. Cobb TK, Dalley BK, Posteraro RH, et al. Anatomy of the flexor retinaculum. *J Hand Surg* 1993;18:91–99.

185. Cobb TK, Cooney WP, An KN. Pressure dynamics of the carpal tunnel and flexor compartment of the forearm. *J Hand Surg* 1995;20:193–198.

186. Bojsen-Moller F, Schmidt L. The palmar aponeurosis and the central spaces of the hand. *J Anat* 1974;117:55.

187. Aggarwal ND, Singh B, Gureja YP. Compression ischaemia of limbs from tight splintage. *J Bone Joint Surg* 1969;51:779–780.

188. Akeson WH, Hargens AR, Garfin SR, et al. Muscle compartment syndromes and snake bites. In: Hargens AR, ed. *Tissue fluid pressure and composition.* Baltimore: Williams & Wilkins, 1981:215.

189. Allen MJ, Steingold RF, Kotecha M, et al. The importance of the deep volar compartment in crush injuries of the forearm. *Injury* 1985;16:273–275.

190. Ashton H. The effect of increased tissue pressure on blood flow. *Clin Orthop* 1975;113:15–26.

191. Bentson LS, Sathy MJ, Port RB. Forearm compartment syndrome due to automated injection of computed tomography contrast material. *J Orthop Trauma* 1996;10:433–436.

192. Burton RI, Miller R. Compartment syndromes. In: Evarts CM, ed. *Surgery of the musculoskeletal system.* New York: Churchill Livingstone, 1983:175.

193. Failla JM. Compartment syndromes and ischemic contracture: hand, wrist, and forearm. In: Cooney WP, Linscheid RL, Dobyns JH, eds. *The wrist: diagnosis and treatment.* St. Louis: Mosby, 1998.

194. Holland DL, Swenson W, Tudor RB, et al. A compartment syndrome of the upper arm: a case report. *Am J Sports Med* 1985;13:363–364.

195. Howie CR, Buxton R. Acute carpal tunnel syndrome due to spontaneous haemorrhage. *J Hand Surg* 1984;9:137–138.

196. Lancourt JE, Gilbert MS, Posner MA. Management of bleeding and associated complications of hemophilia in the hand and forearm. *J Bone Joint Surg* 1977;59:451.

197. Owen CA. Crush syndrome. In: Mubarak SJ, Hargens AR, ed. Compartment syndromes and Volkmann's contracture. Philadelphia: WB Saunders, 1981:166–182.

198. Botte MJ, Rhoades CE, Gelberman RH, et al. Peroneal nerve function in acute anterior compartment syndrome. *Orthop Trans* 1986;10:206.

199. Clark WE, Le Gros. An experimental study of the regeneration of mammalian striped muscle. *J Anat* 1947;80:24.

200. Gelberman RH, Szabo RM, Williamson RV, et al. Tissue pressure threshold for peripheral nerve viability. *Clin Orthop* 1983;178:285–291.

201. Heppenstall RB, Scott R, Sapega A, et al. A comparative study of the tolerance of skeletal muscle to ischemia. *J Bone Joint Surg* 1986;68:820.

202. Heppenstall RB, Sapega AA, Scott R, et al. The compartment syndrome. An experimental and clinical study of muscular energy metabolism using phosphorous nuclear magnetic resonance spectroscopy. *Clin Orthop* 1988;226:138–155.

203. Karwatowska-Prokopczuk E, Czarnowska E, Beresewicz A. Iron availability and free radical-induced injury in the isolated ischaemic/reperfused rat heart. *Cardiovasc Res* 1992;26:58–66.

204. Rydevik B, Lundborg G. Permeability of intraneural microvessels and perineurium following acute, graded experimental nerve compression. *Scand J Plast Reconstr Surg* 1977;11:179.

205. Szabo R, Gelberman RH. Peripheral nerve compression etiology, critical pressure threshold, and clinical assessment. *Orthopedics* 1984;7:1461–1466.

206. Szabo RM, Gelberman RH. The pathophysiology of nerve entrapment syndromes. *J Hand Surg* 1987;12:880–884.

207. Yamaguchi S, Viegas SF. Causes of upper extremity compartment syndrome. *Hand Clin* 1998;14:365–370.

208. Ashton H. Effect of inflatable plastic splints on blood flow. *Br Med J* 1966;2:1427.

209. Bingold AC. On splitting plasters. A useful analogy. *J Bone Joint Surg* 1979;61:294.

210. Greene TL, Louis DS. Compartment syndrome of the arm—a complication of the pneumatic tourniquet: a case report. *J Bone Joint Surg* 1983;65:270–273.

211. O'Neil D, Sheppard JE. Transient compartment syndrome of the forearm resulting from venous congestion from a tourniquet. *J Hand Surg* 1989;14:894–896.

212. Ouellette EA. Compartment syndromes in obtunded patients. *Hand Clin* 1998;14:431–450.

213. Owen CA, Mubarak SJ, Hargens AR, et al. Intramuscular pressure with limb compression. Clarification of the pathogenesis of the drug-induced compartment syndrome/crush syndrome. *N Engl J Med* 1979;300:1169–1172.

214. Palmer AK. Complications from tourniquet use. *Hand Clin* 1986;2:301–305.

215. Patterson S, Klenerman L. The effect of pneumatic tourniquets on the ultrastructure of skeletal muscle. *J Bone Joint Surg* 1979;61:178–183.

216. Perkoff GT, Dioso MM, Bleisch V. A spectrum of myopathy associated with alcoholism. *Ann Intern Med* 1967;67:481–484.

217. Schreiber SN, Liebowitz MR, Bernstein LH, et al. Limb compression and renal impairment (crush syndrome) complicating narcotic overdose. *N Engl J Med* 1971;284:368–369.

218. Sutin KM, Longaker MT, Wahlander S, et al. Acute biceps compartment syndrome associated with the use of a noninvasive blood pressure monitor. *Anesth Analg* 1996;83:1345.

219. McNeill IF, Wilson JS. The problems of limb replacement. *Br J Surg* 1970;57:365–377.

220. Abbott LC, Saunders JB. Injuries of the median nerve in fractures of the lower end of the radius. *Surg Gynecol Obstet* 1933;57:507–516.

221. Better OS, Abassi Z, Rubenstein I, et al. The mechanism of muscle injury in the crush syndrome: ischemic versus pressure stretch myopathy. *Miner Electrolyte Metab* 1990;16:181.

222. Blick SS, Brumback RJ, Poka A, et al. Compartment syndrome in open tibial fractures. *J Bone Joint Surg* 1986;68:1348–1353.

223. Brumback RJ. Compartment syndrome complicating avulsion of the origin of the triceps muscle. *J Bone Joint Surg* 1987;69:1445–1447.

224. Bywaters EG, McMichael J. Crush syndrome. In: Cope Z, ed. History of the Second World War: surgery. London: H. M. Stationery Office, 1953:673–686.

225. Campbell CC, Waters PW, Emans JB, et al. Neurovascular injury and displacement in type III supracondylar humerus fractures. *J Pediatr Orthop* 1995;15:47.

226. Carter PR. Crush injury of the upper limb. Early and late management. *Orthop Clin North Am* 1983;14:719–747.

227. Clement DA. Assessment of a treatment plan for managing acute vascular complications associated with supracondylar fractures of the humerus in children. *J Pediatr Orthop* 1990; 10:97.

228. Cooney WP, Dobyns JH, Linscheid AR. Complication of Colles' fractures. *J Bone Joint Surg* 1980;62:613–619.

229. Dormans JP, Squillante R, Sharf H. Acute neurovascular complications with supracondylar humerus fractures in children. *J Hand Surg* 1995;20:1.

230. Dresing K, Peterson T, Schmit-Neuerburg KP. Compartment pressure in the carpal tunnel in distal fractures of the radius. A prospective study. *Arch Orthop Trauma Surg* 1994;113:285–289.

231. Drury JK, Scullion JE. Vascular complications of anterior dislocation of the shoulder. *Br J Surg* 1980;67:579–581.

232. Elstrom JA, Pankovich AM, Egwele R. Extra-articular low-velocity gunshot fractures of the radius and ulna. *J Bone Joint Surg* 1978;60:335–341.

233. Gardner RC. Impending Volkmann's contracture following minor trauma to the palm of the hand. A theory of pathogenesis. *Clin Orthop* 1970;72:261–264.

234. Gupta A, Sharma S. Volar compartment syndrome of the arm complicating a fracture of the humeral shaft. A case report. *Acta Orthop Scand* 1991;62:77–78.

235. Harris IE. Supracondylar fractures of the humerus in children. *Orthopedics* 1992;15:811.

236. Hernandez J Jr, Peterson HA. Fracture of the distal radial physis complicated by compartment syndrome and premature physeal closure. *J Pediatr Orthop* 1986;6:627.

237. Holden CE. Compartmental syndromes following trauma. *Clin Orthop* 1975;113:95–102.

238. Jenkins NH, Mintowt-Czyz WU. Compression of the biceps brachialis compartment after trivial trauma. *J Bone Joint Surg* 1986;68:374.

239. Joseph FR, Posner MA, Terzakis JA. Compartment syndrome caused by a traumatized vascular hamartoma. *J Hand Surg* 1984;9:904–907.

240. Kikta MJ, Meyer JP, Bishara RA, et al. Crush syndrome due to limb compression. *Arch Surg* 1987;122:1078–1081.

241. Kongsholm J, Olerud C. Carpal tunnel pressure in the acute phase after Colles' fracture. *Arch Orthop Trauma Surg* 1986;105:183–186.

242. Mckee NH, Kuzon WM Jr. Functioning free muscle transplantation: making it work. What is known? *Ann Plast Surg* 1989;23:249.

243. Moed BR, Fakhouri AJ. Compartment syndrome after low-velocity gunshot wounds to the forearm. *J Orthop Trauma* 1991;5:134–137.

244. Olerud C, Lonnquist L. Acute carpal tunnel syndrome caused by fracture of the scaphoid and the 5th metacarpal bones. *Injury* 1984;16:198–199.

245. Peters CL, Scott SM. Compartment syndrome in the forearm following fractures of the radial head or neck in children. *J Bone Joint Surg* 1995;77:1070.

246. Pirone AM, Grahm HK, Drajbich JI. Management of displaced extension-type supracondylar fractures of the humerus in children. *J Bone Joint Surg* 1988;70:641–650.

247. Royle SG. Compartment syndrome following forearm fracture in children. *Injury* 1990;21:73.

248. Savage R. Compartment syndrome caused by false aneurysm. *J Bone Joint Surg* 1990;72:923.

249. Shall J, Cohn BT, Froimson AI. Acute compartment syndrome of the forearm in association with fracture of the distal end of the radius. *J Bone Joint Surg* 1986;68:1451–1454.

250. Stockley I, Harvey IA, Getty CJ. Acute volar compartment syndrome of the forearm secondary to fractures of the distal radius. *Injury* 1986;19:101–104.

251. Calhoun JH, Gogan WJ, Viegas SF, et al. Treatment of high-pressure water gun injection injuries of the foot with adjunctive hyperbaric oxygen: a case report. *Foot Ankle Int* 1989;10:40–42.

252. Gelberman RH, Posch MJ, Jurist JM. High-pressure injection injuries of the hand. *J Bone Joint Surg* 1975;57:935–937.

253. Harte BT Jr, Harter KC. High-pressure injection injuries. *Hand Clin* 1986;2:547–552.

254. Weltmer JB, Pack LL. High-pressure water-gun injection injuries to the extremities: a report of the six cases. *J Bone Joint Surg* 1988;70:1221–1223.

255. Bomberg BC, Hurley PE, Clark CA, et al. Complication associated with the use of an infusion pump during knee arthroscopy. *Arthroscopy* 1992;8:224–228.

256. Fruensgarrd S, Holm A. Compartment syndrome complicating arthroscopic surgery. Brief report. *J Bone Joint Surg* 1988;70:146–147.

257. Halpern AA, Mochizuki R, Long CE. Compartment syndrome of the forearm following radial-artery puncture in a patient treated with anticoagulants. *J Bone Joint Surg* 1978;60:1136–1137.

258. Hastings H II, Misamore G. Compartment syndrome resulting from intravenous regional anesthesia. *J Hand Surg* 1987;12:559–562.

259. Hawkins LG, Lischer CG, Sweeney MN. The main line accidental intra-arterial drug injection. A review of seven cases. *Clin Orthop* 1973;94:268.

260. Horlocker TT, Bishop AT. Compartment syndrome of the forearm and hand after brachial artery cannulation. *Anesth Analg* 1995;81:1092.

261. Mabee JR, Bostwick TL, Burke MK. Iatrogenic compartment syndrome from hypertonic saline injection in bier block. *J Emerg Med* 1994;12:473–476.

262. Macon WL, Futrell JW. Median nerve neuropathy after percutaneous puncture of the brachial artery in patients receiving anticoagulants. *N Engl J Med* 1973;288:1396.

263. Martens MA, Moeyersoons JP. Acute and effort-related compartment syndrome in sports. *Sports Med* 1990;9:62.

264. Merril DG, Brodsky JB, Hent Z. Vascular insufficiency following axillary block of the brachial plexus. *Anesth Analg* 1981;60:162–164.

265. Neviaser RJ, Adams JP, May GI. Complications of arterial puncture in anticoagulated patients. *J Bone Joint Surg* 1976;58:218–220.

266. Nixon RG, Brindley GW. Hemophilia presenting as compartment syndrome in the arm following venipuncture: a case report and review of the literature. *Clin Orthop* 1989;244:176–181.

267. Ott B, Neuberger L, Frey HP. Obliteration of axillary artery after axillary block. *Anaesthesia* 1989;44:773–774.

268. Parziale JR, Maorino AR, Herndon JH. Diagnostic peripheral nerve block resulting in compartment syndrome. *Am J Phys Med Rehab* 1988;67:82–84.

269. Peek RD, Haynes DW. Compartment syndrome as a complication of arthroscopy: a case report and a study of interstitial pressures. *Am J Sports Med* 1984;12:464–468.

270. Sneyd JR, Lau W, McLaren ID. Forearm compartment syndrome following intravenous infusion with a manual bulb pump. *Anesth Analg* 1993;76:1160.

271. Younge D. Haematoma block for fractures of the wrist: a cause of compartment syndrome. *J Hand Surg* 1989;14:194.

272. Bindiger A, Zelnik J, Kuschner S, et al. Spontaneous acute carpal tunnel syndrome in an anticoagulated patient. *Bull Hosp Joint Dis* 1995;54:52–53.

273. Black PR, Flowers MJ, Saleh M. Acute carpal tunnel syndrome as a complication of oral anticoagulant therapy. *J Hand Surg* 1997;22:50–51.

274. Bonatz ED, Seabol K. Acute carpal tunnel syndrome in a patient taking Coumadin: case report. *J Trauma* 1993;35:143–144.

275. Case DB. An acute carpal tunnel syndrome in a haemophiliac. *Br J Clin Pract* 1967;21:254–255.

276. Copeland J, Wells HG Jr, Puckett CL. Acute carpal tunnel syndrome in a patient taking Coumadin. *J Trauma* 1989;29:131–132.

277. Dumontier C, Sautet A, Apoil A. Entrapment and compartment syndromes of the upper limb in hemophilia. *J Hand Surg* 1994;19:427–429.

278. Hay Groves EW. A clinical lecture upon the surgical aspects of haemophilia with special reference to two cases of Volkmann's contracture resulting from this disease. *Br Med J* 1907;1:611–614.

279. Hill RL, Brookes B. Volkmann's ischemic contracture in hemophilia. *Am Surg* 1936;103:444.

280. Kilpatrick T, Leyden M, Sullivan J. Acute median nerve compression by haemorrhage from acute myelomonocytic leukaemia. *Med J Aust* 1985;142:51–52.

281. Molitor PJ, Wimperis JZ. Acute carpal tunnel syndrome in haemophiliacs. *Br J Clin Pract* 1990;44:675–676.

282. Narajna RJ Jr, Chan PS, High K, et al. Treatment considerations in patients with compartment syndrome: an inherited bleeding disorder. *Orthopedics* 1997;20:706.

283. Nkele C. Acute carpal tunnel syndrome resulting from haemorrhage into the carpal tunnel in a patient on warfarin. *J Hand Surg* 1986;11:455–456.

284. Seiler JG III, Valadie AL, Drvaric DM, et al. Perioperative compartment syndrome. *J Bone Joint Surg* 1996;78:600.

285. Thomas WO, Harris CN, D'Amore TF, et al. Bilateral forearm and hand compartment syndrome following thrombolysis for acute myocardial infarction: a case report. *J Emerg Med* 1994;12:467.

286. Flynn JM, Bischoff R, Gelberman RH. Median nerve compression at the wrist due to intracarpal canal sepsis. *J Hand Surg* 1995;20:864–867.

287. Goldie BS, Jones NF, Jupiter JB. Recurrent compartment syndrome and Volkmann's contracture associated with chronic osteomyelitis of the ulna. *J Bone Joint Surg* 1990;72:131–133.

288. Hung LK, Kinninmonth AW, Woo ML. *Vibrio vulnificus* necrotizing fasciitis presenting with compartmental syndrome of the hand. *J Hand Surg* 1988;13:337–339.

289. Schnall SB, Holtom PD, Silva E. Compartment syndrome associated with infection of the upper extremity. *Clin Orthop* 1994;309:128–131.

290. Zielinski CJ, Bora FW. *Vibrio* hand infections: a case report and review of the literature. *J Hand Surg* 1984;9:754–757.

291. Garfin SR, Mubarak SJ, Davidson TM. Rattlesnake bites: current concepts. *Clin Orthop* 1979;140:50–57.

292. Hardy DL, Jeter M, Corrigan JJ Jr. Envenomation by the northern blacktail rattlesnake (*Crotalus molossus molossus*):

report of two cases and the in vitro effects of the venom of fibrinolysis and platelet aggregation. *Toxicon* 1982;20:487–493.

293. Moylan JM, Inge WW, Pruitt BA. Circumferential extremity burns evaluated by the ultrasonic flowmeter, an analysis of 60 thermally injured limbs. *J Trauma* 1971;11:763–768.

294. Roberts RS, Csencsitz TA, Heard CW. Upper extremity compartment syndromes following pit viper envenomation. *Clin Orthop* 1985;196:184–188.

295. Russel FE. Clinical aspects of snake venom poisoning in North America. *Toxicon* 1969;7:33–37.

296. Russel FE. Snake venom poisoning in the United States. *Ann Rev Med* 1980;31:247–259.

297. Salisbury RE, McKeel DW, Matson AD. Ischemic necrosis of the intrinsic muscles of the hand after thermal injuries. *J Bone Joint Surg* 1974;56:1701–1707.

298. Seiler JG III, Sagerman SD, Geller RJ, et al. Venomous snake bite: current concepts of treatment. *Orthopedics* 1994;17:707–714.

299. Vigasio A, Battiston B, De Filippo G, et al. Compartmental syndrome due to viper bite. *Arch Orthop Trauma Surg* 1991;110:175.

300. Axelrod TS, Buchler R. Severe complex injuries to the upper extremity: revascularization and replantation. *J Hand Surg* 1991;16:574–584.

301. Hofmeister EP, Shin AY. The role of prophylactic fasciotomy and medical treatment in limb ischemia and revascularization. *Hand Clin* 1998;14:457–465.

302. Tomai S. Twenty years' experience e of limb replantation—a review of 293 upper extremity replants. *J Hand Surg* 1982;7:549–556.

303. Wang SH, Young KF, Wei JN. Replantation of severed limbs—clinical analysis of 91 cases. *J Hand Surg* 1981;6:311–318.

304. Bird CB, McCoy JW Jr. Weight-lifting as a cause of compartment syndrome in the forearm. A case report. *J Bone Joint Surg* 1983;65:406.

305. Weber AB, Churchill JO. Compartment syndrome after squash. *Aust N Z J Surg* 1996;66:771–772.

306. Dickinson JC, Kleinert JM. Acute carpal tunnel syndrome caused by a calcified median artery. A case report. *J Bone Joint Surg* 1991;73:610–611.

307. Faithfull DK, Wallace RF. Traumatic rupture of the median artery an unusual cause for acute median nerve compression. *J Hand Surg* 1987;12:233–235.

308. Nather A, Chacha PB, Lim P. Acute carpal tunnel syndrome secondary to thrombosis of a persistent median artery (with high division of the median nerve). A case report. *Ann Acad Med Singapore* 1980;9:118–121.

309. Rose RE. Acute carpal tunnel syndrome secondary to thrombosis of a persistent median artery. *West Indian Med J* 1995;44:32–33.

310. Smith R. Non-ischemic contractures of the hand. *J Bone Joint Surg* 1971;53:1313–1331.

311. Lipscomb PR, Burleson RJ. Vascular and neural complications in supracondylar fractures of the humerus in children. *J Bone Joint Surg* 1955;37:487–492.

312. Meyerding HW. Volkmann's ischemic contracture associated with supracondylar fracture of humerus. *JAMA* 1936;106:1139.

313. Royle SG. The role of tissue pressure recording in forearm fractures in children. *Injury* 1992;23:549.

314. Gelberman RH, Szabo RM, Mortensen WW. Carpal tunnel pressures and wrist position in patients with Colles' fractures. *J Trauma* 1984;24:747–749.

315. Lynch AC, Lipscomb PR. The carpal tunnel syndrome and Colles' fracture. *JAMA* 1963;185:363–366.

316. Haasbeek JF, Cole WG. Open fractures of the arm in children. *J Bone Joint Surg* 1995;77:576.

317. Bajpai J, Shinha BN, Srivastava AN. Clinical study of Volkmann's ischemic contracture of the upper limb. *Int Surg* 1975;60:162–164.

318. Ridings P, Gault D. Compartment syndrome of the arm. *J Hand Surg* 1994;19:147–148.

319. Gainor BJ. Closed avulsion of the flexor digitorum superficialis origin causing compartment syndrome. *J Bone Joint Surg* 1984;66:467.

320. McHale KA, Giessele A, Perlik PD. Compartment syndrome of the biceps brachii compartment following rupture of the long head of the biceps. *Orthopedics* 1991;14:787–788.

321. Quigley JT, Colonel L, Popich GA, et al. Compartment syndrome of the forearm and hand: a case report. *Clin Orthop* 1981;161:247–251.

322. Luce EA, Futrell JW, Wilgis EF, et al. Compression neuropathy following brachial arterial puncture in anticoagulated patients. *J Trauma* 1976;16:717–721.

323. Rudoff J, Ebner S, Canepa C. Limb-compartmental syndrome with thrombolysis. *Am Heart J* 1994;128:1267–1268.

324. Love BR. The tourniquet and its complications. *J Bone Joint Surg* 1979;61:239.

325. Dolich BH, Aiache AE. Drug-induced coma: a cause of crush syndrome and ischemic contracture. *J Trauma* 1973;13:223–228.

326. Penn AS, Rowland LP, Fraser DW. Drugs, coma, and myoglobinuria. *Arch Neurol* 1972;26:336–343.

327. Bloom AI, Zamir G, Muggia M, et al. Torture rhabdomyorhexis—a pseudo-crush syndrome. *J Trauma* 1995;38:252–254.

328. Bywaters EG, Beall D. Crush injuries with impairment of renal function. *Br Med J* 1941;1:427–434.

329. Bywaters EG, Delorey GE, Remington C, et al. Myohaemoglobin in urine of air raid casualties with crushing injury. *Biochem J* 1941;35:1164–1168.

330. Chen JC, Bullard MS, Liaw SJ. Crush syndrome—delayed diagnosis due to a lack of apparent injury mechanism. *Chanh Keng I Hsueh (Taiwan)* 1994;17:184–190.

331. Dennis C. Disaster following femoral vein ligation for thrombophlebitis; relief by fasciotomy; clinical case of renal impairment following crush injury. *Surgery* 1945;17:264–269.

332. Burchard KW, Slotman GJ, et al. Crush syndrome with death following pneumatic antishock garment application. *J Trauma* 1984;24:1052–1056.

333. Michaelson M. Crush injury and crush syndrome. *World J Surg* 1992;16:899.

334. Odeh M. The role of reperfusion-induced injury in the pathogenesis of the crush syndrome. *N Engl J Med* 1991;324:1417–1422.

335. Reis ND, Michaelson M. Crush injury to the lower limbs. *J Bone Joint Surg* 1986;68:414–418.

336. Rowland LP, Penn AS. Myoglobinuria. *Med Clin North Am* 1972;56:1233–1256.

337. Schreiber SN, Liebowitz MR, Bernstein LH. Limb compression and renal impairment (crush syndrome) complicating narcotic overdose. *J Bone Joint Surg* 1972;54:1683–1692.

338. Shaposhnikov G, Kozhin NP, Kikogosian RV, et al. The outcomes in crush syndrome of the extremities half a year after the earthquake in Armenia. *Voen Med Zh (USSR)* 1990;4:44–45.

339. Weeks S. The crush syndrome. *Surg Gynecol Obstet* 1968;127:369–376.

340. Shin LA, Chambers H, Wilkins KE, et al. Suction injuries in children leading to acute compartment syndrome of the interosseous muscles of the hand: case reports. *J Hand Surg* 1996;21:675–678.

341. Urbaniak JR. Replantation. In: Green DP, ed. *Operative hand surgery*, 2nd ed. New York: Churchill Livingstone, 1988:1105–1126.

342. Trumble T. Forearm compartment syndrome secondary to leukemic infiltrates. *J Hand Surg* 1987;12:563–565.

343. Mann RJ, Wallquist JM. Early decompression fasciotomy in the treatment of high-voltage electrical burns of the extremities. *South Med J* 1975;68:1103–1108.

344. Parrish HM. Incidence of treated snakebites in the United States. *Public Health Rep* 1966;81:269–276.

345. Phillips JH, Mackinnon SE, Murray JF, et al. Exercise-induced chronic compartment syndrome of the first dorsal interosseous muscle of the hand. A case report. *J Hand Surg* 1986;11:124–127.

346. Puranen J, Alasvaikko A. Intracompartmental pressure increase on exertion in patients with chronic compartment syndrome in the leg. *J Bone Joint Surg* 1981;63:1304–1309.

347. Rydholm U, Werner CO, Ohlin P. Intracompartmental forearm pressure during rest and exercise. *Clin Orthop* 1983;175:213–215.

348. Styf JR. Diagnosis of exercise-induced pain in the anterior aspect of the lower leg. *Am J Sports Med* 1988;16:165.

349. Wise JJ, Fortin PT. Bilateral, exercise-induced thigh compartment syndrome diagnosed as exertional rhabdomyolysis. *Am J Sports Med* 1997;25:126–129.

350. Lee BY, Brancato RF, Park IH, et al. Management of compartmental syndrome. Diagnostic and surgical considerations. *Am J Surg* 1984;148:383–388.

351. McDougall CG, Hohnston GH. A new technique of catheter placement for measurement of forearm compartment pressures. *J Trauma* 1991;31:1404.

352. Russell WL, Apyan PM, Burns RP. An electronic technique for compartment pressure measurement using the wick catheter. *Surg Gynecol Obstet* 1985;161:173–175.

353. Wiig H. Evaluation of methodologies for measurement of interstitial fluid pressure (P_i). Physiological implications of recent P_i data. *Crit Rev Biomed Eng* 1990;18:27–54.

354. Henke J, Becker HP, Gerngrof H. Entwicklung der intrakompartimentellen Meftechnik. In: Willy C, Sterk J, Gerngrof H, eds. *Das Kompartment-Syndrome*. Berlin: Springer-Verlag, 1998:112–118.

355. Zweifach SS, Hargens AR, Evans KL. Skeletal muscle necrosis in pressurized compartments associated with hemorrhagic hypotension. *J Trauma* 1980;20:941–947.

356. Amendola A, Rorabeck CH, Vellett D, et al. The use of magnetic resonance imaging in exertional compartment syndromes. *Am J Sports Med* 1990;18:29–34.

357. Gershuni DH, Gosink BB, Hargens AR, et al. Ultrasound evaluation of the anterior musculofascial compartment of the leg following exercise. *Clin Orthop* 1982;167:185–190.

358. Landi A, DeSantis G, Toricelli P, et al. CT in established Volkmann's contracture in forearm muscles. *J Hand Surg* 1989;14:49–52.

359. Vukanovic S, Hauser H, Wettstein P. CT localization of myonecrosis for surgical decompression. *Am J Rad* 1980;135:1298–1299.

360. Mars M, Hadley GP. Failure of pulse oximetry in the assessment of raised limb intracompartmental pressure. *Injury* 1994;25:379–381.

361. Mars M, Maseko S, Thomson S, et al. Can pulse oximetry detect raised intracompartmental pressure? *S Afr J Surg* 1994;32:48–50.

362. Gelberman RH, Hergenroeder PT, et al. The carpal tunnel syndrome. A study of carpal canal pressures. *J Bone Joint Surg* 1981;63:380–383.

363. Gelberman RH. Acute carpal tunnel syndrome. In: *Operative nerve repair and reconstruction*. Philadelphia: JB Lippincott Co, 1991:939–948.

364. Nylander G, Nordström H, Lewis D, et al. Metabolic effects of hyperbaric oxygen in postischemic muscle. *Plast Reconstr Surg* 1987;79:91–96.

365. Strauss MB, Hargens AR, Gershuni DH, et al. Reduction of skeletal muscle necrosis using intermittent hyperbaric oxygen in a model compartment syndrome. *J Bone Joint Surg* 1983;65:656–662.

366. Strauss MB, Hargens AR, Gershuni DH, et al. Delayed use of hyperbaric oxygen for treatment of a model anterior compartment syndrome. *J Orthop Res* 1986;4:108–111.

367. Caurso DM, King TJ, Tsujimura RB, et al. Primary closure of fasciotomy incisions with a skin-stretching device in patients with burn and trauma. *J Burn Care Rehabil* 1997;18:125.

368. Cohn BT, Shall J, Berkowitz M. Forearm fasciotomy for acute compartment syndrome: a new technique for delayed primary closure. *Orthopedics* 1986;9:1243.

369. Geary N. Late surgical decompression for compartment syndrome of the forearm. *J Bone Joint Surg* 1984;66:745–748.

370. Patman RD, Thompson JE. Fasciotomy in peripheral vascular surgery. Report of 164 patients. *Arch Surg* 1970; 101:663.

371. Sheridan GW, Matsen FA. Fasciotomy in the treatment of the acute compartment syndrome. *J Bone Joint Surg* 1976;58:112–117.

372. Sheridan GW, Matsen FA III. An animal model of the compartmental syndrome. *Clin Orthop* 1975;113:36–42.

373. Idler RS, Mih AD. Soft-tissue coverage of the hand with a free digital fillet flap. *Microsurgery* 1990;11:215–216.

374. Berenbaum MC, Birch CA, Moreland JD. Paroxysmal myoglobinuria. *Lancet* 1953;1:892–895.

375. Cunningham E, Kohli R, Venuto RC. Influenza-associated myoglobinuric renal failure. *JAMA* 1979;242:2428–2429.

376. Paller SM. Hemoglobin and myoglobin induced acute renal failure in the rat: the role of iron nephrotoxicity. *Am J Physiol* 1988;255:539.

377. Zager RA. Studies of mechanisms and protective maneuvers in myoglobinuric acute renal injury. *Lab Invest* 1989; 60:619.

378. Leguit P Jr. Compartment syndrome of the upper arm. *Netherlands J Surg* 1982;34:123–126.

379. Palumbo RC, Abrams JS. Compartment syndrome of the upper arm. *Orthopedics* 1994;17:1144–1147.

380. Rajoo R, Mennen U, Stevanovic M. Compartment syndrome in transferred muscle: an unusual complication. *J Hand Surg* 1991;16:75–77.

381. Gaspard D, Kohl RD Jr. Compartment syndromes in which the skin is the limiting boundary. *Clin Orthop* 1975;113:65–68.

382. Frober R, Linss W. Anatomic bases of the forearm compartment syndrome. *Surg Radiol Anat* 1994;16:341–347.

383. Blomgren I, Blomqvist G, Ejeskar A, et al. Hand function after replantation or revascularization of upper extremity injuries. *Scand J Plast Reconstr Surg* 1988;22:93–101.

384. Boden BP, Buinewicz BR. Management of traumatic cutaneous defects by using a skin-stretching device. *Am J Orthop* 1995;[Suppl 27].

385. Adamson JE, Srouji SJ, Horton CE, et al. The acute carpal tunnel syndrome. *Plast Reconstr Surg* 1971;47:332–336.

386. Bauman TD, Gelberman RH, Mubarak SJ, et al. The acute carpal tunnel syndrome. *Clin Orthop* 1981;156:151–156.

387. Chidgey LK, Szabo RM, Wiese DA. Acute carpal tunnel syndrome caused by pigmented villonodular synovitis of the wrist. *Clin Orthop* 1967;228:254–257.

388. Mack GR, McPherson SA, Lutz RB. Acute median neuropathy after wrist trauma. The role of emergent carpal tunnel release. *Clin Orthop* 1994;300:141–146.

389. Paley D, McMurtry RY. Median nerve compression by volarly displaced fragments of the distal radius. *Clin Orthop* 1987;215:139–147.

390. Weiland AJ, Lister GD, Villarreal-Rios A. Volar fracture dislocations of the second and third carpometacarpal joints associated with acute carpal tunnel syndrome. *J Trauma* 1976;16:672–675.

391. Gaur SC, Kulshreshtha K, Swarup S. Acute carpal tunnel syndrome in Hansen's disease. *J Hand Surg* 1994;19:286–287.

392. Gerardi JA, Mack GR, Lutz RB. Acute carpal tunnel syndrome secondary to septic arthritis of the wrist. *J Am Osteopath Assoc* 1989;89:933–934.

393. Chiu KY, Ng WF, Wong WB, et al. Acute carpal tunnel syndrome caused by pseudogout. *J Hand Surg* 1992;17:299–302.

394. McClain EJ, Wissinger HA. The acute carpal tunnel syndrome: nine case reports. *J Trauma* 1976;16:75–78.

395. Ogilvie C, Kay NR. Fulminating carpal tunnel syndrome due to gout. *J Hand Surg* 1988;13:42–43.

396. Pai CH, Tseng CH. Acute carpal tunnel syndrome caused by tophaceous gout. *J Hand Surg* 1993;18:667–669.

397. Robbins H. Anatomical study of the median nerve in the carpal canal and etiologies of the carpal tunnel syndrome. *J Bone Joint Surg* 1963;45:953–956.

398. Segal LS, Adair DM. Compartment syndrome of the triceps as a complication of thrombolytic therapy. *Orthopedics* 1990;13:90–92.

399. Steinberg DR, Szabo RM. Anatomy of the median nerve at the wrist. Open carpal tunnel release—classic. *Hand Clin* 1996;12:259–269.

400. Verfaillie S, De Smet L, Leemans A, et al. Acute carpal tunnel syndrome caused by hydroxyapatite crystals: a case report. *J Hand Surg* 1996;21:360–362.

401. Szabo R. Peripheral nerve injuries in athletes. *Mediguide Orthop* 1985;5:1–5.

402. Gelberman RH, Szabo RM, Williamson RV. Sensibility testing in peripheral nerve compression syndromes. An experimental study in humans. *J Bone Joint Surg* 1983;65:632–638.

403. Szabo RM, Gelberman RH, Williamson RV, et al. Effects of increased systemic blood pressure on tissue fluid pressure threshold of peripheral nerve. *J Orthop Res* 1983;1:172–178.

404. Sahs AL, Helms CM, DuBois C. Carpal tunnel syndrome. Complication of toxic shock syndrome. *Arch Neurol* 1983;40:414–415.

405. Ford DJ, Ali MS. Acute carpal tunnel syndrome. Complications of delayed decompression. *J Bone Joint Surg* 1986;68:758–759.

406. McDermott AG, Marble AE, Yabsley RH. Monitoring acute compartment pressures with the S.T.I.C. catheter. *Clin Orthop* 1984;190:192–198.

407. Taliesnik J. The palmar cutaneous branch of the median nerve and approach to the carpal tunnel: an anatomical study. *J Bone Joint Surg* 1973;55:1212.

408. Reid RL, Travis RT. Acute necrosis of the second interosseous compartment of the hand. *J Bone Joint Surg* 1973;55:1095–1097.

409. Halpern AA, Mochizuki RM. Compartment syndrome of the interosseous muscles of the hand. A clinical and anatomic review. *Orthop Rev* 1980;9:121–127.

410. Lefer AM, Tsao PS, Lefer DJ, et al. Role of endothelial dysfunction in the pathogenesis of reperfusion injury after myocardial ischemia. *FASEB J* 1991;4:2029–2034.

411. Harris K, Walker PM, Mickle DA, et al. Metabolic response of skeletal muscle to ischemia. *Am J Physiol* 1986;250:213–220.

412. Weiland AJ, Villarreal-Rios A, Kleinert HE, et al. Replantation of digits and hands: analysis of surgical techniques and functional results in 71 patients with 86 replantations. *J Hand Surg* 1977;2:1–12.

413. Bolli R, Patel BS, Zhu WX, et al. The iron chelator desferrioxamine attenuates postischemic ventricular dysfunction. *Am J Physiol* 1987;253:372–380.

414. Fantini GA, Yoshioka T. Deferoxamine prevents lipid peroxidation and attenuates reoxygenation injury in postischemic skeletal muscle. *Am Physiol* 1993;264:1953–1959.

415. Feller AM, Roth AC, Russel RC, et al. Experimental evaluation of oxygen free radical scavengers in the prevention of reperfusion injury to skeletal muscle. *Ann Plast Surg* 1989;22:321–331.

416. Friedl HP, Till GO, Ward PA. Role of oxygen radicals in tourniquet-related ischemia-reperfusion injury of human patients. *Klin Wochenschr* 1991;69:1109–1112.

417. Granger DN. Role of xanthine oxidase and granulocytes in ischemia-reperfusion injury. *Am J Physiol* 1988;363:1269–1275.

418. Green CJ, Dhami L, Prasad S, et al. The effect of desferrioxamine on lipid peroxidation and survival of ischaemic island skin flaps in rats. *Fr J Plast Surg* 1989;42:565–569.

419. Montagnani CA, Simeone FA. Observations on liberation and elimination of myohemoglobin and of hemoglobin after release of muscle ischemia. *Surgery* 1953;34:169.

420. Suzuki S, Matsushita YH, Isshiki N, et al. Salvage of distal flap necrosis by topical superoxide dismutase. *Ann Plast Surg* 1991;27:253–257.

421. Williams RE, Zweier JL, Flaherty JT. Treatment with deferoxamine during ischemia improves functional and metabolic recovery and reduces reperfusion induced oxygen radical generation in rabbit hearts. *Circulation* 1991; 83:1006–1014.

422. Howse AJ, Seddon H. Ischaemic contracture of muscle associated with carbon monoxide and barbiturate poisoning. *Br Med J* 1966;1.

423. Frankenthal L. Über Verschüttungen. *Virchows Arch* 1916; 111:332.

424. Kayser FF. *Von Schjerning's Handbuch der Artzlichen Erfahrugen in Weltkriege.* Leipzig: 1922.

425. Weiting J. Über Wundliegen Druckenkrose und Entlastung. *Münch Med Wochenschr* 1918;36:311.

426. Minami S. Über Nierenveränderungen nach Verschüttung. *Virchows Arch* 1923;245:247.

427. Linton AL, Adams JH, Lawson DH. Muscle necrosis and acute renal failure in carbon monoxide poisoning. *Postgrad Med J* 1968;44:338–341.

428. Orizaga M, Ducharme FA, Campbell JS, et al. Muscle infarction and Volkmann's contracture following carbon monoxide poisoning. *J Bone Joint Surg* 1967;49:965–970.

429. Gordon JD, Newman W. Lower nephron syndrome following prolonged knee-chest position. *J Bone Joint Surg* 1953;35:764–768.

430. Keim HA, Weinstein JD. Acute renal failure: a complication of spine fusion in the tuck position. *J Bone Joint Surg* 1970;52:1248–1250.

431. Leung A, Robson L. Myoglobinuria from child abuse. *Paed Urol* 1987;29:45.

432. Better OS, Stein JH. Early management of shock and prophylaxis of acute renal failure in traumatic rhabdomyolysis. *N Engl J Med* 1990;322:825–829.

433. Honda N. Acute renal failure and rhabdomyolysis. *Kidney Int* 1983;23:888–898.

434. Collins AJ. Kidney dialysis treatment for victims of the Armenian earthquake. *N Engl J Med* 1989;320:1291–1292.

435. Ward MM. Factors predictive of acute renal failure in rhabdomyolysis. *Arch Intern Med* 1988;148:1553.

436. Rergstad A, Hellum C. Volkmann's ischemic contracture of the forearm. *Injury* 1980;12:148.

437. Ranney D, Wells R, Dowling J. Lumbrical function: interaction of lumbrical contraction with the elasticity of the extrinsic finger muscles and its effect on metacarphalangeal equilibrium. *J Hand Surg* 1987;12:100–114.

438. von Schroeder HP, Botte MJ. Functional anatomy of the extensor tendons of the digits. *Hand Clin* 1997;13:51–62.

439. Botte MJ, Keenan MA, Gellman H, et al. Surgical management of spastic thumb-in-palm deformity in adults with brain injury. *J Hand Surg* 1989;14:174.

440. Matsen FA III, Clawson DK. Compartmental syndrome: a unified concept. *Clin Orthop* 1975;113:8–14.

441. Sundoraraj GD, Mani D. Pattern of contracture and recovery following ischemia of the upper limb. *J Hand Surg* 1985;10:155.

442. Zancolli E. Tendon transfers after ischemic contracture of the forearm. Classification in relation to intrinsic muscle disorders. *Am J Surg* 1965;1098:356.

443. Zancolli E. Classification of established Volkmann's ischemic contracture and the program for its treatment. In: *Structural and dynamic bases of hand surgery*, 2nd ed. Philadelphia: JB Lippincott Co, 1979:314–324.

444. Backhouse K, Catton W. An experimental study of the functions of the lumbrical muscles in the human hand. *J Anat* 1954;88:133–144.

445. Midgely RD. Volkmann's ischemic contracture of the forearm. *Orthop Clin North Am* 1973;4:983.

446. Parks A. The treatment of established Volkmann's contracture by tendon transplantation. *J Bone Joint Surg* 1951;33:359.

447. Sasake Y, Sugioka Y. The pronator quadratus sign: its classification and diagnostic usefulness for injury and inflammation of the wrist. *J Hand Surg* 1989;14:80.

448. Peacock EE, Madden JW, Trier WC. Transfer of median and ulnar nerves during early treatment of forearm ischemia. *Ann Surg* 1969;169:748.

449. Botte MJ, Keenan MA, Korchek JI, et al. Modified technique for the superficialis-to-profundus transfer in the treatment of adults with spastic clenched fist deformity. *J Hand Surg* 1987;12:639–640.

450. Page CM. An operation for the relief of flexion-contracture in the forearm. *J Bone Joint Surg* 1923;5:233.

451. Fowler S. Extensor apparatus of the digits. Proceedings of the British Orthopaedic Association. *J Bone Joint Surg* 1949;31:477.

452. Phalen GS, Miller RC. The transfer of wrist and extensor muscles to restore or reinforce flexion poser of the fingers and opposition of the thumb. *J Bone Joint Surg* 1947; 29:993.

453. Burkhalter WE, Christensen RC, Brown PL. The extensor indicis proprius opponensplasty. *J Bone Joint Surg* 1973; 55:725.

454. Huber E. Hilfsoperation bei median Uslahmung. *Dtsch Arch Klin Med* 1921;136:271.

455. Appleby D, Boniface RJ, Fu FH. Isolated contracture of the abductor digiti minimi. *J Hand Surg* 1987;12:290–293.

456. Bilbo J, Stern P. The first interosseous muscle: an anatomic study. *J Hand Surg* 1986;11:748–750.

457. Brand P. *Clinical mechanics of the hand.* St. Louis: CV Mosby, 1985:342.

458. Bunnell S. Ischaemic contracture local in the hand. *J Bone Joint Surg* 1953;35:88–101.

459. Haines RW. The extensor apparatus of the finger. *J Anat* 1951;85:251.

460. Harris C, Riordan DC. Intrinsic contracture in the hand and its surgical treatment. *J Bone Joint Surg* 1954;36:10–20.

461. Kaplan E. Anatomy, injuries and treatment of the extensor apparatus of the hand and digits. *Clin Orthop* 1950;13:24.

462. Landsmeer J. The anatomy of the dorsal aponeurosis of the human finger and the functional significance. *Anat Rec* 1949;104:31.

463. Lee FS, Gellman H. Reconstruction of intrinsic hand deformities. *Hand Clin* 1998;14:499–506.

464. Linscheid RL, An KN, Gross RM. Quantitative analysis of the intrinsic muscles of the hand. *Clin Anat* 1991;4:265.

465. Long C. Intrinsic-extrinsic muscle control of the fingers. *J Bone Joint Surg* 1968;50:973–984.

466. Lister G. *The hand: diagnosis and indications,* 2nd ed. Edinburgh, Scotland: Churchill Livingstone, 1984.

467. Parks A. The "lumbrical plus" finger. *J Bone Joint Surg* 1971;53:236–239.

468. Smith RJ. Intrinsic contracture. In: Green DP, Hotchkiss RN, eds. *Operative hand surgery*, 3rd ed., vol. 1. New York: Churchill Livingstone, 1993:607–626.

469. Spinner M, Aiache A, Silver L, et al. Impending ischemic contracture of the hand. *Plast Reconstr Surg* 1972;50:341–349.

470. Thomas D, Long CI, Landsmeer J. Biomechanical considerations of lumbricalis behavior in the human finger. *J Biomech* 1968;1:107–115.

471. Weinzweig H, Starker I, Sharzer L, et al. Revisitation of the vascular anatomy of the lumbrical and interosseous muscles. *Plast Reconstr Surg Am* 1997;99:785–790.

472. Smith RJ. Intrinsic muscles of the fingers: function, dysfunction, and surgical reconstruction. *AAOS Instr Course Lect* 1975;5:24.

473. Ikuta Y, Kubo T, Tsuge K. Free muscle transplantation by microsurgical technique to treat severe Volkmann's contracture. *Plast Reconstr Surg* 1976;58:407.

474. Tamai S, Komatsu S, Sakamoto H, et al. Free muscle transplants in dogs with microsurgical, neurovascular anastomoses. *Plast Reconstr Surg* 1970;46:219.

475. Taylor GI, Daniel RK. The free flap: composite tissue transfer by vascular anastomoses. *Aust N Z J Surg* 1973;43:1.

476. Bradley EL. The anterior tibial compartment syndrome. *Surg Gynecol Obstet* 1973;136:289–297.

477. Davey JR, Rorabeck CH, Fowler PJ. The tibialis posterior muscle compartment. An unrecognized cause of exertional compartment syndrome. *Am J Sports Med* 1984; 12:391.

478. Fronek J, Mubarak SJ, Hargens AR, et al. Management of chronic exertional compartment syndrome of the lower extremity. *Clin Orthop* 1987;220:217–227.

479. Mohler LR, Styf JR, Pedowitz RA, et al. Intramuscular deoxygenation during exercise in patients who have chronic anterior compartment syndrome of the leg. *J Bone Joint Surg* 1997;79:844–849.

480. Styf JR, Korner LM. Microcapillary infusion technique for measurement of intramuscular pressure during exercise. *Clin Orthop* 1986;207:253.

481. Styf JR, Lysell E. Chronic compartment syndrome in the erector spinae muscle. *Spine* 1987;12:680.

93

VASCULAR DISORDERS: ARTERIOVENOUS MALFORMATIONS

JOE UPTON
JENNIFER J. MARLER
STEPHEN A. PAP

Vascular malformations (VMs) in the upper extremity represent very challenging problems in hand surgery. With adequate experience, these are treatable problems with predictable outcomes (1).

In 1982, Mulliken and Glowacki (1a) proposed a classification of vascular anomalies that described vascular tumors based on cellular biology and natural history (Tables 1 and 2). Compared with vascular tumors, malformations do not involute, and they are classified by the aberrant vessel type and by their flow speed. Change in size can be affected by mechanical factors and cellular changes with aging and hormonal modulation. They may be associated with skeletal overgrowth, and fast-flow lesions, in particular, can cause very challenging, occasionally life-threatening, clinical problems.

PATHOGENESIS

VMs arise from errors in embryogenesis (2). Current research efforts are beginning to provide insight into the pathogenesis of abnormal blood vessel formation, and genetic studies are starting to identify particular chromosome changes in syndromes that include arteriovenous malformations (AVMs), such as Osler-Rendu-Weber syndrome (3).

CUTIS MARMORATA TELANGIECTASIA CONGENITA

Cutis marmorata telangiectasia congenita is a rare vascular anomaly that presents with extensive cutaneous marbling exacerbated by exposure to lower temperatures or when the patient is crying. These skin lesions are depressed, may have ulcerations, and are most frequently found unilaterally in the trunk and extremities. They have a distinctive purple color.

Cutis marmorata telangiectasia congenita must be distinguished from cutis marmorata, in which normal vascularity causes skin mottling when exposed to low temperatures but disappears on rewarming. Almost all affected children with cutis marmorata telangiectasia congenita show some degree of improvement of the skin changes during the first year of life into adolescence (3,4). However, atrophy and pigmentation often persist into adulthood, in association with ectasia of the superficial veins in the involved limb (Fig. 1).

CAPILLARY MALFORMATIONS

Clinical Features

Capillary malformations are capillary- to venule-sized vessels in the superficial and deep dermis of skin and owe their color to erythrocytes. They have also been called "port-wine stain," "angel kiss," and "stork bite" (Fig. 2). These dilated vessels lack a normal smooth muscle layer within their walls and vasa nervorum (5). Extensive cutaneous capillary malformations can be associated with soft tissue and bone hypertrophy. In the upper extremity, capillary malformations are often associated with a deeper VM or lymphatic malformation (LM) (1). They must be distinguished from other benign, common birthmarks of infancy.

Treatment

The tunable pulsed-dye laser can decrease the color of the cutaneous blush, and more dramatic results are obtained on the face and neck than on the trunk and extremities (6). Soft tissue debulking and skeletal procedures required with overgrowth are particular to the other associated VMs, LMs, and AVMs.

TABLE 1. VASCULAR ANOMALIES OF THE UPPER LIMB

Vascular tumors
    Hemangiomas
        Congenital
            Rapidly involuting congenital hemangioma
            Noninvoluting congenital hemangioma
        Infantile
        Hemangiomatosis
    Pyogenic granuloma
    Kaposiform hemangioendothelioma
    Rare tumors
        Hemangiopericytoma
        Hemangioendothelioma
        Giant cell angioblastoma
        Angiosarcoma
Vascular malformations
    Cutis marmorata telangiectasia congenita
    Capillary malformations
    Venous malformations
    Lymphatic malformations
    Arteriovenous malformations
    Combined (eponymous) malformations

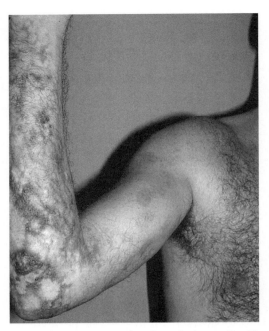

FIGURE 1. Cutis marmorata telangiectasia congenita. The characteristic features of cutis marmorata telangiectasia congenita include a reticulated, marblelike appearance with a typical deep purple color. Involved limbs may have both soft tissue and skeletal atrophy.

VENOUS MALFORMATIONS

Clinical Features

Most VMs are sporadic, although a genetic pattern of susceptibility for certain types of VMs has been suggested. VMs of the upper extremity are all present at birth but may not become clinically evident until school age. They grow commensurately with the child and slowly expand during the adolescent growth spurt.

They most commonly present as a mass, swelling, or cutaneous discoloration. These slow-flow malformations engorge with the limb in a dependent position and decompress with the limb held above the level of the heart. Most VMs are located in the subcutaneous tissue planes external to the muscular fascia in the axilla, arm, and forearm (Fig.

3). Most are solitary lesions, and a small number of patients have extensive lesions that may extend into the axilla and ipsilateral chest wall (Fig. 3C).

Pain and paresthesias are usually the result of local inflammation around intralesional thrombi or nerve compression (1). Areas with phlebothrombosis are swollen, firm, and very painful when compression garments are applied. Most symptoms are aggravated after exercise in which repetitive movements such as lifting, gripping, or pinching are involved.

Intramuscular VMs are found within the flexor and extensor muscles and compartments of the forearm as well as within the hand in the dorsal interossei, thenar, and hypothenar intrinsic muscles. In the absence of phleboliths, nerve compression, or intralesional bleeding, most VMs are asymptomatic. Subtle deficiencies in grip and pinch strength may be measured with extensive intramuscular involvement; however, these generally seem minimal. Despite significant involvement, function of the involved muscles remains surprisingly good.

VMs occasionally involve skeletal structures, showing cortical lucencies where vessels penetrate medullary canals, but no large areas of osteolysis. Pathologic fractures can occur in upper limbs with large diffuse lesions. VMs do not progress from a slow-flow to high-flow state. Enlargement after partial resections represents redirection of flow into adjacent anomalous channels. There is a hormonal modulation in females with medium- and large-sized VMs and lymphatic venous malformations (LVMs), which may

TABLE 2. COMPARISON OF TYPICAL INFANTILE HEMANGIOMAS AND VASCULAR MALFORMATIONS

	Hemangioma	Vascular malformation
Present at birth	No in 70% of cases. 30% of cases have premonitory spot.	Yes (may not be clinically evident).
Growth characteristics	Rapid growth during first year of life followed by spontaneous involution.	Growth commensurate with child. Subject to extrinsic modulation by hormonal and other factors.
Female to male ratio	3:1	1:1

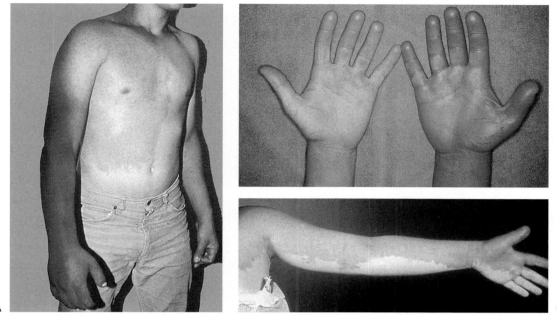

FIGURE 2. Diverse presentations of capillary malformation (CM). CMs can involve any portion of the upper extremity and do not necessarily follow a segmental or dermatologic pattern. **A:** An extensive circumferential lesion of the arm, forearm, and hand. Note the less intense CM of the ipsilateral chest and abdomen. **B:** Diffuse enlargement of the hand is noted in the patient shown in **A**. **C:** CM involving the C3 to C5 distribution of the upper limb.

increase in size during adolescence, menses, and pregnancies and with oral contraceptives.

Large VMs can be coagulopathic, and a coagulation profile should be obtained in all patients. Platelet counts are usually in the range of 100,000 to 150,000 per microliter. Prothrombin time may be increased, with normal activated partial thromboplastin, low fibrinogen levels (150 to 200 mg per dL), and increased fibrin split products.

Evaluation

Magnetic resonance imaging scans provide the gold standard for the evaluation of VMs (Fig. 4). These lesions can involve all tissue layers. On T1-weighted sequences, VMs are isointense, whereas gradient-weighted images show diffuse, homogeneous enhancement. T2-weighted images show septation within the soft tissue mass and signal voids characteristic of phleboliths. Flow-sensitive gradient-weighted sequences show no evidence of high flow. Magnetic resonance venography is very helpful for evaluation of large VMs anywhere in the upper limb. Direct puncture phlebography obtains a more detailed evaluation of the intrinsic anatomy of a VM and visualizes the extrinsic drainage of the limb and is usually obtained before sclerotherapy.

Arterial anatomy is normal in limbs with VMs, LVMs, and capillary-lymphatic-venous malformations, although

there may be some distortion due to a mass effect. Abnormalities on the venous side show puddling of contrast and delayed flow out of the VM. Angiograms are helpful in the preoperative evaluation of large VMs or of lesions in very difficult areas for dissection.

Treatment

Observation

The initial treatment for all VMs is conservative (Fig. 5). Most large and small lesions are asymptomatic. Compression garments are very helpful to control the enlargement of the VM during or after exercise. Low-dose aspirin therapy is helpful in reducing thrombus formation.

Sclerotherapy

The authors' second line of treatment is provided by the interventional radiologist for all but the small, well-localized lesions in the upper limb that can be easily resected. Sclerotherapy is used for functional or aesthetic considerations and is most successful in lesions with large saccular channels. Absolute alcohol (100%) is the preferred sclerosant in the United States (7); Ethibloc (Ethicon, Hamburg, Germany) is used outside of the United States (8).

The passage of sclerosant into the general circulation can be potentially very dangerous if a proximal tourniquet is

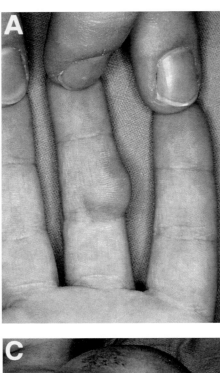

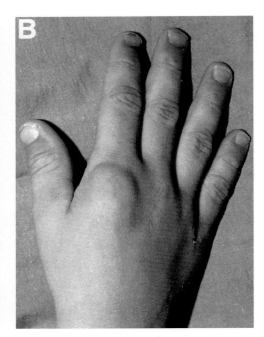

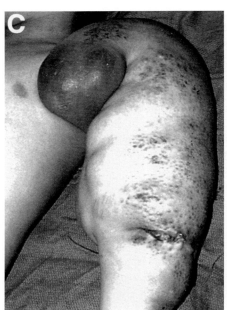

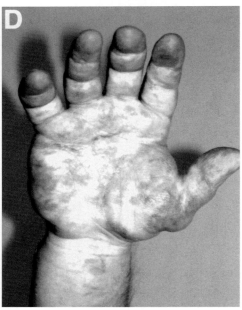

FIGURE 3. Diverse presentations of venous malformation (VM). **A:** An isolated VM along the palmar surface of a digit is symptomatic if intralesional thrombi compress digital nerves. **B:** This dorsal lesion is soft and compressible and symptomatic. **C:** Extensive VMs may involve the entire extremity and chest wall. This patient is septic from an infected phlebothrombosis in the anterior axillary region. **D:** This diffuse VM involves every soft tissue structure of the hand and distal forearm. Surgery is indicated only for symptomatic regions.

not used. The authors' radiologists prefer to treat specific areas in multiple bimonthly intervals (7) and have the best outcomes with large VMs in the arm and proximal forearm (Fig. 6).

Complications extend from ecchymosis, blistering, and, occasionally, full-thickness loss of overlying skin to damage of adjacent soft tissue structures (Fig. 7). Extensive hemolysis may lead to renal toxicity. Excessive intravenous sclerosant may cause cardiac compromise (7). The inflammatory reaction and scar formation after sclerotherapy are significant and cross tissue planes. The surgeon must be available when the interventional radiologist plans to sclerose extensive VMs.

Surgery

The indications for surgical treatment are primarily functional but can be aesthetic (1,9). Judicious resections of VMs are both safe and predictable. Small, well-localized lesions anywhere in the subcutaneous tissue planes, on the dorsum of the hand, or along the sides of a digit or thumb are easily removed.

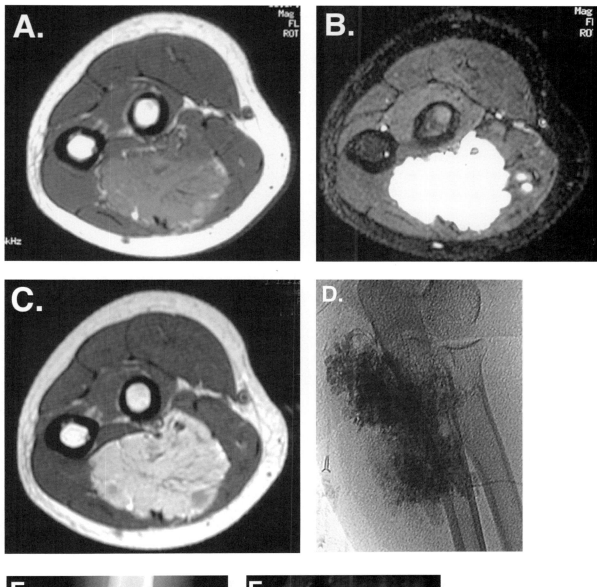

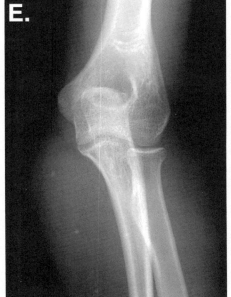

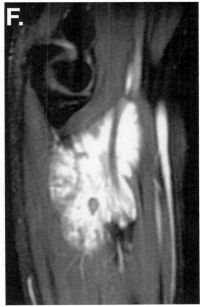

FIGURE 4. Imaging of a venous malformation (VM) in an adult patient with a forearm lesion. **A–C:** Transverse magnetic resonance images of the forearm that are differently weighted highlight characteristic findings of a VM. On a T1-weighted sequence **(A)**, the VM is isointense to adjacent skeletal muscle. On a T1-weighted sequence with gadolinium enhancement **(B)**, there is diffuse enhancement of the VM. On a T2-weighted sequence **(C)**, there is a high signal with signal voids within the VM that represents phleboliths. **D:** Intravenous injection of contrast at the time of sclerotherapy reveals abnormal collection of saccular venous structures. **E:** Phleboliths are seen in soft tissues on a lateral plain radiograph. **F:** T2-weighted sagittal magnetic resonance imaging sequence.

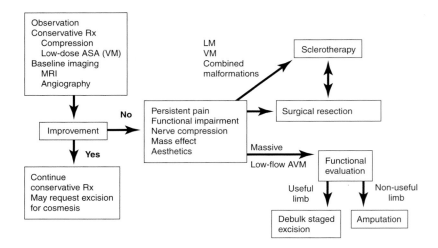

FIGURE 5. Treatment algorithm for slow-flow vascular malformations. ASA, aspirin; AVM, arteriovenous malformation; LM, lymphatic malformation; MRI, magnetic resonance imaging; Rx, treatment; VM, venous malformation.

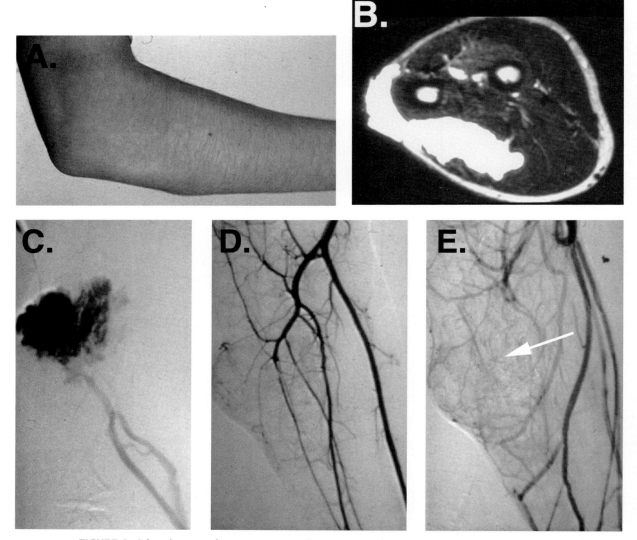

FIGURE 6. Sclerotherapy of an upper extremity venous malformation. **A:** Venous malformation involving the superficial flexor and extensor compartments of the forearm. **B:** T1-weighted magnetic resonance imaging sequence demonstrates the extent of involvement. Physical examination alone may be deceiving. **C:** Injection of contrast material at the time of sclerotherapy demonstrates the abnormal venous vessels. **D:** Arterial phase angiogram after sclerotherapy demonstrates a normal arterial circulation. **E:** Venous phase angiogram after sclerotherapy shows lack of contrast at the site of the sclerosed venous malformation (*white arrow*).

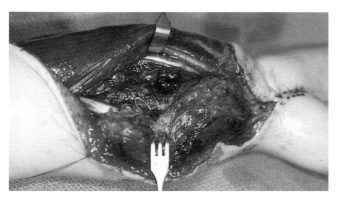

FIGURE 7. Sclerotherapy complication. An acute compartment syndrome developed within hours after this venous malformation was injected. The lesion ran along the interosseous membrane, involving all four superficial flexor muscle bellies and the terminal flexor to the thumb. Clots and thrombi are seen during the fasciotomy. Involved portions of muscles were excised. The only residuum 4 years later was a weak thumb flexor.

Any resection involving the neurovascular structures in the antecubital fossa, pronator tunnel, and deep palmar spaces of the hand requires careful planning. Single or staged debulking on the dorsum of the hand may extend through the intermetacarpal spaces into the deep palmar spaces, a difficult area in which to control bleeding. Loupe magnification is used at all times, and the authors do not hesitate to use the operating microscope if needed (Table 3).

The authors avoid intramuscular dissections unless that particular area is very symptomatic due to phlebothrombosis. Within the arm or forearm, it is often better to completely resect the affected muscle(s) and to restore its function with tendon transfers or replacement. It is impossible to completely excise large, diffuse lesions with or without muscular involvement. Symptomatic, enlarged digits can be debulked in two stages with incisions placed in the midlateral line. Microscopic preservation of digital arteries, including individual vincular branches and nerves, is important (Fig. 8). In dorsal digital debulking, it is unwise to proceed beyond Cleland's ligaments on the

TABLE 3. OPERATIVE PRINCIPLES FOR RESECTION OF UPPER EXTREMITY VASCULAR MALFORMATIONS

Maintain absolute hemostasis under tourniquet control.
Carefully plan dissection within a well-defined region.
Preserve nerves, arteries, and joint cavities. Avoid intraneural dissection.
Avoid reoperation in a previously scarred region by performing a thorough initial dissection.
Avoid combined dorsal and palmar dissections.
Use separate procedures for debulking of digit, hand, forearm, and arm. Debulk axilla and chest wall together.
Perform joint synovectomies and tendon dissections within the digital sheath sparingly.

opposite side of the digit. Forearm debulkings are completed in the same two-staged fashion (Fig. 9). Fortunately, extensive VMs rarely extend through the brachial plexus, a structure that precludes dissection with the aid of a tourniquet. These resections should be avoided in asymptomatic patients with normal distal radial, ulnar, and median nerve function.

Large VMs extending along the entire arm into the axilla and ipsilateral chest wall are challenging, especially when the patient may be septic from localized phlebothrombosis (Fig. 3C). Coagulopathies are often present. Surgical aids include catheters in the subclavian artery and vein, cell saver, hypotensive anesthesia, pneumatic tourniquet for the most distal portion of the VM, and experienced assistants who can compress the lesion while the primary surgeon dissects it off the muscular fascia. One unit of fresh frozen plasma must be replaced with every three units of blood. The authors try to limit total blood replacement to one blood volume in these children.

The complication rate after partial or complete removal of slow-flow VMs is less than 10%. Patients with complications usually have more than one problem directly proportional to the size and specific location of the VM (1). Because postoperative hematomas are common, the authors have used delayed primary closures at 24 to 72 hours postresection after removal of large VMs. Hematomas can be avoided in the upper limb with elevation and good compression dressings and drains. The most common long-term problems have been neuromas-in-continuity, loss of function and contracture after intramuscular resections, and soft tissue losses (1).

LYMPHATIC MALFORMATIONS

Clinical Features

Lymphatic anomalies are usually present at birth, with smaller lesions in less conspicuous regions becoming evident by 4 years of age. In contrast to VMs, these lesions have a rubbery consistency and do not decompress easily. These two characteristics clearly define LMs from VMs. Males and females are affected equally. LMs are most commonly found in the cervicofacial region, where large lesions are often detected by prenatal ultrasound. Although thoracic duct anomalies can occur, they are rarely seen with isolated upper extremity and chest wall LMs.

Clinically, LMs have the appearance of a sponge with large, small, or combined spaces, also referred to as *channels*. In the upper limb, solitary or diffuse lesions in the arm, axilla, and chest wall have both macroscopic and microscopic channels (Fig. 10). Distal to the elbow, almost all LMs are predominantly microscopic, a characteristic that makes them less amenable to sclerotherapy. Diffuse lesions involving the dorsum of the hand, wrist, and forearm usually contain microcystic spaces with large amounts

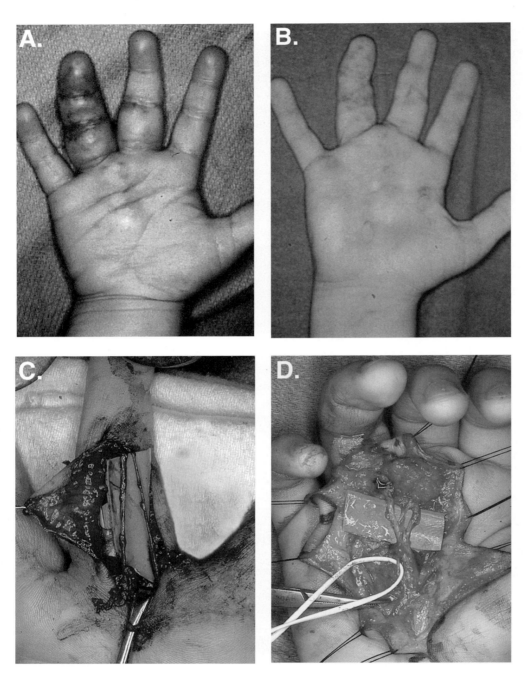

FIGURE 8. Surgical resection of a venous malformation involving the palm and long and ring digits. **A:** Preoperative appearance. The extent of involvement is always much greater than is estimated on physical examination. **B:** The first of multiple staged procedures consisted of debulking one-half of each of the long and ring fingers. Microscopic dissection is invaluable for preservation of neurovascular structures. **C:** The radial digital nerve and artery are seen after microscopic dissection. **D:** All neurovascular structures (except the venae comitantes) are preserved during a full palmar dissection.

of adjacent adipose tissue. Histologically, the walls of lymphatic spaces contain both smooth and skeletal muscle cells and are of variable thickness. The lumens and cystic spaces are filled with protein-rich fluid. In all upper extremity locations, LMs are accompanied by large amounts of fat within the subcutaneous tissue plane.

LMs in the upper limb can also present a dermal capillary malformation component. The skin is thick and may have deep cutaneous puckering as well as a bluish discoloration. LMs in the superficial layers present as single or coalesced vesicles that often weep and provide a portal of entry

for bacterial flora. Dark blue or red nodules represent vesicles filled with blood. Skin involvement is usually patchy in the presence of extensive deep LMs. One variant of LM has a venous component termed *LVM*.

Lymphatic anomalies in the upper limb are most commonly isolated to a specific region in a digit, the hand, forearm, or arm. Axillary LMs typically extend onto the ipsilateral chest wall and into the supraclavicular space and neck. Fortunately, most LMs are confined to the subcutaneous tissue planes and skin and do not penetrate the intermuscular fascia into muscle but can spread along

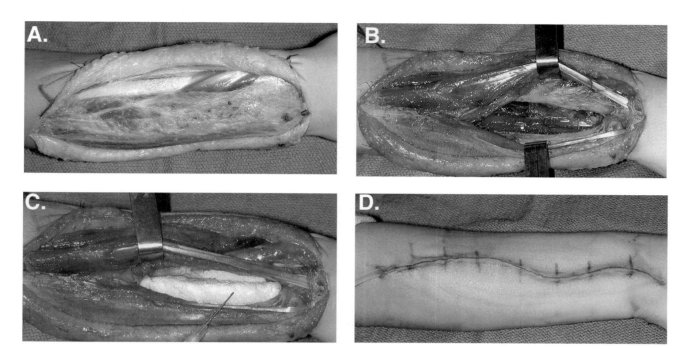

FIGURE 9. Persistent venous malformation after surgical resection. **A:** A 9-year-old boy presented after an unsuccessful excision of a symptomatic venous malformation at another institution, during which the surgeons found themselves "operating in an inkwell." At the time of reoperation at our institution, the skin flaps have been reflected and scarred muscular fascia exposed. **B:** Excision included the interosseous membrane and all involved soft tissue, as well as several distal muscle bellies. **C:** Before closure, gelatin sponge has been placed within the dead space, along with drainage catheters. **D:** An intradermal subcutaneous closure should always be performed on the exposed dorsal surface of the forearm.

these fascial planes. Most symptoms in larger lesions are related to the size, weight, and noncompressibility of the lesion or the weeping, maceration, and ulcers of infected regions. Nerve compression and phlebothrombosis are uncommon.

LMs in the upper and lower extremity can be associated with both skeletal and soft tissue overgrowth that can progress to gigantism. In most of these limbs, there is an accompanying adipose overgrowth, and there is no invasion of the LM into the bone or muscle.

Lymphangiomatosis refers to unique patients who have evidence of disseminated LM. This constellation typically includes diffuse thoracic duct anomalies with recurrent pleural effusions, together with pathognomonic osteolytic bony lesions. These bony lesions were originally described as "Gorham-Stout syndrome," "disappearing bone disease," or "phantom bone disease" (10).

Evaluation

Magnetic resonance imaging T1-weighted images are hypointense, and secondary to the high water content, T2-weighted sequences are hyperintense (Fig. 11). Large macrocysts may have high fluid levels due to protein or blood. Contrast administration may reveal absent or slight rim

enhancement, and gradient-weighted sequences show no evidence of high-flow voids (11).

Treatment

Observation

Small lesions and involved areas of skin are easily observed and treated with local wound care. The two major problems with LMs are infection and intralesional bleeding. Bleeding within a pure LM is not necessarily indicative of a coagulopathy, but a hematologic workup is advised. Bleeding causes the LM to enlarge and to become bluish in color and sometimes painful. Cold compression, elevation, rest, and empiric antibiotic therapy provide effective treatment.

Infection is a more serious problem. Bacteria from a systemic infection may seed channels within an LM. A rapidly progressing cellulitis in children is usually secondary to an upper respiratory infection. Beta-streptococcal organisms are the major pathogens and respond to the prompt administration of penicillin or a broad-spectrum antibiotic. These wildfire infections usually resolve as rapidly as they progress.

Simple aspiration of large cysts provides only temporary relief. Sustained, intermittent compression of large lesions in the upper extremity adequately decompresses one region,

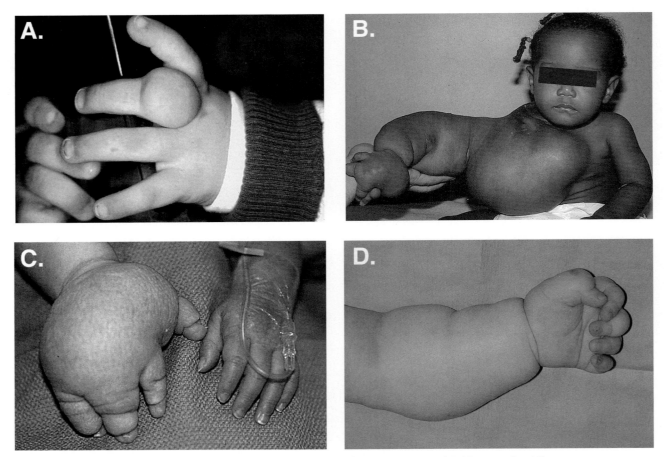

FIGURE 10. Diverse presentations of lymphatic malformations. **A:** Hard, rubbery semimobile mass on the dorsum of the ring finger in an 18-month-old male. **B:** Gross involvement of the upper limb, ipsilateral chest, mediastinum, and neck in a 2-year-old girl. **C:** Lymphatic malformation involving the right hand and wrist of a neonate who was erroneously diagnosed as having an amniotic band syndrome on a prenatal ultrasound, resulting in unnecessary fetal surgery at another institution. The tissue is rubbery and minimally compressible. **D:** The forearm and dorsum of the hand and digits are common presentations for more extensive lymphatic malformations.

displacing fluid into adjacent portions of the LM. Without continuous wear of an elastic garment, the fluid eventually reaccumulates.

Sclerotherapy

The second line of treatment is sclerotherapy by direct injection into the cystic cavities (Fig. 11). Macrocystic LMs respond much more favorably than microcystic lesions, and for this reason, sclerosants are rarely used around the wrist, hand, or digits. Pure ethanol, sodium tetradecyl sulfate, and doxycycline are the most frequently used sclerosants (11). OK-432, derived from group A *Streptococcus pyogenes*, has been used for LMs.

Surgery

Surgical resection is the most predictable way to control LMs. Operative indications for both LMs and LVMs

include pain, intralesional thrombi (venous component present), episodic bleeding, recurrent infection, chronic ulceration and maceration, or functional problems. Local resections in the arm, axilla, and chest wall are often necessary to control excessive drainage (Fig. 5).

Expertise and knowledge of neural and vascular anatomy are essential for dissections of the brachial plexus, antecubital fossa, and palmar spaces of the hand (including the carpal and ulnar tunnels) and along the digits and thumb. The authors have noted most difficulty with extensive lesions within the antecubital fossa and the pronator tunnel, where the multiple motor branches of the ulnar and median nerves must be preserved. Within the palm of the hand, both superficial and deep palmar arches must be preserved with the common digital vessels and all motor branches to intrinsic muscles along the deep motor branch of the ulnar nerve.

The digits and thumb should be approached through midaxial incisions, avoiding zigzag incisions in the glabrous

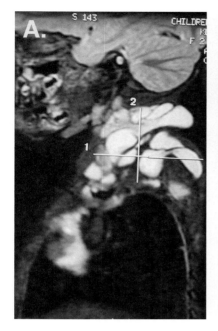

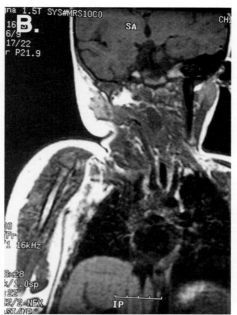

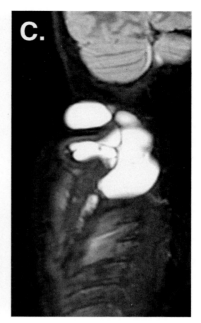

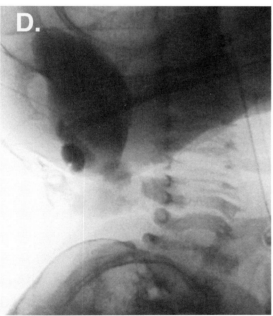

FIGURE 11. Radiologic characteristics of lymphatic malformation. **A:** Multiple macrocysts within a large cervical lymphatic malformation are seen in this T2-weighted magnetic resonance image sagittal view. **B:** In a more anterior T1-weighted coronal plane, the extension of this lesion through the axilla along the chest wall can be appreciated. The areas of high signal intensity represent abnormal fat. **C:** The large macrocysts are the most amenable to sclerotherapy. **D:** The largest cyst is demonstrated on fluoroscopy just before injection of the sclerosant.

skin, as they may hypertrophy. One neurovascular bundle should be left untouched during each of two staged debulkings of a massively enlarged digit (Fig. 12). Cleland's ligaments represent important landmarks during dissection. Dorsal debulking should not extend beyond this ligament to the opposite side of the digit. The adventitia around digital arteries and the epineurium of digital nerves can help to indicate the location of neurovascular structures. All closures must be tension-free. Early use of self-adherent wrapping and continuous passive motion machines decreases postoperative swelling and the residual scar that often develops postoperatively.

The dorsal surfaces of the hand and wrist should be debulked in stages with incisions along the borders of the hand or through a single incision parallel to the third metacarpal (Figs. 12 and 13). When this skin contains deep dermal LM and epidermal vesicles, consider total excision and replacement with either a full-thickness skin graft or a thin fasciocutaneous flap. The tissue over the thumb and thenar muscles and that over the hypothenar muscles are easy to debulk. In contrast, a thorough dissection of LM within the palm is one of the most difficult procedures in all of hand surgery. Postoperative swelling is very difficult to control.

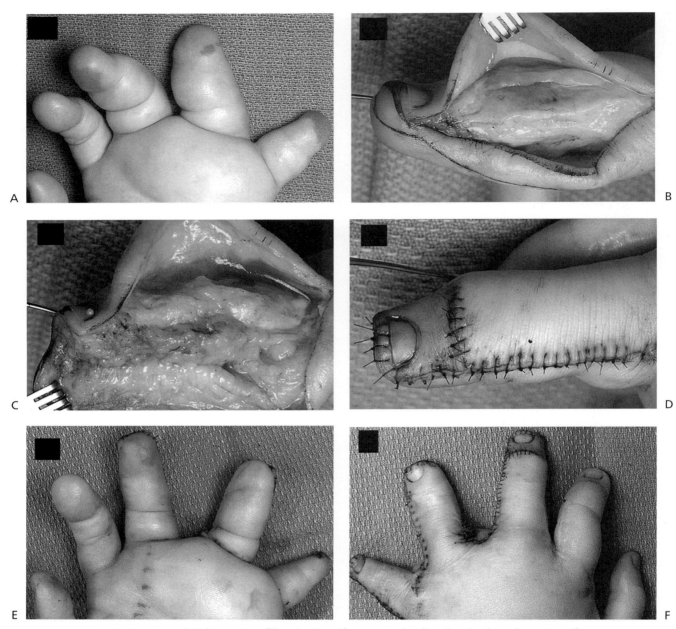

FIGURE 12. A: Digital resection of lymphatic malformation. The digital and palmar dissections of this lymphatic malformation are performed separately. One side of the digit is debulked at a time. **B:** The radial neurovascular bundle, including vincular branches of the artery, has been preserved. An excess amount of fat is admixed with the microcystic lymphatic malformation. The ulnar neurovascular bundle is untouched. **C:** Excess skin is excised through dorsal skin creases. A 2-mm skin bridge is preserved on the distal fingertip for suturing of the palmar flap. Flaps are raised through a high midaxial incision. Estimated regions of skin excision include a large portion of the pulp tissue. There is significant scar tissue from a previous excision. **D:** Postoperative appearance of dorsal surface. **E:** Postoperative appearance of palmar surface. **F:** Dorsal surface closure.

The forearm is ideally approached through a straight medial incision, extending from wrist to elbow. Each stage can extend no more than 200 degrees around the circumference of the forearm. The elbow and arm are best approached medially, and extensive LMs or LVMs are removed in two or more stages. The use of continual compression garments and compression pumps preoperatively and postoperatively makes a tremendous difference in achieving a satisfactory result. Although fluid collection can be partially controlled with compression, most resections proximal to the elbow drain for weeks postoperatively.

After performing separate resections of the chest wall and axilla for many years, the authors now perform this in a single stage during which all neurovascular structures can

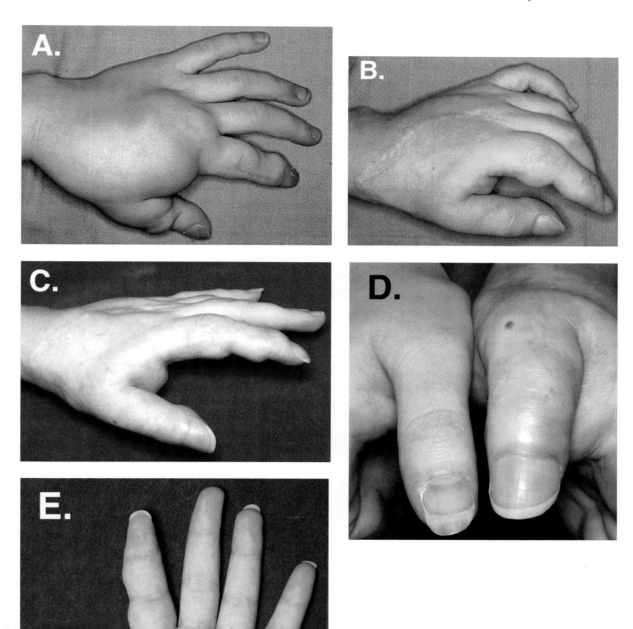

FIGURE 13. Volar hand resection of lymphatic malformation. **A:** This girl is seen at age 6 years after debulking of the index and long digits. Resection of the dorsum of the hand and thumb is planned in two additional procedures. **B:** Postoperative result, 24 years later. **C:** Result 30 years after resection. **D,E:** Regions over the radial side of the index finger and the palmar pulp of the thumb continue to be swollen and hyperhidrotic due to intradermal lymphatic malformation.

be clearly identified (Fig. 14). A thorough preoperative preparation of the entire surgical and anesthesia team is essential for these long, meticulous operations.

The principle of "performing as thorough a resection as possible" is more important in the resection of an LM than with any other vascular anomaly. Hypertrophic scars are common, and swelling may be difficult to control. The bleeding and fibrosis encountered on reentry of these previously dissected regions are unique and profound. Dissect these areas in such a way that reentry is not necessary.

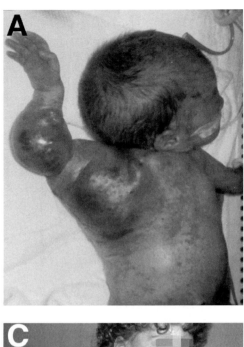

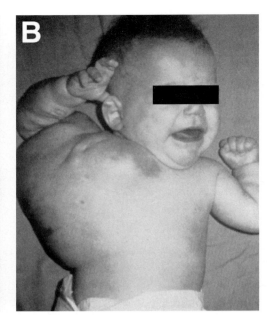

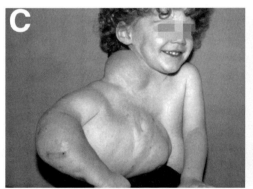

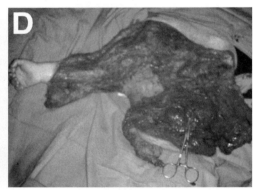

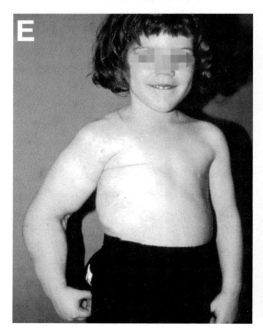

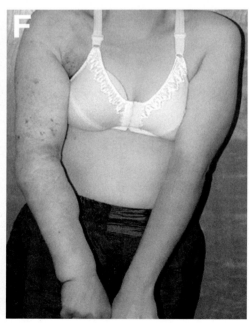

FIGURE 14. Natural history and resection of extensive lymphatic malformation. **A:** At birth, this baby had a rubbery mass with peau d'orange and a bluish hue within the arm and axilla. The diagnosis of lymphatic malformation can be made on physical examination alone. **B:** Over the next 3 months, the mass enlarged and was not compressible. **C:** By 20 months of life, the size and weight of the lesion had become problematic. **D:** The lesion along the chest wall, the axilla including the brachial plexus and arm, was dissected and resected during one procedure. **E:** The chest and arm with residual malformation have been well controlled with compression wrappings at age 5 years. **F:** Despite three additional debulkings of the forearm and arm, it has been difficult to control swelling in this region. Bleeding and maceration from direct dermal involvement within the axilla have necessitated antibiotic treatment for an average of 3 months per year.

Compression pumps augment circumferential wrapping of the wrist, forearm, and axillary regions. With extensive LMs or LVMs, these modalities displace fluid into the mediastinal LM. Thick skin with dermal involvement (either with or without vesicles) contains lymphatic channels and invariably fissures, ulcerates, or becomes infected; it invariably requires surgical replacement. Hypertrophic scar formation can be expected wherever there is LM within the dermis on either side of the wound closure.

The outcomes of aggressive surgery are quite satisfactory, with a complication rate of 22% (1,12). Scar revisions, resection of neuromas, and replacement of drains for persistent drainage in the proximal portions of the limb and chest wall were the most common complications (12). Amputation is often elected for massively enlarged digits, hands, or portions of the arm or after unsuccessful limb salvage attempts. During the past 3 years, the authors have effectively used continuous passive motion machines to maintain motion in released joints at all levels from fingertip to glenohumeral joint.

ARTERIOVENOUS MALFORMATIONS

AVMs are believed to result from errors of vascular development between the fourth and sixth weeks of embryonic gestation. One hypothesis holds that they result from failure of arteriovenous channels in the primitive retiform plexus to regress (13).

Tissue from the epicenter of an AVM, termed the *nidus*, demonstrates close juxtaposition of medium-sized arteries, veins, and vessels. The veins become "arterialized" and exhibit intimal thickening, increased smooth muscle within the media, and dilatation of the vasa vasorum (14). There is also progressive dilatation of the proximal arteries, with fibrosis, thinning of the media, and diminished elastic tissue (14).

Several mechanisms have been proposed to account for the tendency of AVMs to expand to involve previously virgin adjacent tissue. Reid believed that the thin-walled arteries and veins could rupture into one another secondary to increased pressure and flow, forming new fistulous connections (14). Other authors have proposed that local ischemia plays a role, as seen in the "steal phenomenon," producing both pain and ulceration. It is well known that an AVM can enlarge rapidly after proximal ligation (15–17).

Fast-flow malformations are usually present at birth but visible only as a red blush that may be mistaken for a port-wine stain. During childhood, a thrill or bruit and a mass that does not respond to elevation develop. The adolescent growth spurt stimulates growth and expansion by an unknown mechanism; thrills, bruits, and warmth beneath the cutaneous stain become clinically obvious. The pain does not always respond to elevation, especially after exercise. In females, the lesion size increases during the adolescent growth spurt and with menses, oral contraceptives, and preg-

nancy; it does not regress to its previous size after delivery. Symptoms of distal ischemia and discoloration of digits progressing to ulceration may develop with increased shunting through proximal arteriovenous fistulas (AVFs). Children with large lesions with extensive AVFs may go into congestive heart failure. These are the most symptomatic of all vascular anomalies. Severe pain usually precipitates surgery.

Clinical Classification

Type A

Type A malformations are fast-flow anomalies and include single or multiple AVFs, aneurysms, or ectasias on the arterial side of the circulation (Fig. 15) (1). They primarily involve either the radial or ulnar system with or without shunting. Symptoms occur only with exercise.

Type B

Type B malformations consist of more extensive AVMs localized primarily to one axial arterial system in the forearm, hand, or digit (Fig. 16). These fast-flow AVMs have stable flow characteristics and provoke minimal or no distal symptoms. A steal phenomenon can develop after exercise early in life.

Type C

Type C malformations are more diffuse, involving at least two of the three axial systems, with microfistulous and macrofistulous AVFs involving all tissue of the extremity. They are usually evident at a very early age and expand into previously uninvolved areas of the hand. Increased warmth, pain, hyperhidrosis, and a progressive distal steal phenomenon are present.

Radiologic Evaluation

The clinical diagnosis and presence of fast flow are confirmed by ultrasonography and color Doppler studies. Ultrasound of large lesions shows high-flow voids with a low arterial resistance. Arteriovenous shunts are well demonstrated. Type A and B lesions can be easily followed with yearly ultrasound examinations.

Magnetic resonance imaging scans are obtained to gain a baseline with large lesions or lesions involving the palmar spaces of the hand (Fig. 16). Scans are not obtained of AVMs isolated to a single digit. Soft tissue thickening and flow voids are easily detected by T1- and gradient-weighted sequences.

Angiograms are the best way to demonstrate the specific abnormal anatomy of the malformation. Superselective angiography is not used until interventional or surgical treatment is planned. Sequential images demonstrate the size and location of the feeding arteries, the AVM nidus, and early opacification of draining veins (Figs. 15, 16, and 17B).

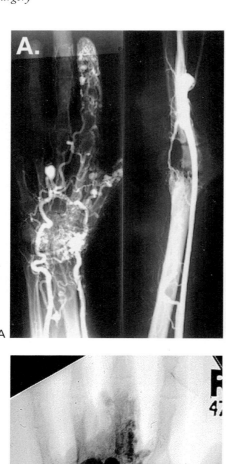

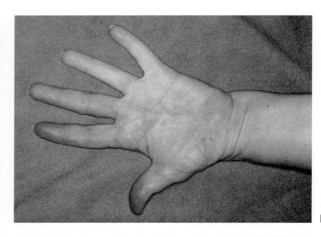

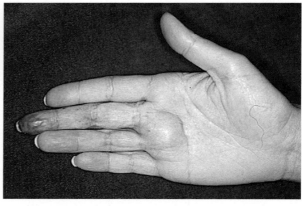

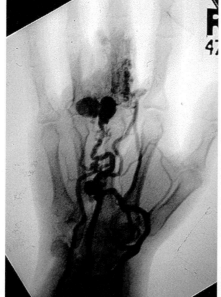

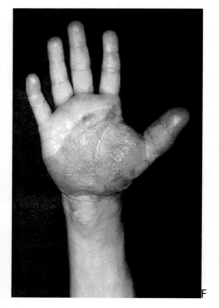

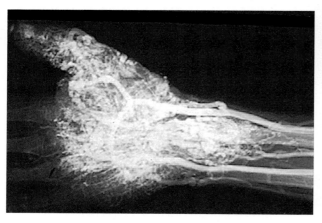

FIGURE 15. Types of fast-flow arteriovenous malformations. **A,B:** Type A consists of single or multiple arteriovenous fistulas, aneurysms on the arterial side of the circulation. **C,D:** Type B lesions are more extensive but localized primarily to one or two of the three axial systems on the arterial side (radial, interosseous, or ulnar). The discoloration of the long fingertip is secondary to the steal phenomenon. **E,F:** Type C malformations are very extensive, involve all three systems, and are very symptomatic. The many microarteriovenous fistulas involve all tissues of the wrist and hand.

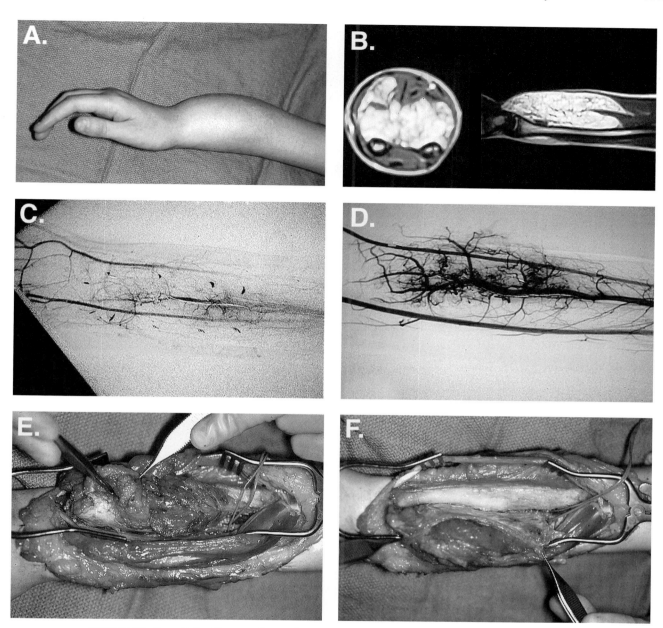

FIGURE 16. Type B fast-flow malformation. **A:** An 8-year-old girl presented with a persistent mass with thrills and bruits over the distal third of the right forearm. **B:** T1-weighted magnetic resonance imaging sequences show flow voids and a mass involving all soft tissue structures dorsal to the interosseous membrane of the forearm. **C:** Early views during angiography demonstrate the many microshunts and arteriovenous fistulas along the interosseous system. **D:** The nidus of the arteriovenous malformation remains along the interosseous membrane, with diffuse extension into the adjacent soft tissue mass. **E:** After preoperative embolization the mass is well visualized. **F:** Resection included the interosseous membrane and involved periosteum of both the radius and ulna. Normal digital and thumb extension was restored postoperatively.

Treatment

Observation

Early in life, observation and compression garments are the mainstays of treatment (Fig. 18). The authors have followed a 67-year-old man conservatively with compression wraps for a type C macrofistulous AVM with multiple AVFs (Figs. 15B, 15E, and 17). Most patients with type B and C lesions develop pain as a result of distention of the lesion and progression of a distal steal phenomenon.

Sclerotherapy

Sclerotherapy can be used to obliterate large tortuous arteries if ligated feeding arteries prevent passage of an embolization catheter. Some well-localized AVMs have been successfully

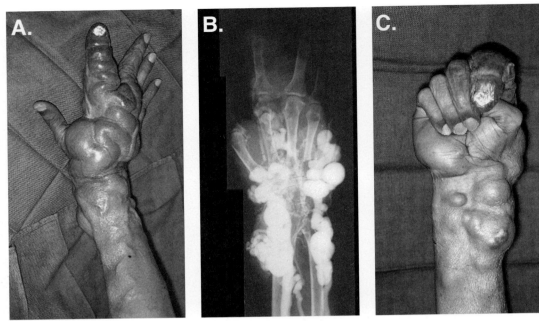

FIGURE 17. Arteriovenous malformation type C, fast-flow. **A:** This 67-year-old executive noted a gradual swelling and pulsation in his hand since his teenage years. Earlier in life, surgical removal of symptomatic regions was aborted due to bleeding that could be controlled only with elevation and pressure. **B:** Early angiographic sequences show macrofistulous shunts involving the radial and ulnar arteries and both palmar arches. With aging, these vascular channels have dilated and become quite tortuous. **C:** He experiences a persistent steal phenomenon in the long and index fingers, and the mass within the palm partially obstructs a functional grasp unless he wears his compression glove. Extrinsic flexion and extension have remained normal. The distorted nail matrix of the index finger has been the source of a chronic paronychia.

treated with a combination of embolization followed by sclerotherapy (11,18), most of these in the head and neck and lower extremity. The risks and morbidity after this combined approach are high (19). The authors have not used this combination in the treatment of upper limb AVMs.

Embolization

The decision to use embolization with or without surgery is made jointly by the surgeon and the interventional radiologist. For minimal to moderately symptomatic type A or B AVMs, embolization is the less traumatic procedure (Fig. 19). Indications include rapid growth of the AVM with increased flow of AVFs, pain, distal discolora-

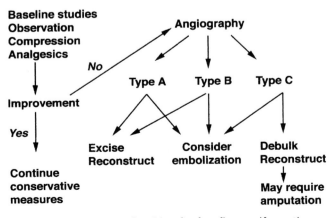

FIGURE 18. Treatment algorithm for fast-flow malformations.

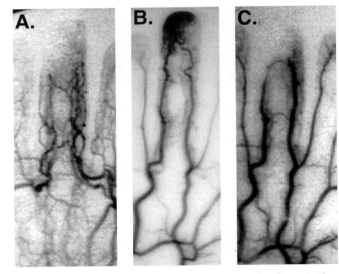

FIGURE 19. Arteriovenous malformation type B, fast-flow. **A:** The angiogram of a 6-month-old child with a swollen, red, tense fingertip. Localized thrills were consistent with a microfistulous arteriovenous malformation involving only the pulp tissue. **B:** Superselective embolization was performed through a catheter that was passed into the ulnar digital artery of this small child. **C:** Follow-up angiography demonstrates complete obliteration of the mass.

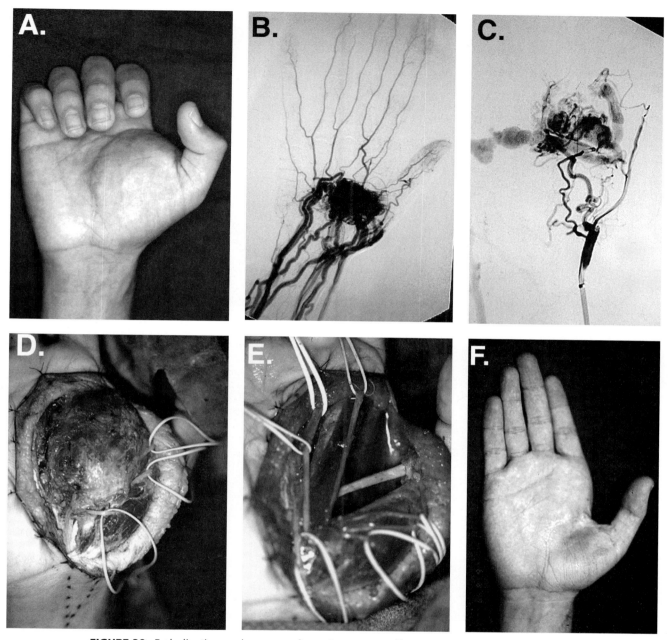

FIGURE 20. Embolization and surgery of arteriovenous malformation type B. **A:** This professional wrestler presented with a painful mass within the thenar muscles. A thrill was first noted during adolescence. There was no history of trauma. **B:** The nidus of the arteriovenous malformation was demonstrated at the level of superficial palmar arch, supplied by radial, interosseous, and ulnar vessels. Distal digital and thumb arterial architecture was shown to be normal. **C:** The postembolization study showed obliteration of most of the arteriovenous malformation with large draining veins. **D:** Two days later, the mass was explored surgically. Yellow vessel loops mark the recurrent motor branch and sensory branches of the median nerve. **E:** All nerves and flexor tendons were preserved during surgical resection. **F:** Five years later, he continued to demonstrate good function. Palmar abduction is present through the abductor pollicis, but key pinch is weak due to the resection of the adductor pollicis muscle.

tion and ulceration, cardiac overload/congestive heart failure, and failure to thrive. The most common symptoms are well localized to specific areas of microfistulous or macrofistulous shunting; these are best controlled with superselective embolization using various types of particles, coils, gelatin sponge packs, and the like. For type C lesions, palliative embolization is often used before surgery (Figs. 20 and 21).

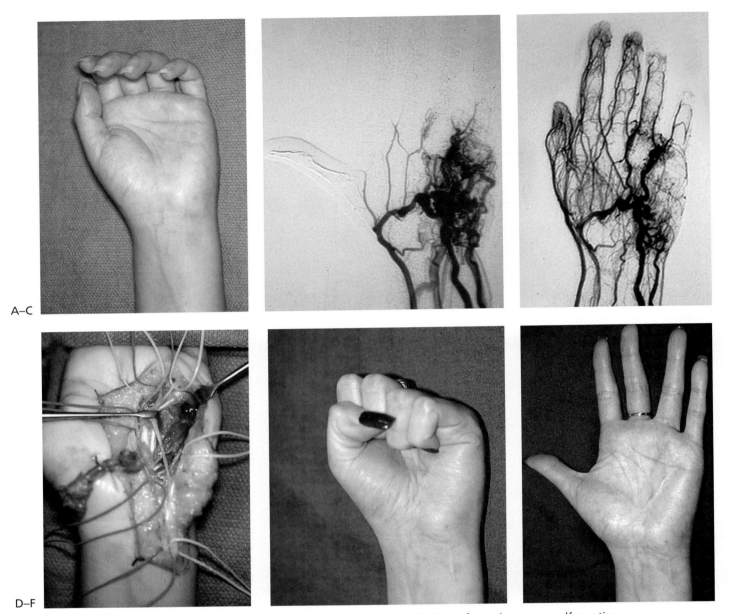

A–C

D–F

FIGURE 21. Embolization, surgery, and repeat embolization of arteriovenous malformation type B. **A:** A pulsatile mass within the hypothenar eminence of this young woman became larger and painful when she started antiovulant medication. **B:** Early angiographic sequences showed a macrofistulous arteriovenous malformation in Guyon's canal fed by both ulnar and interosseous vessels. **C:** A postembolization sequence showed persistence of many shunts. Note the lack of perfusion of the pulp tissue of both ring and long digits, which were most symptomatic. The caliber of the ulnar artery was twice normal. **D:** Surgical excision included removal of ulnar artery and common digital vessel to the fourth web space. Sensory and motor nerves and flexor tendons were preserved and revascularization to the ulnar side of the ring and both sides of the fifth digit performed with autogenous vein grafts. **E:** Normal flexion and extension without claw posturing were noted 2 years postoperatively. **F:** Five years later, she presented with a painful mass at the base of the ring finger. This represented some residual arteriovenous malformation at the margin of the previous resection within the intermetacarpal space and was easily embolized without the need for more surgery.

TABLE 4. CLINICAL STAGING SYSTEM FOR ARTERIOVENOUS MALFORMATIONS

Stage	Description
I Quiescence	Pink-bluish stain, increased warmth, arteriovenous shunting detectable on 20-MHz Doppler
II Expansion	Stage I plus enlargement, pulsations, thrill, and bruits, tortuous/tense veins
III Destruction	Stage II plus dystrophic skin changes, ulceration, bleeding, persistent pain, and soft tissue necrosis
IV Decompensation	Stage III plus cardiac failure

Surgery

In all but the least complicated resections, angiography and superselective embolization precede surgical resection by 24 to 72 hours. Under pneumatic tourniquet control, the embolized regions are easy to find and provide excellent landmarks for the surgeon. With large lesions, embolization alone can be palliative for difficult problems such as congestive heart failure, continued bleeding, and localized pain. Surgery is mandated for uncontrolled intralesional bleeding, compartment syndromes, nerve compressions, chronic ulceration, and gangrene. Table 4 describes staging guidelines based on clinical findings.

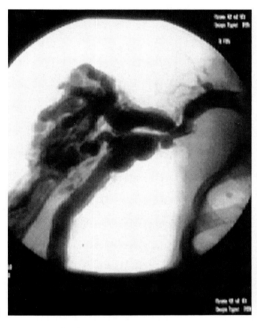
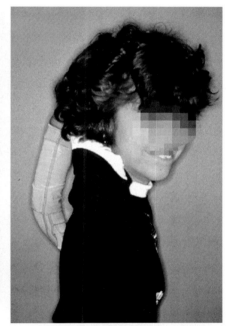

A,B

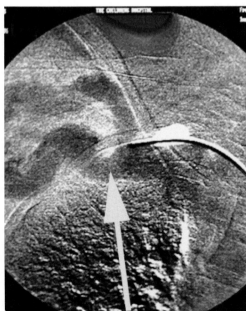
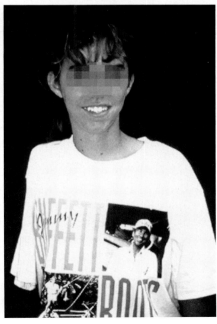

C,D

FIGURE 22. Microfistulous, progressive arteriovenous malformation type C. At age 1 year, this child presented with a capillary malformation of the hand and pulsatile mass of the distal forearm. The diagnosis of Parkes Weber syndrome was made, and she was treated with compression garments. An angiogram at age 6 years showed a progressive microfistulous, painful arteriovenous malformation of the distal forearm. By the time she was 12 years old, she was in continual pain. **A:** Massively enlarged subclavian and axillary arteries were demonstrated, and at the same time, she showed early signs of cardiac compromise. **B:** She learned to control her pain by dislocating her glenohumeral joint and compressing her axillary artery, a position in which she often slept. **C:** Intraarterial balloon catheters were helpful at the time of shoulder disarticulation for removal of her parasitic and extremely painful limb. **D:** Preservation of the scapula helps drape clothing and makes the appearance of these patients less conspicuous. Within 6 months, she gained 20 pounds, became less morose, and excelled in school and cross-country running.

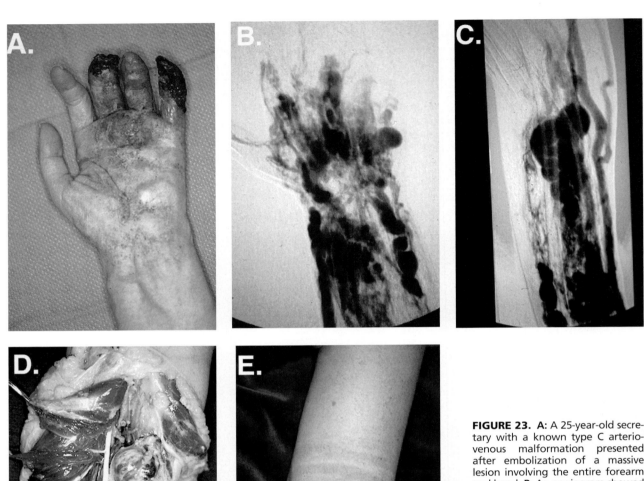

FIGURE 23. A: A 25-year-old secretary with a known type C arteriovenous malformation presented after embolization of a massive lesion involving the entire forearm and hand. **B:** An angiogram showed macrofistulous shunting involving all three arterial systems of the hand. The digital vessels to the ulnar three digits were not visualized at any stage of the study. **C:** The shunts and fistulas with the forearm appeared to be massive. **D:** Appearance during amputation. **E:** With a well-healed, nonpainful below-elbow amputation stump, she functioned very well with and without a myoelectric prosthesis. She regretted that she did not have this procedure performed much earlier in life.

Wound dehiscence, bleeding, and infection are common early sequelae, and neuroma-related pain, sympathetic dystrophies, and contracture often follow the unsuccessful resection. Partial resections of type B and C AVMs are doomed to fail. The need for microvascular revascularization of the hand or individual digits must be addressed. Most of the preoperative pain in these patients is steal phenomenon–related.

The most difficult aspect of these resections lies in defining the limits of the malformation that characteristically cross tissue planes. The authors' approach has been to preoperatively angiograph and embolize the symptomatic portion of the AVM(s) and to anatomically define the resection margins

before an incision has been made. Even in the ideal bloodless field afforded by the tourniquet, the surgeon may not have a clear delineation of the malformation margins (Fig. 21) (1).

Long-term outcomes of type B and C patients after upper extremity resections or amputations are not available. The authors' preliminary experience with approximately 45 patients is that most showed expansion of residual malformations somewhere near the periphery of the resection within 10 years. The majority followed beyond this time became symptomatic in those areas within 10 years. The spread of the malformation into previously uninvolved portions of the extremity has been much greater for microfistulous AVFs and macrofistulous lesions (Fig. 22).

It is difficult for the surgeon to know when not to operate. Some categorically refuse to consider any surgical approach after witnessing colleagues trying to "operate in an inkwell" after uncontrolled hemorrhage from macrofistulas. For upper extremity lesions, tourniquets, embolization, careful planning, good surgical technique, aggressive resections, and reconstructions together provide opportunities that are not readily available in other anatomic regions such as the head and neck, trunk, pelvis, and peritoneum. Symptomatic type A and B lesions are the most amenable to surgery.

The recommendation to amputate is both difficult for the surgeon and exasperating for the patient and his or her par-

ents who, in desperation, often seek multiple additional opinions. If the patient is requesting amputation, he or she is usually right, and the request should not be denied by the surgeon. Pain, impending gangrene, symptoms secondary to severe steal, early cardiac compromise, and a failure of young children and adolescents to maintain normal growth parameters are all indications for selective amputation (Figs. 22, 23, and 24). The authors' outcome study of type C patients showed an amputation rate of more than 90% over a 30-year period of time. In retrospect, with nine of 17 patients eventually requiring amputation at the forearm, arm, or shoulder level, the authors prolonged the inevitable amputation for a

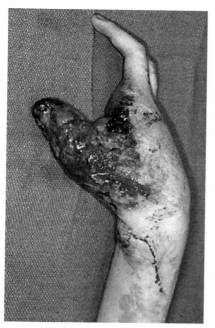
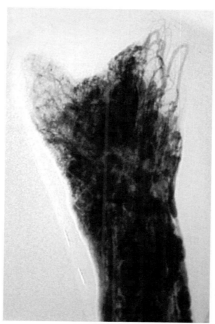
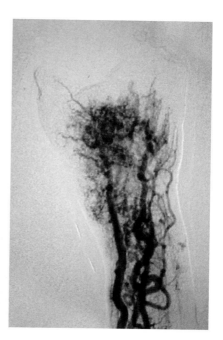

A–C

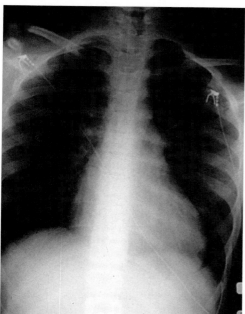

D

FIGURE 24. Type C, microfistulous and macrofistulous, congestive heart failure, and below-elbow amputation. **A:** Both this teenager with a type C arteriovenous malformation and his parents wanted to save this hand. The index ray had been resected for uncontrollable pulsatile bleeding. The thumb then became ulcerated and congested, and the patient became suicidal because of the unrelenting pain. **B:** Angiography showed massively tortuous and enlarged axial vessels feeding microfistulous shunts within the forearm and hand. **C:** A later sequence demonstrated the extent of the shunting and lack of distal digital perfusion. **D:** Chest radiograph and electrocardiogram were consistent with congestive heart failure. A below-elbow amputation was followed by a predictable recovery and normal adolescent growth spurt.

number of reasons. The recovery after ablation of the parasitic part and elimination of the chronic pain are both remarkable and predictable. Rapid weight gain, improved disposition, and increased level of activity are all notable.

REFERENCES

1. Upton J, Coombs CJ, Mulliken JB, et al. Vascular malformations of the upper limb: a review of 270 patients. *J Hand Surg [Am]* 1999;24:1019–1035.

1a. Mulliken JB, Glowacki J. Hemangiomas and vascular malformations in infants and children: a classification based on endothelial characteristics. *Plast Reconstr Surg* 1982;69:412–422.

2. Mulliken J, Young A. *Vascular birthmarks: hemangiomas and malformations.* Philadelphia: WB Saunders, 1988.

3. Guttmacher AE, Marchuk DA, White RI. Hereditary hemorrhagic telangiectasia. *N Engl J Med* 1955;333:918–924.

4. Devillers AC, de Waard-van der Spek FB, Oranje AP. Cutis marmorata telangiectatica congenita: clinical features in 35 cases. *Arch Dermatol* 1999;135:34–38.

5. Smoller BR, Rosen S. Port-wine stains. A disease of altered neural modulation of blood vessels? *Arch Dermatol* 1986;122:177–179.

6. Mulliken J, Boon L, Takahashi K. Pharmacologic therapy for endangering hemangiomas. *Curr Opin Dermatol* 1995;2:109–113.

7. Berenguer B, Burrows PE, Zurakowski D, et al. Sclerotherapy of craniofacial venous malformations: complications and results. *Plast Reconstr Surg* 1999;104:1–11; discussion 12–5.

8. Dubois JM, Sebag GH, De Prost Y, et al. Soft-tissue venous malformations in children: percutaneous sclerotherapy with Ethibloc. *Radiology* 1991;180:195–198.

9. Upton J, Mulliken JB, Murray JE. Classification and rationale for management of vascular anomalies in the upper extremity. *J Hand Surg [Am]* 1985;10:970–975.

10. Gorham L, Stout A. Massive osteolysis (acute spontaneous absorption of bone, phantom bone, disappearing bone): its relation to hemangiomatosis. *J Bone Joint Surg* 1955;37:986–1004.

11. Burrows PE, Laor T, Paltiel H, et al. Diagnostic imaging in the evaluation of vascular birthmarks. *Dermatol Clin* 1998;16:455–488.

12. van der Horst CM, Koster PH, de Borgie CA, et al. Effect of the timing of treatment of port-wine stains with the flash-lamp-pumped pulsed-dye laser [see comments]. *N Engl J Med* 1998;338:1028–1033.

13. Halsted W. Congenital arteriovenous and lymphaticovenous fistulae: unique clinical and experimental observations. *Trans Am Surg Assoc* 1919;37:262.

14. Reid M. Abnormal arteriovenous communications, acquired and congenital. II. The origin and nature of arteriovenous aneurysms, cirsoid aneurysms and simple angiomas. *Arch Surg* 1925;10:601.

15. Braverman I, Keh A, Jacobson B. Ultrastructure and three-dimensional organization of the telangiectases of hereditary hemorrhagic telangiectasia. *J Invest Dermatol* 1990;95:422.

16. Coleman CJ. Diagnosis and treatment of congenital arteriovenous fistulas of the head and neck. *Am J Surg* 1973;47:354.

17. Reinhoff WJ. Congenital arteriovenous fistula: an embryological study with report of a case. *Bull Johns Hopkins Hosp* 1924;35:271.

18. Yakes WF, Rossi P, Odink H. How I do it. Arteriovenous malformation management. *Cardiovasc Intervent Radiol* 1996;19:65–71.

19. Kohout MP, Hansen M, Pribaz JJ, et al. Arteriovenous malformations of the head and neck: natural history and management. *Plast Reconstr Surg* 1998;102:643–654.

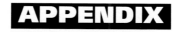

APPENDIX

COMBINED (EPONYMOUS) MALFORMATIONS

SLOW-FLOW COMBINED MALFORMATIONS

Capillary-Lymphatic-Venous Malformation (Klippel-Trénaunay Syndrome)

A capillary-lymphatic-venous malformation (Fig. 25) is associated with skeletal and soft tissue overgrowth (1–5).

In 80%, only the lower limb is involved, mostly unilateral. Upper extremity lesions can extend into the mediastinum and retropleural space but rarely evoke symptoms. Lymphatic hypoplasia is present in more than half of the patients, and generalized lymphedema is common. Upper extremity capillary-lymphatic-venous malformation presents with skeletal overgrowth of the arm, forearm, or hand (Fig. 25). However, undergrowth can occur. Pulmonary embolism may occur in up to 25% of patients.

Proteus Syndrome

Proteus syndrome is a sporadic, progressive vascular, skeletal, and soft tissue condition that truly lies at the interface of vascular anomalies and overgrowth syndromes. The authors do not consider this syndrome as a vascular anomaly.

The 1998 National Institutes of Health workshop diagnostic criteria include three mandatory general criteria: (a) a mosaic or asymmetric distributions of lesions, (b) a progressive course, and (c) sporadic occurrence (6). In addition, some number of "category signs" must be present. These include verrucous (linear) nevus, lipomas and lipomatosis, macrocephaly (calvarial hyperostoses), asymmetric limbs with partial gigantism of the hands and/or feet, and curious cerebriform plantar thickening ("moccasin" feet). As a rule, Proteus syndrome is not present at birth. These features suggest that this syndrome may be the result of a dominant lethal gene that survives by somatic mosaicism (6).

Maffucci's Syndrome

Maffucci's syndrome (Fig. 26) denotes the coexistence of exophytic venous malformations with bony exostoses and enchondromas (7). The osseous lesions appear first, most often in the hands, feet, long bones of the extremity, ribs, pelvis, and cranium (8). There may be a history of recurrent fractures secondary to enchondromatous weakening of bony diaphyses. The VMs involve the subcutaneous tissues and bones and are generally distributed in the extremities (Fig. 26). These patients often develop spindle cell hemangioendotheliomas within the VMs. These are a reactive vascular proliferation rather than a true tumor (9). Malignant transformation, usually chondrosarcoma, occurs in 20% to 30% of patients (10,11). A majority of the chondrosarcomas are of histologically low grade and can often be cured with surgical resection (12,13).

FAST-FLOW EPONYMOUS SYNDROMES

Parkes Weber Syndrome

Parkes Weber syndrome is much less prevalent than capillary-lymphatic-venous malformation. The capillary malformation is usually more diffuse and pink. The major difference is the presence of the AVM with AVFs, which all present early in childhood. These lesions become progressively worse and carry a poor long-term prognosis. With time, the involved regions of the arm and forearm form large macrofistulous shunts. Surgical treatment is helpful only for well-localized symptomatic shunts, compartment syndromes, or compression syndromes. Because many of these upper extremity lesions are so diffuse, surgical resection is unrealistic.

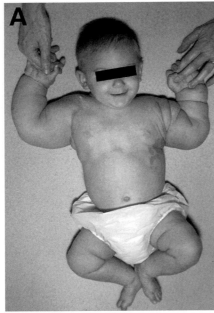

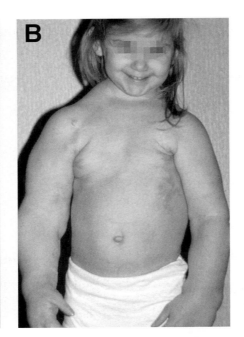

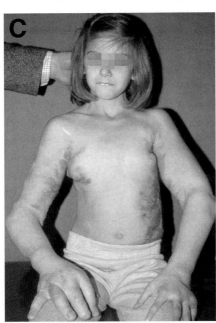

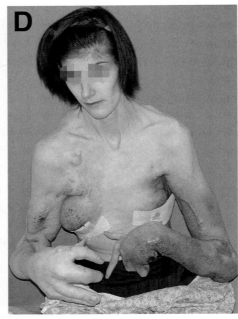

FIGURE 25. Capillary-lymphatic-venous malformation progression. **A–D:** The progression of a combined capillary-lymphatic-venous malformation is seen at ages 6 months, 3 years, 12 years, and 28 years. Manifestations of upper limb involvement included skeletal and soft tissue overgrowth, macrodactyly, development of extensive lymphatic vesicles, and worsening of joint contractures after multiple operations at another local institution. At age 22, she delivered a normal infant, and 6 years later, she died of suspected pulmonary embolus.

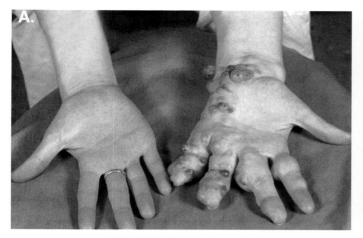
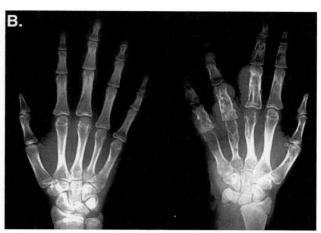

FIGURE 26. Maffucci's syndrome. **A:** The unilateral hand of a girl with Maffucci's syndrome shows the characteristic sessile, pedunculated venous malformations. **B:** Radiographs demonstrate multiple phalangeal and metacarpal lucencies secondary to enchondromas. Her right distal ulnar has been previously resected.

REFERENCES

1. Upton J, Coombs CJ, Mulliken JB, et al. Vascular malformations of the upper limb: a review of 270 patients. *J Hand Surg [Am]* 1999;24:1019–1035.
2. Baskerville PA, Ackroyd JS, Lea Thomas M, et al. The Klippel-Trenaunay syndrome: clinical, radiological and haemodynamic features and management. *Br J Surg* 1985:72:232–236.
3. Gloviczki P, Stanson AW, Stickler GB, et al. Klippel-Trenaunay syndrome: the risks and benefits of vascular interventions. *Surgery* 1991;110:469–479.
4. Jacob AG, Driscoll DJ, Shaughnessy WJ, et al. Klippel-Trenaunay syndrome: spectrum and management. *Mayo Clin Proc* 1998;73:28–36.
5. Samuel M, Spitz L. Klippel-Trenaunay syndrome: clinical features, complications and management in children. *Br J Surg* 1995;82:757–761.
6. Biesecker LG, Happle R, Mulliken JB, et al. Proteus syndrome: diagnostic criteria, differential diagnosis, and patient evaluation. *Am J Med Genet* 1999;84:389–395.
7. Maffucci A. Di un caso di encondroma ed angioma multiplo contribuzione al a genesi embrionale dei tumor. *Movimento Med Chir (Naples)* 1881;3:399.
8. Lewis R, Ketcham A. Maffucci's syndrome: functional and neoplastic significance. *J Bone Joint Surg Am* 1979;55:1469.
9. Perkins P, Weiss SW. Spindle cell hemangioendothelioma. An analysis of 78 cases with reassessment of its pathogenesis and biologic behavior. *Am J Surg Pathol* 1996;20:1196–1204.
10. Kaplan RP, Wang JT, Amron DM, et al. Maffucci's syndrome: two case reports with a literature review. *J Am Acad Dermatol* 1993;29:894–899.
11. Sun TC, Swee RG, Shives TC, et al. Chondrosarcoma in Maffucci's syndrome. *J Bone Joint Surg Am* 1985;67:1214–1219.
12. Coley B, Higinbotham N. Secondary chondrosarcoma. *Ann Surg* 1954;139:1954.
13. Cook P, Evans P. Chondrosarcoma of the skull in Maffucci's syndrome. *Br J Radiol* 1977;50:833.

94

RAYNAUD'S SYNDROME

DAVID T. NETSCHER

Digital vasoconstriction is a normal homeostatic mechanism. It is said that aberrant microvascular flow that is secondary to acute or chronic trauma, systemic processes, congenital abnormalities, or genetic reasons affects more than 10% of the population and 20% to 30% of premenopausal women (1,2). However, inferences regarding the epidemiology of primary Raynaud's disease are tenuous. Recent community-based surveys (3,4) indicate that approximately 12% of patients, regardless of race or gender, report fingertips or toes being unusually sensitive to cold. Nearly 25% of the cold-sensitive population (representing 3% of the adult population in those studies) actually had blanching or cyanosis, or both. In some locales, as many as 20% of people are aware of digital blanching and numbness (5), but most people do not consider themselves to be adversely affected by the disorder.

An otherwise healthy person who has blanching and no other discernible manifestations of systemic illness apparent at initial evaluation is unlikely to develop a systemic disease over time (6). There is probably no value to serologic tests (antinuclear, anticentromere, anti-SCL70 antibodies) (7,8) or even to periungual capillary microscopy (9) in this setting. Thus, many people for whom common sense has taught to avoid a cool ambient temperature need have no concerns about their symptoms boding worsening conditions in terms of digital damage or development of systemic disease. They may, in fact, as has been suggested by some (9), be at one end of a spectrum of normal or exaggerated vascular homeostasis to cold. It is my task, in the course of this chapter, to provide an understanding of the macro- and microanatomy of digital vasculature, to try to elucidate thermoregulatory mechanisms, to put in perspective the clinical features of a potential patient, and to provide an analysis of indications for nonsurgical and surgical treatments.

Vascular *incompetence* occurs when there is an inability to appropriately modulate thermoregulatory and nutritional blood flow to fulfill metabolic requirements, which leads to pain, cold intolerance, and numbness. When vascular *insufficiency* occurs, nutritional blood flow is inadequate to maintain cellular viability; ulceration and gangrene then occur. Symptoms that are caused by abnormal perfusion may occur secondary to congenital or acquired disorders that affect anatomic vascular structures (thrombosis or occlusion), vascular function (abnormal vasomotor control), or both (10).

SURGICAL ANATOMY AND PHYSIOLOGY

In most people, the major blood supply to the hand is provided by the superficial palmar arch (continuation of the ulnar artery) and the deep palmar arch (continuation of the radial artery), but a large median or interosseous artery may be present. The superficial palmar arch is completed by branches from the deep palmar arch in 78.5% of subjects, and the arch is incomplete in 21.5% (11). However, the deep arch is completed on the ulnar side in 98.5% of people (11). The incidence of loss of the hand after ligation of the ulnar artery after war injuries was reported as 1.6% and, when the radial artery was ligated, as 5.1% (12). However, the ulnar artery has long been thought of as the dominant blood supply to the superficial palmar arch and, hence, to the common digital arteries (13). Anatomic dissections provide only a static representation of the potential blood flow to the hand and do not demonstrate the circulation dynamics. Using pulse-volume recording (PVR), a study of the dynamics of hand circulation found that, in normal subjects, only 5% of hands had ulnar artery dominance (pulse-volume amplitude was greater during radial artery compression) in all digits, and 28% had complete radial artery dominance (14). Ulnar artery dominance in three or more digits occurred in 21.5% compared to 57% with radial dominance; 21.5% had equal dominance. Overall, 87% of thumbs were radial dominant (14).

Blood vessels that are smaller than 100 μm in diameter constitute the microcirculation, deliver nutrients to the microvascular beds, and provide adequate capacity for arteriovenous (AV) thermoregulatory blood flow. The microcirculation of the fingertips, volar parts of the fingers, palms, toes, soles, and ear lobes is distinctive from the microcirculation of skin elsewhere. At these locations, the arterioles and venules are not only connected through capillary beds,

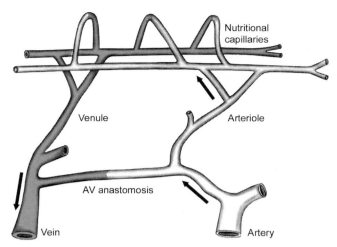

FIGURE 1. Microcirculation of fingertips shows that arterioles and venules are connected through nutritional capillary beds, as well as through heavily innervated thermoregulatory arteriovenous (AV) shunts.

but also through large numbers of heavily innervated, convoluted, muscular-walled AV shunts (15) (Fig. 1). The AV shunts serve a thermoregulatory function and are in parallel with the nutritional capillary beds. Under normal conditions, approximately 80% to 90% of digital blood flow passes through the thermoregulatory beds (16). In response to total body cooling or aerobic exercise, an increase in sympathetic tone closes AV shunts, but leaves capillary nutrient beds patent, thereby preserving digital nutrition. If there is severely diminished total blood flow, or when there

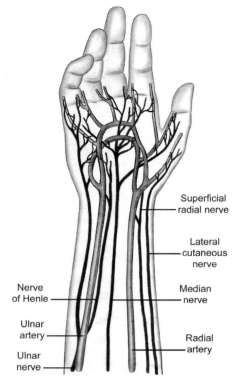

FIGURE 3. Sympathetic nerve connections between main peripheral nerve trunks and forearm and hand arteries.

is excessive microvascular distribution into nonnutritional thermoregulatory beds, flow may be inadequate to sustain cellular viability, thus leading to cell injury or death.

Peripheral nerve function is important for the microvascular control of digital blood flow. Peripheral sympathetic fibers are predominantly group C unmyelinated fibers. They travel variable distances within peripheral nerves before pursuing a perivascular course (17–19). In the hand and digits, common and proper digital nerves have sympathetic fibers that connect to correspondingly sized vessels (20) (Fig. 2). After traveling in perivascular adventitial tissue, these sympathetic fibers penetrate the arterial and venous walls (20). In the forearm, sympathetic fibers reach the perivascular tissue of the radial and ulnar arteries mainly from the ulnar, median, superficial radial, and lateral cutaneous nerves (18). The nerve of Henlé is a branch from the ulnar nerve and supplies large segments of the ulnar artery in the forearm and hand (21) (Fig. 3). In a dissection study of 40 extremities, the nerve of Henlé was not found in 43% (22). In the remaining extremities, the nerve of Henlé was identified more commonly to originate from the ulnar nerve in the proximal forearm and, less frequently, in the distal forearm. This nerve not only carries the sympathetic supply to the ulnar artery, but also provides distal cutaneous sensation to the palm and distal forearm. The palmar cutaneous branch of the ulnar nerve was absent in cadavers with a nerve of Henlé and may, in fact, be a distal variant of that nerve (22).

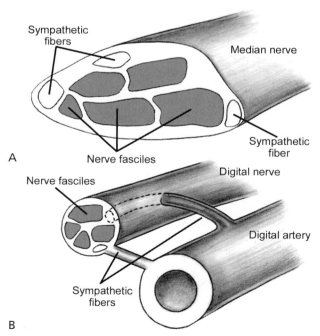

FIGURE 2. A: Peripheral sympathetic nerve fibers in the forearm nerve. **B:** Sympathetic fibers connect the digital nerve and the digital artery.

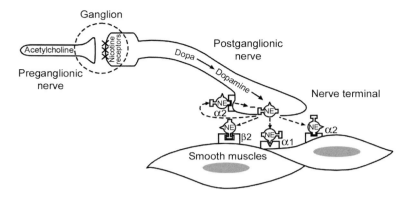

FIGURE 4. Sympathetic control of smooth muscles of the vessel walls. NE, norepinephrine.

Sympathetic control is regulated through ganglionic synapses and motor end plates on the smooth muscle of vessel walls (Fig. 4). Acetylcholine neuroreceptors are broadly divided into muscarinic (smooth muscle and glands) and nicotinic (sympathetic ganglia) (23). Smoking probably has an adverse vasoconstrictor effect on digital blood flow primarily through its nicotinic stimulatory effects on postganglionic sympathetic fibers (24).

Active vasoconstriction is caused by adrenergic neurotransmitters that act on vascular smooth muscle at the motor end plates. There are adrenergic receptors pre- and postsynaptically. Postsynaptic alpha-1 and alpha-2 receptors cause vasoconstriction when they are stimulated by released norepinephrine. Beta-2 receptors cause vascular smooth muscle relaxation. Presynaptic alpha-2 receptor stimulation moderates vasoconstriction by inhibiting norepinephrine release. Unlike alpha-1 receptors, alpha-2 receptors are not widely distributed in the vascular system. The latter are not present in large arteries, but are generally restricted to small arteries and arterioles and to venous circulation (25,26).

In patients with primary Raynaud's disease, there is increased sensitivity or density, or both, of peripheral alpha-adrenergic receptors (27). There is an increased number of alpha-2 receptors on platelets in patients with primary and obstructive Raynaud's syndrome (28). There are subtypes of alpha-2 receptors. In laboratory experiments, cold causes a selective increase in the ability of alpha-2 receptors to induce vasoconstriction, and these receptors seem to function as cutaneous thermosensors (29). The alpha-2C receptors were previously thought to be silent. However, at cold temperatures, the augmented vasoconstrictor response to alpha-2 receptor stimulation is blocked by an alpha-2C receptor antagonist (30). In patients with Raynaud's syndrome, there may be increased sensitivity or density, or both, of peripheral alpha-2 receptors (27, 31). Indeed, the response in Raynaud's syndrome may represent a local fault in alpha-2C receptors (30). Because these receptors appear to be "silent" in normal regulation of vascular function, their selective blockade may potentially provide a highly specific therapeutic intervention for cold-induced vasospastic conditions.

At a local level, there are also metabolic and myogenic autoregulatory effects on blood vessels and microvascular perfusion. Myogenic autoregulation is mediated by transneural pressure and stretch-operated calcium channels (32). The vascular endothelium generates several vasoactive substances, including the potent vasoconstrictor endothelin-1 (33) and the vasodilator nitric oxide (34) (whose production may be stimulated by acetylcholine action on nitric oxide synthase). A temperature-dependent disorder of the endothelium that involves underproduction of nitric oxide or overproduction of endothelin-1 may be a factor in the pathogenesis of Raynaud's syndrome (35).

PATHOPHYSIOLOGY

Normal vasomotor tone directs blood to nutritional capillary beds and also allows appropriate thermoregulatory control. Adequate tissue perfusion requires delivery of blood to nutritional capillary beds to fulfill metabolic requirements and to provide adequate oxygen carrying capacity. Inappropriate vasospasm produces pain and cold intolerance that interfere with quality of life and may result in ulceration or gangrene, or both. Raynaud's syndrome is a spectrum of vasospastic states that may be primary (Raynaud's disease) in the absence of identifiable etiology or secondary (Raynaud's phenomenon) in the presence of a causal condition. The criteria for defining Raynaud's dis-

TABLE 1. CRITERIA FOR RAYNAUD'S DISEASE

Characteristic triphasic digital color changes that are induced by exposure to cold or stress
Bilateral hand involvement
Absence of arterial occlusion that is proximal to the fingers
Absence of gangrene or trophic changes (fingertip trophic changes are permissible)
Absence of underlying disease that may cause vasomotor problems (vascular disorders)
Symptoms of at least 2 years in duration
Female predominance

TABLE 2. DISTINCTIONS BETWEEN RAYNAUD'S DISEASE AND RAYNAUD'S PHENOMENON

	Characteristic	Disease	Phenomenon
History	Triphasic color change	Yes	Yes
	>40 years of age	No	Yes
	Rapid progression	No	Yes
	Underlying disease	No	Yes
	Female predominance	Frequent	Occasional
Physical examination	Trophic findings (ulcer, gangrene)	Infrequent	Frequent
	Abnormal Allen's test	No	Common
	Asymmetric findings	Infrequent	Frequent
Laboratory findings	Blood chemistry	Normal	Frequently abnormal
	Microangiology	Normal	Frequently abnormal
	Angiography	Normal	Frequently abnormal

ease are listed in Table 1 (36), and the distinctions between Raynaud's disease and Raynaud's phenomenon are presented in Table 2 (37).

Symptoms of vasospastic conditions result from inadequate vascular structure or inappropriate vascular control mechanisms, or a combination of the two (2). Presumptive pathologic mechanisms in secondary vasospastic disorders include (a) structural changes that reduce blood vessel radius, (b) impaired vascular tone, (c) changes in blood components and hyperviscosity, and (d) a decrease in pressure gradient (38) (Table 3). Based on pathophysiologic criteria, patients may be categorized into one of four symptomatic Wake Forest groups (39) (Table 4). Categorization of patients into one of these groups helps formulate the treatment strategy. The presence of occlusive disease produces secondary vasospasm (40). The combination of occlusive disease in a patient with a preexisting vasospastic condition often precipitates a crisis that results in ischemic pain, nonhealing ulcers, and gangrene. Often, with occlusive vascular disease, a critical point of ischemic pain and ulceration is reached when two levels of occlusion occur (e.g., ulnar artery and digital artery).

A variety of disorders are associated with Raynaud's syndrome. These all tend to result from a combination of vaso-occlusive disorders and vasospasm:

1. Vibration-induced white finger syndrome is described in those who regularly work with vibratory equipment, such as pneumatic hammers, jackhammers, and riveters. The problem appears to be worse in outdoor workers in cold climates (41). These patients usually do not complain when using the vibratory tool but have greater sensitivity to cold exposure and Raynaud's

TABLE 3. CLASSIFICATION OF PRESUMPTIVE PATHOLOGIC MECHANISMS FOR SECONDARY VASOSPASTIC DISORDERS

Structural changes reducing vessel radius
  Connective tissue diseases
    Scleroderma
    Systemic lupus erythematosus
    Mixed connective tissue disease
    Dermatomyositis
    Sjögren's syndrome
    Rheumatoid arthritis
    Primary biliary cirrhosis
  Other diseases of small vessels
    Cryoglobulinemia
    Infectious diseases
    Malignancies
    Drug-induced vasculitis
    Buerger's disease
    Polyarteritis nodosa
    Thromboembolism
    Occupational trauma
    Occlusive arterial diseases
  Miscellaneous
    Bleomycin
    Vinyl chloride disease
    Heavy metals, uremia

Abnormal vascular tone
  Drug induced
    Ergotamines
    Beta-blocking agents
    Alpha-sympathomimetic agents
  Sympathetic hyperactivity
    Unilateral: invading tumor and thoracic outlet, carpal tunnel, vibration-induced syndromes
    Bilateral: connective tissue disorders
Changes in blood components and hyperviscosity
  Increased plasma viscosity
    Cryoglobulinemia
    Paraproteinemia
    Cold agglutinins
    Hyperfibrinogenemia
  Increased blood viscosity
    Polycythemia
    Thrombocytosis
    Leukemia
Direct decrease in pressure gradient
  Neurovascular compression syndromes
  Arteriosclerosis obliterans
  Thromboembolism
  Arteriovenous shunts

TABLE 4. PATHOPHYSIOLOGIC WAKE FOREST CLASSIFICATION OF VASOSPASTIC AND VASO-OCCLUSIVE DISEASE

Group 1	Raynaud's disease	—	—
Group 2	Raynaud's phenomenon due to collagen vascular disease	Adequate circulation	Inadequate circulation
Group 3	Vasospasm due to vascular injury or occlusion	Adequate collateral circulation	Inadequate collateral circulation
Group 4	Vasospastic disease due to non-vascular injury	—	—

attacks while they are at rest (42). The precise cause is unknown, as investigation has been impeded by the inability to predictably reproduce the syndrome and the presence of other variables, such as tobacco use and underlying connective tissue disorders. Cold provoca-

tion tests for workers with vibration white finger syndromes are reported to be positive from 40% to 97% (43). There does seem to be hypertrophy of vascular smooth muscle, which may also cause vascular lumen constriction (44).

2. Carpal tunnel syndrome has been cited as an associated cause of Raynaud's syndrome (45), but this association is doubted (46).

3. Connective tissue disorders account for no more than 20% of patients with Raynaud's syndrome (47), but these disorders are among the most severe problems and probably represent the majority of patients in a hand surgery practice. Vasospasm occurs in a variety of connective tissue disorders, such as rheumatoid arthritis (11%) (48), scleroderma (95%) (49), systemic lupus erythematosus (40%) (38), dermatomyositis (30%) (48), and mixed connective tissue disease (91%) (50). In these conditions, there is intimal fibrosis and thickening of small vessels, and, conceivably, the Raynaud's phenomenon could be caused by a normal

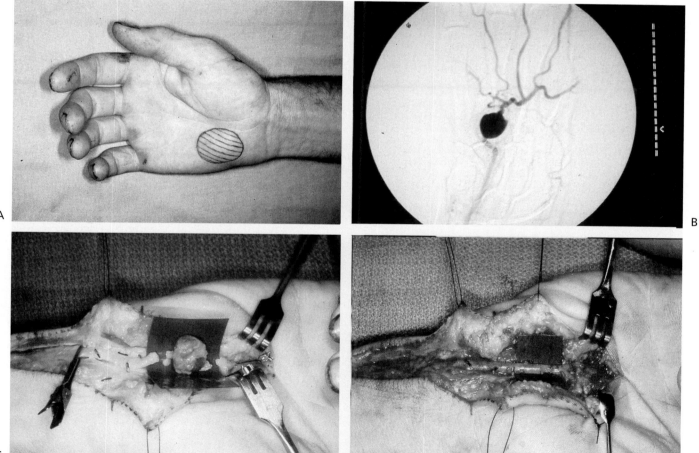

FIGURE 5. A hypothenar hammer syndrome that resulted from repetitive trauma to the proximal palm in an automobile mechanic. **A:** Ulnar artery aneurysm is palpable in a patient with Raynaud's discoloration of the fingertips. **B:** Aneurysm of the ulnar artery. **C,D:** Treatment by aneurysm resection and end-to-end anastomosis of the ulnar artery.

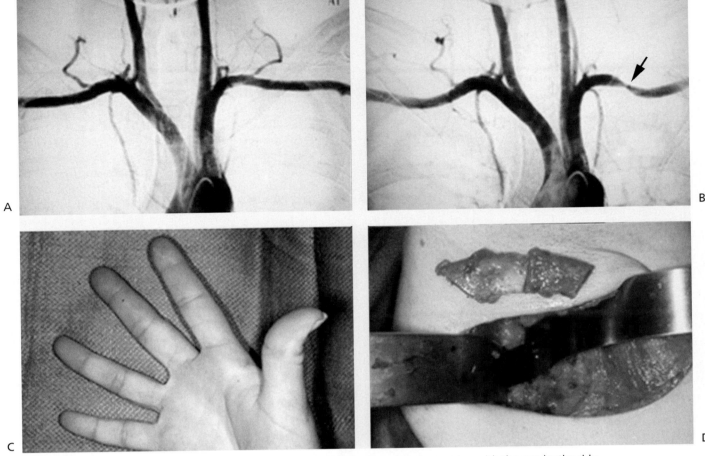

FIGURE 6. Arteriography of a patient with thoracic outlet compression with the arm by the side **(A)** and then with the arm abducted at the shoulder **(B)** that shows subclavian stenosis (*arrow*). This patient presented with severe unilateral Raynaud's phenomenon **(C)** and underwent trans-axillary first rib resection **(D)**.

vasoconstrictor response acting on a structurally diseased and narrowed artery. However, it seems that an abnormal vasoconstrictor response does play a role, and it is also known that successful medical control of the connective tissue disease does not necessarily correlate with improvement in the Raynaud's syndrome (51).

4. Trauma may have wide-ranging effects that result from delayed responses to frostbite, fracture displacement that causes vessel fibrosis (52), and ulnar thrombosis in the palm from *hypothenar hammer syndrome* (Fig. 5). In this latter condition, the digital vasospasm can often be corrected by simple excision of the occluded arterial segment (53). However, with current microvascular techniques, particularly when there appears to be reduced distal back flow, most surgeons now prefer resection and arterial repair or vein graft reconstruction in this situation (54). Raynaud's syndrome may occur as an acute vascular steel phenomenon immediately after the creation of a dialysis shunt. This can be associated with profound motor and sensory loss, as well as vasospasm (46). The treatment for this condition is to reverse the steel phenomenon.

5. Proximal vascular disorders, such as thromboangiitis obliterans (Buerger's disease), atherosclerosis, or thoracic outlet syndrome, must always be excluded, because Raynaud's attacks may result from low-pressure flow or embolic phenomena (Figs. 6 and 7).

EVALUATION

Clinical History and Physical Examination

Important details in patient history are the presence of previous injury, particularly repetitive insults; blood dyscrasias; drug exposure and tobacco use; factors that might be associated with connective tissue disorders; the frequency and severity of the Raynaud's events; the extent of the cold sensitivity, numbness, and associated pain; and stimulation of

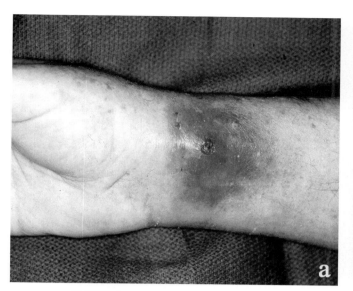
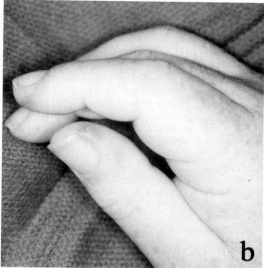

FIGURE 7. A: Patient with infected radial artery pseudoaneurysm at the wrist after radial artery cannulation. **B:** Distal infected emboli to paronychia and pulps of thumb and index finger.

the vasomotor disorder by emotional changes. Raynaud's disease and Raynaud's phenomenon that is associated with systemic illness (e.g., connective tissue disorders or blood dyscrasias) are usually bilateral and may also involve the feet. Unilateral Raynaud's phenomenon nearly always suggests a vascular occlusive disease and, especially when it is combined with necrosis or nonhealing ulcers, should be considered pathognomonic of vascular compromise from thrombosis or embolism (10). Symptomatic complaints may be quantified by using validated questionnaires, such as the McCabe Cold Sensitivity Severity Scale (55). Use of such validated instruments also improves follow-up evaluation of progress.

The physical examination for a vascular disorder of the upper extremity must include a thorough evaluation of the entire upper extremity and neck and also auscultation of the heart. Heart murmurs, as well as auscultatory bruits in the neck or thoracic outlet region, may be supportive evidence for embolic phenomena, as might be an irregular rhythm from atrial fibrillation. The brachial blood pressure is taken bilaterally, and a systolic pressure difference between each side is determined. Palpate for masses along the course of major peripheral vessels. An Allen's test at the wrist and proximal phalanges provides information regarding arterial perfusion to the hand and fingers and may identify occlusive disease (56) (Fig. 8). A handheld Doppler

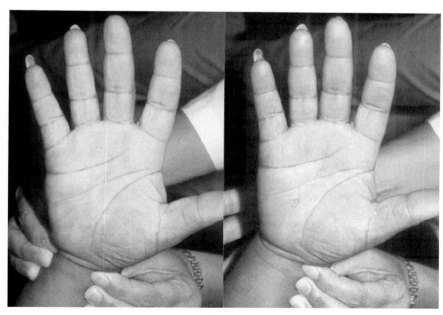

FIGURE 8. Allen's test. **A:** Digits are white, with the radial and ulnar arteries occluded. **B:** Digits are perfused, with pressure released on the ulnar artery but maintained on the radial artery, thus demonstrating an intact palmar arch system.

A,B

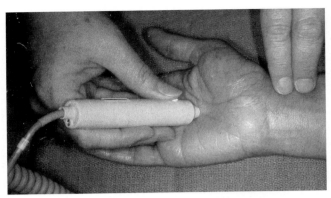

FIGURE 9. The handheld Doppler that is used in the office detects flow in the superficial palmar arterial arch.

flowmeter (Fig. 9) is readily used in the office setting. Careful mapping can identify areas of occlusion, and sequential occlusion of the radial and ulnar arteries may enable Doppler monitoring of collateral arterial inflow. The hands are specifically evaluated for capillary refill, pulp turgor, skin integrity, ulceration or gangrene, fungal or pyogenic infections of the nail and paronychia, the quality and rhythm of the peripheral pulse, and alterations in skin temperature and finger color in response to emotional and cold stimuli, with inspection of the nail folds for evidence of collagen vascular disease by examination with an ophthalmoscope (57) (Fig. 10).

Special Diagnostic Tests

These tests evaluate vascular competency to define the anatomic vascular structure that is involved, as well as the functional flow performance. The functional flow tests may be done under stressed and nonstressed conditions. Thus, a combination of vascular studies may be necessary to arrive at the appropriate anatomic and functional diagnosis, to help differentiate between occlusive and vasospastic disorders and their relative importance when both occur together, and hence to help with a therapeutic plan, as well as to enable objective follow-up and evaluation of the instituted therapy. Most vascular evaluations estimate total blood flow; however, vital capillaroscopy is the only special test that truly evaluates nutritional flow. Laser Doppler fluxmetry evaluates nutritional and thermoregulatory flow (Table 5).

The goal of diagnostic testing is to determine the structural anatomy of the vasculature, as well as the functional capability of the system to respond to stress. In the office, the clinical history and examination, which includes wrist and digital Allen's testing, as well as handheld Doppler mapping, are used as a guide to further testing. Digital blood pressure and digital brachial index (DBI) are calculated, and, then, appropriate tests are chosen to delineate the structural abnormalities and also to determine the quality of the collateral circulation and to define the role of

vasospasm. Anatomic details are best identified by B-mode ultrasonography or contrast arteriography. Arteriography probably still remains the "gold standard" in the majority of cases; however, surgical exploration after noninvasive testing is recommended in a number of circumstances (58). Functional control of vascular supply is studied in various stress situations. Digital temperature and laser Doppler fluxmetry may be used to assess this functional control. Some of these modalities are not universally available, but, nonetheless, a thermal stress response can still be evaluated by using digital plethysmography (PVR).

Doppler, Digital Plethysmography (Pulse-Volume Recordings), Segmental Pressures, and Color Duplex Imaging

PVR should be interpreted in conjunction with other noninvasive studies, such as DBI, Doppler mapping, and temperature measurements. PVR findings can only yield meaningful information if they are correlated with the clinical picture. Some information is garnered from the contour of the pulse recording. Digital pulse contours may be categorized as normal when there is a rapid systolic up-slope with a diastolic down-slope and a dicrotic wave (Fig. 11). An obstructed digital pulse contour has a delayed up-slope with a rounded peak and a convex down-slope that bows away from the baseline (59). No dicrotic wave is found in the down-slope. In the presence of adequate collateral circulation, however, an obstructed pulse contour may not be found. In patients with thoracic outlet compression who have a vascular component, blood pressure measurements and PVR may be done with the upper extremity in various positions in an attempt to elicit the degree of vascular compression.

Segmental systolic arterial pressure determinations enable ratios to be calculated between levels. Thus, a radial brachial index and a DBI can be calculated. A DBI or radial brachial index of less than 0.7 indicates inadequate arterial flow to a hand or digit and necessitates medical or surgical intervention, or both (60). Differences of 15 mm Hg between fingers or a wrist-to-finger difference of 30 mm Hg is said to indicate occlusion at the level of or distal to the palmar arch. Waveform analysis aids in differentiation between symptoms of occlusive disease and vasospastic responses to cold stimuli (19). Pressure differences of greater than 20 mm Hg at the same level between the affected and contralateral extremities may also indicate arterial stenosis or occlusion (19).

Plethysmography and PVR have been compared with arteriography and have been found to have a correlation as high as 97% (61) to 100% (62). Arteriography gives a static picture of the vasculature, whereas dynamic information is provided by the noninvasive studies. PVR provides dynamic information about subclavian, forearm, and digital vessels and even indicates (by alteration of amplitude and shape of the wave) the presence of an occlusion that is

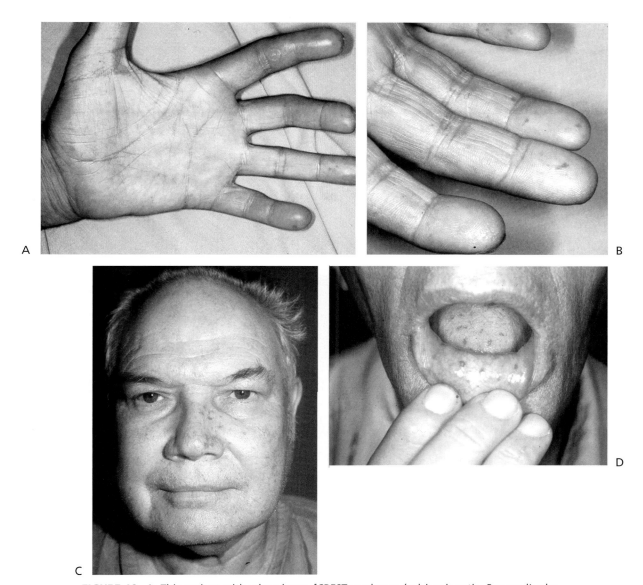

FIGURE 10. A: This patient with scleroderma [CREST syndrome (calcinosis cutis, *R*aynaud's phenomenon, *e*sophageal dysfunction, *s*clerodactyly, and *t*elangiectasia)] presented with severe bilateral Raynaud's phenomenon. **B–D:** He had multiple telangiectasias on the fingertips, on the face, and in the mouth.

TABLE 5. VALUES OF DIFFERENT TYPES OF VASCULAR SPECIAL TESTS

Specific tests	Anatomic delineation	Functional performance	Flow component measured
Digital plethysmography (pulse-volume recording)	None	Good	Total flow
Segmental anterior perfusion	Fair	Good	Total flow
Color duplex imaging	Good	Good	Total flow
Laser Doppler fluxmetry	None	Good	Nutritional and thermoregulatory
Vital capillaroscopy	Excellent	None	Nutritional
Technetium 99m scan	Fair	Good	Total flow
Magnetic resonance angiography	Good	Fair	Total flow
Arteriography	Excellent	Fair	Total flow

Adapted from Koman LA, Ruch DS, Smith VP, et al. Vascular disorders. In: Green DP, Hotchkiss RN, Pederson WC, eds. *Green's operative hand surgery*, 4th ed. New York: Churchill Livingstone, 1999:2254–2302.

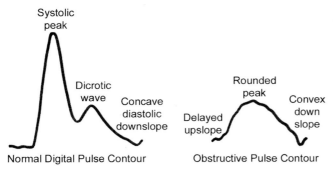

FIGURE 11. Normal and obstructive digital pulse volume contours.

small enough to alter vessel dynamics but not large enough to reduce blood pressure. However, PVR cannot accurately localize subclavian lesions but can demonstrate the hemodynamic significance of such an obstructive lesion. Thus, arteriography has specifically been recommended for proximal vaso-occlusive lesions, embolic diseases, vascular tumors, and vascular malformations (62). PVR has an advantage of providing a noninvasive manner of monitoring the results of medical and surgical treatment and providing long-term follow-up. This noninvasive evaluation has been combined with peripheral nerve block to determine those patients in whom a digital sympathectomy may be likely to be successful (17,18,63) (Figs. 12 and 13). In those patients who had a positive response to peripheral nerve blockade with the local anesthesia and were then subjected to surgical digital sympathectomy, almost all obtained benefit from the operation. However, others have indicated that, although improvement in temperature and PVR after a digital block may confirm increased total flow, it does not indicate any changes in nutritional perfusion (39). Conversely, if nutritional flow is increased without measurable change in total digital blood flow, ulcers heal nonetheless (64). Thus, an increase in digital temperature or plethysmography after digital or sympathetic block may not necessarily be a prerequisite for surgical sympathectomy. Perfusion may be improved in patients with combined vasospastic and occlusive disease without significant increase in digital temperature by redirecting a portion of the thermoregulatory flow to the nutritional vascular beds. Thus, it is the belief of some authors that the precise group of patients who might benefit the most from a peripheral sympathectomy may indeed not be identified without data that more specifically determine nutritional blood flow, such as that which might be derived from an evaluation that uses laser Doppler fluxmetry or vital capillaroscopy (65).

Color duplex imaging (CDI) combines ultrasound imaging techniques and a color-coded Doppler evaluation of flow. Indications in the upper extremity for CDI include the evaluation of masses, the determination of anomalous vasculature, the identification of perfusion abnormalities,

and also a postoperative evaluation. CDI provides less anatomic information than arteriography but has the advantages of lower cost, noninvasiveness, and dynamic acquisition of flow data.

Laser Doppler fluxmetry evaluates the motion of blood cells in the area immediately beneath the probe. Laser Doppler perfusion imaging measures cutaneous perfusion over a 12×12 cm^2 surface and produces a color-coded image. A composite scan is produced by the computer. This technique assesses thermoregulatory and nutritional components of flow. It provides an estimate of cutaneous microvascular perfusion over a significant surface area.

Vital Capillaroscopy

Structural changes in capillary morphology can be evaluated by using this vital capillaroscopy. The nutritional capillaries are oriented parallel to the skin surface at the nail fold, thereby allowing direct assessment of the entire capillary loop. This technique may provide direct clinical information about the pathology of patients with Raynaud's phenomenon and scleroderma.

Dynamic capillary videomicroscopy is the only technique that permits direct assessment of nutritional perfusion. The flow and morphology of nutritional vessels are analyzed by direct, dynamic videophotometric capillaroscopy (2). Resting capillary blood flow varies widely among individuals, and, thus, a dynamic intervention (stress) is required to assess flow response patterns and to permit quantitative comparisons. This technique may be unsuitable in approximately 12% of subjects, because capillary visibility is hampered by vessel orientation, length of the capillary loop, hyperkeratotic skin, or dense pigmentation (2,10). Abnormal capillary morphology may permit the direct diagnosis of systemic diseases.

Bone Scintigraphy

Radionuclide imaging provides an assessment of upper extremity vascular anatomy, documents spatial and temporal alterations of vascular distribution, and quantifies perfusion characteristics. After intravenous injection of technetium 99m pertechnetate, the first phase of a three-phase nuclear bone scan is obtained. Many vascular lesions have a typical radionuclide scan appearance (66). AV malformations may exhibit characteristic patterns. Absence of the radiotracer activity distal to occlusive disease may be a poor prognostic sign for possible pending necrosis.

Magnetic Resonance Angiography

Although this magnetic resonance angiography produces no ionizing radiation, cannot initiate allergic reactions, and provides imaging through radiodense casts or splints, conventional x-ray techniques and angiography currently pro-

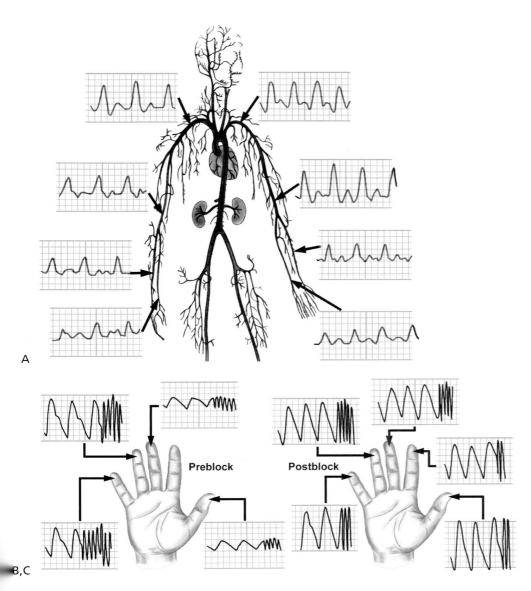

FIGURE 12. A: Pulse volume recordings and pressures are made noninvasively at the brachium, the forearm, the hand, and the digits. **B,C:** Augmentation of flow is seen by larger amplitude digital tracings after digital local anesthetic block in a patient with significant vasospasm.

vide more detailed data, produce higher resolution, and are available at more locations. The use of magnetic resonance angiography continues to evolve.

Arteriography

Contrast arteriography provides the best anatomic structural information on upper extremity vasculature but is nonetheless a static evaluation of the extremity. Information is optimized by using intraarterial vasodilators [e.g., tolazoline hydrochloride (Priscoline hydrochloride)] to identify stenoses that might be secondary to vasospasm and subtraction techniques that minimize background interference. Potential problems with arteriography include catheter-induced vasospasm and the possible failure to observe distal arterial reconstitution because of vasospasm. Consider regional anesthetic block, such as a stellate ganglion block, if vasospasm prevents adequate visualization. Indica-

tions for arteriography include unilateral Raynaud's phenomenon, unexplained clinical escalation of symptoms despite ongoing medical therapy, unexplained progression of ulceration, evidence of occlusive disease by physical examination or noninvasive studies, or anticipation of a surgical intervention to determine feasibility of vascular reconstruction.

Normal collateral blood flow between the radial and ulnar systems exists in multiple anatomic configurations (67). However, all reported variations of arterial anatomy include the presence of three palmar common digital arteries at the level of the metacarpophalangeal joint (68). This observation does help simplify the differentiation of pathologic from normal anatomic variance. The latter should always include a minimum of three palmar common digital vessels (69).

In summary, a complete evaluation of vascular function requires analysis of flow before, during, and after a controlled and repeatable stress. This type of stress may include thermal,

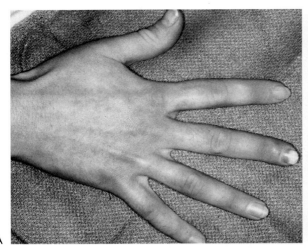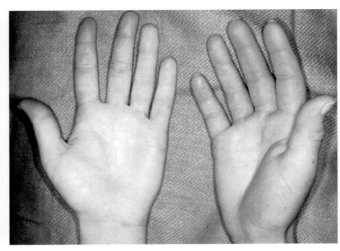

FIGURE 13. **A:** Patient with systemic lupus erythematosus who presented with severe bilateral Raynaud's phenomenon. **B:** Stellate sympathetic block was performed on the right hand, which demonstrates a warm well-perfused hand, and is contrasted with the persistent Raynaud's phenomenon of the left hand.

anoxic, or emotional. The analysis of flow should include an assessment of total flow, as well as its thermal regulatory and nutritional components. In addition to identifying vasospastic conditions, occlusive vascular disorders and their locations must be sought. In particular, occlusion of the distal ulnar artery is common in patients with connective tissue disease and must not be overlooked (2,10).

TREATMENT OPTIONS

Treatment options include the following:

Increase collateral flow by reducing vasoconstrictor tone:
    Eliminate tobacco
    Biofeedback
Increase nutritional flow by use of calcium channel blockers
Sympathectomy:
    Chemical with alpha- and beta-blockers
    Continuous autonomic blockage with sustained brachial plexus block
    Surgical, by one of the following:
        Leriche sympathectomy that resects the thrombosed arterial segment and ligates the artery
        Periarterial adventitial dissection
Restoration of circulation by:
    Resection and repair
    Thrombectomy
    Resection and vein graft
    Arterial bypass
    Thrombolytic therapy
    Omental resurfacing, reversal of AV shunts

Classification of vasospastic disorders that is based on anatomic occlusive sites and functional flow, as well as the sever-

ity of the condition, which includes adequacy of circulation, aids in the selection of appropriate treatment options. Those who have secondary vasospasm and occlusive disease (group 3) and who have adequate collateral circulation (group 3A) require minimal intervention and generally respond to sympatholytic medications or sympathectomy techniques, including resection of a thrombosed vascular segment and arterial ligation. Medical management of these group 3A patients includes biofeedback and pharmacologic interventions, as well as environmental modifications, such as cessation of tobacco use, avoidance of caffeine, and minimization of cold exposure with the use of gloves. Surgical options in these cases include procedures to decrease the vasoconstrictor tone or to restore blood flow. Simple resection and ligation of the thrombosed vessels (Leriche sympathectomy) may be all that is required. When there is otherwise unreconstructable arterial occlusive disease but, nonetheless, adequate collateral flow and symptoms that cannot be controlled by medical management alone, then peripheral periarterial sympathectomy would be considered a salvage procedure. If collateral flow is inadequate (group 3B) with secondary vasospasm, arterial reconstruction is required for maximal recovery.

In contrast, biofeedback alleviates symptoms most effectively in patients with Raynaud's disease, vasospasm from nonneural or nonvascular etiology, and Raynaud's phenomenon with an adequate collateral circulation. The results of biofeedback are much less favorable in patients with inadequate collateral circulation (groups 2B and 3B).

Thus, an algorithm for the management of vasospastic conditions might be as follows:

1. History and physical examination reveal Raynaud's symptoms and severity of the condition with or without gangrene and ulcers.
2. Upper extremity Doppler recordings are performed.

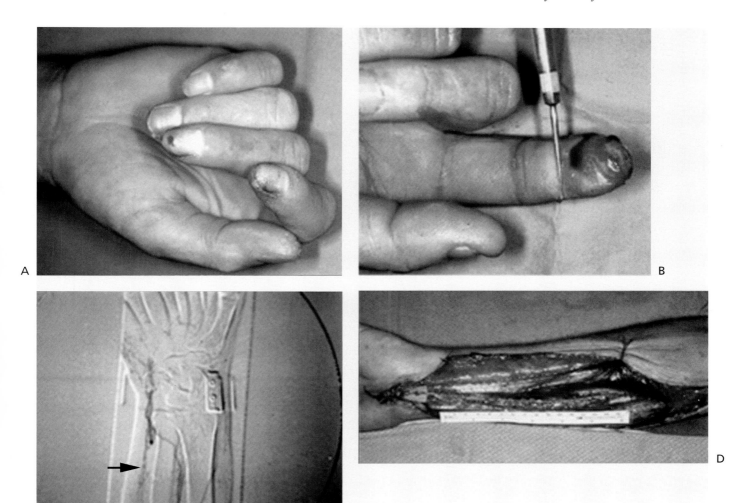

FIGURE 14. A,B: A patient with unilateral atherosclerotic occlusive Raynaud's phenomenon had necrosis and paronychial infection of the index finger and also impending ischemic changes of the middle finger. He had long-segment ulnar artery occlusion in the distal forearm (*arrow*) that was reconstructed **(C)** by resection and vein graft interposition **(D)**. Simultaneous index–fingertip débridement was performed. *(continued)*

3. If the Doppler recordings reveal proximal disease or unilateral symptoms, then arteriography is done in anticipation of revascularization surgery.
4. If the upper extremity Doppler recordings determine that there is distal disease, then noninvasive evaluations with digital Doppler recordings (PVR) and a technetium 99m scan are done.
5. The noninvasive vascular examinations may identify segmental arterial obstruction that would then necessitate arteriography, which leads to the necessity for microvascular reconstruction (probably including extended sympathectomy) (Fig. 14).
6. If there is more diffuse disease, and, in particular, when nerve block and stress responses show digital flow changes, then digital sympathectomy should be considered.
7. Cessation of tobacco products is crucial. Nicotine patches have been used for smoking cessation pro-

grams, and it has been found that they do not affect nutritional microcirculation adversely (10). Total blood flow may be maximized by the use of vasodilators, such as chlorpromazine (Thorazine), and nutritional flow may be enhanced by calcium channel blockers or adrenergic compounds.

Preventive Medical Treatment

Preventive measures can reduce the severity and frequency of attacks in the management of all types and severity of Raynaud's syndrome. The patient should avoid cold exposure, cigarette smoking, caffeinated beverages, vasoconstrictive drugs, and vibrational injury. The patient with Raynaud's syndrome requires great educational effort. The patient should avoid wet hands, wear gloves, use holders for handling cold beverages, keep gloves on a hook at the refrigerator for use when handling frozen foods, and use oil

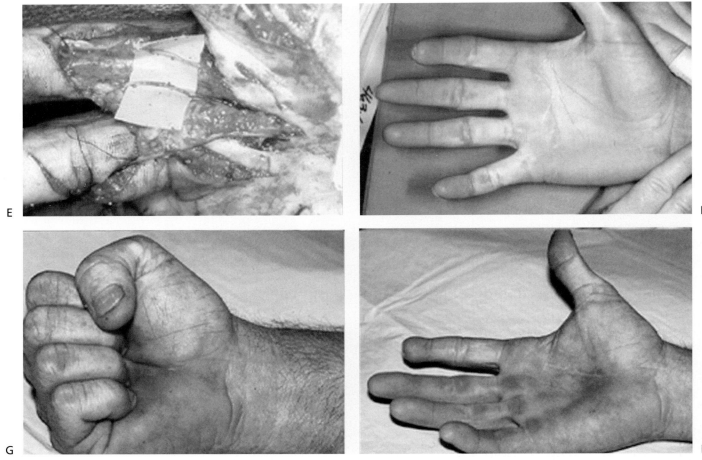

FIGURE 14. (*continued*) **E:** Persistent Raynaud's phenomenon required extended digital sympathectomy, as well. **F:** Allen's test shows patency of ulnar artery reconstruction on release of digital pressure on that artery but with maintenance of radial artery pressure. **G,H:** The patient is back at work as a carpenter. However, a prerequisite to the success of the reconstruction was also an absolute cessation of smoking.

for skin protection from dryness that might cause skin cracking and cellulitis (70).

Biofeedback Therapy

When simple preventive measures fail, biofeedback training may be helpful. This is done by measuring skin temperature while patients observe a visual or audio display of the temperature reading, and the patients imagine themselves in a warming situation. Benefit in 66% to 92% of Raynaud's patients has been found with biofeedback therapy (71). However, these subjects were generally people who did not have associated disease or ischemic ulcerations.

Pharmacologic Management

Pharmacologic management is the best treatment for patients with adequate collateral circulation. In these patients who nonetheless have significant vasospasm, pharmacologic agents may redistribute flow to nutritional capillary beds and may prevent inappropriate shunting (2). Calcium channel blockers are the drugs of choice for vasospastic disorders. They prevent calcium influx in vascular smooth muscle and thus diminish sympathetically driven vasoconstriction. Nifedipine (10 to 30 mg) taken orally three times a day (or 30 to 60 mg per day for the long-acting form) is the drug that is used most frequently. Diltiazem is somewhat less potent than nifedipine but has fewer adverse effects. It is useful in patients who do not tolerate the side effects of nifedipine.

It is interesting that pharmacologic management is the principal treatment for Raynaud's syndrome but has a reported benefit of only 40% to 66% of patients and rarely offers complete relief from the vasospastic disorders (72,73). It is difficult to measure success with pharmacologic management and is usually defined as fewer or less-severe vasospastic attacks, with healing of ischemic ulcers. Because there is a lack of objective parameters to assess treatment, the U.S. Food and Drug Administration has approved no single pharmacologic agent as safe and effective for Raynaud's syndrome (although several are classified as possibly effective) (74).

Tricyclic antidepressants and selective serotonin reuptake inhibitors are efficacious in the management of vasospastic symptoms. The former have analgesic and sedative effects that also help relieve pain and insomnia. Additionally, the tricyclic antidepressants inhibit postganglionic presynaptic reuptake of amine neurotransmitters. Amitriptyline (Elavil) (25 to 75 mg orally at night) is the most common tricyclic antidepressant that is used. Nonetheless, these agents do have some adverse side effects, including orthostatic hypotension, anticholinergic effects, and seizures. Selective serotonin reuptake inhibitors include fluoxetine (Prozac), sertraline (Zoloft), and paroxetine (Paxil). Clonidine (a presynaptic alpha-2 agonist that is sympatholytic) can be administered orally or topically (as a patch) but is often poorly tolerated because of the side effects of dry mouth and drowsiness (75).

Aspirin (80 mg tablet per day) is the most widely accepted method to reduce possible vascular occlusion and to prevent stroke and myocardial infarction. There is no controlled study of its use in Raynaud's syndrome; however, it is recommended in those patients who are at high risk for digital vessel occlusion.

There are some pharmacologic agents that are infrequently used but hold potential in the future for more widespread use. Calcitonin gene-related peptides (CGRPs) are endogenous neurotransmitters that are widely distributed in the nervous system and are especially abundant in perivascular nerve endings. CGRP acts directly on smooth muscle and is a potent vasodilator. A controlled study using intravenous CGRP in scleroderma patients with severe Raynaud's syndrome demonstrated significantly increased blood flow by using a laser Doppler study and showed healing of ulcerations (76). Similarly, drugs affecting prostaglandin metabolism have also proven effective in reversing severe digit-threatening episodes (77). These include prostaglandin E_1 and prostacyclin (prostaglandin I_2). These agents have been reserved for use in patients with threatened digit loss usually due to connective tissue disease, because their use is dose- and time-limited (78). Ketorolac may be a good choice for oral pain management in those patients who have no renal problems because of its known additional antithrombotic activity.

Operative Treatment

Patients in group 4 (with nonvascular injury) seldom require operative procedures to modify vascular tone. Surgical options are aimed at reconstruction of occluded vessels or modification of sympathetic tone, or both. The former is achieved by (a) resection of occluded vessels and end-to-end repair, (b) resection of occluded vessels and reconstruction with graft, and (c) bypass grafting of occluded vascular areas. When possible, an end-to-side proximal venous graft anastomosis may be preferable to an end-to-end technique for restoring arterial flow, because there is less risk to the collateral circulation. In scleroderma patients, there is a high incidence of ulnar artery occlusion, so reconstruction of this vessel is a frequent consideration. Sympathetic tone may be altered by (a) proximal cervicothoracic sympathectomy, (b) Leriche sympathectomy, and (c) peripheral periarterial sympathectomy. Posterior cervicothoracic sympathectomy by phenol injection with computed tomography guidance control is reversible, and it may be of benefit during collateral vessel maturation after acute vascular occlusion.

Early experience revealed that simple amputation of fingertip gangrenous tissue was frequently followed by failed healing and necrosis of the amputation stump, which led to progressively more proximal amputations. However, if digital artery sympathectomy or, sometimes, revascularization is done adjunctively at the time of débridement or amputation, removal of only the devitalized tissue generally leads to predictable healing of the amputation stump (78).

Leriche Sympathectomy

Excision of a thrombosed arterial segment with proximal and distal arterial ligation promotes collateral circulation, provides a distal sympathectomy, and ameliorates symptoms in patients who have adequate collateral flow in conditions in which there is vaso-occlusive disease that is compromised by increased sympathetic tone (40). However, obviously, if there is inadequate collateral circulation, or if there are multiple levels of occlusion, a Leriche sympathectomy alone does not suffice. If the ulnar artery is involved, then it is recommended that the nerve of Henlé, as well as other connections between the ulnar nerve and artery, are transected.

Peripheral Periarterial Sympathectomy

Flatt (79) performed distal sympathectomy at the level of the bifurcation of the common and proper digital arteries, stripping only a 3- to 4-mm segment of adventitia by using loupe magnification. This technique was modified by removing adventitia more distally and extensively for a 2-cm segment of the common and proper digital arteries and by confining the adventitial removal to only the symptomatic digits (17). At first, there was general pessimism regarding the use of this procedure in patients with connective tissue disease. However, more recent reports (49,80) have suggested subjective improvement and healing of ulceration in patients with connective tissue disease as well. The periarterial sympathectomy that is done under these conditions, however, is generally a more extensive procedure. The efficacy of periarterial sympathectomy, particularly in scleroderma patients, results not only from sympathetic denervation but also from decompression of the ischemic vessel through removal of fibrotic and non-compliant adventitia. Because of this extrinsic arterial compression, lack of response to preoperative sympathetic nerve blockade per se is not necessarily a predictor of postoperative outcome (81).

Palmar and Hand Sympathectomy

Koman (82), Jones et al. (49,83), and Merritt (80) have all advocated more wide sympathectomy, including the palm and the hand, particularly when performing sympathectomy that is required in association with connective tissue diseases. Jones et al. have advocated an inverted J-shaped incision starting at the ulnar artery at Guyon's canal in the distal forearm. A digital sympathectomy may be combined with microsurgical revascularization in these circumstances. Koman advocated using three separate incisions, an oblique incision in the distal palm to gain access to the superficial arterial arch and the common digital vessels and then an incision for access to the radial and ulnar arteries in the distal forearm. The adventitia of the radial and ulnar arteries is dissected under the operating microscope for a length of 2 cm. In the palmar incision, the origins of the three common volar digital arteries are located. All connections from the peripheral nerves to these arteries are severed with the aid of an operating microscope, and the adventitia is dissected from the vessels. A fourth incision might be used (particularly if there are significant symptoms in the thumb) (65) to locate the deep branch of the radial artery and the origin of the deep arch through the anatomic "snuff box." Good results have been presented in 15 patients in whom extended digital sympathectomy was performed for patients with Raynaud's phenomenon in association with connective tissue disorders (80). There were no recurrent ulcerations in operated hands after 1 to 5 years of follow-up. Six of those patients returned for surgery on the other hand because of ischemic ulceration. However, after 5 years, four of the original 15 postoperative patients did redevelop painful symptoms. They were found to have ulnar artery occlusion at the hypothenar region and subsequently had vein graft reconstructions. The conclusions from that study were to perform more extensive periarterial sympathectomies to include the three or four locations, as has been described by Koman (82).

Arterial Reconstruction

Arterial reconstruction is required in vaso-occlusive disease to restore arterial inflow. However, reconstitution of distal arterial channels is a necessary prerequisite (39). It is indicated in patients with refractory symptoms and inadequate collateral circulation (groups 2B and 3B). A vascular reconstruction may be indicated for patients in groups 2A and 3A on an individualized basis. The surgical reconstruction increases digital perfusion pressure and therefore enhances nutritional flow in the ischemic digits (2). There is not only enhanced arterial inflow as a consequence of the vascular repair (by graft or simple end-to-end anastomosis), but also functional modification of the sympathetic tone as a result of the peripheral sympathectomy that is associated with the vascular resection. A Leriche resection, even if combined with peripheral digital-palmar sympathectomy, improves nutritional flow by eliminating inappropriate AV shunting but does not increase total flow (84). In patients who have inadequate collateral circulation that is associated with reconstructible proximal occlusive disease (at the ulnar artery and superficial palmar arch), as well as unreconstructable distal occlusion (i.e., both proper digital arteries in a finger), successful reconstruction of the more proximal occlusion may increase total digital flow and nutritional flow sufficiently to diminish symptoms and to allow ulcers to heal (84).

In scleroderma patients, there is a high incidence of ulnar artery occlusion, and, therefore, reconstruction of this vessel is a frequent consideration (Fig. 15). Replacement of the entire superficial vascular arch by a vein graft to the proximal ulnar artery with the common digital vessels has been described (83). After vein graft reconstruction of the arch, recurrent ulcerations occurred in 20%, and occlusion of the graft occurred in 35%.

Microvascular omentum transfer has been described for successful treatment in a small group of patients with severe wrist pain and fingertip ulceration in whom the vascular disease was not amenable to microvascular bypass (65,85). The vascularized omentum is then thought to vascularize the surrounding ischemic tissues.

CONCLUSION

Thus, in summary, treatment modalities that are chosen should be goal specific, and decisions are based on a knowledge of the structural and functional characteristics of Raynaud's syndrome and also on the severity classification of the vasospastic state. Patients with Raynaud's phenomenon and inadequate circulation (group 2B) are the most refractory to treatment and also have the highest incidence of ulceration. However, patients who have secondary vasospasm from a nonvascular injury (group 4) have the best outcome and rarely have ulcerations. They often respond to oral medications and biofeedback. Irrespective of etiology or classification, the goal of treatment is to provide adequate nutritional capillary flow under stressed and nonstressed conditions. Environmental modification, biofeedback, and pharmacologic agents are often effective for Raynaud's disease (group 1), Raynaud's phenomenon with adequate circulation (group 2A), and those patients in group 4. All of these have normal vascular anatomy but abnormal sympathetic vascular reactivity. In patients with Raynaud's phenomenon and inadequate circulation (group 2B) or in those patients with vaso-occlusive disease and compromised collateral flow (group 3B), the prognosis is guarded, and arterial reconstruction is required

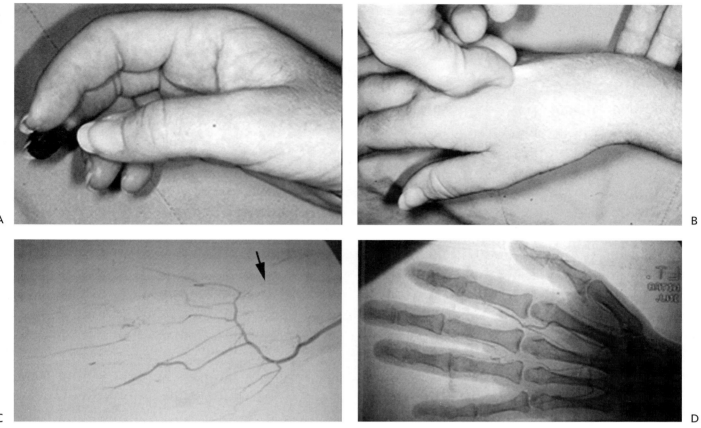

FIGURE 15. A patient with scleroderma and middle-fingertip necrosis **(A)** shows dorsal hand skin thickening **(B)**. She had ulnar artery occlusion **(C)** (*arrow*), as well as small vessel digital disease **(D)**, which is seen better on subtraction angiography. Simultaneous fingertip amputation and ulnar artery inflow reconstruction resulted in a healed wound and abolished the Raynaud's ischemic symptoms.

for successful treatment. There are no specific criteria for the selection of patients who might be best suited to periarterial sympathectomy. Increased digital temperature or PVR and decreased symptoms after peripheral nerve block confirm an abnormal sympathetic tone and that a sympathectomy can provide palliation.

However, in patients with vaso-occlusive disease in the face of adequate collateral circulation, there is unlikely to be a change in digital temperature or PVR (both of which are reflections of total flow), although nutritional flow may be maximized by peripheral nerve block (and, hence, periarterial sympathectomy). In these patients, symptoms decrease, and ulcers heal; it is precisely patients in this group who benefit the most from periarterial sympathectomy, although they are seemingly paradoxically not as responsive to peripheral nerve block and stress testing (65).

REFERENCES

1. Koman LA, Goldner JL, Smith TL. The effect of extremity blood flow on pain and cold intolerance. In: Omer G, Spinner M, Van Beek A, eds. *Management of peripheral nerve problems,* 2nd ed. Philadelphia: WB Saunders, 1998:107–115.

2. Koman LA, Smith VP, Smith TL. Stress testing in the evaluation of upper extremity perfusion. *Hand Clin* 1993;9:59–83.

3. Maricq HR, Weinrich MC, Keil JE, et al. Prevalence of Raynaud phenomenon in the general population. *J Chron Dis* 1986;39:423–427,

4. Maricq HR, Weinrich MC, Keil JE, et al. Prevalence of scleroderma spectrum disorders in the general population of South Carolina. *Arthritis Rheum* 1989;32:998–1006.

5. Maricq HR, Carpentier PH, Weinrich MC, et al. Geographic variation in the prevalence of Raynaud's phenomenon: A five-region comparison. *J Rheumatol* 1997;24:879–889.

6. Fitzgerald O, Hess EV, O'Connor GT, et al. Prospective study of the evolution of Raynaud's phenomenon. *Am J Med* 1988;84:718–726.

7. Sarkozi J, Bookman AAM, Lee P, et al. Significance of anticentromere antibody in idiopathic Raynaud's syndrome. *Am J Med* 1987;83:893–898.

8. Spencer-Green G, Alter D, Welch HG. Test performance in systemic sclerosis: anti-centromere and anti-Scl 70 antibodies. *Am J Med* 1997;103:24–28.

9. Hadler NM. "Primary Raynaud's" is not a disease or even a disorder; it's a trait. *J Rheumatol* 1998;25:2291–2294.

10. Koman LA, Ruch DS, Smith VP, et al. Vascular disorders. In: Green DP, Hotchkiss RN, Pederson WC, eds. *Green's operative hand surgery*, 4th ed. New York: Churchill Livingstone, 1999:2254–2302.

11. Coleman SS, Anson BJ. Arterial patterns in the hand based upon a study of 650 specimens. *Surg Gynecol Obstet* 1961;113:409–424.

12. DeBakey M, Simeone F. Battle injuries of the arteries in World War II. *Ann Surg* 1946;123:434–479.

13. Baker R, Chunprapaph B, Nyhus L. Severe ischemia of the hand following artery catheterization. *Surgery* 1976;80:449–457.

14. Kleinert JM, Fleming SG, Abel CS, et al. Radial and ulnar artery dominance in normal digits. *J Hand Surg* 1989;14:504–508.

15. Edwards EA. Organization of the small arteries of the hand and digit. *Am J Surg* 1960;99:837–846.

16. Conrad MC. *The circulation of the skin in functional anatomy of the circulation to the lower extremities.* Chicago: Yearbook Medical Publishers, 1971:64–95.

17. Wilgis EF. Evaluation and treatment of chronic digital ischemia. *Ann Surg* 1981;193:693–698.

18. Wilgis EF. Digital sympathectomy for vascular insufficiency. *Hand Clin* 1985;1:361–367.

19. Miller LM, Morgan RF. Vasospastic disorders: etiology, recognition, and treatment. *Hand Clin* 1993;9:171–187.

20. Morgan RF, Reisman NR, Wilgis EFS. Anatomic localization of sympathetic nerves in the hand. *J Hand Surg* 1983;8:283–288.

21. Pick J. *The autonomic nervous system.* Philadelphia: JB Lippincott Co, 1990.

22. McCabe SJ, Kleinert JM. The nerve of Henlé. *J Hand Surg* 1990;15:784–788.

23. Ganong WF. Synaptic and junctional transmission. In: Ganong WF, ed. *Review of medical physiology.* Los Altos, CA: Langa Medical Publications, 1963:62–84.

24. Wigoda P, Netscher DT, Thornby J, et al. Vasoactive effects of smoking as mediated through nicotinic stimulation of sympathetic nerve fibers. *J Hand Surg* 1995;20:718–724.

25. Faber JE. In situ analysis of alpha-adrenoceptors on arteriolar and venular smooth muscle in rat skeletal muscle microcirculation. *Circ Res* 1988;62:37–50.

26. Flavahan NA, Cooke JP, Shepherd JD, et al. Human postjunctional alpha-1 and alpha-2 adrenoceptors: differential distribution in arteries of the limbs. *J Pharmacol Exp Ther* 1987;241:361–365.

27. Coffman JD, Cohen RA. Alpha-2 adrenergic and 5-HT receptor hypersensitivity in Raynaud's phenomenon. *J Vasc Med Biol* 1990;2:100–106.

28. Keenan EJ, Porter JM. Alpha-2 adrenergic receptors in patients with Raynaud's syndrome. *Surgery* 1983;94:204–209.

29. Ekenvall L, Linblad LE, Norbeck O, et al. Alpha adrenoceptors and cold-induced vasoconstriction in human finger skin. *Am J Physiol Heart Circ Physiol* 1988;255:1000–1003.

30. Chotani MA, Flaverhan S, Mitra S, et al. Silent alpha-2c adrenergic receptors enable cold-induced vasoconstriction in cutaneous arteries. *Am J Physiol Heart Circ Physiol* 2000;278:1075–1083.

31. Freedman RR, Sabharwall SC, Desai N, et al. Increased alpha-adrenergic responsiveness in idiopathic Raynaud's disease. *Arthritis Rheum* 1989;32:61–65.

32. Faber JE, Meininger GA. Selective interaction of alpha-adrenoceptors with myogenic regulation of microvascular smooth muscle. *Am J Physiol* 1990;259:1126–1133.

33. Yanagisawa M, Kurihara H, Kimura S, et al. A novel potent vasoconstrictor peptide produced by vascular endothelial cells. *Nature* 1988;33:411–415.

34. Furchgott RF, Zawadzki JV. The obligatory role of endothelial cells in the relaxation of arterial smooth muscle to acetylcholine. *Nature* 1980;228:373–376.

35. Leppert J, Ringqvist A, Karlberg BE, et al. Whole-body cooling increases plasma endothelin-1 levels in woman with primary Raynaud's phenomenon. *Clin Physiol* 1998;18:420–425.

36. Allen EV, Brown GE. Raynaud's disease: a clinical study of 147 cases. *JAMA* 1932;99:1472.

37. Campbell PM, LeRoy EG. Raynaud phenomenon. *Semin Arthritis Rheum* 1986;16:92–103.

38. Kallenberg CG. Early detection of connective tissue disease in patient's with Raynaud's phenomenon. *Rheum Dis Clin North Am* 1990;16:11–13.

39. Troum SJ, Smith TL, Koman LA, et al. Management of vasospastic disorders of the hand. *Clin Plast Surg* 1997;24:121–132.

40. Leriche ER, Fontaine R, Dupertuis SM. Arterectomy with follow-up on 78 operations. *Surg Gynecol Obstet* 1937;64:149–155.

41. Fisher M, Grotta J. New uses for calcium channel blockers: therapeutic implications. *Drugs* 1993;46:961–975.

42. Taylor W, Pelmear PL, Hempstock TI, et al. Correlation of epidemiological data and the measured vibration, In: Taylor W, Pelmear PL, eds. *Vibration white finger in industry.* London: Academic Press, 1975:123–133.

43. Greenstein D, Kent PJ, Wilkinson D, et al. Raynaud's phenomenon of occupational origin. *J Hand Surg* 1991;16:370–377.

44. Takeuchi T, Futatsuka M, Imanishih TM, et al. Pathologic changes observed in the finger biopsy of patients with vibration-induced white finger. *Scand J Work Environ Health* 1986;12:280–283.

45. Chatterjeed S, Barwick DD, Petrie A. Exploratory electromyography in the study of vibration-induced white finger in rock drillers. *Br J Ind Med* 1982;39:89–97.

46. Loeve M, Heidrich H. The carpal tunnel syndrome—a disease underlying Raynaud's phenomenon? *Angiology* 1988;39:891–901.

47. Grigg MH, Wolf JH. Raynaud's syndrome and similar conditions. *Br Med J* 1991;303:913–916.

48. McGrath MA, Penny R. The mechanism of Raynaud's phenomenon: part 2. *Med J Aust* 1974;2:367–375.

49. Jones NF, Imbriglia JE, Steen VD, et al. Surgery for scleroderma of the hand. *J Hand Surg* 1987;12:391–400.

50. Kallenberg CG. Connective tissue disorders in patients presenting with Raynaud's phenomenon alone. *Ann Rheum Dis* 1991;50:666–667.

51. Belch JJ, Sturrock RD. Raynaud's syndrome: current trends. *Br J Rheum* 1983;22:50–55.

52. Bouhoutsos J, Morris T, Martin T. Unilateral Raynaud's phenomenon in the hand and its significance. *Surgery* 1977;82:547–551.

53. Barker NW, Hines EA. Arterial occlusion in the hand and finger associated with repeated occupational trauma. *Proc Mayo Clin* 1944;19:345–349.

54. Mehlhoff TL, Wood MB. Ulnar artery thrombosis and the role of interposition vein grafting: patency with microsurgical technique. *J Hand Surg* 1991;16:274–278.

55. McCabe SJ, Mizgala C, Glickman L. The measurement of cold sensitivity of the hand. *J Hand Surg* 1991;16:1037–1040.

56. Allen EV. Thromboangiitis obliterans: methods of diagnosis of chronic occlusive arterial lesions distal to the wrist with illustrative case. *Am J Med Sci* 1929;178:237–244.

57. Maricq HR. The microcirculation in scleroderma and allied diseases. *Adv Microcirc* 1982;10:17–52.

58. Kleinert JM, Gupta A. Pulse volume recording. *Hand Clin* 1993;9:13–46.

59. Sumner DS. Noninvasive assessment of upper extremity ischemia. In: Bergan JJ, Yao JS, eds. *Evaluation and treatment of upper and lower extremity circulatory disorders.* Orlando, FL: Grune & Stratton, 1984:75.

60. Zimmerman NB. Occlusive vascular disorders of the upper extremity. *Hand Clin* 1993;9:139–150.

61. Archie JP, Larson BO. Noninvasive vascular laboratory evaluation of subclavian artery occlusion. *South Med J* 1978;71:482–483.

62. Berger AC, Kleinert JM. Noninvasive vascular studies: a comparison with arteriography and surgical findings in the upper extremities. *J Hand Surg* 1992;17:206–210.

63. Wilgis EF, Jezio D, Stonesifer L, et al. The evaluation of small vessel flow. *J Bone Joint Surg* 1974;56:1199–1206.

64. Pederson WC, Pribaz JJ. Revascularization of the upper extremity with microsurgical omental transfer, when faced with end-stage ischemia. *J Reconstr Microsurg* 1995;11:397.

65. Koman LA, Smith BP, Pollack FE, et al. The microcirculatory effects of peripheral sympathectomy. *J Hand Surg* 1995;20:709–717.

66. Holder LE, Merine DS, Yang A. Nuclear medicine, contrast angiography, and magnetic resonance imaging for evaluating vascular problems in the hand. *Hand Clin* 1993;9:85–113.

67. Lawrence HW. The collateral circulation in the hand after cutting the radial and ulnar arteries at the wrist. *Indust Med* 1937;6:410–411.

68. Parks BJ, Arbelaez J, Horner RL. Medical and surgical importance of the arterial blood supply of the thumb. *J Hand Surg* 1978;3:383–385.

69. Koman LA. Diagnostic study of vascular lesions. *Hand Clin* 1985;1:217–231.

70. Coffman JD. Raynaud's phenomenon: an update. *Hypertension* 1991;17:593–602.

71. Freedman RR. Physiological mechanisms of temperature biofeedback. *Biofeedback Self Regul* 1991;16:95–115.

72. Kiowski W, Erne P, Buhler FR. Use of nifedipine in hypertension and Raynaud's phenomenon. *Cardiovasc Drugs Ther* 1990;4[Suppl 5]:935–940.

73. Coffman JD. New drug therapy in peripheral vascular disease. *Med Clin North Am* 1988;72:259–265.

74. Seibold JR. Serotonin in Raynaud's phenomenon. *J Cardiovasc Pharmacol* 1985;7[Suppl]:95–98.

75. Czop C, Smith TL, Rauck R, et al. The pharmacologic approach to the painful hand. *Hand Clin* 1996;12:633–642.

76. Bunker CB, Reavle YC, O'Shaughnessy DJ, et al. Calcitonin gene-related peptide in treatment of severe peripheral insufficiency in Raynaud's phenomenon. *Lancet* 1993;342:80–83.

77. Seibold JR, Allegar NE. The treatment of Raynaud's phenomenon. *Clin Dermatol* 1994;12:312–321.

78. Merritt WH. Comprehensive management of Raynaud's syndrome. *Clin Plast Surg* 1997;24:133–159.

79. Flatt A. Digital artery sympathectomy. *J Hand Surg* 1980;5:550–556.

80. Merritt WH. Long-term results of digital artery sympathectomy and revascularization in connective tissue patients. In: *Reconstructive Microsurgery Current Trends: Proceedings of the 12th Symposium of the International Society of Reconstructive Microsurgery.* Singapore: Goh Bros Enterprise Humanities Press, 1996:475.

81. Yee AM, Hotchkiss RN, Paget SA. Adventitial stripping: a digit-saving procedure in refractory Raynaud's phenomenon. *J Rheumatol* 1998;25:269–276.

82. Koman LA. *Bohman Grey School of Medicine orthopedic manual.* Winston-Salem, NC: Wake Forest University Orthopedic Press, 1997.

83. Jones NF. Acute and chronic ischemia of the hand: pathophysiology, treatment, and prognosis. *J Hand Surg* 1991;16:1074–1083.

84. Koman LA, Ruch DS, Smith TL, et al. Arterial reconstruction in the ischemic hand and wrist: the effect on microvascular physiology. Advances in vascular imaging photoplethysmography. *Adv Vasc Imaging Photoplethysmogr* 1995;221:71–75.

85. Pederson WC. Management of severe ischemia of the upper extremity. *Clin Plast Surg* 1997;24:107–120.

95

THUMB RECONSTRUCTION

FU-CHAN WEI

Thumb reconstruction in traumatic loss and congenital deficiency has always been a challenge to the reconstructive surgeon because of its functional and aesthetic significance. It is universally agreed that reconstruction of an opposable thumb should be attempted whenever it is possible by using whatever techniques are available. The attributes that make the thumb unique are its position, stability, strength, length, motion, sensibility, and appearance (1). The reconstructive procedure for a deficient thumb that is caused by trauma or developmental deficit should be planned to reflect these qualities. An appropriate realistic plan should be made that considers age, occupation or functional demands, psychology and motivation, and commitment to postoperative therapy. Each case should have an individual assessment and reconstruction planned.

There appears to be some controversy as to the amount of thumb shortening that can exist before significant functional deficit, but the author's experience suggests that amputations up to thumb interphalangeal joint can still provide reasonable function (2), and loss of length proximal to this critical level leads to inadequate residual stump for grasp and pinch functions. Restoration of at least protective sensation after salvage or reconstruction is essential, otherwise thumb usage by the patient is reduced. Irrespective of the technique of reconstruction, the position of the thumb that is achieved should be that of opposition to the digits for key pinch and grasp. Although movement at the metacarpophalangeal or interphalangeal joints is not an absolute prerequisite, the function of the reconstructed thumb improves if the joint movements are present.

The considerations for thumb reconstruction are different in traumatic loss and congenital absence. In cases of amputation, the methods vary according to the level of amputation, whereas in congenital absence, not only are the structures deficient or underdeveloped, but their cortical representation is also impaired.

It is essential that, after amputation of the thumb, replantation be attempted. When successful, replantation provides more functional benefit than any other method of reconstruction. Since the advent of microsurgical techniques, the indications and use of conservative modalities have become limited.

NONMICROSURGICAL RECONSTRUCTION

The deficient thumb has always prompted the surgeon to attempt reconstruction by using the best techniques available or by devising a better method. The current methods of thumb reconstruction have resulted from a gradual progression over the last decades. Before the advent of microsurgical techniques, a number of traditional techniques were described, many with good results. These traditional methods use rearrangement and transfer of bone, joint, and soft tissues.

BONE LENGTHENING

The thumb lengthening can be performed as a single-stage procedure with distraction of the osteotomized bone and immediate bone graft insertion (3) or with continuous distraction at a speed of 0.5 to 1.0 mm per day over 2 to 4 months in cases of subtotal amputation through the proximal phalangeal or metacarpal level (4–6). This new bone organizes into mature bone by an additional 2 to 3 months (7). Lengthening of 2 to 3 cm can greatly enhance general hand function by improving pinch and grasp.

Pin tract infection and fracture of the bone graft are possible complications during the procedure. Failure of bone regeneration can occur along with rotational or angular deformities during the distraction. Proper lengthening device application and adequate immobilization until bone consolidation help prevent these complications.

Good-quality, pliable, sensate skin over the thumb stump is a prerequisite for this procedure. If the soft tissue coverage is not pliable, during distraction, greater resistance is encountered, and, subsequently, flexion contracture or subluxation of the joints, or both, can result. Thumb lengthening is a relatively simple and reliable procedure and can be performed in patients in whom conditions may not permit microvascular reconstruction. However, the thumb lacks joint and nail; therefore, the function and appearance may be far from desirable.

PHALANGIZATION

Phalangization (8) by deepening of the thumb web space creates an illusion of increased length and may also actually augment breadth of the hand, allowing firmer grasp of larger objects. The first metacarpal is converted into a phalanx that protrudes relatively farther from the hand, thereby increasing the space that is available for grasp.

In the absence of soft tissue contracture, the web space can be easily broadened with a large Z-plasty. In the presence of severe contracture, additional skin (local, pedicled, or free flaps) may be required. Resection of a useless index ray may further enlarge the web space. In extreme cases, trapeziometacarpal capsulotomy or even trapeziectomy may be necessary to allow sufficient thumb metacarpal abduction.

Excessive release of the first dorsal interosseous and adductor pollicis is not advised, as it may result in significant flexion-adduction weakness. Proximal migration of origins of the first dorsal interosseous and the adductor pollicis preserves their function (7,9). The function and esthetics of phalangization are always suboptimal.

OSTEOPLASTIC RECONSTRUCTION

Initiated as a Gillies' cocked-hat flap, in which local skin and subcutaneous tissue are mobilized from the dorsal and lateral aspects of first metacarpal to cover as much as 2.5 cm of iliac bone graft, the osteoplastic reconstruction (10,11) provides a useful increase in length for the thumb that is amputated at or proximal to the metacarpophalangeal joint. To improve the results, it has been modified subsequently and is performed in stages. Initially, an iliac crest bone graft is inserted and is covered by a tube pedicled flap, followed by tube division and a neurovascular pedicle transfer for sensibility. There is no interphalangeal joint, and the sensation is referred to the donor finger. Cosmesis is also inferior owing to the lack of nail and bulkiness. In addition, there can be long-term complications such as absorption and fracture of the bone graft.

POLLICIZATION

For traumatic amputations and also for congenital hypoplasia, proximal to metacarpophalangeal joint pollicization is one choice for thumb reconstruction, provided that the other fingers are intact (12). Sometimes, a less damaged digit also can be used (13,14). Pollicization is safe and quick to perform. It provides a stable thumb reconstruction with better sensory recovery. The pollicization of the index finger is easiest and safest and does not require crossover of vessels, nerves, or tendons. The dorsal veins can be preserved; good web space can be formed after removal of the second metacarpal. The long finger covers its place and functions spontaneously, and there are no scars in the palm. However, the long, ring, and little fingers can also be used. Theoretically, only one procedure is involved, although, in practice, most cases require prior flap reconstruction or later secondary procedures such as tenolysis, rotational osteotomy, and first web reconstruction. One of the main advantages of pollicization is that it provides a carpometacarpal joint (basal joint), which may not otherwise exist or has been injured in trauma.

THUMB RECONSTRUCTION USING MICROSURGICAL TECHNIQUE

During the middle and late nineteenth century, surgeons attempted composite tissue pedicle transfer for hand reconstruction. Nicoladani in 1897 (15) first developed pedicle transfer of a toe and foot skin to reconstruct a thumb. The development of precision-operating microscope, needles, and micro instruments and the basic principles of microvascular surgery heralded thumb reconstruction by single-stage transplantation of the toe in the early era of microsurgery. Buncke et al. (16) led the first successful toe-to-hand transplantation in rhesus monkeys in 1966. The first clinical transplantation of a second toe and great toe to reconstruct thumb were reported respectively by Yang (17) and Cobbett (18) in 1966. Based on the dorsal arterial supply, the first toe-to-hand transplantation was performed by O'Brien et al. (19). Gilbert had described in detail the dorsal and planter arterial system, based on cadaveric studies (20).

The 1970s and 1980s witnessed a furious pace of advancements in technical aspects of transplantations, as well as original ideas for thumb reconstruction. Morrison and MacLeod (21) developed the wrap-around flap that uses portions of the great toe without its bony components transplanted on the microvascular pedicle for thumb reconstruction, thus improving thumb cosmesis and reducing donor site morbidity. Wei et al. (22) described trimmed great-toe transplantation for thumb reconstruction in 1988, which provided cosmesis similar to that of the great-toe wrap-around flap but preserved the interphalangeal joint function in the transplant. Thumb reconstruction by means of toe transplantation has become well accepted. It, in general, provides the best reconstruction at all levels.

Because the success rate of toe transplantation to thumb has been high, function and appearance of the reconstructed thumb have become important considerations. Ideal transplantation depends on proper selection of tech-

TABLE 1. COMPARISON OF FUNCTIONAL RESULTS

Function	Total great toe	Wrap around	Trimmed great toe	Second toe
Sensibility	****	***	***	***
Stability	****	***	***	**
Grip strength	****	***	***	**
Pinch power	***	***	***	**
Fine pinch	**	***	***	***
Interphalangeal motion	***	***	**	**

Note: The number of asterisks indicates the level of function that was attained through thumb reconstruction.

TABLE 2. COSMESIS AND DONOR SITE MORBIDITY COMPARISON

	Total great toe	Wrap around	Trimmed great toe	Second toe
Cosmesis	***	****	****	**
Donor site morbidity	***	**	**	*

Note: The number of asterisks indicates the level of function that was attained through thumb reconstruction.

niques. It requires balancing the patient's age and functional needs, the appearance of the reconstructed thumb, and the donor site morbidity. There are numerous advantages of toe transplantation for thumb reconstruction. It offers total reconstruction in a single procedure and provides mobile digits with stable joints and sensibility. Because the toe has a nail, the appearance is similar to the thumb, and near normal appearance of the hand is preserved. With meticulous preoperative planning, the donor site morbidity is low and acceptable. Its disadvantages include comparatively less mobility and incomplete sensory recovery in the new thumb.

A number of options are available for transplantation, including whole great toe, second toe, great-toe wrap-around flap, and trimmed great toe (23–25). Although the choice of the toe and technique is a matter of debate, there are some guidelines regarding selection of the best techniques for optimal thumb reconstruction (2).

In selecting the ideal toe and procedure for the thumb reconstruction, the cosmetic and functional requirements of the hand and the donor site and the preference of the patient must be considered (Tables 1 and 2). The level of amputation, the structures that are preserved, the location and extent of coverage of the defect in the residual hand, the similarity and difference between the normal thumb and the planned toe, and the dominance and growth potential should be all evaluated. The considerations in reconstruction of congenital thumb hypoplasia and deficiency should include the type of deficiency and associated anomalies, the availability of motorizing units (muscles and tendons), the recipient vessels, and the nerves at the time of reconstruction. In traumatic and congenital thumb amputation and deficiency, prior skin coverage might be necessary, as it alleviates the need for extra skin harvest from the foot during subsequent toe transfer.

The timing of thumb reconstruction can be primary, immediately after the injury, or secondary, after definitive coverage. Early, single-stage reconstruction is now advocated. This includes simultaneous reconstruction of the thumb and fingers, if needed, thereby providing functional capacity to the hand at the earliest. The results in terms of survival, immediate and late complications, and the need

for secondary procedures have been shown to be similar for primary, as well as for secondary, reconstruction (26), and the advantages of primary toe transplantation are reduction in overall recovery and rehabilitation period, thus permitting earlier return to work.

RELEVANT SURGICAL ANATOMY

The foot shares many anatomic features with the hand; however, because of different functional roles, they have various anatomic differences. The great-toe transverse diameter is approximately one-third bigger than that of the thumb. All phalanges in the great toe are also slightly longer than those of the thumb. The great-toe nail is also bigger, and there is more subcutaneous tissue in the pulp. Therefore, modified great-toe–harvesting techniques involve a reduction in its size. In contrast, the lesser toes are shorter than the digits and have a square shape at the distal ends. The joints have limited flexion and a tendency to claw. The extensor and flexor mechanisms are similar to those of the hand.

The skin on the dorsum of the foot is thin and mobile, so the veins and tendons are usually visible. The plantar surface or sole of the foot is thick, except on the instep, and contains many sweat glands and much fat in the subcutaneous tissue, especially over the heel.

The dorsal aspect of the foot receives innervation from the sural, superficial, and deep peroneal nerves. The plantar surface of the foot is supplied by the tibial nerve, which divides into the medial and plantar nerves to supply cutaneous branches to the medial three and one-half toes and the lateral one and one-half toes, respectively.

The dorsal digital veins run along the dorsal margins of each toe and unite in their webs to form common dorsal digital veins. These veins join to form a dorsal venous arch on the dorsum of the foot. Veins leave the dorsal venous arch and converge medially to form the great saphenous vein and laterally to form the small saphenous vein. The plantar foot surface has two venous systems, superficial and deep. The deep veins originate from the plantar digital veins and communicate with the dorsal digital veins via perforating veins.

The arteries of the foot are the terminal branches of the anterior and posterior tibial arteries (Fig. 1). The anterior

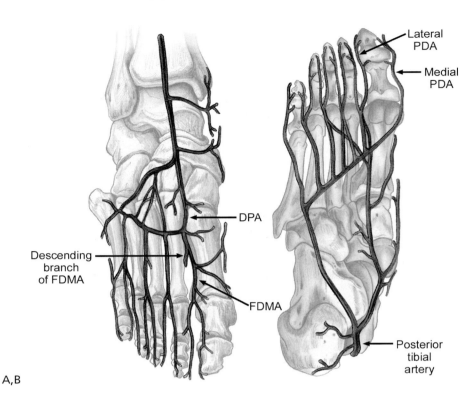

A,B

FIGURE 1. Anterior anatomy of the foot, related to free tissue transfer of the great toe. **A:** Dorsal view. The dorsalis pedis artery (DPA) splits near the proximal end of the first and second intermetatarsal space into the first dorsal metatarsal artery (FDMA) and its descending branch. **B:** Plantar view. The plantar digital artery system, derived from the posterior tibial artery and the descending branch of the FDMA, when present, terminates on the great toe as the medial plantar digital artery (PDA) and the lateral PDA.

tibial artery continues as the dorsalis pedis artery on the dorsum of the foot and runs lateral to the extensor hallucis longus tendon toward the first web space. Proximal to the base of the first and second metatarsals, it gives off the arcuate artery, which provides the second, third, and fourth dorsal metatarsal arteries. Distally, the dorsalis pedis artery bifurcates just past the base of the first and second metatarsal into the deep plantar artery and the first dorsal metatarsal artery (FDMA). The deep plantar artery (also known as the *descending*, *perforating*, or *communicating branch*) courses downward between the first two metatarsals to contribute to the plantar arch. The anatomic variations in the arterial pattern should be kept in mind while harvesting toe transplantation (27–33). The FDMA always passes dorsal to the deep transversal metatarsal ligament. At this point, it divides into medial and lateral branches, which are named as digital arteries to the second and great toes, respectively, and a communicating branch to the first plantar metatarsal artery (FPMA). This is a constant anatomic landmark that is helpful in arterial identification during toe harvesting. In approximately 70% of cases, the FDMA is bigger than the FPMA (dorsal-dominant system); in 20%, the FPMA is bigger than the FDMA (plantar-dominant system); and in the rest, 10%, both arteries can be of similar size (34).

TOE DISSECTION TECHNIQUE

Toe dissection always starts in the dorsal aspect of the first web space, where the junction of the lateral digital artery of

the great toe and the medial digital artery of the second toe is identified. Further dissection of the pedicle is then carried out from this junction proximally. If the arterial system is dorsal dominant, as in 70% of cases (34), the retrograde dissection continues until the required length and diameter of the artery are reached. When a plantar-dominant system is noted, with the FDMA absent or small, the dissection is continued up to the middle metatarsal shaft on the plantar surface. At this point, the union between the FPMA and the dorsalis pedis artery through the proximal communicating artery is located. Because dissection of the communicating branch might be tedious and destructive for the foot, it is better to divide the FPMA at this level and, if required, to use a vein graft for the vascular anastomosis, thus avoiding unnecessary extensive dissection in the foot.

The technique of *retrograde dissection* of the vascular pedicle (35) helps earlier identification of the dominant-dorsal and planter-dominant vascular pedicles (34), eliminates anatomic confusion, alleviates the need for preoperative angiogram, and aids optimal pedicle length dissection (Fig. 2).

Skeletonization of vessels and nerves during toe dissection facilitates osteotomy and skeletal fixation. It also allows passage of the vessels and nerves under the skin bridge to reach recipient vessels at a proximal level without being compressed. This technique is particularly useful in distal digital reconstruction. It is advisable to dissect the artery and nerves several millimeters distal to the osteotomy site, before osteotomy. The extra minutes that it takes to skeletonize the artery and nerves pay dividends later for osteotomy and skeletal fixation.

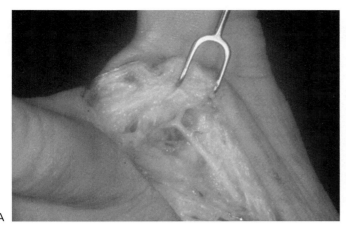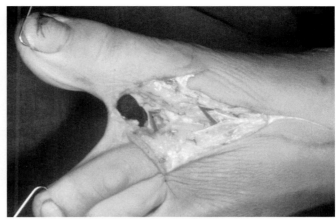

FIGURE 2. **A:** Retrograde dissection with dorsal dominant vascular pedicle. **B:** Retrograde dissection with plantar dominant vascular pedicle.

The *donor site considerations* play an important role in final results of reconstruction and overall patient satisfaction. With meticulous preoperative planning and exact surgical techniques, it is possible to reduce the deformity and to provide a functional foot in the great majority of cases. The planning for reconstruction should ideally start from initial care after trauma, when all viable tissue, especially skin, must be preserved (36). If necessary, further skin coverage should be provided by using pedicled groin flap, as this prevents harvest of extra skin from the foot during toe transplantation and helps primary closure of donor defect. During great-toe harvest, it is advisable to preserve at least 1 cm of the proximal phalanx, to maintain foot span, and the appearance and push-off function of the donor foot, to prevent windlass effect. Skin grafting the donor site should be avoided in toe transplantation, as it seldom takes adequately, therefore delaying foot functional recovery and leaving unstable and painful scars.

RECIPIENT SITE PREPARATIONS

Recipient site preparations generally remain similar irrespective of the type of toe transplantation. The amputation stump is exposed through cross incisions to create four skin flaps (Fig. 3), to prepare the bone, and to identify tendons, nerves, and arterial stumps. The skin flaps are sufficiently undermined, and redundant fat or scar tissue is trimmed off to obtain thin skin flaps for smooth skin closure. The periosteal dissection should be minimal to expose the osteotomy site. The bony surface in the stump is regularized to provide good contact and stability, which are essential for adequate bone union. If composite joint repair with the corresponding joint in the transplanted toe is planned, the joint capsule and ligaments must be carefully dissected while exposing the cartilage surface. Usually, the extensor tendon is localized close to the bony stump, and there is no

need to detach it from the bone. Integrity of the extensor mechanism is essential for finger function. The flexor tendons have different locations in distal and proximal finger amputations, and the pulley system must be preserved while exposing the tendon. It is critical for the functional result to have a good tendon excursion. Therefore, tenolysis is performed if it is necessary. The digital or common digital nerves stumps are identified and are prepared to be coapted to the counterparts of the transplanted toe, after proximal dissection, to the point at which they have a relatively normal appearance. The radial artery in the snuffbox or the princeps pollicis artery is usually the recipient artery and is prepared with a separate incision, creating a subcutaneous tunnel for passage of the pedicle. When the toe pedicle has a short length (for instance, with a plantar dominant system) or the proximal arteries in the hand are required for anastomoses, vein grafts should be considered more liberally instead of trying to increase the length of the donor artery in the foot by a more destructive dissection or by doing vascular anastomoses under tension. Usually, one vein on the dorsal aspect of the hand is prepared as the recipient vessel.

INSETTING OF THE TRANSPLANT

After verifying optimal length, osteosynthesis is performed by using interosseous wires (37) (Fig. 3B). It provides good stability for early mobilization of the joints and thus prevents tendon adhesions and improves the overall range of motion. Because the fixation is not rigid, it permits postoperative correction of slight angulation or malrotation, if necessary. It is a simple and quick method and can be applied to a stump of phalanx that is as short as 5 mm. Next, the extensor tendon is repaired with the interphalangeal and metacarpophalangeal joints in full extension to minimize extension lag and flexion defor-

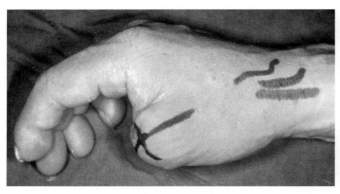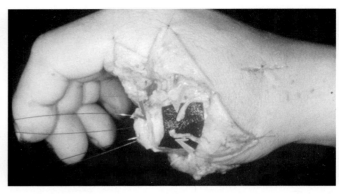

FIGURE 3. **A:** Amputation stump and preparation of recipient vessels. **B:** Exposure of various structures and the proximal phalangeal bone stump. Note the interosseous wiring in the bone stump.

mity. The long flexor tendon is repaired with the flexor pollicis longus. The nerves are anastomosed in an end-to-end fashion with 10-0 nylon sutures. The artery and vein are tunneled to the corresponding recipient site, and the skin is adjusted and temporarily closed, allowing room to do the vascular anastomoses. The four skin flaps that are built in the recipient stump are tailored and interposed with the triangular flaps of the transferred toe, creating a regular surface. The arterial anastomosis is performed, first followed by vein, and the remaining wounds are closed. If there is some tension in closing the skin, partial closure and skin grafting the partially opened surface are advisable, although it should be uncommon with adequate preoperative planning. A small silastic drain is used to prevent a hematoma, avoiding any contact of the drain with the vascular anastomoses.

TOTAL GREAT-TOE TRANSPLANTATION

Anatomic and functional differences between the great toe and the thumb must be analyzed when opting for this procedure. These include circumference, nail width, and phalangeal and joint length and width. On an average, the diameter (transverse) is 13 and 11 mm larger, and the great-toe nail is wider by 4 and 3 mm than the thumb in men and women, respectively (22). The great toe is approximately 20% larger and longer than the thumb. There are 10 to 15 degrees of hallux valgus, and the metatarsophalangeal joint is a hyperextension joint with limited flexion (25,38). Functionally, as the great toe provides the best results by providing stronger pinch and better grasp, it should be considered for thumb reconstruction for amputations between the interphalangeal joint and the base of the metacarpal shaft. It should be used for patients who request better hand function and appearance and who are willing to accept mild to moderate functional disturbance of the foot. It is also indicated in severe injury that involves other parts of the hand, as it provides strong grip and pinch. It is best suited when the size difference between the

thumb and great toe is acceptable. Usually, the left great toe is preferred for transplantation, irrespective of which side of the thumb is to be reconstructed, as the left foot bears less functional stress. The results, including sensibility, stability, grip strength, pinch power, and interphalangeal joint motion, are usually the best for the great toe compared to other toes for thumb reconstruction. However, the appearance of the reconstructed thumb is too big, and the donor foot morbidity is greater, compared with all other toe transplantation techniques (Fig. 4).

TRIMMED GREAT-TOE TRANSPLANTATION

First described by Wei et al. (22), this technique reduces the bony and soft tissue girth of the great toe to make it more equivalent to the thumb while preserving the interphalangeal joint articulation. The trimming of bone, joint, and soft tissues is done on the tibial aspect, as the pedicle is located on the fibular side. This technique combines the better aesthetics of wrap-around procedures with the better function of the total great-toe transfer; therefore, it is most suitable for patients who are concerned about appearance and function. It is indicated for thumb amputations at or distal to the metacarpophalangeal joint when there is an obvious size discrepancy between the thumb and great toe and when movement at the interphalangeal joint is desirable. Trimming does reduce some joint movements, but, overall, usefulness and appearance of the reconstructed thumb are excellent. Initially, this technique was used in adults only, but the long-term results of careful trimming of immature growth plate have been shown to preserve its blood supply and integrity, thereby maintaining the growth potential (39).

Harvesting Technique

The size difference between the thumb and the great toe is determined by measuring the circumference of the thumb at three points: the nail base, the interphalangeal joint, and

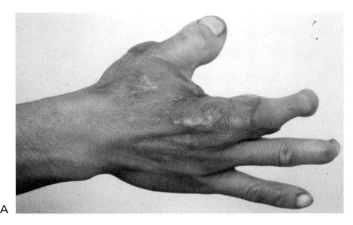
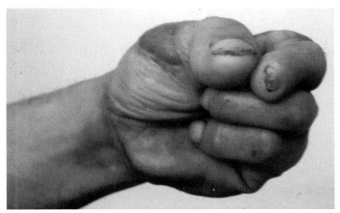
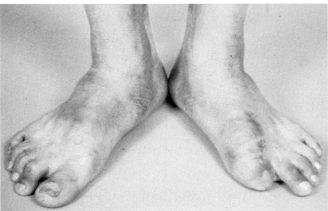
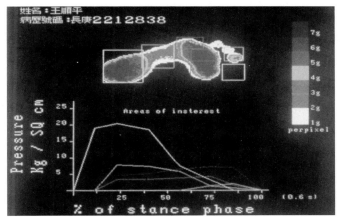

FIGURE 4. A: Total great-toe and second-toe, for thumb and middle finger, reconstruction. **B:** Broad contact surface with total great-toe–to–thumb reconstruction. **C:** Donor site after total great-toe–to–thumb transplantation. **D:** Foot pressure analysis after total great-toe transplantation. Note the even pressure distribution.

the middle of the proximal phalanx. These are transposed onto the great toe, with the excess placed medially (tibial side), taking care to preserve the nail fold. This excess denotes the size difference between the two. The excess medial strip is usually approximately 8 to 15 mm wide and is tapered to a point at the tip of the toe.

After isolating the neurovascular pedicle and tendons, the excess medial skin strip is elevated from distal to proximal, deepening the incision to periosteum at the tip of the distal phalanx. The medial collateral ligament, joint capsule, and periosteum are incised and elevated as a perijoint composite flap to the midplantar surface of the phalanges in the subperiosteal plane. A longitudinal osteotomy is then done with an oscillating saw, with removal of 2 to 4 mm of bone from the phalanges and 4 to 6 mm from the joint. The perijoint composite flap is redraped, and the redundant part is trimmed. The repair of the perijoint composite flap should be tight to maintain interphalangeal joint stability. The proximal phalanx is then osteotomized, leaving only the pedicle intact. The donor site is primarily closed, and, if needed, the proximal portion of medial strip is used for closure (Fig. 5).

GREAT-TOE WRAP-AROUND FLAP

Originally described by Morrison (21,40), the great-toe wrap-around flap was devised as an alternative to total great-toe transplantation. The flap only consists of a nail and soft tissue envelope of the great toe without skeleton and tendons. Thus, the patient retains the great toe. This addresses the donor site concerns as well as the size discrepancy between the great toe and thumb. The thumb skeleton, if not already preserved, needs to be reconstructed with nonvascularized iliac crest graft.

Although not intended originally, this flap is ideally indicated for thumb reconstruction in amputations distal to the interphalangeal joint and for soft tissue avulsion injuries distal to the metacarpophalangeal joint with intact joints, skeleton, and tendons (2). Although the original technique involved harvesting the soft tissue flap without any bone, subsequent modification includes the distal phalanx for nail support, which also prevent swiveling of the wrap-around flap and grafted bone fracture or absorption (41,42). The appearance of the reconstructed thumb is usually excellent, and the great toe need not be sacrificed

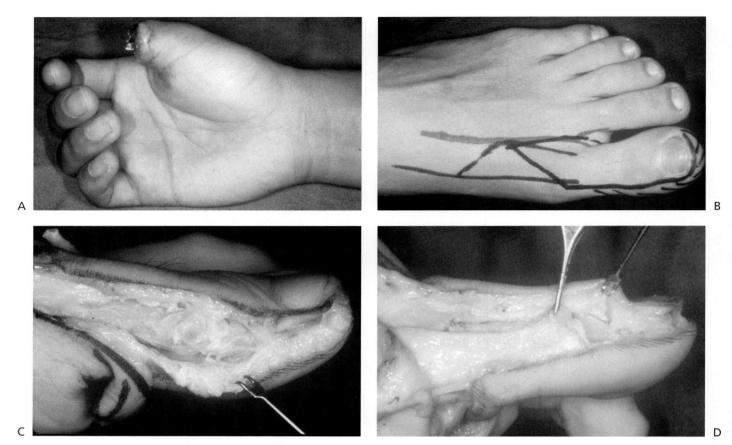

FIGURE 5. A: Thumb amputation through the base of the proximal phalanx in the right hand. **B:** Templating for trimmed great-toe transplantation in left foot. **C:** Medial skin flap elevation. **D:** Elevation of composite perijoint soft tissue envelope. (*continued*)

entirely. Although longer great-toe stump is preserved, and the donor site deformity is less conspicuous, healing may be complicated because the donor site needs skin grafting or cross-toe flaps.

Harvesting Technique

The flap is designed and elevated as described for the trimmed great toe. The distal great toe is disarticulated at the interphalangeal joint, and a longitudinal osteotomy is performed to remove approximately one-third of the width of the distal phalanx. The plantar side of the distal phalanx is burred to reduce its thickness. This technique allows reduction in width, preserving vascularity of distal phalanx on the lateral side and preserving the nail bed and future nail growth. If required, tendons can be included in the flap.

The cartilage surface or several millimeters of the proximal phalanx can be removed to facilitate a tension-free donor site closure. The proximal portion of the medial skin strip sometimes is helpful in wound closure, but skin grafts and cross-toe flaps are usually not necessary (Fig. 6).

SECOND-TOE TRANSPLANTATION

As the second toe (17) has a smaller and bulbous contact surface for opposition, a tendency for claw, a smaller toe nail, and inferior cosmesis with less ideal functions as compared to the trimmed or total great-toe transplantation, it does not make a preferred option for thumb reconstruction. The second toe is also not advisable in cases in which the patient's occupation requires a broad area for opposition, the thenar muscle function is suboptimal, the dominant hand is to be reconstructed, or the patient is a manual laborer.

However, the second toe can be used in cases in which preservation of the great toe is necessary. When the second toe is sizable, matching size of the thumb, it is the best indication for thumb reconstruction. In reconstruction of nondominant hands, or for patients who are satisfied with second-best looks and function, second toe is also a good selection. In proximal thumb amputations that involve the metacarpal shaft, the great-toe transplantation is not advisable because of donor site morbidity considerations; second-toe transplantation at metatarsal level can be used. In children, second toe for thumb transplantation remains the preferred option, except in some cases of severe and

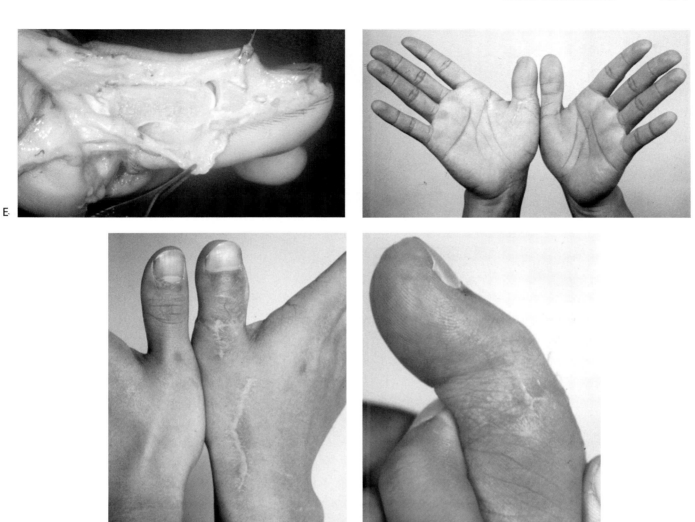

FIGURE 5. (*continued*) **E:** Trimming of phalanges and interphalangeal joint. **F:** Final result, with the reconstructed thumb similar to the opposite one. **G:** Final appearance. **H:** Flexion at the reconstructed interphalangeal joint.

bilateral hand injuries, in which the trimmed great toe (39) or even a total great-toe–to–thumb transfer (43) may be indicated.

Harvesting Technique (for Transmetatarsal Harvest)

The length of the thumb to be reconstructed is decided by measuring the opposite thumb, and, with the help of x-rays, the proposed level of osteotomy on the second metatarsal is marked. The skin flaps on the dorsal and plantar aspects are marked with a V shape to facilitate closure for donor and recipient sites. The vertex of this V shape should be 1 cm proximal to osteotomy, and the divergent limbs suggest the midpoint of the adjacent webs. The dorsal incision is curvilinear or lazy S–shaped, and the incision in the plantar aspect is curved and angulated, avoiding the weightbearing area.

The branches of the deep peroneal nerve to the great toe are preserved. The nerves and extensor and flexor tendons are dissected to required lengths. On the plantar aspect, all but 2 to 3 mm of subcutaneous fat and tissue is discarded under the skin to reduce bulk and to facilitate metacarpophalangeal joint motion in the transferred toe. If a long nerve segment is required, the common digital nerves to the first and third toes are split by interfascicular dissection, preserving supply to these toes. All of the structures except the pedicle are divided carefully, the nerves may be marked with 6-0 sutures, and the tourniquet is released to allow reperfusion of the toe. The donor site is closed primarily without tension. In certain situations, the third toe may have to be used for thumb reconstruction, such as when the second toe is not available or is not suitable, or if the great toe is harvested from the same foot (then the second toe is spared), and when the third toe is a better match for thumb size (44). The flap design and

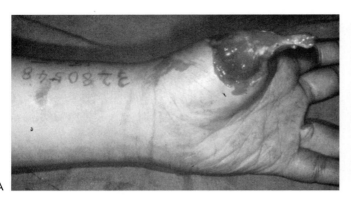

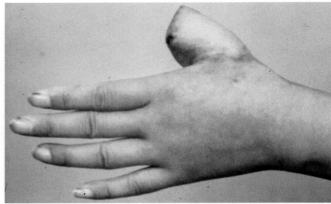

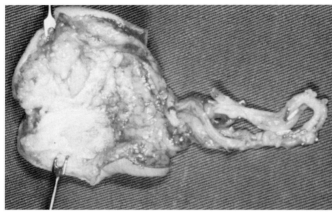

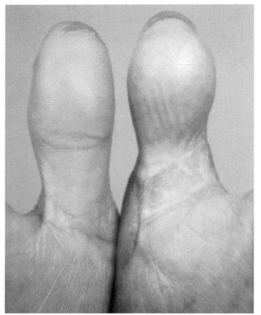

FIGURE 6. A: Soft tissue avulsion injury of the thumb. **B:** Pre–toe transplantation soft tissue cover with pedicled groin flap. **C:** Modified great-toe wrap-around flap: Note the inclusion of the distal phalanx in the flap. **D:** Final appearance of the reconstructed thumb.

harvest are similar to the second toe, and if the first and second toes have previously been transplanted, it can be raised on the third common digital planter artery (Fig. 7).

POSTOPERATIVE MANAGEMENT

The patients receive care for several days in a high-dependency unit in which specialized nurses can closely monitor the transplanted toe. The proximal palm and wrist are gently wrapped with the fingers uncovered for continuous observation. The hand and forearm are kept slightly elevated, resting over a smooth support, to reduce edema. Bulky dressings are not advised, as blood clots can be retained around the wounds, and removal could induce vasospasm. It is not possible to start early postoperative rehabilitation.

An initial bolus of 100 mL of dextran 40 (low molecular weight) is rapidly administered intravenously, 10 min-utes before completion of the arterial anastomosis, followed by continuous infusion (25 mL per hour) during the next 4 to 5 days. Aspirin (325 mg daily) is administered during 2 weeks to reduce platelet aggregation risk. Prophylactic antibiotics are seldom needed, but, in prolonged surgical cases or dirty wounds, antibiotics that cover gram-positive and gram-negative bacteria should be administered.

The vascular conditions in the toe are subjectively monitored by direct observation of the skin color, capillary refilling, and turgor and are objectively monitored by measuring the surface temperature in the toe in comparison to the adjacent normal finger and the opposite hand. Assessing the artery patency with Doppler ultrasonography is helpful when these subjective and objective evaluations are in doubt.

The donor foot is gently covered with Furacin gauze over the wound and a light fluff dressing. No splints are used in the donor foot or the recipient hand. The foot can

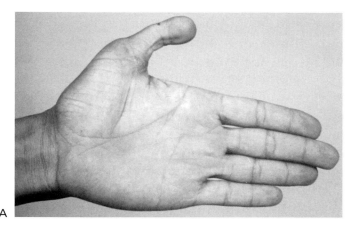
A

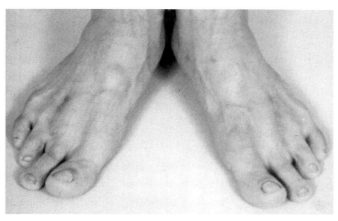
B

FIGURE 7. A: Second-toe transplantation for the nondominant thumb. **B:** Donor feet after bilateral second-toe transplantation.

be uncovered in 2 days without further dressings. The patient is allowed to walk a few steps on the heel of the donor foot after the second week. It must be emphasized that any contact with the anterior plantar weightbearing surface should be avoided during this time. After approximately 6 weeks, the patient is allowed to walk with a normal gait in shoes if the wound heals.

REHABILITATION

Early and intense supervised motor and sensory rehabilitation (45) results in quicker and better recovery of functions after transplantations. An early mobilization regimen consists of a protective stage (first 3 postoperative days), an early mobilization stage (from the third day to the third week), an active motion stage (the fourth to fifth weeks), a training stage in activities of daily living (the fifth to seventh weeks), and a prevocational training stage (after the seventh week). The advantages of early mobilization regimen include less stiffness, fewer tendon adhesions, and early return to activities. The rehabilitation continues from the acute phase to complete recovery and helps enhance surgical results (45).

The incidence of secondary procedures in toe transplantation for the purpose of functional improvement has been shown to be approximately 14% (46). These procedures involve tendons (9%, mainly tenolysis), bones and joints (3.8%, mainly arthrodesis), and soft tissues (3.8%, mainly web space deepening).

INTRA- AND POSTOPERATIVE COMPLICATIONS

One of the most frequent complications is vasospasm, which can occur intraoperatively or immediately postoperatively. Arterial vasospasm during the procedure can be relieved by topical instillation of local anesthetics, such as

lidocaine (Xylocaine, 1% to 2%) or papaverine. Adventitiectomy helps relieve the spasm and should be carried out under suitable magnification. Tension from vascular anastomosis should be avoided, and vein grafts should be used, if required, although, with adequate preoperative planning, its use would be rare. The vessels should be kept moist during the procedure, and the skin closure should not be tight.

Postoperative vasospasm could be precipitated by low room temperature, low blood pressure, anxiety in the patient, or excessive manipulation of the hand. Prevention consists of keeping an optimal blood pressure, supplying adequate fluids, and avoiding oversedation. If vasospasm occurs, some skin sutures should be removed, and vasodilators, such as lidocaine, should be intermittently instilled from the partially opened wounds. Sublingual nitroglycerin or nifedipine (47) and regional blocks (48) may help relieve vasospasm. However, if no improvement of circulation is noted after observation for a reasonable time (1 hour), prompt reexploration in the operating room is mandatory. In some cases, incomplete adventitiectomy or a small hematoma may be responsible for local vasospasm. Once the adventitial layer has been adequately excised or after draining the hematoma, the vasospasm may be relieved. When there is a refractory vasospasm or when the artery is thrombosed, redoing the anastomosis is indicated, with or without an interposed vein graft.

In contrast to arterial thrombosis, the venous thrombosis is less common and is often related to incorrect positioning, such as twisting or kinking or compression by tunnel, hematoma, or tight skin closure. In most instances of vascular compromise, it is possible to salvage the transplanted toe after reexploration. From the author's experience of 103 thumb reconstructions with various types of toe transplantations, 13 cases (12.6%) required exploration for circulatory compromise, with a successful result in 98% of cases (2). Therefore, the attitude toward reexploration should be aggressive.

Other complications that are observed in the first 2 weeks usually involve skin coverage and wound healing problems. In most cases, these are secondary to partial necrosis of thin skin flaps in the transplanted toe or in the scarred recipient site. With exposure of important structures, such as tendons, nerves, and vessels, immediate coverage reconstruction should be performed to prevent desiccation of these structures and subsequent sequelae.

LATE COMPLICATIONS AND THEIR MANAGEMENT

Late complications include reduced range of movement secondary to tendon and joint adhesions, extension lag, and nonunion at the osteosynthesis site. Some of these can be prevented or minimized by using early, supervised, and aggressive postoperative rehabilitation (45).

Tendon Adhesions

If required, tenolysis can be done. In the author's series of 139 toe transplantations (46), the incidence of tendon-related secondary procedures, such as tenolysis, tenorrhaphy, and tendon transfer, was 9% (46).

Extension Lag

Extensor lag usually results from tendon repair under inadequate tightness or loosening of the repair. It can be corrected with reoperation or prolonged splinting in extension. The results of secondary tendon repair are usually poor. Sometimes, the terminal joint can be arthrodesed in an extended position.

Joint Stiffness

Early, intensive, supervised postoperative therapy helps achieve good joint movements. If required, arthrolysis or arthrodesis can be carried out. In the author's experience, the incidence of joint-related secondary procedures was 2.3% (46).

Nonunion

With interosseous wiring, the incidence of nonunion is 1.5% (46). If symptomatic, secondary osteosynthesis or bone grafting can be undertaken.

PITFALLS IN TOE-TO-THUMB TRANSPLANTATIONS AND MANAGEMENT

Suboptimal outcomes usually result from pitfalls that can be related to surgical planning or surgical technique.

Planning-Related Pitfalls

Improper Donor Toe Selection

Various considerations concerning patient requirements, available options, and donor site morbidity, as mentioned previously, must play significant roles in decision making.

It is vital that the patient is fully involved in this process. Factors such as desire for strong hand function, interphalangeal joint motion, and appearance should be balanced against athletic ambitions, donor site concerns, and the surgeon's preference and competence before deciding on a particular toe transplant for thumb reconstruction. An improper toe selection would result in suboptimal thumb reconstruction.

Improper Timing of Surgery

If the wound is not clean and complete débridement can not be assured, it is advisable to perform serial débridements, to delay surgery, or even to perform surgery as a secondary procedure after the wound heals, as the complications, such as infection, are comparatively fewer with secondary toe transfers (26). However, in suitable patients, primary toe transplantation can be considered for early recovery and return to work.

Excess Tissue Harvest from Donor Foot

Harvest of excess tissue for simultaneous coverage reconstruction of the hand in toe transplantation is a major cause of complications at the donor foot. It may result in prolonged wound healing and painful scar formation. Pre–toe-transfer soft tissue augmentation, using pedicled groin flap, can minimize these complications. The redundant skin also helps the smooth transition between the transplanted toe and the amputated stump and provides for an adequate first web. In proximal thumb amputations, the bone length can be augmented by using nonvascular iliac bone graft (if the great toe or its variant is planned) or by using transmetatarsal lesser-toe transplantation.

Improper Length

The length of the reconstructed thumb should not go beyond the interphalangeal joint of the index finger, otherwise the reconstructed thumb looks strange and ugly. A slightly shorter thumb is preferable than a longer one (49).

Improper Position

The reconstructed thumb should be optimally positioned for opposition, especially when the remaining thenar muscles function or when basal joint movements are inadequate. The length and position of the thumb to be reconstructed in this situation can be judged by using a temporary thumb prosthesis.

Technique-Related Pitfalls

Claw Second Toe

The second toe is prone to become clawed because of its anatomic position and its stronger flexor than extensor muscles.

Therefore, during tendon repairs, the extensor tendon should be repaired in full extension, and the flexor tendon should be repaired in appropriate tension. The distal interphalangeal joint can be transfixed in extension with a Kirschner wire for 6 weeks. Furthermore, night splints in maximum extension should be used for at least 12 months. If necessary, fusion, especially of the distal interphalangeal joint, in corrected position can be undertaken to improve function and appearance.

Unstable Interphalangeal Joint in Trimmed Great-Toe Transplantation

Unstable interphalangeal joint can occur after trimming of the interphalangeal joint. It can be prevented by initially elevating a proper composite soft tissue envelope, including periosteum, joint capsule, and collateral ligament, by trimming the excess, and then by repairing under proper tension.

Donor Site Complications

Resection of the great toe, in general, causes more deformity in the foot than removal of the second toe alone. In transplantation of the great toe or its variants, it is advisable to preserve at least 1 cm of the proximal phalanx, as it preserves attachment of plantar aponeurosis, thereby maintaining the medial longitudinal arch, and avoids windlass effect (50).

REFERENCES

1. Lister G. The choice of procedure following thumb amputation. *Clin Orthop* 1985;195:45–51.
2. Wei FC, Chen HC, Chuang CC, et al. Microsurgical thumb reconstruction. Selection of various techniques. *Plast Reconstr Surg* 1994;93:345–351.
3. Fultz FW, Lester DK, Hunter JM. Single stage lengthening by intercalary bone graft in patients with congenital hand deformities. *J Hand Surg* 1986;11:40–46.
4. Matev IB. Thumb reconstruction in children through metacarpal lengthening. *Plast Reconstr Surg* 1979;64:665–669.
5. Matev IB. *Reconstructive surgery of the thumb.* Brentwood, England: Pilgrims Press, 1983.
6. Smith RJ, Gumley GJ. Metacarpal distraction lengthening. *Hand Clin* 1985;1:417–429.
7. Seitz WH Jr, Dobyns JH. Digital lengthening with emphasis on distraction osteogenesis in the upper limb. *Hand Clin* 1993;9:699–706.
8. Bunnel S. Physiologic reconstruction of the thumb after total loss. *Surg Obstet Gynaecol* 1931;52:245.
9. Tubiana R, Roux JP. Phalangisation of the first and fifth metacarpal. Indications, operative techniques and results. *J Bone Joint Surg* 1974;56:447–457.
10. Chase RA. An alternative to pollicization in subtotal thumb reconstruction. *Plast Reconstr Surg* 1969;44:421.
11. Verdan C. The reconstruction of the thumb. *Surg Clin North Am* 1968;48:1033.
12. Brunelli GA, Brunelli GR. Reconstruction of the traumatic absence of thumb in the adult by pollicization. *Hand Clin* 1992;8:41–45.
13. Littler JW. Reconstruction of the thumb in traumatic loss. In: Converse JM, ed. *Reconstructive plastic surgery,* 2nd ed. Philadelphia: WB Saunders, 1977:3350–3367.
14. Cheng MH, Cheng SL, Tung TC, et al. A case report of pollicization of traumatized index finger for reconstruction of traumatic amputation of thumb. *J Surg Assoc Rep China* 1992;30:134–139.
15. Nicoladani C. Daumenplastik. *Wien Klin Wochenshr* 1897;10:663.
16. Buncke HJ, Buncke CM, Schulz WP. Immediate Nicoladani procedure in rhesus monkey, for hallux to hand transplantation, utilizing microminiature vascular anastomosis. *Br J Plast Surg* 1966;19:332.
17. Zhong-wei C, Dony-yue Y, Di-Sheng C. *Microsurgery.* New York: Springer-Verlag, 1982.
18. Cobbett JR. Free digital transfer. Report of a case of transfer of great toe to replace an amputated thumb. *J Bone Joint Surg* 1969;51:677.
19. O'Brien GM, MacLeod AM, Sykes PJ, et al. Hallux-to-hand transfer. *Hand* 1975;7:128.
20. Gilbert A. composite tissue transfer from the foot. Anatomic basis and surgical technique. In: Daniller AI, Strauch B, eds. *Symposium on microsurgery.* St. Louis: CV Mosby, 1976.
21. Morrison WA, MacLeod AM. Thumb reconstruction with a free neurovascular wrap around flap from the big toe. *J Hand Surg* 1980;5:575–583.
22. Wei FC, Chen HC, Chuang CC, et al. Reconstruction of thumb with a trimmed great toe transfer technique. *Plast Reconstr Surg* 1988;82:506.
23. Buncke HJ. Thumb and finger reconstruction by micro vascular and joint auto transplantation. In: McCarthy JG, ed. *Plastic surgery.* Philadelphia: WB Saunders, 1990:4409–4429.
24. May JW. Micro vascular great toe to hand transfer for reconstruction of amputated thumb. In: MC Carthy JG, ed. *Plastic surgery.* Philadelphia: WB Saunders, 1990:5153–5158.
25. Gordon L. Toe to thumb transplantation. In: Green DP, ed. *Operative hand surgery.* Edinburgh: Churchill Livingstone, 1993:1253–1282.
26. Yim KK, Wei FC. A comparison between primary and secondary toe to hand transplantation. Paper presented at: the American Society for Reconstructive Microsurgery, 12th annual meeting; January 13, 1997; FL.
27. Foucher G, Norris RW. The dorsal approach in harvesting the second toe. *J Reconstr Microsurg* 1988;4:185–187.
28. Foucher G, Merle M, Maneaud M, et al. Microsurgical free partial toe transfer in hand reconstruction. A report of 12 cases. *Plast Reconstr Surg* 1980;65:616–627.
29. Leung PC. The Chinese culture and hand reconstruction. In: Landi A, ed. *Reconstruction of the thumb.* London: Chapman and Hall, 1989:11–16.
30. Foucher G, Moss AL. Microvascular second toe to finger transfer: a statistical analysis of 55 transfers. *Br J Plast Surg* 1991;44:87–90.
31. Leung PC. Use of an intramedullary bone peg in digital replantation, revascularization and toe-transfers. *J Hand Surg* 1981;6:281–284.
32. Chen HC, Tang YB, Wei, FC, et al. Finger reconstruction with triple toe transfer from the same foot for a patient with a special job and previous foot trauma. *Ann Plast Surg* 1991;27:272–277.

33. Gordon L. Toe-to thumb transplantation. In: Green DP, ed. *Operative hand surgery.* Edinburgh: Churchill Livingstone, 1993:1253–1282.

34. Wei FC, Santamaria E. Toe to finger reconstruction. In: Green DP, Hotchkiss RN, Pederson WC, eds. *Green's operative hand surgery.* Philadelphia: Churchill Livingstone, 1993.

35. Wei FC, Silverman TS, Hsu WM. Retrograde dissection of the vascular pedicle in toe harvest. *Plast Reconstr Surg* 1995;96:1211–1214.

36. Wei FC. Tissue preservation in hand injury: the first step to toe-to-hand transplantation [Editorial]. *Plast Reconstr Surg* 1998;102:2497–2501.

37. Yim KK, Wei FC. Intraosseous wiring in toe-to-hand transplantation. *Ann Plast Surg* 1995;35:66–69.

38. Strauch B, Yu HL. Free second toe transfer. In: Strauch B, Yu HL, eds. *Atlas of micro vascular surgery.* New York: Thieme Medical Publishers, 1993:356–360.

39. Jain V, Wei FC, et al. Trimmed great toe to thumb transfer in children: long term results. *Plast Reconstr Surg (in press).*

40. Urbaniak JR. Wrap-around procedure for thumb reconstruction. *Hand Clin* 1985;1:259–269.

41. El Gammal TA, Wei FC. Micro vascular reconstruction of the distal digit by partial toe transfer. *Clin Plast Surg* 1997;24:49–55.

42. Foucher G, Binhammer P. Plea to save the great toe in total thumb reconstruction. *Microsurgery* 1995;16:373–376.

43. Wei FC, El Gammal TA, Chen HC, et al. Toe to hand transfer for traumatic digital amputation in children and adolescents. *Plast Reconstr Surg* 1997;100:605–609.

44. Wei FC, Yim KK. Single third toe transfer in hand reconstruction. *J Hand Surg* 1995;20:388–394.

45. Ma HS, El Gammal TA, Wei FC. Current concepts of toe to hand transfer: surgery and rehabilitation. *J Hand Ther* 1996;9:41–46.

46. Yim KK, Wei FC. Secondary procedures to improve function after toe-to-hand transfers. *Br J Plastic Surg* 1995;48:487–491.

47. Nilsson H, Jonasson T, Ringquist I. Treatment of digital vasospastic disease with the calcium-entry blocker, nifedipine. *Acta Med Scand* 1984;215:135–139.

48. Neimkin RJ, May JW, Roberts J, et al. Continuous axillary block trough an indwelling Teflon catheter. *J Hand Surg* 1984;9:830–833.

49. Wei FC, Chen HC, Chuang DC, et al. Aesthetic refinements in toe-to-hand transfer surgery. *Plast Reconstr Surg* 1996;98:485–490.

50. Sammarco GJ. Biomechanics of the foot. In: Jahss MH, ed. *Disorders of the foot.* Philadelphia: WB Saunders, 1982:163.

96

FINGER RECONSTRUCTION
AND RAY RESECTION

GUY G. FOUCHER
JOSÉ MEDINA HENRIQUEZ
ROGER K. KHOURI

To retain parts which can neither be restored as useful members nor can contribute tissues for overall restoration is as ridiculous as indiscriminate amputation without a thorough inventory of parts for possible use in repair.

—Chase RA

Finger reconstruction could encompass a lot of elective procedures, and this chapter concentrates on the difficult issue of reconstruction after finger mutilation. These injuries are frequent, and the decision for abstention or reconstruction as well as the method to be selected is a complex decision based on multiple factors. The desires of the patient are to be clarified not only on a functional basis but also concerning appearance.

It is difficult to define the function of a "normal" hand. Mobility, sensibility, absence of pain, and good strength are only basic requirements. But the hand also plays a role in body language and interaction. As underlined by Verdan et al. (7), the hand is "the instrument of desire, exchanges and pleasure." This introduces an esthetic component that should be taken into account in limited mutilation in which a five- or four-fingered hand could be reconstructed. Indeed, a one-finger mutilation without a visible stump could remain unnoticed, at least during gesture. It is simpler to define the so-called basic hand. Entin defined it "as a hand which has a stable wrist, a radial digit with good sensation and mobility and at least one or two fingers on the ulnar aspect of the hand separated by a deep cleft" (1).

GENERAL CONSIDERATIONS

The function of the radial fingers is relevant in fine pinch [the precision grip of Napier (2)] and depends mainly on the quality of their sensory discrimination, the pulp being, as mentioned by Moberg (111), the eyes of the hand. For the ulnar fingers, the roll up has relevance in the strength of the hand [the power grip of Napier (2)] and mobility with good enduring skin cover has a dominant role. When assessing hand function and considering the manual function of a patient with severe unilateral multidigital mutilations, grip patterns can be simplified into four types. Fine pinch needs at least one ray of sufficient length, sensibility, and mobility to come in contact with the thumb pulp. Only the presence of the nail really allows one to grip tiny objects. "Chuck" pinch, with three converging rays, enhances strength and stability. "Grip" uses the ulnar side of the hand, with the last two rays locking the digito-palmar grasp. Finally, "key-grip" is sometimes the only one that can be restored, with the tip of the thumb joining the lateral side of a finger.

Classification of mutilation takes into account these considerations. It is useful to develop a score, adding the figures for each ray (Fig. 1) from 0 to 9 (0 meaning absence of mutilation). This was found useful for codification in computerized clinical files and makes the comparison of results easier (3,4). Classification has the merit of helping in surgical indications.

Several points are of relevance; namely, location, level and number of amputated fingers, and association to thumb amputation. The authors use a modification of Pulvertaft's classification (5), allowing easy inclusion of the indications for toe transfer. Four groups of amputations may be formed: (a) radial amputations (affecting one to three rays but leaving the little finger intact), (b) central amputations (affecting one to two rays but leaving the index and the little finger intact), (c) ulnar amputations (affecting one to three rays but leaving the index functional), and (d) complete amputations (affecting all four fingers). They could be described as oblique, atypical ("crenelated"), or transverse and can be phalangeal or metacarpal.

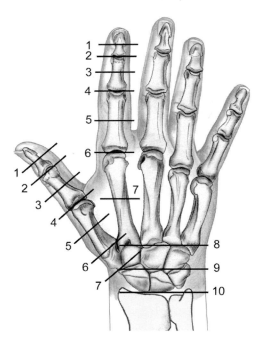

FIGURE 1. Score system for classification of hand mutilation to facilitate computerization of files and comparison of clinical cases.

EVALUATION

History

The patient's history, age, dominance, job, and leisure activities are recorded. Age is a definite limit, and aging is more a problem for nerve surgery than artery repair. It is mandatory to check for any history of associated pathology (vascular and neurologic but also psychological).

A complete history of the trauma and previous surgery is mandatory. For example, an avulsion injury would be a relative contraindication to any technique involving a neurotization (e.g., a toe transfer or a free sensory flap) due to difficulty in assessing the state of the recipient nerves. Crush injuries are responsible for extensive sclerosis and poor vascularization. Any postoperative complication (e.g., infection, reflex sympathetic dystrophy) is useful to know. Any pain has to be clarified to separate nociception from deafferentation, phantom pain, sympathetic maintained pain, or simple cold intolerance.

Physical Examination

A thorough examination of each finger is followed by an assessment of the global function and appearance.

The quality and trophicity of the skin cover are controlled, and any skin blanching of the tip in full extension is noticed as well as any discoloration (venous stasis). Palpation allows assessment of the soft tissue padding and stability and determination of the presence of any tumor

(neuroma or inclusion cyst) or a bone spur. Vascularization of the finger is of outstanding importance, as there are few possibilities for reconstruction in the absence of a good patency of the palmar arteries. An Allen's test is useful, with successive compression of the vascular bundle at the wrist and at the base of each finger.

Sensibility tests (e.g., two-point discrimination and Semmes-Weinstein) and mobility (goniometric) measurements are recorded as well as strength (using the Jamar dynamometer and Preston gauge). The authors also measure the first web span using a custom-made cylinder ranging from 6 to 14 cm in diameter.

Some hidden problems need special emphasis. Limitation of joint motion could be related to joint alteration but also to tendon or intrinsic muscle imbalance. Tightness of intrinsic muscles (using the Finochietto maneuver) and tenodesis effects of extensor and flexor tendons should be checked. Parkes (6) has described the limitation of proximal interphalangeal (PIP) joint active flexion when the flexor profundus tendon is allowed to retract after distal phalanx amputation. Tightening of the lumbrical muscle when trying to flex the finger is followed by "paradoxal" extension of the PIP joint. This phenomenon has been most frequently noticed in the index and middle fingers due to a unilateral origin of the muscle. The other phenomenon that should be well known is the quadriga syndrome described by Verdan (7), which happens when the profundus is stuck to the stump under some traction (frequently noticed after fixation to the stump). In this case, the neighboring fingers present a lack of active flexion. This is essentially observed on the three ulnar fingers due to a common muscle. Finally, limitation of a short segment of proximal phalanx is frequently noticed due to the limited function of intrinsic muscles [45 degrees of flexion, according to Louis (8)].

In case of short segment of phalanx, a tendency to a flexion deformity could be observed due either to imbalance or retraction of muscles. The flexion of the PIP joint in amputation through the proximal part of the middle phalanx is frequently related to the strength of the flexor superficialis. This exposed stump is frequently painful with inadvertent trauma.

After analytic examination, a global assessment of the hand is helpful in selecting some basic daily activity and looking for exclusion with bypassed finger stump(s). For the same purpose, toys are used in children. All types of grips should be checked, and it is more helpful in complex mutilations to assess what is remaining than what is missing.

Office Tests

Based on clinical examination findings, some tests could be useful. Concerning pain related to a palpable neuroma, a test (9) with successive infiltration of serum and then local anesthesia has to be performed. A Doppler probe could be used to assess arterial inflow and venous outflow. If imaging has a limited place, plain radiography is useful to check for a foreign body, an inclusion cyst, a bone spur, or residual signs of reflex sympathetic dystrophy. Joints (and growth plates in children) are to be assessed carefully before deciding on any reconstruction.

In some circumstances, more sophisticated tests should be used, including a work simulation [either on Baltimore Therapeutic Equipment (Baltimore Therapeutic Equipment Company, Hanover, MD) or in the ergotherapy department], a pain clinic consultation, an electromyogram study, or a more precise vascular assessment. A stress test in case of cold intolerance or an arteriogram in case of possibility of performing an island transfer could be of interest. Pictures and, frequently, a video of the hand function and appearance are sometimes advisable. For all complex cases, the authors believe a psychological assessment is of outstanding importance.

Psychological Assessment

The authors have found it useful during 24 years of hand surgery practice to work with a full-time psychoanalyst who is present at each consultation and dressing session (10). Preoperatively, the psychoanalyst assesses the cultural, religious, and psychological background of the patient.

Cultural background is not to be neglected, as surgeons have all heard about Asian patients looking more for a five-fingered hand and refusing any finger sacrifice for functional improvement. As another example, Yoshimura in Japan has a unique series of second toe–to–fifth finger transfer in Yacusa punished by mutilation (94).

A good "contract" is necessary, with good comprehension on both parts: the patient and the surgeon. The psychologist serves as a well-trained neutral person to translate and make clear both the "real" demands of the patient and the "true" answers of the surgeon.

The authors have learned the following about psychological assessments:

1. The absence of patient demand for treatment should be heard and respected, even if the correction is simple and effective. Some patients use the hand's appearance to avoid forgetting the injury; others use it to obtain benefits from their family or employer. There is also the occasional patient who just needs to speak about his or her problem simply to be reassured about the future.

2. Treatment options should be carefully considered even when there is an urgent patient demand. The demand may be related to a time of crisis for the patient, including depression, decreased self-image, or a changed personal situation (e.g., familial or professional) with pending problems. After a major trauma or mutilation, any reconstruction plan should respect the so-called grieving period that the patient must go through, even if experience has demonstrated that some patients have no mourning process and simply adjust after a variable amount of time. Any posttraumatic stress disorder requires some psychological counseling as well as any conflict in compensation claims. The psychologist is a useful guide for fixing the optimal date of surgery, taking into account that early reconstruction provides superior functional integration.

3. Real patient motivations for treatment should be distinguished from advanced reasons. For example, a patient who wants esthetic improvement of his or her hand may not hesitate to hide the real surgical demand by complaining of pain or some functional problem. Pain could be a way for a patient to express unhappiness with the hand's appearance.

4. Brown, in his classic paper "Less Than Ten—Surgeons with Amputated Fingers" (11), has demonstrated the role of high motivation in a group of physicians who had amputations. However, the authors' conclusion differs from Brown, who thought that replantation is not necessary in such patients. The authors' experience has demonstrated that "great performers," such as surgeons or musicians, are ideal candidates for surgical reconstruction.

5. The expectations of the patient could be too high. A patient might secretly hope to erase the injury, not only from the hand, but from their history as well. In other cases, the level of injury and the patient's suffering may be out of proportion. The authors have found that the smaller the objective stigma, or injury, the more perfectionist the patient becomes and the more difficult to satisfy. This is perfectly illustrated by nail surgery.

6. The demand for treatment could come from a patient with a fragile psychological background or from a known or unknown psychiatric patient. Indeed, the hand surgeon taking care of casualties deals with a supposedly "normal" population. But the National Institute of Mental Health has demonstrated that 15% of the random population is affected by mental disorders, and 40% are not identified (12). The percentage could be even larger in trauma cases, and Schweitzer et al., in a series of replantations, found preaccident psychopathology in 21% of patients (13). Surgeons need to avoid the major pitfall of psychotic decompensation. Other and less dramatic pitfalls are dissatisfied patients with dysmorphophobia, or SHAFT syndrome. Patients with phobias or obsessions usually just complain—contrary to the aggressive paranoiac who may put his words into action. Operations on hysteric patients have not been a problem when operating on true disease and not on the conversion symptom. In fact, there are few contraindications to surgery in a good psychological environment.

One word is needed about the well-known "freedom of choice" of the patient so often claimed but not really practical. How could a patient "choose" among different techniques whose results depend on so many factors when the surgeon often has difficulty in making a decision and explaining the choice? Certainly, a surgeon should never avoid explaining a possible technique (e.g., microsurgery) due to his or her own technical insufficiency. In fact, transferring responsibility to the patient frequently reflects a surgeon's own uncertainty. In the authors' opinion, it is much more important to listen to the patient and understand his or her real needs and demands, expose briefly the possibilities, and justify the choice based on the functional and cosmetic desires of the patient.

CONSERVATIVE TREATMENT

Apart from psychological support, some conservative treatments are useful mainly in case of pain or esthetic disorder.

It is not the purpose here to discuss all of the medical treatments of hand pain, but in case of nociceptive pain, desensitization has been helpful. Some therapists use contact with different kinds of tissues and materials for desensitization, whereas others prefer to rely on ultrasound or electrical stimulation. Transcutaneous electrical nerve stimulation is more classically used in deafferentation pain; in such cases, rehabilitation is helpful to allow reintegration of the painful stump in daily activity. Reintegration of a bypassed finger is difficult, but neurologic experiments have demonstrated some brain plasticity, even in adults (14). In the majority of cases, an energetic program of rehabilitation (sensory or motor, or both) is helpful, avoiding any surgery in some cases or preparing for it in others. Scar compression and local massage have a role in skin preparation, as well as dynamic splinting to improve passive range of motion (15).

Concerning improvement of appearance, there is no doubt that esthetic prostheses have a place. However, they have been quite disappointing for isolated nail problems. In such cases, there are two alternatives: acrylic paste reconstruction when the base of the nail plate is sufficient or a "thimblelike" prosthesis in more severe cases. Finger prostheses have some functional role by lengthening the stump to facilitate contact with the thumb; by maintaining sensation, thanks to their thinness; by protecting a sensitive stump; or by supporting, pushing, or holding (elastic memory) light objects. Occasionally, they contribute to saving the whole hand because a patient may be more likely to use the hand if the mutilation remains unnoticed in social life (16,17).

These cosmetic devices could be used as the sole treatment or combined with surgical reconstruction. The authors have found it useful to consult Jean Pillet (16,17) even if surgery is contemplated. When there is any doubt concerning the best solution between a prosthesis and surgery, bear in mind that it is easier to don and doff a prosthetic device than a toe transfer. Surgeons should remember that an esthetic prosthesis should never be used to hide a bad and useless surgical reconstruction.

In a recent review of a series of 178 workers on compensation, Hopper et al. (18) found that 28% never or occasionally used their prosthesis whereas 24% used it more than 4 hours a day. Sixty-two percent reported stump problems, with 21% of those patients saying that it interfered with the use of the prosthesis. Low utilization was associated with male gender, stump problems, ring amputations, and distal amputations. High utilization was related to a shift to nonmanual work activity. But the authors conclude that prediction remains impossible. In a noncompensation population with preoperative common consultation between the surgeon and the prosthetist, the dropoff was much lower, with only 13% of 54 patients not wearing their prosthesis at all. Even when dropped, a prosthesis may help the patient pass the difficult phase of accepting the mutilation.

Currently, use is limited for functional prostheses in unilateral finger mutilation. Functional prostheses have been proposed by Smith and Dworecka (19) in the "one-finger" hand with an isolated thumb or finger when the patient refuses any surgery. A "counter post" could be built to oppose the thumb in metacarpal hands with short segments (20).

SURGICAL TREATMENT

General procedures in hand mutilations, such as correction of contracted scar, improvement of motion and sensibility, or stabilization of unstable skeleton parts, are not discussed in this chapter. Specific reconstructives procedures, ranging from local flap to toe transfer, are discussed in the following sections. The technique selected depends greatly on such local factors as the number of fingers involved, their level of amputation, as well as the state of the thumb.

The type of anesthesia used may be relevant, and Katz and Melzack (21) have stressed the possibility that patients may memorize painful experiences. They suggest decreasing pain associated with surgery by using nerve blocks in the days preceding surgery and during surgery. Nerve blocks have the advantage of acting directly on pain fibers, contrary to general anesthesia. Postoperative infusions by catheter have also proven efficiency (22).

Stump Improvement

Skin Cover

It is impossible to discuss all flaps used to improve the cover of an insufficient stump in this chapter. The authors have devoted a full book to the topic (23). It is sufficient to say that local flaps are preferable to loco-regional or distant flaps. They offer a "like-skin" result with, in the majority of cases, preservation of excellent sensibility. The choice depends on the level of amputation and the necessary advancement. In distal amputation, local flaps include the Tranquilli Leali flap (24), the Atasoy flap (25), and the Ven-

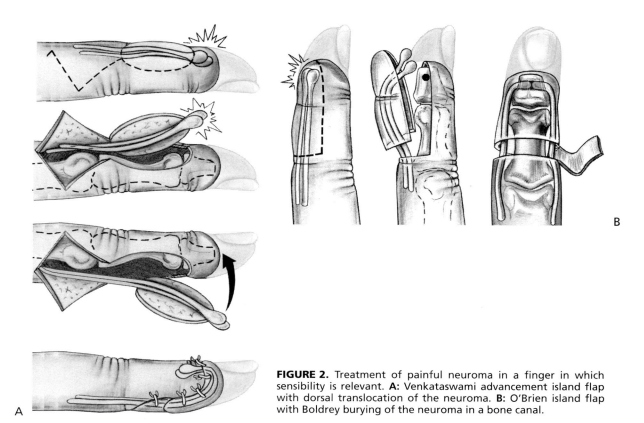

FIGURE 2. Treatment of painful neuroma in a finger in which sensibility is relevant. **A:** Venkataswami advancement island flap with dorsal translocation of the neuroma. **B:** O'Brien island flap with Boldrey burying of the neuroma in a bone canal.

kataswami homodigital island flap (26,27), for which only a small amount of tissue is needed. This last flap has provided at the index level a maximum advancement of 22 mm with preservation of excellent sensibility. This explains why indications for cross-finger flaps and free neurovascular flaps from the toes have decreased. They are currently restricted to huge loss (always harvested from the great toe) in young, healthy, well-motivated patients mainly in cases of composite loss involving some distal nailbed and bone. These flaps are discussed in Nail Surgery. For more proximal amputations, the flaps described by Hueston (28,29) and O'Brien (30,31) are ideal.

Pain related to a painful neuroma is not infrequent, and in a series of 118 amputations, Scott (32) found 13 cases (11%). When resistant to conservative treatment, a neuroma may be treated in more than 100 ways, but, as underlined by Tupper (33), the majority result in 80% improvement. More proximal resection of the digital nerve is the most popular treatment to allow the new neuroma to develop in a well-vascularized bed. This could decrease the sensibility of the distal part of the finger, increasing or triggering some deafferentation pain. When the distal sensibility is not satisfactory, the authors favor *en bloc* advancement of the skin and the nerve (34,35). The dissected neuroma, or the nerve extremity after resection of a large neuroma, is transferred either dorsally in an area at a distance of any stimulus or in a bone hole in the distal aspect of the phalanx (36). When both nerves present a painful neuroma, a

tunnel is created, and the two nerves are introduced inside end to end (Fig. 2).

Nail Surgery

From a functional and esthetic point of view, the nail plays a unique role. Its reconstruction is only possible in distal amputation. When the nail is dystrophic, the authors have found that, after excision of the nail matrix, a skin graft of precise size can mimic a nail. When present but deformed, as in hook nail deformity, conventional techniques have been described. Acrylic resin paste may be used in moderated cases (37). Dufourmentel (38) has proposed withdrawal of the nail on the bone support. The distal skin loss is then covered by two small lateral flaps. The distal scar is a problem, as well as the dorsal "fold" of skin in excess. Atasoy preferred the "antenna" procedure of lifting the nailbed, which is maintained through several Kirschner wires (K-wires); the distal skin defect is covered by a cross-finger flap (39). The authors favor three techniques, according to the bone loss. When the loss is limited, it is possible to perform a progressive bone distraction by a small external fixator. In three cases, the authors have obtained bone healing without any bone graft after a mean lengthening of 6 mm (40,41). However, this technique has many drawbacks that should be emphasized to the patient. It is technically demanding to put three or four K-wires in a tiny piece of bone, time to bone healing is lengthy, and complications are not infre-

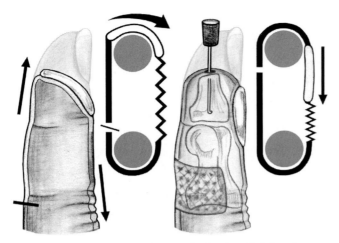

FIGURE 3. Escalator technique for hook nail deformity.

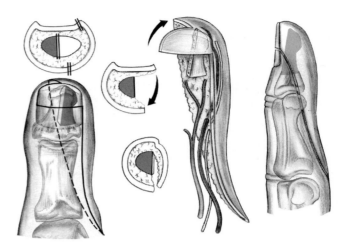

FIGURE 4. Custom-made reconstruction of the distal finger with bone, nail flap, and pulp.

quent even if they were not observed in the authors' short series (40,41).

When the deformity is more pronounced, the authors have described a technique called *escalator* (42). In this technique, all of the distal aspect of the finger is lifted *en bloc* from the distal phalanx, including the palmar skin and the nail (Fig. 3). One of the dorsal branches of the palmar artery that vascularizes the nail complex has to be saved. Then the volar skin is advanced as a bipedicled island O'Brien flap (30) after cutting transversally the skin in the PIP joint crease. The nail is shifted proximally on the bone support, and the skin is pinned to the distal phalanx with a needle. A full-thickness skin graft is put in the secondary volar defect. A dorsal fold is avoided by the extent of dorsal dissection, allowing better repartition of the skin in excess.

When too much distal phalanx is missing, the authors favor a custom-made free transfer from the great toe (43–45,47). A vascularized piece of bone is mandatory to maintain the result on a long-term basis (46). The bone is longitudinally harvested from the distal phalanx of the great toe *en bloc* with the pulp and a flap of the nailbed, which represents the distal half (43). The nailbed flap is turned around the bone and carefully sutured to the finger nailbed (Fig. 4). In two cases, the authors have left exposed the vascular bundle to avoid extensive dissection. The exteriorized bundle is cut at 3 weeks, taking care to protect the nerve repair. This trick decreases the amount of scar and the number of remodelings frequently necessary due to the bulging of fat around the vascular pedicle. The authors have performed four cases of such sophisticated reconstruction on fingers (the indication having been more frequent in the thumb). Three of the patients were cord musicians. The mean two-point discrimination was 9 mm without any difference when the vascular pedicle was severed. Cold intolerance was mentioned in all cases at the hand level and in one case at the donor level.

When the nail matrix was missing, the authors have transferred the nail of the second toe in two musicians (one

harpist and one guitarist) (48). Indeed, the result could not be justified on esthetic grounds, as the nail is small compared to the neighboring fingers. Some authors have used the nail of the great toe (sometimes with arterialization of the venous flap), but the published pictures are not convincing, with some dystrophy being obvious on the resected side of the nail (49).

Among the more recent propositions, Baruchin et al. (50) described anchoring a nail prosthetic device in the distal phalanx through a titanium screw. They had only one failure out of eight cases, but several steps are necessary, with insertion of the implant and cover screw followed by reentry 4 months later to remove the cover screw and fixation of the acrylic nail. The length of treatment was 5 to 6 months.

Finger and Stump Redistribution and Reorientation

In multiple-finger amputation patients who have difficulty with pinch, it can be of benefit when no lengthening is planned to reorient the fingers by rotatory-angulatory osteotomy. It is most frequently applied to the fifth metacarpal in radial finger amputation associated with some shortening of the thumb. When only the index persists and the web has a limited span, an ulnar translocation on the third (or even fourth) metacarpal with removal of ray(s) could be of benefit.

Stump Amputation

In some distal amputations, length preservation has no relevance, and a limited shortening could permit improvement of the soft tissue cover or removal of a painful bone spur. When possible, it is better to save the insertion of the flexor profundus to preserve strength. However, in some cases the flexion of the distal interphalangeal joint is responsible for a painful stump. The same problem could happen at the PIP joint and metaphalangeal (MP) joint level.

In more proximal amputation, shortening could also be proposed. For example, after a disarticulation at the PIP joint of the middle finger, the stump usually is easily hurt, as it is the longest proximal phalanx. Otherwise, there is no contraindication for a disarticulation (with resection of the lateral flare) (51), and there is no more elective site for amputation. When a finger is difficult to use due to stiffness, shortening (distally or during an arthrodesis) makes the finger less cumbersome. When the amputation is performed distally on a finger with preserved pulp and neurovascular bundles, the authors favor isolation of the pulp as a bipedicled island and withdrawal of it on the stump to provide good padding and prevent any neuroma.

Ray resections with or without translocation are more complex operations, presenting the following advantages and drawbacks that should be carefully explained to the patient.

1. Second ray resection improves the esthetic aspect of the hand, resulting in a four-fingered hand, but does not reestablish a normal cascade of the fingers, as the middle finger appears too long. The indication could also be based on functional grounds. A good candidate presents with a painful stump functionally excluded from pinch and grasp and stiff in extension who hurts each time the web grasp is used. The authors have insisted, after reviewing a series of 43 index fingers that had sustained repetitive reconstructive surgery, on the "all or none" response of this finger, especially due to the difficulty of cortical integration of an index finger bypassed for more than 6 months, even when analysis of the active mobility and sensibility is satisfactory (52). One of the best indications for second ray resection remains when part of the index finger could be used for reconstruction of the other fingers (53–57). In isolated index stump with thumb amputation, pollicization of the stump combined with second ray resection (58,59) not only allows lengthening of the thumb but increases the first web span and improves appearance. It has the disadvantage of reducing strength.

2. Technically, Chase (54) has proposed a combined volar and dorsal approach, allowing resection with preservation of the base to protect tendon insertions. Many tendon transfers have been proposed to improve middle finger function (54). The first interosseous and the flexor superficialis could be inserted in the base of the first phalanx of the middle finger (60). The extensor indicis proprius could be transposed on the extensor hood of the middle finger. The authors have proposed a modification of the technique to decrease the scar on the visible dorsal aspect of the hand (61). A purely palmar approach makes the nerve dissection (more proximal) and bone section

(with an oblique dorsal slope) even easier. The authors bury the four neuromas (dorsal and palmar nerves) in the medulla of the base of the second metacarpal. A plasty of the first web avoids having an angulated web and provides a smooth, round shape. There has not been any difference when the extensor proprius and the first interosseous were transferred, as in all cases the patients have developed good pinch and independent extension of the middle finger. If performed, the intrinsic transfer has to be fixed without tension to avoid a flexion deformity of the third MP joint, as it seems to have an essential role in web contouring. In a series of 17 patients operated on through a volar approach, only one developed a painful dorsal nerve neuroma. Murray et al. (62) have published the most pessimistic series, with 26 of 41 patients presenting a drop in strength of 20% during pinch, grasp, and supination (even in absence of hyperesthesia). Strength in pronation was the most affected, with 50% of the predicted values. Thirty-seven percent of the patients presented some hyperesthesia that interfered with activity, and 10% were disabled. However, 21 patients had a painful stump before the operation, and only three of them were entirely relieved by the ray resection. The authors have found in a small group of eight patients that when a second ray resection was performed for an index stump with painful neuroma, seven patients increased their grasp strength an average of 12%. Strength should be measured before ray amputation, and comparison postoperatively with the contralateral normal side should be avoided.

3. For the fifth finger, ray resection could also be performed from the palmar aspect. However, the esthetic benefit is limited due to the abnormal cascade, and no functional benefit has been found by the authors. Indeed, due to the carpometacarpal mobility and the hyperflexion of the MP joint, even a first phalanx could be useful in locking a tool handle.

4. For the third and the fourth rays, the controversy remains concerning the advantages and drawbacks of simple resection versus translocation. The gap in the hand is not just a cosmetic concern, as small objects have a tendency to slip out of the hand, and finger convergence is frequently altered.

5. The technique of resection is simple, and preservation of a short proximal metacarpal segment as well as strong reconstruction of intermetacarpal ligament by a "vest-over-the-pants" technique is mandatory (63). We have modified the technique, proposing a volar approach, again to avoid any conspicuous dorsal scar. The whole dissection is done through the palmar incision, which makes the dissection of the neurovascular bundles and the repair of the intermetacarpal ligament even easier.

6. The techniques of translocation are complex, and multiple variations have been proposed derived from the

Carrol technique (64) for the index to middle ray transfer and from the Slocum technique for ulnar fingers (65). The intrinsic muscles of the removed finger have to be excised, but the intrinsic muscles inserted on the displaced finger are frequently distorted in their normal course. For the third ray, osteotomy at the base allows for faster healing. The authors favor a transverse metaphyseal osteotomy (66). The step-cut, as proposed by Posner (67), does not allow for correcting any rotation deformity during fixation. This fixation is provided by two K-wires, one longitudinal and one transverse through the neighboring metacarpal.

7. For the fourth ray, the classic translocation not only modifies the direction of hypothenar muscles, but also sacrifices the 35 degrees of the fifth carpometacarpal joint mobility and distorts the ulnar supporting border of the hand. Leviet (68) has described a technique consisting of removal of the fourth ray combined with a wedge resection of the radial side of the hamate (Fig. 5). This wedge has to be precisely calculated to avoid any rotation deformity; after removing the opposite cartilage surface of the capitate, fixation is performed either by a transverse screw or by one or two staples. Early motion is permitted.

8. In a series of 13 ray resections, Steichen and Idler (63) have shown excellent functional and esthetic results. Grasp was 70% for third ray resection and 68% for the fourth one. Masmejean et al. (69), in a series of eight cases of fourth ray resection reviewed with a mean follow-up of 47 months, found similar results, with a grip strength of 65% compared to the contralateral side.

9. Colen et al. (70), reviewing 19 classic translocations with a mean follow-up of 10 months, compared strength and mobility to the opposite, normal hand. Pinch strength was 83%, grip strength was 80%, and range of motion of the translocated finger was 78 degrees at the MP joint, 88 degrees at the PIP joint, and 81 degrees at the distal interphalangeal joint levels.

10. Leviet (68) reviewed 17 cases treated with his technique. Seven had some rotation deformity of the fifth ray. Strength was improved in six of the eight cases in which strength was measured before the operation. Among the other complications he observed was one pseudarthrosis and one reduction of fifth MP joint mobility. With a mean follow-up of 24.5 months, none of the patients complained of any pain at the wrist level; this was confirmed by a later review (71) of 46 patients with a mean follow-up of 137 months.

11. The authors have published a comparative study of translocation versus ray resection in a clinical series of 43 patients in which a score based on activities of daily living, pain, esthetic aspect, loss of strength, time off from work, and return to work was described (72). In a series of 43 patients, translocation II–III resulted in better strength than third ray resection, but the global score

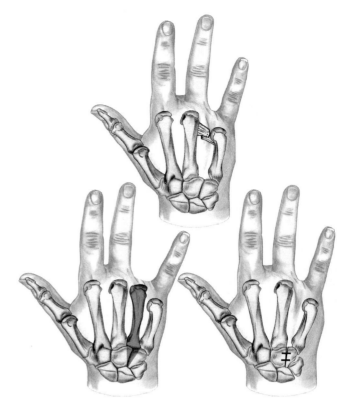

FIGURE 5. Ray resection and Leviet's translocation for the fourth ray.

was favorable to the resection. The x-ray study demonstrated a limited narrowing of the hand. For the fourth ray, Leviet translocation has provided superior results compared to simple ray resection, but some slight residual pain was frequently mentioned by patients. Narrowing of the hand was more limited in fourth ray resection (11% vs. 22%), but the strength loss was superior (37% vs. 17%). Again the indication for such operations is reinforced when the stump is used for reconstruction of the thumb or neighboring fingers.

Stump Lengthening

The "relative" lengthening provided by web deepening is briefly covered. The main indication is to gain the 1.5 cm necessary to fit a cosmetic finger prosthesis.

Fifth metacarpal phalangization with removal of some neighboring metacarpal to create a cleft and increase the mobility of the fifth ray is not used often (73). It remains helpful in cases of contraindication of all other methods due to age or associated pathology.

Osteointegrated prostheses have been proposed (74) based on the principle of titanium bone integration. Manurangsee et al. (75) in a limited number of cases found an indication for use of these prostheses when the segment of proximal phalanx was very short. Indeed, prosthetic fitting in such cases implies making two rings, with one fixed on the normal finger supporting the device as in a dental bridge. The technique is not different than the previously described nail implantation except that the self-tapping titanium screw is inserted in the medulla. Manurangsee et al. (75) claimed an excellent stability (and increased grip strength) with some sensibility transmitted through the bone. The main problem has been frequent skin instability.

Distal bone grafting with iliac crest graft combined with some type of flap has been popularized for the thumb by Gillies and Millard (76) and applied to the metacarpal hand (77). Creation of such a "post" has currently limited application. When toe transfer is contraindicated (due to age, motivation, bilateral amputation, or absence of available toe), a short metacarpal hand with a good thumb could be an indication. The procedure can be performed either by lifting up the existing skin to insert a bone graft or by providing an osteoplastic reconstruction with skin flap and bone graft. A compound, vascularized transfer of skin and adjacent bone, pedicled (e.g., from the groin with iliac crest), in island [compound forearm flap with a piece of radius (78)], or free, reduces the number of operation stages and the risk of bone resorption. These techniques do not improve mobility or growth potential (in children), and the sensibility remains limited.

Free, nonvascularized, toe phalange transfer continues to enjoy some popularity (79) due to absence of resorption when the periosteum is preserved. It is a simple one-stage procedure possible to use in case of presence of skin in excess, a more frequent opportunity in congenital anomalies or tumor resection than in trauma cases.

One-stage lengthening with osteotomy and perioperative distraction of the two fragments with a cervical lamina spreader has been used by a few authors (80). It has the advantage of a one-stage operation, but even in children, it provides only a limited lengthening [12 to 25 cm for Buck-Gramcko (80)].

On-top plasty with an island composite transfer is a time-honored technique (81,82), which has been used more for lengthening the thumb (59) than the fingers. The authors have used this technique to combine two fingers in bad condition to provide a good one. An example is the presence of an index finger distally amputated but presenting a good PIP joint and a middle one with intact distal phalanx but no proximal joint. If one vascular bundle is intact, the distal phalanx of the third finger is isolated in the island and transferred on top of the index finger; at the same stage, a II–III translocation or a third ray resection is performed to avoid a gap in the hand (Fig. 6). The authors have performed three such reconstructions, and, in two cases, neurotization of the donor nerves at the recipient site was necessary; a good discrimination was obtained due to the young age of the patients (13 and 19 years old). A similar technique has been used in some cases of phalangeal hand when a longer segment was

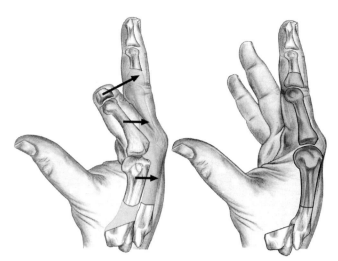

FIGURE 6. Reconstruction of one finger out of two bad ones. Index finger with intact proximal interphalangeal joint, but distally amputated, and middle finger with good distal part, but no proximal interphalangeal joint.

present on the ulnar side. This segment could be isolated on its palmar vessels and transferred in a more radial position to improve pinch.

Progressive bone distraction remains an excellent technique (83). It consists of two (or more) staged operations with transverse osteotomy and lengthening by an external fixator. For finger reconstruction, the authors have limited the indication to some rare cases of nail hook deformities, as already mentioned, and to phalangeal or metacarpal hands.

The principle is to approach the metacarpal bone to lengthen, through a longitudinal dorsal incision, with minimal freeing of the shaft. Insertion of the K-wires or pins is performed through separate, short incisions to retract relevant structures (e.g., tendons and neurovascular bundles). Four bicortical pins (or four threaded pins) are usually necessary and are introduced distally and proximally to the future osteotomy site. After assembling the external apparatus, the bone is cut according to the technique selected and the skin closed. After a variable period of rest, distraction is begun daily until the desired length is obtained. A "stabilization" phase of variable length is respected. Secondary surgery (e.g., bone graft, translocation, web deepening, and hardware removal) is performed according to the indication.

Two techniques are available: (a) bone replacement (graft) or (b) bone regeneration, called *distraction osteogenesis* or *callotasis*. The authors favor the latter in children. In such cases, preservation of the vascularization and periosteum is relevant. After longitudinal incision of the periosteum, a transverse corticotomy with a chisel is done. Before beginning the lengthening, the callus is allowed to form during a rest period of 8 to 10 days. No more than 1 mm per day of lengthening is allowed, and the fixator is maintained until solid bone healing (with visible trabeculation) is obtained.

Bone replacement has been favored in adult patients, with the defect being filled with a bone graft. In such cases, the periosteum is transversally cut as well as the bone and a perioperative lengthening of 1 or 2 mm is performed. After 5 days, lengthening is begun, and a more rapid pace is adopted based on pain and skin blanching. When the desired length is obtained, a rest period of 1 week allows for soft tissue stretching. Bone defect is filled with a bone graft stabilized usually by osteosynthesis after removal of the external fixator. Frequently, a resected metacarpal could be used to avoid an iliac crest bone graft. "Lengthening-translocation" is a an alternative (40,41,84). In a metacarpal or a phalangeal hand with a phalangeal thumb, the second ray could be first lengthened and then the distal part of the second metacarpal translocated onto the third ray. The second ray is proximally sacrificed to deepen the web and provide a "relative" lengthening of the thumb. Some loss of length is always to be anticipated at the time of translocation, but large objects may be grasped in the first web.

The technique provides up to 100% lengthening in young children without perturbation of sensibility. Even in the long term, there is no bone resorption (in absence of infection).

However, if lengthening-translocation appears simple at first glance, it is plagued by numerous complications that are not always easy to avoid. These complications are summarized in Table 1.

Globally speaking, the rate of complications decreases with the experience of the surgeon but increases proportionally to the length obtained. The rate remains inferior to those published for lower limb lengthening [72% of major complications in the 110 patients of Dahl et al. (85)]. In the authors' first published series of 20 cases, the complication rate was 25% (40) and in a more recent combined series, it was 32% (41).

Apart from a quite high rate of complications, lengthening-translocation has some drawbacks. It requires major cooperation from the patient and family. It does not add mobility, adds some scarring, does not improve much

TABLE 1. POTENTIAL COMPLICATIONS OF PROGRESSIVE BONE LENGTHENING

Bad pin placement (tendon or neurovascular injury, epiphyseal injury, pin tract infection, biomechanical failure)
Infection
Pain
Bone protrusion through the skin
Temporary sensory disturbance
Early bone healing
Loss of length
Callus deformation or fracture
Delayed bone healing
Joint stiffness

appearance (except in nail hook deformity), and remains a cumbersome and lengthy procedure (mean, 4.5 months in the authors' trauma series).

Due to all these drawbacks, the authors restrict indications for lengthening-translocation to patients in whom a microsurgical toe transfer is contraindicated or the necessary lengthening is limited. The basic requirement is a sufficient stump with good skin cover, good sensibility, and no pain.

Toe transfer has a long history, as Nicoladoni (86) used the technique in a pedicled fashion, the hand remaining attached to the foot for a few weeks. He did this procedure for thumb reconstruction, and it seems that the first second toe–to–finger pedicled transfer was performed in 1900, two years after Nicoladoni by Von Eiselsberg, as reported by Davies (87). Esser and Ranschburg (88) are credited with transferring four toes in a metacarpal hand. However, only microsurgery has allowed the technique to gain popularity. The second toe is a good substitute for amputated fingers. This is not the place to give all the technical details, but a few original points and some useful tips and tricks follow.

Tactically speaking, it is more efficient to work with only one team, beginning at the donor site to allow for revascularization during the preparation of the recipient finger (89–92). After completion of the transfer, the reconstructed finger is revascularized during closure of the donor site. This succession of phases avoids loss of time and permits a more precise measure of the necessary length for each anatomic structure; indeed, the authors have never found it necessary to insert a nerve graft or a vein graft due to insufficient pedicle length.

Concerning the donor site, the homolateral side is usually selected for having the larger nerve for the more relevant radial side of the finger.

Foot and hand dissections are performed under tourniquet and using magnification. The authors have described a technique using a purely dorsal approach without plantar incision except to harvest a small triangular skin flap (92). The incision is straight centered on the first intermetatarsal space, the classical S-shape incision being prone to marginal necrosis. A dorsal triangular flap is drawn to avoid a circular scar at the base of the thumb. Tributaries of the great saphenous vein are dissected out, maintaining as many as possible. A communicant vein between the superficial and deep network is often present where the dorsalis pedis artery dives into the first interosseous space. This artery (absent in five of the authors' clinical series of 223 toe transfers) is easily found under the extensor hallucis brevis. Then the dissection is performed distally in the first space to seek for the arteries of the first and second toe. If the common artery is found dorsal to the intermetatarsal ligament, it is a dorsal metatarsal artery with either a superficial track or a deeper one passing through the muscles. Then dissection proceeds proximally; a communicating vein between the superficial and deep network usually marks any change in the course of the first dorsal metatarsal artery. If there is no artery dorsal to the ligament, the vascularization is based on the arterial system. Whatever the type of vessels, the authors have found that it is better to harvest at least two or even three arteries to feed the transfer. Indeed, the authors have not seen any postoperative vascular crisis when more than one artery was preserved. The arteries could be either harvested separately or in continuity with the dorsalis pedis and the plantar arch, according to the type of transfer planned and the level of anastomosis at the hand level.

The next step is the proximal section of the long and short extensor tendon and the osteotomy of the second metatarsal close to its base. This section has two advantages: It makes easy the dissection of all plantar anatomic structures, and, after reconstruction of the intermetatarsal ligament, it provides an esthetic closure of the space. When the metatarsal is lifted, it is possible to see immediately the plantar artery of the second space, a vessel overlooked in the classic anatomic descriptions (93). The authors have found it in all dissections passing under the metatarsal, tethered to the fibular aspect of the plantar plate, and supplying the arteries of the second space. A second dorsal metatarsal artery was found of sufficient diameter in only three of the authors' clinical series. After section of the intermetatarsal ligament of the first space, it is possible to proceed with the dissection of the plantar artery of the first space proximal and distal to the metatarsophalangeal (MTP) joint; indeed, at this level one or two small vessels tether the artery to the plantar plate. Gentle traction on the proximal and distal segments allows for hemostasis and total freeing. All of the dissected arteries are maintained in continuity with the dorsalis pedis artery. During this step, the plantar nerves are freed and an endoneurolysis allows harvesting of a segment as long as necessary. A similar dissection is performed in the second space after sectioning the intermetatarsal ligament; if the MTP joint is used for reconstruction, it is not necessary to free the second plantar metatarsal artery from the plantar plate. In this space, the endoneurolysis is more demanding due to the smaller diameter of the nerves. It is easier to perform a thorough defatting at the base of the toe before cutting the vessels of the neighboring toes. When these vessels are cut, the arteries are at risk during the defatting, which is mandatory to avoid a proximal bulging and to improve appearance. When repair is possible at the recipient site, the intrinsic tendons are cut at the musculo-tendinous junction for later transfer. The last step is to gently pull on the isolated toe and retract the adductor hallucis to harvest as much as possible of the flexor tendons.

At the recipient stump, it is necessary to lift two flaps, the larger one to cover the more relevant defect on the fibular side of the toe. The authors use an S-shaped incision, which is prolonged dorsally and volarly. On the dorsum, the incision is limited for cosmetic purposes but allows for extensor repair and accommodation of the triangular dorsal flap harvested from the foot. On the volar aspect, it is prolonged in a Bruner way to approach the palmar nerves, the recipient vessels, and the flexor tendons. The bone and the recipient extensor tendons are prepared. A separated transverse incision is performed on a preoperatively marked dorsal vein. Skin undermining is done between this incision and the distal one to allow delivery of the donor vein; the tunnel has to be ample enough to avoid any compression. Precise measurement of the necessary length of artery and vein is controlled. Two possibilities are to be considered. For a "short" or "long" transfer, according to Yoshimura (94), the recipient arteries are prepared accordingly. The collateral digital arteries are selected for a short transfer and the palmar arcade (or, rarely, the radial artery) for a long one.

The first step after the transfer of the toe to the hand is usually the bone synthesis. Many methods are available. When a segment of the first phalanx is present at the recipient level, the authors like to perform a "ball and socket" penetration and stabilize with two crossed K-wires or one longitudinal wire combined with interosseous loop wiring. A periosteum suture adds to the stability in young patients. The technique does not differ significantly when the MTP joint is incorporated in the transfer, as in case of amputation proximal to the MP joint. This joint moves mainly in hyperextension (with only a limited range of flexion). The authors have described an oblique osteotomy through the metaphysis, allowing the joint to tilt volarly approximately 45 degrees (Fig. 7). This trick prevents a "Z" deformity, with MP joint hyperextension and PIP joint flexion and provides a more useful range of flexion. When a hemijoint reconstruction is contemplated, the whole capsulo-ligamentous apparatus of the MTP joint is harvested to be fixed to the recipient metacarpal bone, taking care to tighten the radial collateral ligament as well as the plantar plate.

The next step is the intrinsic repair by weaving the donor intrinsic tendons into the recipient ones. The extensor tendons are then repaired with a vest-over-the-pants technique, maintaining sufficient tension, as the

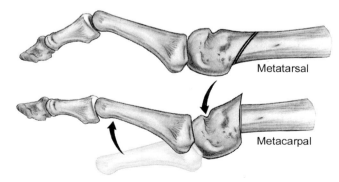

FIGURE 7. Tilting of the metatarsophalangeal joint when transferred with a second toe for reconstruction of a metatarsal hand.

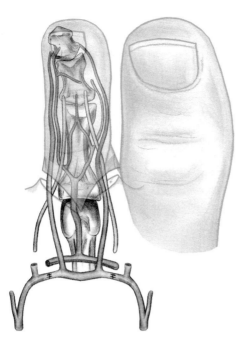

FIGURE 8. Second toe–to–finger transfer with intercalated artery.

mechanism is sometimes unable to compensate for the flexor force. Then the skin around the toe is closed, and the flexor superficialis and profundus are repaired, trying to stagger the two sutures. The microsurgical step begins with the nerve repair (performed as distally as the state of the recipient nerves allows), followed by arterial suture. When a long transfer is performed, the authors favor cutting the superficial arcade and intercalating the segment of dorsalis pedis artery and plantar arch (Fig. 8). Two end-to-end sutures are performed, reestablishing a physiologic flow in both the arcade and the toe (95). The vein, which has been passed in the dorsal subcutaneous tunnel, is sutured end-to-end to the recipient vein, and the skin is entirely closed.

During the revascularization of the hand, the foot is closed after reconstruction of an intermetatarsal ligament and control of the hemostasis.

The patient is hospitalized 4 to 5 days in an intensive care unit. During this period, color and temperature of the reconstructed finger are monitored. A low dose of aspirin is maintained, as well as pain medication if necessary. The authors do not use any anticoagulant. The dressing is not disturbed for 2 weeks, and the K-wires are usually removed at 6 weeks. The authors' attempt to have patients begin early motion has been disappointing, and currently motion is begun at 6 weeks, and a roll-up, dynamic splint is worn several hours during the day. An extension splint is maintained for several months at night to control the tendency to flexion deformity, at least in adult patients.

Secondary surgery may be performed either to improve function (mainly tenolysis) or to improve appearance. A longitudinal central resection was proposed (96) to reduce the bulky pulp.

As for all microsurgical transfers with nerve repair, age is a definite limit except in few cases of bilateral amputations in which no pinch is possible (Fig. 9). The authors found in a statistical analysis (97) that 35 years is a limit for providing a good sensory result. A young, healthy, and motivated patient is necessary for such a complex reconstruction. Due to limited range of flexion, the authors have not performed any transfer for ulnar finger amputations. When one radial finger is amputated, indications are limited to musicians, as the authors do not think that the appearance is good enough to propose it for esthetic purposes. Good mobility is expected when the recipient finger has a normal PIP joint, but in musicians the authors have performed such a transfer even in the absence of a PIP joint. In a 40-year-old pianist, the authors obtained 85 degrees of mobility! With amputation of two radial fingers, pinch remains good between a normal thumb and the ring finger, but in some cases a four-fingered hand could be reconstructed by a ray resection and a toe transfer. Again, it is desirable to transfer the toe on a finger with a good PIP joint. There are more indications when three radial fingers are amputated. The pinch with the remaining auricular is weak, and acceptable function and appearance are obtained by a double second-toe transfer from both feet combined with a ray amputation. Finally, phalangeal or metacarpal hands are excellent indications despite a quite poor final appearance. The authors always offer preoperatively a common consultation with the prosthetist to customize the esthetic glove. A double transfer has the advantage of providing a more stable chuck pinch. We have stopped using an *en bloc* transfer of the second and third toe for metacarpal hand reconstruction, despite a better range of motion at the MP joint level compared with separated double toe transfer from both feet. This is mainly due to poor appearance of the donor site and some worrying about long-term foot tolerance. Leung and Ma (98) prefer to build two fingers, one with a fillet flap from the great toe and the other with a second toe. As could be expected, the bone peg insert in the fillet flap frequently resorbed or fractured (nine cases out of ten at 12-month follow-up) (98).

In the authors' clinical series of 68 toe-to-finger transfers in 55 patients (97), 52 were transferred for mutilation (41 patients). The more frequent ray reconstructed was the middle one. Mean operative time for isolated transfer was 190 minutes with an ischemia time of 55 minutes. The mean follow-up was 6.7 years, the failure rate 6%, and some secondary surgery was deemed necessary in 18% of the patients. Mean active range of flexion was 36 degrees, with a mean extension lack of 33 degrees. A better passive mobility was noticed in children as well as a mean active range of 45 degrees. Two-point discrimination was an average of 11 mm (6 mm in children). Grasp was 47% of the opposite normal side and pinch 38%. Sixty-two percent of the active manual workers were able to return to work.

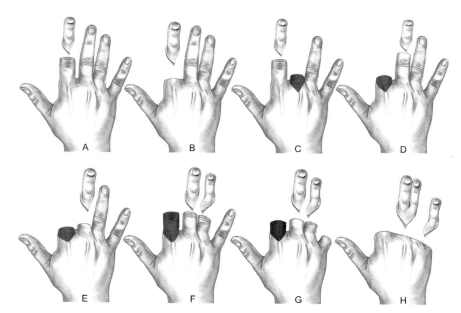

FIGURE 9. Indications for second-toe transfer in finger mutilations. **A:** Isolated amputation distal to the proximal interphalangeal joint. **B:** Isolated amputation distal to the metacarpophalangeal joint. **C–E:** Adjacent amputations with ray resection of one digit. **F:** Three adjacent amputations with double toe transfers and single ray resection. **G:** Quadruple amputations with double toe transfers and single ray resection. **H:** Triple toe transfer for complete loss of all digits.

In a previous computerized statistical analysis (91), the authors isolated several factors influencing the rate of complication and the final outcome (two-point discrimination and range of motion). Higher complication rate was associated with an aging patient, "short" transfer, and long ischemia time. Tobacco (four failures out of six smokers, but the sample was too small for statistical study) and number of arteries feeding the transfer did not reach significance. A strong significant correlation was found between the quality of discrimination and young patient age as well a proximal site of amputation. Compensation injury patients fared worse than patients with other types of trauma. Possibly favorably influential (but not statistically significant) were short ischemia time and multiple feeding arteries, good mobility, and sensory reeducation. The mobility was favorably and significantly influenced by a multiple "set" of arteries and a more proximal level of amputation. It is possible, then, to predict the final result by selecting the indications and taking into account all of these factors. It is impossible to analyze all of the published series, but in fact only a few gave precise data concerning the final outcome.

In their series of 54 transfers, Lister et al. (99) reported 34% of circulatory compromise, which occurred more frequently in "short" transfer with anastomoses to collateral digital arteries (46% vs. 26% for "long" transfers). Secondary surgery was performed in 68% of the patients (mainly tenolysis). Two-point discrimination was less than 10 mm in 75% of the patients reviewed at more than 2 years. In two large series of 300 (100) and 200 (101) toe transfers of all types, the return to operative room was 10% and 14% and the failure rate was 4.5% and 4%, respectively. Gu et al. (100) carefully reviewed their complications and stressed that perioperative problems were spasm and bad selection of feeding vessels. Complications occurring in the first 24 postoper-

ative hours were vascular embolism related to technical problems, and they recommended early reoperation. The most common complication 48 hours postoperatively was vascular spasm, which was treated medically without the need for reoperation. In a consecutive paper, Gu et al. (102) reviewed the 14 failed cases and demonstrated that postoperative states of hypercoagulability could be an important cause of failure.

Results are often difficult to compare, and, for example, 59% of the 61 cases of Koshima et al. (103) were performed for reconstruction distal to the DIP joint when this indication represents only 10% of Buncke's series (101). Inclusion of pediatric population and sensory reeducation also improves sensory results, as demonstrated by Dellon in his literature review (104). In the series of Gu et al. (100), 72% of the patients had a two-point discrimination of less than 10 mm, and 40% returned to their previous jobs. Demirkan et al. (105), in their series of 25 reconstructed fingers, gave precise data concerning the mobility of the transfer. Transfers at the proximal phalanx level provided 29 degrees of active range of motion (AROM). When implanted on the metacarpal bone (two cases), the transferred MTP joint had 28 degrees of AROM. Distal transfers with an intact PIP joint gave a global AROM of 67% compared to a normal finger.

Finally, finger hand-to-hand transfer is an exceptional indication. Edgerton (106) published a case of pedicled, cross–hand-finger transfer but, more recently, free microsurgical transfers have been successfully performed. The authors have reported such an operation in bilateral hand and feet mutilation secondary to a frostbite (107). When there is a short but useful finger on one side and no pinch on the other (dominant) hand, a mutilated finger can be microsurgically transferred. Free transfer of an intact ring, as proposed by Morrison et al. (108) has not gained popularity despite excellent results. However, in case of paralysis (109), the hand could be a unique donor site.

TREATMENT ALGORITHM

After primary hand surgery, the authors usually mention to the patient the possibility of secondary reconstruction without further details. This has a positive psychological effect, decreasing posttraumatic anxiety and preventing the patient from organizing his or her life around the disability.

Elective decision making in finger amputation is based on multiple factors. Any attempt at proposing a treatment algorithm is risky, as the final decision has to be customized to each patient. However, among the factors of relevance are the patient's gender, age, dominance and desires, psychological status, general health conditions, job and leisure activities, and economic situation. Others are related to the trauma as the mechanism of injury, and the problem of avulsion has been stressed. Finally, other factors related to the hand are the number of fingers involved and the level of amputation. Although it is out of the scope of this chapter, the state of the thumb, also frequently involved, could give precedence to its reconstruction.

In unidigital distal amputations, surgical indications for lengthening are exceptional and reserved to demanding manual activity. Any operation based only on cosmetic grounds is to be carefully approached with the patient, and the authors have found patients consulting for minor nail dystrophy difficult to satisfy.

In unidigital proximal finger amputation, stump improvement is frequently indicated in case of insufficient soft tissue or pain related to neuroma. Lengthening is rarely an indication, and ray resection or translocation has some functional and esthetic benefit but at the price of a loss of strength due to narrowing of the hand.

In unilateral multidigital amputations, amputations have a limited place except for deepening a limited first web with a short thumb or to take advantage of useful parts of a useless finger. In patients older than 40 years, there are only rare indications for a microsurgical reconstruction with nerve repair (a nail transfer is possible, as only the artery is repaired). Pinch could be provided or improved by conventional methods such as progressive bone lengthening. In multidigital radial amputations in young, healthy patients, second-toe transfers, single or double from both feet, are frequently indicated. They provide in some cases a good compromise between function and appearance when a four-fingered hand could be built. In the phalangeal and metacarpal hand, the authors find them also rewarding functionally and have combined them with a custom-made cosmetic glove when appearance is a concern.

In bilateral heavy mutilations (110), as seen after blast injury or thermal injuries, the severity is superior to the sum of lost segments, and, frequently, microsurgery has to be combined with conventional techniques and prosthetic devices. The first goal is to struggle to give independence to the patient in as few operations as possible. It is mandatory to avoid immobilizing both hands at the same time by beginning with the less-injured extremity and sometimes waiting to obtain full function of this side. Retaining all available structures is of outstanding importance. Any sacrifice has to be carefully assessed for loss versus benefits. As Moberg stressed, "handling of these difficult cases cannot be learned from books or short papers but only from experience" (111).

CONCLUSION

Microsurgery has added new possibilities to the field of reconstruction in finger mutilation. Acutely, replantations allow complex secondary reconstruction to be avoided. Free transfers have also opened a new field, but more conventional techniques are not to be forgotten, and age remains an ultimate barrier to obtaining good sensory results. In the more extreme mutilation, the goal remains to save the "basic hand," as defined by Entin (1) for independent life. Any operation that does not provide the expected benefit needs careful assessment of remaining motivation before proceeding with surgery. In the less severe cases, remember the esthetic role of the hands and bear in mind that function and appearance are closely linked. Indeed, a hand that is considered ugly by the patient remains buried in a pocket, even if it has some functional potential. As Vilain stressed, "Good appearance is already function."

REFERENCES

1. Entin MA. Salvaging the basic hand. *Surg Clin North Am* 1968;48:1063–1081.
2. Napier JR. The prehensile movements of the human hand. *J Bone Joint Surg* 1956;38B:902–908.
3. Foucher G, Moss ALH. Microvascular second toe to finger transfer: a statistical analysis of 55 transfers. *Br J Plast Surg* 1991;44:87–90.
4. Foucher G, Smith D. Free vascularized toe transfer in post-traumatic hand reconstruction. In: Peimer CA, ed. *Surgery of the hand and upper extremity.* New York: McGraw-Hill, 1995;85, 1911–1917.
5. Pulvertaft GR. Reconstruction of the mutilated hand. *Scand J Plast Reconstr Surg* 1977;11:219–224.
6. Parkes A. The lumbrical plus finger. *Hand* 1970;2:64–167.
7. Verdan CE, Crawford GP, Martini-Benkeddach Y. The valuable role of tenolysis in the digits. In: Cramer LM, Chase RA, eds. *Symposium on the hand,* vol. 3. St. Louis: Mosby, 1971:192–208.
8. Louis DS. Amputations. In: Green D, ed. *Operative hand surgery,* 2nd ed. New York: Churchill Livingstone 1988:55–111.
9. Green TL, Steichen JB. The surgical management of painful neuromas in the hand. In: *Difficult problems in hand surgery.* St. Louis: Mosby, 1982:324–331.

10. Didierjean A, Foucher G. Retentissement psychologique de l'accident de la main. *Journal d'Ergothérapie* 1990;12:105–107.

11. Brown PW. Less than ten—surgeons with amputated fingers. *J Hand Surg* 1982;7:31–37.

12. Sims ACP. Psychogenic causes of physical symptoms, accidents and death. *J Hand Surg* 1985;10B:281–282.

13. Schweitzer J, Rosenbaum MB, Sharzer LA, Strauch B. Psychological reaction and processus following replantation surgery: a study of 50 patients. *Plast Reconstr Surg* 1985;76:97–103.

14. Merzenich M. Somatosensory cortical map changes after digit amputation in adult monkey. In: Sudarsky L, ed. *Pathophysiology of the nervous system.* Boston: Little, Brown, 1990:104–105.

15. Foucher G, Greant P, Ehrler S, et al. Le rôle de l'orthèse dans les raideurs de la main. *Chirurgie* 1989;115:100–105.

16. Pillet J. Esthetic hand protheses. *J Hand Surg* 1983;8:778–781.

17. Pillet J. Aesthetic prostheses. In: *Reconstruction after mutilation of the hand.* London: Martin Dunitz, 1997:169–178.

18. Hopper RA, Griffiths S, Murray J, Manktelow RT. Factors influencing use of digital prostheses in workers' compensation recipients. *J Hand Surg* 2000;25A:80–85.

19. Smith RJ, Dworecka F. Treatment of the one-digit hand. *J Bone Joint Surg* 1973;55A:113–119.

20. Bender LF. Prostheses for partial hand amputations. *Prosthet Orthot Int* 1978;2:8–11.

21. Katz J, Melzack R. Pain memories in phantom limb: review and clinical observation. *Pain* 1990;43:319–336.

22. Fisher A, Meller Y. Continuous post-operative regional analgesia by nerve sheath block for amputation surgery. *Anesth Analg* 1991;72:300–303.

23. Foucher G. *Fingertip injuries.* New York: Churchill Livingstone, 1991:151.

24. Tranquilli Leali E. Ricostruzione dell'apice delle falangi ungueali mediante autoplastica volare peduncolata per scorrimento. *Infort Trauma Lavoro* 1935;1:186–193.

25. Atasoy E, Ioakimidis E, Kasdan ML, et al. Reconstruction of the amputated finger tip with a triangular volar flap. *J Bone Joint Surg* 1970;52A:921–926.

26. Venkataswami R, Subramanian N. Oblique triangular flap: a new method of repair for oblique amputations of the fingertip and thumb. *Plast Reconstr Surg* 1980;66:296–300.

27. Foucher G, Smith D, Pempinello C, et al. Homodigital neurovascular island flap for digital pulp loss. *J Hand Surg* 1989;14B:204–208.

28. Hueston JT. Local flap repair in finger tip injuries. *Plast Reconstr Surg* 1966;2:261–277.

29. Foucher G, Dallaserra M, Tilquin B, et al. The Hueston flap in reconstruction of finger tip skin loss: results in a series of 41 patients. *J Hand Surg* 1994;A:92–126.

30. O'Brien McB. Neurovascular island pedicle flaps for terminal amputations and digital scars. *Br J Plast Surg* 1968;21:258–261.

31. Foucher G, Delaere O, Citron N, Molderez A. Long-term results of neurovascular palmar advancement flaps for distal thumb injuries. *Br J Plast Surg* 1999;52:64–68.

32. Scott JE. Amputation of the finger. *Br J Surg* 1974;61:574–576.

33. Tupper JW. Treatment of painful neuromas of sensory nerves in the hand: a comparison of traditional and newer methods. *J Hand Surg* 1976;2:144151.

34. Foucher G. Le névrome douloureux. In: Tubiana R, ed. *Traité de chirurgie de la main*, Tome 4. Paris: Masson, 1986.

35. Foucher G, Sammut D, Greant P, et al. Indications and results of skin flaps in painful digital neuroma. *J Hand Surg* 1991;16B:25–29.

36. Boldrey E. Amputation neuroma in nerves implanted in bone. *Ann Surg* 1943;118:1052–1057.

37. Schmaman J, Carr L. Acrylic resin finger prosthesis. *J Hand Surg* 1992;17B:673–674.

38. Dufourmentel C. Correction des extrémités digitales en "massue." *Ann Chir Plast* 1963;2:99–102.

39. Atasoy E, Gofrey A, Kalisman M. The "antenna" procedure for the hook-nail deformity. *J Hand Surg* 1983;8A:55–58.

40. Foucher G, Hultgren T, Merle M, Braun JM. L'allongement digital selon Matev. A propos de 2O cas. *Ann Chir Main* 1988;7:210–216.

41. Foucher G, Lamas C, Mir X. Reconstruccion digital segun tecnica de Matev. Estudio de 45 casos. *Rev Iber Cir Mano* 2000;27:31–39.

42. Foucher G, Lenoble E, Goffin D, Sammut D. Le lambeau "escalator" dans le traitement de l'ongle en griffe. *Ann Chir Plast Esth* 1991;36:51–53.

43. Foucher G, Merle M, Maneaud M, Michon J. Microsurgical free partial toe transfer in hand reconstruction: a report of 12 cases. *Plast Reconstr Surg* 1980;65:616–627.

44. Foucher G, Van Genechten F, Morrison WA. Composite tissue transfer to the hand from the foot. In: Jackson IT, Sommerland BC, eds. *Recent advances in plastic surgery.* New York: Churchill Livingstone, 1985.

45. Foucher G. The partial toe flap. In: Serafin D, ed. *Atlas of microsurgical composite tissue translocation.* Philadelphia: Saunders, 1995:144–150.

46. Foucher G. Indication du transfert osseux vascularisé en chirurgie de la main. *Rev Chir Orthop* 1982;68:38–39.

47. Foucher G, Binhammer P. Plea to save the great toe in total thumb reconstruction. *Microsurgery* 1995;16:373–376.

48. Foucher G. Traitement chirurgical des mutilations de la main chez le musicien. *Médecine des Arts* 1995:12–13, 25–27.

49. Nakayama Y, Iino T, Ychida A, et al. Vascualarized free nail grafts nourished by arterial inflow from the venous system. *Plast Reconstr Surg* 1990;85:239–245.

50. Baruchin AM, Nahlieli O, Vizethum F, Sela M. Utilizing the osseointegration principle for fixation of nail prostheses. *Plast Reconstr Surg* 1995;96:1665–1671.

51. Whitaker LA, Graham WP, Riser WH, Kilgore E. Retaining the articular cartilage in finger joint amputations. *Plast Reconstr Surg* 1972;49:542–547.

52. Foucher G, Merle M, Braun FM, et al. La chirurgie de l'index. Attitude de "tout ou rien." *Ann Chir Plast* 1982;27:581–583.

53. Peacock EE. Reconstructive surgery of hands with injured central metacarpophalangeal joints. *J Bone Joint Surg* 1956;38A:291–302.

54. Chase RA. *Atlas of hand surgery.* Philadelphia: Saunders, 1973:61–84.

55. Chase RA. Expanded clinical and research uses of composite tissue transfers on isolated vascular pedicles. *Am J Surg* 1967;114:222–229.

56. Foucher G, Merle M, Michon J. Traitement "tout en un temps" des traumatismes complexes de la main avec mobilisation précoce. *Ann Chir* 1977;31:1059–1063.

57. Foucher G, Braun FM, Merle M, Michon J. Le doigt "banque" en traumatologie de la main. *Ann Chir* 1980;34:693–698.

58. Foucher G, Hoang P, Dury M, et al. La pollicisation en urgence et en secondaire des segments digitaux mutilés. A propos de seize cas. *Ann Chir Plast Esth* 1988;33:54–57.

59. Foucher G, Rostane S, Chammas M, et al. Transfer of a severely damaged digit to reconstruct an amputated thumb. *J Bone Joint Surg* 1996;78-A:1889–1896.

60. Eversmann WW, Burkhalter WE, Dunn C. Transfer of the long flexor tendon of the index finger to the proximal phalanx of the long finger during index-ray amputation. *J Bone Joint Surg* 1971;53A:769–773.

61. Foucher G, Debry R, Braun FM, Merle M. L'abord palmaire dans l'amputation proximale du deuxième rayon de la main. *Rev Chir Ortho* 1982;68:581–583.

62. Murray JF, Carman W, McKenzie JK. Transmetacarpal amputation of the index finger: a clinical assessment of hand strength and complications. *J Hand Surg* 1977;2:471–481.

63. Steichen JB, Idler RS. Results of central ray resection without bony transposition. *J Hand Surg [Am]* 1986;11:466–474.

64. Carroll RE. Transposition of the index finger to replace the middle finger. *Clin Orth* 1959;15:27–34.

65. Slocum DB. Upper extremity amputation. In: Flynn JE, ed. *Hand surgery*, 2nd ed. Baltimore: Williams & Wilkins, 1975.

66. Littler JW. Les principes architecturaux et fonctionnels de la main. *Rev Chir Othop* 1960;46(2):131–138.

67. Posner MA. Ray transposition for central digital loss. *J Hand Surg* 1979;4:242–257.

68. Leviet D. La translocation de l'auriculaire par ostéotomie intracarpienne. *Ann Chir* 1978;32(9):609–612.

69. Masmejean E, Alnot JY, Couturier C, Cadot B. Resection du quatrième rayon pour lésions de l'annulaire: les amputations du quatrième rayon de la main. *Rev Chir Ortho* 1997;83:324–329.

70. Colen L, Bunkis J, Gorden L, Walton R. Functional assessment of ray transfer for central digital loss. *J Hand Surg* 1985;10A:232–237.

71. Leviet D. La translocation de l'auriculaire par ostéotomie intracarpienne. *Ann Chir Main* 1982;1:45–56.

72. Van Overstraeten L, Foucher G. Etude comparative des résections métacarpiennes et des translocations après amputations des doigts médians. *Ann Chir Main* 1995;14:74–83.

73. Tubiana R, Stack GH, Hakstian RW. Restoration of prehension after severe mutilation of the hand. *J Bone Joint Surg* 1966;48B:455–473.

74. Lundborg G, Branemark PI, Rosen B. Osseointegrated thumb prosthesis: a concept for fixation of digit prosthetic devices. *J Hand Surg* 1996;21A:216–221.

75. Manurangsee P, Isariyawut C, Chatuthong V, Mekraksawanit S. Osseointegrated finger prosthesis: an alternative method for finger reconstruction. *J Hand Surg* 2000;25A:86–92.

76. Gillies HD, Millard DR. *The principles and art of plastic surgery*. Boston: Little, Brown; London: Butterworths, 1957.

77. Michon J. Le pouce sans doigt. *Chirurgie* 1970;96:633–638.

78. Foucher G, Van Genechten F. A compound radial artery forearm flap in hand surgery: an original modification of the chinese forearm flap. *Br J Plast Surg* 1984;37:139–148.

79. Goldberg NH, Watson HK. Composite toe transfers in the reconstruction of the aphalangic hand. *J Hand Surg* 1982;7:454–459.

80. Buck-Gramcko D. Wiederherstellungschirurgie bei Gliedverlusten. In: Nigst H, Buck-Gramcko D, Millesi H, eds. *Handchirurgie band II*. Stuttgart: Thieme Verlag, 1983.

81. Soiland. Lengthening finger with the "on the top" method. *Acta Chir Scand* 1961;122:184–186.

82. Kelleher JC, Sullivan JG, Baibak GJ, Dean RK. "On top plasty" for amputated fingers. *Plast Reconstr Surg* 1968;42:242–248.

83. Matev IB. Thumb reconstruction through metacarpal bone lengthening. *J Hand Surg* 1980;5:482–487.

84. Kessler I. Transposition lengthening of a digital ray after multiple amputations of fingers. *Hand* 1976;8:176–178.

85. Dahl MT, Gulli B, Berg T. Complications of limb lengthening. A learning curve. *Clin Orthop* 1994;301:10–18.

86. Nicoladoni C. Daumenplastik und organischer Ersatz der Fingerspitze. (Anticheiropastik und Daktyloplastik). *Archiv Klin Chir* 1900;1;606–628.

87. Davies JE. Toe-to-hand transfers. *Plast Reconstr Surg* 1964;33:422–436.

88. Esser JFS, Ranschburg P. Reconstruction of a hand and four fingers by transplantation of the middle part of the foot and four toes. *Ann Surg* 1940;111:655–659.

89. Foucher G, Braun FM, Merle M, Michon J. Le transfert du 2ème orteil dans la chirurgie reconstructrice des doigts longs. *Rev Chir Orthop* 1981;67:235–240.

90. Foucher G, Van Genechten F, Merle M, et al. Le transfert à partir d'orteil dans la chirurgie reconstructrice de la main. A propos de 71 cas. *Ann Chir Main* 1984;3:124–129.

91. Foucher G, Binhammer P. Free vascularized toe transfer. In: *Reconstruction surgery in hand mutilation*. London: Martin Dunitz, 1997:57–65.

92. Foucher G, Norris RW. The dorsal approach in harvesting the second toe. *Intern J Microsurg* 1988;4;185–187.

93. Gilbert A. Composite tissue transfers from the foot: anatomic basis and surgical technique. In: Daniller AI, Strauch B, eds. *Symposium on microsurgery*. St. Louis: Mosby, 1976.

94. Yoshimura M. Toe to hand transfer. *Plast Reconstr Surg* 1984;73;851–852.

95. Foucher G. Vascularized joint transfer. In: *Operative hand surgery*, 2nd ed. New York: Churchill Livingstone, 1988:1271–1293.

96. Wei FC, Yim KK. Pulp plasty after toe-to-hand transplantation. *Plast Reconstr Surg* 1995;96:661–666.

97. Foucher G. Second toe-to-finger transfer in hand mutilations. *Clin Orthop* 1995;314:8–12.

98. Leung PC, Ma FY. Digital reconstruction using the toe flap. Report of 10 cases. *J Hand Surg* 1982;7A:366–370.

99. Lister GD, Kalisman M, Tsu Min Tsai. Reconstruction of the hand with free microneurovascular toe to hand transfer: experience with 54 toe transfers. *Plast Reconstr Surg* 1983;71:372–384.

100. Gu YD, Zhang GM, Cheng DS, et al. Free toe transfer for

thumb and finger reconstruction in 300 cases. *Plast Reconstr Surg* 1993;91:693–700.

101. Buncke HJ. Discussion of free toe transfer for thumb and finger reconstruction in 300 cases. *Plast Reconstr Surg* 1993;91:701–702.

102. Gu YD, Zhang GM, Chen DS, et al. Toe-to-hand transfer: an analysis of 14 failed cases. *J Hand Surg* 1993;18:823–827.

103. Koshima I, Etoh H, Moriguchi T, Soeda S. Sixty cases of partial or total toe transfer for repair of finger losses. *Plast Reconstr Surg* 1993;92:1331–1338.

104. Dellon AL. Sensory recovery in replanted digits and transplanted toes: a review. *J Reconstr Microsurg* 1986;2:123–129.

105. Demirkan F, Wei FC, Jeng SF, et al. Toe transplantation for isolated index finger amputations distal to the proximal interphalangeal joint. *Plast Reconstr Surg* 1999;103:499–507.

106. Edgerton MT. The cross-hand finger transfer. *Plast Reconstr Surg* 1976;57:281–293.

107. Foucher G, Nagel D. Pinch reconstruction by hand to hand finger transfer associated with hallux transfer after a severe frostbite injury. *J Hand Surg* 1999;24B:617–620.

108. Morrison WA, O'Brien McB, MacLeod AM. Ring finger transfer in reconstruction of transmetacarpal amputations. *J Hand Surg* 1984;9A:4–11.

109. Pederson WC. Digital reconstruction by free microvascular transfer of two fingers as a unit from the contralateral paralyzed hand. *Microsurgery* 1994;15:643–637.

110. Merle d'Aubigné R, Tubiana R. Les mutilations bilatérales des mains. *Chirurgie* 1968;94:224–226.

111. Moberg E. The treatment of mutilating injuries of the upper extremity. *Surg Clin North Am* 1964;44:1107–1113.

97

WRIST AND MID-HAND RECONSTRUCTION

JOHN J. WALSH IV

Restoring useful function to a patient with an amputation between the distal radius and the metacarpal heads is a daunting task. A marked limitation in function is present after an injury at this level. The *Guide to the Evaluation of Permanent Impairment* (1) provides whole-person impairment estimates between 32% and 56% for amputations at this level. The estimates depend on the exact level of the injury and whether the thumb is present or absent in patients who have metacarpal-level amputations. Alterations in body image can be partially addressed by cosmetic prostheses. There is, however, a near inverse relationship between cosmesis and function for the options available after an injury of this nature (2). This chapter initially reviews issues that surround decision making at the time of injury. Late reconstructive options, including tissue transfer and allograft hand transplant, are also discussed.

ACUTE DECISION MAKING

Patients who sustain a multiple digit transcarpal or whole-hand amputation present a dramatic acute clinical picture. Replantation offers significant functional recovery possibilities (3); however, many injuries are incompatible with an acute replant. A working knowledge of salvage, reconstructive, and prosthetic issues guides the treating surgeon's choices during performance of initial wound care and in plans for future surgery. The primary concerns for the limb after amputation involve durable skin cover, avoidance of symptomatic neuromas, maintenance of the length of the digit remnants and muscle–tendon units (4), and regaining motion in whatever joints remain. These allow the patient to recuperate as rapidly as possible and facilitate future reconstructive efforts. Tagging of the ends of nerves and vessels speeds surgical dissection during reconstruction and is especially helpful in children. Small-caliber structures that are exposed by the injury are marked by colored, fine, nonabsorbable suture. They are then more easily located when they are entrapped by scar tissue.

Soft tissue coverage should be gained as rapidly as possible with the minimum degree of invasiveness possible. A nearly complete amputation with a perfused, distal portion of full-thickness tissue may allow use of a fillet graft. This obviously provides an excellent color and tissue-type match, while avoiding additional donor site morbidity. As circumstances allow, any form of coverage should be sized generously to ease closure of later transfer efforts.

The previous discussion suggests a thought process that involves initial evaluation, a decision against complete replantation, and direction of initial treatment toward optimizing later salvage operations. A form of acute, nonanatomic reconstruction that can be used to preserve uninjured parts was described more than 20 years ago in China (5). This report describes the transplantation of two or three uninjured digits to the forearm stump by using microvascular methods at the time of injury. This allows a form of pincer grasp and excellent sensory recovery and avoids any additional donor site morbidity (5). It requires a limited intercalary zone of injury with midcarpal destruction. It also presumes an otherwise healthy patient who is able to tolerate 10 to 12 hours of surgery. The uninjured fingers are then attached to the radial and ulnar stumps after wide débridement to healthy tissue proximally and distally. An alternative is to transplant toes if ipsilateral fingers are not available for reconstruction (Fig. 1). Tendon, nerve, and vessel repair is performed as it is with a conventional replant. Complications, including infection and tendon adhesions, were not uncommon (5).

Choosing the level of amputation for an injury at the midcarpal level (which defies any acute salvage) should be guided by a number of principles. Amputations through the carpus can be treated with shortening to the wrist disarticulation or below the elbow amputation or can be left at the injury length, if soft tissue permits. Preservation of the wrist joint permits a greater arc of forearm rotation (3). It does create a more bulbous stump, which is helpful in suspension of a conventional prosthesis. Conversely, this stump is less amenable to myoelectric prosthesis fitting due

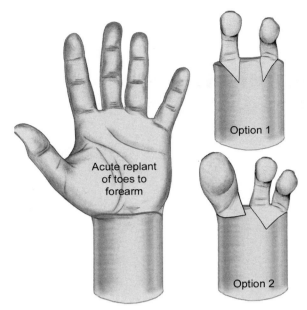

FIGURE 1. Acute replant of the amputated digits to the forearm.

to a number of technical issues (6). If even a small segment of the metacarpal base is present, the segment that is distal to the radius and ulna should be preserved. The intact wrist flexor and extensor attachments allow preservation of some wrist flexion and extension. Use of the stump as a "helper" is improved to a modest degree. If a myoelectric prosthesis can be fitted, the patient can flex the distal portion of the stump inside the prosthesis, improving motor control. This also aids in stabilization of a purely passive device (3,6). More proximal injuries, which preserve carpal bones alone, should be treated with radiocarpal disarticulation. Due to the absence of flexor or extensor attachments at this level, there is little benefit in retaining the carpus, as compared to the benefit of radiocarpal disarticulation.

LATE RECONSTRUCTION

The recreation of prehensile function in a fingerless hand or handless arm can be divided into three broad categories. The first approach involves lengthening of existing structures by using adjacent transfer or distraction lengthening, or both (7). The second approach involves a nonanatomic free tissue transfer or local rearrangement to effect some form of prehension (2,4,8–12). Included in this group is the Krukenberg procedure (13,14). The last option involves allograft hand transplantation, which is currently investigational (15–22).

The simplest method of generating a pincer-type grasp involves distraction lengthening of metacarpals with the creation of a deeper web space and an opposing post for pinch. Karev (7) described a form of this technique by

lengthening a remaining thumb metacarpal, excising the index metacarpal, and transferring it onto the long-finger metacarpal. This was covered by a groin flap. The web space between the thumb and the new metacarpal post was also deepened. This produced a pincer, side-to-side grasp between the thumb stump and the metacarpal post.

The Krukenberg procedure was originally described by the German army surgeon Hermann Krukenberg early in 1917 (13,14). This procedure attempts to develop a form of pincer grasp at the forearm level. This is done by initially separating the radius and ulna, striving for bone lengths of 10 to 15 cm (Fig. 2). A 10- to 12-cm opening between the tips is desirable. Skin flaps are designed and rotated to preserve an innervated space between the bones. Motor control is gained by using muscle groups that originate from the medial epicondyle for grasp between the radius and ulna. Corresponding muscles that originate from the lateral epicondyle function to open the interval. Although this procedure does not preclude later prosthesis fitting, it is generally reserved for patients for whom prostheses are difficult to obtain, such as those in the developing world (13,14). It is particularly useful for a blind double amputee who lacks the visual feedback to control an insensate prosthesis.

More complex methods of hand reconstruction for multiple digit amputations involve toe transplantation. This has been practiced and refined by multiple authors (2,4,8–10,12). Wei et al. (11) have described distal hand injuries as a *metacarpal hand* and classified these in two types. The distinction between types involves the extent of remaining useful thumb length and supporting thumb structures. The two main types are then subclassified based on the extent of

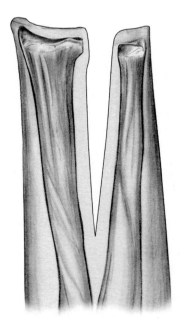

FIGURE 2. Krukenberg procedure.

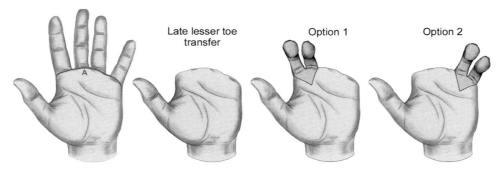

FIGURE 3. Late lesser-toe transfer to recreate opposable posts for grasp or pinch. A, amputation level.

digit injuries (4). A thorough and systematic algorithm has been developed for which toes should be transplanted (and in what order), the level of transplantation relative to the web spaces, and the planning of donor site issues (4,8,10,12). These efforts are directed at the creation of useful tripod pinch, stronger hook grip, lateral stability, and handling precision (Figs. 3 and 4) (4). In addition to the previously mentioned benefits, single toe transplantation to the forearm has been described to improve control of a myoelectric prosthesis (23). This provides for a considerably smaller donor site deficit and substantially improves prosthetic control.

Transplantation of a hand from an unrelated donor for reconstruction of a unilateral or bilateral amputee has received a great deal of media attention after the first transplant in 1998. The topic has also provoked a sometimes contentious debate in the hand surgery community (15,16,18–22,24). As of 2003, 14 hand transplants have been performed in 11 patients, including three bilateral transplants. The first transplant was amputated 2 years and 4 months after the index procedure for chronic rejection (21). Results from the first bilateral hand transplant 21 months after surgery were reported at the 2002 American Society for Surgery of the Hand meeting (18). Two episodes of acute rejection in the skin were treated by

topical and systemic immunosuppressive medication changes. Active wrist and finger range of motion was 30% of normal. Extrinsic muscle activity accounted for the majority of function, but clinical and electromyographic evidence of intrinsic activity had developed. Protective sensation was present; static two-point discrimination was absent. Functional brain magnetic resonance imaging comparisons pre- and posttransplant did show progressive cortical reorganization, and systemic immunosuppression was well tolerated (18).

Strict preoperative screening (20,22), patient advocacy measures (22), and close monitoring of issues that are related to systemic immunosuppression have been used to avoid ill-advised patient selection and postoperative complications. Nevertheless, fundamental issues exist regarding the adequacy of the experimental support for the procedure (17,21). Comparisons to solid organ transplantation and the relative danger of lifelong immunosuppression, expectations for functional recovery, and ethical considerations have all been debated and remain without conclusive answers (16,18–22,24). As such, transplantation from an unrelated donor remains an investigational procedure and the focus of intense study, and caution has been urged by the American Society for Surgery of the Hand.

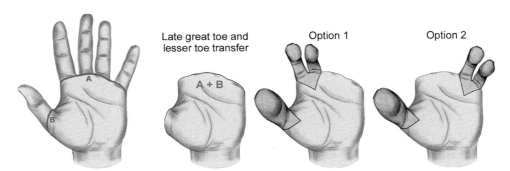

FIGURE 4. Late great-toe and lesser-toe transfers (staged). A, amputation level of fingers; B, amputation level of thumb.

REFERENCES

1. Cocchiarella L, Anderson G. *Guide to the evaluation of permanent impairment,* 5th ed. American Medical Association, 2001.
2. Zhong-Wei C. Reconstruction by autogenous toe transplantation for total hand amputation. *Orthop Clin North Am* 1981;12:835–842.
3. Trumble T. *Principles of hand surgery and therapy.* Philadelphia: WB Saunders, 2000.
4. Green DP, Hotchkiss RN, Peterson WC, eds. *Green's operative hand surgery,* 4th ed. Philadelphia: Churchill Livingstone, 1993.
5. Cheng GL, Pan DD, Qu ZY. Transplantation of severed digits to forearm stump for restoration of partial hand function. *Ann Plast Surg* 1985;15:356–366.
6. Lamb DW, Scott H. Management of congenital and acquired amputation in childhood. *Orthop Clin North Am* 1981;12:992–994.
7. Karev A. Reconstruction of a transmetacarpal amputation by means of a ray transfer and distraction lengthening. *Ann Plast Surg* 1982;8:423–425.
8. Gordon L, et al. Hand reconstruction for multiple amputations by double microsurgical toe transplantation. *J Hand Surg* 1985;10:218–225.
9. Holle J, et al. Grip reconstruction by double-toe transplantation in cases of a fingerless hand and handless arm. *Plast Reconstr Surg* 1982;69:962–968.
10. Tan BK, Wei FC, Chang KJ , et al. Combined third and fourth toe transplantation. *Hand Clin* 1999;15:589–595.
11. Wei FC, El-Gammal TA, et al. Metacarpal hand: classification and guidelines for microsurgical reconstruction with toe transfers. *Plast Reconstr Surg* 1997;99:122–128.
12. Tan BK, et al. Strategies in multiple toe transplantation for bilateral type II metacarpal hand reconstruction. *Hand Clin* 1999;15:607–612.
13. Tubiana R. Krukenberg's operation. *Orthop Clin North Am* 1981;12:819–826.
14. Irmay F, Merzouga B, Vettorel D. The Krukenberg procedure: a surgical option for the treatment of double hand amputees in Sierra Leone. *Lancet* 2000;356:1072–1075.
15. Cooney WP, Hentz PR. Hand transplantation: current status. *J Hand Surg* 2002;27:165.
16. Breidenbach WC III, et al. A position statement in support of hand transplantation. *J Hand Surg* 2002;27:760–770.
17. Daniel RK, Egerzaegi EP, Samulack DD, et al. Tissue transplantation in upper extremity reconstruction. A preliminary report. *J Hand Surg* 1988:1–8.
18. Dubernard JM, Herzberg G, Lanzetta M. Follow-up on the first bilateral hand transplant patient. Paper presented at: ASSH meeting; 2002; Phoenix, AZ.
19. Edgell SE, et al. Different reference frames can lead to different hand transplantation decisions by patients and physicians. *J Hand Surg* 2001;26:196–200.
20. Germann G. Bilateral hand transplantation—indication and rationale. *J Hand Surg* 2001;26:521.
21. Jones NF. Concerns about human hand transplantation in the 21st century. *J Hand Surg* 2002:771–787.
22. Jones JW, Gruber SA, Barker JH, et al. Successful hand transplantation. One year follow-up. *N Engl J Med* 2000;343:468–473.
23. Chen ZW, Hu TP. A reconstructed digit by transplantation of a second toe for control of an electromechanical prosthetic hand. *Microsurgery* 2002;22:5–10.
24. Andrew Lee WP. The debate over hand transplantation. *J Hand Surg* 2002;27:757–759.

98

FOREARM RECONSTRUCTION

FIESKY A. NUÑEZ V.

The forearm represents the anatomic part of the upper extremity that links the elbow and the hand and provides humans with the important movement of forelimb rotation.

The movements of pronation and supination (rotation) of the forearm that have accompanied increase in brain size, and the development of the prehensile thumb, have been considered the most important elements in the evolution and differentiation of the human race, bringing the development of the ability to manage and control beneficially the environment (1,2).

It is well accepted that mangling upper extremity injuries may be treated with early amputation in some patients, thereby avoiding long suffering. However, prostheses in the upper extremity provide poor functional outcomes, and in severe lesions on the forearm, reasonable attempts of salvage and reconstruction represent a challenge that must be tackled.

SURGICAL ANATOMY

Based on the importance of pronation and supination of the forearm (vital for most of our activities of daily living) and the structural complexity of this region (especially its biomechanics), reconstruction must seek to achieve as close to the normal anatomy as possible. This has been affirmed by many authorities (3–5), particularly when compared with diaphyseal fractures of other areas.

The bones of the forearm lie one beside the other but not totally parallel. The radius and ulna are united only at their ends, through the proximal and distal radioulnar joints. The proximal radioulnar joint is a trochoid articulation between the head of the radius and the sigmoid notch of the ulna. This joint is stabilized by the capsule of the elbow and the annular ligament. The distal radioulnar joint is also a trochoid joint and comprises the head of the ulna and the sigmoid notch of the radius; it is stabilized by the triangular fibrocartilage complex. Both joints are functionally very complex and are responsible for the rotation of the forearm. The ulna is a relatively straight bone, but the radius has two curvatures that play an important role in the prono-supination movement. The importance and complexity of

the radial curvatures and angles have been pointed out by Sage (6), especially in the mechanics of pronation and supination. The interosseous space between the radius and the ulna is bridged by the interosseous membrane, which has been known since the classic descriptions of the anatomists of the sixteenth century. Many different descriptions, denominations, and functions have been attributed to this anatomic structure, according to past authors (7–9). Some of the facts that they emphasize are that the fibers are orientated both transversely and obliquely (10,11) and anchored to the interosseous border of the ulna and radius and the membrane is thick and strong proximally and thin and membranous distally. The membrane serves also as surface for muscular origins both on the volar and dorsal aspects. The interosseous membrane also has the following functions:

- It separates the volar and dorsal compartment of the forearm.
- The variation of tension of its fibers participates in the rotational movements of the radius around the ulna (12–15).
- It approximates both bones at the middle of the forearm in pronation.
- It stabilizes forearm bones and the distal radioulnar joint.
- It allows the ascent of the ulnar head in supination and its descent during pronation, a fact that has been demonstrated by Epner et al. (16) and Palmer et al. (17).

PATHOPHYSIOLOGY

Defects of the forearm result from wide resections of tumors by oncology surgery or as consequence of trauma: The defects may be of the soft tissues, by bone loss, or combinations of both.

Forearm fractures are often the sequelae of high-energy injury, and many of those are open fractures, resulting in defects, as mentioned previously. Other consequences of trauma are perfusion problems due to vascular lesions, paralysis caused by nerve injury, compartment syndromes and their consequences, malunion, nonunion, and radioulnar synostosis.

CLASSIFICATION

For many years, the author has used a classification of defects of the forearm to assist and orient surgeons in diagnosis and treatment, as well as to aid in determining the prognosis of the lesions. The lesions have been separated into two major categories: bone defects and soft tissue lesions. The bone defects are classified into three groups:

A: Bone defects less than 2 cm
B: Bone defects between 2 and 8 cm
C: Defects greater than 8 cm

These initial groups are subdivided depending on the bone in which the defect is localized:

- Group A (less than 2 cm): U (ulnar defect), R (radial defect), U + R (ulnar and radial defects)
- Group B (between 2 and 8 cm): U, R, U + R
- Group C (greater than 8 cm): U, R, U + R

To define the location, add 1 if the center of the defect is in the proximal one-third of diaphysis, 2 for the middle third, and 3 for the distal third. For example, a 6-cm proximal defect of the ulna combined with a 2-cm distal of the radius is classified as BU1 + AR3.

Because high-energy transfer is responsible for producing these lesions and most are the sequelae of open fractures, soft tissue defects or lesions are frequently associated with bone defects. Soft tissue defects are classified as follows:

- Type 0: Soft tissues not requiring reconstruction
- Type 1: Skin defects requiring reconstruction
- Type 2: Muscle and tendon defects
- Type 3: Nerve defects or poor vascularity, or both
- Type 4: Multiple defects

Taking into consideration this classification, the author has proposed a scheme (Fig. 1) to be used as an algorithm to facilitate the process of reconstruction in a rational way, serving as a guide for practical use that is considered later in this chapter.

TREATMENT

Most patients with severe lesions of the forearm also have injuries to other parts of the body that must be recognized and treated within the context of polytrauma. Also, a multidisciplinary trauma team is required, and each lesion must be given its priority according to the severity, starting with those that endanger life. Many different protocols have been proposed for the treatment of acute limb lesions.

However, most of them agree on the following: In the acute phase, the importance of consecutive cultures and aggressive débridements with resection of devitalized tissues is well recognized. Immediate bone stabilization is mandatory. As soon as the wounds are biologically stable (no infection and good tissue perfusion), the soft tissue reconstruction must be initiated within 72 hours and no later than 6 days after injury. Any bone reconstruction must be done between the first and the sixth weeks. Depending on the condition of the wounds, these steps may overlap.

Many severe lesions of the limbs have associated vascular damage that must be treated by reimplantation or revascularization, using microvascular anastomoses. However, many authors doubt that this effort is justified, due to the time consumed, the high cost, and the poor functional results that usually supervene (18–20).

In view of this problem, Johansen and colleagues developed the "mangled extremity severity score" (20), taking into consideration the energy dissipation, hemodynamic status, degree and length of warm limb ischemia, and age of the patient. This permits the allocation of a system of points, with the goal of deriving a total score that helps make the decision between immediate ablation and a program of reconstruction. Either way, the treatment of the upper limb differs fundamentally from the treatment of the lower limb. Patients with these kinds of lesions in lower limbs benefit greatly from early amputation, immediate use of prosthesis, and a vigorous program of rehabilitation and vocational reorientation (21,22). This way, the patient may return to daily activities much earlier than expected and with minimum repercussions on his or her social and occupational prospects.

The lower limb is a weight-bearing extremity, whereas the upper extremity's purpose differs fundamentally because it is a synergistically sensitive and mobile extremity with superb harmonic esthetics. That is why all the surgical reconstruction possibilities must be exploited before making the decision of an amputation. Using modern and aggressive reconstructive methods, many mangled upper extremities can be salvaged, and the patient can return early to a productive and social life.

George Omer stated (23) the following:

Before considering any hand amputation, then, one should weigh well the possibility of surgical reconstruction, especially with the idea of restoring natural sensation and strong prehension. Whenever reasonably feasible, surgical reconstruction of a damaged hand or arm should be attempted first. Often the result will be such that a prosthesis will not be necessary. . . . Every useful part of a limb, and every bit of skin that has sensation, should be preserved, thus giving more useful material for reconstruction and, finally, for the fitting, if necessary, of a prosthesis.

Once the decision is made to reconstruct, two important aspects must be considered in the treatment plan: the soft tissues and the bone defects. Only in those cases beyond

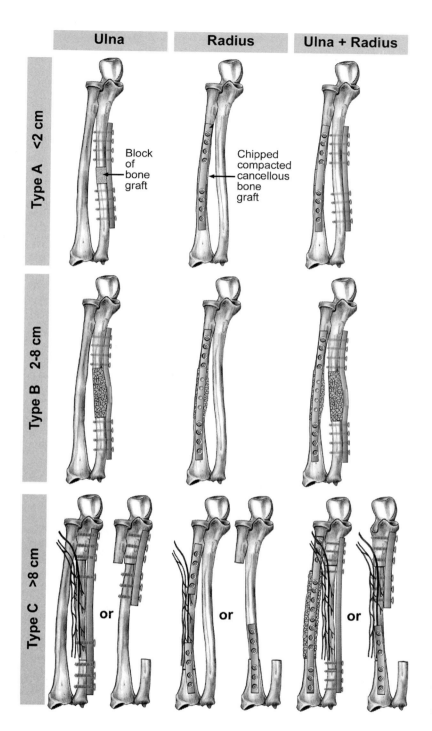

FIGURE 1. Practical scheme recommended for forearm reconstruction according to the bone defect classification. The choice between two-bone reconstruction or one-bone forearm depends on the potential for pronosupination recovery, depending on the muscle state and joint conditions.

any possible reconstruction is the remaining choice to do an amputation and send the patient for prosthetic rehabilitation as soon as possible.

Soft Tissue Lesions

Most traumatic wounds can undergo either delayed primary closure or healing by secondary intention, especially of small defects. Many of those do not result in a functional deficit, and for those, additional treatment is not necessary. Very few require reconstruction for cosmetic reasons, especially in those with emotional dysfunction. Many skin defects can be treated by skin grafting as the initial treatment. When skin grafts are used in the proximal forearm over the muscular tissues, they do not create problems, but when they are used distally over tendons adhesions, they may impair the gliding of the tendons, with consequent limitation of mobility of the wrist and the hand.

A wide variety of possibilities are available to solve this situation, ranging from local pedicle flaps and distant pedicle flaps, to free vascularized tissue transfer. The most-used distant pedicle flap was described in 1972 by McGregor and Jackson (24) as the groin flap. This flap's vascularity derives from the superficial circumflex iliac artery and has the advantage of providing abundant soft tissue for large defect coverage, especially in the middle and distal parts of the forearm, where the tendons are often exposed. The donor site most of the time is closed primarily and usually is well tolerated; however, the forearm must stay united to the flap for a minimum of 3 weeks, and this compromises rehabilitation of the extremity. Abdominal pedicle flaps, which are supplied by the hypogastric or thoracogastric arteries, provide good coverage for large and deep soft tissue loss, as can be seen in Figure 2; however, primary closure of the donor site is not always possible, and split skin graft is very often necessary, with the consequent cosmetic problem. Just as with other pedicle flaps, compromise of the mobility of the hand, elbow, and shoulder impairs the rehabilitation of the hand. Pedicle flaps are also considered parasitic in nature, requiring a vascularized bed at the recipient defect for vascular ingrowth to allow detachment by the third week.

When the damage of the forearm is less extensive, local flaps can be used. These can be one of two different types: random pattern and axial pattern. Random-pattern flaps receive their blood supply not from a single arteriovenous pedicle but from many minute vessels of the subdermal, or subcutaneous, plexus (25). During the design of this type of flap, some general rules related to the width of the base must be followed to avoid impairment of the blood supply. This clearly limits the range of applications for the random-pattern flaps, especially on a severely traumatized forearm.

Axial-pattern flaps receive their blood supply from a single constant vessel larger than those of the subdermal plexus. This anatomic condition allows for the design of flaps with a more predictable vascular territory. There has been increasing interest in axial-pattern flaps for defects in the forearm, and the two most popularly used are the radial artery forearm flap, known as the *Chinese flap* (26,27), and the posterior interosseous artery flap (28,29). The Chinese flap is a fasciocutaneous flap, the blood supply of which is based on the radial artery; it is therefore obvious that the patient needs to have an intact ulnar artery. An Allen's test must be performed to demonstrate the total vascularity of the hand through the palmar arch. The posterior interosseous artery provides the vascularity for the flap with that name, and its popularity has increased since the more detailed description of its vascular anatomy allows its use as a reverse flap (distal to proximal perfusion), increasing the overall potential arc of rotation. Both flaps provide low-profile, nonbulky soft tissue coverage for either dorsal or volar forearm defects. Obviously, the magnitude of the lesion and the vascular damage to the forearm may preclude the use of those flaps. Fortunately, with the possibility of early (within 72 hours) transfer of vascularized tissues into the traumatic defect as a method of reconstruction, many of those severe forearm lesions can be reconstructed, decreasing the complications frequently associated with such pathology (nonunion and osteomyelitis). It also reduces the patient's degree and time of incapacity.

Godina and Lister (30) showed the clear advantages of this treatment strategy (radical débridements and early soft tissue cover using vascularized tissue). This has also been the author's experience dealing with this type of lesion.

All forearm lesions too extensive to be covered by a conventional type of flap or those with an inadequate recipient bed are ideal candidates for free vascularized soft tissue transfer, but the surgeon must be trained in microsurgery to perform the vascular anastomosis. Two major benefits of free tissue transfer are evident; first, the extremity does not need to be immobilized in a dependent position, thereby facilitating rehabilitation. The second advantage is that new vascularity is brought to the area. These two facts greatly influence the healing process.

Free tissue transfer to cover defects in the forearm may be achieved using many different flaps, but the most frequently used are the lateral arm and dorsal pedis flaps for small defects and the scapular flap for medium-sized defects; for more extensive loss, the contralateral radial forearm flap, the groin flap, or the latissimus dorsi flap (31) is recommended. It is also important to mention that some flaps, such as the lateral arm, the radial forearm, and the groin flaps, as well as free vascularized fibula, can provide osteocutaneous tissue for composite tissue loss (combined bone and soft tissues defects).

As mentioned previously, early soft tissue reconstruction (less than 72 hours after the damage occurs) has been emphasized by many authors in the past, mainly for the following reasons:

- Reduced possibility of infection
- Avoidance of dehydration of anatomic elements
- Protection of the neurovascular structures
- Creation of an adequate well-vascularized environment for bone healing
- Facilitation of future reconstructions that are usually necessary in these lesions
- Improvement in the functional recovery of the patient

In conclusion, it can be affirmed that complications are reduced when a well-planned protocol of serial aggressive débridements and reconstruction follows severe open fractures of the forearm, and the selection of the ideal method depends on the following:

- Lesion characteristics
- General condition of the patient
- The extent and type of trauma
- The functional needs of the patient

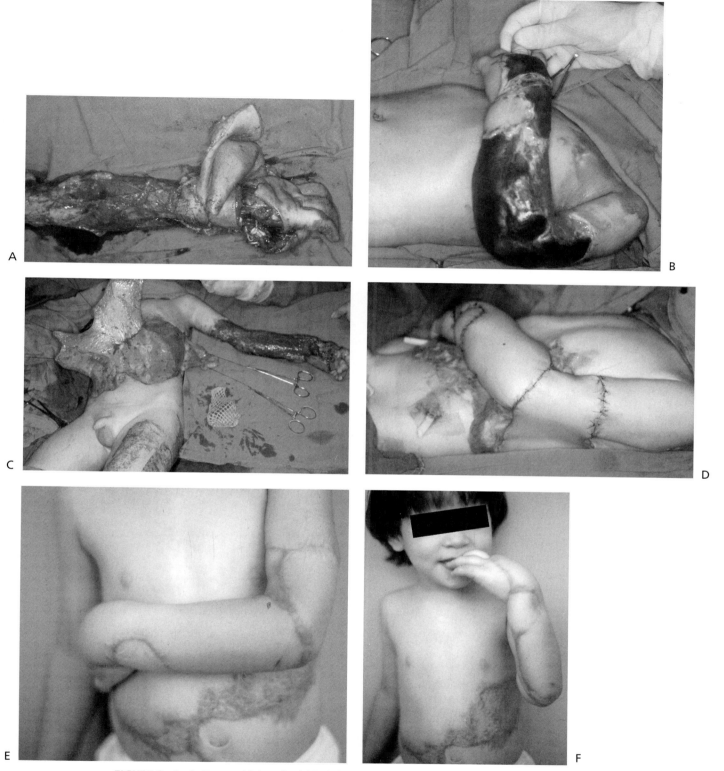

FIGURE 2. A: A 5-year-old boy had his left (nondominant) upper limb caught in a rolling machine of a bakery. He is shown with a severe degloving of the arm, elbow, forearm, wrist, and hand. **B:** After initial attempt at revascularization, the situation was an extensive, noninfected, necrotic lesion. **C,D:** Combined abdominal and thoracoabdominal flap was performed. **E,F:** Final result of excellent coverage of this large soft tissue loss, but primary closure of the donor site was not possible, and skin graft was necessary, with the consequent cosmetic problem.

In general, careful evaluation of the lesion determines the strategy for defect coverage.

Bone Lesions

For many years, forearm fracture treatment comprised close reduction followed by cast immobilization for long periods of time (32–40), and any result of such treatment with less than 10% of nonunion was considered acceptable. With this perspective, less importance was given to the functional outcome, which is now given its true importance for the simple reason that precise movement is the most important task of the upper limb. The literature is full of studies showing malunion, nonunion, and poor functional results, and the most convincing of those were published by Hughston (41) and Charnley (42), reporting 92% unsatisfactory functional results and 27% malunion, nonunion, or synostosis.

In an attempt to avoid shortening while maintaining the reduction, continuous traction and pinning using Kirschner wires above and below the fracture, included in the cast, were recommended (43). Additionally, intramedullary nailing of forearm fractures was widely used in the past, with an unacceptably high rate of complications (44). Even Charnley, in his masterpiece, *Closed treatment of common fractures*, recommended the surgical treatment of forearm fractures (42).

All the initial attempts of treatment with open reduction and internal fixation of forearm fractures developed a plethora of complications, basically due to inadequate fixation and subsequent cast immobilization after the surgery. Seeking to find something to improve the results, Danis (45) introduced the concept of interfragmentary compression using a plate that produced such stability after anatomic reduction that healing of diaphyseal fractures occurred without the formation of callus. Danis' work, and the contributions of the Albin Lambotte, stimulated Maurice Müller to find a better way to treat fractures using rigid internal fixation and immediate functional rehabilitation to improve the results. Finally, in 1958, Müller, with this objective, encouraged a group of Swiss surgical colleagues to investigate, create an armamentarium, and conduct clinical trials to evaluate the benefits of this method. All this led to the creation of the Arbeitsgemeinschaft für Osteosynthesefragen (AO), later to be known in English as the *Association for the Study of Internal Fixation*.

With the use of well-designed plates and screws and the application of AO principles to the treatment of forearm fractures, the results improved dramatically, and this approach emerged as the gold standard for this type of lesion. With anatomic reduction and stable fixation, external immobilization is no longer required, allowing immediate functional aftercare. Open reduction and internal fixation following this philosophy has been demonstrated to produce approximately 96% to 98% of union (46,47) and restitution of satisfactory function in some 90% of patients (48). Complications have been presented over the years, but most of them are caused by the incorrect application of the biomechanical principles of fixation; ignorance of the importance of the biologic milieu of the fracture, especially the correct care and handling of the soft tissues and the preservation of vascularity; the failure to restore the normal curvature of the radius; the loss of reduction of the fractures; and the persisting incongruity of the elbow, radioulnar, and wrist joints.

The more frequent bone-related problems reported in forearm fractures are nonunion, synostosis, and malunion.

Nonunion

Unsuccessful forearm bone healing can produce pain, deformities, instability, pronosupination dysfunction, and disability of manual function. The author has previously mentioned the unacceptable functional results in nonoperative treatment in the fractures of the forearm, which also result in a high percentage of nonunion, reaching 12% in some series (49). Most cases of nonunion are associated with three factors:

1. Loss of bone tissue
2. Fracture comminution (50–55)
3. The surgeon's ignorance of the biologic and biomechanical principles of fixation of the fractures

Even though it is clear that the use of bone graft as a primary treatment reduces the risk of nonunion (52,55), there are nevertheless situations with high potential to develop nonunion. These could be fractures caused by high-energy transfer, with severe lesions of the soft tissue, or sizable bone defects. The disastrous results of early attempts at open reduction and internal fixation using different methods such as sutures, intramedullary nails, and small plates and screws are cited previously (49,56–59). It is also important to mention how results improved with the evolution of plate and screw designs, which made them more reliable (60,61). However, the quantum leap was the use of interfragmentary compression by the AO/Association for Study of Internal Fixation (62).

The nonunion rate reduced to a minimum of 2% (55) by using the right technique, paying attention to detail, and giving importance to the biologic principles of the bone healing process. A competent preoperative plan is essential to the success of treatment of forearm nonunion as it is in fresh fractures (63). Success is achieved by addressing the following questions:

Q: How does the soft tissue affect the bone healing?
A: Fibrotic scar tissue, with poor blood supply, is not conducive to bone healing. The importance of supplying a well-vascularized soft tissue coverage has been emphasized. Exposed bone has little potential to heal and is more likely to become infected and to develop osteomyelitis; the combination of nonunion and infection is one of the most difficult problems to face the fracture surgeon.

Q: How does the blood supply of the bone fragments affect fracture healing?

A: Bone healing is considerably affected by the blood supply of bone tissue. A rational approach to vascular considerations was the focus of the Judet brothers in 1960, when they considered two types of nonunions: avascular nonunion with atrophic bone ends and poor healing potential and hypervascular nonunions with hypertrophic bone ends and high healing potential. These observations have helped other authors in the classification of nonunions according to osteogenic potential, which is directly related to the vascularity of the bone fragments (64). By this approach, the author finds pseudarthrosis with exuberant callus formation with an evident optimal blood supply but with a situation of mechanical instability, affecting the bone healing. In most of these cases, this is caused by a insufficient immobilization, due in turn to inappropriate orthopedic treatment or poor surgical fixation. These cases tend to heal when the stresses on the healing tissues are reduced, usually by producing mechanical stability using appropriate surgical means. In most hypertrophic nonunions, bone grafts are not needed; the problem is mechanical, not biologic, and so the solution is mechanical and not biologic. This has been demonstrated in a study by Schenk et al. (65), which shows how the achievement of mechanical stability leads to the penetration of blood vessels and the consequent calcification of the interposed fibrocartilage in the pseudarthrosis, thereby producing osseous bridging between the fragments and then bone remodeling.

A more difficult situation is present when bone loss and devascularization (atrophic nonunion) are encountered. These cases are common after high-energy open fractures, multiple surgical assaults, or the sequelae of osteomyelitis. This is basically a biologic failure with mechanical consequences. The logical approach is therefore to produce a biologic solution by bone grafting but with an appropriately stable mechanical environment.

When persistence of motion is present at the nonunion site, a fluid-filled, synovial-like cavity can form as a new joint (neoarthrosis). This may occur with hypertrophic vascular callus formation, or more commonly in the atrophic type, with little or no callus. It has also been called a *synovial pseudarthrosis*.

Q: Will bone graft be required?

A: Atrophic nonunions require bone graft, especially when a defect is present. On the other hand, hypertrophic nonunions need only rigid stability.

Q: Which implant is more reliable?

A: Even though at the beginning, the 4.5-mm narrow plates were recommended, today, there is an acceptance of 3.5-mm narrow plates for fractures and pseudarthrosis of the forearm as the ideal size (66).

Q: How important are the bone defects?

A: The size of the bone defect determines the prognosis and the type of treatment that must be used in forearm nonunion; a longer defect means major bone substitution, a carefully planned and biomechanically executed stabilization, and also more potential to develop complications.

Q: Which principle of fixation should be used?

A: Interfragmentary compression and axial compression are the most commonly used techniques for hypertrophic nonunions, but the bridging principle is used for atrophic nonunions, especially in the presence of a segmental defect.

Type A Bone Defects

Type A defects (less than 2 cm) of ulna or radius may be treated with tricortical iliac bone graft, and good contact between the graft and the bone ends permits stabilization using a plate with axial compression. Screw thread purchase in at least eight cortices (four screws) in each main shaft fragment (proximal and distal) must be used. This way, the stability is likely to permit immediate mobilization. It is well known that this type of bone graft goes through a slow incorporation process, characterized by gradual replacement of dead bone by new living bone, described by Barth (67) as "creeping substitution" (68). During this process, the graft is in a weakened condition, and the implants must support sizable forces. Such an implant-dependent fixation exposes the metal to the danger of fatigue failure. However, the length of the creeping process is proportional to the size of the defect (69). Because type A defects are relatively small, the time to healing is relatively short, and the implants remain within their fatigue life.

In type A3 defects, the situation is more unstable, and it is recommended that the defect on the ulna be treated with a stable fixation using a tricortical graft and compression plate. The defect on the radius can be treated with autogenous cancellous fragment grafts, which have the advantages of being osteogenic, osteoinductive, and osteoconductive. Having a very large surface accessible to the surrounding vascularity and a relatively small volume, they are rapidly incorporated. This autograft has been demonstrated to be biologically vastly superior to allograft and any of the currently available bone substitutes (70). The author recommends fragmenting the cancellous graft into very small chips and then compacting them with a mallet inside a syringe (Fig. 3G), a technique learned from Jesse Jupiter, which is graphically shown in a publication of Freeland (71). In this way, more vital bone cells can be concentrated per milliliter, and it is amazing how fast this type of graft incorporates: definitely much faster than structured bone grafts. The stability is achieved with a plate, using the bridge principle. Mobility must start as early as possible to prevent cross-

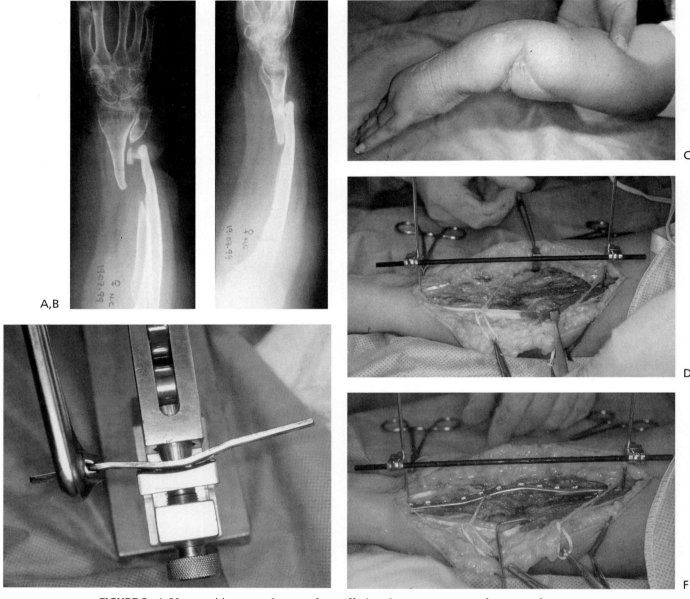

FIGURE 3. A 30-year-old woman 6 years after suffering the consequences of an open forearm fracture, complicated by osteomyelitis, presented with severe incapacity, having had multiple prior surgeries. **A,B:** Anteroposterior and lateral radiographs showing atrophic nonunion of both bones of forearm, with a 7-cm defect of the radius located on mid-diaphysis and a 3-cm bone loss of the ulna in its distal third (BR2 + BU3). **C:** Great instability was evident, but good potential for recovery of rotational movements of forearm was determined after careful evaluation of the soft tissue. **D:** Through a volar approach, the radial nonunion was exposed and intraoperative lengthening was achieved using an external fixator. **E,F:** A wave plate was modeled and used to fix the radius. (*continued*)

union (radioulnar synostosis), especially when the defects are located at the same level.

Type B Bone Defects

In type B defects of ulna or radius (2 to 8 cm), the situation is much more unstable, and the creeping substitution process is slower in big grafts. For that reason, the author rec-

ommends using the compacted bone graft and the "wave plate" bridging principle (Fig. 3E,F) introduced by Weber (72). This technique has the following theoretic advantages: (a) It provides excellent access for the application of the bone graft or transplant; (b) it allows for ingrowth of vessels in the bone graft beneath the plate; (c) it reduces the danger of fatigue fracture of the plate by distributing bending stresses over a longer sector of the plate, thus avoiding

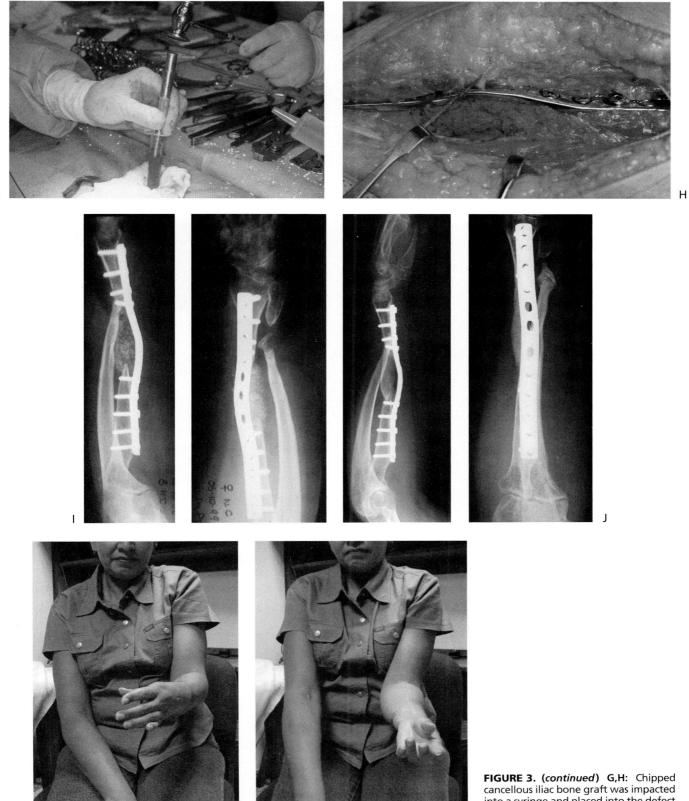

FIGURE 3. (*continued*) **G,H:** Chipped cancellous iliac bone graft was impacted into a syringe and placed into the defect under the plate. **I:** Radiographic result after 1 month and (**J**) 4 months postoperatively. **K,L:** Limited pronation and full supination. (*continued*)

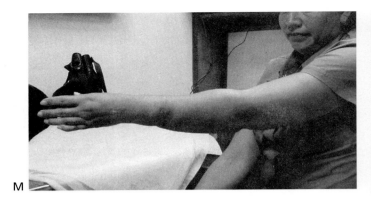

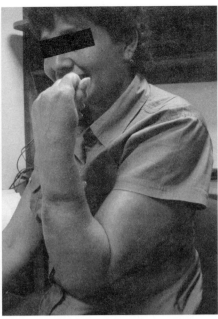

FIGURE 3. (*continued*) **M,N:** Flexion and extension, good stability, and no pain.

local stress concentrations; and (d) it reduces interference with the vascular supply to the bone at the fracture locus by avoiding plate bone contact. The author and colleagues published in 1999 (73) their experience using the wave plate and compacted bone graft in seven poorly vascularized nonunions of the forearms, with defects between 1 and 5 cm, with multiple previous unsuccessful surgeries; in all those patients, the avascular problem and poor quality of the bone were evident. Using this method, bone healing was obtained in all of the patients. Stimulated by these results, the author and colleagues decided to use the same principle in nonunions with longer defects, as can be observed in a patient with a 7-cm radius defect, which healed nicely after having multiples surgeries and a previous osteomyelitis (Fig. 3I,J).

Even greater instability is found in type B defects of both the ulna and radius. In such cases, the ulna must be treated with a tricortical iliac bone graft, stabilized with a plate using the axial compression principle, and the radius with a wave plate and the compacted bone grafts. The mobility must also start as soon as possible.

Type C Bone Defects

The greatest challenge in forearm bone loss is represented by type C defects (more than 8 cm). In this situation, healing is jeopardized by two factors: first, the length of the defect and, second, vascular compromise, which is very frequent in this kind of lesion. Many have previous complications, such as osteomyelitis and previous surgeries, with scarred surrounding soft tissues offering a poor vascular bed for a conventional graft. The most important decision is whether to keep two bones in the forearm, or just one. This decision depends on the conditions of the muscles and other soft tissues. Patients with the potential for rehabilita-

tion of the pronosupination (distal and proximal radioulnar joint mobility and good muscles) on either the ulna or radius must be treated with a vascularized fibula transplant (keeping two bones). This method has proved to be effective in the reconstruction of the forearm (74–76). When a vascularized fibula is used as a reconstructive technique, it must be stabilized with plates. Using this method, the movement of pronosupination can be preserved, which is the ideal situation. In some cases, the joints are not preserved, and the muscular damage is so extensive that the reconstruction of both bones is not possible. In those cases, one-bone forearm surgery must be considered.

The most difficult cases to treat are type C defects of both ulna and radius; many of these have multiple irreparable nerve lesions that cause loss of sensibility in the hand and soft tissue lesions that lead to muscle dysfunction. Some of these cases benefit from an early amputation, immediate use of a prosthesis, and a vigorous rehabilitation with vocational orientation. However, reconstruction is justified in patients with sensibility in the hand or at least a reparable nerve lesion and muscles available for the restitution of hand and wrist function.

One-Bone Forearm

In patients with type C defects who have no chance of recovery of the pronosupination and have great instability, the goal of the treatment is to obtain stability of the forearm to guarantee the function of the elbow, wrist, and, most important, the hand. The procedure recommended in this situation is a one-bone forearm, which was first published by Hey-Grooves in 1921 (77). It was wrongly described as a "forearm arthrodesis." It is based on the creation of a forearm with a single bone, in which the proximal ulna is united to the distal radius. In this way, forearm stability is achieved, but pronosupination is sacrificed. The benefit of this procedure has been demonstrated in traumatic cases (78,79), in congenital abnormalities (80,81), in sequelae of forearm infections (82,83), and also in patients who have undergone oncologic surgeries in which extensive tumor resections have left great bone defects (84,85). This procedure has been recently proposed for patients with neurologic deficit and forearm deformities (supination contracture) caused by muscular imbalance (86).

Three situations in which the one-bone forearm is considered the appropriate solution are ulnar defects, radial defects, and both bone defects. When the defect is of the ulna, the proximal radius must be osteotomized proximally and mobilized to be fixed to the preserved proximal portion of the ulna

(Fig. 1). Fixation must be accomplished by using a plate. If the defect is of the radius, the process is the opposite, the ulna being osteotomized distally and mobilized to be fixed to the distal preserved portion of the radius. The forearm must be fixed in neutral pronosupination, and the movements of the shoulder compensate for the rotational deficiency.

When performing one-bone forearm, end-to-end or end-to-side bone unions can be performed (Fig. 4).

The one-bone forearm procedure can also be performed when the defect is in both bones. In this situation, it is done by using a vascularized fibula (Fig. 5) (87), especially in those type C cases in which the defect is accompanied by a scarred soft tissue bed and the use of conventional bone graft usually fails.

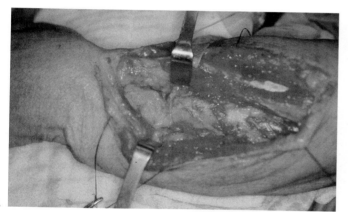
A

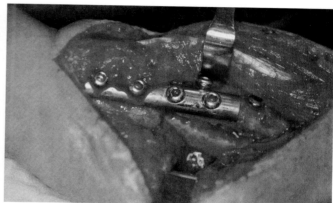
B

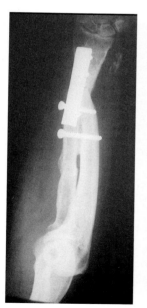
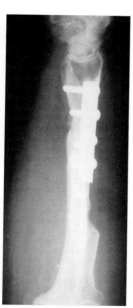
C,D

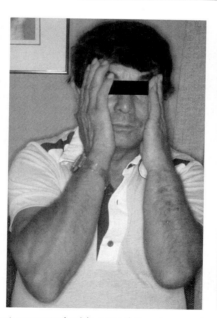

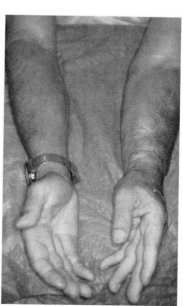
E,F

FIGURE 4. A 47-year-old male patient presented with a recalcitrant nonunion as a sequela of chronic osteomyelitis after a high-energy open fracture of the forearm bones suffered in a car accident. Careful evaluation showed no potential for recovery of pronosupination. **A:** Through a dorsal approach, poor bone conditions were demonstrated on both bones. **B:** A one-bone forearm procedure of an end-to-side union type was performed, and fixation was obtained with plate and screws using the principle of interfragmentary compression. **C,D:** Anteroposterior and lateral radiographs showing solid union. **E,F:** Functional results 6 months after surgery and 2 years of initial injury.

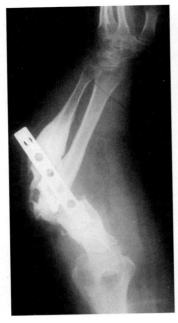
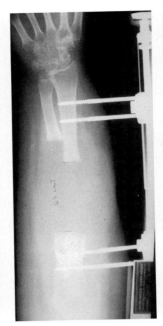
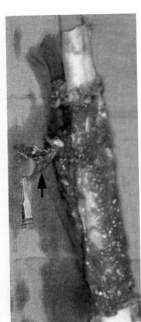

A–C

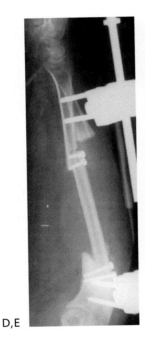
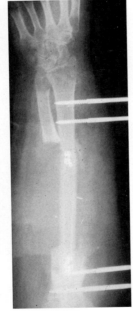

D,E

FIGURE 5. A 52-year-old female patient with a synovial pseudarthrosis who presented after three previous unsuccessful surgeries and 6 months after initial injury suffered in a car accident. **A:** Radiograph shows marked angulation and shortening, with necrotic bone and a failed previous osteosynthesis. **B:** Necrotic bone and osteosynthesis material were removed. During the same operation, a lengthening process was initiated. **C:** Three weeks later, a contralateral fibula was harvested to be used as a vascularized transplant; the black solid arrow indicates the peroneal vessels. **D,E:** A step-cut was performed on the radius and ulna to allow good bone contact with the vascularized fibula. Fixation was performed using screws with the interfragmentary compression principle. A lengthening device was kept as a supplementary immobilization system until the bone showed evidence of consolidation.

In some selected cases with associated defects of radius and ulna but with potential rehabilitation of pronosupination, both bones must be reconstructed. The author recommends vascularized fibula for the ulnar reconstruction and wave plate with the compacted bone grafts for the radius, as previously described.

Vascularized Fibula

Based on Taylor et al.'s proposal of the use of vascularized fibula for reconstruction of limb bone defects (88) and the experience of the last 20 years, this technique has demonstrated its usefulness in extensive long bone defect treatment (89). Even though its most common application has been in the reconstruction of the lower limb, some series report satisfactory results in the upper extremity (90,91). The efficacy of this procedure has been demonstrated by Hurst et al. and Dell and Sheppard in forearm bone defect sequelae of osteomyelitis (75,87). Its benefit has been shown in tumor resection defects, according to Pho (92), and in congenital forearm pseudarthrosis (93).

The procedure is especially indicated in the following situations:

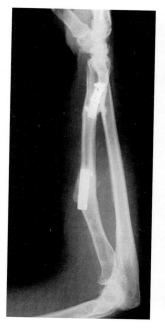
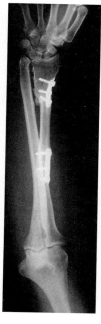
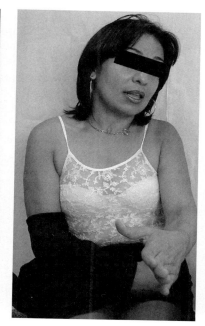
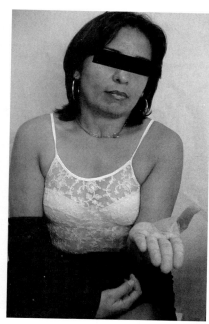

A,B

C,D

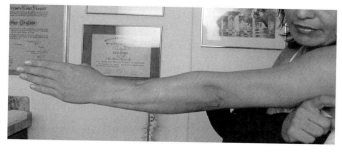

E

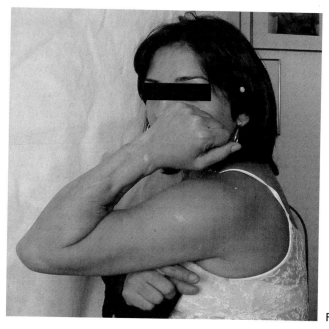

F

FIGURE 6. A 24-year-old woman presented after a gunshot injury, having 8-cm loss from the radius and a soft tissue defect. **A,B:** Radiographic result 6 years after a vascularized, osteocutaneous, fibular free flap. Bone fixation was performed using 3.5-mm plates. **C–F:** Excellent functional and cosmetic results.

- Type C bone defects with poorly vascularized, fibrotic soft tissue, caused by high-energy lesions
- Cases in which conventional bone graft has failed (recalcitrant nonunion)
- Cases that demand energetic early rehabilitation
- Type C defects, products of tumor resection, or sequelae of chronic osteomyelitis
- Congenital pseudoarthrosis of the forearm

In some situations of bone defect associated with soft tissue loss, vascularized fibula can be used as an osteocutaneous free flap to satisfy both deficiencies (Fig. 6).

The rate of successful outcome with this method, from the point of view of bone consolidation, has been calculated at approximately 85%, and the most frequent complications are delayed union, nonunion, sepsis, radial or ulnar nerve palsies in the recipient limb, and peroneal nerve palsy and loss of flexion of the hallux in the donor limb.

With the goal of minimizing the potential complications, the following should be implemented meticulously:

- Thorough evaluation of the forearm vascularity. Pulse or Doppler examinations can be used, and in doubtful cases, an arteriographic assessment must be performed.

- Meticulous preoperative planning, especially in the selection of the most appropriate approach. The volar approach adapts better in many cases, especially because it facilitates the vascular anastomoses.
- Meticulous microsurgical technique to guarantee the patency of the anastomosis.
- Absolute stability is vital. The use of plates is highly recommended. Delayed union and nonunion are related to insufficient stability.
- In the face of any doubt, addition of bone graft is highly recommended.

The reliability of the reconstruction of the forearm with a vascularized fibula transplant is related directly to the experience of the surgeon and the appropriate selection of this technique in the right patient.

Bone Lengthening

In some cases, longitudinal bone deficiencies are accompanied by shortening of the ulna, radius, or both bones, and distraction lengthening has proved to be an effective method of treatment (94,95). It is indicated especially when the shortening is more than 3 cm and dysfunction is present at the wrist or elbow, accompanied by instability and cosmetic deficiency. Figure 7 shows a patient who benefited from progressive distraction followed by a vascularized fibula transplant after multiple unsuccessful surgeries after tumor resections. However, forearm lengthening has been associated with a high rate of complications, such as reflex sympathetic dystrophy, nonunion, nerve irritation, vascular deficiencies, elbow and/or wrist stiffness, pin track infections, and pin hole–related fractures.

With the goal of reducing the risk of complications, it is recommended that these suggestions be followed:

- Pin insertion must be performed very carefully through small incisions to avoid nerve and vascular damage. Daily care of the pins is essential.
- The distraction must not exceed 1 mm per day, and when facing any related complication, the distraction speed must be reduced.
- Bone graft, or vascularized bone transplantation, is highly recommended, once the desired length has been reached.
- Good bone stabilization is essential. Plates are highly recommended.
- The patients must be stimulated to start elbow and wrist movements during the distraction to avoid joint stiffness.

Synostosis

Posttraumatic radioulnar synostosis is a highly disabling complication that is difficult to treat. It can happen at any level of the interosseous membrane, and it consists either of bone bridge formation between the ulna and the radius or of bone contact due to malreduction of fractures, causing cross-union. In either, the interosseous space is occupied by bone tissue, thus blocking the movements of pronation and supination. This problem was first described by Gross as a "vicious union" in 1864 based on results that he found at autopsy.

Any trauma that injures the interosseous membrane or that permits the formation of a hematoma between the two bones can induce a radioulnar synostosis. Radioulnar synostosis has been described in both children and adults, and its incidence is between 2% and 6.6%, according to Vince and Miller and Bauer et al. (96,97).

Risk factors have been described in the development of synostosis (46,96–103) such as the following:

- High-energy trauma with severe soft tissue damage
- Comminuted fractures
- Open fractures
- Fractures of both ulna and radius located at the same level
- Disruption of the interosseous membrane
- Wide surgical dissections, especially in complex fracture reductions
- Large displacements of the bone fragments
- Fracture-related dislocations
- Delayed surgical fixation of forearm fractures
- Long-term immobilization
- Head injuries associated with fractures in polytraumatized patients
- Burn-related trauma

Certain similarities have also been found between this problem and heterotopic ossifications (formation of mature lamellar bone in nonosseous tissues).

Much has been debated about the treatment for synostosis. The basis of the treatment comprises the resection of the abnormal bone union between the ulna and the radius, with interposition of some kind of material to try to avoid recurrence, which happens in approximately 30% of the cases. The most frequently used materials are fatty tissue, cellophane, fascia, and silicone. However, the results have been of variable degrees of success, and none of the publications has analyzed a sufficient number of cases to recommend any specific option.

The following are some important aspects to remember during synostosis surgery to minimize the risk of recurrence:

- Many cases have had previous surgery and must be carefully planned and approached via the previous incisions.
- Careful dissection must be performed to avoid greater stimulation of bone formation.
- Avoid subperiosteal dissection when possible.
- The bone bridge must be totally resected.
- Protection of the neurovascular elements is essential in proximal synostosis because of the risk of damage to the posterior interosseous nerve and the risk of damaging the interosseous artery at any level.

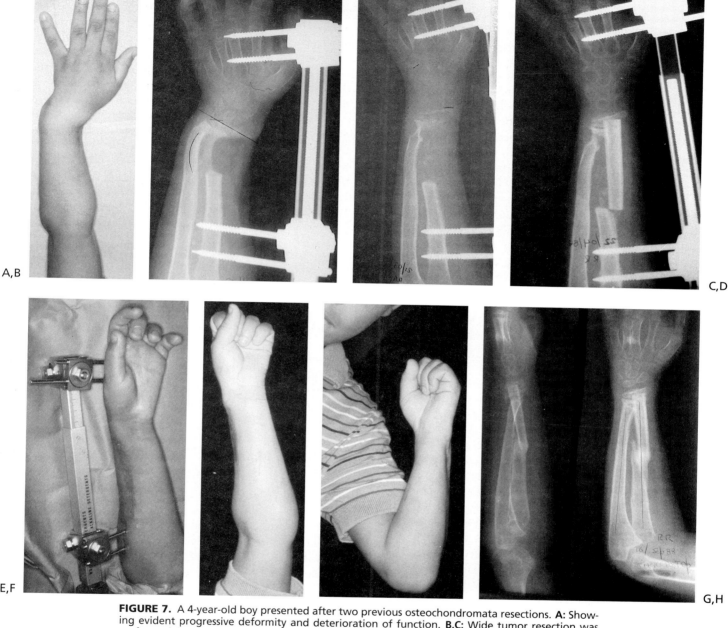

FIGURE 7. A 4-year-old boy presented after two previous osteochondromata resections. **A:** Showing evident progressive deformity and deterioration of function. **B,C:** Wide tumor resection was performed, leaving a considerable bone defect and 4-cm shortening of the radius. A lengthening process was initiated immediately, using the Wagner technique. **D,E:** After 45 days of lengthening, a vascularized fibular procedure was performed. The lengthening device was kept in place until evidence of healing was present radiographically. **F,G:** Clinical results. **H:** Radiographic results.

- An exhaustive and meticulous hemostasis is recommended.
- Simultaneous procedures are not recommended.
- The range of mobility must be determined intraoperatively.
- Energetic rehabilitation must be started immediately after surgery.

Even though these precautions are taken, the risk of recurrence is high, and synostosis can behave like heterotopic ossification, for which reason the use of nonsteroidal antiinflammatory drugs (indomethacin) (103) has been proposed. The mechanism by which these drugs act is unknown, but it has been considered that they may stop the synthesis of prostaglandin E_2. What has certainly been observed is the inhibition of precursor differentiation to osteoblasts while under the influence of these drugs (104). Diphosphonates have also been used; they act by preventing or inhibiting the crystallization of hydroxyapatite, which in turn diminishes the mineralization of osteoid (105). However, its use has been discontinued due to gastrointestinal problems and the production of osteomalacia. Perhaps the most used method to prevent recurrence is radiation in low doses (106–108); its clinical use is based on the prevention of cell proliferation and bone growth in rat femur models (109). Hastings and Graham (110) have recommended a single dose of 700 to 800 cGy administered within 48 to 72 hours of the surgery. It is also important to determine the portal of radiation with great precision.

Another determining factor is the time of surgery. Later surgery is commonly advocated, with the object of allowing the maturation of the ectopic bone formation, thereby decreasing the recurrence rate of synostosis. However, surgery done too late may lead to a contraction of soft tissue, causing limitation of movement (103,107). Other authors recommend early resection followed by postoperative radiation (106–108).

The success in dealing with a radioulnar synostosis depends on an early identification of risk factors, a good knowledge of the pathophysiology and local anatomy, and, most important, well-conducted surgery after the above recommendations. Finally, it is very important to evaluate the needs and expectations of the patient in planning a rational treatment regimen.

Malunion

Malunion is a frequent complication in forearm fractures when treated by nonsurgical means and external immobilization. Maintaining the bone fragments inside the immobilization devices (casts, splints) is difficult, especially because of the transmission of force via the muscular insertions of the biceps brachii, pronator teres, and pronator quadratus. Malunion of the forearm bones associated with long periods of immobilization may cause important limitations of pronosupination, with the consequent inability to perform daily activities of life. In 1945, Evans (38) had already observed the problem of limitation of these movements associated with rotational malunion of forearm fractures, and Patrick (111) in 1946 observed the same problem with angular malunions. Even worse is a combination of both deformities or major angulation of both bones converging to the interosseous space creating impingement. The disastrous results that may follow immobilization treatment of these fractures have previously been mentioned. Some authors, however, insist on this method of treatment, claiming that some degree of deformity is tolerable. The question is how much angulation can be tolerated and still be compatible with a good function. These same authors have demonstrated in a model (112–114) a direct relationship between the angular deformity and the loss of rotation of the forearm. The conclusion is that an almost anatomic reduction (less than 10 degrees of combined deformity of both bones) is needed to guarantee satisfactory function.

The poor results obtained by intramedullary nailing of forearm fractures, especially due to a straightening of the normal anatomic radial bow, which is quintessential to guaranteeing the movements of rotation, have already been mentioned (111,115). Although the results after the use of plating of these fractures are better than the other methods mentioned previously, malunion has also been reported with plate fixation when the surgeon does not have the skills to obtain a precise reduction of the fractures, affecting the final functional result and reducing grip strength (116).

Malunion of metaphyseal forearm fractures associated with dislocations of proximal and distal radioulnar joints (Monteggia's and Galeazzi's injuries, respectively) has been known to have poor results, but this falls outside the scope of this chapter. Malunion of forearm diaphyseal fractures may also be related to distal radioulnar joint instability. Bowers (117) mentions five situations of instability of that joint related to diaphyseal malunion:

1. Radius—malunited fractures with volar apex angulation
2. Radius—malunited fractures with dorsal apex angulation
3. Radius—malunited fractures with medial apex angulation
4. Ulna—malunited fractures with volar apex angulation
5. Malunited fractures with shortening of either of the forearm bones

Each of these situations is consistently associated with incompetence of the joint capsuloligamentous supporting elements (triangular fibrocartilage complex).

From all of these data, one can conclude that restoration of normal skeletal anatomy after forearm lesions is essential to the maintenance of normal function of the upper limb, paying special attention to restoration of rotational movements. Also, in all of these situations in which symptomatic functional limitations are present, affecting the activities of normal daily life, reconstructive procedures are mandatory. These interventions may involve corrective osteotomy to restore the anatomy to its normal form.

These procedures are highly complex, require a detailed knowledge of the normal anatomy, and must be performed with a very precise technique.

The success in dealing with forearm malunion depends on the following recommendations:

■ Meticulous examination of the patient. This is necessary to determine the degree of incapacity, and a discussion with the patient is needed to define individual needs.
■ Determination of the degree of deformity. When only angular malunion is present, conventional comparative anteroposterior and lateral radiographs, showing the elbow and the wrist, are enough to plan the treatment. However, when rotational or combined deformities are present, a comparative computed tomography scan, which must show the biceps tuberosity and the radial styloid as references, is needed to quantify the deformity.
■ Meticulous preoperative planning using information obtained by the previous studies. It is important to anticipate the type of osteotomy and any bone graft needs.

- Osteotomy stabilization using plating and following the AO principles.
- Early energetic rehabilitation.

APPROACHES

Q: Which approach should be used in forearm reconstruction?

A: The approach depends on the bone and is determined by the soft tissue surrounding it.

Often, the approaches for forearm reconstruction are determined by the extent and location of the soft tissue lesions. The following approaches may be used:

- Usually, the radius can be approached dorsolaterally, especially when the defect is located in the middle third. This approach is not recommended when the lesion is located in the proximal third because it has risk of damaging the radial nerve; it also is not recommended when the lesion is distal due to the possible interference with the gliding surface of the extensor tendons. The preferred approach for the radius is volar, as described by Henry (118). This is a very anatomic route that allows exposure of the whole radius from proximal to distal, and it offers the flat side, which makes the plating much easier. Also, the radial artery and the comitant veins can be dissected in cases of vascularized fibula transplantation for radius reconstruction. The median nerve can also be repaired through this approach.
- The ulna can be completely exposed via the dorsomedial approach using a straight incision; however, a volar approach can also be used, especially for more distal defects. The approach should be between the ulnar artery and nerve and flexor carpi ulnaris medially and the flexor tendons and medial nerve laterally.
- When trying to reconstruct both bones, two well-separated incisions are recommended to avoid skin necrosis. Trying to reconstruct both bones with a single incision may increase considerably the risk of radioulnar synostosis and nerve lesions (96,97).

Q: What rehabilitation protocol is recommended?

A: The early start of movement depends on the degree of stability obtained with the osteosynthesis.

Postoperative Treatment

From the first day, the operated arm must be kept elevated while the patient is motivated to perform active digital movements. In cases in which the osteosynthesis is stable, the postoperative treatment is totally functional, allowing the patient to move the elbow and the wrist and especially encouraging the movements of forearm rotation. This protocol helps prevent radioulnar synostosis and joint stiffness. In cases in which the stability is doubtful, especially in cases

of osteoporosis or extensive bone loss, immobilization for 4 or 5 weeks is recommended using a volar splint or a sugar-tong splint.

AMPUTATION

Amputation of the forearm and the use of prostheses can be the best option in severe lesions in which not even modern reconstructive methods can provide the functional recovery needed for daily activities. Fortunately, the modern prostheses can provide the basic functions, and they can certainly satisfy the esthetic aspect. The surgeon must offer this option as the best way to be reincorporated into social and productive activities, especially in the unfortunate situation in which the disability negatively affects the patient. The amputee must be treated by a multidisciplinary team with enough experience with these types of patients. There are now units that specialize in these matters. In these institutes, they have resources and strategies that can provide patients with a functional recovery and help them through the emotional experience of losing a limb (119). The amputee must be the center of attention of a team comprising physiatrists, occupational therapists, physical therapists, prosthetists, psychologists, and vocational rehabilitation counselors. However, amputations have a higher incidence in young, working adult males and most frequently affect the dominant hand because the lesions are work related (120,121). Finally, it is important to emphasize that the results in these patients must be measured in terms of community interrelations, emotional adaptation, and the level of functional recovery.

Amputation Surgery

The success of amputation surgery depends on the following:

- The maximum length possible must be preserved to maximize pronosupination (122–124).
- Both flaps must be of the same length and must be designed distal to the amputation level in the bone to permit the cover of the stump.
- The nerve ends must be buried deep in the muscle tissues to avoid troublesome neuromata.
- The use of pneumatic tourniquets is recommended; the ulnar and radial arteries must be ligated and the interosseous vessels cauterized. At the end of the surgery, the tourniquet is released, and hemostasis is performed to avoid hematomas. Suction drainage is recommended.
- The bone ends must be rounded off to avoid irritation of the overlying skin.
- The skin flaps must close without tension to avoid necrosis or delayed healing. Excessive soft tissue bulk of the stump can interfere with the fit of the prosthesis.
- Elastic bandages are recommended to avoid edema.

- Early movement is recommended to avoid joint stiffness and contractures.

The goal of the amputation surgery must be focused on crafting a good stump with the following characteristics:

- More cylindrical than conical
- Full-thickness, mobile soft tissue cover over bone ends
- Free of pain

All of these features must be achieved to adapt better to the new socket types and prosthesis designs.

Once the amputation is done, the logical option is the use of a prosthesis, and even though this field continues to evolve rapidly, offering better designs almost daily, the problem of sensibility remains unanswered. The distinction between coldness and warmth and light and coarse touch and the ability to appreciate textures and to identify the size and shape of objects, also known as *stereognosis*, at a cerebral cortical level, is a phenomenon that cannot be replaced by any artificial hand available at this time. This means that patients wearing prostheses must use sight as a poor substitute. The problem is magnified when the patient is in the dark or when the patient has impaired vision. A possible solution to this problem is the procedure described by Krukenberg in 1919, which consists in dividing the forearm into two stumps, a radial stump and an ulnar stump, and transforming the forearm into two "fingers" or "lobster claws" (forearm digitalization). Those stumps are moved by the pronator teres muscle. Much has been debated in the literature about the indications for the procedure (125,126), and one can conclude that the only strong indication is in blind patients with bilateral forearm amputations, such as mine explosion victims. However, it may be practiced in patients with normal sight. When the procedure is performed on the dominant limb, sight is not needed, and patients can perform tasks in the dark. This method does not preclude the use of a standard prosthesis. De Santolo (127,128) has extended his indications by proposing the adaptation of a special design of prosthesis that is moved by the two stumps. The major criticism of the Krukenberg procedure is the somewhat grotesque appearance of the limb. A detailed description of the technique and its modification has been published by Nathan and Trung (129) and Swanson and Swanson (126).

Prosthesis

There has been much debate on the subject of the ideal time when the patient should initiate the use of a prosthesis after a forearm amputation, but in amputations below the elbow, as at other levels, the immediate use of a provisional prosthesis is undoubtedly beneficial. This provisional prosthesis can be either body-powered or myoelectric (130). The specific benefits of this strategy are the following:

- There is better control of edema.
- There is promotion of the healing process of the wounds.
- There is reduction of pain.
- There is acceleration of the rehabilitation process.
- The amputee has the optimal opportunity of becoming a good prosthesis user after early fitting and training.

Approximately 3 to 4 weeks after ablation, after the wounds show evidence of healing, is the time to choose the definite prosthesis. Among the current, available options, the following are worthy of mention:

- Purely cosmetic prosthesis
- Passive-hand prosthesis
- Body-powered prosthesis
- Myoelectric hand
- Electrically powered type

The selection of the most appropriate prosthesis depends on the patient's wishes and needs. The body-powered prosthesis is the most-used design around the world (119,131). This prosthesis is mostly recommended for patients whose jobs require heavy activity, such as carpenters, mechanics, gardeners, or those who participate in sports activities. This design has proved to be the longest-lasting, lightest, most affordable, and, in general terms, simplest for training purposes. However, it has some disadvantages, including the following: (a) There is more exaggerated movement of the body, especially the shoulder girdle (by scapular abduction and humeral flexion), to activate the hook; (b) it requires a more complex harnessing system; and (c) the cosmetic appearance (perhaps the greatest disadvantage).

Alternatively, the myoelectric prostheses provide more power, are more esthetic, and require less harnessing; however, they are much more expensive, they are heavier, their maintenance is more complex, and optimal contact between the skin of the stump and the socket is required, particularly at the level of the electrodes. In these prostheses, patients must learn to moderate the tension of the muscles in the stump to stimulate the electrodes and trigger the electrical impulses that drive the motor of the prosthesis and create the desired movement. Generally, patients expect much better results than the prosthesis is capable of providing. This has been strongly influenced by modern cinema and the media, in which an amputee, such as Robocop, is able to perform amazing feats. In relation to the fitting of the stump to the socket, it is clear that thermoplastic materials and modern techniques offer advantages, especially in comfort and stability.

Passive cosmetic prostheses are the lightest. They satisfy esthetic expectations; it is now possible to simulate color, shape, and details of the limb, which transforms them into virtual works of art. However, they are also the most expensive, shortest-lasting, and least functional. For these reasons many of them end up in a closet.

In conclusion, each day, new hybrid designs are seen that combine the best characteristics of the different types of prostheses, with the goal of offering a prosthesis that satisfies all of the patient's wishes and needs. A detailed analysis of the advantages and disadvantages can be found in the publication of Esquenazi and collaborators (132).

In the process of determining the best option available, the patient must be informed of the advantages and disadvantages of each design and should also share the experiences of other amputees. Success depends on the most appropriate selection for each individual. Whichever type of prosthesis is selected, the outcome depends on the training and the periodic visits to a specialized center for amputees. To evaluate the functional success of the prosthesis, it is recommended that the following checklist be used, as proposed by Meier (133), which serves as a guide to define the achievable goals:

- Dons and doffs the prosthesis independently
- Is independent in the activities of daily living
- Can write legibly with the remaining hand
- Has comfortably switched dominance if necessary
- Drives a motor car
- Has returned to work (same or modified occupation)
- Can tie shoelaces with one hand
- Uses a button hook easily
- Can prepare a meal in the kitchen
- Has been shown adaptive equipment for kitchen and activities of daily living
- Has performed carpentry and automotive maintenance (if desired)
- Wears prosthesis during all waking hours
- Uses prosthesis for bimanual activities representing at least 25% of activities

Dealing with severe forearm lesions always presents a challenge that obliges us to use all our knowledge, skills, and experience to achieve a good reconstruction.

The success of the outcome in severe forearm lesion relies on the influence of the following "ten commandments":

1. Prior determination of patient needs
2. Meticulous preoperative planning
3. Prior evaluation of neurologic status of the limb
4. Prior evaluation of the vascular status of the limb
5. Precise evaluation of soft tissue condition
6. Evaluation of the bone condition and magnitude of any defect
7. Bone stabilization
8. Amputation considered as a last resort
9. Early use of prosthesis (when amputation is done)
10. Early energetic rehabilitation

The main goal of forearm reconstruction is to return the patient as soon as possible to occupational, recreational, and social activities with the minimal socioeconomic repercussions.

REFERENCES

1. Almquist EA. Evolution of the distal radioulnar joint. *Clin Orthop* 1992;275:5–13.
2. Linscheid RL. Biomechanics of the distal radioulnar joint. *Clin Orthop* 1992;275:46–55.
3. Ralston EL. *Handbook of fractures.* St. Louis: Mosby, 1967.
4. Sage FP. Fractures of the shaft of the radius and ulna in adult. In: Adams JP, ed. *Current practice in orthopaedic surgery,* vol. 1. St. Louis: Mosby, 1963.
5. Watson-Jones R. *Fractures and joint injuries,* vol. 1, 4th ed. Edinburgh: E&S Livingstone, 1952.
6. Sage FP. Medullary fixation of fractures of the forearm. A study of the medullary canal of the radius and a report of fifty fractures of the radius treated with a pre-bent triangular nail. *J Bone Joint Surg Am* 1959;41:1489–1516.
7. Weibrecht J. *Syndesmologia sive historia ligamentorum corporis humani, quam secundum observationes anatomicas concinnavit, et figuris and objecta resentía abumbratis illustravit.* Petropoli: Academy of Sciences, 1742.
8. Poirier P, Charpy A. *Traité d'anatomie humaine.* Paris: Masson, 1899.
9. Winslow JB. *Exposition anatomique de la structure du corps humain,* 2nd ed. Amsterdam: 1746.
10. Boyes M. *Traité complet d'anatomie ou description de toules les parties du corp humain.* Paris: Migneret, 1815.
11. Rouviére H. *Anatomie humaine descriptive et topographique,* vol. 2, 3rd ed. Paris: Masson, 1932.
12. Bichart MFX. *Traité d'anatomie descriptive.* Paris: Goben & Cie, 1801–1803.
13. Gerdy PN. *Physiologie medicale didactique et critique.* Paris: Crochard, 1833.
14. Cruveilhier J. *Traité d'anatomie descriptive,* 4th ed. Paris: 1862.
15. Testut L. *Traité d'anatomie humaine.* Paris: Octave Doin, 1893.
16. Epner RA, Boyes WH, Gilford WB. Ulnar variance: the effect of wrist position and roentgen filming technique. *J Hand Surg [Am]* 1982;7:298.
17. Palmer AK, Glisson RR, Werner FW. Ulnar variance determination. *J Hand Surg [Am]* 1982;7:376.
18. Gregory RT, Gould RJ, Peclet M, et al. The mangled extremity syndrome (M.E.S): a severity grading system for multisystem injury to the extremity. *J Trauma* 1985;25:1147–1150.
19. Howe HR, Poole GV, Hansen KJ, et al. Salvage of lower extremities following combined orthopaedic and vascular trauma: a predictive salvage index. *Am J Surg* 1987;53:205–208.
20. Johansen K, Daines M, Howie T, et al. *Objective criteria for amputation after lower extremity trauma.* Paper presented at Orthopaedic Trauma Association annual meeting, Dallas, Oct. 27–29, 1988.
21. Caudle RJ, Stern PJ. Severe open fractures of the tibia. *J Bone Joint Surg Am* 1987;69:801–807.
22. Hansen ST. The type III-C fracture: salvage or amputation [editorial]. *J Bone Joint Surg Am* 1988;69:799–800.
23. Omer GE. Amputation. In: Hunter JM, ed. *Rehabilitation of the hand.* St. Louis: Mosby, 1978:541–573.
24. McGregor IA, Jackson IT. The groin flap. *Br J Plast Surg* 1972;25:3.

25. McGregor IA, Morgan G. Axial and random pattern flap. *Br J Plast Surg* 1973;26:202–213.

26. Song R, Gao Y, Song Y, et al. The forearm flap. *Clin Plast Surg* 1982;9:21.

27. Muhlbauer W, Herndl E, Stock W. The forearm flap. *Plast Reconstr Surg* 1982;70:336–340.

28. Penteato CV, Masquelat AC, Chevrel JP. The anatomic basis of the fascio-cutaneous flap of the posterior interosseous artery. *Surg Radio Anat* 1986;8:209–215.

29. Zancolli EA, Angrigianni C. Colgajo dorsal del antebrazo (en "Isla" con pediculos de vasos interoseos posteriores). *Rev Assoc Arg Ortop Traumat* 1986;51:161–168.

30. Godina M, Lister G. Early microsurgical reconstruction of complex trauma of the extremities. *Plast Reconstr Surg* 1986;78:285.

31. Tansini I. Sopra il mio nuovo processo di amputazione della mamella. *Riforma Medica* 1906;12:757; *Gas Med Ital* 1906;57:141.

32. Magnuson PB. Mechanics of treatment of fractures of the forearm. *JAMA* 1922;78:789–794.

33. Buxton JD. Discussion of the treatment of fractures of the forearm, excluding fractures of the olecranon and those of the lower end of the radius of the Colles type. *J R Soc Med* 1025;19:17–30.

34. Buxton JD. Treatment of closed fractures of the radius and ulna. *BMJ* 1939;2:795–799.

35. Bagley CH. Fracture of both bones of the forearm. *Surg Gynecol Obstet* 1926;42:95–102.

36. Eliason EL, Brown RB, Kaplan L. Fractures of the forearm—except Colles. *Am J Surg* 1937;38:511–525.

37. Carrell WB. Fractures of both bones of the forearm excluding those at the elbow joint and wrist joint. *Surg Gynecol Obstet* 1938;66:506–511.

38. Evans EM. Rotational deformities in the treatment of fractures of both bones of the forearm. *J Bone Joint Surg* 1945;27:373–379.

39. Compere EL. The treatment of fractures of both bones of the forearm. *Surg Clin North Am* 1948;25:48–58.

40. Bolton H, Quinlan AG. The conservative treatment of fractures of the shaft of the radius and ulna in adults. *Lancet* 1952;1:700–705.

41. Hughston JD. Fractures of the distal radial shaft, mistakes in management. *J Bone Joint Surg Am* 1957;39:249–264.

42. Charnley J. *Closed treatment of common fractures*, 3rd ed. Edinburgh: Livingstone, 1961.

43. Böhler J. *Treatment of fractures*. Bristol, England: Wright, 1936.

44. Smith H, Sage FP. Medullary fixation of forearm fractures. *J Bone Joint Surg Am* 1957;39:91–98.

45. Danis R. *Théorie et pratique de l'ostéosynthése*. Paris: Masson, 1979.

46. Anderson LD, Sish TD, Tooms RE, et al. Compression plate fixation in acute diaphyseal fractures of radius and ulna. *J Bone Joint Surg Am* 1975;57:287–297.

47. Hadden WA, Reschauer R, Seggl W. Results of AO plate fixation of forearm shaft fractures in adults. *Injury* 1983;15:44–52.

48. Tile M, Petrie D. Fractures of the radius and ulna. *J Bone Joint Surg Br* 1969;51:193.

49. Knight RA, Pulvis GD. Fracture of both bones of the forearm in adults. *J Bone Joint Surg Am* 1949;31:755–764.

50. Naiman PT, Schein AJ, Siffert RS. Use of ASIF compression plates in selected shaft fractures of the upper extremity. A preliminary report. *Clin Orthop* 1970;71:208–216.

51. Dodge HS, Cady GW. Treatment of fractures of the radius and ulna with compression plates. A retrospective study of one hundred and nineteen fractures in seventy-eight patients. *J Bone Joint Surg Am* 1972;54:1167–1176.

52. Anderson LD, Sisk TD, Tooms RE, et al. Compression-plate fixation in acute diaphyseal fractures of the radius and ulna. *J Bone Joint Surg Am* 1975;57:287–297.

53. Grace TG, Eversmann WW Jr. The management of segmental bone loss associated with forearm fractures. *J Bone Joint Surg Am* 1976;58:283–214.

54. Teipner WA, Mast JW. Internal fixation of forearm fractures: double plating verses single compression (tension band) plating—a comparative study. *Orthop Clin North Am* 1980;11:381–391.

55. Chapman MW, Gordon JE, Zissimos AG. Compression plate fixation of acute fractures of the diaphysis of the radius and ulna. *J Bone Joint Surg Am* 1989;71:159–169.

56. Smith H, Sage FP. Medullary fixation of forearm fractures. *J Bone Joint Surg Am* 1957;39:91–98.

57. Sage FP. Medullary fixation of fractures of the forearm: a study of the medullary canal of the radius and a report on 50 fractures of the radius treated with a pre-bend triangular nail. *J Bone Joint Surg Am* 1982;64:857–863.

58. Caden JG. Internal fixation of fractures of the forearm. *J Bone Joint Surg Am* 1961;43:1115–1121.

59. Street DM. Intramedullary forearm nailing. *Clin Orthop* 1986;212:219–230.

60. Jinking WJ, Lockhart LD, Eggers GWN. Fracture of the forearm in adults. *South Med J* 1960;53:669–679.

61. Baker GI, Burkhalter WE, Barclay WA, et al. Treatment of forearm shaft fractures by long slotted plates. *J Bone Joint Surg Am* 1969;51:1035.

62. Muller ME, Allgower M, Willenegger H. *Technique of internal fixation of fractures*. New York: Springer-Verlag, 1965.

63. Mast J, Jakob R, Ganz R. *Planning and reduction technique in fracture surgery*. Berlin: Springer-Verlag, 1989.

64. Weber BG, Cech O. *Pseudarthrosis pathophysiology, biomechanics, therapy, results*. Bern: Huber, 1976.

65. Schenk RK, Muller ME, Willenegger H. [Experimental histological contribution to the development and treatment of pseudarthrosis.] *Hefte Unfallheilkd* 1968;94:15–24.

66. Rüedi TP, Murphy WM. *AO principles of fracture management*. Stuttgart: Thieme, 2000.

67. Barth H. Histologische Untersuchungen uber Knochentransplantation. *Beitr Path Anat Allg Path* 1895;17:65–142.

68. Phemister DB. The fate of transplanted bone and regenerative power of various constituents. *Surg Gynecol Obstet* 1914;19:303–333.

69. Enneking WF, Burchardt H, Puhl JJ, et al. Physical and biological aspects of repair in dog cortical bone transplants. *J Bone Joint Surg Am* 1975;57:237–251.

70. Goldberg VM, Stevenson S, Shaffer JW. Bone and cartilage allografts: biology and clinical application. In: Friedlander GE, ed. *Biology of autografts and allografts*. Park Ridge, Ill.: American Academy of Orthopaedic Surgeons, 1989.

71. Freeland AE. Hand fractures. *Repair, reconstruction, and rehabilitation*. New York: Churchill Livingstone, 2000.

72. Weber BG. *Special techniques in internal fixation.* Berlin: Springer-Verlag, 1981.

73. Nuñez FA, et al. Tratamiento de las pseudoartrosis del antebrazo con utilización de la placa en onda más autoinjerto óseo. *Rev Venez Cir Mano* 1999;1:63–69.

74. Olekas J, Guobys A. Vascularised bone transfer for defects and pseudarthroses of the forearm bones. *J Hand Surg [Br]* 1991;16:406–408.

75. Hurst LC, Mirza MA, Spellman W. Vascularized fibular graft for infected loss of the ulna: case report. *J Hand Surg [Am]* 1982;7:498–501.

76. Weiland A, Moore JR, Daniel RK. Vascularized bone autografts, experience with 41 cases. *Clin Orthop* 1983;174:87–95.

77. Hey-Groves EW, ed. *Modern methods of treating fractures*, 2nd ed. Bristol, England: John Wright & Sons, 1921:320–323.

78. Murray RA. The one-bone forearm: a reconstructive procedure. *J Bone Joint Surg Am* 1955;37:366–370.

79. Castle ME. One-bone forearm. *J Bone Joint Surg Am* 1974;56:1223–1227.

80. Vitale CC. Reconstructive surgery for defects in the shaft of the ulna in children. *J Bone Joint Surg Am* 1952;34:804–809.

81. Rodgers WB, Hall JE. One-bone forearm as a salvage procedure for recalcitrant forearm deformity in hereditary multiple exostoses. *J Pediatr Orthop* 1993;13:587–591.

82. Greenwood HH. Reconstruction of forearm after loss of radius. *Br J Surg* 1932;20:58–60.

83. Jones RW. Reconstruction of the forearm after loss of the radius. *Br J Surg* 1934;22:23–26.

84. Reid RL, Baker GI. The single-bone forearm—a reconstructive technique. *Hand* 1973;5:214–219.

85. Haddad RJ, Drez D. Salvage procedures for defects in the forearm bones. *Clin Orthop* 1974;104:183–190.

86. Wang AA, Hutchinson DT, Coleman DA. One bone forearm fusion for pediatric supination contracture due to neurologic deficit. *J Hand Surg [Am]* 2001;26:611–616.

87. Dell PC, Sheppard JE. Vascularized bone grafts in the treatment of infected forearm nonunions. *J Hand Surg [Am]* 1984;9:653–658.

88. Taylor GI, Miller GDH, Ham FJ. The free vascularized bone graft: a clinical extension of microvascular techniques. *Plast Reconstr Surg* 1975;55:533–544.

89. Wood MB, Cooney WP III, Irons GB Jr. Skeletal reconstruction by vascularized bone transfer: indications and results. *Mayo Clin Proc* 1985;60:729–734.

90. Wood MB. Upper extremity reconstruction by vascularized bone transfers: results and complications. *J Hand Surg [Am]* 1987;12:422–427.

91. Weiland AJ, Kleinert HE, Kutz JE, et al. Free vascularized bone grafts in surgery of the upper extremity. *J Hand Surg [Am]* 1979;4:129–144.

92. Pho RWH. Free vascularized fibular transplant for replacement of the lower radius. *J Bone Joint Surg Br* 1979;61:362–365.

93. Allieu Y, Gomis R, Yoshimura M, et al. Congenital pseudarthrosis of the forearm—two cases treated by free vascularized fibular graft. *J Hand Surg [Am]* 1981;6:475–481.

94. Cheng JCY. Distraction lengthening of the forearm. *J Hand Surg [Br]* 1991;16:441–445.

95. Lamoureux J, Verstreken L. Progressive upper limb lengthening in children: a report of two cases. *J Pediatr Orthop* 1986;6:481–485.

96. Vince KG, Miller JE. Cross-union complicating fracture of the forearm. Part I: adults. *J Bone Joint Surg Am* 1987;69:640–652.

97. Bauer G, Arand M, Mutschler W. Post-traumatic radioulnar synostosis after forearm fracture osteosynthesis. *Arch Orthop Trauma Surg* 1991;110:142–145.

98. Botting TDJ. Post-traumatic radio-ulnar cross-union. *J Trauma* 1970;10:16–24.

99. Watson FM Jr., Eaton RG. Post-traumatic radio-ulnar synostosis. *J Trauma* 1978;18:467–468.

100. Garland DE, Dowling V. Forearm fractures in the head-injured adult. *Clin Orthop* 1983;176:190–196.

101. Maempel FZ. Post-traumatic radioulnar synostosis. A report of two cases. *Clin Orthop* 1984;186:182–185.

102. Breit R. Post-traumatic radioulnar synostosis. *Clin Orthop* 1983;174:149–152.

103. Jupiter JB. Heterotopic ossification about the elbow. In: *Instructional course lectures*, vol. XL. American Academy of Orthopaedic Surgeons, 1991.

104. Rosenoer LML, Gonsalves MR, Roberts WE. Indomethacin inhibition of preosteoblast differentiation associated with mechanically induced osteogenesis. *Trans Orthop Res Soc* 1989;14:64.

105. Russel R, Fleisch H. Pyrophosphate and diphosphonates in skeletal metabolism. *Clin Orthop* 1975;108:241.

106. Abrams RA, Simmons BP, Brown RA. Treatment of post-traumatic radioulnar synostosis with excision and low-dose radiation. *J Hand Surg [Am]* 1993;18:703–707.

107. Cullen JP, Pellegrini VD, Miller RJ, et al. Treatment of traumatic synostosis by excision and postoperative low-dose irradiation. *J Hand Surg [Am]* 1994;19:394–401.

108. Failla JM, Amadio PC, Morrey BF. Post-traumatic proximal radio-ulnar synostosis: results of surgical treatment. *J Bone Joint Surg Am* 1989;69:1208–1213.

109. Tonna EA, Cronkite EP. Autoradiographic studies of cell proliferation in the periosteum of intact and fractured femoral of mice utilizing DNA labeling with H3 thymidine. *Proc Soc Exp Biol Med* 1961;107:719.

110. Hastings H, Graham TJ. The classification and treatment of heterotopic ossification about the elbow and forearm. *Hand Clin* 1994;10:417–437.

111. Patrick J. A study of supination and pronation, with especial reference to the treatment of forearm fractures. *J Bone Joint Surg Br* 1946;28:737–748.

112. Matthews LS, Kaufer H, Garver DF, et al. The effect on supination-pronation of angular malalignment of fractures of both bones of the forearm. An experimental study. *J Bone Joint Surg Am* 1982;64:14–17.

113. Sarmiento A, Ebramzadeh E, Brys D, et al. Angular deformities and forearm function. *J Orthop Res* 1992;10:121–133.

114. Tarr RR, Garfinkel AL, Sarmiento A. The effects of angular and rotational deformities of both bones of the forearm. *J Bone Joint Surg Am* 1984;66:65–70.

115. Sage FP. Medullary fixation of fractures of the forearm: a study of the medullary canal of the radius and a report on 50 fractures of the radius treated with a pre-bend triangular nail. *J Bone Joint Surg Am* 1982;64:857–863.

116. Schemitsch EH, Richards RH. The effect of malunion on functional outcome after plate fixation of fractures of both bones of the forearm in adults. *J Bone Joint Surg Am* 1992;74:1068–1078.

117. Bowers WH. Instability of the distal radioulnar articulation. *Hand Clin* 1991;7:311–327.

118. Henry AK. *Exposures of long bones and other surgical methods.* Bristol, England: John Wright, 1927.

119. Meier RH. Amputation and prosthetic fitting. In: Fisher SV, Helm PA, eds. *Comprehensive rehabilitation of burns.* Baltimore: Williams & Wilkins, 1984.

120. Kay HW, Newman JD. Relative incidences of new amputations: statistical comparisons of 6,000 new amputees. *Orthot Prosthet* 1975;29:3.

121. Glattly HW. A statistical study of 12,000 new amputees. *South Med J* 1964;57:1373.

122. Stack HG. Amputations. In: Rob C, Smith R, Pulvertaft G, eds. *Operative surgery: the hand*, 3rd ed. London: Butterworths, 1977:353.

123. Tooms RE. Amputation surgery in the upper extremity. *Orthop Clin North Am* 1972;3:383–395.

124. Tooms RE. Amputations through upper extremity. In: Edmonson AS, Crenshaw AH, eds. *Campbell's operative orthopaedics*, 6th ed. St. Louis: Mosby, 1980:857–867.

125. Swanson AB. The Krukenberg procedure in the juvenile amputee. *J Bone Joint Surg Am* 1964;46:1540–1548.

126. Swanson AB, Swanson GD. The Krukenberg procedure in the juvenile amputee. *Clin Orthop* 1980;148:55–61.

127. De Santolo A. A new approach to the use of the Krukenberg procedure in unilateral wrist amputations. An original functional-cosmetic prosthesis. *Bull Hosp Jt Dis Orthop Inst* 1984;44:177–187.

128. De Santolo A. *La digitalización del antebrazo (Krukenberg) nueva prótesis funcional-cosmetica. Monogram.* Caracas: 1982.

129. Nathan PA, Trung NB. The Krukenberg operation: a modified technique avoiding skin grafts. *J Hand Surg [Am]* 1977;2:127–130.

130. Malone JM, Childers SJ, Underwood J, et al. Immediate postsurgical management of upper extremity amputation: conventional, electric and myoelectric prosthesis. *Orthot Prosthet* 1981;35:1.

131. Fryer CM. Body powered components. In: Bowler JH, Michael JW, eds. *Atlas of limb prosthetics: surgical, prosthetic and rehabilitation principles*, 2nd ed. St. Louis: Mosby, 1992.

132. Esquenazi A, Leonard JA, Meier RH, et al. Prosthetics, orthotics, and assistive devices. 3. Prosthetics. *Arch Phys Med Rehabil* 1989;70(Suppl):206–209.

133. Meier RH. Upper limb prosthetic: dosing, prescription, and application. In: Peiner CA, ed. *Surgery of the hand and upper extremity.* New York: McGraw-Hill, 1996.

99

TUMORS: GENERAL PRINCIPLES

EDWARD A. ATHANASIAN

The optimal treatment of bone and soft tissue tumors of the hand and forearm requires disease-specific knowledge as well as a thorough understanding of the principles of patient evaluation and management. Knowledge of general treatment principles should be considered part of the complete and required preparation for the care of a given patient, as it helps to achieve the best possible outcome. Lack of preparation can result in inadequate treatment, which has implications not only for the patient's limb, but also for the patient's life in the event of a malignant diagnosis.

The efforts of the hand surgeon usually focus on preservation or restoration of function and the appearance of the hand. When treating primary malignant tumors, the focus must be eradication of the disease. Within the context of the malignant potential of the disease, concerns of patient function and reconstruction must be given secondary consideration. An elegant reconstruction may be useless in the setting of a local recurrence that may be the result of insufficient resection. At times, a two-team approach may be best, with a resection team concentrating on eradication and a reconstruction team responsible for reconstruction. This helps the surgeon performing the resection avoid the temptation to spare functional tissues at the risk of leaving residual disease. The reader is encouraged to frequently review the principles of evaluation, diagnosis, biopsy, and treatment on a regular basis. This is most important when caring for a patient with a malignant tumor.

PATIENT ASSESSMENT

History

A thorough history and physical examination remain the cornerstones of initial patient assessment. The patient should be asked the duration of symptoms, swelling, or mass. A history of pain or recent growth may give information regarding the aggressive potential of the lesion. It is important to remember that soft tissue sarcomas are often painless. These lesions may be present for long periods with little or no growth. History of exposure to radiation, herbicides, or other carcinogens may help in generating a differ-

ential diagnosis (1,2). The family history may provide insight into hereditary diseases or genetic syndromes that predispose to sarcoma.

Physical Examination

Physical examination includes the assessment of the lesion in question, including swelling, color, size, warmth, consistency, tenderness, mobility, and proximity to fascia, tendons, nerves, and vessels. Transillumination can demonstrate fluid or myxomatous tissue, as seen with a ganglion or soft tissue myxoma. The location of the lesion is important in formulating a differential diagnosis. If a diagnosis of ganglion cyst is considered, the lesion should be in a typical or well-described location. An unusual location should raise the suspicion of an alternate diagnosis. The nerve and blood supply to the hand should be carefully assessed. Allen's testing has important implications for the use of pedicle flaps during reconstruction. Regional lymph nodes should be initially assessed by palpation and, subsequently, with radiographic studies or biopsy, if indicated.

Radiographs

Plain x-ray remains the most specific test for developing a differential diagnosis of bone lesions and should be obtained during the assessment of nearly all bone and soft tissue tumors. Calcifications present in soft tissue tumors may aid in making a diagnosis. Phleboliths aid in the diagnosis of a soft tissue hemangioma. Plain x-rays of soft tissue sarcomas may demonstrate calcifications and, more important, may give the first sign of bone invasion. Chest x-rays may demonstrate a primary tumor or metastasis from an extremity lesion and should be done when suspicion of malignancy is high or after malignancy has been documented.

Computed tomography (CT) is particularly useful in determining the cortical integrity of bone lesions. High-resolution or thin cut sections may aid in localizing an occult osteoid osteoma. CT scans are necessary for systemic staging, as most bone and soft tissue sarcomas metastasize to the lungs when metastasis occurs. Axillary lymph nodes can also be assessed on chest CT scan.

Radioisotope bone scan may give insight into bone turnover in lesions but has limited benefit in predicting aggressiveness of the lesion under consideration. It is most useful for systemic staging when trying to identify other lesions in the bony skeleton and should be done for all primary bone sarcomas and may be considered for soft tissue sarcomas, as these can spread to bone.

The value of magnetic resonance imaging (MRI) is dependent on the quality of the study obtained. A high-quality MRI can demonstrate the pathologic local anatomy in exquisite detail. This is particularly beneficial in determining the local extent of disease and in planning surgical resection. MRI is less specific than plain x-ray for bone lesions but may be useful in confirming or narrowing the differential diagnosis. It is important for the ordering physician to be certain that the appropriate equipment, personnel, and expertise are available to obtain the information desired from the study. A dedicated wrist and hand coil and closed machine may yield higher-quality images. The entire lesion must be imaged. Either sagittal or coronal images are needed to rule out proximal skip metastasis for malignant bone lesions. Axial images through at least one adjacent joint are imperative to localize the lesion within the anatomic region. This aids in preoperative planning of bone transection sites during resection and while using clinical landmarks during surgery. Axial T1-weighted images are particularly useful for determining the relation of the lesion to large vessels and nerves. This information has implications for whether a lesion can be resected.

Ultrasound can be useful for the identification and delineation of fluid-filled structures. This test may be most useful in the low-cost detection of suspected occult ganglia. Aspiration, injection, and even needle biopsy can be accurately performed with ultrasound guidance.

STAGING

Staging of patients with both benign and malignant tumors may be beneficial in assessing patient prognosis and directing patient treatment. Although there may be disease-specific staging systems, it is important for hand surgeons to be familiar with general staging systems for benign bone tumors, malignant bone tumors, and malignant soft tissue sarcomas.

The staging of benign bone tumors has been described by Enneking (3) and is depicted in Figure 1. This system is based on the plain radiographic appearance of the lesion in question. Stage I, or "latent," lesions are entirely confined to bone. There is no thinning or expansion of the cortex and no soft tissue extension. There the bone may react to the lesion with surrounding sclerosis and sharply defined borders. Stage II, or "active," lesions have an effect on the overlying or surrounding cortex. Endosteal erosion or

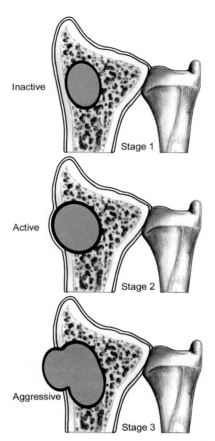

FIGURE 1. Staging of benign bone lesions.

destruction may be present. Expansion or distention of the cortex without soft tissue extension may be seen. The intramedullary borders of the lesion may be less distinct, with a broader zone of transition. Stage III, or "aggressive," lesions can have the features previously described for stage I and II but must have, in addition, cortical destruction, perforation, and soft tissue extension.

The staging of malignant bone lesions was described by Enneking and has been adopted by the American Musculoskeletal Tumor Society (MSTS) (4). This system is depicted in Figure 2. The primary determinant of stage is the histologic grade of the lesion, with all patients with metastasis, regardless of grade, assigned to stage III. Low-grade lesions are considered stage I (A or B). High-grade lesions are considered stage II (A or B). The relation of the lesion to the involved anatomic compartment or compartments is also assessed and categorized as either A or B. Those lesions that are confined to a single anatomic compartment are considered intracompartmental (A). Tumors that extend out of a single compartment or involve multiple compartments are considered extracompartmental (B). This system was developed with bone sarcoma as the model disease.

The MSTS system for the staging of bone sarcomas has been applied to soft tissue sarcoma, but other systems are commonly used outside the field of orthopedics. The

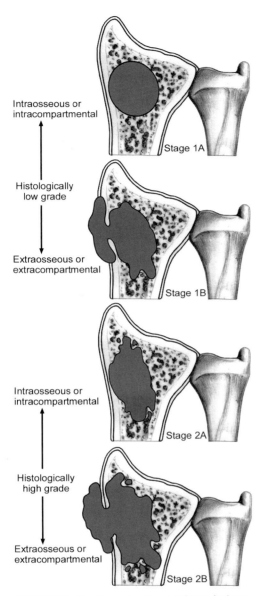

FIGURE 2. Staging of malignant bone lesions.

Labels within figure:
Intraosseous or intracompartmental — Stage 1A
Histologically low grade
Extraosseous or extracompartmental — Stage 1B
Intraosseous or intracompartmental — Stage 2A
Histologically high grade
Extraosseous or extracompartmental — Stage 2B

TABLE 1. AMERICAN JOINT COMMITTEE ON CANCER STAGING SYSTEM FOR SOFT TISSUE SARCOMA

Stage I	A (Low-grade, small, superficial, and deep)
	B (Low-grade, large, superficial)
Stage II	A (Low-grade, large, deep)
	B (High-grade, small, superficial, and deep)
	C (High-grade, large, superficial)
Stage III	High-grade, large, deep
Stage IV	Any metastasis

Memorial Sloan-Kettering Cancer Center system and the American Joint Committee on Cancer system (Table 1) incorporate data regarding tumor grade (high or low), size (smaller than or larger than 5 cm), relation to superficial fascia (superficial or deep), and the presence or absence of metastasis (5). Those patients with metastasis are considered stage IV. When considering soft tissue sarcomas, staging using these systems is more predictive of patient prognosis than the MSTS system (6).

BIOPSY

Many bone and soft tissue lesions in the hand do not require biopsy. Bone lesions that are readily recognized on

x-ray as benign and asymptomatic can be observed as long as the mechanical integrity of the bone is not compromised and the expected natural history of the lesion is not aggressive. In many cases, osteochondromas and enchondromas can simply be observed if the x-ray is classic for the lesion under consideration and there is no functional impairment, symptom, or significant fracture risk. If observation is chosen as the appropriate course, periodic reassessment is necessary to be certain that there is no progressive change, which may suggest an alternate diagnosis or indicate the need for biopsy.

Soft tissue lesions that can be confidently and clearly diagnosed on clinical grounds can be observed, provided they are asymptomatic and not progressively enlarging. A lesion suspected of being a soft tissue ganglion that arises in a classic location, clearly transilluminates, and yields gelatinous fluid on aspiration does not require biopsy. Suspected superficial lipomas can be observed, provided that physical examination and MRI characteristics are diagnostic. If a lesion is large, deep to fascia, painful, or growing, it should be submitted for biopsy (7). If a single accurate clinical diagnosis cannot be made, biopsy or specialist referral must be considered, even for lesions that are painless and do not appear to be growing. Soft tissue sarcomas can present as painless lesions that have been present for many years without apparent growth. Even small, painless lesions must be approached as if they are potentially malignant and not simply observed, unless a specific benign clinical diagnosis can be made.

There are two classes of biopsies that can be done in the extremity: open biopsy and closed, or needle, biopsy. The compact anatomies of the forearm and hand limit the role of core needle biopsy. Open biopsy is known to have greater diagnostic accuracy than needle biopsy, largely due to the increased size of the tissue sample obtained. The diagnostic accuracy of open biopsy on permanent analysis at a major tumor center is 96% (8,9). The disadvantages of this more invasive procedure include greater cost, complication risk, and greater degree of soft tissue contamination. The greatest risk of open biopsy is improper execution by the operating surgeon. Inappropriate incision placement or orientation may render standard limb-salvage incisions or amputation flaps impossible and may result in the need for soft tissue coverage at the definitive

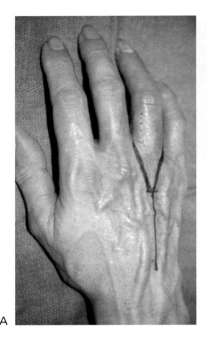 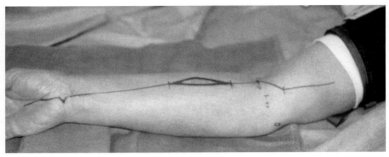

FIGURE 3. A: Longitudinal finger incision biopsy site placed within the ray amputation field, with skin flaps marked. **B:** Longitudinal forearm incision biopsy site placed within the limb-salvage incision needed for definitive resection. Biopsy site is marked with an ellipse and will be excised en bloc with the tumor.

resection. Contamination of major nerves and vessels during biopsy may render limb-salvage impossible. These concerns highlight the need for a well-planned and well-executed biopsy that results in the least amount of soft tissue contamination consistent with the possibility of subsequent definitive limb-salvage.

Incision Biopsy

Incision biopsy refers to the procedure in which an incision is placed directly into the tumor and a piece of tissue or sample is taken directly from the lesion while leaving the lesion in place. During the planning of this type of biopsy, a limb-salvage incision or amputation flaps are drawn on the patient. If limb-salvage is to be performed, the biopsy incision should be placed in line with or immediately parallel to the salvage incision so that the biopsy tract can be removed en bloc with the tumor (Fig. 3). Because the tumor is entered directly, anything the surgeon touches during the procedure may be contaminated with tumor cells. In the event of a final malignant diagnosis, the entire prior operative field, including drain and suture sites, must be excised en bloc with the major tumor mass. Incision biopsy is probably the best type of biopsy for those lesions in the distal forearm and hand that are larger than 2 cm. Incision biopsy should be used in the proximity of major nerves, vessels, or tendons that do not need to be exposed for incision biopsy but are contaminated by excision biopsy or gross total excision. This is a particularly safe type of biopsy when performed well. The crucial step is to place the incision so that it can be incorporated into a limb-sparing incision or amputation flap in the event of a sub-

sequent malignant diagnosis. Soft tissue contamination is limited to the soft tissues immediately superficial to the lesion, whereas the risks to surrounding nerves or vascular structures are minimized.

Excision Biopsy

Excision biopsy is the term used to describe a biopsy in which the entire lesion is removed. This type of biopsy is considered a marginal excision. The plane of dissection is at the edge of the capsule or pseudocapsule and transects the reactive zone surrounding the lesion. The advantages of this type of biopsy include large sample size and a single-stage procedure in the event of a benign diagnosis. The major disadvantage of this biopsy is that in the event of a malignant diagnosis, there is extensive soft tissue contamination with malignant cancer cells due to the biopsy itself. Microscopic residual disease that is at a minimum will be left in the patient. This has major implications in the forearm and hand. The subsequent definitive treatment of a malignant lesion requires an amputation or wide excision in which the entire operative field must be removed while cutting through a surrounding cuff of normal, nonreactive tissue. In areas where functional tissues are compactly arranged, this may require sacrifice of blood vessels, nerves, tendons, and skin that may not have been required had an incision biopsy been performed. This can increase the need for distant soft tissue coverage or amputation and might increase the risk of positive margins and local recurrence after definitive resection (10).

Excision biopsy should be used with great caution. It is particularly dangerous in the carpal tunnel, palm, and

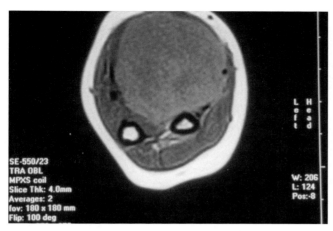

FIGURE 4. Axial magnetic resonance image of synovial sarcoma in the proximal forearm. Excision biopsy produces extensive soft tissue contamination.

antecubital fossa (Fig. 4). It should be limited to lesions smaller than 2 cm in the hand and 3 cm in the forearm. It should be reserved for those lesions in which malignancy is not considered likely or where amputation would be the next procedure in the event of a malignant diagnosis.

Primary Wide Excision

Primary wide excision is a form of biopsy in which the entire lesion is definitively removed en bloc with a surrounding cuff of normal, nonreactive, uninvolved tissue. The lesion is removed as if it were malignant, and healthy tissue is sacrificed to provide adequate margins of resection. This approach is used when the suspicion of malignancy is high and the lesion is in close proximity to major functional tissues such as nerves, vessels, and tendons. This procedure should be considered when the risk of contamination of soft tissues at the time of biopsy with other techniques outweighs the functional and cosmetic deficit produced by the sacrifice of normal, uninvolved tissue. This is a safe form of biopsy and an excellent oncologic procedure. It may be most appropriate for lesions in areas with limited compartmentalization, such as the palm, carpal tunnel, and antecubital fossa. The risks of this procedure are significant. The decision of whether to perform this type of biopsy is difficult and may be best made after consultation with a musculoskeletal oncologist.

Special Considerations

Specific tumors require specific approaches for biopsy. Nerve lesions, such as suspected schwannoma and neurofibroma, are biopsied by performing a marginal excision under magnification. In the event of a subsequent unanticipated malignant diagnosis, such as intraneural synovial sarcoma, the patient will require a subsequent staged wide

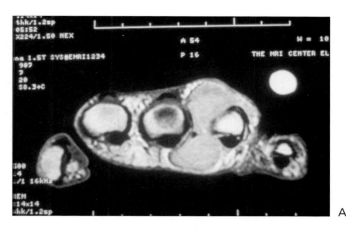
A

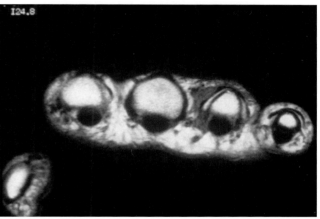
B

FIGURE 5. Malignant fibrous histiocytoma of the finger and web space at presentation **(A)** and after preoperative radiation **(B)** to improve resectability and allow only single ray amputation.

excision incorporating all structures exposed at the time of biopsy.

Incision biopsy should be considered in the setting of a suspected soft tissue sarcoma in which the use of adjuvants (radiation or chemotherapy) before the definitive resection may improve limb-salvage options or reduce the extent of required amputation (Fig. 5).

Biopsy Incisions

Finger

Incisions that do not compromise subsequent proximal or single ray amputation are generally acceptable in the finger. Longitudinal dorsal or lateral incisions may be useful for phalanx lesions. Limited palmar zigzag incisions are acceptable in the finger but usually produce contamination, which precludes any attempt at a finger-sparing option should it be considered possible. Definitive wide excision for malignant finger lesions generally requires amputation at a more proximal level or ray amputation. Definitive amputation flaps should be drawn at the time of biopsy as a reminder to avoid proximal contamination (Fig. 6).

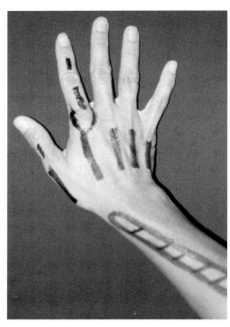

FIGURE 6. Potential sites for finger and metacarpal biopsy, dorsum of hand. Finger incisions should be drawn within potential amputation flaps in the event a malignant diagnosis is made.

Hand: Dorsum

Straight dorsal longitudinal incisions are most appropriate for biopsy in the dorsum of the hand. The incision should be planned such that it does not compromise a subsequent amputation flap or limb-salvage incision in the event of a malignant final diagnosis. Definitive amputation flaps or the potential limb-salvage incision should be drawn on the patient at the time of biopsy. The biopsy incision should be in line with or immediately parallel to the limb-salvage incision or within the amputation flaps.

Hand: Palm

The palm and carpal tunnel are unquestionably among the most dangerous regions in which to perform biopsy. The risk of contamination of skin and important functional tissues is extremely high. Any contamination produced by biopsy may limit limb-salvage options or commit the patient to a major amputation. Excision biopsy is extremely dangerous in this location (Fig. 7). Standard zigzag incisions should be avoided. Short longitudinal incisions, with limited oblique extension if needed, are usually best until the benign nature of the lesion can be assured. Incision biopsy, even for small lesions, should be more frequently considered in the hand. Primary wide excision may be most appropriate for certain carpal tunnel lesions. Definitive amputation flaps or the potential limb-salvage incision should be drawn at the time of biopsy to limit the potential for contamination.

Distal Radius

A longitudinal incision in line with or immediately parallel to a limb-salvage incision is most appropriate for

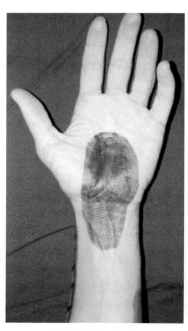
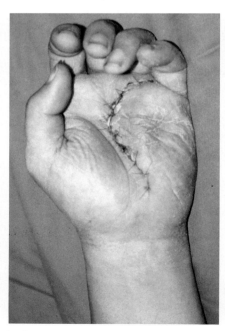
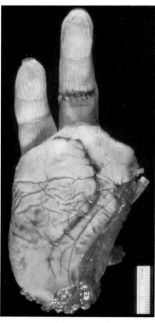

FIGURE 7. A: Danger zone for biopsy of palm lesions is marked. **B:** Excision biopsy of a synovial sarcoma through a long curved incision results in contamination of all structures contacted. **C:** Hemi-hand amputation is required for definitive wide excision.

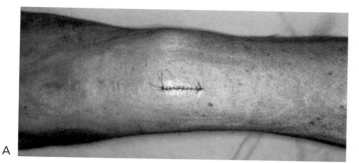

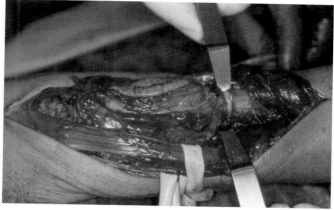

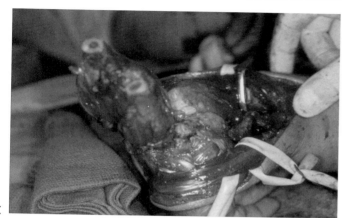

FIGURE 8. Dorsal incision biopsy of the distal radius through Lister's tubercle **(A)** limits access to palmar structures during definitive tumor resection **(B)**. **C:** Transection of the radius and ulna proximal to the tumor and flexion of the distal radius and ulna allow dissection of the palmar structures.

biopsy of the distal radius. Dorsal incisions may be centered over Lister's tubercle; however, there is typically only 4 mm between the second and third compartments. If these compartments are violated, there is extensive spread of hematoma proximally and distally along the course of tendon sheaths, which may increase the risk of local recurrence. Subsequent definitive resection may require a second palmar incision or transection of both the radius and the ulna, with flexion of the distal segment to allow palmar exposure and dissection at definitive treatment (Fig. 8).

A palmar radial incision may be particularly useful for the treatment of giant cell tumor of bone (Fig. 9). There is a window of approximately 8 mm between the first dorsal compartment and the radial artery 1.5 cm proximal to the radial styloid of an average adult. A palmar branch of the superficial radial nerve may be encountered. Distal radius biopsy is done at the edge of the radial insertion of the pronator quadratus. This approach is particularly useful for resecting lesions with palmar extension or when intralesional treatment of giant cell tumor of bone is considered.

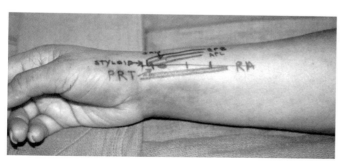

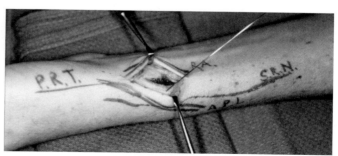

FIGURE 9. **A,B:** Palmar radial biopsy of the distal radius 1.5 cm proximal to the radial styloid in the interval between the radial artery and the first dorsal compartment allows excellent exposure of the distal radius tumors with palmar extension. APL, abductor pollicis longus; EPB, extensor pollicis brevis; PRT, pronator teres; RA, radial artery; SRN, superficial radial nerve.

Forearm

A longitudinal incision that can be incorporated into a subsequent limb-salvage incision is most appropriate for forearm biopsy. Major nerves should not be exposed at the time of biopsy unless primary wide excision is done.

TREATMENT

Classification of Surgical Procedures

The use of accepted oncologic terminology is imperative when planning or describing the treatment of a patient with a tumor. Enneking's descriptive terminology should be used, as it clearly conveys to other physicians exactly what has been done (3). Terms such as *local excision*, *total excision*, and *complete excision* are ambiguous and should be avoided.

Intralesional

During intralesional treatment, the tumor is directly entered and removed in a piecemeal fashion. For bone lesions, this is commonly known as *curettage*. After this type of treatment, tumor cells are invariably left in the tumor cavity. With lesions such as enchondroma, this is sufficient treatment with a low risk of local recurrence (Fig. 10). Adjuvants may be used after intralesional treatment to "extend" the zone of curettage and reduce the number of remaining viable cells. Common adjuvants include phenol, liquid nitrogen, and methylmethacrylate cement and may be considered in the treatment of an aneurysmal bone cyst or giant cell tumor of bone.

Marginal Excision

During marginal excision, dissection is done directly along the border of the lesion. The plane of dissection is through the reactive zone produced by the lesion. The reactive zone is commonly called a *capsule* or *pseudocapsule*. Excision biopsy is typically a marginal excision. Marginal excision is usually adequate treatment for benign lesions such as giant cell tumors of tendon sheath and lipoma. It is insufficient treatment for malignant lesions, as malignant tumor cells extend beyond the pseudocapsule and are left in the patient. The use of external beam radiation as an adjuvant after this type of procedure is not sufficient treatment for primary malignant tumors, with few exceptions.

Wide Excision

Wide excision is the term used to describe the procedure in which a tumor is removed while cutting through a layer of normal, nonreactive tissue, leaving a cuff of healthy tissue surrounding the lesion. The tumor is never seen or touched, although it may be palpable through the covering

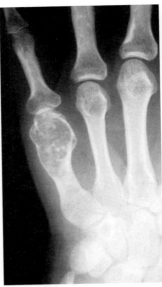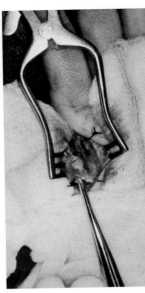

A,B

FIGURE 10. A,B: Enchondroma of the fifth metacarpal treated with curettage and bone grafting.

tissue. There is no prescribed "width" of a wide excision for most tumors. Specific tumors, such as dermatofibrosarcoma protuberans, low-grade myxofibrosarcoma, and epithelioid sarcoma, are known to require particularly wide margins (2 to 3 cm) to reduce the risk of local recurrence. Wide excision is the procedure of choice for most primary bone and soft tissue sarcomas. In many instances in the hand, this is best achieved with some form of amputation.

Radical Resection

Radical resection refers to the complete removal of a tissue compartment in an effort to remove a tumor within it. This procedure minimizes the risk of local recurrence after tumor removal but is seldom clinically indicated. Local recurrence risk is reduced by the excision of potential skip metastases that may be present within a soft tissue compartment. An example of a radical resection is the removal of the entire ray for an intraosseous tumor of the phalanx, such as a chondrosarcoma. Radical resection in the form of above-elbow amputation may be indicated for malignant primary hand tumors with extensive soft tissue involvement and proximal skip metastases. This procedure may be indicated for some epithelioid sarcomas of the hand with proximal spread along tendon sheaths.

Treatment of Malignant or Benign Aggressive Tumors by Location

Distal or Middle Phalanx Lesions

Malignant or aggressive benign lesions involving the distal phalanx or overlying soft tissues are usually best treated

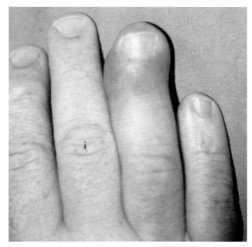
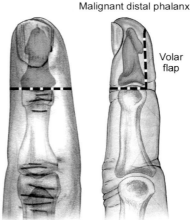
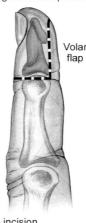
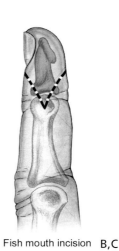

Malignant distal phalanx

Volar flap

Transverse incision   Fish mouth incision

A

B,C

FIGURE 11. A: Metastatic thymic carcinoma to the distal phalanx. **B:** Transverse incision with palmar flap for distal phalanx disarticulation. **C:** Fish mouth incision for distal phalanx tumors with palmar extension.

with excision, which, in virtually all instances, means some form of amputation. The level of amputation chosen must ensure that wide margins are achieved. If the required amputation would leave a functionless residual finger, ray amputation may even be required (Fig. 11).

Proximal Phalanx Lesions

Malignant tumors of the proximal phalanx are best treated with at least single ray amputation. Soft tissue extension to adjacent rays may require multiple ray amputation (Fig. 12). In some circumstances, a lesion that appears to require double ray amputation can be treated with a preoperative adjuvant (chemotherapy or radiation) that may then allow a single ray amputation. There are isolated case reports of giant cell tumor of bone involving a phalanx treated with wide excision and toe phalanx transfer (11). On rare occasions, wide excision of the proximal thumb phalanx may be considered if wide margins can be achieved.

Metacarpal Lesions

Bone and soft tissue sarcomas involving the metacarpal are usually treated with wide excision as a single or multiple ray amputation (Fig. 13). On rare occasions, wide excision of the metacarpal and reconstruction can be considered for intracompartmental lesions for which an effective adjuvant is available. This approach may be better suited for low-grade lesions. In selected cases, giant cell tumor of bone, without or with only limited soft tissue extension, may be treated in this manner. Reconstructive options include bone graft and fusion, allograft, and fibula reconstruction with implant arthroplasty (12) (Fig. 14). If wide excision without amputation is considered,

the goal of wide margins must not be compromised. Local recurrence is associated with the subsequent development of systemic metastasis with many types of bone and soft tissue sarcomas (13–15).

Hand: Dorsum

Soft tissue sarcomas involving the dorsum of the hand are best treated with wide excision, possibly with the use of radiation as an adjuvant (Fig. 15). The anatomy of the dorsum of the hand is less complex than that of the palm, with fewer vital structures and functional tissues. There appears to be a relatively high risk of local recurrence for soft tissue sarcomas occurring in this location (14). The reason for this finding is unclear and may be related to the relatively loose areolar tissue in the subcutaneous space without fascial septa or compartments, which may limit microscopic extension. Wide excision in this region often requires both tendon reconstruction and soft tissue coverage.

Hand: Palm

Malignant soft tissue tumors involving the superficial palm may be treated with wide excision, possibly in combination with ray or multiple ray amputation (Fig. 16). In most cases, soft tissue coverage is needed. On occasion, amputation of the hand may be required, particularly if there is extension of the tumor into the deeper soft tissues.

Carpus

Malignant primary tumors involving the carpus with soft tissue extension palmarly often require distal forearm-

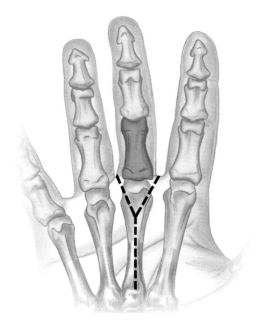

A,B

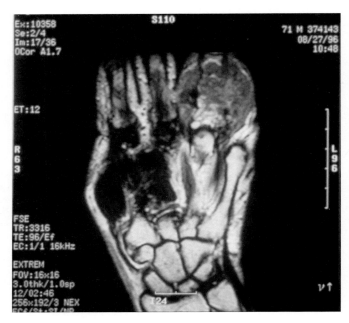

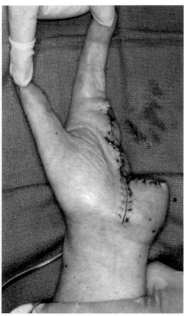

C,D

FIGURE 12. Malignant proximal phalanx lesions usually require single **(A)** or multiple ray amputation **(B–D)** as in this case of a proximal phalanx osteogenic sarcoma.

level amputation. If there is limited soft tissue extension or lack of extension into the carpal tunnel, wide excision of the carpus, including the radiocarpal articulation and distal radioulnar joint, may be considered. Reconstruction may be done most predictably with arthrodesis using a fibula graft.

Carpal Tunnel

All lesions of the carpal tunnel should be approached with great caution. Any contamination produced by excision biopsy or marginal excision may eliminate the possibility of sparing the patient's hand. Lesions are often best approached with incision biopsy or primary wide excision before a histologic diagnosis has been established. Some soft tissue sarcomas, such as synovial sarcoma, may be reduced in size with preoperative chemotherapy or radiation before definitive resection. This type of approach can render a previously unresectable lesion resectable. Extensive tendon nerve and vessel reconstruction can be performed after wide excision, if indicated. Large tumors in the carpal tunnel, tumors with extensive soft tissue con-

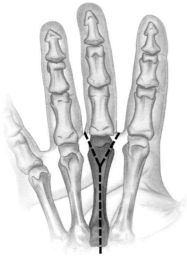
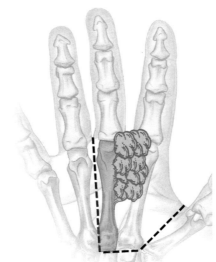

A,B   Malignant metacarpal lesion requiring single ray amputation   Malignant metacarpal and soft tissue tumor requiring double ray amputation

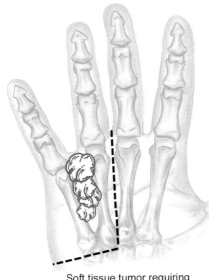
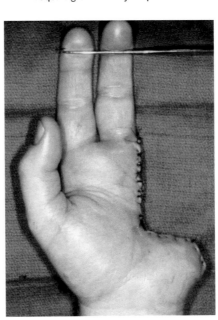

C,D   Soft tissue tumor requiring double ray amputation

FIGURE 13. Malignant bone and soft tissue tumors at the metacarpal level usually require single **(A)** or multiple ray amputation **(B–D)**.

tamination, and those tumors not commonly responsive to adjuvants are often best treated with either below-elbow amputation or, in rare instances, above-elbow amputation.

Distal Radius

Distal radius lesions are readily treated with wide excision. If there is extension of the tumor into the carpus or pathologic fracture into the carpus, the wide excision can incorporate the entire carpus and distal radioulnar joint (extraarticular wide excision) (Fig. 17). Lesions limited to the radius can be treated with intraarticular wide excision.

On rare occasions, segmental resection of the distal radius can be done while sparing the articular surface. Reconstruction can be done with intercalary allograft, arthrodesis with vascularized or nonvascularized fibula, articular radius allograft, articular fibula autograft, or transposition of the carpus to the ulna with arthrodesis.

Distal Ulna

Wide excision of the distal ulna can be readily done, incorporating portions of the distal radius or carpus as needed. Distal ulna replacement is not necessary, although stabilization of the carpus with soft tissue

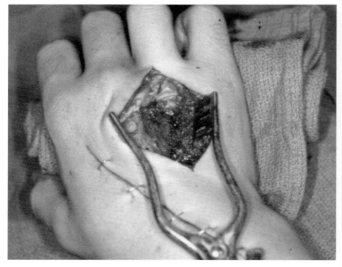

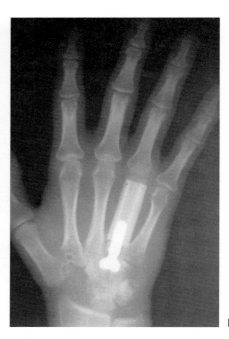

FIGURE 14. A,B: Silicone implant arthroplasty and fibula grafting for metacarpal reconstruction after wide excision of a ring finger metacarpal multifocal malignant hemangioendothelioma. Involved scaphoid and trapezium were also excised en bloc.

reconstruction or partial arthrodesis may be indicated (Fig. 18) (16,17).

Principles of Soft Tissue Coverage for Tumor Reconstruction

Reconstruction of defects produced after tumor extrication differs significantly from that which is normally encountered in the treatment of traumatic defects. Imme-

diate reconstruction should be anticipated and planned in most instances. The use of two surgical teams is advantageous. This avoids the tendency of the surgeon to compromise the resection or remove less tissue out of concern for maintaining reconstruction options. Operating room personnel must adhere to strict precautions to prevent cross contamination of operative fields. This includes the use of separate draping, instruments, operative clothing, and personnel. The planning for reconstruction should

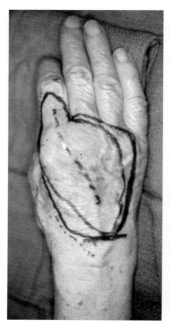

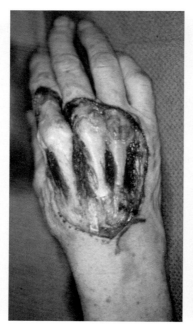

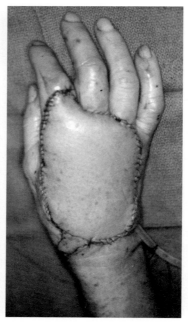

FIGURE 15. Wide excision soft tissue sarcoma from the dorsum of the hand **(A,B)** with radial forearm flap for soft tissue coverage **(C)**.

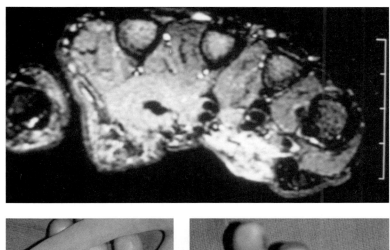

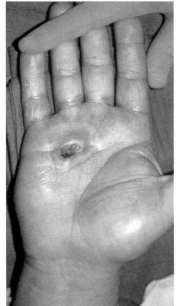
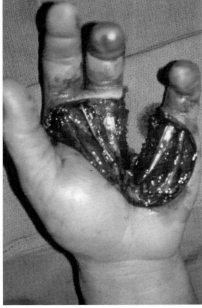

FIGURE 16. A–C: Wide excision of an epithelioid sarcoma with palm ulceration in combination with ray amputation. Methylene blue has been injected to facilitate sentinal lymph node biopsy.

include the possibility that the margins of resection might be positive. If a local or rotation flap is to be performed, the potential for spread of the tumor to the donor site must be considered. Groin flaps should be avoided. The use of distant or free tissue transfer increases reconstruction complexity but reduces the risk of donor field contamination and is more frequently used after tumor reconstruction. Vascularized bone transfer or soft tissue coverage may be particularly beneficial and may improve healing in those patients who need postoperative chemotherapy or radiation.

Adjuvants to Surgical Treatment

Adjuvants are more commonly used in the setting of malignant lesions but may also be used for benign lesions to reduce local recurrence risk. Phenol, liquid nitrogen, methylmethacrylate cement, and high-speed burring all have been postulated to reduce the risk of local recurrence for specific benign tumors and should be considered in the treatment of aneurysmal bone cyst and giant cell tumor of bone.

Chemotherapy is indicated for specific high-grade bone sarcomas, including osteogenic sarcoma and Ewing sarcoma. Although the primary benefit is control of systemic disease, extremity lesions often decrease in size, which can facilitate limb-sparing surgery. The use of effective adjuvants significantly decreases the risk of local recurrence when wide excision is performed for high-grade malignant bone or soft tissue tumors.

The use of chemotherapy for soft tissue sarcomas is more controversial. Primary tumor size has been found to be a predictor of prognosis. Chemotherapy is usually recommended for those patients with high-grade soft tissue sarcomas larger than 10 cm. Patients with high-grade lesions between 5 and 10 cm may be considered for

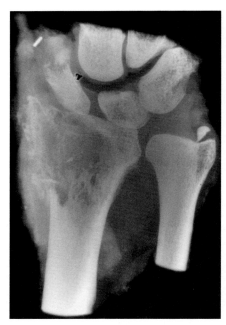

FIGURE 17. X-ray of an extraarticular wide excision of the distal radius for giant cell tumor of bone with pathologic fracture and intraarticular extension.

adjuvant chemotherapy. High-grade lesions smaller than 5 cm are not usually treated with chemotherapy unless the histology is known to be particularly sensitive to chemotherapy or the potential for decreasing the size of the primary lesion may significantly affect limb-sparing options.

Radiation is usually used to reduce the risk of local recurrence of soft tissue sarcomas larger than 5 cm. It may be considered for smaller lesions if a subsequent local recurrence will result in the need for amputation. External beam radiation may be used preoperatively to decrease tumor size and reduce the extent of resection or amputation. Such an approach may convert a double ray amputation to a single ray amputation. Whereas external beam radiation can be successfully used for either high- or low-grade soft tissue sarcomas, brachytherapy is only effective for high-grade lesions. Brachytherapy radiation uses thin catheters placed in the operative field at the time of surgery, after resection. These catheters are then loaded 5 days after surgery to deliver a high dose of radiation to a limited field over a short period. This method is only effective for high-grade lesions.

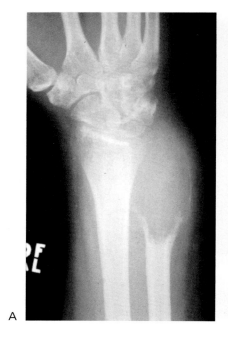

A

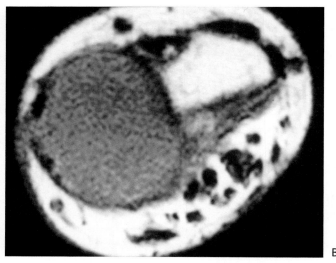

B

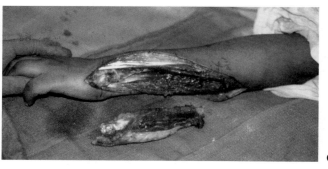

C

FIGURE 18. Giant cell–rich osteogenic sarcoma of the distal ulna **(A,B)** treated with wide excision **(C)**.

REFERENCES

1. Brady MS, Gaynor JJ, Brennan MF. Radiation-associated sarcoma of bone and soft tissue. *Arch Surg* 1992;127:1379–1385.
2. Hardell L, Sandstrom A. Case-control study: soft-tissue sarcomas and exposure to phenoxyacetic acids or chlorophenols. *Br J Cancer* 1979;39:711–717.
3. Enneking WF. *Musculoskeletal tumor surgery*. New York: Churchill Livingstone, 1983.
4. Enneking WF, Spanier SS, Goodman MA. A system for the surgical staging of musculoskeletal sarcoma. *Clin Orthop* 1980;153:106–120.
5. *AJCC cancer staging handbook*. Philadelphia: Lippincott-Raven, 1998:139–146.
6. Wunder J, Healey JH, Davis AM, et al. A comparison of staging systems for localized extremity soft-tissue sarcoma. *Cancer* 2000;88:2721–2730.
7. Athanasian EA. Biopsy of musculoskeletal tumors. *Orthopaedic knowledge update: musculoskeletal tumors*. American Academy of Orthopaedic Surgery, 2002.
8. Skyzynski MC, Biermann JS, Montag A, et al. Diagnostic accuracy and charge-savings of outpatient core needle biopsy compared with open biopsy of musculoskeletal tumors. *J Bone Joint Surg* 1996;78:644–649.
9. Simon MA. Biopsy of musculoskeletal tumors. *J Bone Joint Surg* 1982;64:1253–1257.
10. Athanasian EA. Biopsy adequacy upon referral of malignant or aggressive tumors of the forearm and hand. Presented at: American Association for Hand Surgery, 2001, San Diego.
11. Torpey B, Faierman E, Lehmann O. Phalangeal transfer for recurrent giant cell tumor of the phalanx of a finger in a nine year old child. A case report with forty-one year follow-up. *J Bone Joint Surg* 1994;76A:1864–1869.
12. Athanasian EA, Bishop AT, Amadio PC. Autogenous fibular graft and silicone implant arthroplasty following resection of giant cell tumor of the metacarpal. A report of two cases. *J Hand Surg [Am]* 1997;22:504–507.
13. Wunder JS, Paulian G, Huvos AG, et al. The histologic response to chemotherapy as a predictor of the oncologic outcome of operative treatment of Ewing sarcoma. *J Bone Joint Surg* 1998;80:1020–1033.
14. Brien EW, Terek RM, Greer RJ, et al. Treatment of soft-tissue sarcomas of the hand. *J Bone Joint Surg* 1995;77A:564–571.
15. Terek RM, Brien EW. Soft tissue sarcomas of the hand and wrist. *Hand Clin* 1995;11:287–305.
16. Cooney WP, Damron TA, Sim FH, et al. En bloc resection of tumors of the distal end of the ulna. *J Bone Joint Surg* 1997;79:406–412.
17. Wolf SW, Mih AD, Hotchkiss RN, et al. Wide excision of the distal ulna: a multicenter case study. *J Hand Surg [Am]* 1998;23:222–228.

100

SOFT TISSUE TUMORS OF THE HAND: MALIGNANT

RICHARD M. TEREK

Hand sarcomas are exceedingly rare, life-threatening diseases that must be managed according to oncologic principles to maximize the chance of cure and preserve hand function. Soft tissue sarcomas encompass a wide range of tumor types that display a broad spectrum of clinical behavior. These tumors originate from the mesenchyme and involve soft tissues of the musculoskeletal system: muscle, fat, nerve, vessels, synovium, joint capsule, and tendons. They occur in both extremity and nonextremity sites, and approximately 25% of extremity sarcomas have metastatic potential. The unique aspects of hand sarcomas are discussed.

REVIEW OF SOFT TISSUE SARCOMA

Soft tissue sarcomas encompass diverse cell types, some of which have normal correlates. Examples include liposarcoma, which resembles fat, and rhabdomyosarcoma, which resembles muscle. Presumably, these tumors arose from normal fat or muscle cells or from a primitive cell, which differentiated down the fat or muscle lineage while undergoing malignant transformation. Other soft tissue sarcomas do not have obvious normal correlates. Examples include malignant fibrous histiocytoma (MFH) and alveolar soft-part sarcoma. Table 1 lists some of the histologic types of soft tissue sarcomas and their normal correlates. The two most common are MFH and liposarcoma. Additional tumors are synovial sarcoma, fibrosarcoma, rhabdomyosarcoma, epithelioid sarcoma, malignant peripheral nerve sheath tumors, and leiomyosarcoma (mostly retroperitoneal). In the hand, there are a disproportionate number of synovial and epithelioid sarcomas. There are approximately 4,000 extremity soft tissue sarcomas per year in the United States. There are 16 major categories of soft tissue sarcoma (1), each with histologic subtypes, and because each anatomic location has its own special features, it has been difficult to establish the unique behavior of each tumor type for each location. However, several variables are consistently identified in multivariate analyses as significant predictors of how patients with soft tissue sarcoma fare with respect to survival, development of metastatic disease, and local recurrence (LR). Those variables are grade, size, and depth and are the variables used in current staging systems (2–6). Histologic subtype is not usually a significant variable, although in some series malignant peripheral nerve sheath tumor and leiomyosarcoma have a worse prognosis (3). Overall, approximately 75% of patients are cured with surgical resection and, in some cases, radiation therapy and chemotherapy, and 25% ultimately succumb to metastatic disease. Now that the overall behavior of soft tissue sarcomas is fairly well described, some investigators are reporting small series of specific histologic subtypes (7–10) or anatomic locations (11–21) and comparing them to the aggregate historical data in an attempt to cull out information about tumors or locations that one would suspect are somehow different than the average soft tissue sarcoma. The small numbers of cases being reported, the lack of consistent treatment protocols, and their oftentimes retrospective nature limit the conclusions one can draw from these studies. Although specific information about soft tissue sarcomas of the hand is even more limited, it appears that most of the principles that apply to soft tissue sarcomas of the extremity also apply to hand sarcomas. The main surgical principles are to not cause undue contamination at the time of biopsy or unplanned resection and to obtain a wide surgical margin at the time of definitive resection.

CLINICAL PRESENTATION

The majority of patients with soft tissue sarcomas present with a chief complaint of a painless mass (19,22–24). Occasionally, patients with hand sarcomas may also present with either a painful mass or neurologic symptoms. It is not uncommon for a hand sarcoma to be initially mistaken for a more common disease of the hand. Epithelioid sarcoma has been mistaken for Dupuytren's disease (25), spindle-cell

TABLE 1. COMMON TYPES OF SOFT TISSUE SARCOMAS

Normal tissue correlate	Sarcoma type	Subtypes
Fat	Liposarcoma	Myxoid Round cell Pleomorphic Well differentiated
Nerve	Malignant peripheral nerve sheath tumor	—
Vascular	Angiosarcoma	—
Smooth muscle	Leiomyosarcoma	
Striated muscle	Rhabdomyosarcoma	Alveolar Embryonal
Fibrous tissue	Fibrosarcoma Malignant fibrous histiocytoma	Storiform-pleomorphic Giant cell
	Epithelioid sarcoma	Inflammatory
	Synovial sarcoma	Myxoid
	Clear cell sarcoma	Angiomatoid
	Alveolar soft part sarcoma	Mono-, biphasic

sarcoma as a benign recurrent nodule (26), sarcoma as a ganglion, malignant eccrine poroma as callus (27), and carpal tunnel syndrome secondary to benign and malignant space-occupying lesions of the carpal canal as idiopathic carpal tunnel syndrome. Carpal tunnel syndrome has been reported to result from synovial sarcoma (28), epithelioid sarcoma (29), giant cell tumor of tendon sheath (30), and chondrosarcoma (31). It is commonly taught that an important symptom to elicit in the history of present illness in the evaluation of a patient with musculoskeletal pain is night pain, which suggests pain of nonmechanical etiology (i.e., tumor or infection). However, it is well known that patients with carpal tunnel syndrome often have discomfort and pain in the hand at night, so that the history is less helpful in determining if hand symptoms are a result of sarcoma. Sarcoma of the carpal canal does occur, but is a rare cause of carpal tunnel syndrome. Unless an obvious mass is present, one must be aware that occult tumors can present as more common hand syndromes, and when encountered intraoperatively, a biopsy should be properly performed.

The duration and time course of symptoms are also important. Children with a mass present since infancy most likely have hamartomas, hemangiomas, or infantile fibrosarcoma (32,33). Rapidly growing lesions usually represent sarcoma or inflammation, but can occasionally be a benign lesion like nodular fasciitis, which is a rapidly growing benign lesion commonly misdiagnosed as a soft tissue sarcoma (34). Fluctuation in size may help differentiate a ganglion cyst or hemangioma from a soft tissue sarcoma. A history of trauma or penetrating injuries may suggest a foreign body granuloma, epidermoid cyst, or traumatic aneurysm as the etiology of a mass. In older patients, particularly those with a significant history of tobacco use or known history of lung carcinoma, metastatic disease

from bronchogenic carcinoma of the lung to the hand is a possibility. Although metastases below the elbow are rare, osseous metastases with a soft tissue mass are usually from lung or renal cell carcinoma (35). Epidemiologic studies have identified cancer syndromes in some families. Risk factors include a first- or second-degree relative with a history of a sarcoma, herbicide exposure, radiation exposure, and long-standing lymphedema in the upper extremity, usually a result of axillary node dissection and/or radiation to the axillary lymph nodes for breast cancer (36).

Important aspects of the physical examination include the size, shape, mobility, site, and consistency of the mass and color of the overlying skin. Swelling of the dorsal wrist, volar wrist, and proximal digital crease are common locations for ganglion cysts, by far the most common lesion causing swelling or a mass (37). Swelling over a distal phalanx is often due to a mucous cyst. The second most common soft tissue tumor in the hand is giant cell tumor of tendon sheath, or pigmented villonodular synovitis, which originates from the synovium of a tendon sheath or joint. Fluctuation of size with palpation and position of the limb is characteristic of hemangioma. If abnormal pigmentation is present, melanoma, nevi, or squamous cell carcinoma (which typically ulcerates) should be suspected. Persistent lesions demonstrating characteristics of a callus (firm, woody hard with or without ulceration) must be evaluated for epithelioid sarcoma, viral wart, pyogenic granuloma, squamous carcinoma, and sweat gland tumor and other tumors of the skin and appendages. Lesions should be assessed for pulsation and bruit to rule out aneurysm. A patient with pain under the nailbed, cold intolerance, and exquisite tenderness, with or without a mass and purple patch, should be evaluated for a glomus tumor. Epitrochlear and axillary lymph nodes should be palpated in all patients with a potential soft tissue sarcoma because epithelioid sarcoma, embryonal rhabdomyosarcoma, synovial sarcoma, and angiosarcoma are at increased risk for lymph node metastasis (38).

IMAGING

The role of magnetic resonance imaging (MRI) for detection of soft tissue sarcomas of the extremity has been well established (39,40). Although both computed tomography (CT) and MRI can demonstrate cross-sectional anatomy, MRI does so with equal or greater spatial resolution and superior contrast resolution. The improved contrast resolution is critical for evaluation of soft tissues. CT remains a better method in assessing calcification and ossification within a lesion and for evaluating cortical changes, although MRI has also been successfully used to detect bone invasion (41). The ideal imaging modality for masses suspected to be sarcoma is MRI. Gadolinium contrast can be helpful, particularly in postoperative studies in trying to distinguish scar from recurrent tumor. MRI can define the local extent of the tumor and is of immense help with preoperative planning. When a mass is initially encountered, there are several options for initial evaluation. If a ganglion is suspected, a simple aspiration will confirm the diagnosis. If clear, highly viscous fluid cannot be aspirated, consideration should be given to MRI, particularly for deep masses. If a mass is in a finger and attached to a tendon sheath, the most likely diagnosis is a giant cell tumor of tendon sheath, for which a primary excision can be performed, particularly if it is in the finger. If by chance the mass happens to be a sarcoma, a finger or ray amputation could be performed. Before excising a mass without a pathologic diagnosis, one should always consider whether one can recoup if the pathology report indicates sarcoma. If irreparable harm is done by the excision such that it will be difficult to obtain a wide margin during a reexcision without sacrificing important functional structures, then one should not be excising the mass. Instead, a biopsy should be performed. Much depends on where the mass is anatomically located. If a small, superficial mass is encountered on the extensor surface, a primary excision can probably be performed. If a reexcision is necessary, extensor tendons can be resected and compensated for with tendon transfers. For large

masses, deep masses, or clinically suspicious masses, MRI should be performed before excision or biopsy. A patient with a rapidly enlarging mass had the radiograph shown in Figure 1A and MRI scan (Fig. 1B), which demonstrate dorsal and volar involvement of bone and soft tissues. Therefore, amputation for a histologically confirmed rhabdoid sarcoma (Fig. 1C) was performed. MRI can be used to diagnose an intramuscular lipoma (Fig. 2). A homogeneous bright mass on T1, of the same signal intensity as subcutaneous fat, and without septations is most likely a lipoma and can be primarily excised (42). Any deep, heterogeneous mass that is not obviously a giant cell tumor of tendon sheath should be biopsied first. If frozen pathology confirms a benign entity, the incision can be extended and the mass resected; however, if there is any doubt about the pathologic diagnosis, one should return after the final pathology has been determined because it is not infrequent for the final pathologic diagnosis to differ from the intraoperative assessment.

In the initial evaluation of a patient with a hand mass, a plain radiograph can sometimes be useful. Radiographs can show bone tumors with associated soft tissue masses or soft tissue masses eroding into bone. Figure 3 shows a radiograph of a finger from a patient with swelling of the fifth

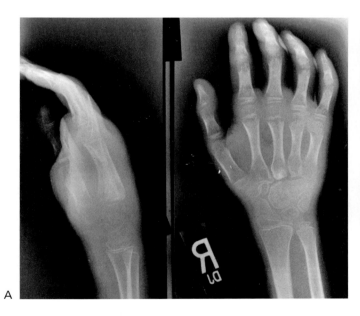

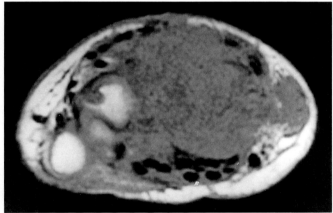

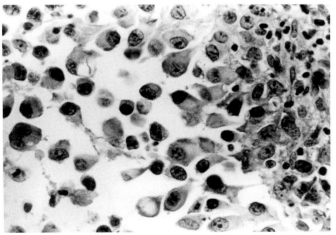

FIGURE 1. A: Hand radiographs showing a soft tissue mass with bone destruction and osteopenia. **B:** Magnetic resonance imaging shows a soft tissue tumor involving volar and dorsal compartments with displacement of the carpal canal structures and bone destruction. **C:** Histology reveals large, pleomorphic, anaplastic cells consistent with rhabdoid sarcoma. (From Terek R, Brien C. Soft tissue sarcomas of the hand and wrist. *Hand Clin* 1995;11, with permission.)

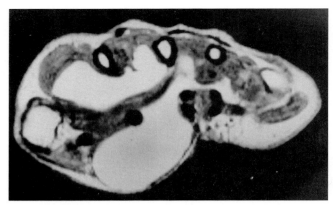

FIGURE 2. T1-weighted magnetic resonance image showing a soft tissue mass in the palmar aspect of the hand, which is lobulated, homogeneous, and bright. Pathology showed a lipoma. (From Terek R, Brien C. Soft tissue sarcomas of the hand and wrist. *Hand Clin* 1995;11, with permission.)

digit, which resulted from an osteoid osteoma of the middle phalanx. The patient whose hand radiograph is shown in Figure 4 had a dorsal soft tissue mass from a Ewing's sarcoma of the fourth metacarpal. Calcification within the mass can be seen in both benign and malignant soft tissue masses. Hemangiomas often have phleboliths. Other benign entities with calcification or ossification include tumoral calcinosis and myositis ossificans. Malignancies include 10% to 30% of patients with synovial sarcoma (Fig. 5), myxoid chondrosarcoma, epithelioid sarcoma, and

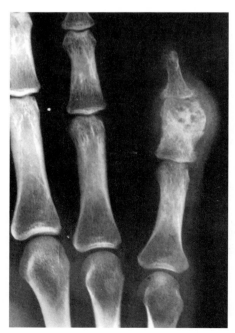

FIGURE 3. Plain radiograph of an adult hand shows a blastic bone lesion with associated soft tissue swelling in the middle phalanx of the fifth digit from an osteoid osteoma. (From Terek R, Brien C. Soft tissue sarcomas of the hand and wrist. *Hand Clin* 1995;11, with permission.)

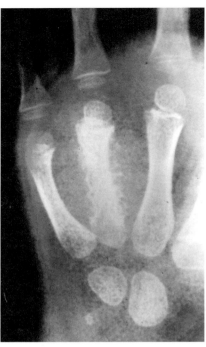

FIGURE 4. Plain radiographs of the hand of a 4-year-old girl with swelling and pain show periosteal reaction and destructive changes of the fourth metacarpal from Ewing's sarcoma. (From Terek R, Brien C. Soft tissue sarcomas of the hand and wrist. *Hand Clin* 1995;11, with permission.)

liposarcoma (43,44). Tumors that erode into bone may also be seen on plain radiographs and are characteristic of pressure from long-standing lesions such as giant cell tumor of tendon sheath, inclusion cyst, and glomus tumor. If both sides of a joint show involvement, pigmented villonodular synovitis, gout, and infection should be considered.

STAGING

The purpose of staging is to give a prognosis and to guide treatment (45,46). Too many variables, and the system would be cumbersome and unwieldy, and what would be the point of dividing patients into too many groups? Our therapies are limited to surgery, radiation, and chemotherapy, so basically we need to divide patients into enough groups to help guide treatment. A staging system with too few variables would lack the ability to discriminate between high- and low-risk patients. The current American Joint Committee on Cancer (AJCC) staging system, modified in 1997 (fifth edition) (47), and the Memorial Sloan-Kettering system (48) both use the following variables (Table 2): grade, tumor size, tumor depth relative to the investing fascia, and metastases, and are considered superior to the Enneking system (49–51).

In a study of patients with small, high-grade soft tissue sarcoma (stage IIB), the estimated 5-year overall survival was 91% (14,52,53). In another study with longer term

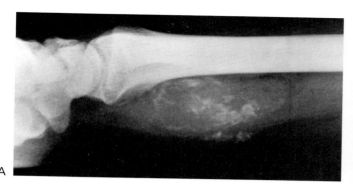

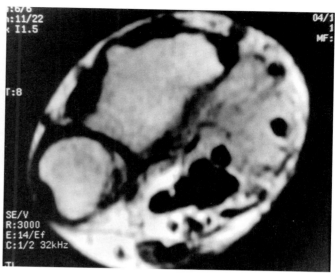

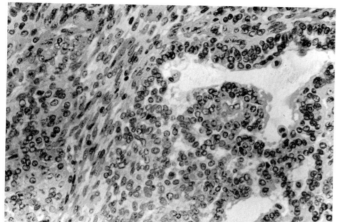

FIGURE 5. A: Lateral view of the wrist shows calcification within a volar soft tissue mass. **B:** Magnetic resonance imaging demonstrates an extensive soft tissue mass in the radial aspect of the wrist, which has encased the radial wrist flexors, is juxtaposed to the carpal canal, and involves the periosteum. **C:** A biphasic synovial sarcoma with epithelial-like and spindle cell components. (From Terek R, Brien C. Soft tissue sarcomas of the hand and wrist. *Hand Clin* 1995;11, with permission.)

follow-up, 5-year overall survival was 83%, although the survival for those with positive margins was only 43% (54). Generally speaking, patients with small, high-grade tumors that can be resected with negative margins have a good prognosis and in some centers are treated with surgery only. In contrast, patients with stage III (large, deep, high-grade) tumors have a much worse prognosis: approximately a 50% 5-year survival (55). Many of the early studies assessing chemotherapy for soft tissue sarcoma patients included all stages. The results were diluted by the inclusion of low-risk patients, so that it has been difficult to prove that chemotherapy makes a difference. Now that the AJCC system has been modified in a way that more reliably separates patients into groups with meaningful differences in survival, current

clinical trials are attempting to include only high-risk patients (stage III) to determine if adjuvant chemotherapy improves survival.

Staging studies include local imaging to determine anatomic extent, size, and depth. This is best accomplished with an MRI scan. The vast majority of metastases are to the lungs. Chest radiographs and chest CT scan are used to detect pulmonary metastases. The latter is more sensitive, and the former is used for routine postoperative monitoring (56,57). Approximately 10% of patients present with detectable metastatic disease. CT scan of the abdomen and pelvis is performed in those patients with myxoid liposarcoma, which has a greater propensity to metastasize to the retroperitoneum and mesentery (56,57). Nodal metastases are detected with clinical examination and biopsy of clinically suspicious nodes, except for patients with rhabdomyosarcoma, who have lymph node biopsy of regional lymph nodes as part of their staging. Sentinel node biopsy has not become routine in the management of soft tissue sarcoma as it has in melanoma. Bone scans are not needed, as bone metastases are rare. Occasionally, CT scan of the primary tumor is useful to assess cortical invasion of an adjacent bone; however, this can usually be determined by clinical examination and the MRI scan (41).

The final step in staging is to biopsy the lesion to establish a diagnosis and grade of the tumor. The final grade may change after the tumor is resected and the entire specimen examined.

TABLE 2. STAGING OF SOFT TISSUE SARCOMA

Stage	Description
IA	Low grade, <5 cm, superficial or deep
IB	Low grade, >5 cm, superficial
IIA	Low grade, >5 cm, deep
IIB	High grade, <5 cm, superficial or deep
IIC	High grade, >5 cm, superficial
III	High grade, >5 cm, deep
IV	Nodal or other metastatic disease

Adapted from Soft tissue sarcoma. In: Fleming ID, Cooper JS, Henson DE, et al., eds. *American Joint Committee on Cancer (AJCC) staging manual.* Philadelphia: Lippincott, 1997:149–156.

Grading

Grade is the most important variable in staging, at least for short-term outcome (6). Tumor size seems more important in determining long-term outcome (58). Grade is determined by the pathologist based on histologic variables and indicates the degree of malignancy or aggressiveness of the tumor. The histologic variables are cellularity, cellular pleomorphism, mitotic activity, nuclear atypia, necrosis (which indicates growth so rapid that the tumor is outgrowing its blood supply), and infiltrative growth (59). Vascular invasion has also been found to portend a poor prognosis (60). The number of grades used varies from 2 to 3 to 4. Most commonly, soft tissue sarcomas are divided into low and high grade or low, intermediate, and high grade. Molecular genetics have identified reproducible translocations that occur with specific soft tissue sarcomas (61,62). Some of these translocations appear identical at the cytogenetic level, but have slightly different breakpoints if one sequences the DNA. Some of these breakpoints result in fusion proteins with different biologic activities and tumors with different degrees of aggressiveness. For example, synovial sarcoma have a translocation resulting in a fusion of the *SYT* and *SSX1* or *SSX2* genes. Patients with *SYT-SSX2* have a better prognosis than those with *SYT-SSX1* (63). These two fusion proteins differ by only 13 amino acids. Nuances such as these have not yet been incorporated into grading of soft tissue sarcomas, although one can expect that these molecular markers will be increasingly used for diagnosis and grading (prognosis), and as treatment targets.

Biopsy and Histology

The majority of patients presenting with a soft tissue mass have benign lesions (37), many of which can be treated with excisional biopsy. However, one must always have an index of suspicion for malignancy before biopsy. This is determined by the history, physical examination, plain radiographs, and, sometimes, MRI. If a lesion presents in an uncommon location for the presumptive benign diagnosis, imaging studies, particularly MRI, may help guide the differential diagnosis (Figs. 2 and 5B). For small, superficial soft tissue tumors in the extremity outside the hand, excisional biopsy may often be performed without jeopardizing future margins and contaminating important structures. The difficulty with excisional biopsy in the hand for unknown lesions is that significant contamination of important nerves and vessels may occur, with the possible exception of very small, superficial tumors or tumors involving the digits. Tumors larger than 3 cm should be evaluated with a biopsy, which can either be a fine needle aspirate, core needle biopsy, or incisional biopsy. Core needle biopsy can be easily performed in the office and usually provides adequate tissue to make a diagnosis of sarcoma. If the mass is deep and a needle biopsy cannot be safely per-

formed without jeopardizing important structures, then an incisional biopsy should be performed. Biopsy incisions should be longitudinal and excised at the time of definitive resection, being left in continuity with the underlying tumor. Dissection and hence contamination of surrounding structures should not be performed. Careful hemostasis and use of a drain exiting close to and in line with the biopsy incision should be used if necessary to prevent contamination of the extremity with postoperative hematoma and tumor (64,65). Marginal excisional biopsy should be avoided in any case that may represent a sarcoma because reexcision may require a more ablative procedure than would have been required if an incisional biopsy had been performed. Most soft tissue sarcomas can be accurately diagnosed with routine histologic sections; however, tissue should be available for immunohistochemistry and electron microscopy. When analyzing sections, one must determine the pathologic diagnosis and grade of the sarcoma. In several studies, grade of tumor is the most important variable in determining overall survival (66–68), although in some studies, long-term survival is more related to size, and grade is more related to LR (58).

Epithelioid sarcoma is one of the most common soft tissue sarcomas of the hand (21,69), which can be confused with granulomatous diseases, squamous cell carcinoma, and monophasic synovial sarcoma. Epithelioid sarcomas have a calluslike consistency and often appear as a nodular or ulcerated lesion (8). Males are more commonly affected (2:1), and the peak incidence is between the ages of 10 and 35 years. It may be present in the subcutis or deeper structures and has a firm consistency, tends to grow along fascial and tendinous structures, and on at least two occasions has been mistaken for Dupuytren's disease (25). Therefore, all tissue excised from the hand should be sent for pathologic review. The microscopic features of cells have an epithelioid appearance in a nodular arrangement, a tendency to undergo central necrosis, and eosinophilia (Fig. 6). Immunohistochemical findings include expression of vimentin, cytokeratin, and epithelial membrane antigen. More than 40% of patients develop lymph node metastases, 40% develop pulmonary metastases, and a very high rate of LR and satellite lesions in the skin are common (8). The recommended treatment is wide resection and radiation therapy for tumors larger than 5 cm and those with positive margins.

Synovial sarcoma is most prevalent in patients between 15 and 40 years old and is also more common in males. It is a common soft tissue sarcoma of the hand (70), and the typical presentation is a deep, firm, tender soft tissue mass. Radiographs may reveal calcification (Fig. 5A). As with all soft tissue sarcomas, MRI demonstrates the extent of tumor involvement with tendons, nerves, and blood vessels (Fig. 5B). Microscopic findings include either a biphasic pattern, which demonstrates fibrosarcoma-like spindle cells and carcinoma-like epithelial cells, or a monophasic pattern with uniform, plump cells with scant cytoplasm and dark-stain-

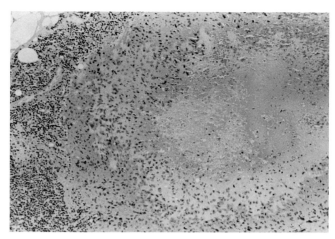

FIGURE 6. Histology of an epithelioid sarcoma showing central necrosis, epithelial-like cells, and inflammatory cells. (From Terek R, Brien C. Soft tissue sarcomas of the hand and wrist. *Hand Clin* 1995;11, with permission.)

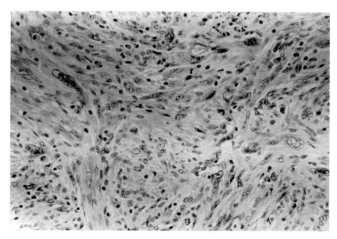

FIGURE 7. Malignant fibrous histiocytoma. (From Terek R, Brien C. Soft tissue sarcomas of the hand and wrist. *Hand Clin* 1995;11, with permission.)

ing nuclei (Fig. 5C). Calcification and mast cells may be seen, and vascularity varies. Monophasic epithelial and poorly differentiated synovial sarcomas are less commonly seen. Molecular genetic analysis of the type of translocation can aid in diagnosis and prognosis (63).

MFH is the most common malignant adult soft-tissue sarcoma, and the overall incidence has increased as many liposarcomas and fibrosarcomas are now categorized as MFH (71). However, the pendulum may be swinging back to using the diagnosis of MFH more discriminately (72). The majority of the tumors occur in patients between the fifth and seventh decades. The histologic appearance can be categorized into several subtypes: storiform-pleomorphic (most common), giant cell, inflammatory, myxoid, and angiomatoid. Histologic findings in the storiform pattern include pleomorphic areas of sheets of bizarre plump spindle cells with slitlike vessels and occasional histiocytic cells with typical and atypical mitotic activity (Fig. 7). The majority of MFHs are high grade, but low-grade tumors do exist. Immunohistochemical findings and electron microscopy are best used for exclusion of other types of sarcomas. Patients with MFH of the upper extremity had a higher LR than those in the lower extremity, and those with tumors below the elbow or knee had a higher LR than those with more proximal tumors (9), probably reflecting difficulties obtaining clear margins as one moves distal in the extremity.

Rhabdomyosarcoma is the most common soft tissue sarcoma in children and young adults (73). It most commonly occurs in locations outside the limb; however, if the extremity is involved, hands, feet, and forearms are the most common locations. Alveolar and embryonal rhabdomyosarcoma are the two most common subtypes to involve the extremity. Histologically, the alveolar subtype has round or oval cells and "alveolar spaces" with central necrosis. Fibrous septa surrounding vascular channels may be present. Prominent giant cells are also seen in the alveolar

subtype in contrast to the embryonal type, which resembles development of skeletal muscle and often has varied cellularity, small amounts of interstitial collagen, and hyperchromatic nuclei with eosinophilic cytoplasm (Fig. 8). Rhabdomyosarcoma, similar to other malignant blue, small, round cell tumors, responds to chemotherapy. The Intergroup Rhabdomyosarcoma Study revealed that the 5-year survival for the entire cohort was 55% when treatment consisted of conservative excision followed by chemotherapy (vincristine, dactinomycin, and cyclophosphamide) and radiation if tumor remained after excision (73). Results vary with stage of the tumor, which is in part determined by resectability of the tumor. If clear surgical margins are obtained, 5-year survival is approximately 80%. If gross residual tumor is present after surgery, combination chemotherapy and radiation therapy can result in approxi-

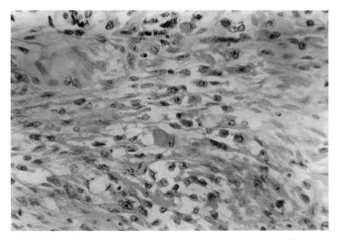

FIGURE 8. Rhabdomyosarcoma, the most common soft tissue sarcoma in childhood, with malignant rhabdomyoblast. (From Terek R, Brien C. Soft tissue sarcomas of the hand and wrist. *Hand Clin* 1995;11, with permission.)

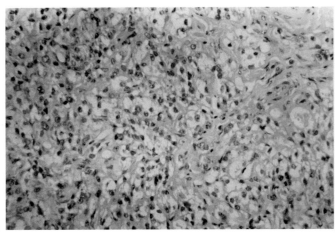

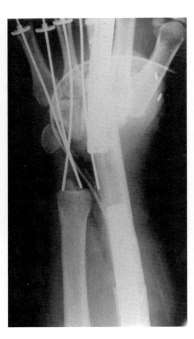

FIGURE 9. This patient had a recurrent clear-cell sarcoma **(A)** on the dorsum of the wrist with invasion of the distal radius. **B:** Postoperative radiograph demonstrates a wrist fusion performed with a vascularized fibula autograft, which included overlying muscle and skin. Brachytherapy catheters used to deliver radiotherapy to the tumor bed are also shown. (From Terek R, Brien C. Soft tissue sarcomas of the hand and wrist. *Hand Clin* 1995;11, with permission.)

mately 60% long-term survival. Unlike other soft tissue sarcomas, lymph node biopsy is part of the staging of rhabdomyosarcoma, as many patients have metastatic disease in lymph nodes that are clinically normal (74). Lymph node metastases significantly worsen the prognosis.

Clear cell sarcoma or malignant melanoma of soft parts is often juxtaposed to aponeuroses and tendons. It most commonly occurs in the foot and ankle but also may occur in the hand and other extremity sites. Young adults, more often female, are afflicted with this tumor that is principally composed of round or fusiform cells with clear cytoplasm (Fig. 9) that are immunoreactive for S-100 protein. The nuclei are round or ovoid with prominent basophilic staining. Recurrence and metastases are common despite resection, and the prognosis is poor.

TREATMENT

Surgery

Local treatment of soft tissue sarcomas of the hand consists of surgical resection with or without radiation therapy (56,57,75,76). Surgical margins, described by Enneking et al. (77), are classified into intralesional, marginal, wide, and radical. Radical resection can be achieved by compartment excision or amputation above the origin of muscles where the tumor is located. Wide excision is the removal of tumor surrounded by an intact cuff of normal tissue, usually 2 cm in thickness. Tumor should not be visualized during the resection. Overall survival is not improved with radical resection or amputation compared to wide excision (18,78,79); however, local control is improved with the former. With radio-

therapy in conjunction with wide excision, local control rates of 80% to 90% can be achieved (76,80). The difficulty with wide surgical excision in the hand is that important nerves, blood vessels, bone, and tendons may need to be sacrificed for deep tumors. In fact, to achieve wide margins, amputation is often required. Although amputation may seem required when strictly following the guidelines for a wide margin, it does not seem that amputation results in any better survival (17,78,79). As a practical matter, some areas of the resection may actually be marginal (e.g., along nerves and vessels), in which case radiation therapy should be used (17,18). Encased nerves and vessels should be resected and reconstructed. The most important risk factor for LR is a positive margin (3,18,20,54,78,81). If a patient has a positive margin after inadequate surgery, which usually occurs during an unplanned resection or shell-out procedure, the tumor bed should be reexcised (82). LRs do cause morbidity, so a reasonable attempt should be made to perform an adequate resection.

Radiation

Radical resection results in the lowest incidence of LR (83,84); however, several reports showed that radical surgery did not improve overall survival when compared to local wide excision (85,86). Because of the significant functional impairment after radical excision or amputation, wide excision and radiation treatment either preoperatively (87,88) or postoperatively (89) are usually used and can achieve local control rates of 85% to 90% for large, high-grade sarcomas. Wide excision has become the preferred method of treatment. Radiotherapy can be administered either as external beam or as brachytherapy, or as a combination of the two. External beam radiotherapy can be given pre- or postoperatively, or both. The rationale for preoperative as opposed to postoperative radiation therapy is that a smaller volume of normal tissue is radiated with preoperative therapy, and sterilizing the tumor bed before surgical manipulation may be more effective at preventing LR. Also, "unresectable" tumors can be made "resectable," or safer to resect, with preoperative radiation therapy (90). The advantages of preoperative radiation therapy are at least partly outweighed by a much higher wound complication rate compared to when radiation is used postoperatively. There has been one prospective study comparing the complications and functional outcome of preoperative and postoperative radiotherapy. That study showed a higher wound complication rate, but better function with preoperative radiotherapy, largely because of less extremity edema and fibrosis.

Brachytherapy can be particularly advantageous in the hand because the catheters can be placed under flaps and radiation limited to the tumor bed, thereby minimizing the side effects of radiating the flap and uninvolved portions of the hand. Brachytherapy catheters are implanted at the time of surgery in the tumor bed and loaded with a radiation source 4 to 5 days postoperatively. Brachytherapy has been shown to decrease LR rates in a prospective randomized trial for the treatment of high-grade sarcomas (80); however, there is no effect on LR for low-grade sarcomas (91). The authors suggest that external beam radiation may be more efficacious for low-grade sarcomas, as these tumors grow more slowly and external beam radiotherapy is delivered over a longer period of time than is brachytherapy (91). The role of radiation therapy for low-grade sarcomas has not been established. Because truly wide margins are difficult to achieve in the hand, even small high- or low-grade tumors may benefit from radiation therapy in contrast to other extremity sites, in which small, high-grade tumors can sometimes be treated with surgery alone (52).

Radiation therapy has been shown to decrease LR in patients with high-grade sarcomas when margins are both positive or negative. However, the recurrence rate is higher when margins are positive (92). When margins are positive, reexcision is recommended (82). Local control in patients with positive margins is not as good as in those with negative margins (92,93).

Several studies have shown that the hand tolerates radiation therapy and that functional results are quite good (15–18). Both pre- and postoperative radiation therapy has been used.

Chemotherapy

The role of chemotherapy has not yet been resolved. Because of the small numbers of patients with what is a heterogeneous disease, it has been difficult to demonstrate that chemotherapy makes a difference.

There have been nine prospective studies evaluating chemotherapy for soft tissue sarcoma of the extremity. Most of the studies were conducted in the 1970s and 1980s and used doxorubicin alone or in combination with other agents that are now known not to have activity against sarcoma (94). None of the trials used ifosfamide, an agent that does have activity against sarcoma. An unpublished metaanalysis showed a small improvement in overall survival for those receiving chemotherapy. There are many caveats, limitations, and shortcomings in the trials composing the metaanalysis, so the conclusion is not considered definitive. The results from two nonprospective trials using doxorubicin-based treatment without ifosfamide did not show any clear benefit (55,95). The two agents with the most activity against sarcoma are doxorubicin and ifosfamide, and only one prospective randomized trial using these agents in high-risk patients (stage III) has been performed. The trial was closed early because of a clear advantage in disease-free and overall survival for patients receiving chemotherapy (96). Chemotherapy is primarily used in an investigational setting (97), to shrink unresectable tumors, for metastatic disease, and in individual high-risk situations. Other investigators advocate isolated or nonisolated limb perfusion with chemotherapy in an attempt to make unresectable tumors resectable or to kill the tumor cells before surgical manipulation with the hope of decreasing LR or metastases. These laudable goals have not been achieved in prospective randomized trials. Improved survival for hand sarcomas, particularly for patients with metastatic disease, will require better systemic treatment than is currently available.

For patients who present with or develop metastatic disease, treatment also entails resection of the pulmonary metastases and chemotherapy. Approximately 25% of these patients will be long-term survivors (98).

IMPACT AND ETIOLOGY OF LOCAL RECURRENCE

Eighty percent of patients who have an LR or develop metastases will do so within the first 2 to 3 years after treatment of the primary tumor. The causal relationship between LR and development of metastatic disease is not entirely clear (99). A positive margin is associated with both a higher rate of LR and distant metastasis (100), although LR does not negatively impact on survival, as similar patients who underwent amputation and had a much lower rate of LR had the same mortality as those with a positive margin and LR, suggesting that most positive margins and LRs are markers for more biologically aggressive tumors. An LR may indicate that the initial treatment was inadequate, or more likely, that despite standard treatment, the tumor is more aggressive than average and has a propensity to recur and metastasize. There are two categories of patients who develop an LR: those who despite implementation of what is considered to be standard, adequate treatment, develop an LR and those who develop an LR after a positive margin. In the former case, an LR is a marker for a tumor that is somehow more biologically aggressive or resistant to treatment. The tumor either invades local and distant tissues to a greater extent than average or the biology of the tumor makes it resistant to radiation therapy so that local treatment is less effective. All of these explanations would fall under the rubric of biologic determinism: There are some tumors for which the die is already cast before local treatment is undertaken.

The other group of patients comprises those who have an LR after having had a positive margin. Again, those with a positive margin can be broken down into two groups: those who received standard treatment, but the tumor extended further than anticipated, and those who had inadequate surgery. The positive margin in the former group is again a proxy for a more aggressive tumor. Patients who have positive margins at the time of resection are at increased risk of LR, and it is not possible to "cover up" a positive margin with radiation therapy. If a margin is positive, particularly if the surgery was inadequate, a repeat resection should be performed (82). At the very least, a positive margin increases the risk of LR; however, stage for stage, it has not been possible to show that an LR actually causes death, as patients with similar tumors who underwent amputation have similar mortality (17,85,100). This suggests that the vast majority of LRs and positive margins are markers for more aggressive tumors. The treatment of an LR is repeat excision and additional radiation therapy, usually administered as brachytherapy.

Theoretically, there may be a small subset of patients for whom an LR does affect survival. One can postulate that a genetically unstable tumor, which is initially nonmetastatic, undergoes additional genetic mutations and acquires the metastatic phenotype between the time when the original tumor is resected and the time the LR is clinically detected. It has not been possible to statistically prove that this actually occurs.

Taken together, one should not take a casual approach to local treatment. An LR is not a benign event and will require a repeat resection and additional radiation therapy with their attendant morbidity, or even an amputation if there is not enough tissue to work with. An LR therefore has a significant functional impact on the patient. This is obviously even more true for hand tumors, as there is little expendable tissue to work with, in contrast to the thigh, for instance, where there is often additional expendable muscle that can be reresected. The standard of attempting to achieve a wide margin should be adhered to, although there are times when marginal margins are tolerated to preserve vital structures. One must keep in mind that if an LR occurs, the repeat resection may have more morbidity than if a wide margin had been achieved the first time around. Given the dubious nature of LR (99), it is a clinical decision that must be made with the patient regarding how much function to sacrifice to maximize the chance of obtaining local control.

METASTATIC DISEASE

Estimated survival of patients treated for pulmonary metastases from soft tissue sarcomas was 25% at 3 years and for those with complete resection of their pulmonary metastasis was 46% at 3 years (98,101). Poor prognostic variables include older age, high-grade sarcoma, short time interval between initial diagnosis of the primary sarcoma and development of metastases, incompletely resectable metastases, liposarcoma, and malignant peripheral nerve sheath tumor. Some patients can be salvaged with serial metastectomies. Such patients are usually treated with chemotherapy if possible.

SPECIFIC DATA ON HAND SARCOMA

Of the 4,000 extremity sarcomas per year in the United States, approximately 3% occur in the hand. The most common histologic type varies from series to series and include epithelioid sarcoma (21), synovial sarcoma (19), MFH (17), and rhabdomyosarcoma (12). Some series have shown that patients with hand sarcomas fare worse than patients with comparable tumors in other extremity sites (19). Other series have shown that the results are similar to other extremity sarcomas (17) and that patients with upper extremity sarcomas fare better than those with lower extremity tumors (14,20). In a retrospective clinical review of soft tissue sarcomas of the hand covering an 8-year period at Memorial Sloan-Kettering Cancer Center (19), 23 patients with hand sarcomas were compared to 152 patients with similar extremity tumors. The most common presentation for patients with hand sarcomas was a painless mass. The majority of the tumors were high grade (20), smaller than 5 cm (18), and deep (15). The most common histologic diagnosis was synovial sarcoma. Two patients presented with lymph node metastases, two patients presented with lung metastases, and four patients developed lymph node metastases after treatment. Eighteen patients had attempted wide local excision, four had amputation, and one patient refused surgery. Adjuvant therapy included radiation treatment (10), chemotherapy (4), and chemotherapy and radiation treatment (4). Positive margins and LR were common. Of the 64% of patients who had negative margins, eight received radiation and one had an LR, whereas six did not have radiation and three had recurrence. Of the 36% who had positive margins, six received radiation and four had LR, whereas two did not receive radiation and one had recurrence. Five-year survival was 50% for hand sarcomas that were high grade, smaller than 5 cm, superficial or deep, and nonmetastatic, whereas 5-year survival for small, high-grade sarcomas in nonhand extremity sites was 91% percent. The authors concluded that soft tissue sarcomas of the hand have a worse prognosis than tumors in other extremity sites because of the high rate of positive margins, the anatomy of the hand, or the biology of the sarcomas that occur in the hand (19).

In another series of 24 hand sarcomas from the Roswell Park Cancer Institute (17), patients who underwent amputation had a lower rate of LR but no difference in survival, again suggesting that LR does not affect survival and that the series reporting a worse survival for hand sarcomas is probably related to the biology of the histologic types in that series.

Thirty-one cases of soft tissue hand sarcomas over 23 years at the Mayo Clinic were comprised of epithelioid sarcoma (10), rhabdomyosarcoma (6), synovial sarcoma (5), and fibrosarcoma (5,21). Of the patients with epithelioid sarcoma, all but one patient had LR. The authors recommended radical excision as the primary procedure and at least a forearm amputation for LR.

Conservative surgery and radiation therapy have been advocated by Talbert et al. (16) for soft tissue sarcomas of the distal extremity. Thirty-nine patients over a 28-year period had soft tissue sarcomas involving the wrist and hand. Rate of failure in sarcomas involving the hand was 52%, involving the wrist was 21%, and involving the finger was 0%. The majority of failure was from LR (15%). Talbert et al. (16) pointed out that recurrence does not impact on overall survival and therefore recommended local excision and radiation.

A literature review of 90 synovial sarcomas of the hand covering a 50-year period (23) showed that the majority of patients were younger than 30 years, and the most frequent symptom was a mass about the carpus. Local excision was performed in 89% and primary amputation in 9% of patients. LRs (54%) and secondary amputations (50%) were common. Radiotherapy was given in 30% and chemotherapy in 5% of patients. The 5-year survival was 18% and 10-year survival was 9%.

Series of soft tissue sarcomas of the hand consistently have high LR rates and poor survival. Secondary procedures for LRs are often amputations, some of which could be avoided if an adequate resection is performed initially.

FUNCTION

Functional analysis of 23 patients who underwent limb salvage surgery, 20 of whom also received radiation therapy, revealed that the vast majority had good to excellent results using a validated, patient-rated outcome instrument and were able to return to occupational and everyday activities (18).

To summarize, limb-sparing surgery, usually in combination with radiation therapy, is possible for most patients with soft tissue sarcoma of the hand.

SPECIFIC RESECTIONS AND RECONSTRUCTIONS

The majority of soft tissue hand sarcomas occur in the web space, dorsal or palmar hand, and wrist (19). These are challenging cases in which to achieve local control and maintain function. Wide excision should be attempted, but sometimes marginal excision and radiation may be an acceptable trade-off. Several articles have shown that LR does not statistically alter overall survival (76,102) and that high salvage rates of locally recurrent disease can occur with aggressive surgery after local surgery and radiation (68,89,103). However, to achieve local control with surgery after LR after marginal excision, a more ablative procedure may be required than what would have been necessary to achieve the same margin at the initial surgery. For instance, the first surgery could have been a partial hand amputation; however, the second surgery for an LR might be a mid-forearm amputation. One must also keep in mind that a positive margin cannot be salvaged with postoperative radiotherapy. There will be a higher recurrence rate than if a negative margin and radiotherapy had been used (81). There may also be a small subset of patients whose tumors recur as more aggressive lesions that are more invasive and have greater metastatic potential for whom an LR will adversely affect survival; however, this has not been definitively demonstrated. To maximize oncologic results, wide excision, including nerves, arteries, and tendons if necessary, should be performed (19). Reconstruction can be performed with a combination of vascular and nerve grafting, tendon transfers, and local and free flaps (27,104–106).

Soft tissue sarcomas involving the digits distal to the metacarpophalangeal joint and web space are best managed with amputation at the metacarpophalangeal joint or ray resection. Attempts at local excision and radiation of finger sarcomas have an unacceptably high LR rate and loss of function. The hand of a patient who underwent a fifth ray amputation for an epithelioid sarcoma of the little finger demonstrates excellent cosmesis, and the patient had excellent function (Fig. 10). A fifth ray amputation should preserve the base of the fifth metacarpal and insertion of the extensor carpi ulnaris.

Resection of one or more rays may be necessary for a hand sarcoma resection and yields excellent local control and function (18,107). Pollicization of the index to the thumb can be used after thumb ray resection. Index ray amputation and small ray amputation do not require transposition but may cause loss of power grip. Important aspects of the index ray amputation include preservation of

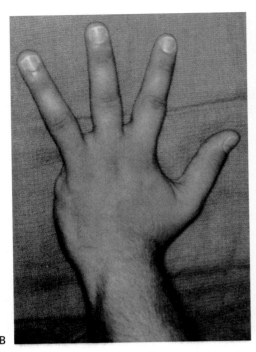
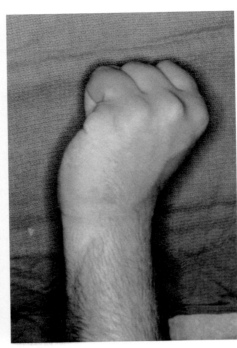

A,B

FIGURE 10. A,B: Hand of a patient who had a fifth ray amputation for epithelioid sarcoma of the little finger.

the base of the index metacarpal where the extensor carpi radialis longus inserts, transfer of the first dorsal interosseous muscle to the radial lateral band of the middle finger for improved abduction of the middle finger and cosmesis of the web space, and transfer of the extensor indicis proprius to the extensor hood of the middle digit to strengthen pinch and independent extension. Middle finger and ring finger ray amputations can be managed with index metacarpal transfer and little finger metacarpal transfer, respectively, to close an unsightly space, improve function, and avoid late deformity. Osteotomy of the index metacarpal and transposition to the osteotomy site of the base of the middle phalanx preserve the insertion of the extensor carpi radialis longus and brevis. For the small finger, either osteotomy or allowing the entire metacarpal of the fifth finger to transpose can be successfully performed, and control of rotation in both transpositions should be performed using Kirschner wire fixation. Resection of the central three rays has been performed for clear cell sarcoma without reconstruction. The patient had functional opposition with the two remaining fingers (108).

Sarcomas occurring on the volar aspect of the wrist and hand are particularly difficult to treat because of potential involvement of the median and ulnar nerves and flexor tendons. Sacrificing the median and ulnar nerve, tendons, and blood vessels for palmar lesions to achieve wide margins may result in unacceptable functional outcome. Vascular reconstruction, reinnervated free muscle transplantation (104), and nerve grafting (109–111) have been reported after tumor resection, but cold intolerance and functional recovery after grafting remain problems. Whether an amputation is a better alternative is difficult to say. Free tissue flaps and local flaps for soft tissue coverage may be required after resection that cannot be closed primarily. Myocutaneous and fasciocutaneous flaps have been used to achieve coverage. The distally based radial artery fasciocutaneous flap (27) can be used to cover defects anywhere in the hand (Fig. 11). Radiation can be delivered as brachytherapy to minimize radiation exposure to the flap and surrounding normal tissues. These treatment modalities should be considered and consultation obtained before resection of the tumor.

For sarcomas involving the dorsum of the wrist, resection of the tumor with the extensor tendons as well as the underlying bone if necessary can be performed and easily reconstructed. A patient with a recurrent synovial sarcoma on the dorsum of the hand that involved the extensor tendons of the fifth digit is shown in Figure 12. Reconstruction was performed by transferring the extensor indicis proprius to the fifth finger extensor, and soft tissue coverage was performed with a distal radial artery–based fasciocutaneous flap. The patient shown in Figure 9A had a recurrent amelanotic melanoma invading the dorsum of the distal radius. The overlying soft tissues, including the extensor carpi radialis longus and brevis, and distal radius were resected. Bone and soft tissue reconstruction was performed with a vascularized fibula graft with fusion of the wrist. One reason for using a vascularized fibula graft (112) instead of a nonvascularized autograft or allograft was that radiation therapy was to be administered postoperatively, which can significantly interfere with healing of nonvascularized grafts. Brachytherapy catheters were placed intraoperatively and are shown in the postoperative radiograph (Fig. 9B).

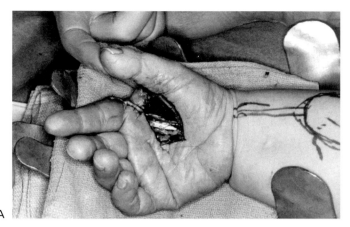

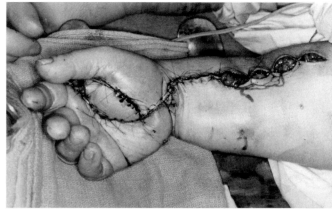

A

B

FIGURE 11. Soft tissue reconstruction volar defect. **A:** Defect after excision of a malignant poroma of the palm. **B:** Reconstruction with a distal radial artery–based fasciocutaneous forearm flap. (From DaSilva MF, Terek R, Weiss AP. *J Hand Surg [Am]* 1997;22, with permission.)

SUMMARY

Soft tissue sarcomas of the hand are rare, difficult problems to treat. The clinical presentation and pathologic analysis are difficult. One should consider diagnostic imaging and biopsy before excision of hand masses, and, while operating on the hand, be prepared to unexpectedly encounter a sarcoma. Avoidance of unnecessary contamination during excision and biopsy is of paramount importance so as to not preclude limb salvage. Once

diagnosed, the most important aspect of treatment is wide surgical resection with negative margins. This can usually be accomplished without amputation. Radiation therapy is frequently used for high-grade tumors and any tumor with a marginal or positive margin. Chemotherapy remains investigational, and patients with high-risk tumors should be given the opportunity to participate in clinical trials. Referral to centers with multidisciplinary cancer programs should be strongly considered before embarking on treatment (113,114).

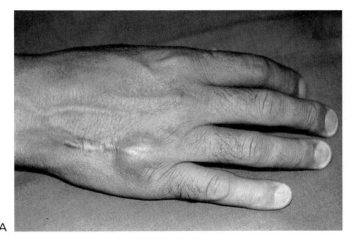

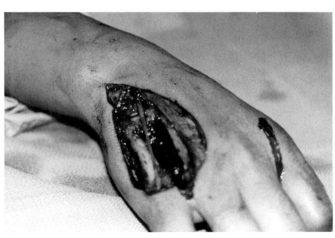

A

B

C

FIGURE 12. A: Patient with a recurrent synovial sarcoma over the dorsum of the fifth metacarpal. **B:** Intraoperative photograph showing the soft tissue defect and the transferred extensor indicis proprius tendon to the extensor tendon of the fifth digit. **C:** Soft tissue reconstruction was performed with a distal radial artery–based fasciocutaneous flap. (From Terek R, Brien C. Soft tissue sarcomas of the hand and wrist. *Hand Clin* 1995;11, with permission.)

REFERENCES

1. Enzinger FM, Weiss SW. *Soft tissue tumors*. St. Louis: Mosby, 1988.
2. Rydholm A, Gustafson P, Alvegard TA, et al. Prognostic factors in soft tissue sarcoma. A review and the Scandinavian Sarcoma Group experience. *Acta Orthop Scand Suppl* 1999;285:50–57.
3. Pisters PW, Leung DH, Woodruff J, et al. Analysis of prognostic factors in 1,041 patients with localized soft tissue sarcomas of the extremities. *J Clin Oncol* 1996;14:1679–1689.
4. Pisters PW, Pollock RE. Staging and prognostic factors in soft tissue sarcoma. *Semin Radiat Oncol* 1999;9:307–314.
5. Brooks AD, Heslin MJ, Leung DH, et al. Superficial extremity soft tissue sarcoma: an analysis of prognostic factors. *Ann Surg Oncol* 1998;5:41–47.
6. Gaynor JJ, Tan CC, Casper ES, et al. Refinement of clinicopathologic staging for localized soft tissue sarcoma of the extremity: a study of 423 adults. *J Clin Oncol* 1992;10:1317–1329.
7. Evans HL, Baer SC. Epithelioid sarcoma: a clinicopathologic and prognostic study of 26 cases. *Semin Diagn Pathol* 1993;10:286–291.
8. Ross HM, Lewis JJ, Woodruff JM, Brennan MF. Epithelioid sarcoma: clinical behavior and prognostic factors of survival. *Ann Surg Oncol* 1997;4:491–495.
9. Salo JC, Lewis JJ, Woodruff JM, et al. Malignant fibrous histiocytoma of the extremity. *Cancer* 1999;85:1765–1772.
10. Vauthey JN, Woodruff JM, Brennan MF. Extremity malignant peripheral nerve sheath tumors (neurogenic sarcomas): a 10-year experience. *Ann Surg Oncol* 1995;2:126–131.
11. Talbert ML, Zagars GK, Sherman NE, Romsdahl MM. Conservative surgery and radiation therapy for soft tissue sarcoma of the wrist, hand, ankle, and foot. *Cancer* 1990;66:2482–2491.
12. Gross E, Rao BN, Pappo AS, et al. Soft tissue sarcoma of the hand in children: clinical outcome and management. *J Pediatr Surg* 1997;32:698–702.
13. Creighton JJ, Clayton AP, Mindell ER, et al. Primary malignant tumors of the upper extremity: retrospective analysis of one hundred twenty-six cases. *J Hand Surg* 1985;10A:805–814.
14. Karakousis CP, De Young C, Driscoll DL. Soft tissue sarcomas of the hand and foot: management and survival. *Ann Surg Oncol* 1998;5:238–240.
15. Johnstone PA, Wexler LH, Venzon DJ, et al. Sarcomas of the hand and foot: analysis of local control and functional result with combined modality therapy in extremity preservation. *Int J Radiat Oncol Biol Phys* 1994;29:735–745.
16. Talbert ML, Zagars GK, Sherman NE, et al. Conservative surgery and radiation therapy for soft tissue sarcomas of the wrist, hand, ankle, and foot. *Cancer* 1990;66:2482.
17. McPhee M, McGrath BE, Zhang P, et al. Soft tissue sarcoma of the hand. *J Hand Surg [Am]* 1999;24:1001–1007.
18. Bray PW, Bell RS, Bowen CV, et al. Limb salvage surgery and adjuvant radiotherapy for soft tissue sarcomas of the forearm and hand. *J Hand Surg [Am]* 1997;22:495–503.
19. Brien EW, Terek RM, Geer RJ, et al. Treatment of soft-tissue sarcomas of the hand. *J Bone Joint Surg [Am]* 1995;77:564–571.
20. Gustafson P, Arner M. Soft tissue sarcoma of the upper extremity: descriptive data and outcome in a population-based series of 108 adult patients. *J Hand Surg [Am]* 1999;24:668–674.
21. Bryan RS, Soule EH, Dobyns JH, et al. Primary epithelioid sarcoma of the hand and forearm. *J Bone Joint Surg* 1974;56A:458–465.
22. Campanacci M, Bertoni F, Laus M. Soft tissue sarcoma of the hand. *Ital J Orthotraumatol* 1981;7:313.
23. Dreyfus UY, Boome RS, Kranold DH. Synovial sarcoma of the hand: a literature review. *J Hand Surg* 1986;11B:471.
24. Owens JC, Shiu MH, Smith R, et al. Soft tissue sarcomas of the hand and foot. *Cancer* 1985;55:2010.
25. Erdmann MW, Quaba AA, Sommerlad BC. Epithelioid sarcoma masquerading as Dupuytren's disease. *Br J Plast Surg* 1995;48:39–42.
26. Power RA, Manek S, McCullough CJ. Spindle-cell sarcoma of the hand may present as a benign recurrent nodule. *J Bone Joint Surg [Br]* 1992;74:316–317.
27. DaSilva MF, Terek R, Weiss AP. Malignant eccrine poroma of the hand: a case report. *J Hand Surg [Am]* 1997;22:511–514.
28. Weiss AP, Steichen JB. Synovial sarcoma causing carpal tunnel syndrome. *J Hand Surg [Am]* 1992;17:1024–1025.
29. Patel MR, Desai SS, Gordon SL. Functional limb salvage with multimodality treatment in epithelioid sarcoma of the hand: a report of two cases. *J Hand Surg [Am]* 1986;11:265–269.
30. McClain EJ, Wissinger HA. The acute carpal tunnel syndrome: nine case reports. *J Trauma* 1976;16:75–78.
31. Steffens K, Koob E. [Compression of the median nerve by chondrosarcoma of the hand]. *Handchir Mikrochir Plast Chir* 1988;20:220–222.
32. Kurkchubasche AG, Halvorson EG, Forman EN, et al. The role of preoperative chemotherapy in the treatment of infantile fibrosarcoma. *J Pediatr Surg* 2000;35:880–883.
33. Kimura C, Kitamura T, Sugihara T. A case of congenital infantile fibrosarcoma of the right hand. *J Dermatol* 1998;25:735–741.
34. Katz MA, Beredjiklian PK, Wirganowicz PZ. Nodular fasciitis of the hand: a case report. *Clin Orthop* 2001;108–111.
35. Healey JH, Turnbull ADM, Miedema B, Lane JM. Acrometastases. A study of twenty-nine patients with osseous involvement of the hand and feet. *J Bone Joint Surg* 1986;68-A:743.
36. Olsson H. A review of the epidemiology of soft tissue sarcoma. *Acta Orthop Scand Suppl* 1999;285:8–10.
37. Evers B, Klammer H. Tumors and tumorlike lesions of the hand: analysis of 424 surgically treated cases. *Arch Am Acad Orthop Surg* 1997;1:34–43.
38. Fong Y, Coit DG, Woodruff JM, Brennan MF. Lymph node metastasis from soft tissue sarcoma in adults. *Ann Surg* 1993;217:72–77.
39. Tung GA, Davis LM. The role of magnetic resonance imaging in the evaluation of the soft tissue mass. *Crit Rev Diagn Imaging* 1993;34:239–308.
40. Capelastegui A, Astigarraga E, Fernandez-Canton G, et al. Masses and pseudomasses of the hand and wrist: MR findings in 134 cases. *Skeletal Radiol* 1999;28:498–507.
41. Panicek DM, Go SD, Healey JH et al. Soft-tissue sarcoma involving bone or neurovascular structures: MR imaging prognostic factors. *Radiology* 1997;205:871–875.

42. Hosono M, Kobayashi H, Fujimoto R, et al. Septum-like structures in lipoma and liposarcoma: MR imaging and pathologic correlation. *Skeletal Radiol* 1997;26:150–154.

43. Cadman NL, Soule EH, Kelly PJ. Synovial sarcoma: an analysis of 134 tumors. *Cancer* 1965;18:613.

44. Horwitz AL, Resnick D, Watson RC. The roentgen features of synovial sarcomas. *Clin Radiol* 1973;24:481.

45. Peabody TD, Gibbs CP Jr, Simon MA. Evaluation and staging of musculoskeletal neoplasms. *J Bone Joint Surg [Am]* 1998;80:1204–1218.

46. Peabody TD, Simon MA. Principles of staging of soft-tissue sarcomas. *Clin Orthop* 1993;19–31.

47. Soft tissue sarcoma. In: Fleming ID, Cooper JS, Henson DE, et al., eds. *American Joint Committee on Cancer (AJCC) staging manual.* Philadelphia: Lippincott, 1997:149–156.

48. Hadju SI. History and classification of soft tissue tumors. Pathology of soft tissue tumors. Philadelphia: Lea & Febiger, 1979:1–55.

49. Wunder JS, Healey JH, Davis AM, Brennan MF. A comparison of staging systems for localized extremity soft tissue sarcoma. *Cancer* 2000;88:2721–2730.

50. Enneking WF. A system of staging musculoskeletal neoplasms. *Clin Orthop* 1986;204:9–24.

51. Peabody TD, Monson D, Montag A, et al. A comparison of the prognoses for deep and subcutaneous sarcomas of the extremities. *J Bone Joint Surg [Am]* 1994;76:1167–1173.

52. Geer RJ, Woodruff J, Casper ES, Brennan MF. Management of small soft-tissue sarcoma of the extremity in adults. *Arch Surg* 1992;127:1285–1289.

53. Weiser MR, Lewis JJ, Leung DH, Brennan MF. Management of small, high-grade extremity soft tissue sarcoma. *Surg Oncol* 1999;8:215–218.

54. Fleming JB, Berman RS, Cheng SC, et al. Long-term outcome of patients with American Joint Committee on Cancer stage IIB extremity soft tissue sarcomas. *J Clin Oncol* 1999;17:2772–2780.

55. Pisters PW, Patel SR, Varma DG, et al. Preoperative chemotherapy for stage IIIB extremity soft tissue sarcoma: long-term results from a single institution. *J Clin Oncol* 1997;15:3481–3487.

56. Pollack R, Brennan M, Lawrence W Jr. Society of Surgical Oncology practice guidelines. Soft-tissue sarcoma surgical practice guidelines. *Oncology (Huntingt)* 1997;11:1327–1332.

57. Demetri GD, Pollock R, Baker L, et al. NCCN sarcoma practice guidelines. National Comprehensive Cancer Network. *Oncology (Huntingt)* 1998;12:183–218.

58. Lewis JJ, Leung D, Casper ES, et al. Multifactorial analysis of long-term follow-up (more than 5 years) of primary extremity sarcoma. *Arch Surg* 1999;134:190–194.

59. Broders AC, Hargrave R, Meyerding HW. Pathological features of soft tissue fibrosarcoma with special reference to the grading of its malignancy. *Surg Gynecol Obstet* 1939;69:267.

60. Gustafson P. Soft tissue sarcoma. Epidemiology and prognosis in 508 patients. *Acta Orthop Scand Suppl* 1994;259:1–31.

61. Mandahl N, Mertens F, Mitelman F. Genetic changes in bone and soft tissue tumors. *Acta Orthop Scand Suppl* 1999;285:30–40.

62. Bell RS, Wunder J, Andrulis I. Molecular alterations in bone and soft-tissue sarcoma. *Can J Surg* 1999;42:259–266.

63. Kawai A, Woodruff J, Healey JH, et al. SYT-SSX gene fusion as a determinant of morphology and prognosis in synovial sarcoma. *N Engl J Med* 1998;338:153–160.

64. Mankin HJ, Mankin CJ, Simon MA. The hazards of the biopsy, revisited. Members of the Musculoskeletal Tumor Society. *J Bone Joint Surg [Am]* 1996;78:656–663.

65. Simon MA, Biermann JS. Biopsy of bone and soft-tissue lesions. *J Bone Joint Surg [Am]* 1993;75:616–621.

66. Mandard AM, Petiot JF, Marnay J, et al. Prognostic factors in soft tissue sarcomas. A multivariate analysis of 109 cases. *Cancer* 1989;63:1437.

67. Myhre-Jensen O, Kaae S, Madsen EH, et al. Histopathologic grading in soft-tissue tumors. Relation to survival in 261 surgically treated patients. *Acta Pathol Microbiol Immunol Scand* 1983;91:145.

68. Tsujimoto M, Aozasa I, Ueda T. Multivariate analysis for histologic prognostic factors in soft tissue sarcomas. *Cancer* 1988;62:994–998.

69. Ahmed MN, Feldman M, Seemayer TA. Cytology of epithelioid sarcoma. *Acta Cytol* 1974;18:459.

70. Ariel M, Pack GT. Synovial sarcoma: review of 25 cases. *N Engl J Med* 1963;268:1272.

71. Weiss SW, Enzinger FM. Malignant fibrous histiocytoma: an analysis of 200 cases. *Cancer* 1978;41:2250.

72. Fletcher CD, Gustafson P, Rydholm A, et al. Clinicopathologic re-evaluation of 100 malignant fibrous histiocytomas: prognostic relevance of subclassification. *J Clin Oncol* 2001;19:3045–3050.

73. Maurer HM, Beltangady M, Gehan EA, et al. The Intergroup Rhabdomyosarcoma Study-1. *Cancer* 1988;61:209.

74. Neville HL, Andrassy RJ, Lobe TE, et al. Preoperative staging, prognostic factors, and outcome for extremity rhabdomyosarcoma: a preliminary report from the Intergroup Rhabdomyosarcoma Study IV (1991–1997). *J Pediatr Surg* 2000;35:317–321.

75. Brennan MF. Management of soft tissue sarcoma. *Br J Surg* 1996;83:577–579.

76. Brennan MF, Casper ES, Harrison LB, et al. The role of multimodality therapy in soft-tissue sarcoma. *Ann Surg* 1991;214:328–338.

77. Enneking WF, Spanier SS, Goodman MA. A system for the surgical staging of musculoskeletal sarcomas. *Clin Orthop* 1980;153:106–120.

78. Heslin MJ, Woodruff J, Brennan MF. Prognostic significance of a positive microscopic margin in high-risk extremity soft tissue sarcoma: implications for management. *J Clin Oncol* 1996;14:473–478.

79. Rosenberg SA, Tepper J, Glatstein E, et al. The treatment of soft-tissue sarcomas of the extremities. *Ann Surg* 1982;196:305–315.

80. Pisters PW, Harrison LB, Leung DH, et al. Long-term results of a prospective randomized trial of adjuvant brachytherapy in soft tissue sarcoma. *J Clin Oncol* 1996;14:859–868.

81. Bell RS, O'Sullivan B, Liu FF, et al. The surgical margin in soft-tissue sarcoma. *J Bone Joint Surg* 1989;71-A:370–375.

82. Noria S, Davis A, Kandel R, et al. Residual disease following unplanned excision of soft-tissue sarcoma of an extremity. *J Bone Joint Surg [Am]* 1996;78:650–655.

83. Abbas JS, Holyoke ED, Moore R. The surgical treatment and outcome of soft-tissue sarcoma. *Arch Surg* 1981;116:765.

84. Eilber FR, Mirra JJ, Grant TT. Is amputation necessary for sarcomas? *Ann Surg* 1980;192:431.

85. Rosenberg SA, Kent H, Costa J, et al. Prospective randomized evaluation of the role of limb-sparing surgery, radiation therapy, and adjuvant chemoimmunotherapy in the treatment of adult soft-tissue sarcomas. *Surgery* 1978;84:63–69.

86. Rosenberg SA, Tepper J, Glatstein E, et al. Prospective randomized evaluation of adjuvant chemotherapy in adults with soft tissue sarcomas of the extremities. *Cancer* 1983;52:424–434.

87. Sadoski C, Suit HD, Rosenberg A, et al. Preoperative radiation, surgical margins, and local control of extremity sarcomas of soft tissues. *J Surg Oncol* 1993;52:223–230.

88. Suit HD, Proppe KH, Mankin HJ, et al. Preoperative radiation therapy for sarcoma of soft tissue. *Cancer* 1994;47:2269.

89. Lindberg RD, Martin RG, Romsdahl MM, et al. Conservative surgery and postoperative radiotherapy in 300 adults with soft-tissue sarcomas. *Cancer* 1981;47:2391.

90. Robinson MH, Keus RB, Shasha D, Harrison LB. Is preoperative radiotherapy superior to postoperative radiotherapy in the treatment of soft tissue sarcoma? *Eur J Cancer* 1998;34:1309–1316.

91. Pisters PW, Harrison LB, Woodruff JM, et al. A prospective randomized trial of adjuvant brachytherapy in the management of low-grade soft tissue sarcomas of the extremity and superficial trunk. *J Clin Oncol* 1994;12:1150–1155.

92. Alektiar KM, Velasco J, Zelefsky MJ, et al. Adjuvant radiotherapy for margin-positive high-grade soft tissue sarcoma of the extremity. *Int J Radiat Oncol Biol Phys* 2000;48:1051–1058.

93. Alekhteyar KM, Leung DH, Brennan MF, Harrison LB. The effect of combined external beam radiotherapy and brachytherapy on local control and wound complications in patients with high-grade soft tissue sarcomas of the extremity with positive microscopic margin. *Int J Radiat Oncol Biol Phys* 1996;36:321–324.

94. Tierney JF, Mosseri V, Stewart LA, et al. Adjuvant chemotherapy for soft-tissue sarcoma: review and meta-analysis of the published results of randomised clinical trials. *Br J Cancer* 1995;72:469–475.

95. Casper ES, Gaynor JJ, Harrison LB, et al. Preoperative and postoperative adjuvant combination chemotherapy for adults with high grade soft tissue sarcoma. *Cancer* 1993;73:1644–1651.

96. Benjamin RS. Evidence for using adjuvant chemotherapy as standard treatment of soft tissue sarcoma. *Semin Radiat Oncol* 1999;9:349–351.

97. Verweij J, Seynaeve C. The reason for confining the use of adjuvant chemotherapy in soft tissue sarcoma to the investigational setting. *Semin Radiat Oncol* 1999;9:352–359.

98. Billingsley KG, Burt ME, Jara E, et al. Pulmonary metastases from soft tissue sarcoma: analysis of patterns of diseases and postmetastasis survival. *Ann Surg* 1999;229:602–610.

99. Brennan MF. The enigma of local recurrence. The Society of Surgical Oncology. *Ann Surg Oncol* 1997;4:1–12.

100. Lewis JJ, Leung D, Heslin M, et al. Association of local recurrence with subsequent survival in extremity soft tissue sarcoma. *J Clin Oncol* 1997;15:646–652.

101. Billingsley KG, Lewis JJ, Leung DH, et al. Multifactorial analysis of the survival of patients with distant metastasis arising from primary extremity sarcoma. *Cancer* 1999;85:389–395.

102. Brennan MF, Hilaris B, Shiu MH, et al. Local recurrence in adult soft tissue sarcoma—a randomized trial of brachytherapy. *Arch Surg* 1987;122:1289.

103. Potter DA, Kinsella T, Gladstein E, et al. High-grade soft tissue sarcomas of the extremities. *Cancer* 1986;58:190.

104. Doi K, Sakai K, Ihara K, et al. Reinnervated free muscle transplantation for extremity reconstruction. *Plast Reconstr Surg* 1993;91:872–883.

105. Visuthikosol V, Kruavit A, Nitiyanant P, et al. Salvage treatment for sarcomas of the hand. *Ann Plast Surg* 1998;40:637–640.

106. Osaka S, Hoshi M, Sano S, et al. Description of new composite tissue transfer for salvage of a complex hand defect. *Clin Orthop* 1996;91–93.

107. Troum S, Floyd WE III. Alveolar soft-part sarcoma of the hand. *J Hand Surg [Am]* 1993;18:1016–1018.

108. Miller SJ, Rayan GM. Triple central ray amputation for clear cell sarcoma of the hand. *Am J Orthop* 2000;29:226–228.

109. Kallio PK, Vastamaki M. An analysis of the results of late reconstruction of 132 median nerves. *J Hand Surg* 1993;18B:97–105.

110. Novak CB, Kelly L, Mackinnon SE. Sensory recovery after median nerve grafting. *J Hand Surg* 1992;17A:59–68.

111. Singh R, Mechelse K, Hop WCJ, Braakman R. Long-term results of transplantation to repair median, ulnar, and radial nerve lesions by a microsurgical interfascicular autogenous cable graft technique. *Surg Neurol* 1992;37:425–431.

112. Duffy GP, Wood MB, Rock MG, Sim FH. Vascularized free fibular transfer combined with autografting for the management of fracture nonunions associated with radiation therapy. *J Bone Joint Surg Am* 2000;82:544–554.

113. O'Sullivan B, Wylie J, Catton C, et al. The local management of soft tissue sarcoma. *Semin Radiat Oncol* 1999;9:328–348.

114. Gustafson P, Dreinhofer KE, Rydholm A. Soft tissue sarcoma should be treated at a tumor center. A comparison of quality of surgery in 375 patients. *Acta Orthop Scand* 1994;65:47–50.

101

PRIMARY BONE TUMORS

PETER M. MURRAY

Primary bone tumors are unusual, accounting for only a small portion of all neoplasms. The actual number of newly diagnosed benign bone neoplasms is unknown, but it is estimated that approximately 3,000 new malignant bone tumors are diagnosed each year (1). Of particular rarity are primary bone tumors of the hand, wrist, and forearm. According to the Leeds Regional Bone Tumor Registry, bone tumors of the hand and wrist region accounted for only 3.9% of all bone tumors in their registry. In a review of the Mayo Clinic Pathology Department files, only 44 primary bone tumors of the carpus were identified among 26,800 bone tumors, for a relative incidence among the carpal bones of 0.16% (2).

The challenge to the hand surgeon is to stay abreast of the clinical and radiographic characteristics of primary bone neoplasms of the hand, wrist, and forearm. These lesions are seen so infrequently that their diagnosis can evade even the most astute and conscientious surgeon. This requires at the very least a formal yearly review of musculoskeletal oncology. Most practicing hand surgeons are presented with one or two malignant bone tumors during their careers. Benign bone neoplasms are encountered with greater frequency. The potential devastating consequences of missing the diagnosis of a malignant bone tumor obligates the hand surgeon to stay well informed about the characteristics of benign and malignant bone tumors. He or she must always consider the diagnosis, despite the rarity of presentation, and be able to obtain a comprehensive tumor workup whenever necessary. In most situations, the community hand surgeon is encouraged to refer malignant bone tumors to medical centers prepared to provide the complex care needed by these patients.

Although many cancer centers prefer to obtain their own biopsy, in some instances, the hand surgeon may obtain the initial biopsy as part of the tumor workup. Nothing is more important to the ultimate outcome than the original biopsy. The specifics of the tumor workup, surgical staging, individual tumor characteristics, as well as the important aspects of obtaining a biopsy are discussed in this chapter.

PHYSICAL EXAMINATION

As with the diagnosis of any musculoskeletal affliction, the physical examination of the patient with a suspected bone tumor must be thorough and complete. Patients with bone tumors may present to the hand surgeon's office by direct referral from a primary care physician or as a consultation from an orthopedic or general surgeon. The patient may already have radiographs and a suspected diagnosis. Alternatively, the patient may occasionally be self-referred with only vague complaints of discomfort or a discrepancy in limb size. Not too infrequently, the patient, having been in denial, may present with a large mass that he or she has tried to ignore. The limb with the bone lesion must be carefully inspected for size differences and any overlying skin changes. In contrast, some patients can be quite astute at identifying subtle changes in limb size. These complaints should serve as a red flag for potential neoplasms and should not be discounted. Too often, these patient concerns are ignored by the examining physician.

An enlargement of any portion of the upper extremity can be subtle. However, a mass or any upper extremity enlargement is easily determined by circumferentially measuring the extremity with a tape measure. When a mass is identified, it should be examined, then characterized for the medical record by outlining its size, mobility, and firmness.

A careful neurologic examination of the entire extremity should also be performed. Malignant and benign bone tumors alike can have significant soft tissue extensions that can subtly affect distal neurologic function. The slow-growing nature of some tumors can cause insidious neurologic compromise, frequently missed by cursory examination. The patient may complain of weakness or paresthesias and present with signs of peripheral nerve compression. Muscle testing of all upper extremity muscle groups is recommended, making comparison with the contralateral extremity. Careful examination of hand sensibility is performed using Semmes-Weinstein monofilaments, with the 2.83 filament considered normal. The volar surface of each digit is touched with the end of the selected monofilament. The patient is asked to keep eyes closed and identify which digit is being touched. Progressively larger filaments are used until the patient can perceive a touch. Deep tendon reflexes should also be examined.

The radial, ulnar, and brachial pulses are palpated to assess the vascular inflow to the extremity. A handheld Doppler device may be helpful to auscultate the pulses in some patients. Increased pulse intensity compared to the contralateral extremity can represent the accentuated perfusion seen in the proximity of malignant bony tumors. The skin is inspected for signs of either chronic or acute venous obstruction. An asymmetric dilatation of peripheral veins or a bluish skin hue can indicate acute venous outflow problems. Nonhealing skin wounds or ulcers are indicative of chronic venous obstruction.

As a part of a complete and thorough tumor workup, the patient with an identified bone tumor should have a complete physical examination (beyond the musculoskeletal examination) by an internal medicine physician. The hand surgeon is responsible for an initial, detailed musculoskeletal examination that includes the patient's height and weight. Routine blood studies should be drawn, including complete blood cell count, chemistry panel, liver function studies, and a urinalysis. In patients with lytic primary bone lesions, a serum and urine protein electrophoresis should be obtained.

IMAGING

The initial workup of the bone tumor patient includes biplaner radiographs of the lesion in question. The radiographs should image the entire affected extremity, including the joints above and below the bone tumor. The radiographs should be carefully inspected for size and extent of the lesion as well as the presence of intralesional or periosteal new bone formation (Fig. 1). The radiographs should also be evaluated for presence or absence of a distinct lesion border. Of greater importance, however, is the ominous sign of lesion expansion beyond cortical boundaries, also known as *cortical break-through* (Fig. 2B). Such characteristics are typically identified in the malignant bone tumor but may also be observed in locally aggressive benign tumors such as the giant cell tumor of bone (Fig. 3C). Any lesion that has destroyed 50% or more of the cortex has traditionally been considered at high risk for pathologic fracture (3). This has been supported by clinical studies (4,5). However, there are a variety of factors that may affect the load sharing capability of diseased bone. These factors include the thickness of the cortex, the formation of new bone within the tumor, indistinct or permeative tumor borders, and nearby or adjacent tumor involvement (6). Therefore, accurately quantifying the risk of pathologic fracture is undoubtedly more complicated than once thought. Midshaft defects with 50% cortical destruction may have a decrease in compressive strength of up to 90%

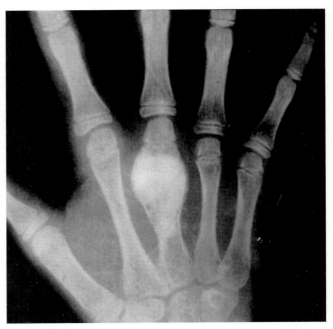

FIGURE 1. Osteogenic sarcoma of the third metacarpal displaying blastic features.

(6). These data have primarily been determined for weight-bearing long bones and have uncertain significance for the bones of the hand and wrist. Whatever criteria are chosen, tumors with impending pathologic fracture require prompt prophylactic treatment.

The patient whose differential diagnosis includes a malignant lesion or a giant cell tumor of bone should have standard screening posteroanterior and lateral radiographs of the affected part, a computed tomography (CT) scan of the chest, a contrast-enhanced abdominal/pelvic CT scan, and a bone scan. These additional studies are necessary to identify possible metastatic involvement, thereby establishing the diagnosis and facilitating appropriate early treatment. Consultation with a medical oncologist, if appropriate, is also obtained during this phase of the patient's workup.

Before biopsy and definitive surgical management, further imaging studies of the bone tumor are required. Non-contrast CT scans of the affected extremity are helpful in preoperative planning and in clarifying the anatomic details of the bone tumor. It is incumbent on the hand surgeon to specify the necessary anatomic limits of the CT scan. All too often, the study ordered does not image the entire tumor. The scan should be obtained in the axial and the coronal planes with 1-mm cuts. Sagittal and three-dimensional reconstruction images should also be ordered. Larger than 1-mm cuts may miss cortical break-through or pathologic fracture. The surgeon should specify to the radiology technician the bone landmarks that define the extent of the desired study. It is never possible to obtain too much information during this stage of the workup. Alternatively, the

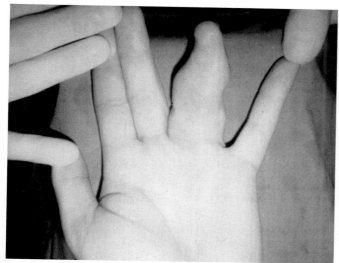

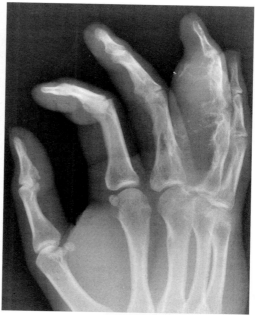

FIGURE 2. A: Fifty-three-year-old woman with slowly enlarging, painful chondrosarcoma of the ring finger. **B:** Oblique radiographic projection demonstrating cortical perforation with invasion of the tumor into the soft tissues.

hand surgeon can confer with the musculoskeletal radiologist for CT scan parameters.

If the bone tumor has a suspected soft tissue extension, magnetic resonance imaging (MRI) may be the imaging technique of choice. Although CT scanning is the classic study for imaging bone, sufficient bone detail is obtainable using MRI. The extent of the soft tissue extension is imaged using the following sequences: T1 axial and best long axis, T2 axial, proton density, short tau inversion recovery, and post gadolinium T1 with fat suppression (axial and best long axis). Malignant bone tumors show signal enhancement on T2 sequencing (7). Blood and pus can also show signal enhancement on T2 imaging. Fat will be bright (enhanced) on both T1 and T2 (7). The MRI should be reviewed directly with a musculoskeletal radiologist, the orthopedic pathologist, and the medical oncologist before proceeding with biopsy and definitive surgical management.

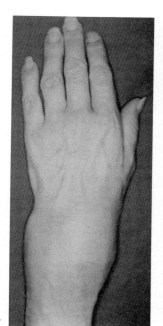

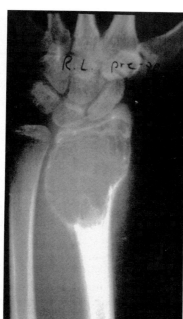

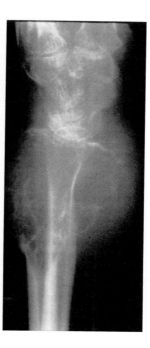

FIGURE 3. A: Forty-eight-year-old woman with enlarging, painful distal wrist mass diagnosed as giant cell tumor of bone. **B:** Posteroanterior wrist view of the tumor demonstrating cortical expansion. **C:** Lateral wrist view showing cortical breakthrough with soft tissue extension of the tumor.

BIOPSY

Unequivocally, the most important step in both the diagnosis and the ultimate treatment of any bone tumor is biopsy. As mentioned previously, many cancer centers prefer obtaining the biopsy in their respective institutions. Studies support the notion that fewer errors in diagnosis occur when the entire workup is performed at the same institution, enabling coordination among the musculoskeletal radiologist, the medical oncologist, the orthopedic pathologist, and the orthopedic musculoskeletal tumor oncologist (8,9). These studies also suggest long-term survival is improved and recurrence more frequent when the biopsy is not obtained at the center performing the definitive treatment (8,9). For practical reasons, for efficiency, and depending on training and experience, the community hand surgeon who first saw the patient may perform the biopsy.

After the tumor workup is complete, the most appropriate anatomic site for the biopsy is chosen. Generally, the ideal anatomic site for biopsy is an area most representative of the lesion. In cases with metastatic involvement, the most accessible area of the bone tumor requiring the least soft tissue dissection is preferred. For example, if a metastatic peripheral lung field tumor is identified, consultation with a thoracic surgeon is obtained.

Surgical Principles

Several surgical principles must be followed in any biopsy. First, the biopsy incision is linear and diminutive. Large, transverse biopsy incisions are to be condemned (1,9,10). It must be remembered that the biopsy tract is considered contaminated. If the biopsy yields a diagnosis of malignant bone tumor, the entire contaminated biopsy tract must be excised during the definitive tumor surgery. Second, impeccable hemostasis is achieved during the tumor biopsy in an attempt to prevent the local spread of tumor cells. Third, the surgeon must plan a biopsy incision that can be incorporated within the incision necessitated by the definitive tumor surgery. To do otherwise can severely jeopardize limb salvage procedures and, potentially, patient survival.

Surgical Technique

General anesthesia is preferred for the patient undergoing biopsy. Regional anesthesia is discouraged because needle penetration in the affected extremity could disseminate tumor cells due to contamination of vascular or lymphatic structures. The patient is positioned supine on the operating room table. An upper arm tourniquet is applied and well padded. The entire upper extremity is prepped and draped free and placed on a hand table. Before incision, the arm is elevated for 10 minutes and the tourniquet inflated to 250 mm Hg. The arm is not exsanguinated because this could also disseminate tumor cells, leading to local recur-

rence or distant metastasis. The arm elevation time can actually commence during prepping and draping, thereby proceeding in an efficient fashion.

Preoperatively, the biopsy incision is planned for ultimate incorporation into the incision to be used for the definitive surgery. A small, longitudinal incision is made, and the soft tissues are carefully dissected to expose the bone tumor in question. Once exposed, the cortex is scored with an appropriately sized drill. For most small bones of the hand as well as the forearm bones, a 2-mm drill bit is adequate. The cortex overlying the lesion is then perforated by multiple drill holes, placed in an oval. This creates a defect with the least stress on the remaining bone. If the lesion is cartilaginous in nature, small curettes or microcurettes are used to remove an ample bone specimen. If the lesion is liquid, a syringe may be used. If the lesion is nonosseous, the biopsy should be sent for frozen preparation and a diagnosis rendered before closing the wound. It is helpful for the surgeon to personally deliver the specimen to the pathology laboratory while an assistant irrigates the wound, obtains hemostasis, and begins closure. The author prefers to personally deliver the specimen to the pathologist to avoid any chance of loss or misplacement. It also allows the author to personally describe the patient's history and to review with the pathologist representative imaging studies. The author can also directly answer any inquiries about the gross appearance of the lesion as well as the feasibility of obtaining more specimens should the pathologist deem this necessary. In most circumstances, no definitive management is performed until the results of the permanent tumor histologic preparations are reviewed. If the lesion is of osteogenic origin, a small rongeur or Kerrison rongeur is used to obtain a specimen for permanent pathology examination. The specimen is prepared using a decalcification technique, typically delaying final diagnosis for several days. A frozen section cannot be obtained on tumors of osteogenic origin.

Meticulous homeostasis is achieved and the wound irrigated and closed. In some situations, the defect created by the bone tumor biopsy destabilizes the bone or puts the bone at risk for pathologic fracture. In these situations, the bone must be prophylactically stabilized using appropriate internal, percutaneous, or external fixation.

STAGING

Enneking et al. (11,12) proposed a surgical staging system for the treatment of musculoskeletal neoplasms. This widely accepted system uses three basic criteria to categorize musculoskeletal neoplasms into stages IA, IB, IIA, IIB, or III. The criteria for surgical staging are tumor grade (G), location of the tumor with respect to its compartment of origin (T), and the presence (or absence) of metastasis (M).

The grade given a neoplasm is subject to agreement between the pathologist and the surgeon. Several factors are taken into consideration when grading a neoplasm; the most important of which is the histology. Benign lesions are G_0, whereas malignancies are either G_1 (low grade) or G_2 (high grade) (11,12). The decision to assign one of these grades to a tumor is based primarily on the histologic characteristics of the lesion. However, the clinical, radiographic, and gross appearance of the lesion is also considered in the designation of the tumor grade (13).

Benign bone tumors (G_0), can be further classified as *latent*, *active*, or *locally aggressive*. Latent tumors seldom change from initial presentation. Active benign tumors may continue to grow, confined by natural barriers. Locally aggressive benign tumors also continue to grow but frequently expand beyond anatomic barriers (10–12).

The location of the tumor is defined as either *intracompartmental* (T_1) or *extracompartmental* (T_2) (11,12). The value of identifying a tumor location as intra- or extracompartmental is that the boundaries of musculoskeletal compartments act as barriers to tumor spread. The relationship of the tumor to its compartment of origin also has a certain prognostic value (13). However, in the hand, compartmental barriers are not as helpful in the control of tumor spread as they are in the lower extremity. A malignant lesion in the proximal phalanx of the index finger, for instance, will most likely spread into the digital flexor tendon sheath. Because the index flexor tendon sheath is continuous with the other flexor tendons at the carpal canal level and because these tendons are contiguous with the flexor compartment in the forearm, tumor spread in this region is difficult to control (14).

The presence or absence of tumor metastasis is the final factor in determining the surgical grade of a tumor. If a distant metastatic lesion is present, the surgical stage of the tumor is defined as III. With tumors having distant metastasis, this surgical stage III is assigned irrespective of tumor grade or location. The full definition of the surgical stages described by Enneking et al. (11,12) are listed in Table 1.

Surgical procedures for extirpation of bone tumors are of four different types: intralesional, marginal, wide, and radi-

TABLE 1. SURGICAL STAGES OF THE MUSCULOSKELETAL SARCOMAS

Stage	Grade (G)	Site
IA	Low (G_1)	Intracompartmental (T_1)
IB	Low (G_1)	Extracompartmental (T_2)
IIA	High (G_2)	Intracompartmental (T_1)
IIB	High (G_2)	Extracompartmental (T_2)
III	Any (G)	Any (T)
	Regional or distant metastasis	Regional or distant metastasis

T, tumor.
Adapted from Enneking WF, Spanier SS, Goodman MA. A system for the surgical staging of musculoskeletal sarcoma. *Clin Orthop* 1980;106–120, with permission.

cal (12). Intralesional tumor resection creates a plane of tumor dissection and removal that is within the tumor itself. After intralesional tumor resection, tumor is found microscopically at all margins. Marginal resection implies that the entirety of the tumor was removed through the tumor's reactive or inflammatory zone. Histologically, the surgical margins can display microscopic extensions of the tumor and possibly skip lesions. A wide surgical excision completely removes the tumor, leaving normal tissue. However, the compartment of tumor origin still remains. Microscopically, the surgical margins display normal tissue, but skip lesions may be present. The radical surgical excision removes the entire compartment that harbors the tumor. Histologically, the tumor margins show only normal tissue, and skip lesions should not be seen (11,12).

BENIGN BONE TUMORS

The majority of all primary bone tumors of the hand and wrist are benign. According to the Leeds Regional Bone Tumor Registry, a review of 80 such tumors found 86% (69 tumors) benign (15). In a strikingly similar series, a review of 300 hand and wrist primary bone tumors from the Westphalian Bone Tumor Register identified 87.3% (248 tumors) as benign (16). The more common benign primary bone tumors found in the hand are reviewed in this section.

Aneurysmal Bone Cyst

Aneurysmal bone cysts (ABCs) can arise alone or in association with another tumor (17), but ABCs are not considered to be of neoplastic origin (17,18). The etiology of ABCs is uncertain, although some have suggested that the lesion arises due to a hemodynamic disturbance (19).

Approximately 80% of all ABCs present within the first two decades of life, with the male to female incidence roughly equal (20). The hand and wrist account for only 5% of all ABCs, with the predominant hand location the metacarpals and the proximal phalanges (Fig. 4) (18). Consistently, the patient with an ABC presents to the hand surgeon for persisting pain and swelling. Presentation due to pathologic fracture has also been reported (18). Radiographically, the lesion markedly expands the cortex of the involved bone, with the common appearance of a sclerotic rim and periosteal new bone formation. Calcification of the matrix is not typically seen (Fig. 5).

Histologically, the lesion is characterized by blood-filled spaces lined with fibroblasts and multinucleated giant cells (20). Both clinically and histologically, the ABC must be distinguished from simple cysts and giant cell tumors.

Success in treatment has been reported with marginal curettage of the lesion and bone grafting. Despite the presumed nonneoplastic nature of ABC, notable recurrence rates have been reported and attributed to incomplete

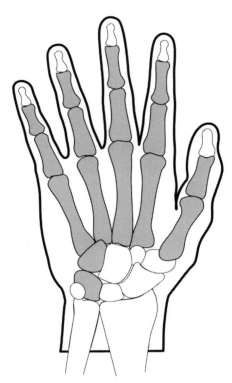

FIGURE 4. Darkened areas depict the more common locations for aneurysmal bone cysts of the hand and wrist region.

curettage of the lesion (18,19). Enhancement of the overall cure rate has been reported using adjuvant cryosurgery. In a series of 44 patients, Marcove et al. (19) reported improvement of overall cure rate from 59% to 82% using curettage

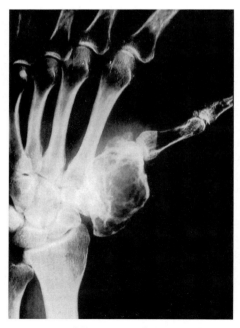

FIGURE 5. Aneurysmal bone cyst of the thumb proximal phalanx with marked cortical expansion.

and cryosurgery as opposed to simple curettage and bone grafting. Cryosurgery relies on the principle of tissue necrosis by rapid freezing. This can be accomplished by the use of liquid nitrogen spray, direct pour, or synthetic probe (10). ABC recurrence rates are also low with the use of adjuvant radiation therapy. Radiation therapy, however, is not recommended due to reports of radiation-induced sarcoma (19). Once the histologic diagnosis of ABC is established by biopsy, surgical treatment should entail thorough curettage of the lesion followed by cryosurgery and iliac crest cortico-cancellous bone grafting (10,18).

Chondroblastoma

Chondroblastoma is a benign cartilage lesion of bone, typically diagnosed in the second decade of life and having a male predominance (17,18). Patients typically present with longstanding mild to moderate pain and localized tenderness on physical examination. The typical radiographic appearance of the chondroblastoma is a lytic lesion located in the epiphysis of a tubular bone. The lesion is typically rimmed by sclerotic bone. Approximately 50% of the lesions show intralesional calcifications (21). This tumor is, however, exceedingly rare in the hand, with fewer than 20 reported cases (17,20). Its presence is relatively more common in the carpus. In a review of 44 primary carpal bone tumors from the Mayo Clinic, six chondroblastomas were identified, accounting for approximately 14% of the carpal bone tumors in this series (2).

Histologically, the chondroblastoma is characterized by the classic "chickenwire calcification" scattered throughout the histologic field of view. In this lesion, multinucleated giant cells are sprinkled throughout the sheets of chondroblasts (20). In general, chondroblasts are treated by curettage and bone grafting (17).

Chondromyxoid Fibroma

Much like the chondroblastoma, the chondromyxoid fibroma is exceedingly rare in the hands and wrist, with fewer than 20 reported cases worldwide (10). Pain is the presenting complaint in chondromyxoid fibroma. Patients typically present in the second and third decades of life and have a male predominance (20). Radiographically, the majority of tumors are lytic, eccentric, and metaphyseal. These lesions are typically not calcified. Histologically, the chondromyxoid fibroma has a myxoid stroma with scattered multinucleated giant cells. Curettage with bone grafting is the treatment of choice (20).

Enchondroma

Enchondroma is the most common bone tumor in the hand and wrist. It is diagnosed in all ages and has a relatively equal male to female distribution (10,16,17,20). Largely asymptomatic, these benign tumors may present due to a pathologic

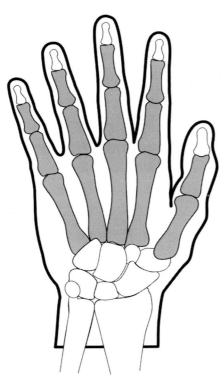

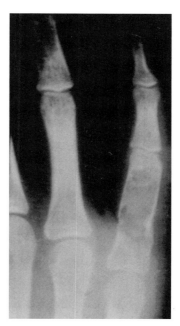

FIGURE 7. Enchondroma of the proximal phalanx of the small finger demonstrating punctate calcification.

FIGURE 6. Darkened areas depict the more common locations for enchondromas of the hand and wrist region.

fracture or may be observed incidentally on routine hand radiographs obtained for other reasons. It has been suggested that the cause of this tumor is proliferation of intraosseous cartilage remnants (22). Analysis of more than 5,500 bone tumors from the Westphalian Tumor Register found enchondromas comprising approximately 45% of all primary bone tumors of the hand (16). In a review by Bauer et al. (23), nearly 90% of all primary hand tumors were enchondromas. The most common location of enchondromas is the proximal phalanx, followed by the metacarpal and the middle phalanx (Fig. 6) (10,23). In a review of 44 primary bone tumors of the carpus, no enchondromas were identified (2).

Radiographically, enchondromas are predominantly medullary in origin, showing sharp, sclerotic margins. The lesions are often expansile, with distortion of the cortex and punctate calcification of the matrix (Fig. 7). Histologically, these lesions are hypocellular, with a cartilaginous matrix and inconspicuous, uniform nuclei. The diagnosis of multiple enchondromas in the same extremity is known as the nonhereditary condition *Ollier's disease*. The enchondromas in Ollier's disease are typically large, causing notable cosmetic and functional compromise. Growth of enchondromas is not likely after skeletal maturity. The growth of an enchondroma after skeletal maturity, particularly when associated with radiographic progression and the onset of pain, should raise the question of malignant transformation. The incidence of malignant transformation from solitary enchondroma is probably overestimated and much

rarer than originally thought (24). Malignant transformation (to chondrosarcoma or osteosarcoma) of lesions in Ollier's disease is much more likely than solitary enchondroma, and is considered to be approximately 30% (10).

Maffucci's syndrome is an extremely rare nonhereditary condition composed of multiple enchondromas and associated hemangiomata. Radiographically, the enchondromas in Maffucci's syndrome appear identical to the solitary enchondromas. Hemangiomas may be identified on plain film radiography as phleboliths. Fewer than 200 cases of Maffucci's syndrome have been reported; the lesions are most common in the hands, the condition is typically identified in childhood, and the male to female ratio is essentially equal (25). Similar to Ollier's disease, patients with Maffucci's syndrome have a notable risk of malignant transformation. Malignant transformation rates have been reported from 23% to 37%, with chondrosarcoma developing in as many as 30% of cases (25,26). Due to the high malignant transformation rates, patients with both Ollier's disease and Maffucci's syndrome require periodic reevaluation.

Incidentally recognized, small, asymptomatic enchondromas require no specific treatment. Should these lesions show enlargement and become painful, formal biopsy should be performed. For the lesion compromising more than 50% of the bone's cortical integrity, impending pathologic fracture must be considered and enchondroma excision planned. Pathologic fractures occurring through enchondromas are treated as fractures first, using whatever means necessary. Once fracture healing has occurred, formal treatment of the enchondroma is initiated. In some instances, skeletal fixation, either percutaneous or internal, is necessary. In these instances, subsequent treatment of the enchondroma is considered on a case-per-case basis. Traditionally, enchondroma removal has involved thorough curettage followed by packing the defect with cancellous bone graft obtained from the anterior iliac crest. The digital enchondroma is generally approached dorsally and the tumor removed by curettage. Using the principles of tumor surgery, cancellous bone from the anterior iliac crest is harvested using separate instruments to prevent cross-contamination. Using the method of treatment, recurrence is approximately 4.5% (10). Alternatives to this method of removal include the use of allograft bone (23) or simply curettage alone without bone grafting (22). Bauer et al. (23) have reported no recurrences, no fractures, and no complications in a series of 19 enchondromas treated with curettage and packing with allograft bone. In a series of 28 consecutive patients, Hasselgren et al. (22) reported that simple curettage without bone grafting is also safe and effective.

Giant Cell Reparative Granuloma

Giant cell reparative granuloma is a lesion of unknown etiology, which is seen more commonly in females in the second and third decades of life (17). Similar to ABCs, this lesion is not considered a true neoplasm and is considered more of a reactive process (17). Approximately 50% of patients present due to local pain and swelling (20). Only one giant cell reparative granuloma was identified among 300 cases in the Westphalian Bone Tumor Register (16).

Radiographically, this process is purely lytic, with cortical thinning, expansion, and occasional cortical break-through (Fig. 8). When cortical break-through does occur, periosteal new bone formation may be seen. Histologically, this lesion displays many clusters of multinucleated giant cells among spindle cells all within a fibrous stroma (20). Unlike giant cell tumors, giant cell reparative granuloma is treatable with curettage, when necessary, and bone grafting. Recurrence of this lesion after curettage is virtually nonexistent.

Giant Cell Tumor

Although these lesions are traditionally regarded as benign tumors, the giant cell tumor of bone can be locally aggressive and even metastasize (10,27,28). More than 85% of giant cell tumors are diagnosed after 20 years of age, with the lesions occurring slightly more often in females (20,29). Only 2% of giant cell tumors arise in the bones of the hand, whereas approximately 14% originate in the distal radius or ulna (20,29,30). Giant cell tumors of bone have been reported in all the carpal bones (10) and account for more than 11% of all primary bone tumors of the carpus (Fig. 9) (2). The patient with a giant cell tumor of the hand or wrist presents with pain and localized swelling.

Radiographically, this tumor is purely lytic with cortical expansion and indistinct borders; the latter often indicate soft tissue expansion (Fig. 3). Histologically, multinucleated giant

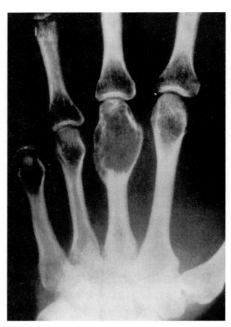

FIGURE 8. Giant cell reparative granuloma of the third metacarpal, with thinning and expansion.

cells scattered within a background of mononuclear cells characterize the lesion. The nuclei of the mononuclear cells appear similar to the nuclei of the multinuclear giant cells. Mitotic activity is quite common.

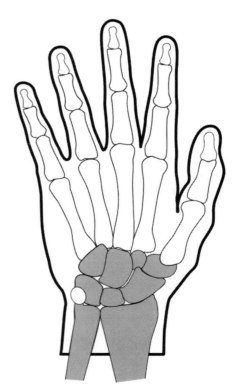

FIGURE 9. Darkened areas depict the more common locations for giant cell tumors of the hand and wrist region.

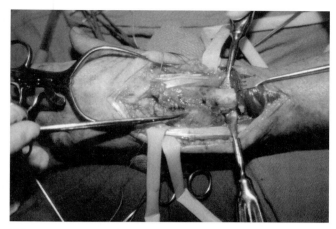

FIGURE 10. Forty-eight-year-old woman from Figure 3 undergoing *en bloc* resection of giant cell tumor with wide surgical margins. The pronator quadratus is used as the volar tumor barrier.

If giant cell tumor is suspected, it is important to perform a "malignancy workup" owing to the locally aggressive nature and metastatic potential of this tumor. Giant cell tumors of the bones of the hand and wrist, including the distal radius, should be treated with wide excision and reconstruction or even amputation. Regarding giant cell tumors of the distal radius, it is important to remember that the pronator quadratus serves as an excellent tumor barrier. In giant cell tumors that have violated the volar distal radius cortex, the pronator quadratus can conveniently be used as a resection margin. A recurrence rate of 79% has been reported with intralesional curettage and bone grafting; this cannot be recommended (29). For nonperforating lesions of the distal radius, success has been reported with curettage supplemented by either cryosurgery (30) or cementation (31). In giant cell tumors of the distal radius with notable soft tissue extension, wide excision and wrist arthrodesis using fibular or iliac crest intercalary autografting and internal fixation are considered the preferred treatment (Fig. 10) (31). Sheth et al. (30) reported local recurrence in 3 of 12 patients treated with curettage and cryosurgery. No recurrences were reported in ten patients treated with *en bloc* excision and wrist arthrodesis (30). Vander Griend et al. (31) reported on a series of five patients treated with curettage and cementation, and 17 patients were treated by wide excision and reconstruction. In this series, no recurrences were reported, and the better functional results were reported in patients who underwent reconstruction by wrist arthrodesis (31) compared to radiocarpal joint preservation.

Osteochondroma

The proportion of osteochondromas arising in the hand was only 1% in the Mayo Clinic pathology files (20) but accounted for nearly 20% of the primary bone tumors of the hand and wrist in the Westphalian Bone Tumor Regis-

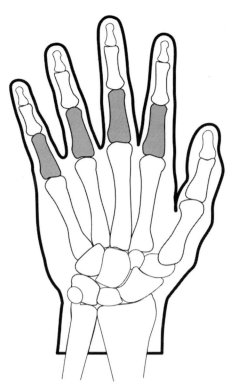

FIGURE 11. Darkened areas depict the more common locations for osteochondroma of the hand and wrist region.

ter. These lesions typically form in the hand about the distal aspect of the proximal phalanges (Fig. 11) (10). These growths form about the physis and possess a cartilage cap. Malignant degeneration, although reported elsewhere in the skeleton, has not been reported in the hand (10). Osteochondromas present in the second or third decade and have a male predominance. Patients may seek medical attention due the tumor's mass effect causing localized pain or cosmetic concerns.

These lesions appear radiographically as bony projections having cortical continuity with the native bone (Fig. 12). Osteochondromas are typified microscopically by the presence of a thin cartilage cap. The younger the patient, the larger the cartilage cap. Symptomatic lesions are removed by simple excision at the base of the lesion, protecting otherwise normal structures. Recurrence of osteochondromas is not seen.

Osteoid Osteoma/Osteoblastoma

The osteoid osteoma often causes pain of increasing severity, typically more intense at night. These patients may also relate relief of symptoms with the use of nonsteroidal anti-inflammatory agents. However, approximately 1% to 5% of the lesions can be painless, with the proximal phalanx the most common painless location (32). Rarely seen in patients older than 40 years of age, patients with osteoid

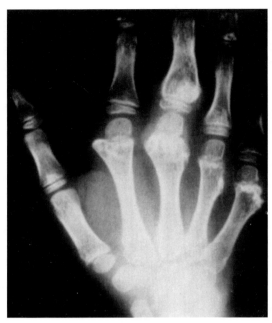

FIGURE 12. Osteochondroma of the index metacarpal illustrating cortical continuity with the native bone.

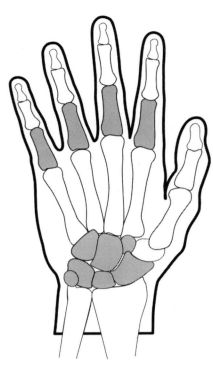

FIGURE 13. Darkened areas depict the more common locations for osteoid osteoma/osteoblastoma of the hand and wrist region.

osteoma are generally seen in their early 20s, with men predominating 2:1 (20,32–34). In a series of 19 patients with osteoid osteoma, Ambrosia et al. (33) identified the proximal phalanx as the most common location in the hand and wrist (Fig. 13). In a Mayo Clinic series, the osteoid osteoma was the most common primary bone neoplasm of the carpus, accounting for 25% of all bone tumors (2). Only approximately 2% of osteoid osteomas appear in the hand and wrist. Due to this low incidence, these lesions are often misdiagnosed or overlooked entirely (33). Doyle et al. (35) reported an average 13.5-month delay in diagnosis of osteoid osteoma.

The osteoid osteoma is identified on plain film radiography as a small round lucency (the nidus), situated within the cortex, surrounded by a sclerotic, reactive rim of bone (Fig. 14). Twenty-five percent of osteoid osteomas cannot be identified using plain radiography and can only be imaged using bone scan or CT scan (36). Microscopically, a nidus is composed of osteoid with a variable amount of mineralization. Within the osteoid of the nidus itself is fibrovascular connective tissue and a rim of sclerotic bone surrounds, but is distinct from, the nidus.

Surgical excision of the osteoid osteoma is the favored treatment. At an average follow-up of 27 months, 34 osteoid osteomas of the upper extremity were treated with excision and curettage. A persisting nidus occurred in six patients; five were in the hand and wrist. Localization of the nidus, therefore, can be difficult in the hand and wrist. In another series of 19 patients, persistence after surgical excision occurred in four phalangeal osteoid osteomas. It is important to obtain adequate preoperative imaging studies

before surgical excision is performed. Preoperative imaging frequently requires a CT scan of the involved area. Alternatively, long-term treatment success has been reported with the prolonged use of nonsteroidal antiinflammatory agents

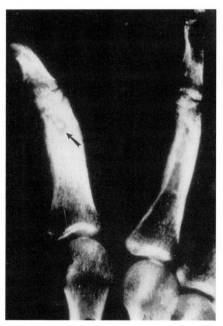

FIGURE 14. Osteoid osteoma of the proximal phalanx (*arrow*). Note the relatively lucent nidus surrounded by sclerotic bone.

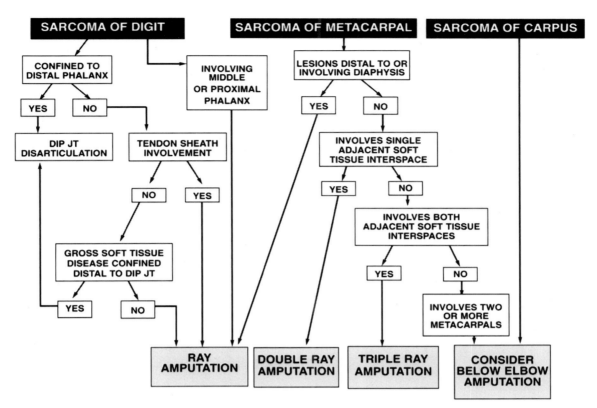

FIGURE 15. Algorithm for the surgical management of high-grade bone sarcomas of the hand and wrist region. This algorithm may be subject to modification, depending on neoadjuvant chemotherapy or postoperative radiation therapy. The adequacy of the surgical margin is also dependent on tumor grade. DIP JT, distal interphalangeal joint.

(37). Medical management alone for the treatment of osteoid osteoma can be considered in those patients in whom operative intervention is not medically feasible, or the lesion is surgically inaccessible.

Osteoblastoma is histologically indistinguishable from osteoid osteoma. Lesions with a radiographic nidus larger than 1.5 cm are considered osteoblastomas. Additionally, osteoblastomas typically do not have periosteal new bone formation. Therefore, the primary diagnostic criterion distinguishing osteoid osteoma from osteoblastoma is size.

MALIGNANT TUMORS

Only approximately 3% to 4% of hand and wrist bone tumors are malignant (15,16). Considering just 2% to 4% of all bone tumors arise in the hand and wrist (15,21), malignant bone tumors of the hand and wrist are, therefore, rare. When diagnosed, malignant bone tumors of the hand and wrist present challenging surgical problems. Compartment separations in the forearm, wrist, and hand do not provide the same convenient barriers as other regions of the body, often making wide excisions impossible without amputation. Fascial compartments are continuous from the digit to the forearm, making amputation above

the wrist the only alternative if a radical margin is sought (11,12,14). Given the devastating functional and cosmetic effects that may occur from obtaining radical surgical margins, removal of less tissue can be facilitated when appropriate adjuncts, such as chemotherapy and radiation therapy, are used. This is helpful in the hand and wrist where convenient compartmental barriers do not exist. For bone sarcomas of the hand and wrist, the ray amputation is the "work-horse" procedure (Fig. 15).

Because these lesions are so rare and due to the special problems encountered with surgical excision, the hand surgeon must maintain an ever-vigilant suspicion for these tumors. This requires at least yearly review of the common characteristics of each malignant bone tumor.

Chondrosarcoma

Chondrosarcoma is a slow-growing malignancy of cartilage, which is commonly regarded as the most common malignant bone tumor of the hand (38). Its production from malignant degeneration from solitary enchondroma is probably overstated but has been clearly reported (24). Malignant degeneration from multiple enchondromatosis (Ollier's disease) is more commonly recognized (10). Chondrosarcoma presents as a slow-growing, painful mass gener-

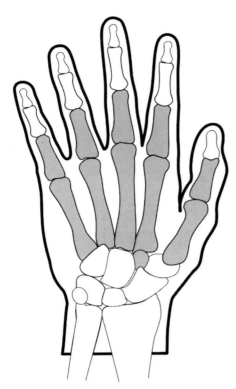

FIGURE 16. Darkened areas depict the more common locations for chondrosarcoma of the hand and wrist region.

ally affecting patients in the fifth and sixth decades of life (10,20). Some present due to episodes of a painful, recently enlarged, long-standing, asymptomatic mass. Others present due to repeated recurrences of a previously removed or misdiagnosed lesion. The most common locations for chondrosarcomas of the hand are the metacarpals and the proximal phalanges (Fig. 16). The tumor is seen equally among males and females (10,20,21,39,40). Although these are malignant lesions with metastatic potential, the majority of them do not metastasize (10). When chondrosarcoma of the hand does metastasize, the most common destination is the lung (10).

Radiographically, these lesions are primarily lytic, but the majority possesses some element of stippled calcifications. The cortex is typically thinned, eroded, and often perforated, making tumor borders indistinct (Fig. 2). Microscopically, chondrosarcomas show blue chondroid matrix production with a wide range of cellularity. The higher grade lesions have greater cellularity, with increasing amounts of pleomorphism. These are cartilage cells typically displaying pyknotic binucleation.

Chondrosarcomas do not respond to radiation or chemotherapeutic intervention, and surgery is the only effective treatment (39). Recommended surgical treatment for the chondrosarcoma is a wide *en bloc* excision (10,41). In the distal digits, this requires digital amputation, whereas in the proximal digits or the hand, ray or double ray amputa-

tion is often necessary. For chondrosarcoma of the wrist or the forearm, wide excision may require below-elbow amputation. Curettage procedures for hand chondrosarcomas have demonstrated unacceptably high local recurrence rates as well as metastatic disease (14,40,41). In a review of 18 consecutive chondrosarcomas of the metacarpals and phalanges treated by ray amputation, local recurrence occurred in only 11% and metastatic involvement did not occur (38). Once treated, it is important to follow these patients for several years, as latent local recurrence or distant metastasis can occur (10).

Ewing's Sarcoma

Much like the other malignant bone tumors, Ewing's sarcoma arises less commonly in the hand and wrist than in the remainder of the skeleton. The hand and wrist account for less than 1% of all diagnosed Ewing's sarcomas (42). Originally described by Ewing in 1921 (43), Ewing's sarcoma presents in the first or second decade of life (20). In the hand, unlike the remainder of the body, a 2:1 male predominance has been reported (44). Pain, swelling, fever, local tenderness, leukocytosis, and an elevated sedimentation rate are often present, diverting the clinician toward a diagnosis of infection. A soft tissue mass is also frequently present. This misdiagnosis of infection is responsible for the frequent delay in diagnosis of Ewing's sarcoma. In a 1990 literature review by Euler et al. (42), only 20 cases of Ewing's sarcoma had been reported in the hand and wrist, with all but three of the cases arising from either the proximal phalanx or the metacarpals.

Ewing's sarcoma is typified radiographically by a destructive, poorly marginated, lytic, diaphyseal lesion. Although marked periosteal reactions are seen in Ewing's sarcoma at other sites, periosteal reactions are seen much less frequently in the hand (44). Conversely, the incidence of cortical expansion has been reported with greater frequency in the hand compared to Ewing's sarcoma located elsewhere (44). The most common location for hand Ewing's sarcoma is the metacarpal and the proximal phalanges (Fig. 17). Histologically, Ewing's sarcoma is a round cell lesion with no identifiable matrix. The nuclei are round with a dispersed chromatin pattern and abundant mitotic figures. The cytoplasm of the round cells in Ewing's sarcoma is periodic acid-Schiff-positive, indicating the presence of glycogen (20).

An autopsy study published by Telles et al. (45) showed notable persisting pulmonary metastatic disease in patients treated with external beam radiation, underscoring the highly malignant nature of this tumor. Wide excision of the tumor or amputation is the preferred surgical treatment, followed by adjuvant chemotherapy. Improved survival with adjuvant chemotherapy has been reported, with the protocols including doxorubicin (Adriamycin), vincristine, dactinomycin, and cyclophosphamide (46). The addition

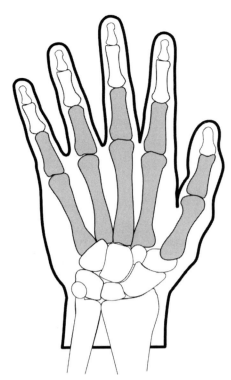

FIGURE 17. Darkened areas depict the more common locations for Ewing's sarcoma of the hand and wrist region.

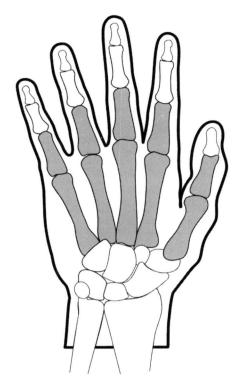

FIGURE 18. Darkened areas depict the more common locations for osteosarcoma of the hand and wrist region.

of neoadjuvant chemotherapy is recommended by many who contend that tumor size is reduced, thereby facilitating the index surgical procedure (10,47,48). Although Ewing's sarcoma displays radiosensitivity (49), its use in the hand and wrist region for local control is less than ideal, owing to the potential radiation complications of soft tissue contracture and radiation-induced sarcoma. The combination of wide surgical excision and neoadjuvant/adjuvant chemotherapy has produced 5-year disease-free survival in excess of 70% (46). If postoperative radiation therapy is used, aggressive hand therapy should be initiated early.

Osteogenic Sarcoma

The incidence of osteogenic sarcoma in the hand and wrist is 0.18%, according to a Mayo Clinic series (50). Although osteogenic sarcoma is the most common primary malignant bone tumor seen in children and adolescents, lesions affecting the hand are seen in older adults (10). Okada et al. (50) reported an average age of 45 years in a review of 11 patients with hand osteosarcoma. Nine of the 11 tumors occurred in either the proximal phalanx or the metacarpal (Fig. 18) (50). Radiation exposure is a possible etiologic factor in adults (51). A firm, painful, and enlarging mass is the usual presenting complaint in hand osteogenic sarcomas.

These lesions may present radiographically as lytic, blastic, or mixed in appearance (Fig. 1). The tumors are poorly marginated, and extensive cortical destruction is often seen. Peri-

osteal new bone formation is common, with the formation of Codman's triangles. Histologically, osteosarcoma comes in several different types: parosteal, periosteal, high-grade surface, low-grade central, and telangiectatic (20). Conventional osteosarcoma is known microscopically for sarcomatous, osteoid-producing stroma. The amount of osteoid production is variable. Additionally, the tumor is composed of spindle cells showing pronounced pleomorphism.

Treatment for osteogenic sarcoma of the hand should be initiated promptly once diagnosed. The use of adjuvant chemotherapy is preferred by most (10,52), although one series has shown no particular advantage to the administration of postoperative chemotherapy (53). Alternative adjuvant chemotherapeutic agents include methotrexate, doxorubicin, bleomycin, and cisplatin (52). Delays in the initiation of adjuvant chemotherapy have been shown to decrease survival (10). Based on reports of extremely rare metastasis rates in hand osteogenic sarcomas (54), the need for neoadjuvant chemotherapy has been questioned, though others contend that its use diminishes tumor size preoperatively, aiding the ultimate tumor resection. Similar to the treatment of other malignant tumors, a wide excision or amputation is the treatment of choice for osteogenic sarcomas of the hand and wrist (55). The intricate anatomy of the hand and wrist region can make upper extremity limb-sparing reconstruction difficult once wide surgical excision has been performed. In these instances, amputation should be considered.

METASTATIC TUMORS

A metastatic tumor to the bones of the hand and wrist may be the initial presentation of a previously undiagnosed malignancy (56) and can be misdiagnosed as an infection (57). In a review by Healy et al. (58), more than one-third of patients with acrometastases presented without a previous diagnosis of cancer. In a review of 41,000 cancer patients, Wu and Guise (59) reported only three patients with metastatic involvement to the hand. Considering that 27% of all cancers develop metastasis to bone, this small number of hand lesions emphasizes the rarity of hand metastatic involvement (6,60,61).

Patients with hand and wrist metastatic tumors may complain of primary bone pain or pain from pathologic fracture. However, metastatic lesions of the hand and wrist may be completely asymptomatic and identified incidentally on hand and wrist radiographs. The lung, kidney, and head/neck comprise the majority of primary sites for hand metastasis, with the lung responsible for more than 40% of all reported metastatic lesions of the hand (62). Other reported primary sites include the esophagus, colon, breast, ovary, prostate, bladder, uterus, and thyroid (58). Metastatic lesions may appear radiographically as blastic or lytic, depending on the tumor histology (Fig. 19).

Considering the majority of patients diagnosed with metastatic hand lesions have a life expectancy of 6 months or less (62), the primary goals of treatment in these patients are pain relief and restoration of function. Nearly 50% of all the hand metastases in a series by Healey et al. (58)

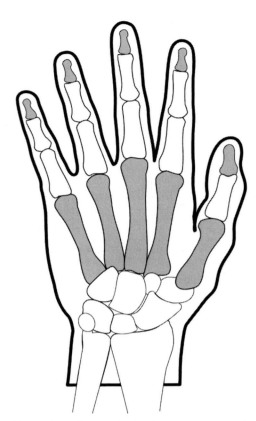

FIGURE 20. Darkened areas depict the more common locations for metastatic bone tumors of the hand and wrist region.

occurred in the metacarpals; the distal phalanx is also considered a common location (Fig. 20). For lesions in this location, the most expeditious treatment for relieving pain and regaining function is ray amputation. For more distal lesions in the phalanges, transverse amputation is appropriate. In terminally ill patients with easily accessible lesions, marginal excision, internal fixation, and radiation therapy can be considered (62). For those lesions that are relatively asymptomatic but have notable bony involvement, risk of pathologic fracture exists. The prophylactic treatment for pathologic fracture is much more effective than any post-fracture treatment.

SUMMARY

Primary bone tumors of the hand and wrist are rare, accounting for less than 4% of all tumors in this region (2,15,21). The hand surgeon must consider primary bone tumors of the hand and wrist when patients present with unexplained pain in this region. The physical examination must be thorough and complete, and biplanar radiographs of the affected area must be obtained initially. The majority of all primary bone lesions in the hand arise in the metacarpals or the proximal phalanges (15,16), whereas most bone tumors of the carpus occur in the scaphoid (2). Subse-

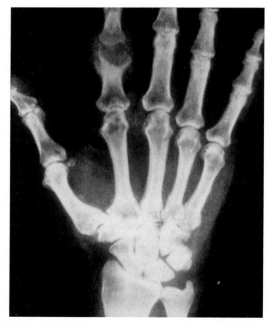

FIGURE 19. Metastatic esophageal carcinoma involving the middle phalanx of the index finger. A metastatic lesion of the hand may be the initial presentation of a systemic metastatic disease, as was the case in this 58-year-old man.

quently, the tumor workup should include a chest CT, bone scan, pelvic CT, and laboratory work if a malignancy is suspected. The biopsy is the single most important step in patients' staging workup, having a direct bearing on the outcome. The biopsy should, in most circumstances, be performed in the same institution where the definitive tumor surgery will be accomplished. The tumor is appropriately staged based on the criteria of Enneking et al. (11,12). Depending on the surgical stage of the tumor, an intralesional, marginal, wide, or radical excision should be performed.

Nearly 90% of all primary bone tumors of the hand and wrist are benign (15,16). The enchondroma accounts for more than 50% of all primary bone tumors of the hand, whereas the osteoid osteoma is the most common primary bone tumor of the carpal bones (2,15,16,23). Chondrosarcoma is the most common malignant bone tumor of the hand (38). Patients with Ollier's or Maffucci's syndrome have notable risk of malignant transformation from hand enchondromas to hand chondrosarcomas (10,25,26). Surgical excision is the only reliable treatment for chondrosarcoma (39). Long-term survival is, however, enhanced with the use of adjuvant chemotherapy in patients with osteosarcoma or Ewing's sarcoma.

The lung, kidney, and head/neck represent the vast majority of primary sites for lesions metastatic to the hand, with the most common location being the metacarpals (62). It is also important to remember that a metastatic tumor to a bone of the hand may be the initial presentation of previously undiagnosed malignancy.

It must not be forgotten that among all the facts and figures, the most important thing that can be learned is compassion for the tumor patient and the family. These patients are being affected both physically and emotionally. In many instances, their lives and their family's lives have been forever changed. Compassion is one of the basic tenets of our profession. As physicians, we owe it to our patients to be ever vigilant for hand and wrist neoplasms. This requires all of us to periodically review the basic characteristics of benign and malignant tumors. The consequences of not recognizing and appropriately treating these lesions are devastating.

REFERENCES

1. Musculoskeletal neoplasms. In: Kasser J, ed. *Orthopaedic knowledge*, vol. 5. Rosemont, IL: American Academy of Orthopaedic Surgeons, 1996:133–148.
2. Murray PM, Berger RA, Inwards CY. Primary neoplasms of the carpal bones. *J Hand Surg [Am]* 1999;24:1008–1013.
3. Harrington K. The role of surgery in the management of pathologic fractures. *Orthop Clin North Am* 1977;8:841–859.
4. Parrish FF, Murray JA. Surgical treatment for secondary neoplastic fractures. A retrospective study of ninety-six patients. *J Bone Joint Surg [Am]* 1970;52:665–686.
5. Fidler M. Incidence of fracture through metastases in long bones. *Acta Orthop Scand* 1981;52:623–627.
6. Hipp JA, Springfield DS, Hayes WC. Predicting pathologic fracture risk in the management of metastatic bone defects. *Clin Orthop* 1995;120–135.
7. Kransdorf MJ, Murphey MD. MR imaging of musculoskeletal tumors of the hand and wrist. *Magn Reson Imaging Clin N Am* 1995;3:327–344.
8. Simon MA. Biopsy of musculoskeletal tumors. *J Bone Joint Surg [Am]* 1982;64:1253–1257.
9. Mankin HJ, Lange TA, Spanier SS. The hazards of biopsy in patients with malignant primary bone and soft-tissue tumors. *J Bone Joint Surg [Am]* 1982;64:1121–1127.
10. Athanasian EA. Bone and soft tissue tumors. In: Green D, ed. *Operative hand surgery*, 4th ed. New York: Churchill Livingstone, 1998:2223–2253.
11. Enneking W. Staging of musculoskeletal neoplasms. In: Uhthoff HK, Stahl E, et al., eds. *Current concepts of diagnosis and treatment of bone and soft tissue tumors.* Berlin/New York: Springer-Verlag, 1984:1–24.
12. Enneking WF, Spanier SS, Goodman MA. A system for the surgical staging of musculoskeletal sarcoma. *Clin Orthop* 1980;106–120.
13. Athanasian EA. Principles of diagnosis and management of musculoskeletal tumors. In: Green D, ed. *Operative hand surgery*, 4th ed. New York: Churchill Livingstone, 1998:2206–2223.
14. Frassica FJ, Amadio PC, Wold LE, et al. Primary malignant bone tumors of the hand. *J Hand Surg [Am]* 1989;14:1022–1028.
15. Campbell DA, Millner PA, Dreghorn CR. Primary bone tumours of the hand and wrist. *J Hand Surg [Br]* 1995;20:5–7.
16. Besser E, Roessner A, Brug E, et al. Bone tumors of the hand. A review of 300 cases documented in the Westphalian Bone Tumor Register. *Arch Orthop Trauma Surg* 1987;106:241–247.
17. Feldman F. Primary bone tumors of the hand and carpus. *Hand Clin* 1987;3:269–289.
18. Frassica FJ, Amadio PC, Wold LE, Beabout JW. Aneurysmal bone cyst: clinicopathologic features and treatment of ten cases involving the hand. *J Hand Surg [Am]* 1988;13:676–683.
19. Marcove RC, Sheth DS, Takemoto S, Healey JH. The treatment of aneurysmal bone cyst. *Clin Orthop* 1995;157–163.
20. Wold LE. Atlas of orthopedic pathology. In: *Atlases in diagnostic surgical pathology*. Philadelphia: Saunders, 1990:xii, 276.
21. Dahlin DC, Unni KK. *Bone tumors: general aspects and data on 8543 cases*, 4th ed. Springfield, 1986.
22. Hasselgren G, Forssblad P, Tornvall A. Bone grafting unnecessary in the treatment of enchondromas in the hand. *J Hand Surg [Am]* 1991;16:139–142.
23. Bauer RD, Lewis MM, Posner MA. Treatment of enchondromas of the hand with allograft bone. *J Hand Surg [Am]* 1988;13:908–916.
24. Nelson DL, Abdul-Karim FW, Carter JR, Makley JT. Chondrosarcoma of small bones of the hand arising from enchondroma. *J Hand Surg [Am]* 1990;15:655–659.
25. Kaplan RP, Wang JT, Amron DM, Kaplan L. Maffucci's syndrome: two case reports with a literature review. *J Am Acad Dermatol* 1993;29:894–899.

26. Lewis RJ, Ketcham AS. Maffucci's syndrome: functional and neoplastic significance. Case report and review of the literature. *J Bone Joint Surg [Am]* 1973;55:1465–1479.

27. Bertoni F, Present D, Enneking WF. Giant-cell tumor of bone with pulmonary metastases. *J Bone Joint Surg [Am]* 1985;67:890–900.

28. Lopez-Barea F, Rodriguez-Peralto JL, Garcia-Giron J, Guemes-Gordo F. Benign metastasizing giant-cell tumor of the hand. Report of a case and review of the literature. *Clin Orthop* 1992;270–274.

29. Athanasian EA, Wold LE, Amadio PC. Giant cell tumors of the bones of the hand. *J Hand Surg [Am]* 1997;22:91–98.

30. Sheth DS, Healey JH, Sobel M, et al. Giant cell tumor of the distal radius. *J Hand Surg [Am]* 1995;20:432–440.

31. Vander Griend RA, Funderburk CH. The treatment of giant-cell tumors of the distal part of the radius. *J Bone Joint Surg [Am]* 1993;75:899–908.

32. Bednar MS, Weiland AJ, Light TR. Osteoid osteoma of the upper extremity. *Hand Clin* 1995;11:211–221.

33. Ambrosia JM, Wold LE, Amadio PC. Osteoid osteoma of the hand and wrist. *J Hand Surg [Am]* 1987;12:794–800.

34. Bednar MS, McCormack RR Jr, Glasser D, Weiland AJ. Osteoid osteoma of the upper extremity. *J Hand Surg [Am]* 1993;18:1019–1025.

35. Doyle LK, Ruby LK, Nalebuff EG, Belsky MR. Osteoid osteoma of the hand. *J Hand Surg [Am]* 1985;10:408–410.

36. Swee RG, McLeod RA, Beabout JW. Osteoid osteoma. Detection, diagnosis, and localization. *Radiology* 1979;130:117–123.

37. Kneisl JS, Simon MA. Medical management compared with operative treatment for osteoid-osteoma. *J Bone Joint Surg [Am]* 1992;74:179–185.

38. Palmieri TJ. Chondrosarcoma of the hand. *J Hand Surg [Am]* 1984;9:332–338.

39. Dick HM, Angelides AC. Malignant bone tumors of the hand. *Hand Clin* 1989;5:373–381.

40. Dahlin DC, Salvador AH. Chondrosarcomas of bones of the hands and feet—a study of 30 cases. *Cancer* 1974;34:755–760.

41. Roberts PH, Price CH. Chondrosarcoma of the bones of the hand. *J Bone Joint Surg [Br]* 1977;59:213–221.

42. Euler E, Wilhelm K, Permanetter W, Kreusser T. Ewing's sarcoma of the hand: localization and treatment. *J Hand Surg [Am]* 1990;15:659–662.

43. Ewing J. Diffuse endothelioma of bone. *Proc N Y Pathol Soc* 1927;21:17–24.

44. Shirley SK, Askin FB, Gilula LA, et al. Ewing's sarcoma in bones of the hands and feet: a clinicopathologic study and review of the literature. *J Clin Oncol* 1985;3:686–697.

45. Telles NC, Rabson AS, Pomeroy TC. Ewing's sarcoma: an autopsy study. *Cancer* 1978;41:2321–2329.

46. Nesbit ME Jr, Perez CA, Tefft M, et al. Multimodal therapy for the management of primary, nonmetastatic Ewing's sarcoma of bone: an Intergroup Study. *Natl Cancer Inst Monogr* 1981;255–262.

47. Bacci G, Picci P, Gitelis S, et al. The treatment of localized Ewing's sarcoma: the experience at the Istituto Ortopedico Rizzoli in 163 cases treated with and without adjuvant chemotherapy. *Cancer* 1982;49:1561–1570.

48. Rosen G. Neoadjuvant chemotherapy for osteogenic sarcoma: a model for the treatment of other highly malignant neoplasms. *Recent Results Cancer Res* 1986;103:148–157.

49. Nesbit ME Jr, Gehan EA, Burgert EO Jr, et al. Multimodal therapy for the management of primary, nonmetastatic Ewing's sarcoma of bone: a long-term follow-up of the First Intergroup study. *J Clin Oncol* 1990;8:1664–1674.

50. Okada K, Wold LE, Beabout JW, Shives TC. Osteosarcoma of the hand. A clinicopathologic study of 12 cases. *Cancer* 1993;72:719–725.

51. Carroll R. Osteosarcoma in the hand. *J Bone Joint Surg [Am]* 1957;39:325–331.

52. Meyers PA, Heller G, Healey J, et al. Chemotherapy for nonmetastatic osteogenic sarcoma: the Memorial Sloan-Kettering experience. *J Clin Oncol* 1992;10:5–15.

53. Edmonson JH, Green SJ, Ivins JC, et al. A controlled pilot study of high-dose methotrexate as postsurgical adjuvant treatment for primary osteosarcoma. *J Clin Oncol* 1984;2:152–156.

54. Mirra JM, Kameda N, Rosen G, Eckardt J. Primary osteosarcoma of toe phalanx: first documented case. Review of osteosarcoma of short tubular bones. *Am J Surg Pathol* 1988;12:300–307.

55. Bickerstaff DR, Harris SC, Kay NR. Osteosarcoma of the carpus. *J Hand Surg [Br]* 1988;13:303–305.

56. Kerin R. Metastatic tumors of the hand. A review of the literature. *J Bone Joint Surg [Am]* 1983;65:1331–1335.

57. Rose BA, Wood FM. Metastatic bronchogenic carcinoma masquerading as a felon. *J Hand Surg [Am]* 1983;8:325–328.

58. Healey JH, Turnbull AD, Miedema B, Lane JM. Acrometastases. A study of twenty-nine patients with osseous involvement of the hands and feet. *J Bone Joint Surg [Am]* 1986;68:743–746.

59. Wu KK, Guise ER. Metastatic tumors of the hand: a report of six cases. *J Hand Surg [Am]* 1978;3:271–276.

60. Chung TS. Metastatic malignancy to the bones of the hand. *J Surg Oncol* 1983;24:99–102.

61. Tubiana-Hulin M. Incidence, prevalence and distribution of bone metastases. *Bone* 1991;12:S9–10.

62. Amadio PC, Lombardi RM. Metastatic tumors of the hand. *J Hand Surg [Am]* 1987;12:311–316.

102

METASTATIC LESIONS

KEITH A. GLOWACKI

Metastatic lesions to the hand are very uncommon. A review of the literature reveals the incidence among metastatic lesions to be less than 0.1% (1–38). For every 10,000 patients presenting with metastatic disease, one has a lesion in the hand. This shows the extremely rare incidence reported in the literature (1,3,5,6,7,10,15,20,27,31,34,37,38). Lesions involving the hand are much less common than metastatic lesions to the proximal or axial skeleton. This represents a new patient presenting to a hand surgeon once every 8 to 10 years with a metastatic lesion that involves the hand. In the lifetime of most practicing orthopedic hand surgeons, this would represent only a very few number of patients. The paucity of cases contributes to the difficulty in using standard staging systems and classifications for treating these tumors (1,5,8,20,25,27,30,32,38).

Bony metastases develop in approximately 10% to 20% of all patients with a malignancy (1,5,6,7,8,10,12,15,38). This overall number of patients is much greater than those presenting with primary bone tumors. Chapters 100 and 101 deal with soft tissue and primary bone tumors. The same general principles apply when treating hand metastases. Lung carcinoma metastases leads the list of primary sites and accounts for almost half of cases involving the hand. The kidney and breast account for most of the remaining. In this chapter, the author discusses the pathology and the incidence and review the clinical findings along with diagnosis and treatment, both operative and nonoperative, for metastatic lesions involving the hand from the carpus to the distal phalanx.

BACKGROUND

The terminal phalanges are involved most frequently as the site of metastases. In a review of the literature, Kerin reported 163 cases: 77 involved the distal phalanx, 52 the metacarpals, and 44 the proximal phalanx (1,5,7). One-half of all metastatic lesions found in the upper extremity are usually found in the humerus. Of these, 3% to 10% of all upper extremity metastatic lesions have an unknown primary site of origin (1,5,7,10). Autopsies and case reports

have shown that the metastatic process seldom crosses into the adjacent joints, sparing the cartilage. Although soft tissue involvement and bony destruction may occur, the true pathology as to why the cartilage is spared is unknown. The known theories for dissemination of metastatic lesions include two routes: One is by hematogenous spread and the other by lymphogenous spread (4,10).

The avascularity of articular cartilage would support the hematogenous theory, especially due to its being spared from disease. The rarity of hand involvement has also been attributed to the paucity of red marrow in these parts of the skeleton. Despite the hands and feet representing nearly half of all the bones in the human body in both, metastases are extremely rare in both. Most metastases are numerous in bones that are rich in red marrow. The most common sites are the vertebrae, pelvic bones, femur, and ribs (1,5,7,38). Most of these lesions represent preterminal events, often part of more widespread metastatic involvement. The lung is the site in more than 40% of reported primary tumors that metastasize to the hand. Primary tumors of the lung can shed cells directly into the systemic arterial circulation, allowing tumor cells to reach parts of the hand distal with very little red marrow as opposed to other visceral primary lesions, which must first pass through the capillary bed of the liver or the lung before reaching the systemic arterial circulation (1,4,5,15,38).

Chemotactic factors that influence the migration and adherence of these cells to the skeleton have been found (1). Prostaglandins may also facilitate this process. Several studies have drawn attention to the relative sparing of the articular surface mentioned (1,7,12). The question has been posed as to whether the cartilage contains some property that insulates against the invasive process or does not allow metastasis to occur simply by being devoid of blood supply (1,4). This question remains to be answered.

INCIDENCE

The first recorded case was in the British literature in 1906 (1,15). The clinical significance of these tumors is that, due to their rarity, they are most often confused with infection and/or osteomyelitis. It is generally recognized that metastases may also masquerade as a distal tip infection or a tumor that is lytic in nature. These are sometimes found in psoriatic arthritis, gout, and rheumatoid arthritis. This is a relatively frequent occurrence in those who are terminally ill. Due to the poor vascularity to the digits, tip necrosis may occur. In Kerin's (5) study, males outnumbered females almost two to one, with a median age of 52. Of 22 lesions in a study from the Mayo Clinic, three involved the carpus, one the metacarpals, two the proximal phalanx, and 12 the distal phalanx. Four were limited to the soft tissues of the wrist or palm (10).

Examination of lesions of the digits and hand is not usually included in a standard postmortem evaluation. The incidence therefore may be somewhat unnoticed and underreported due to lesions that may be subclinical. The presentation of a metastasis to the hand usually occurs when there is already a generalized dissemination. This connotes a very poor prognosis and high morbidity rate.

PATHOLOGY

The pathology of metastatic deposits may mimic certain nonneoplastic conditions such as Sudeck's atrophy, osteomyelitis, septic arthritis, gout, or other osteoarthritic conditions. Evaluation of blood serum chemistry and cultures assists in ruling out some of these causes. In addition to masquerading as a benign disease clinically, acrometastases may present a diagnostic challenge to histopathologists. The morphologic appearance on light microscopy is similar to that of other malignant tumors such as renal cell carcinoma, adrenocortical carcinoma, alveolar rhabdomyosarcoma, clear cell sarcoma, alveolar soft tissue sarcoma, and malignant melanoma. Careful immunohistochemical and ultrastructural studies have to be done to find the histogenesis of the tumor. Of critical importance in aiding the pathologist is an appropriate biopsy sample of tissue. Very often, the biopsy specimen dictates further limb salvage attempts or necessary life-saving amputation (13).

DIAGNOSIS

The principles of managing tumors of the upper limb do not differ essentially from those of managing tumors in other areas of the musculoskeletal system (18,21,25,30,38). The importance of maintaining a high index of suspicion when dealing with a presumed chronic infection of the hand and obtaining specimens not only for culture but also for histologic study cannot be overemphasized (Fig. 1). Most of the patients in all the series studied died within a 6-month period of the diagnosis of a hand metastasis (1,5,7,10,12,15). These patients are often chronically

debilitated, and palliation is usually the most important goal. A thorough evaluation of the patient's clinical and family history, including the physical characteristics of the lesion and diagnostic images, provides information to determine whether this is an aggressive lesion and to allow staging to be performed.

Physical Examination

Assessment of the mass is very important, especially if it is painful or in an uncommon location for a typical benign lesion. A firm, nonmobile tender mass that does not allow the passage of light and that is growing rapidly should also heighten suspicion that the lesion may be malignant. A thorough history should include the length of time that this lesion has been present and the relative rapid growth or slow growth associated. Determination of symptoms as well as any family incidence and/or family history is necessary. A history of coexistent cancer is an obvious but often overlooked fact. Examination should include sensation, swelling, and mobility as well as possible axillary or regional lymphadenopathy present throughout the upper extremity. Clinically, these patients present with a swollen, erythematous, painful, and warm digit typical of acute inflammation or infection. Most have a known malignancy, usually carcinoma, but occasionally, they may have no history of malignancy and seek medical attention only for their digit. Initial workup should include a standard complete blood count, serum alkaline phosphatase, myeloma studies, and sedimentation rate. These studies are only early screens that are sensitive to most neoplastic and inflammatory problems but not specific to certain tumors. Imaging further aids in determining the extent, location, and involvement of the tumor.

Imaging

Plain radiography, magnetic resonance imaging, and computed tomography scans aid in diagnosing these lesions. Radiographs are indicated in symptomatic cases to identify the cause of localized pain to the hand. In some cases, a bone scan may help to identify and/or localize the area of involvement. Appearance on radiograph differs dramatically from that of benign cystic or pseudocystic erosions commonly found in the usual benign osseous neoplasms (Fig. 2). Metastatic lesions are more destructive but difficult to distinguish from osteomyelitis. There is often a large associated soft tissue mass with reactive periosteal bone (Fig. 3). Distal phalangeal metastases usually do not cross the articular surface. In fact, they characteristically preserve a thin margin of the subcortical bone, sometimes appearing as a blown-out cortical shell. Osteomyelitis, on the contrary, may cross a joint. This would aid in a differential diagnosis. It is possible, however, to have an infection in a metastatic distal phalanx lesion.

include an appropriate amount of normal tissue and an appropriate decision can be made as to whether limb salvage or amputation is necessary.

TREATMENT

The imaging studies discussed and a biopsy of the tumor are vital to the outcome of aggressive lesions. In primary malignant tumors, the possibility of limb-sparing procedures and long-term survival is much more likely than in the metastatic case. This is due to the high incidence of morbidity and the frequent delay in presentation of the metastatic lesions to the hand. Despite this, however, carefully planned preimaging studies and an appropriate biopsy should follow the standard principles described previously (Fig. 5). The biopsy should be planned to allow a pathologist to handle the fresh tissue right from the operating room for appropriate and extensive studies if necessary. Before the biopsy, it is important to discuss these issues directly with the pathologist to avoid common biopsy pitfalls. Staging studies should be done before the biopsy to plan the appropriate area for the incision and tissue acquisition. The incision should be placed in a location that can then be excised in the definitive surgical procedure to be performed later. The compartments violated by the biopsy should be contained, and no contamination of other compartments should occur. The violation of additional compartments may cause inadvertent seeding of tumor cells elsewhere. All the appropriate studies that may be necessary such as immunofluorescence and different biochemical assays should be known before obtaining the tissue so that appropriate handling can be performed. A team approach whereby everyone who is involved is aware of the goals is a priority. Mankin et al., in a case review, reported how often the biopsy is performed poorly (30).

The choices of biopsy include incisional, excisional, and needle or fine-needle aspiration. The choice is usually dictated by the clinical situation and the size, extent, and location of the tumor. Although fine-needle aspiration has been shown to be effective at diagnosing certain types of malignant metastases, it provides, for the most part, a very limited amount of tissue to study (11). Most biopsies occur with a pathologist available for a fresh frozen sectioning to make sure that an adequate quantity of tissue is obtained. The procedure should be performed under tourniquet control without exsanguination so as not to drive further malignant cells into the blood stream with the Esmarch. Excisional biopsy removes a portion of the tumor without a significant margin of normal tissue. This is done so as not to compromise subsequent surgical procedures in most small tumors. Correct incisions are usually longitudinal, avoiding any contamination of adjacent soft tissue planes. This parallel approach with adequate hemostasis allows for the most effective removal of a biopsy (Fig. 6). Mankin et al. studied the error rate in biopsies and found it to be as high as 18% (30). There is also a high incidence of infection and skin problems with inappropriately performed biopsies. The conclusion is therefore to treat the biopsy as a crucial and carefully planned

portion of the definitive surgery. An accurate diagnosis is the desired end result so that appropriate surgical planning can be performed.

Surgery

Metastatic tumors to the upper extremity present a different surgical management course. Although they are extremely rare, most reports have described metastases to the hand that occur primarily from lung, breast, kidney, and colon (1,4,5,7,15). Sarcomas and squamous cell are also found. In general, the prognosis is dismal. Most series found that nearly all of the patients died within 6 months to a year from the appearance of the metastatic tumor in the hand (1–38). The concepts of limb salvage with delayed reconstruction, marginal excision, wide excision, and/or amputation all apply to metastatic tumors. Most patients with metastatic disease in the hand are often chronically debilitated. If the lesion is symptomatic, causing pain and/or infection, amputation through the joint proximal to the level of involvement usually provides relief of pain and elimination of open, draining wounds to preserve maximum function. When the lesion is more proximal, local excision either alone or with local radiation is often effective. Radiation therapy is also helpful in treating symptoms of isolated pain from interosseous metastases without surgical intervention being necessary.

In most tumor literature, a 5-cm cuff is the definition of a wide resection clear of any tumor cells. In using limb salvage techniques in the upper extremity, this wide margin frequently cannot be achieved. This is clearly the case in the digits, where 5 cm may represent the entire digit; amputation must be considered in situations in which a wide margin cannot be obtained. Limb salvage combines a wide resection with neoadjuvant chemotherapy and radiotherapy for improved results. If negative margins cannot be obtained with local wide excision, amputation is the next step. With the development of neoadjuvant chemotherapy for soft tissue sarcomas, continued investigation into attempted limb sparing is needed (28,29,34,38). Improvement in results due to new prosthetic devices and better allograft or autograph reconstruction is possible in the future. Metastatic lesions involving the hand are rare. Malignant soft tissue tumors of the upper extremity involving the skin are much more common than malignant bone tumors, as indicated in previous chapters. A concerted effort to diagnose accurately and treat to give the greatest chance of survival is the ultimate goal.

CONCLUSION

Treatment of this type of tumor remains mostly palliative. Treatment is a team effort involving the medical oncologist and both the orthopedic hand and oncologic surgeons. Some patients have survived long term with appropriate treatment of these destructive lesions. It is hoped that con-

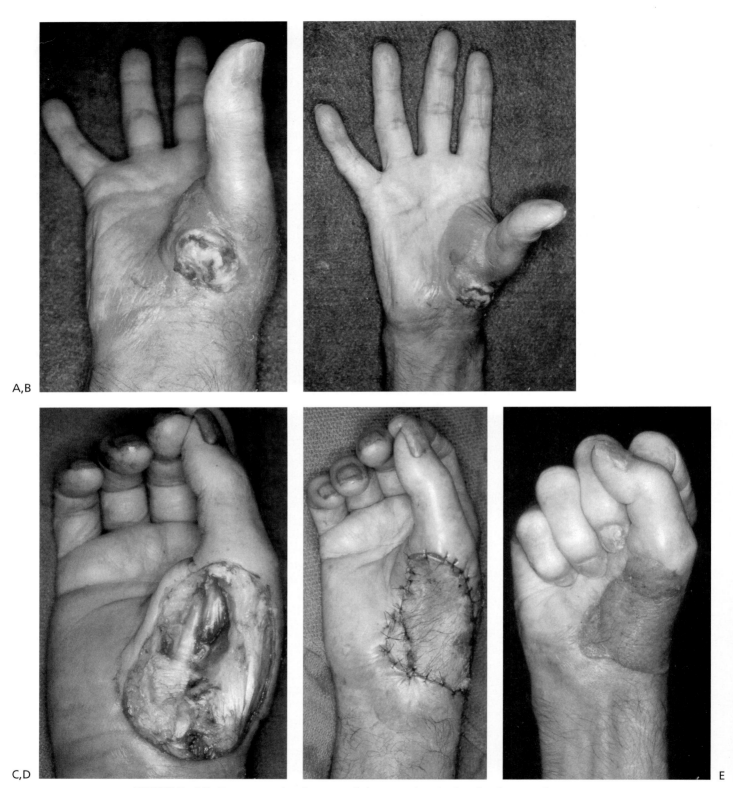

FIGURE 5. A,B: Gross tumor involvement of thenar region. Patient has lung carcinoma. **C,D:** A wide resection of the tumor leaves a soft tissue defect that is treated with skin grafting. **E:** Clinical result 6 months postoperation. (Reproduced with permission from Charles Eaton, M.D.)

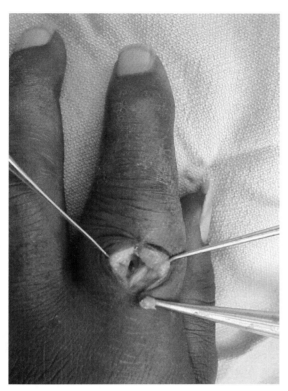

FIGURE 6. Biopsy of proximal phalanx tumor through a longitudinal approach. Ray resection was the end result in this case.

tinued clinical and basic science studies will help those numbers increase.

The lung, kidney, head, and breast are the most common sites of primary lesions that metastasize to the hand. A history of malignancy is usual, but some patients are seen without clinical evidence of malignancy. Although the average time from diagnosis to death is usually short, prolonged survival is possible. Treatment is usually palliative, but in patients with an apparently isolated metastatic lesion, wide excision may produce long disease-free intervals (38).

REFERENCES

1. Kerin R. The hand in metastatic disease. *J Hand Surg [Am]* 1987;12:77–83.
2. Hankin FM, Hankin RC, Louis DS. Malignant fibrous histiocytoma involving a digit. *J Hand Surg [Am]* 1987;12:83–86.
3. Chirodian N, Dickson MG, Kerr PS. Fingertip metastasis presenting with a history of trauma. *Hosp Med* 1998;59:819–821.
4. Adegboyega PA, Adekunle A, Viegas SF. Acrometastasis in renal cell carcinoma. *South Med J* 1999;92:1009–1012.
5. Kerin R. Metastatic tumors of the hand. *J Bone Joint Surg Am* 1983;65:1331–1335.
6. Monsees B, Murphy WA. Distal phalangeal erosive lesions. *Arthritis Rheum* 1984;27:449–455.
7. Kerin R. Metastatic tumors of the hand. *J Bone Joint Surg Am* 1958;40:263–278.
8. Mulvey RB. Peripheral bone metastases. *AJR Am J Roentgenol* 1964;91:155–160.
9. Calo RA, Torricelli P, Squarzina PB, et al. The value of computed tomography in the diagnosis of soft-tissue swellings of the hand. *J Hand Surg [Br]* 1990;15:229–232.
10. Amadio PC, Lombardi RM. Metastatic tumors of the hand. *J Hand Surg [Am]* 1987;12:311–316.
11. Knapp D, Abdul-Karim FW. Fine needle aspiration cytology of acrometastasis. *Acta Cytol* 1994;38:589–591.
12. Healy JH, Turnbull ADM, Miedama B, et al. Acrometastases. *J Bone Joint Surg Am* 1986;68:743–746.
13. Johnston AD. Pathology of metastatic tumors in bone. *Clin Orth Rel Res* 1970:73:8–32.
14. Vaezy A, Budson DC. Phalangeal metastases from bronchogenic carcinoma. *JAMA* 1978;239:226–227.
15. Wu KK, Guise ER. Metastatic tumors of the hand: a report of six cases. *J Hand Surg* 1978;3:271–276.
16. Gall RJ, Sim FH, Pritchard DJ. Metastatic tumors to the bones of the foot. *Cancer* 1976;37:1492–1495.
17. Greene MH. Metastasis of pulmonary carcinoma to the phalanges of the hand. *J Bone Joint Surg Am* 1957;39:972–975.
18. Bevan DA, Ehrlich GE, Gupta VP. Metastatic carcinoma simulating gout. *JAMA* 1977;237:2746–2747.
19. Cabanela ME, Sim FH, Beabout JW, et al. Osteomyelitis appearing as neoplasms: a diagnostic problem. *Arch Surg* 1974;109:68–72.
20. Mangini V. Tumors of the skeleton of the hand. *Bull Hosp Jt Dis Orthop Inst* 1967;28:61–103.
21. Brien EW, Terek RM, Geer RJ, et al. Treatment of soft-tissue sarcoma of the hand. *J Bone Joint Surg Am* 1995;77:564–571.
22. Serra JM, Muirragui A, Tadjalli H. Extensive distal subcutaneous metastases of a "benign" giant cell tumor of the radius. *Plast Reconstr Surg* 1985;75:263–267.
23. Lewin JS, Cleary KR, Eicher SA. An unusual metastasis to the thumb in a laryngectomized tracheoesophageal speaker. *Arch Otolaryngol Head Neck Surg* 1997;123:1007–1009.
24. Heymans M, Jardon-Jeghers C, Vanwijck R. Hand metastases from urothelial tumor. *J Hand Surg [Am]* 1990;15:509–511.
25. Enneking WF, Spanier SS, Goodman MA. The surgical staging of musculoskeletal sarcoma. *J Bone Joint Surg Am* 1980;62:1027–1030.
26. Gottschalk RG, Smith RT. Chondrosarcoma of the hand: report of a case with radioactive sulphur studies and review of the literature. *J Bone Joint Surg Am* 1963;45:141–150.
27. Hicks MC, Kalmon EH, Glasser SM. Metastatic malignancy to phalanges. *South Med J* 1964;57:85–88.
28. Jaffe N, Frei E, Trageis D, et al. Adjuvant methotrexate and citrovorum factor treatment of osteogenic sarcoma. *N Engl J Med* 1974;291:994–997.
29. Malawer MM, Dunham W. Cryosurgery and acrylic cementation as surgical adjuncts in the treatment of aggressive (benign) bone tumors. Analysis of 25 patients below the age of 21. *Clin Orthop* 1991;262:42–57.
30. Mankin JH, Lange TA, Spanier SS. The hazards of biopsy in patients with malignant primary bone and soft tissue tumors. *J Bone Joint Surg Am* 1982;64:1121–1127.
31. Mason ML. Tumors of the hand. *Surg Gynecol Obstet* 1937;65:129–148.
32. Simon, MA. Biopsy of musculoskeletal tumors. *J Bone Joint Surg Am* 1982;64:1253–1257.

33. Smith, RJ. Tumors of the hand: who is best qualified to treat tumors of the hand? *J Hand Surg* 1977;2:251–252.

34. Smith RJ, Waldo EF. Surgical treatment of aggressive lesions of the hand and forearm. In: Green DP, ed. *Operative hand surgery*, vol. 3, 2nd ed. New York: Churchill Livingstone, 1988:2363–2389.

35. Weiland AJ, Kleinert HE, Kutz JE, et al. Free vascularized bone grafts in surgery of the upper extremity. *J Hand Surg [Am]* 1979;4:129–144.

36. Yajima H, Tamai S, Mizumoto S, et al. Vascularized fibular graft for reconstruction after resection of aggressive benign and malignant bone tumors. *Microsurgery* 1992;13:227–233.

37. Yasko AW, Lane JW. Management of metastatic lesions. In: Bogumill GP, Fleegler EJ, eds. *Tumors of the hand and upper limb*. Edinburgh: Churchill Livingstone, 1993:403–412.

38. Putnam MD, Cohen M. Malignant bony tumors of the upper extremity. *Hand Clin* 1995;11:265–286.

103

HAND INFECTIONS

DONALD H. LEE
RANDOLPH J. FERLIC
ROBERT J. NEVIASER

Hand and upper extremity infections have a wide range of clinical manifestations. They vary from simple superficial infections (e.g., mild cellulitis) treatable by oral antibiotics to limb- or life-threatening infections (e.g., necrotizing fasciitis) requiring a combination of surgical débridement and intravenous antibiotics. They can also present as indolent, chronic infections (e.g., mycobacterial infection) in which the diagnosis is either delayed or missed. The hand being constantly exposed to the environment provides a wide variety of pathogens (bacteria, fungi, viruses, *Mycoplasma*) ample opportunity to invade it. With the rise of immunosuppression secondary to a variety of conditions—including human immunodeficiency virus (HIV) infections; use of posttransplantation immunosuppressants, chemotherapy, or chronic steroids; hematologic malignancies; chronic renal failure; diabetes; advanced age; alcohol abuse; and rheumatologic conditions—a simple hand infection can rapidly become a serious health problem (1). An understanding of infectious pathogens, the clinical conditions they produce, and the appropriate treatment helps limit these potential debilitating conditions.

GENERAL PRINCIPLES

Several factors may predispose the hand or extremity to an infection. These include local wound conditions (crush injuries, contaminated puncture wounds, chronic edema), altered immune states, or host conditions (diabetes, poor nutritional status, tobacco dependency). A careful medical history and physical examination should identify any additional infection risk factors, which may determine the need for more aggressive treatment. The successful treatment of hand and upper extremity infections requires an early recognition of the infection; the initiation of empiric and subsequent culture-directed antibiotic coverage; surgical débridement and irrigation of contaminated, devitalized tissues; and adequate follow-up care (2–9). Prompt recognition and initiation of treatment increase the chance of a favorable outcome (10–12). Delay in treatment, especially in conjunction with severe contamination, can lead to an increased incidence in wound infections (1).

Although diabetes mellitus has not been shown to be an independent risk factor for postoperative wound infection, it is a host risk factor for established upper extremity infections (13–17). The prevalence of diabetic comorbidities, including vasculopathy and neuropathy, increases as the duration of the disease process progresses. These poor host factors are often adversely complemented with other additional factors of poor prognostic value, including tobacco abuse and malnutrition. This combination of host factors is manifested by a higher incidence of diabetes in patients requiring inpatient admission for hand infection, ranging between 7% and 58% (9,15).

Diabetic patients presenting with an infection have predominately gram-negative or mixed cultures rather than the typical predominance of gram-positive organisms seen in nondiabetic patients. In addition, surgical outcomes and rates of reoperation, amputation, and mortality are higher (13–16,18,19).

PATHOPHYSIOLOGY

Pathogens are microorganisms capable of invading the body and causing disease. An *infection* is the disease caused by replicating pathogens, usually in the presence of tissue damage. The ability of a pathogen to produce an infection in a given host depends on the organism's pathogenicity and virulence (20–24). The *pathogenicity*, or likelihood of producing a disease, is determined by several factors, including the organism's ability to survive in the environment, to be transmitted between hosts, to attach to body surfaces, to defend itself against the host's immunologic attack and reproduce, and to damage the host (e.g., by toxin production). *Virulence* is the ability of an organism to cause severe disease. *Infectiousness* is the ease with which a pathogen can spread within a given population.

There are several routes of transmission of an infection. *Fomites* are inanimate environmental objects acting as intermediaries, transporting pathogens from source to host (e.g., towels or bedding transmitting an infection between hospital patients). *Vectors* are living creatures that can transmit infection from one host to another [e.g., arthropods (mosquito, flea, tick)]. Infections can also be spread through direct contact, inhalation, ingestion, and inoculation.

A pathogen can produce host damage through a variety of mechanisms, including the direct action of the microorganism or production of bacterial toxins. *Endotoxins* are the intracellular and cell-associated toxic components of gram-negative organisms, including the lipopolysaccharide antigen of the bacterial cell wall. It partly protects the bacteria against the bactericidal activity of serum and can also activate the complement cascade. *Exotoxins* are toxic substances excreted by the organism. These toxins can be classified in a variety of ways. For instance, they can be classified according to the symptoms produced (neurotoxin, enterotoxin, cytotoxin), their mode of action (extracellular or transmembrane toxins, membrane-damaging toxins, deregulating toxins), their intracellular targets, their biologic effects (hemolytic toxin, edema-producing toxins), and the producing organism (pertussis toxin, cholera toxin).

Microbes also work synergistically to help establish an infection, facilitate tissue invasion, reduce the host's immune response, and enhance the virulence of the various pathogens. Such polymicrobial infections include necrotizing fasciitis and gangrene. HIV infections, by diminishing the host's virulence, allow other pathogens to invade the host.

Pathogens can be classified into five main groups: bacteria, fungi, viruses, protozoa, and metazoa (20). Bacteria are grouped by four characteristics: Gram's stain reaction (gram-positive and gram-negative), shape (cocci, bacilli, spiral), atmospheric requirements (obligate aerobes, microaerophilic, capnophiles, facultative anaerobes, obligate anaerobes), and the presence of spores. Other varying structural characteristics of bacteria include the cell wall, plasma membrane, bacterial capsule, extracellular slime, fimbriae (pili), flagella, and pathogenicity islands (genomic regions that determine pathogenicity and virulence). Fungi are classified in different ways, including the means of reproduction and morphology or the type of infection produced (superficial and subcutaneous, systemic, or fungi associated with immunocompromised patients). Viruses are classified according to the type of nucleic acid and means of transcription (DNA, RNA), the structure and symmetry of the structural proteins (capsids), and the presence or absence of an envelope. Protozoa are classified according to spore production (sporozoa), flagellate (flagellates), ameboid, and ciliate. Metazoa or helminths are classified into nematodes or roundworms, platyhelminths or flatworms, cestodes or tapeworms, and flukes.

Resistance to infection occurs through several mechanisms, including nonspecific, or innate, immunity and specific immunity (20,24,25). Nonspecific immunity includes normal mechanical and physiologic properties of the host (e.g., skin, mucosae, gastric acid, complement system, phagocytosis). Specific immunity includes a variety of defensive responses by the host to microorganisms (antigens, cell-mediated and humeral immune responses).

The manifestations of infection include fever, inflammation, and rashes (20,22). Fevers occur due to a release of cytokines and interferon-alpha by activated mononuclear phagocytes, which act on specialized endothelial cells in the hypothalamic blood vessels. The subsequent release of prostaglandins causes a resetting of the body temperature that is controlled by the hypothalamus. Inflammation occurs as a combination of several events: vasodilatation at the affected site, exudation of tissue fluid from dilated capillaries, accumulation of neutrophils and macrophages at the site, and the release of active chemicals (lysozymes, free radicals, lactoferrin, leukotrienes) from neutrophils. These events cause local heat and redness. Rashes are a particular form of inflammation or tissue affecting the skin. They may be generalized or localized. The characteristics of rashes (e.g., appearance, method of spread) are frequently typical of the organism(s) producing the infection.

CLINICAL EVALUATION

Bacterial infections usually produce the normal signs of infection, including erythema, edema, and tenderness. Dorsal, as opposed to palmar, hand swelling may be noted due to the relative pliability of the dorsal skin as compared with the thickened, glabrous palmar skin. Certain infections (e.g., pyogenic tenosynovitis) present with classic clinical findings, including fusiform digital swelling and a flexed finger position (see below). However, nonbacterial infections (e.g., mycobacterial infections) may present with innocuous swelling without significant erythema or pain. Included in the differential diagnosis of hand infections are gout, inflammatory conditions (e.g., tenosynovitis, rheumatoid arthritis), collagen vascular diseases, foreign body reactions, soft tissue calcifications, and neoplasm (26).

An appropriate history includes the location and quality of pain, the duration of the process, any systemic manifestations (fever, chills), the mechanism of injury (if applicable), any previous antibiotic or surgical treatment, and a complete medical history. The physical examination includes inspection and palpation of the involved area, evaluation of lymphadenopathy, neurovascular examination, and use of provocative maneuvers (e.g., passive finger extension for pyogenic tenosynovitis). The presence of fever should be noted.

IMAGING STUDIES

Diagnostic studies should include radiographs to rule out a fracture, foreign body, periosteal reaction, osteomyelitis, or implant loosening (28,29). Soft tissue shadows, indicative of edema, may be seen. Computed tomography can help determine the presence of septic arthritis and adjacent osteomyelitis. Magnetic resonance imaging is helpful in the evaluation of musculoskeletal infections, providing excellent soft tissue contrast, multiplanar capability, and improved assessment of bone marrow and joint involvement. Early changes in the bone marrow space in the early stages of acute osteomyelitis can be defined by magnetic resonance imaging scan. A decreased signal intensity in the bone marrow density is seen on T1-weighted images and increased signal intensity on T2-weighted images (21,22, 24,27). These images can help define distended joint spaces and periarticular extensions of infections. Ultrasound can be used to evaluate areas of edema, fluid accumulation, abscess formation, pyarthrosis, and osteomyelitis (27). Nuclear imaging is used to detect abscesses, septic arthritis, and osteomyelitis (20,22).

LABORATORY STUDIES

Complete Blood Cell Count with Differential

The complete blood cell count with differential white blood cell count is frequently used to detect signs of infection. Leukocytosis (white blood cell count of more than 12,000) and a left shift showing more immature polymorphonuclear leukocytes are signs of an infectious process (22,23,27).

Acute-Phase Proteins

The concentration of several plasma proteins rises in the presence of inflammation. C-reactive protein, a commonly monitored acute-phase reactant, is produced in the liver. Its levels are rapidly elevated during the acute inflammatory phase in many bacterial and viral infections (20). Serum levels increase from 1 µg per milliliter by 100 to 1,000 times within hours due to an induction in hepatic synthesis (22,27). It is a disc-shaped pentameric molecule that readily binds a number of substances, including the C fraction of pneumococcal lysates, hence its name (20,22). In its bound form, it activates the complement cascade.

Erythrocyte Sedimentation Rate

The viscosity of plasma is altered during inflammation secondary to protein changes. The erythrocyte sedimentation rate (ESR) is the rate that red blood cells settle in anticoagulated blood left standing. The normal ESR is less than 20 mm per hour, rises to 30 to 50 mm per hour in acute infections, and can rise to 70 to 100 mm per hour in certain conditions (abscesses, immunologic diseases, atypical pneumonias) (20). It can also be elevated

with recent surgery or fractures; malignancies; myocardial infarction; and gastrointestinal, thyroid, renal, and collagen vascular diseases (29). Both the ESR and C-reactive protein level are nonspecific indicators of inflammatory changes, with the ESR rising more slowly than the C-reactive protein levels.

NONOPERATIVE MANAGEMENT OF HAND INFECTIONS

Uncomplicated simple lacerations of the hand do not require the use of prophylactic antibiotic therapy (30). Cleansing these simple lacerations with povidone-iodine (Betadine) solution, followed by loose primary suture approximation, is adequate (31). The use of prophylactic antibiotic coverage for more complex (contaminated wounds or those involving bone, tendon, or neurovascular structures) lacerations or for elective hand surgery is controversial and currently is best decided at the treating surgeon's discretion (32–39).

The initial medical treatment of open contaminated wounds should include the use of relatively broad-spectrum antibiotics covering the more commonly found aerobic pathogens (e.g., *Staphylococcus*, *Streptococcus*, *Haemophilus*) and anaerobic organisms (e.g., *Eikenella*, *Bacteroides*, *Enterobacter*) (26). In general, penicillin (anaerobic coverage) with nafcillin or a first-generation cephalosporin [e.g., cefazolin (Ancef) (gram-positive coverage, penicillinase resistance)] is used (26). Gentamicin is added for broader coverage for gram-negative infections (40). Table 1 includes a list of common types of infections, commonly involved pathogens, and the recommended initial antibiotic coverage until culture results and sensitivities can be obtained.

SURGICAL MANAGEMENT OF HAND INFECTIONS

A biopsy is indicated in cases of persistent signs of infections failing to respond to splinting, elevation, and antibiotics; in cases of obvious infections (e.g., abscesses); and in cases in which a definitive diagnosis is needed. The initial biopsy should include a deep wound sample of the infected area. An adequate surgical field and setup, with use of a tourniquet and appropriate anesthesia, should be used to allow for formal débridement and irrigation should an obvious infection be found. Sufficient tissue samples should be obtained for multiple cultures, including aerobic, anaerobic, mycobacterial, atypical mycobacterial, and fungal cultures. A specimen is sent for Gram's stain, and in cases of suspected mycobacterial and fungal infections, appropriate stains (acid-fast bacillus stain and potassium hydroxide preparation) should also be sent.

TABLE 1. EMPIRIC ANTIBIOTIC RECOMMENDATIONS FOR HAND INFECTIONS

Infection	Organisms	Antibiotic	Alternative antibiotic
Paronychia/felon	*Staphylococcus aureus*, oral anaerobes	Nafcillin, cefazolin, clindamycin, dicloxacillin	Cephalexin, erythromycin
Flexor tenosynovitis	*S. aureus, Streptococcus*, gram-negative rods	Cefazolin	Nafcillin or vancomycin plus gentamicin, imipenem
Deep space infection	*S. aureus*, anaerobes, gram-negative rods	Cefazolin, ampicillin/sulbactam (Unasyn)	Nafcillin, vancomycin plus gentamicin, imipenem
Cellulitis/lymphangitis	*S. aureus*, beta-hemolytic streptococci	Nafcillin, cephalexin, dicloxacillin	Cephalexin, erythromycin
Human bite	*S. aureus*, coagulase-negative staphylococci, *Eikenella corrodens, Streptococcus* spp., *Bacteroides* spp., *Peptostreptococcus*, anaerobes	Cefazolin plus penicillin, clindamycin plus ciprofloxacin, trimethoprim-sulfamethoxazole (Bactrim/Septra), ampicillin/clavulanate (Augmentin)	Nafcillin plus penicillin, amoxicillin-clavulanate (Augmentin), ampicillin/sulbactam (Unasyn), cefoxitin
Animal bite	Gram-positive cocci, *S. aureus*, anaerobes, *Pasteurella multocida*	Cefazolin plus penicillin, amoxicillin-clavulanate (Augmentin)	Nafcillin plus penicillin, amoxicillin-clavulanate (Augmentin), ampicillin/sulbactam (Unasyn), clindamycin plus ciprofloxacin, trimethoprim-sulfamethoxazole (Bactrim/Septra)
Septic arthritis	*S. aureus, Streptococcus, Neisseria gonorrhoeae*	Cefazolin, ceftriaxone	Nafcillin, vancomycin, clindamycin, doxycycline
Osteomyelitis	*S. aureus, Streptococcus*, gram-negative rods	Cefazolin plus gentamicin	Nafcillin, vancomycin, clindamycin, doxycycline
Traumatic/contaminated wounds	*S. aureus, Streptococcus*, anaerobes, gram-negative rods	Imipenem	Cefazolin plus gentamicin
Intravenous drug abuse–related	Gram-positive, gram-negative methicillin-resistant *S. aureus*	Nafcillin plus gentamicin	Vancomycin plus gentamicin, imipenem
Diabetes-related	Gram-positive cocci, gram-negative rods	Cefazolin plus gentamicin	Cefoxitin, ampicillin/sulbactam
Herpetic whitlow	Herpes simplex virus	Acyclovir	Valacyclovir, famciclovir

Data from references 21, 24, 26, 27, and 97.

ALGORITHM FOR THE EVALUATION AND MANAGEMENT OF HAND INFECTIONS

Figure 1 provides an algorithm for the evaluation and management of hand infections.

INFECTIONS

Paronychia

The *perionychium* is defined as the paronychium (border tissue around the nail) and the nailbed (germinal and sterile matrix). A paronychia is an infection of the lateral nail fold (Fig. 2). When the infection extends to the *eponychium* (defined as the thin membrane distal to the nail wall at the base of the nail), it is properly termed an *eponychia*. When infection involves both lateral nail folds and eponychium, it is called a *run-around infection* (41,42).

In adults, *Staphylococcus aureus* is the most common pathogen (43). Infection occurs when there is violation of the seal between the nail plate and nail fold, allowing the inoculation of bacteria. Hangnails, manicures, penetrating trauma, constant exposure to a wet or moist environment, and nail biting or sucking are common inciting events for an infection (44). Initial swelling, erythema, tenderness

with progression to fluctuance, and abscess formation are the typical clinical presentation. Spontaneous decompression can occur, including tracking beneath the nail plate (subungual abscess). Deeper infections can involve the nailbed, pulp space, and bone, producing nailbed destruction, felon, or osteomyelitis. In children, there is often a mix of aerobic and anaerobic organisms believed to be related to the finger-sucking and nail-biting habits of this young population (45).

Infections in the early stages can be treated with oral antibiotics, warm soaks, rest, and observation. Otherwise, surgical decompression is the treatment of choice for acute, established paronychia. With simple infections, a digital or metacarpal local anesthetic block may not be needed. Decompression is performed by carefully entering the abscess cavity between the nail plate and nail fold with a scalpel blade or hemostat (Fig. 3) (41,43,46). A small wick is placed for 24 to 48 hours to prevent the incision from closing and recurrence of the infection. The wick is removed, and saline warm soaks are begun.

Aggressive decompression is needed with more established or resistant infections. A digital or metacarpal block with local plain lidocaine (Xylocaine) is used. Depending on the extent of the infection, a partial or complete nail plate removal with or without lateral nail fold relief inci-

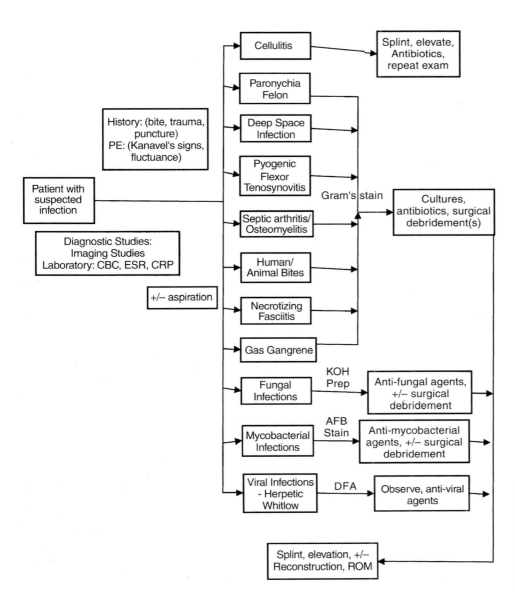

FIGURE 1. Algorithm for the evaluation and management of hand infections. AFB, acid-fast bacillus; CBC, complete blood cell count; CRP, C-reactive protein; DFA, direct fluorescent antibody; ESR, erythrocyte sedimentation rate; KOH, potassium hydroxide; PE, physical examination; ROM, range of motion.

sion(s) is performed. The incision should be made perpendicular to the edge of the nail fold (Fig. 4). A single or double incision is used depending on the location of the infection. As before, the wound is packed with a wick and subsequently changed, and intermittent warm saline soaks are started.

Subungual abscesses are treated with removal of a portion of or the entire nail. The abscess is carefully débrided while protecting the sterile and germinal matrices. Cultures should be obtained at the time of decompression, with initiation of empiric oral antibiotic therapy. Wound care, including splinting of the distal interphalangeal joint, warm saline or Epsom salt soaks, and serial observation, should be continued until wound healing. The antibiotic coverage is adjusted based on the results of the wound cultures. The majority of these infections resolve without permanent sequelae, including nail dystrophy.

Chronic paronychia occurs more commonly in individuals constantly exposed to moist environments. Infections may be intermittent; clinically, the eponychial fold is thickened and painful. *Candida albicans* is a frequent offending organism (see the section Fungal Infections).

Marsupialization of the nail may be needed with chronic paronychias (47). After digital block anesthesia, a small, crescent-shaped portion of the eponychial fold is removed and made proximal to the distal edge of the eponychial fold without injuring the germinal matrix. A 5-mm wedge of skin, extending to lateral margins of the nail fold, is removed (Fig. 5). The nail plate is removed if severely deformed or if there are signs of infection. Xeroform or similar nonadhering gauze is placed under the nail fold and changed at 24 to 48 hours. Wound epithelialization gradually occurs over 2 to 3 weeks. Topical antifungal ointments are generally used 4 to 6 weeks.

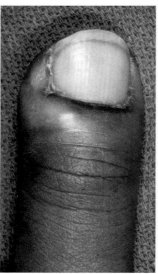
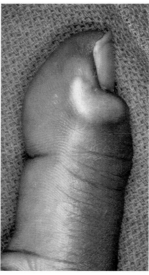

A,B

FIGURE 2. A,B: A paronychia, or infection of the lateral and eponychial nail fold.

Felon

A felon is a deep space infection or abscess of the distal pulp of the finger or thumb. It differs from the superficial apical infection involving the distal portion of the pulp skin, which often responds to a small, deroofing incision (41,43,46). The hyponychium, the region of keratinized skin beneath the distal nail plate, is normally very resistant to infection.

The pulp is composed of multiple vertical septae extending from the skin to the palmar distal phalanx, creating multiple small enclosed compartments in the pulp. Penetrating trauma, such as that from a splinter, often, but not always, serves as the

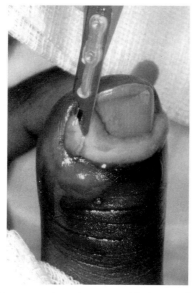

FIGURE 3. Decompression of a paronychia by entering the abscess cavity between the nail plate and nail fold with a scalpel blade.

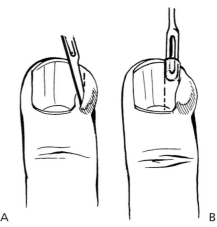

A   B

FIGURE 4. A: An infected lateral and proximal nail fold can be elevated by an elevator or scalpel. **B:** For extensive infections, a relief incision(s) is made perpendicular to the edge of the nail fold to allow for removal of a portion or all of the nail plate. (Reprinted from Seiler JG. *Essentials of hand surgery*. Philadelphia: Lippincott Williams & Wilkins, 2002, with permission. Copyright American Society of Surgery of the Hand.)

event introducing a bacterial load. The infection can progress to produce a sinus, skin sloughing, or osteomyelitis. With further progression, the infection can produce a septic arthritis of the distal interphalangeal joint or pyogenic tenosynovitis. The organism most frequently cultured from a pulp space infection is *S. aureus* (43,48). Clinical presentation includes throbbing pain and tense swelling localized to the pulp (Fig. 6).

Surgical decompression of a felon is performed when an obvious infection with fluctuance is noted. One of several incisions can be used, including a preferred unilateral longitudinal incision, a J-shaped or hockey-stick incision, a through-and-through incision, or a volar longitudinal incision. A fishmouth incision should be avoided (Fig. 7) (6,7,46,49–53). Although the site of maximal induration often dictates the location of the incision, a unilateral longitudinal incision is ideally performed on the noncontact surface of the involved digit. This includes the ulnar sides of the index and long fingers and the radial sides of the ring finger,

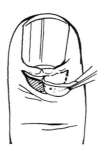

FIGURE 5. Eponychial marsupialization is performed by removing a small, crescent-shaped portion of the eponychial fold proximal to the distal edge of the eponychial fold. Care is taken to not injure the underlying germinal matrix. (Reprinted from Seiler JG. *Essentials of hand surgery*. Philadelphia: Lippincott Williams & Wilkins, 2002, with permission. Copyright American Society of Surgery of the Hand.)

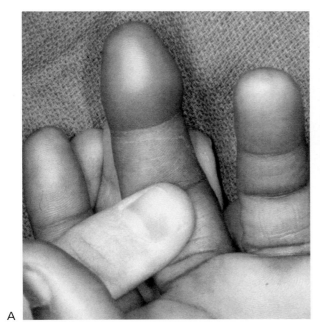

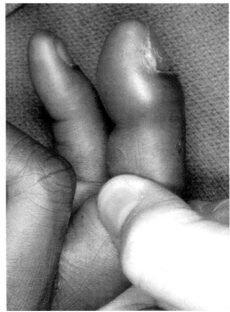

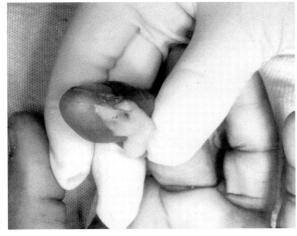

FIGURE 6. A,B: A felon, or abscess of the distal finger pulp. Note the smaller, normal-sized adjacent finger. **C:** A unilateral longitudinal incision is used to decompress the felon.

small finger, and thumb. The incision begins dorsal and distal to the distal interphalangeal joint flexion crease and extends distally toward, but does not include, the hyponychium. This incision parallels the lateral nail fold with a 5-mm interval of separation. Sharp dissection is carried out in line with the skin incision to the volar cortex of the distal phalanx. A small hemostat is then gently spread to allow complete decompression by disrupting the vertical septae.

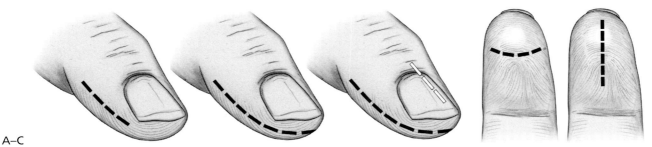

FIGURE 7. Incisions used for decompression of a felon. **A:** A midlateral incision is preferred. **B:** A J-shaped or hockey-stick incision. **C:** A through-and-through incision. **D,E:** A volar transverse or longitudinal incision.

A longitudinal central midline incision (43,52) is advocated in an attempt to avoid skin slough, digital nerve injury, or creation of an unstable fat pad. This incision is preferred in the presence of a sinus track, allowing incorporation of the sinus track with the incision. The hockey-stick, fishmouth, and transverse palmar incisions are to be avoided due to their potential iatrogenic morbidity. With any of these incisions, care is taken not to injure the neurovascular structures or introduce an infection into the flexor tendon sheath. A common problem is using too small an incision to adequately decompress the infection.

After appropriate lavage irrigation, a small wick is placed for 24 to 48 hours, with initiation of appropriate wound care and allowance of secondary wound closure. As with paronychias, cultures should be obtained at the time of decompression, and empiric oral antibiotics should be started. The antibiotics are adjusted according to the results of the deep wound cultures.

Deep Space Infections

The appropriate treatment of deep space infections requires careful surgical planning and drainage, acquiring intraoperative cultures to direct the antibiotic coverage needed, and allowing wound closure by secondary intention. Postoperative wound care, edema control, splinting, and motion optimization are preferably pursued with therapy supervision (54). Initial empiric antibiotic coverage with a second-generation cephalosporin, such as cefazolin, while awaiting culture identification and sensitivity is usually adequate. Addition of gram-negative coverage is recommended in an immunocompromised individual.

Web Space Infections

A web space infection, also known as a *collar button abscess* or *hourglass abscess*, involves the subfascial palmar space between the digits. The infection begins as an infected blister, an open wound, or a palmar callus or from the adjacent subcutaneous area (55). An abscess subsequently develops and extends either volarly or usually dorsally to include the contiguous subcutaneous space of the dorsal hand. The involved adjacent digits are held apart from one another in a characteristic abducted posture. This clinical presentation, combined with prominent dorsal hand swelling and a tender palmar web space, usually makes the diagnosis clear. Incisional drainage is performed with separate dorsal or volar or combined approaches (Fig. 8) (46,50,55–58). The type of incision(s) used depends on the location of the abscess. A combined approach is used in cases in which the infection is noted both dorsally and volarly. A transverse incision in the web space itself should be avoided to prevent possible web space scar contracture (46,57). After formal débridement and irrigation of the wound, a 16-gauge polyethylene catheter can be sutured into an open wound to

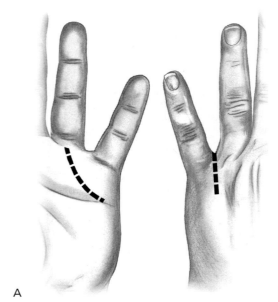

FIGURE 8. Incisions used for decompression of a web space infection. **A:** A curved volar incision. **B:** A dorsal longitudinal incision.

allow for subsequent saline irrigation (100 mL per hour) of the wound for 24 to 48 hours (46).

Dorsal Subaponeurotic Space Infections

The dorsal subaponeurotic space is a potential space located deep to the extensor tendons and dorsal to the metacarpals. Penetrating trauma usually introduces bacteria to this space, which can subsequently become an abscess (55). Although it is difficult clinically to discern from subcutaneous edema with overlying cellulitis, aggressive surgical incision and débridement are recommended if in doubt. Two dorsal longitudinal incisions are preferable rather than a single central one, which may result in tendon desiccation. One incision is centered over the second metacarpal; the other is in the fourth-fifth intermetacarpal region to allow an adequate intervening skin bridge. Care is taken to protect the dorsal veins to minimize hand swelling. The wounds are allowed to heal by secondary intention, and early hand motion is instituted to minimize extensor tendon adhesions (26).

Palmar Space Infections

The deep palmar spaces are potential spaces in the hand and are divided into the midpalmar space, thenar space, hypothenar space, and posterior adductor space (Fig. 9) (26,46,57,59). The midpalmar space is located deep to the flexor tendons and lumbricals and extends dorsally to the volar fascia, investing the second and third volar interossei and the third and fourth metacarpals. Radially, it is bordered by the midpalmar or oblique fascial septum. This septum extends from the third metacarpal to the sheath, enclosing the long-finger flexor ten-

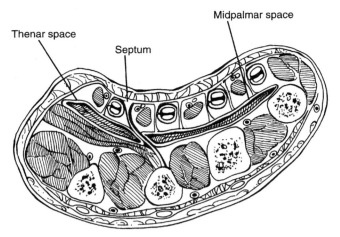

FIGURE 9. Diagram of palmar spaces. (Reprinted from Seiler JG. *Essentials of hand surgery*. Philadelphia: Lippincott Williams & Wilkins, 2002, with permission. Copyright American Society of Surgery of the Hand.)

dons (ulnar bursa in some people). The midpalmar space extends distally to the level of the vertical septa of the palmar fascia, ending approximately 2 cm proximal to the web spaces. Proximally, the space extends to the distal edge of the carpal canal.

The thenar space is bordered ulnarly by the vertical midpalmar septum and posteriorly and radially by the adductor pollicis fascia, and it lies deep to the flexor pollicis longus. The hypothenar space is located ulnar to the midpalmar space, contains the hypothenar muscles, and is enclosed by their investing fascia. This space is bordered radially by a fibrous hypothenar septum coursing between the fifth metacarpal and palmar aponeurosis. The posterior adductor space is another potential space located dorsal to the adductor pollicis and palmar to the first dorsal interosseous.

The clinical presentation of palmar space infections typically includes pain, erythema, swelling, and guarding with tenderness at the focus of abscess. It is not unusual for a patient to present 48 to 72 hours after a penetrating injury with signs of infection.

Several possible surgical incisions can be used for midpalmar space infections (Fig. 10A–D) (6,50,55,58,60–62).

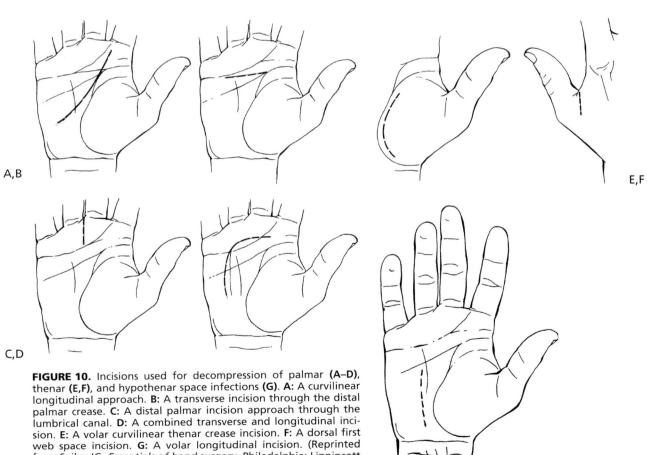

FIGURE 10. Incisions used for decompression of palmar **(A–D)**, thenar **(E,F)**, and hypothenar space infections **(G)**. **A:** A curvilinear longitudinal approach. **B:** A transverse incision through the distal palmar crease. **C:** A distal palmar incision approach through the lumbrical canal. **D:** A combined transverse and longitudinal incision. **E:** A volar curvilinear thenar crease incision. **F:** A dorsal first web space incision. **G:** A volar longitudinal incision. (Reprinted from Seiler JG. *Essentials of hand surgery*. Philadelphia: Lippincott Williams & Wilkins, 2002, with permission. Copyright American Society of Surgery of the Hand.)

These options include a preferred curvilinear longitudinal approach, a transverse incision through the distal palmar crease, a distal palmar incision approach through the lumbrical canal, and a combined transverse and longitudinal incision.

A thenar space infection may require a volar and a separate dorsal first web space incision if dorsal extension has occurred around the adductor pollicis and first dorsal interosseous muscles (Fig. 10E,F). This is the so-called dumbbell, or pantaloon, abscess. Hypothenar space infections can be drained using a volar longitudinal incision along the medial aspect of the hypothenar eminence (Fig. 10G). Alternately, an incision along the medial aspect of the hypothenar eminence can be used. Continuous or intermittent irrigation of the infected space can also be used (46,63).

Pyogenic Flexor Tenosynovitis

Pyogenic flexor tenosynovitis, or suppurative flexor tenosynovitis, is a bacterial infection of the digital flexor sheath. The majority of these infections are secondary to traumatic penetrating injuries; therefore, skin flora, including *S. aureus*, is the source of the most common infecting organisms (46,64–67).

The flexor sheath is an intricate continuous synovial sheath originating at the level of the metacarpal neck and ending at the insertion of the flexor digitorum profundus. It separates into an outer parietal and an inner visceral layer. The parietal layer thickens at different intervals, consistently forming discrete annular and cruciform pulleys.

The visceral layer is the epitenon. Between the two layers is the synovial space, which is essentially a closed space.

The flexor sheath of the little finger flexor digitorum profundus tendon (and, on occasion, the ring, long, and index fingers) communicates with the ulnar bursa, which extends proximal to the wrist level. The flexor sheath of the flexor pollicis longus communicates with the radial bursa, which extends proximal to the wrist level as well. The radial and ulnar bursa can communicate at the level of the transverse carpal ligament through Parona's space (57,67), producing a horseshoe abscess. Parona's space is a potential space in the distal forearm located between the pronator quadratus muscle and the flexor digitorum profundus tendons.

The clinical findings of pyogenic tenosynovitis include Kanavel's four cardinal signs: pain with passive extension of the digit (the most reproducible clinical sign), symmetric digital swelling (sausage digit), tenderness along the flexor sheath, and a semiflexed resting posture of the involved digit (Fig. 11) (62).

Nonoperative treatment may be possible if the infection is detected and treated early (e.g., within 24 to 48 hours) (46). Treatment includes the use of intravenous antibiotics (Table 1), splint immobilization of the hand, elevation, and serial observations for 48 hours. With continued signs of infection, surgery should be performed.

Surgery is the mainstay of treatment for pyogenic tenosynovitis. Several surgical techniques can be used, including the preferred two-incision, closed–tendon sheath, irrigation method (Fig. 12) (46,64,66,67–73); open drainage of the tendon sheath (60,61,74,75); single palmar incision for antibiotic instillation (76); distal digital drainage with proxi-

A–C

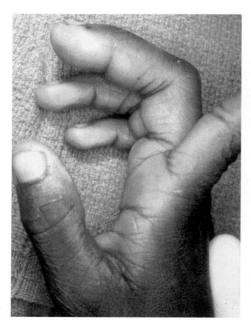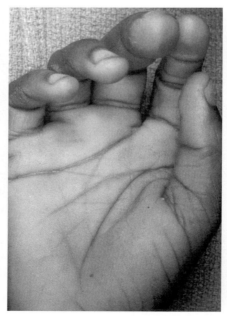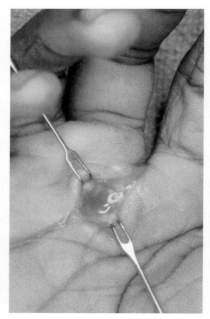

FIGURE 11. A,B: A digit with pyogenic flexor tenosynovitis showing symmetric digital swelling and a flexed resting posture. **C:** Palmar incision revealing purulent drainage from the flexor sheath.

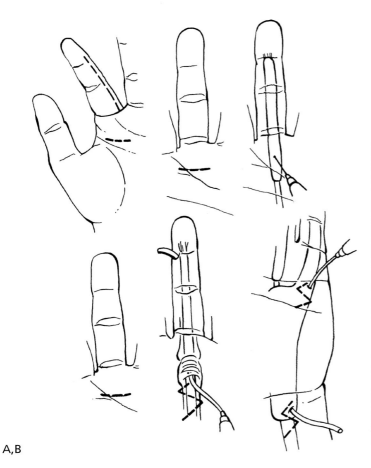

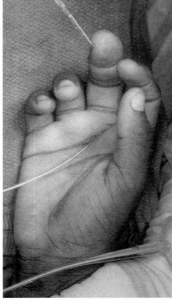

A,B

FIGURE 12. A: Diagram of incisions used for decompression of flexor sheath infections. (Reprinted from Seiler JG. *Essentials of hand surgery.* Philadelphia: Lippincott Williams & Wilkins, 2002, with permission. Copyright American Society of Surgery of the Hand.) **B:** Intraoperative photograph of irrigation fluid being flushed through a pediatric feeding tube. The tube has been passed from the proximal palmar incision through the flexor sheath and out distally through a midlateral incision. The distal end of the tube is withdrawn into the sheath to irrigate the flexor sheath.

mal antibiotic instillation with a needle (77); and a through-and-through (two-incision) intermittent irrigation (68,73).

Pyogenic flexor tenosynovitis has been classified into three stages (Table 2) (64,69,78). The type of surgical treatment varies with the clinical stage of the infection. Stages I and II can be effectively treated with the preferred two-incision, closed–tendon sheath, irrigation technique (Fig. 12). With this technique, the A1 pulley is approached proximally through a preferred transverse, versus a longitudinal

TABLE 2. THREE STAGES OF PYOGENIC FLEXOR TENOSYNOVITIS

Intraoperative stage	Characteristic findings	Treatment
Stage I	Increased fluid in sheath, primarily a serous exudate	Minimal invasive drainage and catheter irrigation
Stage II	Cloudy/purulent fluid, granulomatous synovium	Minimal invasive drainage with or without indwelling catheter irrigation
Stage III	Septic necrosis of the tendon, pulleys, or tendon sheath	Extensile open débridement, possible amputation

or zigzag palmar, incision at the level of the metacarpal head. After entrance into the flexor sheath, cloudy fluid or pus should be identified and cultured. A No. 5 French pediatric feeding tube is inserted into the incised sheath and advanced distally. Alternatively, a 16-gauge polyethylene catheter can be used. A separate midlateral incision is made distal to the A4 pulley, where a small section of the sheath is resected. An alternate palmar incision can be used. This incision allows a through-and-through irrigation of sterile saline solution. The sheath is irrigated with 500 to 1,000 mL of saline. A small drain can be sutured in the distal incision to keep the wound patent. Postoperatively, the hand is dressed in a bulky dressing and elevated. The catheter is either manually flushed with 50 mL of sterile saline solution every 2 hours or attached to a continuous infusion pump infusing sterile saline at approximately 25 to 30 mL per hour. Care must be taken to avoid direct extravasation of fluid into the adjacent tissue. This is ensured by having the tube visibly exit the distal sheath or placing a small, separate Penrose drain in the distal incision.

The radial and ulnar bursas can be drained and irrigated through the use of an open technique (50) or the through-and-through irrigation technique (46,72). The distal end of the radial bursa is exposed at the level of the proximal end of the flexor sheath near the metacarpophalangeal flexion sheath or, more proximally, at the level of the thenar flexion crease. The proximal end of the bursa is approached with an incision just radial to the flexor carpi radialis tendon. The ulnar bursa is exposed with a distal incision at the distal palmar flexion crease and a proximal incision ulnar to the flexor carpi ulnaris. The tendon and ulnar neurovascular bundle are retracted ulnarly during the exposure. With the open technique, after irrigation of the bursa, Penrose drains are left in wounds and removed in 24 to 48 hours. With the irrigation technique, a 16-gauge polyethylene catheter or pediatric feeding tube is used in a similar fashion for the digital sheath infections. A horseshoe abscess requires simultaneous drainage of both the radial and ulnar bursas.

To minimize the most common complication of digital stiffness, early active digit range of motion is initiated postoperatively as soon as the catheter is removed. Initial empiric parenteral antibiotic is administered, usually a second-generation cephalosporin, such as cefazolin. Patients typically can leave the hospital after 48 hours on culture-directed oral antibiotic therapy for a total of 7 to 14 days.

Stage III infections with tissue necrosis require a more aggressive regimen, including an extensile surgical approach with surgical débridement versus ultimate salvage amputation. A midaxial incision, made dorsal to the neurovascular bundle, may be preferred in an effort to limit tendon and tendon sheath exposure and desiccation (79). A synovectomy is performed, leaving the annular ligaments intact. A separate palmar incision is made to complete the synovectomy proximally. A prolonged parenteral (4 to 6 weeks) antibiotic course is not unusual. Initial broad-spectrum antibiotic coverage is preferable until culture identification, especially if the patient is immunocompromised (64).

Septic Arthritis

Septic arthritis is infection of a joint space that, if left untreated, progresses to joint destruction and osteomyelitis (80,81). The most common infecting organism is *S. aureus*, whereas *Streptococcus* species are the second most prevalent bacterial isolates in the hand and wrist (81). Organisms can gain entry to a joint either by a penetrating event or by hematogenous seeding (80).

Patients present with a painfully swollen joint with guarded limited motion. The ESR and C-reactive protein level are sensitive laboratory indicators of inflammation, although they are not specific for infection. The white blood cell count is elevated in less than one-half of these patients (81). The definitive diagnosis is made with a joint aspiration. The aspirate typically has a white blood cell count of more than 100,000, with polymorphonuclear leukocytes comprising more than 75% of the total field (27). The specimen should also be evaluated (a) for the presence of crystals; (b) for glucose and uric acid levels; and (c) with Gram's stain, aerobic, anaerobic, fungal, and mycobacterial cultures. Local anesthetic often has an antiseptic preserva-

tive; therefore, the aspirate should be obtained with a separate syringe. A wrist aspirate is performed 1 cm distal to Lister's tubercle at the 3-4 (between the third and fourth extensor compartments) arthroscopic portal. The small joints of the hand are typically aspirated dorsally as well.

Favorable outcomes are directly dependent on early diagnosis and prompt surgical drainage (80–82). Wrist arthrotomy is performed through the third dorsal extensor compartment. The metacarpophalangeal joint is approached dorsally as well, often requiring splitting of the proximal extensor hood for exposure. The sagittal band is incised, and a capsulotomy is performed. The interphalangeal joints are best approached through midaxial incisions, with release of the accessory collateral ligament(s), thereby avoiding dorsal disruption of the central slip (83). Alternately, the joint can be exposed through a dorsal incision between the central slip and lateral band, preserving the collateral ligament. The wounds are then packed open with a drain, which is removed in 24 to 48 hours. Alternatively, an 18- or 20-gauge angiocatheter is sutured into the wound with a drain sutured into the opposite end of the wound. The catheter is used postoperatively to irrigate the joint for 24 to 48 hours (46). Intraoperative cultures are obtained, and the wounds are frequently left open to heal by secondary intention. Conversely, loose closure over suction drains can be performed if adequate joint débridement can be obtained. Supervised early motion improves ultimate composite digit flexion.

Osteomyelitis

Osteomyelitis infections occur secondary to an infection from an adjacent wound abscess, penetrating trauma (e.g., bites), septic arthritis, pyogenic tenosynovitis, hematogenous seeding, or open fractures or after open treatment of closed fractures (26,46,80,84). The hematogenous spread of an infection is uncommon (46). Osteomyelitis secondary to open fractures occurs in 1% to 11%, with a higher rate of infection occurring with severe contamination and soft tissue injury (80,85). The infection can involve any of the bones in the hand. The most common pathogens are *S. aureus* and *Streptococcus* spp. (20,26,46).

Clinically, signs of infection, including pain, erythema, swelling, and warmth, are usually present. Fever and elevated white blood cell count, C-reactive protein level, and ESR are variably present. Radiographs, depending on the stage of the infection, may reveal lucencies, periosteal reaction or bone formation, osteolysis, or sequestrum formation. Computed tomography and magnetic resonance imaging can help determine the extent of the infection (21,22,27). Nuclear imaging is helpful in detecting the infection earlier than in plain radiographs.

Treatment includes performing a biopsy to identify the pathogens, using antibiotics empirically until culture sensitivities have been obtained, and surgically draining the infection (26,46,84). The surgical incision(s) depends on the location of the infection and the bone involved. A midaxial incision is used for phalangeal infections, and a dorsal incision is used for metacarpal and carpal infections. Distal radius infections can be approached dorsally or volarly. Surgery should include removal of all of the infected bone and sequestra. A cortical window may be needed to access the area of infection. After irrigation of the area of infection, the wound can be left open and treated with wet-to-dry or whirlpool dressing changes or closed over a drain. Repeat surgical débridement and antibiotic impregnated cement spacers may be needed. Severe infections may require an amputation. Late reconstruction may require flap coverage or skin grafting.

Animal Bites

Animal bites are common, requiring more than 1 million medical visits per year, or approximately 1% of all emergency room visits, and $30 million in health care costs annually. Eighty percent to 90% of these bites are dog bites, and cat bites comprise another 5% (1,26,86,87). The dominant hand is the most frequently involved, and children are susceptible to animal bites (86,88).

Animal bites are similar to human bites in the polymicrobial aerobic-anaerobic nature of the wounds. However, the normal animal oral flora is less pathogenic than human flora (86). This is reflected by the higher number of isolates per wound in human bites, which is subsequently reflected by a higher incidence of infections and complications in human bite wounds. Anaerobes still outnumber aerobes 10:1 in both floras (86).

Wound cultures of dog and cat bites usually consist of multiple aerobic or facultative anaerobic [*Pasteurella* (*multocida* and *canis*), *Streptococcus, Staphylococcus* (*aureus* and *epidermidis*), *Moraxella, Neisseria, Bacillus, Haemophilus, Proteus, Pseudomonas, Eikenella*] and anaerobic (*Peptostreptococcus, Bacteroides, Fusobacterium, Porphyromonas, Prevotella, Propionibacterium, Veillonella, Actinomyces*) organisms (26,27,86,88–94). *P. multocida*, a gram-negative coccobacillus, is isolated in approximately 16% to 26% of dog bites (86,92).

Cat-scratch disease can follow a cat, dog, or monkey bite or scratch. An erythematous lesion and primary papule form 3 to 5 days postinjury, with adenopathy developing 5 to 50 days later. *Bartonella henselae* and *Afipia felis*, both gram-negative bacteria, have been implicated as causative pathogens (1,20,95,96). The disease is generally self-limiting but has been treated with ciprofloxacin, azithromycin, and trimethoprim-sulfamethoxazole (95,97).

Most animal bites have a high infection potential due to the nature of the penetrating injury, inoculation of a high number of bacterial flora, and local tissue devitalization secondary to the crushing nature of the injury. Risk factors for infection include a delay in treatment (more than 12 hours), advanced patient age, and more severe and deeper wounds. Cat scratches and bites are more likely to become infected than dog bites due to their needle-sharp teeth creating a deep-seated puncture, rather than avulsion, wound (98). Insect, snake, and arthropod bites are less likely to become infected than are cat and dog bites (87). Snake venom is sterile, although snake oral flora reflects the fecal flora of its prey. Venom is inhibitory to aerobic, but not anaerobic, flora.

Clinically, animal bite infections produce cellulitis, lymphangitis, and subsequently purulent drainage. The estimated cumulative incidence of infection after a dog bite without medical treatment is 16%. The incidence decreases to 9% in a patient population treated with prophylactic antibiotic use (99). Broad-spectrum antibiotic coverage is initially used and subsequently tailored according to culture sensitivities. A puncture wound secondary to an animal bite in the hand should be cleansed topically with an antiseptic solution and evaluated clinically and radiographically. In general, the antibiotics used should include a beta-lactam antibiotic and a beta-lactamase inhibitor, a second-generation cephalosporin with anaerobic activity, or combination therapy with penicillin and a first-generation cephalosporin or clindamycin and a fluoroquinolone (94). Penicillin is used for *Pasteurella* infections. Tetracycline and cephalosporin can be alternately used. Augmentin (combination of amoxicillin and clavulanate, a beta-lactamase inhibitor) is commonly used.

Surgical débridement and irrigation are indicated in those cases with an obvious infection, purulent drainage, joint (pyarthrosis) or tendon (pyogenic tenosynovitis) involvement, or osteomyelitis. Cultures for both aerobic and anaerobic organisms should be obtained. The wounds should be left open and allowed to heal by secondary intention.

Rabies prophylaxis may be indicated with wild animal bites. Emergency rooms should have a protocol in place to notify the Humane Society to verify animal identification versus capture and help assess the need for rabies immunization.

Human Bites

Human bite injuries can be classified into four different types: self-inflicted, traumatic amputations, full-thickness bite wounds to the hand or digits, and clenched-fist (e.g., blow to the mouth producing a knuckle-tooth wound) injuries (Fig. 13A) (100). They have a higher number of different bacterial, especially anaerobic (e.g., *Peptostreptococcus* and *Bacteroides* species), isolates than do animal bites (1,86,88,90,93,101,102). The most common pathogens found in human bite infections include *Streptococcus* and *Staphylococcus* (*aureus* and *epidermidis*) (1,46,86,88,90,93,103). Other isolated aerobic or facultative anaerobic organisms include *Neisseria, Corynebacterium, Eikenella,* and *Haemophilus.* The incidence of *Eikenella corrodens,* an anaerobic gram-negative rod, as a pathogen varies from 2% to 29% (104). It is more commonly cultured from

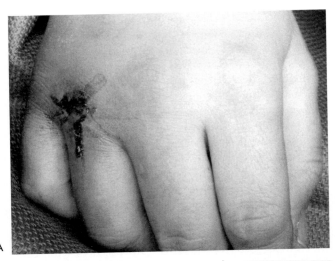

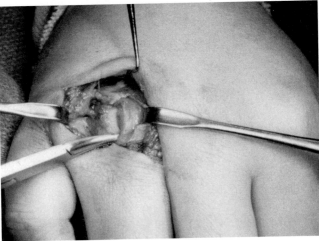

FIGURE 13. A: Typical example of a human bite wound (knuckle-tooth wound). **B:** The wound extends to the metacarpophalangeal joint, requiring open irrigation and débridement of the wound.

dental scrapings than saliva, which may explain the higher incidence of this organism in clenched-fist injuries (91,100, 105,106). Anaerobic organisms include *Bacteroides*, *Peptostreptococcus*, *Propionibacterium*, *Fusobacterium*, *Eubacterium*, *Veillonella*, and *Clostridium*. The presence of anaerobic spirochetes and fusiform bacilli correlates with a worse prognosis (1). Penicillin-resistant gram-negative rods have been reported in approximately one-third of bite wound cultures. Additionally, infectious diseases can be transmitted via human bites, including hepatitis B infection, tuberculosis, scarlet fever, actinomycosis (107–116).

The treatment of human bites depends on several factors, including the time from the occurrence of the bite, the wound location, and the presence or absence of an infection. A history is taken and physical examination performed. The mechanism and timing of the injury and any previous treatment should be known. With clenched-fist injuries, the penetrating tooth track is effectively sealed with digital extension, creating a closed-space environment. Three potential spaces may be entered: the dorsal subcutaneous space between the skin and extensor mechanism, the subtendinous space between the extensor mechanism and joint capsule, and the joint space itself (100).

The physical examination should determine the presence and location of erythema and swelling, purulent discharge, joint or tendon involvement (e.g., septic arthritis and pyogenic tenosynovitis), and lymph node enlargement. Radiographs are taken to rule out fractures, foreign bodies, the presence of subcutaneous gas, retained tooth remnant, or osteomyelitis (28).

Bites that are seen early, within 24 hours and without an obvious infection, and those not involving a joint or tendon may be treated with local wound care and oral antibiotics (117). Gram's stain and cultures are obtained before antibiotic administration. Local irrigation and débridement of open wounds should be performed and the wound left open to heal secondarily. Oral antibiotics and tetanus prophylaxis are given and the hand appropriately splinted. Repeat examination should be performed in 12 to 24 hours, with follow-up therapy if needed (e.g., whirlpool and range-of-motion exercises).

Formal surgical débridement under tourniquet hemostasis is indicated in cases of obvious infection, tendon or joint involvement, or tendon and nerve injury (86,101,118–120). Clenched-fist injuries demand surgical exploration to document depth of entry and to perform a thorough irrigation and débridement (Fig. 13) (11,121). Associated structures, including the extensor mechanism and chondral surfaces, can be assessed and addressed primarily or secondarily, depending on the cleanliness of the wound. The wound is left open to heal by secondary intention, including the capsular rent if present.

Hospitalization is indicated in cases in which formal surgical débridement is indicated, as well as in those cases involving sepsis, extensive cellulitis, and patient noncompliance. Serial débridements may be needed to obtain control of the infection. The type of antibiotic used is ultimately determined by the results of culture and sensitivities. With the presence of beta-lactamase–producing isolates (e.g., *P. multocida*, *E. corrodens*) and anaerobes, antibiotics should include a beta-lactamase inhibitor and penicillin. Tetracycline may be used in patients with a penicillin allergy. *E. corrodens* is resistant to oxacillin, methicillin, nafcillin, most aminoglycosides, and clindamycin. It is usually sensitive to penicillin G, ampicillin, carbenicillin, and tetracycline (100). Empiric initial coverage must take this into consideration while also providing coverage for gram-positive aerobes, such as *Staphylococcus* and *Streptococcus*, as well as anaerobes.

Necrotizing Fasciitis

Necrotizing fasciitis is a severe limb- and life-threatening infection caused by a variety of organisms. A combination of aerobic and anaerobic bacteria spreads rapidly along fascial planes (1,27,40,122–124). The most common pathogens are streptococcal and staphylococcal organisms, but these infections can also be caused by a mixture of facultative and anaerobic organisms.

Two types of necrotizing fasciitis have been described based on the pathogens involved (125). The more common type I infections are caused by a combination of pathogens, including anaerobic bacteria and facultative anaerobic bacteria (e.g., *Enterobacter* and non–group A streptococci), whereas type II infections include group A streptococci combined with *S. aureus* or *S. epidermidis*. Others have reported a single pathogen (group A beta-hemolytic streptococci), instead of multiple pathogens, as the cause of the infection. The mechanism of infection appears to be the production of bacterial enzymes (e.g., hyaluronidase, lipase), which facilitates tissue necrosis (124,126).

Predisposing factors include diabetes mellitus; advanced age; obesity; arteriosclerosis; poor nutrition; peripheral vascular disease; alcoholism; malignancy; compromised immune system; polymyositis; intravenous drug use; postpartum state; and infections of the chest, trunk, or perineum (1,26,122,124,127–130). Infections may result from minor abrasions and lacerations, insect bites, hypodermic needle injections, or surgical incisions.

The clinical findings are variable and include some combination of pain, fever, cellulitis, soft tissue edema, crepitus, skin bullae, skin necrosis, and rapidly expanding margins of infection that are nonresponsive to antibiotic therapy if initially misdiagnosed as cellulitis. Lymphangitis and lymphedema are limited (131). Leukocytosis may be present (40). Sepsis may occur with progression to acute respiratory distress syndrome, hemodynamic instability, and multiple organ system failure (122,128,132). Reported mortality rates vary from 8.7% to 73.0%, with a mean rate of 32.2% (1,122,130).

The surgical findings can include fascial necrosis, possible underlying myositis, and myonecrosis. Treatment includes radical surgical débridement of all necrotic structures (40,122,124). A fasciotomy should be performed. The fascia appears gray or grayish-green; a watery, thin exudate may be encountered, known as *dishwater pus*. Multiple surgical débridements and secondary wound closure or reconstruction are usually required. Amputation may be required in severe cases.

Broad-spectrum antibiotics, including penicillin, clindamycin, or metronidazole, and an aminoglycoside are used initially and adjusted pending cultures. Fluid resuscitation and hemodynamic monitoring are required. Mortality rates are increased with older age, peripheral vascular disease, and diabetes (1).

Gas Gangrene

Gas gangrene is a rare, although potentially deadly, infectious process that can arise not only after open fractures and farm injuries, but it has also been reported after minor medical procedures, such as injection or venipuncture. *Clostridium perfringens* is cultured in 50% to 100% of all gas gangrene infections, although more than 150 species exist (20,27,123,124,133). Clostridia are gram-positive, anaerobic, spore-forming, encapsulated bacilli and are soil contaminants. When cultured, they often require 48 to 72 hours for growth (133).

Exotoxins produced by *Clostridium* cause muscle necrosis and hemolysis. The wound typically is edematous and has a gray discoloration. A brown, watery discharge occurs, with expanding marginal erythema and hemorrhagic bullae. Palpable crepitance is a late finding. Systemically, the patient may be hypotensive and tachycardic, with multiple system organ failure progressing to death if left untreated. Early recognition with aggressive serial surgical débridements, antibiotic coverage (penicillin remains the antibiotic of choice, or metronidazole), and consideration for hyperbaric oxygen therapy optimize potential results (20,134,135).

Fungal Infections

Fungal infections of the hand can occur in normal hosts or in immunocompromised patients, such as transplant patients, patients taking immunosuppressive agents, diabetics, HIV patients, chronic renal failure patients, and patients with myeloproliferative disorders (136,137). These infections can occur as cutaneous, subcutaneous, or deep wound or systemic infections (137–141). Cutaneous infections occur in three anatomic areas: the paronychium, nail, and skin (140). These infections include chronic paronychia, onychomycosis (fingernail infection), tinea manuum (palmar interdigital area infection), and tinea corporis (glabrous skin infection).

Chronic Paronychia

Chronic paronychia is usually caused most commonly by *C. albicans* infections (142–145) of the nail and usually presents with a chronically indurated eponychium, nail thickening, and episodes of inflammation and drainage (42,143,146,147). A secondary bacterial infection can occur, resulting in the appearance of acute infection. There is often a history of frequent exposure to water or moisture (e.g., as with housekeeping personnel) (144). Potassium hydroxide smears help identify spores, branching mycelia, hyphae, or budding yeast. Fungal (Sabouraud's medium), aerobic, and anaerobic cultures should be taken to identify fungal and bacterial infections. Treatment of chronic paronychia consists of the use of topical antifungal agents (e.g., tolnaftate or clotrimazole) (Table 3) with or without nail removal or nail removal and marsupialization (42,47,140,148) of the nail fold (see the section Paronychia).

TABLE 3. DRUGS USED TO TREAT FUNGAL INFECTIONS

Infection	Organisms	Drug	Alternative drug
Chronic paronychia	*Candida albicans*	Nystatin, imidazoles, tolnaftate	Ketoconazole, fluconazole, itraconazole, griseofulvin
Onychomycosis	Dermatophytes, *Candida albicans*	Nystatin, imidazoles, terbinafine	Fluconazole, itraconazole, griseofulvin
Tinea manuum	Dermatophytes, *Candida albicans*	Nystatin, imidazoles	Ketoconazole, fluconazole
Sporotrichosis	*Sporothrix schenckii*	Amphotericin B, itraconazole, potassium iodide	Fluconazole, ketoconazole
Histoplasmosis	*Histoplasma capsulatum*	Amphotericin B, itraconazole	Ketoconazole, fluconazole
Blastomycosis	*Blastomyces dermatitidis*	Amphotericin B, itraconazole	Ketoconazole, fluconazole
Coccidioidomycosis	*Coccidioidomycosis immitis*	Amphotericin B, itraconazole	Ketoconazole, fluconazole
Aspergillosis	*Aspergillus fumigatus*	Amphotericin B, voriconazole	Itraconazole

Data from references 21–24.

Onychomycosis

Onychomycosis, or tinea unguium, is caused by a fungal infection of the nail plate resulting in destruction of the nail. The most common pathogens include dermatophytes, especially *Trichophyton rubrum*. The infection can also be caused by *C. albicans* (138,141,149–151). The infection can start in the hyponychium, in the eponychium, or on the nail plate surface (152). The infection can begin with localized white or yellowish discoloration of the nail, progressing to involve the entire nail and gradual nail thickening. Further nail discoloration (green, black, brown) occurs with subsequent bacterial colonization of the nail (Fig. 14) (152).

The infection can be treated with topical agents [e.g., nystatin, imidazoles (miconazole, clotrimazole, econazole, ketoconazole), tolnaftate] or oral agents [e.g., the triazoles (fluconazole, itraconazole), terbinafine, or griseofulvin] (Table 3) (141,150,151,153–158). These systemic medications should be used with caution due to potential liver, renal, and bone marrow toxicity.

Extensively involved nails are removed using digital block anesthesia. Care is taken to protect the germinal and sterile matrix, which are gently scraped with a curette or scalpel. Scrapings should be sent for a potassium hydroxide smear and fungal, aerobic, and anaerobic cultures. Topical antifungal agents are applied to the nailbed once or twice per day until a new nail grows (approximately 120 to 160 days) (140,150).

Skin Infections

Tinea manuum and tinea corporis are fungal infections of the interdigital areas of the palm and the glabrous skin of the hand, respectively. All dermatophytes (*Epidermophyton*, *Microsporum*, and especially *T. rubrum*) and *C. albicans* are the usual pathogens. The fungal infection usually occurs between the digits and varies from scalelike, hyperkeratotic lesions to areas of acute inflammation and vesicles. Infections frequently occur in patients with spasticity with moist palms and fingers due to a clenched-fist posture (140).

Treatment includes addressing the cause of the cutaneous infection (e.g., decrease exposure to moisture, correct finger flexion contractures) and the use of keratolytic agents (e.g., Whitfield's ointment), topical imidazoles, and antifungal agents (Table 3) (31,156).

Subcutaneous Infections

Subcutaneous infections include sporotrichosis caused by *Sporothrix schenckii*, commonly involving the lymphocutaneous system, although deep wound infections, including septic arthritis, can occur (138,159–164). The organism is commonly found in North America in soil and plants. The infection is noted in farmers, gardeners, florists, and forest and nursery workers. The infection commonly involves the upper extremity (160). A history of a penetrating injury (rose thorn scratch, animal bite, foreign body) is frequently noted. The infection appears as a papule at the site of the initial infection and the spreads along the lymphatic system. Secondary lesions form, appearing indurated and cordlike, and occasionally form seropurulent draining abscesses. Cultures (Sabouraud's agar) may take days to weeks to become positive. A saturated solution of potassium iodide has been used

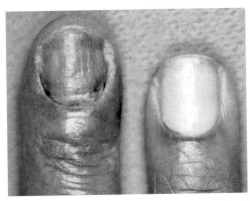

FIGURE 14. An example of onychomycosis. Note the discoloration and deformity of the nail compared with the adjacent nail.

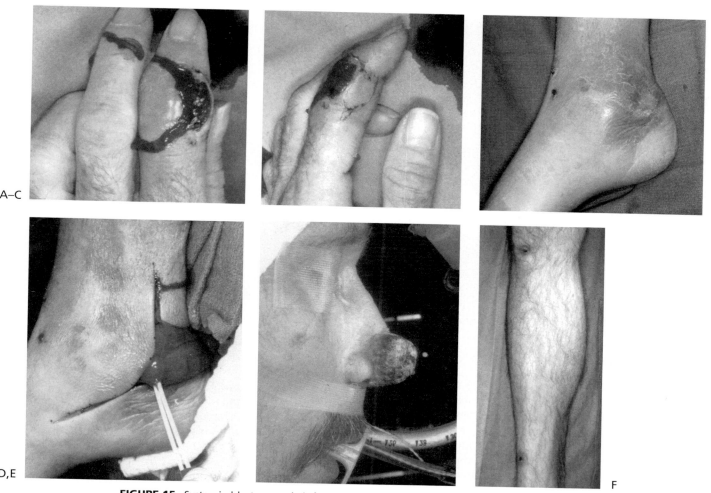

A–C

D,E

F

FIGURE 15. Systemic blastomycosis infection involving the index finger distal interphalangeal joint **(A,B)** and ankle joint **(C,D)**. Cutaneous lesions are noted on the nose **(E)** and leg **(F)**.

to treat cutaneous sporotrichosis. Itraconazole is used to treat lymphocutaneous sporotrichosis (Table 3).

Deep Infections

Deep infections can present as chronic tenosynovial infections, septic arthritis, or osteomyelitis and are secondary to histoplasmosis, blastomycosis, sporotrichosis, coccidioidomycosis, and paracoccidioidomycosis. Infections in immunocompromised individuals can be caused by aspergillosis, candidiasis, mucormycosis, and cryptococcosis.

Histoplasmosis is caused by *Histoplasma capsulatum*, found commonly in the Mississippi-Ohio River valley. It commonly produces pulmonary infections but is also found as tenosynovial infections or septic arthritis (165–167). Blastomycosis, caused by *Blastomyces dermatitidis* and found in the same region, produces cutaneous lesions, subcutaneous draining abscesses, septic arthritis, and systemic infections. It can produce infections of the hand (Fig. 15) (168–175). Lymphangitis and lymphadenitis and skin ulcerations can occur. Coccidioidomycosis, caused by *Coccidioidomycosis immitis*, is endemic to the southwestern United States and northern Mexico. It commonly produces pulmonary infections that can spread hematogenously to the upper extremity. It can cause osteomyelitis, septic arthritis, and especially tenosynovitis (176–180). Dorsal or volar hand and wrist swelling secondary to synovial thickening is frequently noted. Aspergillosis, caused by *Aspergillus fumigatus*, is found in immunocompromised patients, producing hemorrhagic vesicles, blebs, and ulcerations of the hand and upper extremity (181–185).

In general, the treatment of deep fungal infections includes surgical débridement and antifungal agents (e.g., amphotericin B) (Table 3) (137–139). Systemic medications include griseofulvin, amphotericin B, various azole derivatives, and flucytosine (e.g., ketoconazole) (cryptococcosis, disseminated candidiasis, aspergillosis), fluconazole (cryptococcal, coccidioidal infections), itraconazole (sporotrichosis, histoplasmosis, blastomycosis, paracoccidioidomycosis, chromomycosis), or terbinafine, can be used with caution due to potential liver, renal, and bone marrow toxicity.

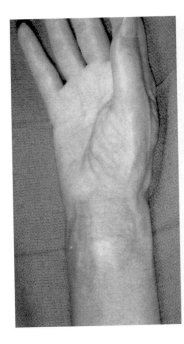 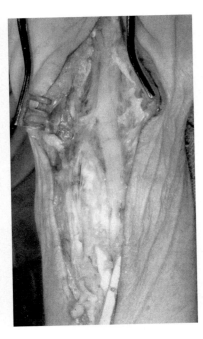

FIGURE 16. Typical example of atypical mycobacterial infection involving the forearm with encasement of the flexor tendons by the infection.

Mycobacterial Infections

Mycobacterial infections involve the skin, subcutaneous tissues, tenosynovium, joints, bone, or a combination of these structures. These infections have a predilection for synovium and produce caseating and noncaseating granulomas (140). Although mycobacterial infections can simulate the appearance of rheumatoid tenosynovitis, the other clinical findings of rheumatoid arthritis are absent. The infections produced by typical and atypical mycobacterial infections are clinically similar. The diagnosis is confirmed by biopsy for histopathologic examination and cultures. Cutaneous infections are generally caused by inoculation and produce nodular or pustular lesions and abscesses draining clear liquid. Lymphangitis is commonly present, but erythema, swelling, and cellulitis are less common.

Tuberculous tenosynovitis involving the hand and forearm is the most common tuberculous infection of the hand and has the similar appearance of chronic tenosynovitis seen with rheumatoid tenosynovitis. The flexor tendons are more commonly involved than the extensor tendons. Constitutional symptoms and local inflammatory signs (erythema, warmth, and pain) are frequently absent. Coexisting pulmonary or extrapulmonary tuberculosis is uncommon. Rice bodies or melon seeds are noted within the synovial mass. A chronic draining sinus may occur. Tendon rupture or fraying occurs in long-standing infections. Osteomyelitis or septic arthritis can occur as the infection spreads.

Tuberculous arthritis most frequently involves the wrist joint. The infection can occur primarily or as the result of untreated tenosynovitis. Infections of the finger joints and elbow can also occur. Painless joint swelling and limited range of motion are noted. Periarticular tenosynovitis or osteomyelitis may be noted. Chronic joint infections can result in joint deformities (dislocation, ankylosis).

Tuberculous osteomyelitis most commonly involves the phalanges and metacarpals. Concurrent pulmonary tuberculosis is uncommon. Painless digital or hand swelling without local inflammatory signs is noted. Pathologic fractures can occur. In chronic cases, abscesses and draining sinuses can occur. Adjacent soft tissue infections can occur.

Mycobacterium tuberculosis Infections

Mycobacterium tuberculosis infection is a slow, insidious process involving the hand and upper extremity (186–209). The infections present as cutaneous infections (194,203–205), chronic tenosynovitis (Fig. 16) (186,188–191,196,197,200,206,207, 210), digital infections (dactylitis) (192,198), or septic arthritis (189,190,193,201,202). Acute inflammatory signs (e.g., warmth and erythema) are usually not present. Radiographs are usually unremarkable except for soft tissue swelling. In cases of tuberculous arthritis or osteomyelitis, radiographic findings of osteopenia and bone and joint destruction may be noted. The Mantoux (tuberculosis) skin test is variably positive, and the ESR may be slightly elevated. Regional lymphadenopathy is usually absent (26,140).

Risk factors for a mycobacterial infection include immunosuppression, malnutrition, advanced age, alcohol abuse, and history of pulmonary tuberculosis (21,23,24,25,97,195). Acid-fast bacilli can be seen on smears. Histologically, caseating granulomas are noted. Cultures using Löwenstein-Jensen medium may take up to 10 weeks to become positive (23,140).

Cutaneous infections are treated with chemotherapy (199,203–205). The treatment of tuberculous tenosynovitis includes culture confirmation of the infection, complete tenosynovectomy (especially if the synovium is heavily affected), and use of antituberculous combination chemotherapy (21–24,26,97,140,200,210). The most commonly used first-line

TABLE 4. RUNYON CLASSIFICATION OF *MYCOBACTERIUM* SPECIES

Type	Characteristic	Natural habitat	Common diseases in humans
Group I	Photochromogens (cream-colored colonies turn-ing yellow on exposure to light)		
M. marinum		Water, fish	Skin, soft tissue
M. kansasii		Water, cattle	Skeletal
Group II	Scotochromogens (produce orange pigment independent of light)		
M. gordonae		Water	Pulmonary (rare)
M. szulgai		Unknown	Bronchopulmonary
Group III	Nonchromogens (white colonies that do not develop pigment)		
M. avium-intra-cellulare		Ubiquitous (soil, water, swine, cattle, birds)	Pulmonary, lymphadenitis, disseminated
M. terrae		Water, soil	Pulmonary (rare)
Group IV	Rapid growers (form cream-colored colonies in ≤1 wk vs. 10–28 d for other groups); resistant to most antituberculous drugs but often sus-ceptible to amikacin, doxycycline, erythromy-cin, kanamycin		
M. fortuitum		Water, soil, animals, marine life	Skin, soft tissue, disseminated
M. chelonae		Water, soil, animals, marine life	Skin, soft tissue, disseminated, skeletal
Others			
M. tuberculosis		Humans	Bronchopulmonary, soft tissue
M. bovis		Humans, cattle	Soft tissue, gastrointestinal
M. leprae		Humans, armadillos	Skin, soft tissue, disseminated (rare)

Data from Schulman ST, Phair JP, Peterson LR, et al. *The biological and clinical basis of infectious diseases*, 5th ed. Philadelphia: WB Saunders, 1997; and Resnick D, Pineda CJ, Weisman MH, et al. Osteomyelitis and septic arthritis of the hand following human bites. *Skeletal Radiol* 1985;14:263–266.

agents include ethambutol, isoniazid, pyrazinamide, rifampin, and streptomycin. Second-line agents include amikacin, capreomycin sulfate, ciprofloxacin, clofazimine, cycloserine, ethionamide, kanamycin, ofloxacin, para-aminosalicylic acid, and rifabutin (21,23–25,97,140). Tuberculous arthritis and osteomyelitis are treated with combination chemotherapy with or without surgical débridement (187).

Atypical Mycobacterial Infections

Atypical *Mycobacterium* infections frequently involve the hand, wrist, and upper extremity (67,139,195,209–287). Hand and upper extremity infections are more commonly produced by atypical mycobacteria rather than *Mycobacterium tuberculosis*. The most common pathogen is *Mycobacterium avium*, but others include *Mycobacterium marinum*, *Mycobacterium kansasii*, *Mycobacterium bovis*, *Mycobacterium chelonae*, *Mycobacterium fortuitum*, among others.

The various types of atypical mycobacteria have been classified according to their growth and pigmentation characteristics (Table 4) (24,288). These organisms are found widely in nature and usually occur as an infection after a puncture wound or trauma and in immunocompromised individuals (23,24,97,190,210,214). The infection frequently involves the flexor tendon, producing a flexor tenosynovitis that inhibits finger motion. Pain may be present, but most patients do not develop systemic symptoms. Skin infections are often associated with subdermal or dermal granulomas (245). Fistulae may be present, and bone and joint infections can also occur (139,212,223,224,226,229,247,254). Tuberculin skin testing is usually not positive with these infections (140).

Mycobacterium avium-intracellulare is an organism found in soil, water, and domestic poultry. The clinical presentation of this infection can also vary from skin and subcutaneous infections, pulmonary disease, arthritis, osteomyelitis, and sepsis (256,257,275,279,282). It is frequently noted in patients with acquired immune deficiency syndrome. Risk factors include puncture wounds, closed trauma, treatment with oral corticosteroids, local steroid injections, and immunodeficiency. The organism is resistant to multiple drugs and is difficult to eradicate.

M. marinum is found in both fresh and salt water fish, snails, crabs, and shrimp. The organism can be found in fish tanks, aquariums, and fish farms. *M. marinum* infections can have a variable presentation, including subcutaneous granulomas with sinus tracks, sporotrichinlike nodules, chronic tenosynovitis, bursitis, arthritis, and osteomyelitis (210,218,223–226,245,251,253,260,284,285). A history of a puncture wound or some form of trauma within a few months is typical. Most patients are healthy and are not immunocompromised. Patients may present with carpal tunnel–like symptoms in the presence of flexor tendon involvement.

The diagnosis of an atypical mycobacterial infection requires a biopsy for histopathologic examination and cultures (23,24,140,195). Cultures should be taken for aerobic, anaerobic, fungal, mycobacterial, and atypical mycobacterial infections. Histology should show evidence of inflammatory changes, noncaseating granulomas, fibrous exudates, and acid-fast bacilli (Ziehl-Neelsen stain). Findings of epithelioid histiocytes cells, multinucleated giant cells, and granulomas may be seen with synovial biopsies. Special media are frequently required to culture atypical mycobacterium (e.g.,

Löwenstein-Jensen medium for 4 to 6 weeks at 20°C for *M. fortuitum* and at 30° to 32°C for *M. marinum*). Cultures frequently take several weeks to become positive.

In general, the treatment of atypical mycobacterial infections requires biopsy confirmation of the infection and antituberculous medications, with or without surgical débridement (26,140,185,209,210,215,222,223,242,256,260,286). Subcutaneous lesions and abscesses may require drainage; joint and tendon involvement requires débridement and synovectomy (140,210,227). An infectious disease consultation is generally used for appropriate antibiotic and dosing regimens. In general, two antibiotic agents (e.g., isoniazid, ethambutol, and rifampin) are used for several months (see above). Clarithromycin and azithromycin in addition to first- or second-line agents have been used for *M. avium* infections. Minocycline, doxycycline, and trimethoprim-sulfamethoxazole, also in addition to first- and second-line agents, have been used for *M. marinum* infections (97,140,248).

Viral Infections

Herpes Infections and Herpetic Whitlow

Herpetic whitlow is a cutaneous viral infection of the digital tip caused by herpes simplex virus type 1 or type 2 (20). Herpes simplex virus type 2 typically presents in patients older than 20 years, whereas patients younger than 20 years tend to have herpes simplex virus type 1. Health workers, such as dental and medical personnel, are at particular risk (289,290). Adults with genital herpes, all age groups with gingivostomatitis, and immunocompromised patients are also at-risk populations (291–293).

Clinically, the digit becomes painful and erythematous. Cutaneous clear vesicular lesions occur and can coalesce and form bullae. A direct fluorescent antibody test, if pursued, may support the diagnosis, although it may be falsely negative (294). The definitive diagnosis is made by direct viral culture of the vesicular fluid, although it is not usually necessary (290,293).

The treatment of herpetic whitlow is nonoperative; therefore, distinction from paronychia or felon is important (289,290,294). Deep surgical drainage has the potential for secondary bacterial superinfection and the theoretical risk of viral encephalitis. Limited deroofing of the vesicles may provide pain relief, although it does not shorten the duration of involvement. Herpetic whitlow is self-limiting, resolving over a course of 3 to 4 weeks. Antibiotics are given in the rare presence of secondary infection, which tends to be cellulitic (293). In the unusual circumstance of a coinciding bacterial abscess, surgical decompression should be considered in conjunction with administration of either oral or intravenous acyclovir (293).

Human Immunodeficiency Virus

HIV can be transmitted via inoculation (e.g., intravenous drug abusers using contaminated needles), blood transfu-

sions, open wound contact, or mucous membranes. The estimated risk of disease transmission via a contaminated needle stick is 0.4% to 0.5% (approximately 1 in 200). The estimated risk of infection for a surgeon over a 30-year career in New York is 1% to 2% and 4% for a surgeon in San Francisco (295). Universal surgical precautions include double gloves; masks; face shields; hourly check of gloves, masks, and gowns for penetration; and minimizing the number of personnel involved in high-risk patients. A minimum number of instruments should be used, with scalpels passed between the nurse and surgeon using a basin (296).

The risk of HIV transmission via blood transmission varies from 1 in 140,000 to 1 in 250,000. The risk of disease transmission with bone allograft use is approximately 1 in 10,000. There is minimal risk when using fibrin glue due to its processing. There is only one reported case of disease transmission from a health care worker (dentist) to five patients (1).

Hand and upper extremity infections are common in HIV-infected patients and include bacterial, viral infections (herpes simplex and cytomegalovirus), fungal infections (candidiasis, cryptococcosis, histoplasmosis, aspergillosis), protozoal infections, or mycobacterial infections (140,297–301). Infections include pulmonary, gastrointestinal, and disseminated infections, as well as cellulitis and osteomyelitis. The treatment for hand infections is similar to other forms of infection (e.g., débridement and intravenous antibiotics) (298). HIV-infected patients with a reduced CD4 lymphocyte count are at a higher risk for postoperative infections (302,303).

COMPLICATIONS

Complications arising from the treatment of infections include surgical complications and complications related to antibiotic use (26). Surgical complications include inadequate drainage of the infection resulting in continued infection or spread of the infection, complications related to the poor selection of incisions (skin flap necrosis, scar contractures), and unnecessary surgery producing a secondary infection (herpetic whitlow). Complications related to the use of antibiotics include inadequate antibiotic coverage resulting in residual infection and toxicity secondary to use of the antibiotics (e.g., renal and ototoxicity with aminoglycosides). Joint stiffness, loss of motion, and deformity occur with long-standing bone, joint, or soft tissue infections. Prolonged immobilization or inadequate therapy can also contribute to the loss of hand function.

REFERENCES

1. Bishop A. Infections. In: Manske P, ed. *Hand surgery update. American Society for Surgery of the Hand.* Rosemont, IL: American Academy of Orthopedic Surgeons, 1996:395–404.

2. Abrams RA, Botte MJ. Hand infections: treatment recommendations for specific types. *J Am Acad Orthop Surg* 1996;4:230.

3. Hausman MR, Lisser SP. Hand infections. *Orthop Clin North Am* 1992;23:171–185.

4. Kilgore ES. Jr. Hand infections. *J Hand Surg [Am]* 1983; 8:723–726.

5. Leddy PJ. Infections of the upper extremity. *J Hand Surg [Am]* 1986;11:294–297.

6. Linscheid RL, Dobyns JH. Common and uncommon infections of the hand. *Orthop Clin North Am* 1975;6:1063–1104.

7. Robins RHC. Infections of the hand. A review based on 1000 consecutive cases. *J Bone Joint Surg Br* 1952;34:567–580.

8. Spiegel JD, Szabo RM. A protocol for the treatment of severe infections of the hand. *J Hand Surg [Am]* 1988;13:254–259.

9. Stern PJ, Staneck JL, McDonough JJ, et al. Established hand infections: a controlled, prospective study. *J Hand Surg [Am]* 1983;8:553–559.

10. Glass KD. Factors related to the resolution of infections of the hand. *J Hand Surg* 1982;7:388–394.

11. Patzakis MJ, Wilkins J. Factors influencing infection rate in open fracture wounds. *Clin Orthop Rel Res* 1989;243:36–40.

12. Swanson TV, Szabo RM, Anderson DD. Open hand fractures: prognosis and classification. *J Hand Surg [Am]* 1991;16:101–107.

13. Connor RW, Kimbrough RC, Dabezies MJ. Hand infections in patients with diabetes mellitus. *Orthopedics* 2001;24:1957–1060.

14. Francel TJ, Marshall KA, Savage RC. Hand infections in the diabetic and the diabetic renal transplant recipient. *Ann Plast Surg* 1990;24:304–309.

15. Gunther SF, Gunther SB. Diabetic hand infections. *Hand Clin* 1998;14:647–656.

16. Kour AK, Looi KP, Phone MH, et al. Hand infections in the diabetic and the diabetic renal transplant recipient. *Clin Orthop Rel Res* 1996;331:238–244.

17. McMurry JF Jr. Wound healing with diabetes mellitus. *Surg Clin North Am* 1984;64:769–778.

18. Lagaard SW, McElfresh EC, Premer RF. Gangrene of the upper extremity in diabetic patients. *J Bone Joint Surg Am* 1989;71:257–264.

19. Mann RJ, Peacock JM. Hand infections in patients with diabetes mellitus. *J Trauma* 1977;17:376–380.

20. Bannister BA, Begg NT, Gillespie SH. *Infectious disease*, 2nd ed. Oxford, UK: Blackwell Science, 2000.

21. Mandell GL, Bennett JE, Dolin R, eds. *Mandell, Douglas, and Bennett's principles and practice of infectious diseases*, 5th ed. Philadelphia: Churchill Livingstone, 2000.

22. Root RK, Waldvogel F, Corey L, et al. *Clinical infectious disease*. New York: Oxford University Press, 1999.

23. Schulman ST, Phair JP, Peterson LR, et al. *The biological and clinical basis of infectious diseases*, 5th ed. Philadelphia: WB Saunders, 1997.

24. Wilson WR, Sande MA. *Current diagnosis and treatment in infectious diseases*. New York: Lange Medical Books/ McGraw-Hill, 2001.

25. Peloquin CA, Iseman MD. *Antimycobacterial drugs. Clinical infectious diseases. A practical approach*. New York: Oxford University Press, 1999:327–335.

26. Szabo R, Palumbo C. Infections of the hand. In: Chapman M, ed. *Chapman's orthopedic surgery*, 3rd ed. Philadelphia: Lippincott Williams & Wilkins, 2001:1989–2008.

27. Lahiji A, Esterhai JL Jr. Principles of treatment of infection and antimicrobial therapy. In: Chapman M, ed. *Orthopedic surgery*, 3rd ed. Philadelphia: Lippincott Williams & Wilkins, 2001:3505–3532.

28. Resnick D, Pineda CJ, Weisman MH, et al. Osteomyelitis and septic arthritis of the hand following human bites. *Skeletal Radiol* 1985;14:263–266.

29. Covey DC, Albright JA. Clinical significance of the erythrocyte sedimentation rate in orthopedic surgery. *J Bone Joint Surg Am* 1987;69:148.

30. Grossman JAI, Adams JP, Kunec J. Prophylactic antibiotics in simple hand lacerations. *JAMA* 1981;245:1055–1056.

31. Roberts AHN, Roberts FEV, Hall RI, et al. A prospective trial of prophylactic povidone iodine in lacerations of the hand. *J Hand Surg [Br]* 1985;10:370–374.

32. Calkins ER. Nosocomial infections in hand surgery. *Hand Clin* 1998;14:531–545.

33. Classen DC, Evans RS, Pestotnik SL, et al. The timing of prophylactic administration of antibiotics and the risk of surgical wound infection. *N Engl J Med* 1992;326:281–286.

34. Fitzgerald RH, Cooney WP, Washington JA, et al. Bacterial colonization of mutilating hand injuries and its treatment. *J Hand Surg [Am]* 1977;2:85–89.

35. Hoffman RD, Adams BD. The role of antibiotics in the management of elective and post-traumatic hand surgery. *Hand Clin* 1998;14:657–666.

36. Norden CW. Antibiotic prophylaxis in orthopedic surgery. *Rev Infect Dis Rev Infect Dis* 1991;13(Suppl 10):S842–S846.

37. Platt AJ, Page RE. Post-operative infection following hand surgery. *J Hand Surg [Br]* 1995;20:685–690.

38. Sloan JP, Dove AF, Maheson M, et al. Antibiotics in open fractures of the distal phalanx? *J Hand Surg [Br]* 1987;12:123–124.

39. Waldvogel FA, Vaudaux PE, Pittet D, et al. Perioperative antibiotic prophylaxis of wound and foreign body infections: microbial factors affecting efficacy. *Rev Infect Dis* 1991;13(Suppl 10):S782–S789.

40. Schecter W, Meyer A, Schecter G, et al. Necrotizing fasciitis of the upper extremity. *J Hand Surg [Am]* 1982;7:15–20.

41. Jebson PJL. Infections of the fingertips. Paronychia and felons. *Hand Clin* 1998;14:547–555.

42. Keyser J, Littler J, Eaton R. Surgical treatment of infections and lesions of the perionychium. *Hand Clin* 1990;6:137–153.

43. Canales FL, Newmeyer WL, Kilgore ES Jr. The treatment of felons and paronychias. *Hand Clin* 1989;5:515–523.

44. Rockwell PG. Acute and chronic paronychia. *Am Fam Physician* 2001;63:1113–1116.

45. Brook I. Bacteriologic study of paronychia in children. *Am J Surg* 1981;141:703–705.

46. Neviaser R. Acute infections. In: Green D, Hotchkiss R, Pederson W, eds. *Green's operative hand surgery*, 4th ed. New York: Churchill Livingstone, 1999:1033–1047.

47. Bednar MS, Lane LB. Eponychial marsupialization and nail removal for surgical treatment of chronic paronychia. *J Hand Surg [Am]* 1991;16:314–317.

48. Perry A, Gottlieb I, Zachary L. Fingerstick felon. *Ann Plast Surg* 1988;20:249.

49. Bolton H, Fowler PJ, Jepson RP. Natural history and treatment of pulp space infection and osteomyelitis of the terminal phalanx. *J Bone Joint Surg Br* 1949;31:499–504.

50. Boyes JH. *Bunnell's surgery of the hand*, 5th ed. Philadelphia: JB Lippincott Co, 1970:613–642.

51. Brown H. Hand infections. *Am Fam Physician* 1978;18:79–84.

52. Kilgore ES Jr, Brown LG, Newmeyer WL, et al. Treatment of felons. *Am J Surg* 1975;130:194–197.

53. Milford LW. The hand. Pyogenic infections. In: Crenshaw AH, ed. *Cambell's operative orthopaedics*, 5th ed. St. Louis: Mosby, 1971:390–397.

54. Peterson TH, Oliver L, Schmidt G. Treatment and results of palmar space infections. *Handchir Mikrochir Plast Chir* 1994;26:144–149.

55. Burkhalter WE. Deep space infections. *Hand Clin* 1989;5:553–559.

56. Crandon JH. Lesser infections of the hand. In: Flynn JE, ed. *Hand surgery*. Baltimore: Williams & Wilkins, 1966:803–814.

57. Jebson PJL. Deep subfascial space infections. *Hand Clin* 1998;14:557–566.

58. Shamblin WR. The diagnosis and treatment of acute infections of the hand. *South Med J* 1969;62:209–212.

59. Kaplan EB. *Functional and surgical anatomy of the hand*, 2nd ed. Philadelphia: JB Lippincott Co, 1965.

60. Bingham DIC. Acute infections of the hand. *Surg Clin North Am* 1960;40:1285–1298.

61. Flynn JE. Modern considerations of major hand infections. *N Engl J Med* 1955;252:605–612.

62. Kanavel AB. *A guide to the surgical treatment of acute and chronic suppurative processes in the fingers, hand, and forearm*, 7th ed. Philadelphia: Lea & Febiger, 1943.

63. Gosain AK, Markison RE. Catheter irrigation for treatment of pyogenic closed space infections of the hand. *Br J Plast Surg* 1991;44:270–273.

64. Boles SD, Schmidt CC. Pyogenic flexor tenosynovitis. *Hand Clin* 1998;14:567–578.

65. Flynn JE. Acute suppurative tenosynovitis of the hand. *N Engl J Med* 1950;242:241–244.

66. Neviaser RJ, Gunther SF. *Tenosynovial infections of the hand. Part I: acute pyogenic tenosynovitis of the hand*, 29th ed. Park Ridge, IL: American Academy of Orthopedic Surgeons, 1980:108–117.

67. Neviaser R. Tenosynovitis. *Hand Clin* 1989;5:525.

68. Carter SJ, Burman SO, Mersheimer WL. Treatment of digital tenosynovitis by irrigation with peroxide and oxytetracycline. *Ann Surg* 1966;163:645–650.

69. Juliano PJ, Eglseder WA. Limited open tendon sheath irrigation in the treatment of pyogenic flexor tenosynovitis. *Orthop Rev* 1991;20:1065–1069.

70. Lee D, Neviaser R. Complications of trauma surgery and reconstructive surgery of the hand. In: Epps C Jr, ed. *Complications in orthopedic surgery*, 3rd ed. Philadelphia: JB Lippincott Co, 1994:403–442.

71. Lille S, Hayakawa T, Neumeister M, et al. Continuous postoperative catheter irrigation catheter is not necessary for the treatment of suppurative tenosynovitis. *J Hand Surg [Br]* 2000;35:304–307.

72. Neviaser R. Closed tendon sheath irrigation for pyogenic flexor tenosynovitis. *J Hand Surg [Am]* 1978;3:462.

73. Pollen AG. Acute infections of tendon sheaths. *Hand* 1974;6:21–25.

74. Entin MA. Infections of the hand. *Surg Clin North Am* 1964;44:981–993.

75. Flynn JE. The grave infections. In: Flynn JE, ed. *Hand surgery*. Baltimore: Williams & Wilkins, 1966:815–832.

76. Besser MIB. Digital flexor tendon irrigation. *Hand* 1976;8:72.

77. Loudon JB, Miniero JD, Scott JC. Infections of the hand. *J Bone Joint Surg Br* 1948;30:409–429.

78. Michon J. Phlegmon of the sheaths. *Ann Chir* 1974;28:272–280.

79. Stern PJ. *Selected acute infections*, 39th ed. Park Ridge, IL: American Academy of Orthopedic Surgeons, 1990:539–546.

80. Freeland AE, Senter BS. Septic arthritis and osteomyelitis. *Hand Clin* 1989;5:533–552.

81. Murray PM. Septic arthritis of the hand and wrist. *Hand Clin* 1998;14:579–587.

82. Rashkoff ES, Burkhalter WE, Mann RJ. Septic arthritis of the wrist. *J Bone Joint Surg Am* 1983;65:824–828.

83. Wittels NP, Donley JM, Burkhalter WE. A functional treatment method for interphalangeal pyogenic arthritis. *J Hand Surg [Am]* 1984;9:894–898.

84. Barbieri RA, Freeland AE. Osteomyelitis of the hand. *Hand Clin* 1998;14:589–603.

85. McLain RF, Steyers C, Stoddard M. Infections in open fractures of the hand. *J Hand Surg [Am]* 1991;16:108.

86. Brook I. Human and animal bite infections. *J Fam Pract* 1989;28:713–718.

87. Snyder CC. Animal bite infections of the hand. *Hand Clin* 1998;14:691–711.

88. Goldstein E. Bite wounds and infections. *Clin Infect Dis* 1992;14:633–638.

89. Arons M, Fernando L, Polayes I. *Pasteurella multocida*—the major cause of hand infections following domestic animal bites. *J Hand Surg [Am]* 1982;7:47.

90. Brook I. Microbiology of human and animal bite wounds in children. *Pediatr Infect Dis* 1987;6:29–32.

91. Goldstein EJC, Barones MF, Miller TA. *Eikenella corrodens* in hand infections. *J Hand Surg [Am]* 1983;8:563–567.

92. Goldstein JC, Citron DM, Feingold SM. Dog bite wounds and infections: prospective clinical study. *Ann Emerg Med* 1980;9:508–512.

93. Goldstein JC, Citron DM, Wield B, et al. Bacteriology of human and animal bite wounds. *J Clin Microbiol* 1978;8:667–672.

94. Talan D. Bacteriologic analysis of infected dog and cat bites. *N Engl J Med* 1999;340:85–92.

95. Dolan MJ, Wong MT, Regenery RL. Syndrome of *Rochalimaea henselae* adenitis suggesting cat scratch disease. *Ann Intern Med* 1993;118:331–333.

96. Hainer BL. Cat-scratch disease. *J Fam Pract* 1987;25:497–499.

97. Schlossberg D. *Current therapy of infectious disease*, 2nd ed. St. Louis: Mosby, 2001:479–482.

98. Synder C. Animal bite wounds. *Hand Clin* 1989;5:571.

99. Cummings P. Antibiotics to prevent infection in patients with dog bite wounds: a meta-analysis of randomized trials. *Ann Emerg Med* 1994;23:535–540.

100. Faciszewski T, Coleman DA. Human bite infections of the hand. *Hand Clin* 1998;14:683–690.

101. Farmer CB, Mann RJ. Human bite infections of the hand. *South Med J* 1966;59:515–518.
102. Griego RD, Rosen T, Orengo IF, et al. Dog, cat, and human bites: a review. *J Am Acad Dermatol* 1995;33:1019–1029.
103. Shields C, Patzakis MJ, Meyers MH, et al. Hand infections secondary to human bites. *J Trauma* 1975;15:235–236.
104. Bayan GM, Putnam JL, Cahill SL, et al. *Eikenella corrodens* in human mouth flora. *J Hand Surg [Am]* 1988;13:953–956.
105. Bilos ZJ, Kucharchuk A, Metzger W. *Eikenella corrodens* in human bites. *Clin Orthop Rel Res* 1978;134:320–324.
106. Rayan GM, Flournoy DJ. Microbiologic flora of human fingernails. *J Hand Surg [Am]* 1987;12:605–607.
107. Blinkhorn R, Strumbu V, Effron D. "Punch" actinomycosis causing osteomyelitis of the hand. *Arch Intern Med* 1988;148:2668–2670.
108. Fasciszewski T, Coleman D. Human bite wounds. *Hand Clin* 1989;5:561.
109. Fayman M, Schein M, Braun S. A foreign body related actinomycosis of the finger. *J Hand Surg [Am]* 1985;10:411–412.
110. Humphreys HF. Notes on three cases of specific infections of the hand in dental surgeons. *Br Dental J* 1946;80:367–368.
111. Mendelsohn BG. Actinomycosis of a metacarpal bone: report of a case. *J Bone Joint Surg Br* 1965;47:739–742.
112. Reiner SL, Herrelson JM, Miller, SE. Primary actinomycosis of an extremity. A case report and review. *Rev Infect Dis* 1987;9:581–589.
113. Robinson RA. Actinomycosis of the subcutaneous tissue of the forearm secondary to a human bite. *JAMA* 1945;142:1049–1051.
114. Rushforth G, Susannah JE. Actinomycosis of the hand. *Hand* 1982;14:194–197.
115. Southwick GJ, Lister GD. Actinomycosis of the hand: a case report. *J Hand Surg* 1979;4:360–363.
116. Winner H. Punch actinomycosis. *Lancet* 1960;2:907–908.
117. Zubowicz V, Gravier M. Management of early human bites of the hand: a prospective randomized study. *Plast Reconstr Surg* 1991;88:111–114.
118. Chuinard RG, Ambrosia RD. Human bite infections of the hand. *J Bone Joint Surg Am* 1977;59:416–418.
119. Mann RJ, Hoffeld TA, Farmer CN. Human bites of the hand: twenty years of experience. *J Hand Surg* 1977;2:97–104.
120. Mennen U, Howells C. Human fight-bite injuries of the hand. A study of 100 cases within 18 months. *J Hand Surg [Br]* 1991;16:431–435.
121. Chadaev AP, Jukhtin VI, Butkevich AT, et al. Treatment of infected clench-fist human bite wounds in the area of the metacarpophalangeal joints. *J Hand Surg [Am]* 1996;21:299–303.
122. Fontes RA Jr, Ogilvie CM, Miclau T. Necrotizing soft-tissue infections. *J Am Acad Orthop Surg* 2000;8:151–158.
123. Gonzalez MH. Necrotizing fasciitis and gangrene of the upper extremity. *Hand Clin* 1998;14:635–645.
124. Gonzalez M, Kay T, Weinzweig N, et al. Necrotizing fasciitis of the upper extremity. *J Hand Surg [Am]* 1996;21:689–692.
125. Giuliano A, Lewis F Jr, Hadley K, et al. Bacteriology of necrotizing fasciitis. *Am J Surg* 1977;143:52–56.
126. McKay D, Pascarelli E, Eaton R. Infections and sloughs in the hands of drug addicts. *J Bone Joint Surg Am* 1973;55:741.
127. Atiyeh B, Zaatari A. Necrotizing fasciitis of the upper extremity. *J Emerg Med* 1994;12:611.
128. Bleton R, Oberlin C, Alnot JY, et al. Necrotising fasciitis of the upper limb: report of twelve cases. *Ann Chir Main Memb Super* 1991;10:286–296.
129. Orangio G, Pitlick S, Della Latta P, et al. Soft tissue infections in parenteral drug abusers. *Ann Surg* 1984;199:97.
130. Sudarsky L, Laschinger M, Coppa G, et al. Improved results from a standardized approach in treating patients with necrotizing fasciitis. *Ann Surg* 1987;206:661–665.
131. Janevicius R, Hann S, Blatt M. Necrotizing fasciitis. *Surg Gynecol Obstet* 1982;54:97.
132. Bisno AL, Stevens DL. Streptococcal infections of skin and soft tissues. *N Engl J Med* 1996;334:240–245.
133. Hart GB, Lamb RC, Strauss MB. Gas gangrene: a collective review. *J Trauma* 1983;23:991–1000.
134. Altemeier WA, Fullen WD. Prevention and treatment of gas gangrene. *JAMA* 1971;217:806–813.
135. DeHaven K, Evarts C. The continuing problem of gas gangrene: a review and report of illustrative cases. *J Trauma* 1971;11:983–991.
136. al-Qattan MM. Opportunistic mycotic infections of the upper limb. A review. *J Hand Surg [Br]* 1996;21:148–150.
137. Hitchcock T, Amadio P. Fungal infections. *Hand Clin* 1989;5:599–611.
138. Amadio PC. Fungal infections of the hand. *Hand Clin* 1998;14:605–612.
139. Meier JL, Beekmann SE. Mycobacterial and fungal infections of bone and joints. *Curr Opin Rheumatol* 1995;7:329–336.
140. Patel M. Chronic infections. In: Green D, Hotchkiss R, Pederson W, eds. *Green's operative hand surgery*, 4th ed. New York: Churchill Livingstone, 1999:1048–1093.
141. Rippon J. *Medical mycology*, 2nd ed. Philadelphia: WB Saunders, 1982.
142. Marten R. Chronic paronychia. A mycological and bacteriological study. *Br J Dermatol* 1959;71:422–426.
143. Stone O, Mullins J. Chronic paronychia. *Arch Dermatol* 1962;86:324–327.
144. Stone O, Mullins J. Incidence of chronic paronychia. *JAMA* 1963;186:71–73.
145. Stone O, Mullins J. Role of *Candida albicans* in chronic disease. *Arch Dermatol* 1965;91:72.
146. Barlow A, Chattaway F, Holgate M, et al. Chronic paronychia. *Br J Dermatol* 1970;82:448–453.
147. Hellier, F. Chronic perionychia: aetiology and treatment. *BMJ* 1995;2:1358–1360.
148. Keyser J, Eaton R. Surgical cure of chronic paronychia by eponychial marsupialization. *Plast Reconstr Surg* 1976;58:66–70.
149. Gupta AK. Types of onychomycosis. *Cutis* 2001;68:4–7.
150. Khosravi AR, Mansouri P. Onychomycosis in Tehran, Iran: prevailing fungi and treatment with itraconazole. *Mycopathologia* 2001;150:9–13.
151. Mercantini R, Marsella R, Moretto D. Onychomycosis in Rome, Italy. *Mycopathologia* 1996;136:25–32.
152. Zaias N. Onychomycosis. *Dermatol Clin* 1985;3:445–460.
153. Cullen SI. Cutaneous candidiasis: treatment with miconazole nitrate. *Cutis* 1977;19:126–129.

154. De Doncker P, Decroix J, Pierard GE, et al. Antifungal pulse therapy for onychomycosis. A pharmacokinetic and pharmacodynamic investigation of monthly cycles of 1-week pulse therapy with itraconazole. *Arch Dermatol* 1996;132:34–41.

155. Hersle K, Mobacken H, Moberg S. Long-term ketoconazole treatment of chronic acral dermatophyte infections. *Int J Dermatol* 1985;24:245–248.

156. Roberts DT. Oral terbinafine (Lamisil) in the treatment of fungal infections of the skin and nails. *Dermatology* 1997;194(Suppl 1):37–39.

157. Stevenson C, Djavahiszwili N. Chronic ringworm of the nails. Long term treatment with griseofulvin. *Lancet* 1961;1:373–374.

158. Wong E, Hay R, Clayton Y. Comparison of the therapeutic effect of ketoconazole tablets and econazole lotion in the treatment of chronic paronychia. *Clin Exp Dermatol* 1984;9:489–496.

159. Atdjian M, Granda JL, Inberg HO, et al. Systemic sporotrichosis polytenosynovitis with median and ulnar nerve entrapment. *JAMA* 1980;243:1841–1842.

160. Bullpitt P, Weedon D. Sporotrichosis: a review of 39 cases. *Pathology* 1978;10:249–256.

161. Carr MM, Fielding JC, Sibbald G, et al. Sporotrichosis of the hand: an urban experience. *J Hand Surg* 1995;20:66.

162. Kedes LH, Siemienski J, Braude AI. The syndrome of the alcoholic rose gardener. Sporotrichosis of the radial tendon sheath. Report of a case cured with amphotericin B. *Ann Intern Med* 1964;61:1139–1141.

163. Liu X, Lin X. A case of cutaneous disseminated sporotrichosis. *J Dermatol* 2001;28:95–99.

164. Rowe JG, Amadio PC, Edson RS. Sporotrichosis. *Orthopedics* 1989;12:981–985.

165. Omer GE Jr, Lockwood RS, Travis LO. Histoplasmosis involving the carpal joint. A case report. *J Bone Joint Surg Am* 1963;45:1699–1703.

166. Perlman R, Jubelirer RA, Schwartz J. Histoplasmosis of the common palmar tendon sheath. *J Bone Joint Surg Am* 1972;54:676–678.

167. Pfaller MA, Kyriakos M, Weeks PM, et al. Disseminated histoplasmosis presenting as an acute tenosynovitis. *Diagn Microbiol Infect Dis* 1985;3:241–243.

168. National Institute of Allergy and Infectious Disease Study Group. Treatment of blastomycosis and histoplasmosis with ketoconazole: result of a prospective randomized trial. *Ann Intern Med* 1985;103:861–872.

169. Bayer AS, Scott VJ, Guze LB. Fungal arthritis IV. Blastomycotic arthritis. *Semin Arthritis Rheum* 1979;9:66–74.

170. Bergman BA, Brown RE, Khardori N. Blastomycosis infection of the hand. *Ann Plast Surg* 1994;33:330–332.

171. Gelman MI, Evarts CS. Blastomycotic dactylitis. *Radiology* 1973;107:331–332.

172. MacDonald PB, Black GB, MacKenzie R. Orthopedic manifestations of blastomycosis. *J Bone Joint Surg Am* 1990;72:860–864.

173. Monsanto EH, Johnston AD, Dick HM. Isolated blastomycotic osteomyelitis: a case simulating a malignant tumor of the distal radius. *J Hand Surg [Am]* 1986;11:896–898.

174. Pappas PG, Pottage JC, Powderly WG. Blastomycosis in patients with acquired immunodeficiency syndrome. *Ann Intern Med* 1992;116:847–853.

175. Pappas PG, Threlkeld MG, Belsole GD. Blastomycosis in immunocompromised patients. *Medicine* 1993;72:311–325.

176. Danzig LA, Fierer J. Coccidioidomycosis of the extensor tenosynovium of the wrist. A case report. *Clin Orthop Rel Res* 1977;129:245–247.

177. Gropper PT, Piesky WA, Bowen V, et al. Flexor tenosynovitis caused by *Coccidioides immitis*. *J Hand Surg [Am]* 1983;8:344–347.

178. Iverson RE, Vistnes LM. Coccidioidomycosis tenosynovitis in the hand. *J Bone Joint Surg Am* 1973;55:413–416.

179. Walker OR, Hall RH. Coccidioidal tendosynovitis. Report of a case. *J Bone Joint Surg Am* 1954;36:391–392.

180. Winter WG, Larson RK, Honnegar MM, et al. Coccidioidal arthritis and its treatment—1975. *J Bone Joint Surg Am* 1975;57:1152–1157.

181. Goldberg B, Eversmann WW, Eitzen EM Jr. Invasive aspergillosis of the hand. *J Hand Surg* 1982;7:38–42.

182. Jones NF, Conklin WT, Albo VC. Primary invasive aspergillosis of the hand. *J Hand Surg [Am]* 1986;11:425–428.

183. Meyer JT, Dunn AD. Aspergillus infection of the hand. *JAMA* 1930;95:794–796.

184. Prystowsky SD, Vogelstein B, Ettinger DS, et al. Invasive aspergillosis. *N Engl J Med* 1976;295:655–658.

185. Young RC, Bennett JE, Vogel CL, et al. Aspergillosis. The spectrum of the disease in 98 patients. *Medicine* 1970;49:147–173.

186. al-Qattan MM, Bowen V, Manktelow RT. Tuberculosis of the hand. *J Hand Surg [Br]* 1994;19:234–237.

187. Benkeddache Y, Gettesman H. Skeletal tuberculosis of the wrist and hand: a study of 27 cases. *J Hand Surg [Am]* 1982;7:593–600.

188. Borgsmiller WK, Whiteside LA. Tuberculous tenosynovitis of the hand ("compound palmar ganglion"): literature review and case report. *Orthopedics* 1980;3:1093–1096.

189. Brashear HR, Winfield HG. Tuberculosis of the wrist: a report of ten cases. *South Med J* 1975;68:1345–1349.

190. Bush D, Schneider L. Tuberculosis of the hand and wrist. *J Hand Surg [Am]* 1984;9:391–398.

191. Ekerot L, Eiken O. Tuberculosis of the hand. *Scand J Plast Reconstr Surg* 1981;15:77–79.

192. Feldman F, Auerbach R, Johnston A. Tuberculosis dactylitis in the adult. *Am J Roentgenol Radium Ther Nuclear Med* 1971;112:478.

193. Garrido G, Gomez-Reino JJ, Fernandez-Depica P, et al. A review of peripheral tuberculous arthritis. *Semin Arthritis Rheum* 1988;18:142–149.

194. Hooker RP, Eberts TJ, Strickland JA. Primary inoculation tuberculosis. *J Hand Surg [Am]* 1979;4:270–273.

195. Hoyen HA, Lacey SH, Graham TJ. Atypical hand infections. *Hand Clin* 1998;14:613–634.

196. Jackson RH, King JW. Tenosynovitis of the hand: a forgotten manifestation of tuberculosis. *Rev Infect Dis* 1989;11:616–618.

197. Kanavel AB. Tuberculosis tenosynovitis of the hand: a report of 14 cases of tuberculous tenosynovitis. *Surg Gynecol Obstet* 1923;37:635–647.

198. Leung PC. Tuberculosis of the hand. *Hand* 1978;10:285–291.

199. Minkowitz S, Brandt LJ, Rapp Y, et al. "Prosector's wart" (cutaneous tuberculosis) in a medical student. *Am J Clin Pathol* 1969;51:260–263.

200. Pimm LH, Waugh W. Tuberculous tenosynovitis. *J Bone Joint Surg Br* 1957;39:91–101.

201. Pinstein ML, Scott RL, Sebes JI. Tuberculous arthritis of the wrist: differential diagnosis and case report. *Orthopedics* 1981;4:1016–1018.

202. Robins RHC. Tuberculosis of the wrist and hand. *Br J Surg* 1967;54:211–218.

203. Rytel MW, Davis ES, Prebil KJ. Primary cutaneous inoculation tuberculosis. Report of two cases. *Am Rev Respir Dis* 1970;102:264–267.

204. Sahn SA, Pierson DJ. Primary cutaneous inoculation drug-resistant tuberculosis. *Am J Med* 1974;57:676–678.

205. Sehgal VN, Wagh SA. Cutaneous tuberculosis. Current concepts. *Int J Dermatol* 1990;29:237–247.

206. Suso S, Peidro L, Ramon R. Tuberculosis synovitis with "rice bodies" presenting as carpal tunnel syndrome. *J Hand Surg [Am]* 1988;13:574–576.

207. Visuthikosol V, Aung PS, Navykarn T, et al. Tuberculous infection of the hand and the wrist. *J Med Assoc Thailand* 1992;75:45–48.

208. Walker GF. Failure of early recognition of skeletal tuberculosis. *BMJ* 1968;1:682–683.

209. Wang CT, Sun JS, Hou SM. Mycobacterial infections of the upper extremity. *J Formos Med Assoc* 2000;99:710–715.

210. Gunther S, Levy C. Mycobacterial infections. *Hand Clin* 1989;5:592.

211. Adams RM, Remington JS, Steinberg J, et al. Tropical fish aquariums. A source of *Mycobacterium marinum* infections resembling sporotrichosis. *JAMA* 1970;211:457–461.

212. Alloway JA, Evangelisti SM, Sartin JS. *Mycobacterium marinum* arthritis. *Semin Arthritis Rheum* 1995;24:382–290.

213. Anouchi YS, Froimson I. Hand infections with *Mycobacterium chelonei*: a case report and review of the literature. *J Hand Surg [Br]* 1988;13:331–332.

214. Ara M, Seral C, Baselga C, et al. Primary tuberculous chancre caused by *Mycobacterium bovis* after goring with a bull's horn. *J Am Acad Dermatol* 2000;43:535–537.

215. Bagatur E, Bayramicli M. Flexor tenosynovitis caused by *Mycobacterium bovis*: a case report. *J Hand Surg [Am]* 1996;21:700–702.

216. Bailey JP, Stevens SJ, Bell WM, et al. *Mycobacterium marinum* infection. A fishy story. *JAMA* 1982;247:1314.

217. Barrow GI, Hewitt M. Skin infection with *Mycobacterium marinum* from a tropical fish tank. *BMJ* 1971;2:505–506.

218. Beckman EN, Pankey GA, McFarland GB. The histopathology of *Mycobacterium marinum* synovitis. *Am J Clin Pathol* 1985;83:457–462.

219. Berman LB. Infection of synovial tissue by *Mycobacterium gordonae. Can Med Assoc J* 1983;129:1078–1079.

220. Breathnach A, Levell N, Munro C, et al. Cutaneous *Mycobacterium kansasii* infection: case report and review. *Clin Infect Dis* 1995;20:812–817.

221. Brown J, Kelm M, Bryan LE. Infection of the skin by *Mycobacterium marinum*: report of five cases. *Can Med Assoc J* 1977;117:912–914.

222. Brutus JP, Baeten Y, Chahidi N, et al. Atypical mycobacterial infections of the hand: report of eight cases and literature review. *Chir Main* 2001;20:280–286.

223. Chow S, Ip FK, Lau JHK, et al. *Mycobacterium marinum* infection of the hand and wrist. Results of conservative

treatment in twenty-four cases. *J Bone Joint Surg Am* 1987;69:1161–1168.

224. Clark RB, Spector H, Friedman DM, et al. Osteomyelitis and synovitis produced by *Mycobacterium marinum* in a fisherman. *J Clin Microbiol* 1990;28:2570–2572.

225. Collins R, Chow S, Ip F, et al. Synovial involvement by *Mycobacterium marinum*. A histopathological study of 25 culture-proven cases. *Pathology* 1998;20:340–345.

226. Cortez LM, Pankey GA. *Mycobacterium marinum* infections of the hand. Report of three cases and review of the literature. *J Bone Joint Surg Am* 1973;55:363–370.

227. Deenstra W. Synovial hand infection from *Mycobacterium terrae. J Hand Surg [Br]* 1988;13:335–336.

228. DeMerieux P, Keystone EC, Hutcheon M, et al. Case report. Polyarthritis due to *Mycobacterium kansasii* in a patient with rheumatoid arthritis. *Ann Rheum Dis* 1980;30:90–94.

229. Dillon J, Millson C, Morris I. Case report. *Mycobacterium kansasii* infection in the wrist and hand. *Br J Rheumatol* 1990;29:150–153.

230. Dixon JH. Non-tuberculous mycobacterial infection of the tendon sheaths in the hand. A report of six cases. *J Bone Joint Surg Br* 1981;63:542–544.

231. Donta ST, Smith PW, Levitz RE, et al. Therapy of *Mycobacterium marinum* infections. Use of tetracyclines vs rifampin. *Arch Intern Med* 1986;146:902–904.

232. Dorff GJ, Frerichs L, Zabransky RJ, et al. Musculoskeletal infections due to *Mycobacterium kansasii. Clin Orthop Rel Res* 1978;36:244–246.

233. Edelstein H. *Mycobacterium marinum* skin infections. Report of 31 cases and review of the literature. *Arch Intern Med* 1994;154:1359–1364.

234. Elston RA. Missed diagnosis mycobacterial infection. *Lancet* 1989;1:1144–1145.

235. Engbaek HC, Thormann J, Vergmann B. Aquarium-borne *Mycobacterium marinum* granulomas. *Scand J Infect Dis* 1980;12:74–78.

236. Enzenauer RJ, McKoy J, Vincent D, et al. Disseminated cutaneous and synovial *Mycobacterium marinum* infection in a patient with systemic lupus erythematosus. *South Med J* 1990;83:471–474.

237. Even-Paz Z, Haas H, Saks T, et al. *Mycobacterium marinum* skin infections mimicking cutaneous leishmaniasis. *Br J Dermatol* 1976;94:435–442.

238. Fisher AA. Swimming pool granulomas due to *Mycobacterium marinum*: an occupational hazard of lifeguards. *Cutis* 1988;41:397–398.

239. Flowers DJ. Human infection due to *Mycobacterium marinum* after a dolphin bite. *J Clin Pathol* 1970;23:475–477.

240. Fodero J, Chung KC, Ogenovski VM. Flexor tenosynovitis in the hand caused by *Mycobacterium terrae. Ann Plast Surg* 1999;42:330–332.

241. Forsgren A. Antibiotic susceptibility of *Mycobacterium marinum. Scand J Infect Dis* 1993;25:779–782.

242. Foulkes GD, Floyd JC, Stephens JL. Flexor tenosynovitis due to *Mycobacterium asiatica. J Hand Surg [Am]* 1998;23:753–756.

243. Girard DE, Bagby GC Jr, Walsh JR. Destructive polyarthritis secondary to *Mycobacterium kansasii. Arthritis Rheum* 1973;16:665–669.

244. Gunther SF, Elliott RC. *Mycobacterium kansasii* infection in the deep structures of the hand. Report of two cases. *J Bone Joint Surg Am* 1976;58:140–142.

245. Gunther S, Elliott R, Brand R, et al. Experience with atypical mycobacterial infections in the deep structures of the hand. *J Hand Surg* 1977;2:90.

246. Halla JT, Gould JS, Hardin JG. Chronic tenosynovial hand infection from *Mycobacterium terrae*. *Arthritis Rheum* 1979;22:1386–1390.

247. Harth M, Ralph ED, Faraawi R. Septic arthritis due to *Mycobacterium marinum*. *J Rheumatol* 1994;21:957–960.

248. Hellinger WC, Smilack JD, Greider JL Jr, et al. Localized soft-tissue infections with *Mycobacterium avium/Mycobacterium intracellulare* complex in immunocompetent patients: granulomatous tenosynovitis of the hand or wrist. *Clin Infect Dis* 1995;21:65–69.

249. Hoffman GS, Myers RL, Stark FR, et al. Septic arthritis associated with *Mycobacterium avium*: a case report and literature review. *J Rheumatol* 1978;5:199–209.

250. Huminer D, Pitlik SD, Block C, et al. Aquarium-borne *Mycobacterium marinum* skin infection. Report of a case and review of the literature. *Arch Dermatol* 1986;122:698–703.

251. Hurst LC, Amadio PC, Badalamente MA, et al. *Mycobacterium marinum* infections of the hand. *J Hand Surg [Am]* 1987;12:428–435.

252. Johnston JM, Izumi AK. Cutaneous *Mycobacterium marinum* infection ("swimming pool granuloma"). *Clin Dermatol* 1987;5:68–75.

253. Jones EJ, Mlisana KP, Peer AK. *Mycobacterium marinum* hand infection. *Br J Plast Surg* 2000;53:161–165.

254. Jones MW, Wahid IA, Matthews JP. Septic arthritis of the hand due to *Mycobacterium marinum*. *J Hand Surg [Br]* 1988;13:333–334.

255. Kaplan H, Clayton M. Carpal tunnel syndrome secondary to *Mycobacterium kansasii* infection. *JAMA* 1969;208:1186–1188.

256. Kelly PJ, Karlson AG, Weed LA, et al. Infection of synovial tissues by mycobacteria other than *Mycobacterium tuberculosis*. *J Bone Joint Surg Am* 1967;49:1521–1530.

257. Kelly PJ, Weed LA, Lipscomb PR. Infections of tendon sheaths, bursae, joints, and soft tissues by acid-fast bacilli other than tubercle bacilli. *J Bone Joint Surg Am* 1963;45:327–336.

258. Kelly R. *Mycobacterium marinum* infection from a tropical fish tank. Treatment with trimethoprim and sulphamethoxazole. *Med J Australia* 1976;2:681–682.

259. Kullavanijaya P, Sirimachan S, Bhuddhavudhikrai P. *Mycobacterium marinum* cutaneous infections acquired from occupations and hobbies. *Int J Dermatol* 1993;32:504–507.

260. Lacy J, Viegas S, Calhoun J, et al. *Mycobacterium marinum* flexor tenosynovitis. *Clin Orthop Rel Res* 1989;238:288–293.

261. Lakhanpal VP, Tuli SM, Singh H, et al. *Mycobacterium kansasii* and osteoarticular lesions. *Acta Orthop Scand* 1980;51:471–473.

262. Lau JH-K. Hand infection with *Mycobacterium chelonei*. *BMJ (Clin Res Ed)* 1986;292:444–445.

263. Leader M, Revell P, Clarke G. Synovial infection with *Mycobacterium kansasii*. *Ann Rheum Dis* 1984;43:80–82.

264. Love GL, Melchior E. *Mycobacterium terrae* tenosynovitis. *J Hand Surg [Am]* 1985;10:730–732.

265. Maberry JD, Mullin JF, Latore OJ. Cutaneous infection due to *Mycobacterium kansasii*. *JAMA* 1965;194:1135–1136.

266. Maher DP. *Mycobacterium fortuitum* infection following treatment of a ganglion cyst: case report and literature review. *Orthop Rev* 1989;18:1193–1196.

267. Maloney JM, Gregg CR, Stephens DS, et al. Infections caused by *Mycobacterium szulgai* in humans. *Rev Infect Dis* 1987;9:1120–1126.

268. May DC, Kutz JE, Howell RS. *Mycobacterium terrae* tenosynovitis: chronic infection in a previously healthy individual. *South Med J* 1983;76:1445–1447.

269. Minkin BI, Mills CL, Bullock DW, et al. *Mycobacterium kansasii* osteomyelitis of the scaphoid. *J Hand Surg [Am]* 1987;12:1092–1094.

270. Parker MD, Irwin RS. *Mycobacterium kansasii* tendinitis and fascitis. Report of a case treated successfully with drug therapy alone. *J Bone Joint Surg Am* 1975;57:557–559.

271. Paul D, Gulick P. *Mycobacterium marinum* skin infections: two case reports. *J Fam Pract* 1993;36:336–338.

272. Petrini B, Svartengren G, Hoffner SE, et al. Tenosynovitis of the hand caused by *Mycobacterium terrae*. *Eur J Clin Microbiol Infect Dis* 1989;8:722–724.

273. Prevost E, Walker EM Jr, Kreutner A Jr, et al. *Mycobacterium marinum* infections: diagnosis and treatment. *South Med J* 1982;75:1349–1352.

274. Prince H, Ispahani P, Baker MA. *Mycobacterium malmoense* infection of the hand presenting as carpal tunnel syndrome. *J Hand Surg [Br]* 1988;13:328–329.

275. Raffi F, Mainard D, Drugeon HB. Non-tuberculous mycobacterial tenosynovitis. *Lancet* 1990;335:613–614.

276. Ries KM, White GL, Murdock RT. Atypical mycobacterial infection caused by *Mycobacterium marinum*. *N Engl J Med* 1990;322:633–634.

277. Sanger JR, Stampfl DA, Franson TR. Recurrent granulomatous synovitis due to *Mycobacterium kansasii* in a renal transplant recipient. *J Hand Surg [Am]* 1987;12:436–441.

278. Scutchfield SB, Hay EL. *Mycobacterium marinum* infections in hands. *Orthop Rev* 1980;9:83–88.

279. Stark RH. *Mycobacterium avium* complex tenosynovitis of the index finger. *Orthop Rev* 1990;19:345–347.

280. Stern PJ, Gula DC. *Mycobacterium chelonei* tenosynovitis of the hand: a case report. *J Hand Surg [Am]* 1986;11:596–599.

281. Straus WL, Ostroff SM, Jernigan DB, et al. Clinical and epidemiologic characteristics of *Mycobacterium haemophilum*, an emerging pathogen in immunocompromised patients. *Ann Intern Med* 1994;120:118–121.

282. Sutker WL, Lankford LL, Tompsett R. Granulomatous synovitis: the role of atypical mycobacteria. *Rev Infect Dis* 1979;1:729–735.

283. Swift S, Cohen H. Granulomas of the skin due to *Mycobacterium balnei* after abrasions from a fish tank. *N Engl J Med* 1962;267:1244–1246.

284. Wendt JR, Lamm RC, Altman DI, et al. An unusually aggressive *Mycobacterium marinum* hand infection. *J Hand Surg [Am]* 1986;11:753–755.

285. Williams CS, Riordan DC. *Mycobacterium marinum* (atypical acid-fast bacillus) infections of the hand. A report of six cases. *J Bone Joint Surg Am* 1973;55:1042–1045.

286. Woods GL, Washington JL II. Mycobacteria other than

Mycobacterium tuberculosis: review of microbiologic and clinical aspects. *Rev Infect Dis* 1987;9:275–294.

287. Zvetina JR, Foster J, Reyes CV. *Mycobacterium kansasii* infection of the elbow joint. A case report. *J Bone Joint Surg Am* 1979;61:1099–1102.

288. Runyon EH. Anonymous mycobacteria in pulmonary disease. *Med Clin North Am* 1959;43:273–290.

289. LaRossa D, Hamilton R. Herpes simplex infections of the digits. *Arch Surg* 1971;102:600–603.

290. Louis DS, Silva J Jr. Herpetic whitlow: herpetic infections of the digits. *J Hand Surg [Am]* 1979;4:90–94.

291. Behr JT, Daluga DJ, Light TR, et al. Herpetic infections in the fingers of infants. *J Bone Joint Surg Am* 1987;69:137–139.

292. Cengizlier R, Uysal G, Guven A, et al. Herpetic finger infection. *Cutis* 2002;69:291–292.

293. Hurst LC, Gluck R, Sampson SP, et al. Herpetic whitlow with bacterial abscess. *J Hand Surg [Am]* 1991;16:311–313.

294. Fowler JR. Viral infections. *Hand Clin* 1989;5:613–627.

295. Lowenfels A, Wormser G, Jain R. Frequency of puncture injuries in surgeons and the estimated risk of HIV infection. *Arch Surg* 1989;124:1284–1286.

296. Bessinger CD Jr. Preventing transmission of human immunodeficiency virus during operations. *Surg Gynecol Obstet* 1988;167:287–289.

297. Ching V, Ritz M, Song C, et al. Human immunodeficiency virus infection in an emergency hand service. *J Hand Surg [Am]* 1996;21:696–699.

298. Glickel S. Hand infections in patients with acquired immunodeficiency syndrome. *J Hand Surg [Am]* 1988;13:770–775.

299. Gonzalez MH, Nikoleit J, Weinzweig N, et al. Upper extremity infections in patients with the human immunodeficiency virus. *J Hand Surg [Am]* 1998;23:348–352.

300. McAuliffe JA, Seltzer DG, Hornicek FJ. Upper-extremity infections in patients seropositive for human immunodeficiency virus. *J Hand Surg [Am]* 1997;22:1084.

301. Seltzer DG, McAuliffe JA, Campbell DR, et al. AIDS in the hand patient: the team approach. *Hand Clin* 1991;7:433.

302. Greene W, Gnore L, White G. Orthopedic procedures and prognosis in hemophilic patients who are seropositive for human immunodeficiency virus. *J Bone Joint Surg Am* 1990;72:2–11.

303. Hoekman P, Van de Perre P, Nelissen J, et al. Increased frequency of infection after open reduction of fractures in patients who are seropositive for human immunodeficiency virus. *J Bone Joint Surg Am* 1991;73:675–679.

104

OPEN-WOUND, INJECTION, AND CHEMICAL INJURIES

LAM-CHUAN TEOH

In injuries of the hand, it is the open wound with bleeding and pain that drives the patient to seek treatment urgently. The first doctor from whom the patient seeks treatment may not be a hand surgeon. It is usually the family doctor or the emergency room doctor with whom the patient first comes into contact. The clinician involved in treating the patient should understand the importance of prompt and definitive treatment of such injuries. Severe injuries are obvious and referral to the hand surgery unit is then expedited. However, it is the seemingly minor injuries that require emphasis. Many such injuries can have concomitant injury of deeper vital structures. The attending clinician should have the necessary basic knowledge of hand injuries and be able to conduct a proper assessment (1).

Hand injuries carry a tremendous negative economic impact to the patient and society (2,3). In a hand surgery unit, the hand surgeon should give his or her personal attention to every individual patient. Treating the open injury or damaged tissues alone is not adequate. The surgeon is responsible for providing the best treatment and rehabilitation therapy; he or she must also attend to patients' fears and emotional needs and finally see them through a successful integration back into society and gainful employment (4–6).

SURGICAL ANATOMY

The hand is a multitissue organ made up of five different tissue components: the skin and subcutaneous tissues; nerve fibers and nerve end organs; a vascular network; tendons and muscles; and skeletal structures, with their bones and joints. In a finger, these five tissues are packed closely together. A small, sharp penetrating injury lacerates not only the skin but can also easily transect the tendons, nerves, or arteries. In an injury of greater magnitude, the five tissue structures can be damaged in any combination. Furthermore, the five tissue structures are interrelated and interdependent in providing intricate motion and function of the hand. Injury to any tissue component, particularly the tendons, can significantly affect the function of the hand.

The palmar skin is glabrous, has ample sweat glands, and is hairless. This makes it ideal for contact function. Hence, in situations in which there is loss of palmar skin, one needs a sensate like-for-like reconstruction. The dorsal skin, seemingly ample and loose on digital extension, will be all taken up and stretched with digital flexion. Therefore, the need to resurface the dorsal skin loss should not be underestimated. The subcutaneous tissue on the palmar surface in particular provides a padding important in distributing the forces during grasping. In a crush injury, loss of subcutaneous tissue results in a deep scar and immobile skin. A finger has two digital arteries, one on each side of the finger, with palmar and dorsal communicating branches (7). With division of both digital arteries, random arterial supply via the subdermal plexus may continue to perfuse the finger distally. This perfusion alone is usually inadequate and may subsequently lead to partial necrosis or atrophy.

The surgical anatomy of the tendon sheaths and palmar spaces is important in the understanding of penetrating and injection injuries. On the palmar site of the finger, the flexor tendon is covered by a fibrous flexor sheath that extends from the head of the metacarpal to the base of the distal phalanx. For the thumb and little finger, the synovial lining of the flexor tendons extends proximally as the bursae into the palm, across the carpal tunnel, and into the distal forearm. Penetrating or injection injuries over the fingertip pulp can easily enter the flexor sheath. In the former, the injury may result in flexor tendon sheath infection. In the latter, the injected substance can spread through the synovial bursae to reach its proximal extent (8).

OPEN-WOUND INJURIES

Pathophysiology

The injury can be defined as something that occurs from "outside in." The extent of the injury is dependent on the nature of the object causing the injury, duration of contact, magnitude of force, and the manner in which the force is applied.

The injury could be caused by a blunt or sharp small object or by heavy machinery with a large surface area. The former results in a superficial, limited zone of laceration and the latter results in a broad zone of crushing injury. The machinery causing the injury could be heated, causing additional thermal damage. The object could be a high-speed rotating electrical saw, causing an irregular segmental loss of tissue (Fig. 1A,B).

The duration of contact is relevant if the object is contaminated or heated; in chemical injuries, the damage increases with increasing duration of contact. The severity of the injury is related to the magnitude of the force applied. A small penetrating injury with sufficient force could have lacerated the flexor tendon and digital nerves (9). A direct crushing by a heavy punch press could have completely pulverized all the five tissues of the hand (Fig. 2A,B).

The extent of damage in avulsion injuries is dependent on how the force is applied. An example is roller injury. The injury is due to the patient's reflex to withdraw from the insult. The hardness of the rollers and the size of the gap between them also influence the extent of the damage. A gloved hand caught in the rotating part of a machine can result in avulsion of the glove together with the skin that it was protecting. In a ring avulsion injury of the finger, the external force is static and the movement of the patient's hand causes the avulsion. It is also important to understand that in avulsion injuries, each of the five tissue components can fail at different levels. The skin disruption is usually more proximal than the skeletal disruption. The disruption of the neurovascular structures can occur at varying levels, and the flexor tendons can be avulsed from the tenomuscular junction (10–12).

In crush injuries, due to different viscoelasticity of the tissues, the severity of damage to the different tissues over the same zone of injury varies greatly. The flexor tendon and digital nerves can still be in continuity despite circumferential skin laceration, disrupted blood vessels, and comminuted fractures of the bone (Fig. 3A–C).

The attitude of the hand in function at the time of injury is important. The level of injury to deeper structures, particularly the flexor tendon and the extensor tendon, could be a significant distance away from the skin wound when the hand is explored in full extension.

Damaged tissues provide an excellent culture medium, and the skin flora, especially *Staphylococcus aureus*, can infect the wound. An open wound is also exposed to the external environment and therefore runs the risk of bacterial infection from external sources. In contaminated environments such as farm, sewage, and construction sites, these injuries, if improperly treated, have a high risk of developing wound infection (13). Animal and raw meat product handlers can develop unusual atypical infection. Infection with *Mycobacterium marinum* has been reported in fishermen and fish handlers (14,15). Injuries in contact with river water may run the risk of *Aeromonas hydrophila* infection (16). Human bites are associated with the risk of

Eikenella corrodens infection and animal bites are associated with *Pasteurella multocida* infection (17,18).

Evaluation

Evaluation is directed toward establishing as comprehensively and as precisely as possible the extent and severity of the injury to the five tissue components of the hand. The injuries can then be categorized and treatment plans formulated accordingly.

History

A good history is aimed at eliciting the details regarding the nature of the offending objects and mechanism of the injury, the time of occurrence, any other associated injuries, and the patient's previous medical history and relevant social history.

What the patient was doing then, how the injury was sustained, and what the working environment was when the injury occurred are pertinent questions to answer. An industrial worker may use some technical jargon to describe the machinery, and the examiner may need to ask for details to understand the implication of the injury. By the time the patient is being assessed by a hand surgeon, many hours may have lapsed since the time of injury. In vascular injuries, the ischemic damage, if prolonged, could be irreversible and negate the chance of a successful revascularization or replantation (19). In evaluating open-wound injuries of the hand, the examiner must always explore the possibility of injury to other parts of the body. It is most unfortunate to treat the hand, where damage is most obvious, but miss a life-threatening injury to a covered part of the body.

Cardiovascular, renal, hematologic, and endocrine diseases are significant elements of the medical history that will influence the treatment plan. The repair and reconstruction may be complicated and require prolonged operative time; hence the patient should be assessed as to suitability for prolonged anesthesia. In a patient with diseased vessels, complex microvascular procedure may not be advisable.

Social history must always be included. Replantation of a single digit may be indicated for a patient who plays musical instruments that require the use of that finger. There is much controversy over the age of the patient and level of economic productivity. Suffice it to say that for a relatively young patient who still has a long period of contribution to society, one is more inclined to offer major reconstructive surgery needed to restore better function. In contrast, for elderly retired persons, rather than to subject them to a higher surgical and anesthetic risk, the plan is to see them through this acute episode and aim for a fast, smooth recovery. The decreased function in one finger may not affect their ability to cope with the activities of daily living (20).

Physical Examination

The patient usually presents to the examiner with the injured hand covered up in a bulky dressing. This could completely

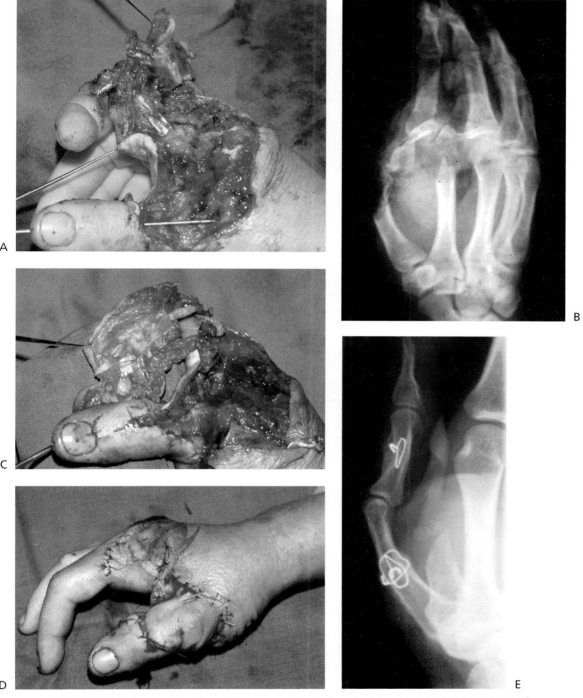

FIGURE 1. A,B: A carpenter injured by a power circular saw. An irregular 3-cm segmental loss of multiple tissue components. The index finger had a near complete amputation through the metacarpophalangeal joint, attached only by a narrow skin bridge. The thumb had loss of dorsal skin, extensor tendon, and metacarpophalangeal joint, but the flexor tendon and both neurovascular bundles were intact. **C–E:** The severely damaged index finger was salvaged for a free composite "fillet flap" of bones, proximal interphalangeal joint, extensor tendon, and skin to reconstruct the corresponding segmental defect over the thumb as a free composite microvascular tissue transfer. The proximal interphalangeal joint of the index finger replaces the metacarpophalangeal joint of the thumb.

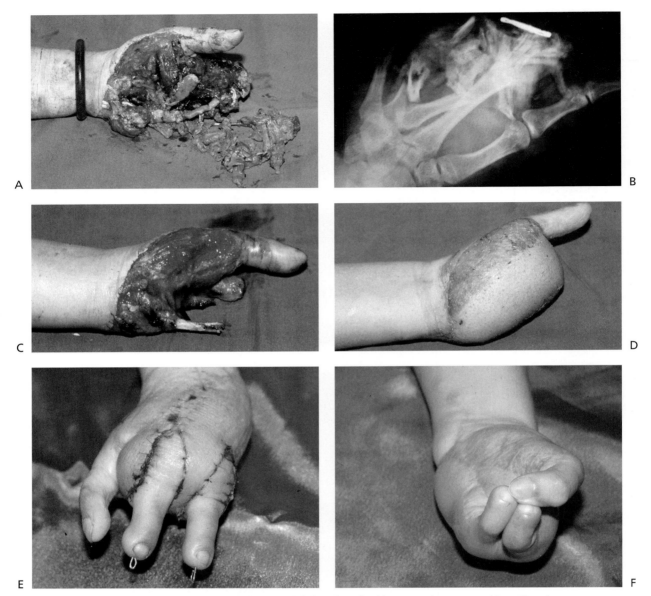

FIGURE 2. A,B: A mould maker had her left hand crushed by a punch press machine. The ulnar four digits and the palm were completely pulverized. The thumb was viable with both neurovascular bundles still intact, but there was loss of thenar muscles and skin. **C:** A meticulous débridement was performed to her hand, removing all the nonviable and contaminated tissues. The thumb was preserved. **D,E:** The large metacarpal defect was immediately resurfaced with a 27-cm by 6-cm free lateral arm flap. Opposition reconstruction with two second-toe transfer to the hand was performed 4 months after the injury. **F:** Sufficient recovery of function and dexterity at 12 months' follow-up. She returned to her original occupation.

conceal the hand from the tip of the digit to the wrist. Blood may have soaked through the dressing, indicating active bleeding. The dressing should not be removed before the necessary preparation for the examination is in place. In severe injury, premature removal of the dressing results in unwelcome bleeding, with the patient in pain and the examiner flustered and unrehearsed for the necessary examination to be completed. The examination should be carried out in a well-lit room. A pressure-regulated tourniquet should be placed over the arm and inflated to 100 mm Hg above the systolic blood pressure for a bloodless examination to be carried out. For the less experienced examiner, the examination steps should be rehearsed to minimize the total time of exposing the hand. The necessary dressing implements should be available and ready to redress the hand on completion of the examination. If there is an exposed distal part not covered by the dressing, the examiner should capitalize on examining these parts before the dressing is removed. Much information can be obtained from the examination, in particular, sensation and circulation. Completely separated parts

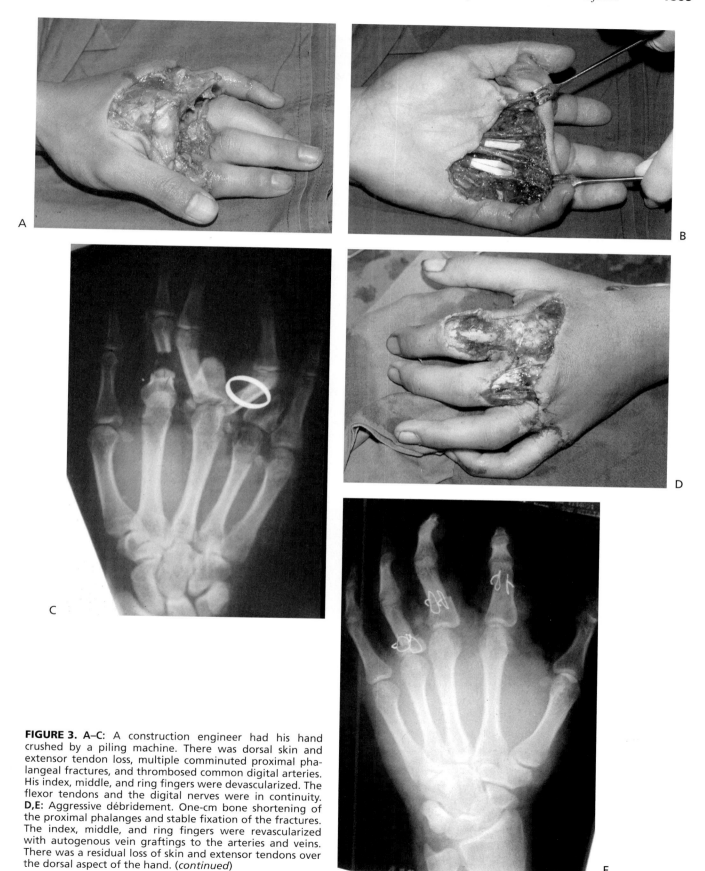

FIGURE 3. A–C: A construction engineer had his hand crushed by a piling machine. There was dorsal skin and extensor tendon loss, multiple comminuted proximal phalangeal fractures, and thrombosed common digital arteries. His index, middle, and ring fingers were devascularized. The flexor tendons and the digital nerves were in continuity. **D,E:** Aggressive débridement. One-cm bone shortening of the proximal phalanges and stable fixation of the fractures. The index, middle, and ring fingers were revascularized with autogenous vein graftings to the arteries and veins. There was a residual loss of skin and extensor tendons over the dorsal aspect of the hand. (*continued*)

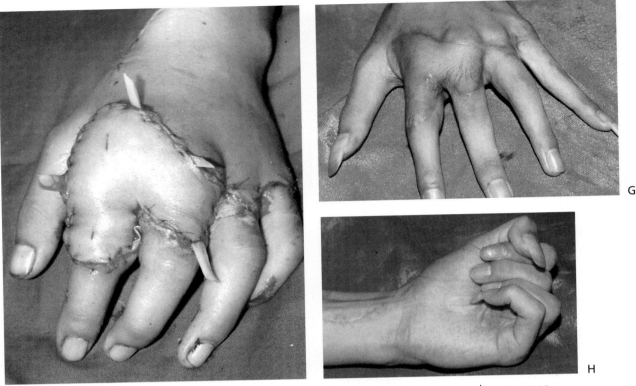

F   G   H

FIGURE 3. *(continued)* **F:** The dorsal combined defect of skin and extensor tendon was reconstructed 7 days later with a free composite tenocutaneous dorsalis pedis flap. **G,H:** Uncomplicated wound healing and recovery of good function with full restoration of finger flexion and extension at 6 months.

should also be examined first to determine the level of the amputation and provide prior information to the corresponding part of the hand from which it came.

The physical examination is directed at assessing and documenting the severity of the five tissue components that are transected or damaged. The examination is carried out in the order of inspection, testing of functions, and assessment of perfusion.

The posture of the hand and digits should be obvious with inspection. A transected flexor tendon results in loss of the natural palmar cascade of the fingers. With the hand raised and the wrist in dorsiflexion, a drop finger indicates a transected extensor tendon. Swellings and deformities can be from bony fractures and joint dislocations. The nature of the open wound must be carefully inspected. It can be a clean, tidy, small laceration or untidy large wound like those resulting from a crush or avulsion mechanism. The wound could be of small dimension or circumferential. The deeper structures can in some cases be visible through the wound. With a good knowledge of anatomy, the anatomic site of the wound should lead one to suspect the possible deeper structures that may be injured. The severity of crushing and the zone of damage should be appreciated during inspection. Extensively flattened and bruised skin with muscles bursting through multiple small lacerations is an indication of a severe crushing injury.

Testing of functions should be carried out to further determine neural and tendon injuries. Test for touch sensation by running a blunt paper clip over the tip of the fingers. The patient can easily appreciate the difference of touch sensation between the fingers with intact digital nerves versus injured digital nerves. A proper two-point discrimination test is time consuming, and a patient in pain is often not easily cooperative with the test (21,22). The patient should perform active motion of the finger. For the patient to cooperate better with the examination, voluntary active motion should start with the uninjured finger followed by the injured finger. The inability to actively flex a finger indicates a transected flexor tendon, and inability to extend a finger, a transected extensor tendon.

If the examination was performed under tourniquet, it should be deflated to enable assessment of perfusion by use of the three clinical parameters of color, refill, and turgidity. In an adequately perfused digit, its color should be pink and comparable to the uninjured adjacent finger. The refill should be well visualized within 1 second. The turgidity should not be flaccid or too tense; it should just be firm and return to its original shape quickly once the pressure is released.

In severe mutilating injuries, a large part of the hand is pulverized, leaving few functional intact parts. The approach in evaluation is a reversal of the above (i.e., to assess what is still intact).

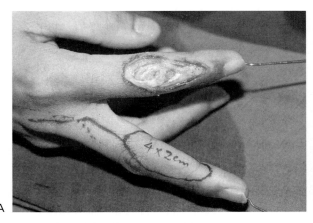

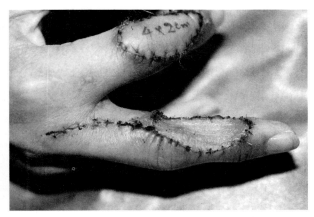

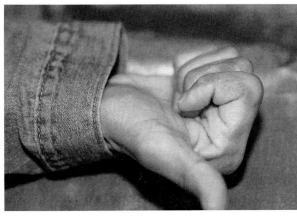

FIGURE 4. A: Shaving injury to the dorsoradial aspect of the index finger. There was a 4-cm by 2-cm loss of skin, with exposed proximal interphalangeal joint and partial loss of extensor tendon. **B,C:** The skin loss was resurfaced with a digital island flap harvested from the middle finger. Uncomplicated wound healing of the finger, with recovery of normal joint motion at 2 months.

Once the examination is completed, the hand is redressed with a firm, bulky dressing. If troublesome bleeding occurs, a local pressure dressing should be applied and the hand elevated to control the bleeding. Blind application with hemostat forceps should be avoided, as this can crush a nerve running close to the artery.

Investigations

The most useful ancillary tools in the evaluation of open-wound injuries are plain radiographs of the hand. The radiographs of the hand in posteroanterior and oblique views and of the fingers in posteroanterior and lateral views should be routinely performed in all the cases. The amputated parts should also be similarly imaged. The radiographs are necessary in assessing bony fractures and joint dislocations. They are also very useful in locating radiopaque foreign bodies. Computed tomography, magnetic resonance imaging, and angiography are seldom indicated.

Examination under Anesthesia

The evaluation is not final without examination under anesthesia. The hand is further evaluated with exploration under a bloodless field and the patient under anesthesia.

The exploration is performed both macroscopically and, if necessary, microscopically.

Classification of Open-Wound Injuries

The classification is based on the five tissue components that are injured. The injury can be a transection of the tissue or loss of the tissue, resulting in a defect. The injury becomes more complex with an increasing number of tissues injured. A single-tissue transection is the easiest to treat and its outcome is most favorable. With each additional tissue injured, the treatment becomes increasingly more complex and the results less favorable (23,24).

Single-Tissue Transection

In single-tissue transection, any of the five tissue components are injured (e.g., a transected tendon, nerve, or artery or a bone fracture). The skin is lacerated but there is no skin loss; after repair of the injured tissue, primary closure is possible.

Single-Tissue Loss

In the category of single-tissue loss, any of the five tissue components is lost in the injury. There is a tissue defect or loss of length. As direct repair is not possible, replacement is required.

The commonest injury in this category is loss of skin. If the defect is superficial, skin grafting will suffice. Flap coverage is indicated if there is exposed bare bone, joint, or tendon (Fig. 4A). In a comminuted fracture, there is bone loss and stability can be achieved only with bone grafting. In some cases of vascular injury, a segment of the blood vessel is thrombosed or missing and a vein graft is needed to bridge the gap.

Multiple-Tissues Transection

The five tissue components can be transected in any combination. It is common to have two to three tissue components transected in the same injury. Many injuries fall into this category such as a lacerated extensor tendon in association with a bone fracture or a lacerated flexor tendon associated with lacerated digital arteries and nerves. However, there is no skin loss, and direct closure after the repair is usually possible (Fig. 5A,B).

Multiple-Tissues Loss

Two or three tissues can be lost in a severe injury (Fig. 3D,E). Usually, there is skin loss associated with loss of tendon and bone (Fig. 6A,B). It can also be a skin loss associated with loss of tendon and digital nerve and artery. These are injuries of greater severity. It is possible to graft the tendon, bone, nerve, and artery defects. The skin defect may require flap coverage. All nonvascularized tissue grafts constitute an ischemic load to the reconstruction. Bone and tendon grafts may take a long time before they are incorporated. As such, the result of multiple-tissue grafting is not very favorable.

All-Tissues Transection (Amputation)

Complete amputation falls into the category of all-tissues transection. The treatment is replantation surgery. In a clean, sharp amputation, end-to-end repair of all the transected tissues is attempted (Fig. 7A,B).

All-Tissues Loss (Mutilating Injury)

Severe, mutilating injuries fall into the category of all-tissues loss. Multiple digits or the whole hand with all five tissue components are completely lost. In the zone of injury, no anatomic units can be salvaged for any possible reconstruction. In the worst situation, all of the tissues in the zone of injury are pulverized (Fig. 2A,B). The damaged tissues must be excised. Other than amputation, the treatment is a complex total reconstruction of the hand with free flaps and multiple toe transfers (25,26).

Treatment

In open-wound injuries of the hand, there is no role for conservative treatment. All open-wound injuries must be promptly treated surgically. Tetanus immunization, both active and passive, is mandatory in all open injuries. The routine use of prophylactic antibiotics in minor, clean, open injuries has not been shown to be beneficial (27,28). How-

ever, the use of prophylactic antibiotics is indicated in complex open injuries with wound contamination (29,30). The use of prophylactic antibiotics is well justified in human and animal bites (17,18,31). The selection of the prophylactic regimen is left to the individual surgeon's choice. The addition of penicillin is recommended for human or animal bites.

Surgical Débridement

The first important step of the surgical treatment is surgical débridement of the wound. This procedure applies to all categories of open-wound injuries.

All open-wound injuries are assumed to be contaminated. Damaged tissues with contamination develop infection very quickly. Therefore, wound débridement must be emphasized. All open wounds, regardless of their size, must go through the routine procedure of débridement. The ideal technique of débridement is excision of the tissues until a healthy and clean margin is achieved. In a heavily soiled wound, excision of a thin layer of tissue may effectively remove the contamination. Excision of damaged skin should be more thorough. The mistake is inadequate excision of nonviable skin. Débridement of tendons, nerves, and blood vessels follows a different approach. The length of these structures has to be preserved as much as possible. The soiling is carefully stripped and removed from them, and only the obviously damaged part is excised (Fig. 2C).

Wound irrigation should be performed only after the débridement procedure. Copious irrigation with saline solution dilutes the residual contamination. Pulse irrigation lavage delivers a large volume of irrigation fluid over a short time and is useful in heavily contaminated wounds (32). The addition of an antibiotic to the irrigation solution has been shown to be beneficial (33).

Repair of Single-Tissue Transection

In the single-tissue transection category, repairs should include those of the flexor tendon, those of the extensor tendon, fixation of the fracture, and microsurgical repair of an injured nerve or artery. All transected tissues should be repaired during the initial emergency surgery. In this category, direct primary wound closure is easily accomplished. Incisions are carefully planned and should incorporate the open wound. There must be adequate exposure for deeper tissue repairs without devascularizing the overlying skin. A transverse wound should be extended with Z-extensions. This improves closure of the wound and minimize scarring. Techniques for individual repair of flexor tendon, extensor tendon, fracture, nerve, and artery are comprehensively discussed in Chapters 8, 9, 37, 40, 45, and 90.

Replacement of Single-Tissue Loss

In open-wound injuries, loss of skin is a frequent occurrence, as it is the most superficial of all the five tissue components. It is usually associated with shaving injuries but can also occur in injuries caused by other mechanisms. Except for treatment of

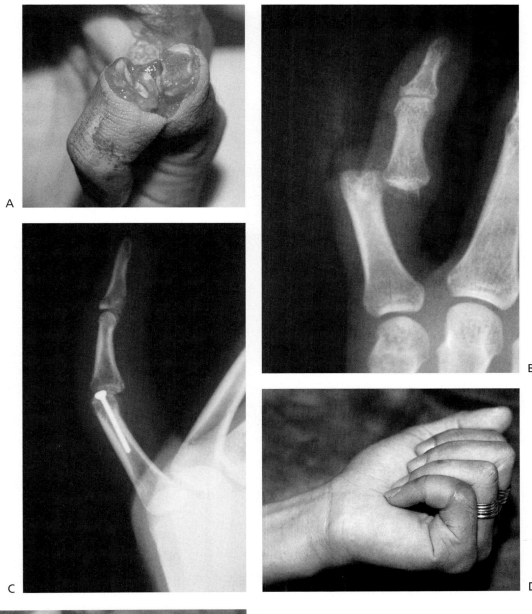

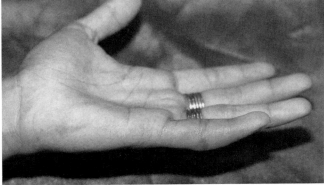

FIGURE 5. A,B: A mechanical paper-cutting machine caused a guillotine injury to the index finger. There was a sharp transection through the proximal interphalangeal joint, with lacerations of the dorsal skin, extensor tendon, and ulnar neurovascular bundle and a condylar fracture. **C–E:** Stable fixation of the fracture with 1.5-mm intraarticular screw. Direct repair of ulnar neurovascular bundle under magnification. Direct repair of extensor tendon and wound closure. The patient had a successful preservation of the proximal interphalangeal joint with good recovery of joint motion.

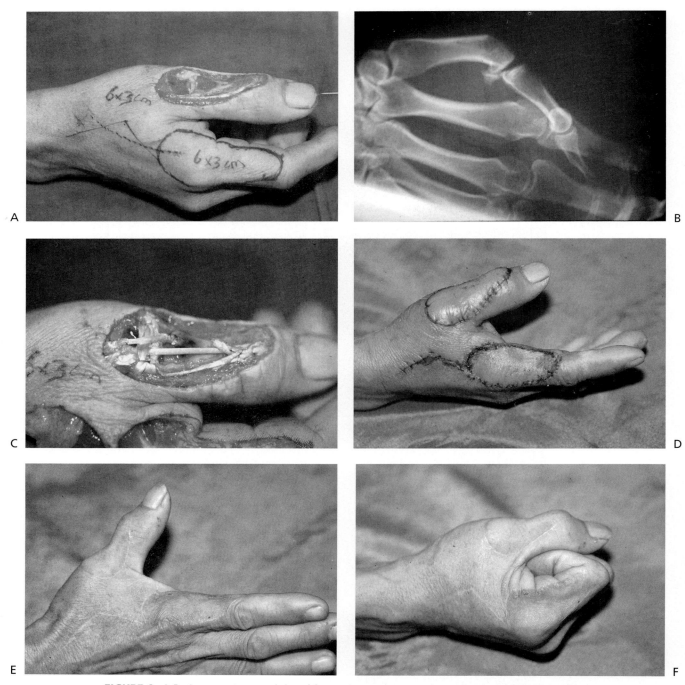

FIGURE 6. A,B: A carpenter was injured by a power planer and sustained multiple-tissue loss over the dorsum of the thumb. There was a 6-cm by 3-cm skin defect associated with loss of extensor tendon and bone over the metacarpophalangeal joint. **C,D:** The extensor tendon defect was reconstructed with a palmaris longus tendon graft. The 6-cm by 3-cm skin defect was resurfaced with a Foucher's first dorsal intermetacarpal artery flap. The joint was stable and no bone grafting was necessary. **E,F:** He had a successful reconstruction, with uncomplicated wound healing, restoration of thumb extension, and metacarpophalangeal joint motion.

some fingertip injuries, secondary intention healing with simple dressing method is not recommended (34,35).

Skin grafting is indicated when there is a well-vascularized soft tissue bed with no exposed bare bone, joint, or tendon remains. Full-thickness grafting is preferred for hand resurfacing, as it provides better padding and durability and less scarring (36,37). The graft can be harvested from the groin or, if small, from the medial aspect of proximal forearm. For a full-thickness skin grafting to take successfully, a meticulous tie-over of the graft is necessary.

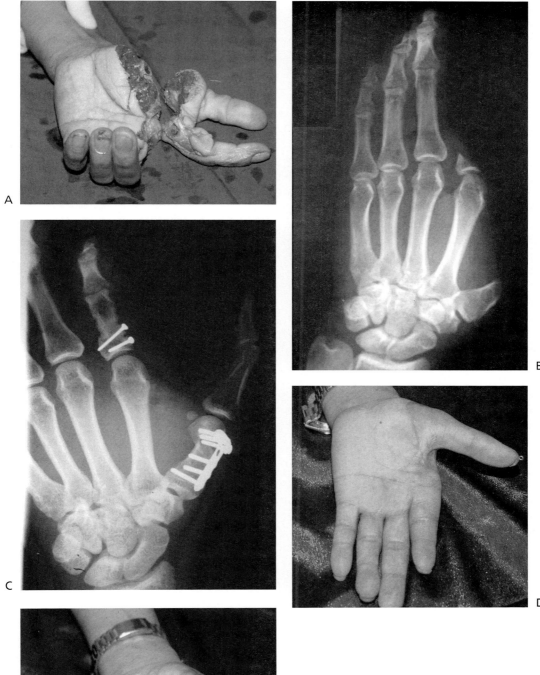

FIGURE 7. A,B: Power saw injury amputating the thumb and index finger. **C–E:** The patient had a reconstructive replantation of the thumb and index finger. Stable internal fixation of the bone with joint preservation. Meticulous repair of all the tissue components. He recovered good functional use of the hand and returned to his original occupation 6 months later.

Flap resurfacing is indicated when there is exposed bare bone, joint, and tendon (Fig. 4B,C). For smaller skin defects, local advancement flaps and regional flaps are adequate (38–43). In a more complex injury due to concomitant injury, donor sites on the same hand for these local or regional flaps may not be available. These defects may also be larger and not suitable for such limited resurfacing. These defects require resurfacing with distant flaps or free tissue transfers (44–50).

An open-wound injury itself is an indication for stable fixation of the associated fracture. To allow early postoperative mobilization, the fracture must be treated with stable fixation. Isolated loss of bone can occur with comminuted phalangeal fractures. Bone loss can result in failure of the fixation construct, leading to a delayed union or nonunion of the fracture. Bone grafting is indicated when there is insufficient contact between the bone ends from excessive bone loss. If the soft tissue injury is not severe, conventional bone grafting is sufficient (51–53).

A tendon gap may be bridged with a tendon graft taken from the palmaris longus tendon or the plantaris tendon. The long extensor tendons of the second and third toes are another source of graft if greater length and bulk of tendon grafts are needed.

Excision of the damaged segment of a crushed nerve results in loss of length. The digital nerve must be repaired with the wrist and fingers placed flat in neutral position. The repair should be possible with 10-0 microsuture. If the tension is excessive, the repair will not be successful and nerve grafting is indicated.

Similarly, excision of thrombosed or damaged artery results in loss of length. Microsurgical repair of the artery should be done without excessive tension, with the wrist and fingers placed in a neutral position on the hand table. Vein grafting to the artery is indicated when the two ends of the artery cannot be brought together without tension on the repair.

Repair of Multiple-Tissues Transection

The repair technique of the individual tissues in multiple transected tissues is similar to that in single-tissue transection. However, the approach in the repair is in the order of deeper tissue first and superficial tissue last. In this category, there is no role for nonoperative treatment of the fracture. Fracture stabilization is mandatory and precedes repair of tendons. Microsurgical repair of nerves and blood vessels is last in the order of the repairs (Fig. 5C–E).

Replacement of Multiple-Tissues Loss

The common combinations encountered in this category of injury are (a) loss of skin and tendon; (b) loss of skin and one neurovascular bundle; and (c) loss of skin, tendon, and bone. These combined injuries can be situated mainly over the dorsum, palmar, ulnar, or radial aspect of the hand.

Tendon, nerve, and bone loss can be replaced with nonvascularized grafts. However, the skin coverage must be a flap that carries its own blood supply. The technique of individual tissue replacement is similar to the category of single-tissue loss replacement, but the reconstruction of a combined injury requires careful planning (54). The injury can be reconstructed in a combined single-stage or multistaged approach. The reconstruction may involve fracture stabilization and bone grafting, tendon grafting, and skin flap cover (Fig. 6C–F). Microvascular free flaps and composite-tissue transfers have become acceptable techniques for reconstruction of these defects (Fig. 3F–H) (55–59). Emergency free tissue transfer has also been shown to be acceptable if it is feasible (60,61).

In a severe combined injury, salvage of a viable digit may not regain sufficient useful function. It requires experience and judgment in deciding whether to salvage or amputate a severely damaged digit. Generally, if three of the five tissue components are lost and required to be replaced, the functional outcome result is unfavorable. In a multiple-digit injury, before a nonreconstructible digit is amputated, salvage for spare grafts to reconstruct the remaining digits should always be considered (Fig. 1C–E) (62,63).

Repair of All-Tissues Transection (Amputation)

See Chapter 90 for specific recommendations regarding replantation in amputations. The approach is an extension of repair of multiple-tissues transection. After surgical débridement of the damaged tissues in the zone of injury, the individual tissues are brought together for repair. Replantation is therefore a repair and reconstruction of all tissues in a complete total transection (Fig. 7C–E).

Replantation requires many hours of arduous microsurgery. Replantation is indicated for multiple digits, thumb, and proximal amputation. The functional outcome result of a single-digit replant justifying the many hours of surgery, cost, and prolonged medical leave remains controversial. The functional outcome result of a major limb replantation is better than prosthetic fitting. In children, there is great potential for functional recovery, justifying the replantation (64–68).

Reconstruction of All-Tissues Loss (Mutilating Injury)

The category of all-tissues loss injury is the most severe and difficult to treat (69). It is often not possible to replace all the tissue components lost in the injury. The approach in managing these injuries should start with formulation of a comprehensive reconstruction plan. In formulating the plan, the reconstructive surgeon should critically review the following questions:

- What is the possible functional goal?
- What has to be done and what can be done with the tissues that remain?
- What tissues must be added on?
- What is the reconstruction "game plan," a combined single-staged or a multistaged reconstruction?

The functional goal must be realistic. This could be aimed toward reconstructing a "basic hand," or "opposable hand," which is a two-digit hand capable of simple pinch function (70–73).

A more functional hand is a three-digit hand, in which there is a thumb opposable to two other digits. This type of hand is capable of a more stable chuck pinch and some grasping function. This approach in reconstruction may require multistage microvascular free tissue transfer. In a typical reconstruction, the first stage is to resurface the huge defect over the hand with a large skin flap, and the second stage involves two toe-to-hand transfers a few months later (Fig. 2D–F) (74–77).

Postoperative Rehabilitation

The rehabilitation can be divided into early and late phases. The early phase occurs during the first 6 weeks after the injury and is aimed at restoring and maintaining the "gliding planes" between the five tissue components. The therapy program should be instituted after the surgery as soon as the wound and vascular status is safe for mobilization. Mobilization should be started early, while the tissues are still in the healing phase. Therefore, mobilization during the initial 6 weeks is most effective in restoring the tissue gliding planes. This window of opportunity must not be missed. With a delay of 6 weeks, the tissue adhesion and scarring would have set in, risking an even greater chance of functional failure. Rehabilitation after 6 weeks is to stretch the scars; it misses the opportunity to restore the gliding planes.

In the late phase, the therapy program should continue for 3 to 6 months and longer if indicated. The rehabilitation is aimed at scar management, sensory reeducation, adhesion stretching, contracture correction, power training, work hardening, and job placement.

INJECTION INJURIES

Pathophysiology

High-pressure industrial appliances and equipment such as water guns, grease guns, paint guns, fuel injection apparatus, and machinery with hydraulic systems can cause injury to the hand. In an injection injury, the severity is dependent on the volume and nature of the injectant (78–80).

These injuries can be further divided into two main groups: those caused by inert materials such as air or water and those caused by irritant and toxic materials such as grease, mineral solvent, and paint. Air or water injection is rather inert and except for the pressure effect it does not cause tremendous soft tissue destruction (81,82). In contrast, irritant and toxic materials such as grease, mineral solvent, and paint can cause extensive destruction. There is a combination of ischemia and direct toxic effect of the injected material. Ischemia is due to local acute vasoconstriction and from increased pressure due to tissue edema. Some mineral solvents have direct toxic effect, causing acute tissue necrosis. Grease provokes chronic inflammatory

response, which is characterized by infiltration of lymphocytes and formation of foreign body giant cells (83–85). This leads to fibrosis and deep tissue scarring. Occasionally, the injectant is successfully walled off by the surrounding tissue to form a foreign body granuloma. In the case of a lubricant, it forms the oleoma.

The entry wound can appear rather innocuous, ranging from one to several millimeters in diameter. There is often associated subcutaneous emphysema from the air accompanying the injection. Foreign material introduced follows the least resistant tissue planes. The foreign material can be injected quite a distance from the original entry point. Injection over the tip of the finger can easily enter the tendon sheath to reach the palm. In the thumb and small finger, their bursae anatomy allows the injectant to easily reach the distal forearm.

Infection can easily occur in any injection injury. Although the product used may be considered "clean," this does not ensure sterility, as contamination may be introduced from soiling of the equipment and the film of dirt on the hand.

Evaluation

A careful history should be obtained of the type of equipment, the operating pressure, and the nature of the injectant. It can be very surprising that many workers have no knowledge of the exact nature of the injectant with which they were inflicted. However, it is generally possible to distinguish the less harmful water injection from that with the more toxic mineral lubricants and solvents.

Clinical examination starts with inspection for the point of entry of the injection. The degree of swelling, inflammation, and associated tenderness proximal to that point are carefully assessed. Palpation should also be conducted to assess the associated subcutaneous emphysema. One should assume that the injected substance reaches the most proximal site of the symptom.

Plain radiographs of the hand and more proximally to the site of the most proximal symptom or sign should be done. The presence of air and radiopaque substances is easily visible (Fig. 8). Large volumes of space-occupying radiolucent substances can also be distinguished easily (86).

Treatment

In the treatment of injection injuries, it is important to recognize that over an apparently small and innocuous puncture wound actually lies an extensive lesion deeper and proximal to it. The need for prompt treatment to avoid debilitating complications can never be overemphasized. All injection injuries should be treated urgently with surgical decompression and débridement (87,88).

The surgical decompression and exploration involve thorough exposure of all the involved tissue compartments. The incision starts from the entry point and extends proxi-

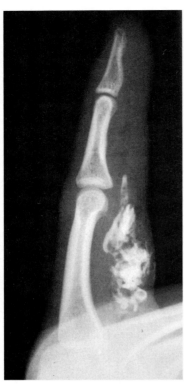

FIGURE 8. Paint injection injury to the index finger. Radiographs showing presence of air and radiopaque paint in the flexor tendon sheath and subcutaneous tissue.

mally over the digits, the palmar spaces, the carpal tunnel, and the forearm. The incision should reach the most proximal site of the injection identifiable by the presence of the injected substance.

Débridement is directed at a complete removal of the injected substance and preservation of the vital anatomic structures. Liquid substance can be easily drained, whereas more solid substances must be débrided or excised. The tendon sheaths should be opened at the less critical regions, preserving the second (A2) and fourth (A4) annular pulleys. The neurovascular bundles are carefully preserved while meticulously removing the injected substance from their surfaces. Excision of the subcutaneous tissue infiltrated with the injected substance can be more generous to ensure its complete removal. The skin is usually not damaged, except for the small entry wound, which should also be débrided. It should be emphasized that chemical solvents should never be used for removal of the injected substances.

The wound is then irrigated with copious amounts of saline solution. The wound is left open and dressed in a bulky dressing. The wound is inspected and dressing changed daily. Repeat débridement may be necessary in a more extensive injury. The wound is planned for closure as soon as it is clean and dry. Direct closure of the wound is usually possible; otherwise, other resurfacing procedures according to the requirement of the wound should be planned (89,90).

CHEMICAL INJURIES

Pathophysiology

A multitude of corrosive chemicals is used in the industry for cleansing processes and for production of other commercial end products. Many household cleansers also contain corrosive chemicals. The hand is exposed to these chemicals due to inadvertent contact or spillage from a major accident in the workplace. Many household users may be unaware of the potential corrosive nature of the cleanser and suffer injury from unprotected handling or chronic exposure (91). These chemicals can be broadly classified into two distinct categories: acids and alkalis.

Acids

Acids are proton donors. After penetrating through the protective stratum corneum, the hydrogen ions from the acid cause amide bond hydrolysis, which in turn causes protein structural collapse. Some acids are also exothermic, producing heat as they dissociate, hence giving rise to a thermal injury in addition to the destructive chemical effects. This results in liquefaction necrosis of the soft tissues. The depth of the tissue damage is limited by the buffering capacity present within the damaged tissues. However, with a large volume of concentrated acid, the destructive necrosis can reach the bone. Two of the most common acids encountered are hydrochloric acid and sulfuric acid, the latter of which is commonly used in vehicle batteries and drain cleaners (92).

Hydrofluoric acid is widely used in semiconductor industries. It is also present in smaller concentration in common rust removers and degreasers. The fluoride ions in this acid cause progressive liquefaction necrosis and bony decalcification (93).

Alkalis

Alkalis accept protons and cause hydroxylation. The alkaline bases combined with tissue elements form soaps. Alkali injuries are clinically more latent than acid injuries. However, with the limited buffering capacity for alkalis, there is further penetration of the lipophilic alkali, resulting in extensive deeper tissue destruction. This reaction may continue for many days (94).

The severity of the injury depends on various factors such as the physical properties of the chemical, its concentration and volume, duration of exposure, and the local skin characteristics (95).

Evaluation

The offending chemical is usually easily ascertained in an industrial injury. The manager of the factory should be able to assist in identifying the chemical that the worker was

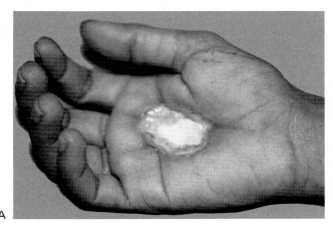
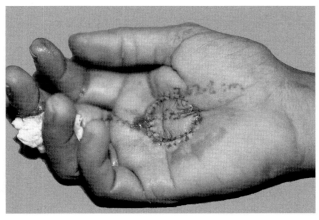

FIGURE 9. **A:** A leaking glove causing accidental hydrofluoric acid burn to the mid-palm. Delay in seeking treatment resulted in full-thickness skin burn, exposing neurovascular bundles and flexor tendons. **B:** The necrosis was débrided and the defect resurfaced with a pedicled digital vascular island flap harvested from the middle finger.

handling. For household injury, the suspected offending chemical may be identified from the labels. The time of injury, the symptom that follows, and the initial treatment should be noted.

The depth and extent of the chemical injury should be carefully assessed. The burn could be superficial with skin erythema, or it could be a full-thickness skin liquefaction with destruction of deeper tissues.

Treatment

Immediate shower water lavage should be instituted. As prehospital water lavage may be inadequate, this treatment should be repeated for all the patients. The water lavage treatment could take more than 1 hour. It should be continued until the burning symptoms have improved and the substance is diluted to harmless concentrations. If the burning pain is too severe for the treatment, a regional nerve block may be indicated. Neutralization therapy is not recommended. Shower water lavage is clinically very effective. It is far superior compared with neutralization therapy in rodent experiments (96–98).

In hydrofluoric acid burns, the patient should be given calcium gluconate therapy immediately (99). Ten percent calcium gluconate is given as a subdermal injection to the affected area. The recommended volume is 0.5 mL per cm². A topical form of calcium gluconate gel should also be applied over the affected area (100). The use of intraarterial and intravenous calcium gluconate infusion has been reported with varying degrees of success (101–103).

The wound should be cleansed with chlorhexidine solution and dressed in a bulky dressing. For a larger area of burn, 1% silver sulfadiazine dressing is recommended. The wound should be inspected and dressings changed daily to detect any extension of the burn. Prophylactic antibiotics are necessary to prevent infection, which further complicate healing. Well-demarcated necrosed skin should be

débrided down to good tissue bed. The defect is covered with skin graft or skin flap as indicated (Fig. 9).

REFERENCES

1. Smith RJ. Education in hand surgery. *J Hand Surg [Am]* 1983;8:655–659.
2. Kelsey JL, Pastides H, Kreiger N, et al. *Upper extremity disorders. A survey of their frequency and cost in United States.* St. Louis: Mosby, 1980.
3. O'Sullivan ME, Colville J. The economic impact of hand injuries. *J Hand Surg [Br]* 1993;18:395–398.
4. Pulvertaft RG. Twenty five years of hand surgery. Personal reflections. *J Bone Joint Surg Br* 1973;55:32–55.
5. Kaplan I. The management of injuries of the hand. *Surg Ann* 1974;6:283–308.
6. Lister G. *The hand: diagnosis and indications*, 3rd ed. Edinburgh: Churchill Livingstone, 1993.
7. Strauch B, de Moura W. Arterial system of the fingers. *J Hand Surg [Am]* 1990;15:148–154.
8. Kaplan EB. *Functional and surgical anatomy of the hand.* Philadelphia: JB Lippincott Co, 1968.
9. Irwin LR, Daly JC, James JH, et al. "Through-glass" injuries. *J Hand Surg [Br]* 1996;21:788–791.
10. McGregor IA. Degloving injuries. *Hand* 1970;2:130–133.
11. Sanguinetti MV. Reconstructive surgery of roller injuries of the hand. *J Hand Surg [Am]* 1977;2:134–140.
12. Kupfer DM, Eaton C, Swanson S, et al. Ring avulsion injuries: a biomechanical study. *J Hand Surg [Am]* 1999;24: 1249–1253.
13. Cooney WP III, Fitzgerald RH Jr., Dobyns JH, et al. Quantitative wound cultures in upper extremity trauma. *J Trauma* 1982;22:112–117.
14. Kullavanijaya P, Sirimachan S, Bhuddhavudhikrai P. Mycobacterium marinum cutaneous infections acquired from occupations and hobbies. *Int J Derm* 1993;32:504–507.
15. Phillips SA, Marya KS, Dryden MS, et al. Mycobacterium marinum infection of the finger. *J Hand Surg [Br]* 1995;20:801–802.

16. Liseki EJ, Curl WW, Markey KL. Hand and forearm infections caused by Aeromonas hydrophila. *J Hand Surg [Am]* 1980;5:605.

17. Arons MS, Fernando L, Polayes IM. Pasteurella multocida—the major cause of hand infections following domestic animal bites. *J Hand Surg [Am]* 1982;7:47–52.

18. Mann RJ, Hoffeld TA, Farmer CB. Human bites of the hand: twenty years of experience. *J Hand Surg [Am]* 1977;2:97–104.

19. Dell PC, Seaber AV, Urbaniak JR. The effect of systemic acidosis on perfusion of replanted extremities. *J Hand Surg [Am]* 1980;5:433–442.

20. Holmberg J, Lindgren B, Jutemark R. Replantation-revascularization and primary amputation in major hand injuries. *J Hand Surg [Br]* 1996;21:576–580.

21. Dellon AL. The moving two-point discrimination test: clinical evaluation of the quickly adapting fiber/receptor system. *J Hand Surg [Am]* 1978;3:474–481.

22. Moberg E. Evaluation and management of nerve injuries in the hand. *Surg Clin North Am* 1964;44:10–19.

23. Tonkin M. Hand surgery: the skin and its contents. *J Hand Surg [Br]* 1992;17:381–382.

24. Campbell DA, Kay SPJ. The hand injury severity scoring system. *J Hand Surg [Br]* 1996;21:295–298.

25. Midgley RD, Entin M. Management of mutilating injuries of the hand. *Clin Plast Surg* 1976;3:99–109.

26. Wei FC, Epstein MD, Chen HC, et al. Microsurgical reconstruction of distal digits following mutilating hand injuries: results in 121 patients. *Br J Plast Surg* 1993;46:181–186.

27. Grossman JA, Adams JP, Kunec J. Prophylactic antibiotics in simple hand lacerations. *JAMA* 1981;245:1055–1056.

28. Peacock KC, Hanna DP, Kirkpatrick K, et al. Efficacy of perioperative cefamandole with postoperative cephalexin in the primary outpatient treatment of open wounds of the hand. *J Hand Surg [Am]* 1988;13:960–964.

29. Madsen MS, Neumann L, Andersen JA. Penicillin prophylaxis in complicated wounds of hands and feet: a randomized, double-blind trial. *Injury* 1996;27:275–278.

30. Hoffman RD, Adams BD. The role of antibiotics in the management of elective and post-traumatic hand surgery. *Hand Clin* 1998;14:657–666.

31. Chadaev AP, Jukhtin VI, Butkevich ATS, et al. Treatment of infected clench-fist human bite wounds in the area of metacarpophalangeal joints. *J Hand Surg [Am]* 1996;21:299–303.

32. Gross A, Cutright DE, Bhaskar SN. Effectiveness of pulsating water jet lavage in treatment of contaminated crushed wounds. *Am J Surg* 1972;124:373–377.

33. Scherr DD, Dodd TA. In vitro bacteriological evaluation of the effectiveness of antimicrobial irrigating solution. *J Bone Joint Surg Am* 1976;58:119–122.

34. Allen MJ. Conservative management of fingertip injuries in adults. *Hand* 1980;12:257–265.

35. Upton J, Havlik R J, Khouri R K. Refinements in hand coverage with microvascular free flaps. *Clin Plast Surg* 1992;19:841–857.

36. Holevich J. Early skin grafting in the treatment of traumatic avulsion injuries of the hand and fingers. *J Bone Joint Surg Am* 1965;47:944–957.

37. Rudolph R. Inhibition of myofibroblasts by skin grafts. *Plast Reconstr Surg* 1979;63:473–481.

38. Cronin TD. The cross finger flap—a new method of repair. *Ann Surg* 1951;17:419–425.

39. Atasoy E, Ioakimidis E, Kasdan M, et al. Reconstruction of the amputated fingertip with a triangular volar flap. *J Bone Joint Surg Am* 1970;52:921–926.

40. Foucher G, Braun JB. A new island flap transfer from the dorsum of the index to the thumb. *Plast Reconstr Surg* 1979;63:344–349.

41. Teoh LC, Khoo D, Lim BH, et al. *Digital vascular island flap to resurface difficult small and medium sized defects of the hand.* Forty-Ninth Annual Meeting of the American Society for Surgery of the Hand, Kansas City, MO, 1994.

42. Bertille JA. Neurocutaneous island flaps in upper limb coverage: experience with 44 clinical cases. *J Hand Surg [Am]* 1997;22:515–526.

43. Brunelli F, Vigasio A, Valenti P, et al. Arterial anatomy and clinical application of the dorsoulnar flap of the thumb. *J Hand Surg [Am]* 1999;24:803–811.

44. Lister GD, McGregor IA, Jackson IT. The groin flap in hand injuries. *Injury* 1973;4:229–239.

45. Ohmori K, Harii K. Free dorsalis pedis sensory flap to the hand, with microneurovascular anastomoses. *Plast Reconstr Surg* 1976;58:546–554.

46. Katsaros J, Schusterman M, Beppu M, et al. The lateral upper arm flap: anatomy and clinical applications. *Ann Plast Surg* 1984;12:489–500.

47. Upton J, Rogers C, Durham-Smith G, et al. Clinical applications of free temporoparietal flaps in hand reconstruction. *J Hand Surg [Am]* 1986;11:475–483.

48. Kuek LB, Teoh LC. The extended lateral arm flap: a new modification. *J Reconstr Microsurg* 1991;7:167–173.

49. Braun RM, Rechnic M, Neil-Cage DJ, et al. The retrograde radial fascial forearm flap: surgical rationale, technique, and clinical application. *J Hand Surg [Am]* 1995;20:915–922.

50. Woo SH, Jeong JH, Seul JH. Resurfacing relatively large defects of the hand using arterialized venous flaps. *J Hand Surg [Br]* 1996;21:222–229.

51. Freeland AE, Jabaley ME, Burkhalter WE, et al. Delayed primary bone grafting in the hand and wrist after traumatic bone loss. *J Hand Surg [Am]* 1984;9:22–28.

52. Bengoechea-Beeby MP, Pellicer-Artigot JL, Abascal-Zuloaga A. Vascularized bone graft from the second metacarpal to the thumb: a case report. *J Hand Surg [Am]* 1998;23:541–544.

53. Stahl S, Lerner A, Kaufman T. Immediate autografting of bone in open fractures with bone loss of the hand: a preliminary report. Case reports. *Scand J Plast Reconstr Surg Hand Surg* 1999;33:117–122.

54. Beasley RW. Principles of soft tissue replacement for the hand. *J Hand Surg [Am]* 1983;8:781–784.

55. Chow JA, Bilos ZJ, Hui P, et al. The groin flap in reparative surgery of the hand. *Plast Reconstr Surg* 1986;77:421–425.

56. Yoshimura M, Shimada T, Matsuda M, et al. Double peroneal free flap for multiple skin defects of the hand. *Br J Plast Surg* 1989;42:715–718.

57. Teoh LC, Khoo DB, Lim BH, et al. Osteocutaneous lateral arm flap in hand reconstruction. *Ann Acad Med Singapore* 1995;24:15–20.

58. Tropet Y, Brientini JM, Garbuio P, et al. Reconstruction of a complex defect of the dorsum of the hand. *J Hand Surg [Br]* 1995;20:591–595.

59. Ninkovic MM, Schwabegger AH, Wechselberger G, et al. Reconstruction of large palmar defects of the hand using free flaps. *J Hand Surg [Br]* 1997;22:623–630.

60. Godina M. Early microsurgical reconstruction of complex trauma of the extremities. *Plast Reconstr Surg* 1986;78:285–292.

61. Ninkovic M, Deetjen H, Öhler K, et al. Emergency free tissue transfer for severe upper extremity injuries. *J Hand Surg [Br]* 1995;20:53–58.

62. Gainor BJ. Osteocutaneous digital fillet flap. A technical modification. *J Hand Surg [Br]* 1985;10:79–82.

63. Libermanis O, Krauklis G, Kapickis M, et al. Use of the microvascular finger fillet flap. *J Reconstr Microsurg* 1999;15:577–580.

64. Morrison W, O'Brien B, MacLeod A. Digital replantation and revascularization. A long term review of one hundred cases. *Hand* 1978;10:125–134.

65. Kleinert HE, Jablon M, Tsia TM. An overview of replantation and results of 347 replants in 245 patients. *J Trauma* 1980;20:390–398.

66. Graham B, Adkins P, Tsai TM, et al. Major replantation versus revision amputation and prosthetic fitting in the upper extremity: a late functional outcome study. *J Hand Surg [Am]* 1998;23:783–791.

67. Tan AB, Teoh LC. Upper limb digital replantation and revascularisation in children. *Ann Acad Med Singapore* 1995;24:32–36.

68. Cheng GL, Pan DD, Zhang NP, et al. Digital replant in children: a long-term follow-up study. *J Hand Surg [Am]* 1998;23:635–646.

69. Brown HC, Williams HB, Woolhouse FM. Principles of salvage in mutilating hand injuries. *J Trauma* 1968;8:319–332.

70. Burkhalter WE. Complex injuries of the hand. In: Sandzen SC Jr, ed. *The hand and wrist: current management of complications in orthopaedics.* Baltimore: Williams & Wilkins, 1986.

71. Vilkki SK. [Free toe transfer to the forearm stump following wrist amputation—a current alternative to the Krukenberg operation.] *Handchir Mikrochir Plast Chir* 1985;17:92–97.

72. Wei FC, Coessens B, Ganos D. Multiple microsurgical toe-to-hand transfer in the reconstruction of the mutilated hand. A series of fifty-nine cases. *Ann Chir Main Memb Super* 1992;11:177–187.

73. Yu ZJ, Huang YC, Yu S, et al. Thumb reconstruction in a bilateral upper extremity amputee: an alternative to the Krukenberg procedure. *J Hand Surg [Am]* 1999;24:194–197.

74. Koshima I, Etoh H, Moriguchi T, et al. Sixty cases of partial or total toe transfer for repair of finger losses. *Plast Reconstr Surg* 1993;92:1331–1338.

75. Wei FC, el-Gammal TA, Lin CH, et al. Metacarpal hand: classification and guidelines for microsurgical reconstruction with toe transfers. *Plast Reconstr Surg* 1997;99:122–128.

76. Wei FC, Chen HC, Chuang CC, et al. Simultaneous multiple toe transfers in hand reconstruction. *Plast Reconstr Surg* 1998;81:366–377.

77. Yu Z, Huang Y. Sixty-four cases of thumb and finger reconstruction using transplantation of the big toe skin-nail flap combined with the second toe or the second and third toes. *Plast Reconstr Surg* 2000;106:335–341.

78. Gelberman R, Posch JL, Jurist JM. High-pressure injection injuries of the hand. *J Bone Joint Surg Am* 1975;57:935–937.

79. Couzens G, Burke FD. Veterinary high pressure injection injuries with inoculations for large animals. *J Hand Surg [Br]* 1995;20:497–499.

80. Sena T, Brewer BW. Natural gas inflation injury of the upper extremity: a case report. *J Hand Surg [Am]* 1999;24:850–852.

81. Klareskov B, Gebuhr P, Rordam P. Compressed air injuries of the hand. *J Hand Surg [Br]* 1986;11:436–437.

82. Weltmer JB, Pack LL. High pressure water gun injection injuries to the extremities. *J Bone Joint Surg Am* 1988;70:1221–1223.

83. Kaufman HD. High pressure injection injuries, the problem, pathogenesis and management. *Hand* 1970;2:63–73.

84. Dickson RA. High pressure injection injuries of the hand. A clinical, chemical and histological study. *Hand* 1976;8:189–193.

85. Failla JM, Linden MD. The acute pathologic changes of paint-injection injury and correlation to surgical treatment: a report of two cases. *J Hand Surg [Am]* 1997;22:792–800.

86. Crabb DJM. The value of plain radiographs in treating grease gun injuries. *Hand* 1981;13:39–42.

87. Stark HH, Ashworth CR, Boyles JH. Grease gun injuries of the hand. *J Bone Joint Surg Am* 1961;43:485–491.

88. Scher C, Schun FD, Harvin JS. High-pressure paint gun injuries of the hand: a report of two cases. *Br J Plast Surg* 1973;26:167–171.

89. Schoo MJ, Scott FA, Broswick JA. High-pressure injection injuries of the hand. *J Trauma* 1980;20:229–238.

90. Lewis HG, Clarke P, Kneafsey B, et al. A 10-year review of high-pressure injection injuries to the hand. *J Hand Surg [Br]* 1998;23:479–481.

91. Bentivegna PE, Deane LM. Chemical burns of the upper extremity. *Hand Clin* 1990;6:253–259.

92. Bond SJ, Schnier GC, Sundine MJ, et al. Cutaneous burns caused by sulfuric acid drain cleaner. *J Trauma* 1998;44:523–526.

93. Anderson WJ, Anderson JR. Hydrofluoric acid burns of the hand: mechanism of injury and treatment. *J Hand Surg [Am]* 1988;13:52–57.

94. Erdmann D, Hussmann J, Kucan JO. Treatment of a severe alkali burn. *Burns* 1996;22:141–146.

95. Davidson DC. Treatment of acid and alkali burns: an experimental study. *Ann Surg* 1927;85:481–490.

96. Bromberg BE, Sung CI, Walden RH. Hydrotherapy of chemical burns. *Plast Reconstr Surg* 1965;35:85–91.

97. Gruber RP, Laub DR, Vistnes LM. The effect of hydrotherapy on the clinical course and pH of experimental cutaneous chemical burns. *Plast Reconstr Surg* 1975;55:200–204.

98. Yano K, Hata Y, Matsuka K, et al. Effects of washing with a neutralizing agent on alkaline skin injuries in an experimental model. *Burns* 1994;20:36–39.

99. Blunt CP. Treatment of hydrofluoric acid burns by injection with calcium gluconate. *Industrial Med Surg* 1964;33:869–875.

100. Dowbak G, Rose K, Rohrich RJ. A biochemical and histologic rationale for the treatment of hydrofluoric acid burns with calcium gluconate. *J Burn Care Rehabil* 1994;5:323–327.

101. Vance MV, Curry SC, Kunkel DB, et al. Digital hydrofluoric acid burns: treatment with intraarterial calcium infusion. *Ann Emerg Med* 1986;15:890–896.

102. Ryan JM, McCarthy GM, Plunkett PK. Regional intravenous calcium—an effective method of treating hydrofluoric acid burns to limb peripheries. *J Accid Emerg Med* 1997;14:401–404.

103. Isbister GK. Failure of intravenous calcium gluconate for hydrofluoric acid burns. *Ann Emerg Med* 2000;36:398–399.

105

PAIN MANAGEMENT

FREDERICK W. BURGESS

This chapter presents a framework for guiding the evaluation and treatment of pain in the hand surgery patient. Pain is often difficult to define, as it represents a conceptual experience rather than a purely sensory signal. The International Association for the Study of Pain defines *pain* as "an unpleasant sensory and emotional experience associated with actual or potential tissue damage, or described in terms of such damage" (1). By any definition, pain is a subjective experience based on prior experiences and, in the human patient, flavored by apprehension and the fear of dependency. It is therefore not surprising that we are often at a loss to eliminate pain with the administration of a medication or the performance of a surgical procedure. Difficulties in detecting and quantifying pain are a recurring source of frustration for physicians and their patients and are likely to remain so. In most circumstances, the patient is the most reliable evaluator of his or her pain and should be relied on to guide therapy. Judicious application of pharmacologic therapy, physical measures, and compassionate concern yield the best outcome.

NEUROBIOLOGY OF PAIN

Painful sensations originate with damage to tissue, bone, or nerves, usually resulting in local inflammation. Direct physical stimulation of peripheral nociceptive nerve endings or chemical sensitization of the surrounding neural sensors begins a process of peripheral and central sensitization. The formation of bradykinin, prostaglandins, and peptides at the site of injury results in the recruitment of C-type nociceptive fibers, activating a barrage of excitatory neurotransmitters onto the second-order neurons in the dorsal horn of the spinal cord. Local liberation of excitatory neurotransmitters, particularly glutamate and substance P, activates ligand-gated sodium and calcium channels on the surface of the wide-dynamic-range neurons in the dorsal horn, which contribute to a reduction in the discharge threshold (Fig. 1) (2). Sensitization of the wide-dynamic-range neuron facilitates discharge of the cell, leading to an amplification of peripheral pain signals. This process has been referred to as *windup*. In the postoperative pain setting, peripheral and central sensitization expands the painful area, creating a regional zone of hypersensitivity beyond the traumatized tissue.

ANALGESIC PHARMACOLOGY

The sequence of events described above identifies several areas for analgesic intervention to prevent escalation of the pain signal. Animal data and several human clinical trials have offered compelling evidence for early and aggressive efforts to block the activation of the pain pathways (3–5). Furthermore, early intervention and sustained pain control may contribute to shortening the period of postoperative pain and disability and may aide in preventing the development of chronic pain in the operative area (6). Perioperative pain treatment strategies should include the use of regional anesthesia, using local infiltration, or neural blockade to prevent sensitization of the nervous system. Neural blockade or field block before incision may substantially reduce the amount of pain experienced during the early postoperative period, independent of other interventions. With the addition of a nonsteroidal antiinflammatory drug (NSAID) and an opioid, further improvements in pain control may be attained. The ideal strategy includes the administration of a regional anesthetic, preoperative administration of an NSAID, and intraoperative administration of an opioid with continued administration on a regular interval during the first 3 to 5 postoperative days.

Nonsteroidal Antiinflammatory Drugs

NSAIDs are an important mainstay of analgesic therapy in orthopedic medicine. Since the synthesis of acetylsalicylic acid in 1899, the NSAIDs have evolved into the most widely prescribed oral analgesic medications. However, the value of this analgesic class is all too often forgotten in the management of the acute trauma and postoperative patient. Avoidance of NSAIDs in these settings is directly attributable to concerns over the potential for bleeding complications.

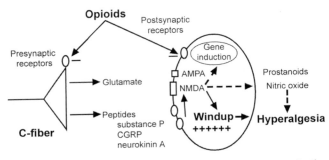

FIGURE 1. Activation of the wide-dynamic-range neuron in the dorsal horn by excitatory neurotransmitters released from the peripheral C-fiber nociceptor. AMPA, alpha-amino-3-hydroxy-5-methyl-4-isoxazole propionic acid; CGRP, calcitonin gene-related peptide; NMDA, N-methyl-D-aspartate. (From Dickenson AH. Spinal cord pharmacology of pain. *Br J Anaesth* 1995;75:193–200, with permission.)

These concerns are largely overstated, as demonstrated in the postmarketing surveillance data collected for 10,272 courses of therapy with ketorolac (7). The data revealed minimal risk of perioperative bleeding at the surgical site. Despite this, many physicians and surgeons continue to advise their preoperative patients to discontinue using their NSAIDs before surgery. As indicated above, there may be a clear rationale to prescribe oral NSAIDs on the morning of surgery.

NSAIDs produce their analgesic action through the inhibition of cyclooxygenase (COX) synthetase at the site of injury in the periphery and possibly through actions within the central nervous system. Tissue trauma liberates phospholipids from damaged cellular membranes, which are in turn converted by regional phospholipase enzymes to arachidonic acid. COX converts the arachidonic acid into prostaglandin precursors responsible for the development of regional pain, edema, and vasodilatation. Recent animal and clinical data have demonstrated a potent central effect of NSAIDs when delivered intraspinally (8). Prostaglandins appear to play a role in the transmission of nociception within the dorsal horn of the spinal cord. The importance of this central mechanism to the analgesic effects of most NSAIDs is uncertain but may provide a useful target for future analgesic directions.

A large number of different NSAIDs are currently on the market. Fortunately, it is not necessary to become familiar with every agent. NSAID selection may be primarily on the basis of duration of action desired and on the side effect tolerance profile. The most potent antiinflammatory effect is provided by indomethacin; however, adverse reactions and side effects have led to a decline in the use of this compound. For short-term therapy, ibuprofen remains one of the least expensive and best-tolerated NSAIDs. The one disadvantage of ibuprofen is its short duration of action, requiring multiple daily doses (Table 1). Compliance with analgesics, as with most medications, can be a problem; however, pain provides an easily recognized reminder. Longer-acting NSAIDs, such as naproxen or piroxicam, offer greater convenience of dosing but appear to carry a greater risk of gastrointestinal bleeding and ulceration (9). This increased risk of gastric perforation and bleeding complications may be related to the sustained inhibition of COX enzyme provided by the prolonged half-lives. Ketorolac deserves mention, as it is available for parenteral delivery, making it convenient for intraoperative and postoperative administration. However, ketorolac has received a black box warning by the U.S. Food and Drug Administration to limit parenteral administration to not more than 5 days (7). This resulted from postmarketing surveillance data that revealed an increase in gastrointestinal bleeding when

TABLE 1. NONSTEROIDAL ANTIINFLAMMATORY AGENTS

Agent	Dose range (mg)	Dosing interval (h)	Maximum dose (mg)	Half-life
Salicylates				
Acetylsalicylic acid	325–650	4–6	4,000–6,000	20–30 min
Choline magnesium trisalicylate	1,000–1,500	12	2,000–3,000	9–17 h
Nonselective COX inhibitors				
Ibuprofen	200–800	4–8	2,400	2.0–2.5 h
Naprosyn	250–500	6–8	1,250	12–15 h
Naproxen sodium	275–550	6–8	1,375	12–15 h
Ketoprofen	25–50	6–8	300	1.5 h
Indomethacin	25–50	8–12	100	2 h
Ketorolac	15–60 i.m.; 10 p.o.	6	120	6 h
Diclofenac	50	8	150	1–2 h
Piroxicam	20–40	24	40	50 h
Etodolac	200–500	6–12	1,000	7 h
Nabumetone	500–2,000	12–24	2,000	24 h
COX-2–selective compounds				
Celecoxib	100–200	12	400	11 h
Rofecoxib	25–50	12–24	50	17 h
Meloxicam	7.5–15.0	24	15	20–24 h

COX, cyclooxygenase.

ketorolac was administered parenterally for more than 5 days. Identified risk factors included age older than 70 years and concomitant medical illness (7).

Selective Inhibition of Cyclooxygenase

COX exists in at least two isoenzyme forms (10). COX-1 is a constitutive enzyme that is continuously expressed in many tissues, including the gastric mucosa, the platelets, and the kidney. A second isoenzyme, COX-2, is an inducible enzyme usually associated with inflammation and healing. It is now possible to selectively target the COX-2 enzyme for inhibition, which greatly reduces unwanted effects on platelet function and the mucosal integrity of the gastrointestinal tract (11). Preliminary data from studies on two new COX-2–selective compounds, celecoxib and rofecoxib, reveal a much lower risk of gastric erosion and ulceration relative to nonselective COX inhibitors such as ibuprofen and naproxen (11–14). Furthermore, celecoxib and rofecoxib do not appear to impact on platelet function. They are devoid of the antiplatelet effects that are associated with COX-1 inhibition. The COX-2 inhibitors may be particularly advantageous during the perioperative period, as they do not need to be discontinued and may be administered on the day of surgery to provide perioperative analgesia. Reuben and Connelly demonstrated a substantial reduction in opioid use after the preoperative administration of rofecoxib to patients undergoing spinal fusion surgery (15). There were no differences in blood loss among the recipients of rofecoxib, celecoxib, or placebo in this trial. Parecoxib, the prodrug form of valdecoxib, is a parenteral COX-2 inhibitor currently under study and its use may eventually supplant the use of ketorolac during the perioperative period.

Although the COX-2 inhibitors represent a major step forward in safety, several important points must be emphasized. It is important to recognize that although the COX-2 inhibitors are safer than the nonselective COX inhibitors, they do not necessarily provide better analgesic or antiinflammatory effects. Thus, in circumstances in which a less expensive nonselective agent for a short-term course of therapy could suffice, the nonselective COX inhibitors remain the best choice for the sake of economy. Also, the selective COX-2 inhibitors are not entirely devoid of the potential for gastrointestinal ulceration. Among patients with known peptic ulcer disease, the COX-2 inhibitors should be avoided. COX-2 is a component of the healing response and is found expressed in healing peptic ulcers. Administration of a COX-2 inhibitor in this setting interferes with the healing process and can cause worsening. The COX-2 inhibitors cannot be used with impunity, particularly in the long-term setting. Finally, the COX-2 inhibitors do have the potential to impair renal function (16). This is most pronounced in the elderly or volume-depleted patient. Peripheral edema and renal failure may accompany their use and should be carefully monitored in the high-risk patient.

For the perioperative patient, combining an NSAID with an opioid can result in a 30% to 40% reduction in opioid requirement (17). Rarely does an NSAID provide adequate analgesia as a solitary analgesic; however, as a component of a combined analgesic regimen, it can improve the quality of pain relief and reduce opioid-related side effects. The opioid-sparing effect is most evident in the orthopedic and dental surgery populations. The advantage of combining an NSAID with an opioid may become evident in a faster return of bowel function, less constipation, less nausea, and improved analgesia. Parenteral ketorolac has been shown to be a useful adjuvant to epidural opioid analgesia (18–21). With the availability of the COX-2 inhibitors, more widespread use of NSAIDs during the perioperative period should result in improved analgesia. The lack of platelet interference allows the COX-2 inhibitors to be administered very early in the treatment of the orthopedic trauma patient, provided careful consideration of renal perfusion and volume resuscitation issues has occurred.

Nonsteroidal Antiinflammatory Drug Hazards

Two forms of gastrointestinal problems are associated with the NSAID class. Many patients encounter dyspepsia on starting a course of NSAID therapy. This effect represents a topical irritant effect of the medication and does not herald peptic ulcer formation or gastric perforation. In most cases, this effect fades with continued use and adaptation. It can also be reduced by encouraging patients to consume food along with their NSAID. More serious gastrointestinal damage is not often heralded by dyspepsia but instead may present as a perforated viscus without prodrome or as spontaneous hemorrhage. The NSAIDs interfere with the protective generation of mucus and bicarbonate, leading to ulceration of the duodenal region. Concomitant administration of histamine antagonists, proton inhibitors, and misoprostol appear to be somewhat helpful but cannot completely prevent ulcerations (22). As a general statement, patients with known peptic ulcer disease should not be treated with an NSAID. Patients with a history of peptic ulcer disease without active ulcers must be treated cautiously. Perhaps the combination of a COX-2–selective inhibitor in conjunction with a cytoprotective agent, such as misoprostol, may be a reasonable approach. At present, there are no data on this.

Adverse renal effects of the NSAID class include impaired renal perfusion, sodium retention secondary to reduced glomerular filtration, peripheral edema, congestive heart failure, hyperkalemia, interstitial nephritis, and nephrotic syndrome. Acute renal failure, peripheral edema, and heart failure are all interrelated and can often be anticipated from the patient's past medical history. Treating any patient with hypertension, a known history of congestive heart failure, or a preexisting renal impairment must be undertaken with caution. Some assessment of renal function should be made before initiating therapy.

Although chemically very different, the NSAIDs as a class appear to carry some risk of hepatotoxicity. Two agents in particular have been linked to hepatic injury, necessitating routine monitoring. Bromfenac, which has been withdrawn from the U.S. market, was linked to hepatic failure. Diclofenac has been associated with a hepatitis-type picture. Other NSAIDs have been associated with hepatic injury; however, as with many drugs undergoing clinical trials, it is not always clear if there is a direct relationship. Any patient at risk or having a history of liver disease should be periodically evaluated.

As a class, the NSAIDs may contribute to aggravation of asthma. Individuals sensitive to aspirin-induced bronchospasm and nasal polyps should probably avoid the NSAIDs.

The well-known potential for aspirin and the NSAIDs to interfere with platelet aggregation has been exploited as a means to prevent perioperative thrombotic complications. However, in the wrong setting this anticoagulant effect may be disastrous. With the availability of the COX-2–selective NSAIDs, these bleeding concerns have been eliminated. There is still some slight potential for modest elevations in the prothrombin time in patients receiving warfarin for anticoagulation; however, this effect appears to be small and can be readily compensated for if necessary.

Opioids

Opioids, a term that refers to the naturally occurring alkaloids (e.g., morphine) and to synthetic opiate analogues (e.g., fentanyl) continue to be the mainstay of analgesic therapy. Opioids provide analgesia by binding to opiate receptors located primarily within the central nervous system and on peripheral nerves. By occupying the opiate receptor, an opioid activates an ion channel, producing a hyperpolarization of the nerve cell membrane, and inhibits depolarization. At least four opiate receptors (mu, delta, kappa, sigma) have been identified. All of the current clinically used opioid analgesics show considerable overlap in their binding to these distinct receptors and are not capable of selectively targeting a single receptor type.

Selection of an opioid analgesic often appears confusing because of the numerous preparations and dose forms currently marketed. Surprisingly, there is actually very little difference between most opioid compounds. All of these agents act on the opiate receptors, their side effects and adverse reactions stem directly from the effects produced at the opiate receptor, and most have an elimination half-life of 3 to 4 hours. Important differences exist in potency, but this is only of relevance in determining a conversion dose between one opioid to another. It is also important to recognize that multiple dose forms are now available, such as the sustained-release formulations. The half-life of the opioid remains the same, but continued liberation of the drug from the dose form produces a sustained effect, necessitating an adjustment (prolongation) of the administration interval.

When choosing from the myriad of opioid preparations, several considerations must be made. Is the pain constant or intermittent? Is this an acute injury that will improve in a short time frame, or is this a chronic pain problem? What is the patient's history of opioid use, side effects, and history of chronic opiate use or abuse? As indicated above, most side effects are directly attributable to the binding of the opioid to the various opiate receptors. Nevertheless, many patients exhibit individual differences in their tolerance of one opioid over another. Expectations and prior experience often lead the patient to avoid an opioid or request a specific treatment. Meeting the patient's expectations may provide the best result in most circumstances. In dealing with a patient suffering from chronic pain, individual biases are often more pronounced and potentially problematic.

Recently, numerous sustained-release opioid products have entered clinical practice and are being heavily marketed for acute and chronic pain treatment. Sustained-release products are available for morphine, oxycodone, and hydromorphone. These products provide gradual liberation of the active drug as the tablet transits the gastrointestinal tract, providing sustained blood levels for periods of 8 to 24 hours. Crushing of these tablets should be avoided, as immediate release of the contents can occur, resulting in exposure to potentially lethal doses. Despite their considerable expense, these products can offer substantial improvement in quality of life and less focus on pain by avoiding the need to ingest a tablet every 4 hours. It should be remembered that many patients experience some variation in their pain relief with these fixed-interval agents. Concomitant delivery of an immediate-release opioid or opioid/acetaminophen combination for breakthrough pain should be a routine practice.

Most opioids have relatively short half-lives ranging from approximately 3 to 4 hours. Two exceptions include methadone and levorphanol, which have half-lives ranging from 12 to 150 hours. Despite their long half-lives, both of these agents are administered on a 4- to 8-hour schedule for analgesia and must be monitored for accumulation. They are predominantly used in the treatment of chronic or cancer pain. Fentanyl transdermal patches have also found limited use in treating acute pain but are best suited for the management of chronic or cancer pain. The patches provide a controlled release of fentanyl onto the skin via an occlusive dressing. Eventually, a reservoir develops in the subcutaneous tissue, providing for gradual absorption into the systemic circulation. The advantage of this delivery system is that it bypasses the gastrointestinal tract, which may contribute to less constipation (23). However, the disadvantages include difficulty in titrating the dose, difficulty with patch adherence in some patients, and expense.

CHRONIC PAIN SYNDROMES AND TREATMENT

Pain complaints affecting the upper extremity are a common reason for patients to seek orthopedic attention. In many individuals, the source of the pain is evident and is amenable to surgical correction; however, many continue to experience pain and limitation in their ability to use the limb despite corrective measures. Additionally, a percentage of patients undergoing any type of surgical intervention develops persistent pain complaints. Persistent pain and dysfunction complaints are more common among workers' compensation injuries. Some of the dysfunction may be attributable to degenerative changes involving the joint, restrictive scar tissue, and nerve injury. A common theme noted in many patients with chronic pain dysfunction is a history of immobilization imposed by the surgeon or patient. Immobilization may contribute to a sequence of events leading to muscle atrophy, tendon shortening, and the development of restrictive adhesions. In addition to the physical changes in the supporting structures, there may be an associated pattern of neuroplastic reorganization within the central nervous system contributing to a loss of descending inhibition or enhanced afferent signal transmission.

COMPLEX REGIONAL PAIN SYNDROMES

In 1994, Merskey and Bogduk introduced the use of the complex regional pain syndrome (CRPS) classification as an alternative to the classically used and rather misleading terminology, *reflex sympathetic dystrophy* (RSD) and *causalgia*. In this review, RSD is identified as CRPS type I and causalgia as CRPS type II, in accordance with the guidelines provided in 1994 by the International Association for the Study of Pain Task Force on Taxonomy (24).

Definitions

CRPS type I is a syndrome that usually develops after an initiating noxious event, is not limited to the distribution of a single peripheral nerve, and is disproportionate to the inciting event. It is associated at some point with evidence of edema, changes in skin blood flow, abnormal sudomotor activity in the region of the pain, or allodynia or hyperalgesia. CRPS type I encompasses the previous definition of RSD.

CRPS type II is a syndrome defined as "burning pain, allodynia, and hyperpathia usually in the hand or foot after partial injury of a nerve or one of its major branches." CRPS type II previously was referred to as *causalgia*.

Clinical Presentation

As defined above, CRPS type I typically accompanies some form of trauma to an extremity. Often, the inciting event is a relatively innocuous injury, such as a sprain, and may often be overlooked on reviewing the patient's history. Other causative events may include visceral events, such as a stroke or myocardial infarct, with manifestations of CRPS

developing in an extremity. Painful symptoms, classically described as burning, usually predominate in a nondermatomal pattern, often resulting in immobilization of the extremity. Discoloration, swelling, and relative temperature changes (either increased or decreased relative to the unaffected extremity) may be present; however, by definition, they need not be present continuously or simultaneously. Evidence of altered autonomic nervous system function may also be present. This is usually noted as altered circulation, such as mottling of the skin, rubor, or cyanosis, and hyperhidrosis. Over time, many patients develop evidence of chronic changes in nail and hair growth or skin texture. These changes often occur quite rapidly in some patients, whereas others may show intermittent rubor, cyanosis, and swelling without progression to the more chronic dystrophic appearance. Extension of the disease to more proximal regions of the extremity is common. Thus, involvement of the hand, arm, shoulder, and cervical areas is often noted after a relatively minor peripheral injury. Motor manifestations, such as tremor, weakness, and dystonia, may also be noted (25). Considerable difficulty may be encountered in attempting to sort out the unwillingness to move the extremity secondary to pain versus an inability to move. A typical patient presenting with CRPS involving the upper extremity enters the examination room holding the involved arm in an elevated and protected position. The hand is often covered by a glove or sleeve. Efforts to examine the extremity are met with an almost reflex guarding by the patient, twisting to avert contact.

CRPS type II differs from CRPS type I in that there is a defined neural injury. Most CRPS type II patients manifest evidence of a localized neuropathy but also show extension of the disease beyond the distribution of the injury, presenting as a burning discomfort, hypersensitivity, or allodynia of the skin. Edema, discoloration, and motor dysfunction are also likely to be present, as with CRPS type I.

Laboratory and Diagnostic Evaluation

Currently, there is no gold standard test available to confirm the diagnosis of CRPS. One reason for this is the heterogeneity allowed by the current working definitions. CRPS is a conglomeration of symptoms and signs that probably do not represent a single entity but instead reflect an amplified common response pathway whereby the nervous system reacts to a variety of injuries. Furthermore, the recognition of CRPS is frequently delayed and confused with the normal healing response to injury (26). Therefore, most patients present at differing stages along a continuum of progression or resolution.

Diagnostic evaluation of both CRPS types involves the use of triple-phase bone scans, thermography, plain radiographs, and in some centers, specialized testing of the sympathetic nervous system. The triple-phase bone scan is considered suggestive of CRPS if the early bone uptake

TABLE 2. COMPLEX REGIONAL PAIN SYNDROME I [REFLEX SYMPATHETIC DYSTROPHY (RSD)] DIAGNOSTIC SCALE

Clinical signs and symptoms
   Burning pain
   Hyperpathia and allodynia
   Temperature and color changes
   Edema
   Hair and nail changes
Laboratory studies
   Thermometry or thermography >1°C
   Radiographic demineralization of affected limb
   Triple-phase bone scan consistent with RSD
   Quantitative sweat test asymmetry
   Response to sympathetic nerve block
Interpretation
   1 point for each criterion, maximum of 10
   >6: probable RSD
   3–5: possible RSD
   <3: RSD unlikely

Adapted from Gibbons JJ, Wilson PR. RSD score: criteria for the diagnosis of reflex sympathetic dystrophy and causalgia. *Clin J Pain* 1992;8:260–263.

phase shows evidence of increased pooling (27). Plain radiographs may show patchy demineralization and periarticular bone loss. Thermography is also considered helpful. Noncontact thermography showing greater than 1.1°C differential is considered supportive evidence. Repeated thermography is often considered, as temperature fluctuations are often unstable depending on environmental, stress-related, and positional factors (28). Stress infrared thermography may improve the predictive value of thermography by demonstrating autonomic dysfunction after a thermal challenge (29).

Diagnostic Criteria

The International Association for the Study of Pain criteria for making a diagnosis of CRPS type I include the following:

- The presence of an initiating noxious event or cause of immobilization.
- Continuing pain, allodynia, or hyperalgesia. The pain is disproportionate to any inciting event.

- Evidence at some time of altered skin blood flow, edema, or abnormal sudomotor changes in the region of pain.
- The exclusion of any other condition that might account for the degree of pain or dysfunction.

The criteria for CRPS type II are similar to the above, except for the causal relationship to a documented nerve injury. These criteria are helpful in defining the disorder; however, in many ways, this has contributed to increased confusion in that the definition is too encompassing. In an effort to quantify the reliability of a CRPS type II diagnosis, Gibbons et al. proposed a diagnostic scale for evaluating patients (Table 2) (30). However, there have been no rigorously controlled trials to track the natural history of this disorder, correlating the symptoms, signs, and laboratory findings with the treatment and eventual outcome. Much of our clinical knowledge of CRPS is anecdotal.

One of the difficulties in evaluating CRPS is that many patients may develop symptoms months and years before the disorder is recognized. CRPS may progress through several stages referred to as *acute, dystrophic,* and *atrophic.* The response to treatment, particularly sympathetic nerve blocks, may become less effective the longer the disorder persists. It is not unusual for the acute phase to be completely missed. Another confusing issue is the variable rate at which each patient progresses through the stages of the disease. Some patients rapidly progress into the dystrophic and atrophic phases, whereas others may persist with intermittent "acute" findings. Whether these differences represent the same disease process or different disorders manifesting with similar signs and symptoms of nervous system injury is unclear. Furthermore, many patients have been partially treated with various pharmacologic and physical therapy interventions. The net result is often a confused picture. A comparison of the three stages is shown in Table 3.

For many years, the CRPS disorders were believed to be directly attributable to abnormal sympathetic nervous system activity. Many anesthesiologists considered pain relief with a sympathetic nerve block to be the hallmark of this disorder (30). A positive benefit from sympathetic blockade was believed to confirm the diagnosis of CRPS. The sympathetic nervous system certainly may have a contributory role in maintaining or potentiating the pain, hence the coining of the

TABLE 3. CLINICAL STAGES OF COMPLEX REGIONAL PAIN SYNDROME I (REFLEX SYMPATHETIC DYSTROPHY)

	Stage I (acute)	Stage II (dystrophic)	Stage III (atrophic)
Onset	Weeks	Months	Months to years
Duration	Weeks to months	Months	Years
Pain	Spontaneous pain in a peripheral nerve distribution	Extension of pain beyond injured area	Pain may abate
Skin	Red, edematous, warm	Cool, mottled, cyanotic, hyperesthetic	Pale, cold, cyanotic, shiny appearance
Bones	No change; bone scan may show early increased uptake	Patchy osteoporosis	Diffuse osteoporosis
Function	Decreased	Loss of function extends beyond area of injury	Atrophy and contractures

phrase *sympathetically maintained pain*. Current impressions have begun to deemphasize the value of sympathetic nerve blocks in establishing the diagnosis of CRPS (31,32). Sympathetically maintained pain may exist in a variety of neurologic disease states, such as diabetic and ischemic neuropathy, indicating a lack of specificity. Furthermore, nerve blocks may carry a very high potential for placebo responses. To avoid this, the administration of an intravenous phentolamine test may have a role in establishing an adrenergic contribution to the pain sensation and support a treatment plan using alpha$_1$-adrenergic blockers or sympathetic nerve blocks (33).

Pathogenesis

The etiology of CRPS is as yet poorly understood. Experimental models involving incomplete nerve injuries have provided some insight into the pathogenesis of CRPS type II. The partial sciatic nerve injury model and the chronic constriction injury model have provided evidence of neuroplastic changes taking place at the level of the dorsal horn and ganglia.

After a partial nerve injury collateral sprouting of adrenergic neurons can be demonstrated in the involved levels of the dorsal root ganglion proximal to the site of injury (34). Sprouting large fibers may also extend into level II of the dorsal horn, causing aberrant connections with the nociceptive pathways (35). Discharge of the sympathetic efferents may then stimulate ectopic activity and spontaneous discharge among the large afferent fibers of the injured neuron, either directly or via sensitization. Sensitization of the nociceptive secondary neurons via the *N*-methyl-D-aspartate receptors has been found to contribute to the pain process. *N*-methyl-D-aspartate receptor antagonists have been helpful in some clinical case reports and in animal models (2). However, the side effects of the currently available antagonists have limited this application.

Concomitant factors such as the expression or upregulation of adrenergic receptors located on the injured primary neuron distal to the site of injury may also contribute to the pain process. Clinical evidence showing increased sensitivity of the vasculature to locally administered catecholamines supports the concept of peripheral denervation rather than increased sympathetic efferent activity (37,38). Kurvers et al. found evidence of autonomic denervation distal to the site of injury in RSD stage I patients (39). Patients in stages II and III show increased evidence of autonomic sensitivity distal to the injury. Their assertion is that CRPS may develop secondary to a peripheral neuropathy, leading to sensitization of the peripheral nervous system to catecholamines, which contribute to persistent pain. It appears that a combination of peripheral and central nervous system changes might contribute to the pain process.

Treatment

An extensive array of treatments have been applied to CRPS patients. The long list of pharmacologic and therapeutic interventions is an indication that no single intervention has proved consistently effective (39). Traditionally, sympathetic and somatic nerve blocks have been the treatment of choice. However, many patients obtain only partial or temporary improvement after a series of sympathetic nerve blocks, causing some to question whether there is a role for sympathetic blockade in treating this disorder. Due to the lack of consistent results with any single treatment, a treatment plan involving a multimodality approach is recommended.

For most patients, the initial approach to therapy of CRPS should include a physical therapy program involving desensitization, active range of motion, and work hardening. Sympathetic and somatic nerve blocks may be used in selected patients to reduce pain and facilitate progress with the physical therapy program. Nerve blocks may be helpful even for individuals who do not exhibit evidence of a strong sympathetic component to their pain (40). Manipulation of the extremity under the influence of a somatic block may help to improve joint flexibility and capsular adhesions, thus allowing faster progress. Continuous nerve block techniques, such as continuous epidural, brachial plexus, or interpleural anesthesia, may reduce complications and provide a more intensive therapy program.

In deciding on the role of sympathetic blockade in the management of the CRPS patient, the following approach can serve as a useful paradigm. If a nerve block is to be the initial approach, it should be pure sympathetic nerve block (stellate or lumbar sympathetic ganglion block). Anesthetic blocks, such as intravenous regional anesthesia, brachial plexus block, or epidural block, may confound the interpretation by producing frank anesthesia of the extremity. The analgesia provided by the anesthesia may lead to improved pain control independent of the sympatholysis. Second, the systemic levels of local anesthetic obtained with these large-volume high-concentration blocks may provide analgesia via systemic mechanisms. The placebo response to a nerve block may also be rather pronounced. Many patients are so relieved that the procedure is complete that their relative anxiety may rapidly decline, leading to an improved pain score secondary to a relaxation effect. The end result is often that every patient experiences some improvement in his or her symptoms. One way around this may be to consider the use of modest sedation in conjunction with the block. Intravenous propofol works extremely well. Many patients are never even aware the procedure was performed.

An alternative to the use of a nerve block is intravenous phentolamine. Phentolamine (1 mg per kg) is delivered intravenously over a 10-minute period in a blinded fashion (33,41). Baseline and continuous pain scores are obtained throughout the infusion and after completion. This may be conducted with the patient blinded to avoid anticipatory responses. A positive response to either the sympathetic block or the phentolamine trial supports a continued trial of nerve blocks for pain control (42).

How many blocks are enough? This question has never been answered. Bonica originally recommended frequent, daily in some patients, blocks until the pain was gone (43). Another approach has been to perform a series of three blocks on alternate days. The patient is then monitored for continued improvement with physical therapy and the resolution of discoloration, edema, and pain. If the patient's progress is stalled or begins to regress, another series is considered. In refractory cases, a more continuous block technique may be sought.

Pharmacologic therapy for neuropathic pain should also be considered simultaneously with other modalities (Table 4). The addition of amitriptyline or nortriptyline (25 to 150 mg) at bedtime can improve sleep patterns, reduce pain, and possibly treat depressive symptoms. Corticosteroids have also been found effective in certain circumstances. It may be worth considering a trial of corticosteroids in patients with early symptoms in whom nerve blocks have not been successful in reversing the pain or in whom a plateau has been reached. Oyen et al. provided evidence of a regional inflammatory response in early-stage CRPS patients, as indicated by indium 111–immunoglobulin G scintigraphy, supporting a role for corticosteroids (32).

Those with CRPS type II often benefit from treatment with an anticonvulsant (43). See Table 4 for suggested agents and doses. Gabapentin, by virtue of its less serious spectrum of adverse reactions, has found a place in the management of neuropathic pain (44). Data supporting the use of gabapentin in neuropathic pain have become available for post–herpetic neuralgia and diabetic neuropathy (44–46). The mechanism of action of gabapentin has not been established. Inhibition of the *N*-methyl-D-aspartate receptor and a global increase in gamma-aminobutyric acid levels have been suggested. Gabapentin should be started by gradually escalating the dose from 300 mg at bedtime, up to 1,200 mg per day. Further escalations may be helpful, but if no response is noted at 1,200 mg, further escalation is unlikely

to help. Carbamazepine, valproate, and phenytoin are well-established alternatives for neuropathic pain and are reasonable second-line agents. When one agent fails to provide relief at reasonable levels or further dose escalations are hampered by side effects, an alternative anticonvulsant should be pursued. Anticonvulsant blood levels do not necessarily correlate with a therapeutic response but can be helpful in determining if additional dose escalations are possible. It is important to remember that carbamazepine induces its own metabolism. Thus, many patients may have a recrudescence of symptoms after a few weeks of good relief. Simply checking a blood level and escalating the dose may be adequate to restore analgesia.

The antiarrhythmic mexiletine is another sodium-channel blocker that may provide analgesia for patients with neuropathic pain (47). This agent, along with intravenous lidocaine, may be effective in reducing allodynia. Anecdotal reports have suggested that long-term (weeks) lidocaine infusions may be beneficial in treating refractory neuropathic pain patients (48).

In those individuals with evidence of sympathetically maintained pain as determined by an intravenous phentolamine test or selective sympathetic nerve block, systemic administration of an alpha-adrenergic blocker may provide improved analgesia. Phenoxybenzamine has been effective in reducing sympathetically maintained pain but may be associated with limiting side effects, particularly sedation and orthostatic hypotension. Terazosin, a long-acting alpha-blocker, may be a reasonable alternative to phenoxybenzamine and does not carry the risk of tumor promotion. Terazosin is started as a single dose at bedtime, gradually escalating the dose up to 2 to 5 mg daily (49). By administering the majority of the dose at night, many of the side effects may be minimized.

Surgical sympathectomy has been recommended for individuals obtaining good analgesia with sympathetic blocks but limited duration of the effect. Most patients obtain only transient improvement in their pain symptoms. Recurrent pain often appears after a few weeks, supporting the concept that sympathetic efferent activity is an aggravating factor but not necessarily causally related to the CRPS process. Failure of a surgical sympathectomy may be due to an inadequate sympatholysis or a contribution from the contralateral sympathetic chain. Some have advocated exploring this possibility by performing contralateral sympathetic blocks to confirm this hypothesis (50).

The antihypertensive agent clonidine, an alpha$_2$-adrenergic agonist, has been shown to be helpful in treating neuropathic pain in cancer patients and in CRPS patients (51). However, the benefits of clonidine in CRPS are often of short duration. Epidural delivery appears most effective, but substantial side effects, including bradycardia, sedation, and hypotension, may be limiting.

For the refractory patient, spinal cord and peripheral nerve stimulation may provide significant relief (52,53).

TABLE 4. ADJUVANT ANALGESICS

Agent	Dose (mg)	Target dose range (mg)	Dosing interval (h)	Half-life (h)
Anticonvulsants				
Gabapentin	100–300	900–2,400	6–8	6
Topiramate	25–200	200–400	12	21
Carba-mazepine	100–200	600–1,200	8	15
Valproate	250	500–1,000	8	10–12
Phenytoin	100	300	8	22
Antidepressants				
Nortriptyline	25–100	50–100	24	31
Amitriptyline	25–100	50–150	24	15
Desipramine	25–100	50–150	24	18

Spinal cord stimulators do not provide complete analgesia, are expensive devices, and are associated with significant mechanical and technical failure rates. Serious adverse reactions can occur, requiring repeat surgeries and the risk for additional nerve injuries. Despite rigorous psychological and temporary stimulator screening efforts, a good outcome cannot be guaranteed. Nevertheless, there is a role for spinal cord stimulation in the treatment of difficult cases, but it should be reserved to salvage situations in which more conservative options have been exhausted.

Recent Developments

Motor dysfunction, although poorly understood, is commonly seen in many CRPS type I patients. Galer and associates pointed out a "neglect-like" syndrome in a group of CRPS type I patients with an apparent sense of disconnection from their injured extremities (25). In these patients, active volitional movement was impaired and required considerable effort and concentration on the part of the patient. Comments such as "the hand" or "if I try to use it, I never know what it will do" illustrate this sense of disconnection. Minnesota Multiphasic Personality Inventory testing did not identify any unexpected personality traits to distinguish their patients from other chronic pain patients. The authors hypothesize the development of a central nervous system origin to this dysfunction; however, factors contributing to its development remain to be determined.

In conclusion, CRPS remains poorly understood. The definition of this pain syndrome is exceedingly broad and will encompass a variety of pain problems having varying etiologies. There is no single effective treatment strategy for managing pain dysfunction problems. However, early and aggressive pain management, early mobilization, and continued physical therapy may offer the best chance of restoring function. Nerve blocks, opioids, NSAIDs, antidepressants, and anticonvulsants should be exploited in an effort to encourage participation in the rehabilitation process.

REFERENCES

1. Merskey H, Bogduk N. *Classification of chronic pain*, 2nd ed. Seattle: IASP Press, 1994:10.
2. Woolf CJ. Evidence for a central component of postinjury pain hypersensitivity. *Nature* 1983;303:686–688.
3. Gordon SM, Dionne RA, Brahim J, et al. Blockade of peripheral neuronal barrage reduces postoperative pain. *Pain* 1997;70:209–215.
4. Tverskoy M, Cozacov C, Ayache M, et al. Postoperative pain after inguinal herniorrhaphy with different types of anesthesia. *Anesth Analg* 1990;70:29–35.
5. Woolf CJ, Wall PD. Morphine sensitive and morphine insensitive actions of C-fibre input on the rat spinal cord. *Neurosci Lett* 1986;64:221–225.
6. Perkins FM, Kehlet H. Chronic pain as an outcome of surgery: a review of predictive factors. *Anesthesiology* 2000;93:1123–1133.
7. Strom BL, Berlin JA, Kinman JL, et al. Parenteral ketorolac and risk of gastrointestinal and operative site bleeding. A postmarketing surveillance study. *JAMA* 1996;275:376–382.
8. Lauretti GR, Reis MP, Mattos AL, et al. Epidural nonsteroidal antiinflammatory drugs for cancer pain. *Anesth Analg* 1998;86:117–118.
9. Silverstein FE, Faich G, Goldstein JL, et al. Gastrointestinal toxicity with celecoxib vs. nonsteroidal anti-inflammatory drugs for osteoarthritis and rheumatoid arthritis. *JAMA* 2000;284:1247–1255.
10. Smith WL, Dewitt DL. Prostaglandin endoperoxide H synthases-1 and -2. *Adv Immunol* 1996;62:167–215.
11. Hawkey CJ. Cox-2 inhibitors. *Lancet* 1999;353:307–313.
12. Griffin MR, Piper JM, Daugherty JR, et al. Nonsteroidal antiinflammatory drug use and increased risk for peptic ulcer disease in elderly persons. *Ann Intern Med* 1991;114:257–263.
13. Lanza FL, Rack MF, Simon TJ, et al. Specific inhibition of cyclooxygenase-2 with MK-0966 is associated with less gastroduodenal damage than either aspirin or ibuprofen. *Aliment Pharmacol Ther* 1999;13:761–767.
14. Simon LS, Weaver AL, Graham DY, et al. Anti-inflammatory and upper gastrointestinal effects of celecoxib in rheumatoid arthritis. *JAMA* 1999;282:1921–1928.
15. Reuben SR, Connelly NR. Postoperative analgesic effects of celecoxib or rofecoxib after spinal fusion surgery. *Anesth Analg* 2000;91:1221–1225.
16. Rossat J, Maillard M, Nussberger J, et al. Renal effects of selective cyclooxygenase-2 inhibition in normotensive salt-depleted subjects. *Clin Pharmacol Ther* 1999;66:76–84.
17. Malmberg A, Yaksh TL. Pharmacology of the spinal action of ketorolac, morphine, ST-91, U50488H, and L-PIA on the formalin test and an isobolographic analysis of the NSAID interaction. *Anesthesiology* 1993;79:270–281.
18. Burgess FW, Anderson DM, Colonna D, et al. Ipsilateral shoulder pain following thoracic surgery. *Anesthesiology* 1993;78:365–368.
19. Singh H, Bossard RF, White PF, et al. Effects of ketorolac versus bupivacaine coadministration during patient-controlled hydromorphone epidural analgesia after thoracotomy procedures. *Anesth Analg* 1997;84:564–569.
20. Gillies GWA, Kenny GNC, Bullingham RES, et al. The morphine sparing effect of ketorolac tromethamine. *Anaesthesia* 1987:42:727–731.
21. Wong HY, Carpenter RL, Kopacz DJ, et al. A randomized double-blind evaluation of ketorolac tromethamine for postoperative analgesia in ambulatory surgery patients. *Anesthesiology* 1993;78:2–14.
22. Graham DY, White RH, Moreland LW, et al. Duodenal and gastric ulcer prevention with misoprostol in arthritis patients taking NSAIDs. *Ann Intern Med* 1993;119:257–262.
23. Donner B, Zenz M, Tryba M, et al. Direct conversion from oral morphine to transdermal fentanyl: a multicenter study in patients with cancer pain. *Pain* 1996;64:527–534.
24. Merskey H, Bogduk N. *Classification of chronic pain*, 2nd ed. Seattle: IASP Press, 1994:40–43.
25. Galer BS, Butler S, Jensen MP. Case reports and hypothesis: a neglect-like syndrome may be responsible for the motor

1832   *Hand Surgery*

disturbance in reflex sympathetic dystrophy. *J Pain Symptom Manage* 1995;10:385–392.

26. Zyluk A. The natural history of post-traumatic reflex sympathetic dystrophy. *J Hand Surg [Br]* 1998;23:20–23.

27. Greyson ND, Tepperman PS. Three-phase bone studies in hemiplegia with reflex sympathetic dystrophy and the effect of disuse. *J Nucl Med* 1984;25:423–429.

28. Sherman RA, Karstetter KW, Damiano M, et al. Stability of temperature asymmetries in reflex sympathetic dystrophy over time and changes in pain. *Clin J Pain* 1994;10:71–77.

29. Gulevich SJ, Conwell TD, Lane J, et al. Stress infrared telethermography is useful in the diagnosis of complex regional pain syndrome, type I. *Clin J Pain* 1997;13:50–59.

30. Gibbons JJ, Wilson PR. RSD score: criteria for the diagnosis of reflex sympathetic dystrophy and causalgia. *Clin J Pain* 1992;8:260–263.

31. Schurmann M, Gradl G, Andress H-J, et al. Assessment of peripheral sympathetic nervous function for diagnosing early post-traumatic complex regional pain syndrome type I. *Pain* 1999;80:149–159.

32. Oyen WJG, Arntz IE, Claessens RM, et al. Reflex sympathetic dystrophy of the hand: an excessive inflammatory response? *Pain* 1993;55:151–157.

33. Raja SN, Treede RD, Davis KD, et al. Systemic alpha-adrenergic blockade with phentolamine: a diagnostic test for sympathetically maintained pain. *Anesthesiology* 1991;74:691–698.

34. Devor M, Janig W, Michaelis M. Modulation of activity in dorsal root ganglion neurons by sympathetic activation in nerve-injured rats. *J Neurophysiol* 1994;71:38–47.

35. Woolf CJ, Shortland P, Coggeshall RE. Peripheral nerve injury triggers central sprouting of myelinated afferents. *Nature* 1992;355:75–78.

36. Reference deleted.

37. Nelson KA, Park KM, Robinovitz E, et al. High-dose oral dextromethorphan versus placebo in painful diabetic neuropathy and postherpetic neuralgia. *Neurology* 1997;48:1212–1218.

38. Arnold JMO, Teasell RW, Macleod AP, et al. Increased venous alpha-adrenoceptor responsiveness in patients with reflex sympathetic dystrophy. *Ann Intern Med* 1993;118:619–621.

39. Kurvers HAJM, Hofstra L, Jacobs MJHM, et al. Reflex sympathetic dystrophy: does sympathetic dysfunction originate from peripheral neuropathy? *Surgery* 1996;119:288–296.

40. Kingery WS. A critical review of controlled clinical trials for peripheral neuropathic pain and complex regional pain syndromes. *Pain* 1997;73:123–139.

41. Gibbons JJ, Wilson PR, Lamer TJ, et al. Interscalene blocks for chronic upper extremity pain. *Clin J Pain* 1992;8:264–269.

42. Arner S. Intravenous phentolamine test: diagnostic and prognostic use in reflex sympathetic dystrophy. *Pain* 1991;46:17–22.

43. Bonica JJ. Causalgia and other reflex sympathetic dystrophies. In: Bonica JJ, ed. *The management of pain*. Philadelphia: Lea & Febiger, 1990:220–243.

44. Mellick GA, Mellick LB. Reflex sympathetic dystrophy treated with gabapentin. *Arch Phys Med Rehabil* 1997;78:98–105.

45. Backonja M, Beydoun A, Edwards KR, et al. Gabapentin for the symptomatic treatment of painful neuropathy in patients with diabetes mellitus. *JAMA* 1998;280:1831–1836.

46. Rowbotham M, Harden N, Stacey B, et al. Gabapentin for the treatment of postherpetic neuralgia. *JAMA* 1998;280:1837–1842.

47. Chabal C, Jacobson L, Mariano A, et al. The use of oral mexiletine for the treatment of pain after peripheral nerve injury. *Anesthesiology* 1992;76:513–517.

48. Brose WG, Cousins MJ. Subcutaneous lidocaine for treatment of neuropathic cancer pain. *Pain* 1991;45:145–148.

49. Stevens DS, Robins VF, Price HM. Treatment of sympathetically maintained pain with terazosin. *Reg Anesth* 1993;18:318–321.

50. Valley MA, Rogers JN, Gale DW. Relief of recurrent upper extremity sympathetically-maintained pain with contralateral sympathetic blocks: evidence for crossover sympathetic innervation? *J Pain Symptom Manage* 1995;10:396–400.

51. Eisenach JC, DuPen S, Dubois M, et al. The Epidural Clonidine Study Group. *Pain* 1995;61:391–399.

52. Hassenbusch SJ, Stanton-Hicks MJ, Schoppa D, et al. Long-term results of peripheral nerve stimulation for reflex sympathetic dystrophy. *J Neurosurg* 1996;84:415–423.

53. Kumar K, Nath RK, Toth C. Spinal cord stimulation is effective in the management of reflex sympathetic dystrophy. *Neurosurgery* 1997;40:503–509.

INDEX

Page numbers followed by *t* indicate tables; those followed by *f* indicate figures.